Contemporary Cardiology

Compliments of Panasonic Corporation

For other titles published in this series, go to
www.springer.com/series/7677

Asymptomatic Atherosclerosis

Pathophysiology, Detection and Treatment

Edited by

Morteza Naghavi, MD
Society for Heart Attack Prevention and Eradication (SHAPE)
Houston, Texas
USA

Humana Press

Editor
Morteza Naghavi, MD
Society for Heart Attack Prevention and Eradication (SHAPE)
710 North Post Oak, Suite 400 Houston, Texas 77024
mn@vp.org

ISBN 978-1-60327-178-3 e-ISBN 978-1-60327-179-0
DOI 10.1007/978-1-60327-179-0
Springer New York Dordrecht Heidelberg London

Library of Congress Control Number: 2009930357

Printed on acid-free paper

Humana Press is part of Springer Science+Business Media (www.springer.com)

Dedications and Acknowledgments

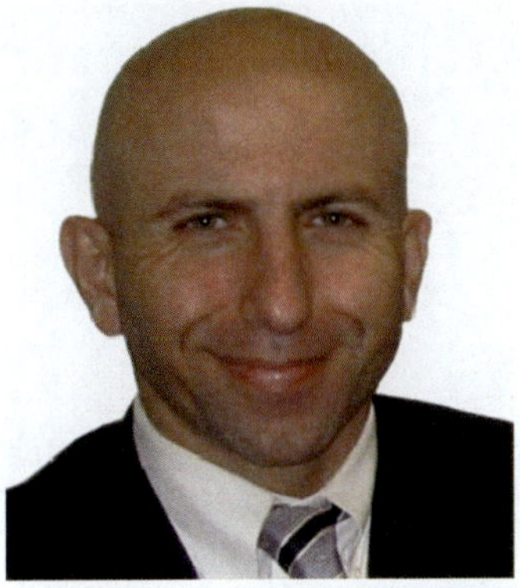

They say that dedicating a book is one of the most exquisite acts of love and generosity one can perform. I would agree, and would like to dedicate my efforts in realizing this book to the following:

To my father, Mohsen Naghavi, who grew up in a hardworking farmer family with 13 children who were fighting poverty and did not have the luxury of going to school. Nonetheless, he always inspired his children with stories of successful people and encouraged them to have great ambitions. He lived a difficult life as a bus driver, but brought up his 7 children to be thriving doctors, engineers, and teachers.

To my mother, Khadijeh Naghavi, whose countless sacrifices and never-ending patience have kept our family warm with love.

To my first mentors, Drs S. Ward Casscells and James T. Willerson, whose integrity and ingenuity taught me priceless lessons and enabled me to realize my "American Dream".

To my respectful advisors, Drs P.K. Shah and Valentin Fuster whose generous support further helped me establish my career.

To my academic colleagues, Drs Erling Falk, Harvey Hecht, Mathew Budoff, Craig Hartley, Ralph Metcalfe, and Ioannis Kakadiaris for their friendship, trust and continued support.

To my collaborators at SHAPE, especially Dr. Khurram Nasir for editorial assistance, Dr. Khawar Gul and Lisa Brown for management assistance, Mark Johnson for graphic illustrations and Princess Fazon for administrative support, whose work made this book possible.

To my past and present associates, especially those I have not had a chance to thank and express my heartfelt appreciation.

And to you who will somehow be inspired by this book and its mission to eradicate heart attacks; you will become an important link in the long causal chain of heart attack eradication.

Do not doubt the cause; our mission is truly achievable.

Cheers to a heart attack-free future for mankind!

Houston, TX — *Morteza Naghavi, MD*

Preface

In the past century, preventive cardiology has been in a defensive mode. Since James Herrick first reported Clinical Features of Sudden Obstruction of the Coronary Artery Disease in JAMA 1912, and Paul Dudley White wrote the textbook of Heart Disease in 1930 and helped create cardiac care units, cardiovascular medicine for the most part has focused on the detection and treatment of symptomatic coronary artery disease. Although Dr. White recognized the importance of preventive cardiology by championing the Framingham Heart Study and establishing the American Heart Association, his dream of "mastering presenile atherosclerosis" is still unrealized. Over the past 50 years, the Framingham study defined the traditional cardiovascular risk factors of smoking, high serum cholesterol, high blood pressure, diabetes and lack of exercise, and the American Heart Association raised public awareness for early detection and treatment of these risk factors. However, atherosclerotic cardiovascular disease has remained the number one killer, diabetes and obesity have wildly increased, and out-of-hospital sudden cardiac deaths is still high and is increasing in women.

New multipronged preventive strategies must be adopted to address these failures, beginning with a change in mindset from a passive defensive to an active offensive mode. The war against sudden coronary death must be shifted from hospitals to homes, and from advanced cardiac care units to primary care offices. In making such a shift, we must walk the walk, as we talk the talk. Attention must shift from the less effective and more expensive treatment of symptomatic atherosclerosis to the early detection and aggressive treatment of asymptomatic atherosclerosis.

Existing risk factor based stratifications e.g., the Framingham Risk Score, have proven grossly inadequate, particularly in identifying the vulnerable patients who are at risk of a near term future event. The traditional methods must be replaced with the more accurate, yet underutilized, measures of subclinical atherosclerosis, notably coronary artery calcium scanning and carotid intima-media thickness measurement. Treatment of asymptomatic patients must be based on the severity of atherosclerosis regardless of the risk factors. The SHAPE initiative is an effort to move in this direction.

In this book, leading cardiovascular physicians and investigators present the latest developments that illuminate the path to translating Dr. White's dream into reality. We must, and I believe we can, master asymptomatic atherosclerosis to accomplish the mission of eradicating heart attacks in the twenty-first century.

Houston, TX — Morteza Naghavi, MD

Foreword

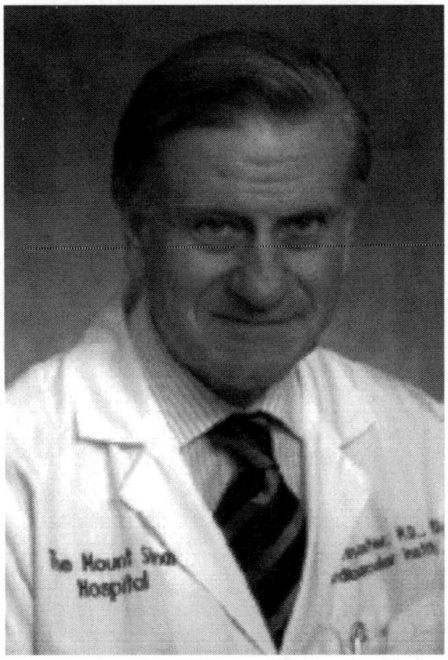

Since the landmark Framingham Heart Study introduced the concept of cardiovascular risk factors 50 years ago, the prediction and prevention of adverse cardiac events have been based primarily on the identification and treatment of these risk factors. Nonetheless, cardiovascular disease has remained the primary cause of mortality and morbidity in developed countries, and is rapidly increasing in the developing world. It is now obvious that new strategies, in addition to the traditional methods, are needed to fight the growing epidemic of atherosclerotic cardiovascular disease. In my view, early detection and treatment of high-risk asymptomatic atherosclerosis is a leading candidate to fulfill that role.

I would like to congratulate Dr. Naghavi and colleagues at the Society for Heart Attack Prevention and Eradication (SHAPE) for their pioneering efforts to advance the early detection and treatment of asymptomatic atherosclerosis. Despite the many challenges ahead, this is a worthy and timely effort that goes beyond traditional risk assessment, and has the potential to transform preventive cardiology. The driving passion and commitment of the members of the SHAPE Task Force is commendable; it serves as an example to all of us who are devoted to eradicating the epidemic of atherosclerotic cardiovascular disease particularly sudden heart attacks and strokes.

I am delighted to welcome "Asymptomatic Atherosclerosis" and look forward to its positive impacts on improving the knowledge and practice of preventive cardiology.

Valentin Fuster, M.D., Ph.D.
Director of the Cardiovascular Institute and Center for Cardiovascular Health
Mount Sinai Medical Center – New York, NY
President of the World Heart Federation
Past President of the American Heart Association

Contents

Contributors

NASER AHMADI, MD • *Los Angeles Biomedical Research Institute at Harbor-UCLA Medical Center, Torrance, CA, USA*

MATTHEW A. ALLISON, MD • *Department of Family and Preventive Medicine, Moores Cancer Center, University of California San Diego, La Jolla, CA, USA*

DAN ARKING, PHD • *McKusick-Nathans Institute of Genetic Medicine, Johns Hopkins University School of Medicine, Baltimore, MD, USA*

BENOIT J. ARSENAULT, MSC • *Department of Anatomy and Physiology, Université Laval, Quebec, QC, Canada*

MICHAEL AVIRAM, DSC • *Technion Institute of Technology, Rappaport Faculty of Medicine, Haifa Israel*

JUAN JOSE BADIMON, PHD • *Cardiovascular Biology Research Laboratory, Cardiovascular Institute, Mount Sinai School of Medicine, New York, NY, USA*

RAYMOND D. BAHR, MD, FACC • *St. Agnes Healthcare, Baltimore, MD, USA*

JACOB FOG BENTZON, MD, PHD • *Department of Cardiology, Research Unit, Aarhus University Hospital, Aarhus, Denmark*

DANIEL S. BERMAN, MD • *Department of Cardiac Imaging and Nuclear Cardiology, Cedars-Sinai Medical School, Los Angeles, CA, USA*

RON BLANKSTEIN, MD • *Department of Radiology, Cardiac MRI-PET-CT Program, Massachusetts General Hospital and Harvard Medical School, Boston, MA, USA*

ROGER S. BLUMENTHAL, MD • *Preventive Cardiology Center, Johns Hopkins Hospital, Baltimore, MD, USA*

S. MATTHIJS BOEKHOLDT, MD • *Department of Vascular Medicine, Academic Medical Center, Amsterdam, The Netherlands*

MATTHEW J. BUDOFF, MD • *BioMed CT Reading Center, Harbor-UCLA Medical Center, Torrance, CA, USA*

MERCEDES R. CARNETHON, PHD • *Department of Preventive Medicine, Northwestern University Feinberg School of Medicine, Chicago, IL, USA*

YIANNIS S. CHATZIZISIS • *Cardiovascular Division, Brigham and Women's Hospital, Harvard Medical School, 75 Francis Street, Boston, MA 02115*

KUANG-YUH CHYU, MD, PHD • *Division of Cardiology, Cedars-Sinai Medical Center, Los Angeles, CA, USA*

GIOVANNI CIMMINO, MD • *Cardiovascular Biology Research Laboratory, Cardiovascular Institute, Mount-Sinai School of Medicine, New York, NY, USA*

JAY N. COHN, MD • *Division of Cardiology, Department of Medicine, University of Minnesota Medical Center, Minneapolis, MN, USA*

AHMET U. COSKUN • *Cardiovascular Division, Brigham and Women's Hospital, Harvard Medical School, 75 Francis Street, Boston, MA 02115*

RICARDO C. CURY, MD • *Department of Radiology, Cardiac MRI-PET-CT Program, Massachusetts General Hospital and Harvard Medical School, Boston, MA, USA*

GEORGE DANGAS, MD, PHD • *Center for Interventional Vascular Therapy, Columbia University Medical Center and New York Presbyterian Hospital, New York, NY, USA*

JASENKA DEMIROVIC, MD, MSC, PHD • *Division of Epidemiology, School of Public Health, The University of Texas Health Science Center, Houston, TX, USA*

DAMINI DEY, PHD • *Department of Imaging, Cedars-Sinai Medical Center, Los Angeles, CA, USA*

JEAN-PIERRE DESPRÉS, PHD, FAHA • *Québec Heart Institute, Montreal, Quebec, QC, Canada*

GEORGE A. DIAMOND, MD • *Division of Cardiology, Cedars-Sinai Medical Center, Los Angeles, CA, USA*

PAMELA S. DOUGLAS, MD, FACC • *Cardiovascular Imaging Center, Duke University Medical Center, Durham, NC, USA*

DANIEL A. DUPREZ, MD, PHD • *Division of Cardioloy, Department of Medicine, University of Minnesota Medical Center, Minneapolis, MN, USA*

ERLING FALK, MD, PHD • *Department of Cardiology Research, Aarhus University Hospital, Skejby, Aarhus, Denmark*

OLE FAERGEMAN, MD, MDSC • *Section of Preventive Cardiology, Department of Medicine and Cardiology, Aarhus Amtssygehu University Hospital, Aarhus, Denmark*

ZAHI A. FAYAD, PHD • *Department of Radiology and Department of Cardiology, Mount-Sinai School of Medicine, New York, NY, USA*

CHARLES L. FELDMAN • *Cardiovascular Division, Brigham and Women's Hospital, Harvard Medical School, 75 Francis Street, Boston, MA 02115*

GARY P. FOSTER, MD • *Texas Cardiovascular Consultants, P.A., Austin, TX, USA*

GUNILLA N. FREDRIKSON, PHD • *Department of Medicine, University Hospital MAS, Malmo, Sweden*

JAMES A. GOLDSTEIN, MD • *Division of Cardiology, William Beaumont Hospital, Royal Oak, MI, USA*

HEIDI GRANSAR, MS • *Departments of Imaging and Medicine and the Burns and Allen Research Institute, Cedars-Sinai Medical Center and the Department of Medicine, David Geffen School of Medicine, University of California at Los Angeles, Los Angeles, CA, USA*

METTE KALLESTRUP HAGENSEN, MSC • *Department of Zoophysiology, Institute of Biological Sciences, University of Aarhus, Aarhus, Denmark*

YASMIN S. HAMIRANI, MD • *St. Agnes Healthcare, Baltimore, MD, USA*

CRAIG J. HARTLEY, PHD • *Department of Medicine, Section of Cardiovascular Sciences, Baylor College of Medicine, Houston, TX, USA*

TOM HATSUKAMI, MD • *Department of Radiology, Vascular Imaging Lab, University of Washington, Seattle, WA, USA*

HARVEY S. HECHT, MD • *Department of Interventional Cardiology, Lenox Hill Hospital, New York, NY, USA*

KEVIN S. HEFFERNAN, PHD • *Department of Kinesiology /Exercise Physiology, University of Illinois at Urbana-Champaign, Urbana, IL, USA*

VICTORIA L.M. HERRERA, MD • *Department of Medicine, Section of Molecular Medicine, Boston University School of Medicine, Boston, MA, USA*

BORJA IBANEZ, MD • *Cardiovascular Biology Research Laboratory, Cardiovascular Institute, Mount-Sinai School of Medicine, New York, NY, USA*

SAE YOUNG JAE, PHD • *The Health and Integrative Physiology Laboratory, Department of Sports Informatics, University of Seoul, Seoul, South Korea*

CRAIG JAMIESON • *Endothelix Inc., Houston, TX, USA*

MICHAEL J. JAMIESON, MD • *Senior Director, RMRS Cardiovascular, Pfizer Inc., Houston, TX, USA*

K.E. JUHANI AIRAKSINEN, MD • *Cardiovascular Laboratory, Department of Medicine, University of Turku, Turku, Finland*

IOANNIS A. KAKADIARIS, PHD • *Department of Engineering, University of Houston, Houston, TX, USA*

JOHN J.P. KASTELEIN, MD, PHD • *Academic Medical Center, Amsterdam, The Netherlands*

SANJAY KAUL, MD • *Division of Cardiology, Cedars-Sinai Medical Center, Los Angeles, CA, USA*

MORTON KERN, MD • *Division of Cardiology, Department of Medicine, University of California at Irvine, Orange, CA, USA*

AMIT KHERA, MD, MSC • *Division of Cardiology, Department of Internal Medicine, University of Texas Southewestern Medical Center, Dallas, TX, USA*

NATALIE KHUSEYINOVA, MD • *Department of Internal Medicine, Cardiology, University of Ulm Medical Center, Ulm, Germany*

WOLFGANG KOENIG, MD, PHD • *Department of Internal Medicine, Cardiology, University of Ulm Medical Center, Ulm, Germany*

KONSTANTINOS C. KOSKINAS • *Cardiovascular Division, Brigham and Women's Hospital, Harvard Medical School, 75 Francis Street, Boston, MA 02115*

IFTIKAR J. KULLO, MD • *Department of Cardiovascular Diesease, Gonda Vascular Center, Mayo Clinic, Rochester, MN, USA*

JEFFREY T. KUVIN, MD • *Cardiovascular Imaging and Hemodynamics Laboratory, Tufts Medical Center, Boston, MA, USA*

EDWIN LEE, MD, PHD • *Center for Interventional Vascular Therapy, Columbia University Medical Center, New York, NY, USA*

STAMATIOS LERAKIS, MD • *Division of Cardiology, Department of Medicine, Emory University School of Medicine, Atlanta, GA, USA*

MICHEL DE LORGERIL, MD • *Cardiovascular Stress and Associated Pathology Laboratory, Joseph Fourier University, Grenoble, France*

A. RAUOOF MALIK, MD • *Division of Cardiovascular Diseases, Mayo Clinic, Rochester, MN, USA*

MARY M. MCDERMOTT, MD • *Division of General Internal Medicine, Northwestern Medical Faculty Foundation, Chicago, IL, USA*

ROXANA MEHRAN, MD • *Center for Interventional Vascular Therapy, Columbia University Medical Center, New York, NY, USA*

ROBERT A. MENDES, MD • *Division of Vascular Surgery, Department of Surgery, The University of North Carolina at Chapel Hill, Chapel Hill, NC, USA*

RALPH METCALFE, MD • *Department of Mechanical Engineering, University of Houston, Houston, TX, USA*

JAMES E. MULLER, MD • *Department of Medicine, Cardiac Unit, Massachusetts General Hospital and Harvard Medical School, Boston, MA, USA*

JONATHON R. MURROW, MD • *Division of Cardiology, Department of Internal Medicine, Emory University School of Medicine, Atlanta, GA, USA*

MORTEZA NAGHAVI, MD • *Society for Heart Attack Prevention and Eradication (SHAPE) 710 North Post Oak, Suite 400 Houston, Texas 77024*

ANUJA NAIR, PHD • *Department of Biomedical Engineering, Cleveland Clinic Foundation, Cleveland, OH, USA*

TASNEEM Z. NAQVI, MD • *Department of Medicine, University of Southern California, Los Angeles, CA, USA*

KHURRAM NASIR, MD • *Cardiac MR-PET-CT Program, Massachusetts General Hospital and Department of Radiology, Harvard Medical School, Boston, MA, USA*

STEPHEN NICHOLLS, MD, PHD • *Department of Cardiovascular Medicine, Cleveland Clinic Foundation, Cleveland, OH, USA*

JAN NILSSON, MD, PHD • *Department of Medicine, University Hospital MAS, Malmo, Sweden*

SEAN O'MALLEY, MD • *Department of Engineering, University of Houston, Houston, TX, USA*

HIDEKI OTA, MD, PHD • *Department of Radiology, Vascular Imaging Lab, University of Washington, Seattle, WA, USA*

SHIVDA PANDEY, MD • *Department of Radiology, Cardiac MRI-PET-CT Program, Massachusetts General Hospital and Harvard Medical School, Boston, MA, USA*

ARSHED A. QUYYUMI, MD • *Division of Cardiology, Department of Internal Medicine, Emory University School of Medicine, Atlanta, GA, USA*

PAOLO RAGGI, MD • *Division of Cardiology, Department of Medicine, Emory University School of Medicine, Atlanta, GA, USA*

Ward A. Riley, PhD • *Department of Neurology, Wake Forest University, Winston-Salem, NC, USA*

Ariel Roguin, MD, PhD • *Department of Cardiology, Rambam Medical Center, Haifa, Israel*

Mira Rosenblat, MSc • *Technion Institute of Technology, Rappaport Faculty of Medicine, Haifa, Israel*

Alan Rozanski, MD • *Department of Cardiology, St. Luke's Roosevelt Hospital Center, New York, NY, USA*

Yoram Rudy, PhD • *Cardiac Bioelectricity and Arrhythmia Center, Washington University in St. Louis, St. Louis, MO, USA*

John A. Rumberger, MD, PhD • *The Princeton Longevity Center, Princeton, NJ, USA*

Patricia Salen, BSc • *Faculté de Médecine, Domaine de la Merci, Université de Grenoble, La Tronche, France*

Raul D. Santos, MD • *Cardiovascular Specialists, P.A., Lewisville, TX, USA*

Paul Schoenhagen, MD • *Department of Diagnostic Radiology and Cardiovascular Medicine, Cleveland Clinic Foundation, Cleveland, OH, USA*

Robert S. Schwartz, MD • *Minneapolis Heart Institute and Abbott Northwestern Hospital, Minneapolis, MN, USA*

Prediman K. Shah, MD • *Director, Division of Cardiology and Atherosclerosis Research Center, Cedars-Sinai Medical Center, Los Angeles, CA, USA*

Leslee J. Shaw, PhD • *Department of Medicine, Emory University School of Medicine, Atlanta, GA, USA*

Anand Soni, MD • *Department of Radiology, Cardiac MRI-PET-CT Program, Massachusetts General Hospital and Harvard Medical School, Boston, MA, USA*

Peter H. Stone • *Cardiovascular Division, Brigham and Women's Hospital, Harvard Medical School, 75 Francis Street, Boston, MA 02115*

Hirofumi Tanaka, PhD • *Department of Kinesiology and Health Education, The University of Texas at Austin, Austin, TX, USA*

Allen J. Taylor, MD • *United States Army Cardiology Service, Walter Reed Army Medical Center, Washington, DC, USA*

Troels Thim, MD • *Atherosclerosis Research Unit, Department of Cardiology, Aarhus University Hospital, Skejby, Aarhus, Denmark*

Arturo G. Touchard, MD • *Minneapolis Heart Institute, Minneapolis, MN, USA*

Manolis Vavuranakis, MD • *Department of Cardiology, Hippokration Hospital, Athens Medical School, Athens, Greece*

Venkatesan Vidi, MD • *Department of Cardiovascular Medicine, Lahey Clinic, Burlington, MA and Tufts University School of Medicine, Boston, MA, USA*

Todd C. Villines, MD • *United States Army Cardiology Service, Walter Reed Army Medical Center, Washington, DC, USA*

GEOFFREY VINCE, PHD • *Department of Biomedical Engineering, Cleveland Clinic Foundation, Lerner Research Institute, Cleveland, OH, USA*

JOSEPH A. VITA, MD • *Department of Medicine, Section of Cardiovascular Medicine, Boston University School of Medicine, Boston, MA, USA*

SERGIO WAXMAN, MD • *Department of Cardiovascular Medicine, Lahey Clinic, Burlington, MA and Tufts University School of Medicine, Boston, MA, USA*

NATHAN D. WONG, PHD, MPH • *Heart Disease Prevention Program, University of California at Irvine, Irvine, CA, USA*

ALBERT A. YEN, MD • *Endothelix Inc., Houston, TX, USA*

CHUN YUAN, PHD • *Department of Radiology, Vascular Imaging Lab, University of Washington, Seattle, WA, USA*

MICHAEL J. ZELLWEGER, MD • *Department of Cardiology, University Hospital, Basel Switzerland*

XIHAI ZHAO, MD, PHD • *Department of Radiology, Vascular Imaging Lab, University of Washington, Seattle, WA, USA*

DAMING ZHU, MD • *Department of Internal Medicine, Johns Hopkins Bayview Medical Center, Baltimore, MD, USA*

1 Preventive Cardiology: The SHAPE of the Future

Morteza Naghavi

CONTENTS

ABSTRACT

In the twentieth century, atherosclerotic cardiovascular disease (ACVD) manifesting as a "heart attack," has claimed millions of lives every year, and killed more people than all wars combined. An epidemic of this magnitude makes it very difficult to imagine a future in which heart attacks are eradicated. Nonetheless, the mission of eradicating heart attacks is no more challenging than the mission of landing humans on Mars. The vision for a heart attack-free future can become a reality in the twenty-first century and can significantly increase human life expectancy. This goal is achievable if we, including academia, industry, health-care providers, payers, and policymakers, invest in the detection and treatment of *asymptomatic* atherosclerotic as much as we have invested in the treatment of symptomatic atherosclerosis. Primary prevention of ACVD, through treatment of risk factors of atherosclerosis, public education, and promotion of heart-healthy life style, has been the main focus of cardiovascular organizations such as the American Heart Association. However, the continued overwhelming burden of ACVD and disappointing trends in the prevalence of ACVD risk factors, particularly obesity and diabetes, have made it clear that traditional methods are inadequate and new strategies are urgently needed. Recent discoveries have created paradigm shifts in our understanding of the underlying mechanisms of ACVD and the sequence of events that result in athero-thrombotic events. These scientific discoveries, along with new diagnostic and therapeutic developments, have opened the way to unprecedented opportunities including (1) screening for early detection and aggressive treatment of the "vulnerable patient" based on noninvasive imaging of asymptomatic atherosclerosis, (2) monitoring therapies and evaluating progression or regression of the disease based on structural, functional, and molecular markers of ACVD, (3) development of safe and

From: *Asymptomatic Atherosclerosis: Pathophysiology, Detection and Treatment*
Edited by: M. Naghavi (ed.), DOI 10.1007/978-1-60327-179-0_1

effective "Polypills" for preemptive population-based therapy, (4) development of safe and effective focal therapies, such as bio-absorbable drug-eluting stents, for rapid stabilization of the "vulnerable plaque," and (5) immune modulation and vaccination strategies for prevention of atherosclerosis at an early age and halting its progression later in life. Simultaneously, the fast evolving IT and communication technologies, as well as low-cost home health-monitoring devices, will facilitate rapid dissemination of new information, empower consumers, and help shift cardiovascular care from hospitals to the home. Through the above, our modern preventive cardiology will shape the future and will lead to the eradication of heart attack in the twenty-first century.

Key words: Preventive cardiology; Asymptomatic atherosclerosis; Subclinical atherosclerosis; Primary prevention; Heart attack; Stroke, Coronary artery disease; Coronary heart disease; Carotid IMT – Carotid intima media thickness; Coronary calcium score; Vulnerable plaque; Vulnerable patient; Coronary risk assessment; Cardiovascular risk assessment; Healthcare policy; Atherosclerosis vaccination; PolyPill

INTRODUCTION

Atherosclerotic cardiovascular disease (ACVD), caused by ischemic complications of arterial atherosclerotic plaques manifested primarily through sudden cardiac death, acute coronary syndromes (ACS) and stroke, is the leading cause of death and disability in most developed countries, and is dramatically increasing in the developing nations. It is projected that by the year 2025 approximately 80–90% of all the cardiovascular diseases in the world will be occurring in low and middle income countries [1]. Despite many satisfactory statistical trends presented by the American Heart Association [2] and celebratory comments by opinion leaders [3] (as if we have conquered heart attacks), more Americans are dying from heart attacks now than they were 50-years ago. This statement is not true about polio and smallpox. While other areas of science and technology have witnessed incredible advances, ACVD and sudden cardiac death still kill apparently healthy people, and claim millions of lives and billions of dollars worldwide. Ironically, despite such a huge loss of lives and dollars every year, most cases of heart attacks and mortality or morbidity associated with ACVD can be prevented by early detection and aggressive treatment of asymptomatic atherosclerosis. Since 1960, a myriad of articles have been added to the medical literature offering insights into this major public health dilemma. However, a very unique opportunity to ease the dilemma, namely early detection and aggressive treatment of high-risk asymptomatic or presymptomatic atherosclerotic individuals (the vulnerable patients), has received little attention. It is well known that ACS do not occur without a preceding atherosclerotic plaque and that atherosclerosis remains hidden (asymptomatic) until too late (myocardial infarction and stroke) [4]. Nonetheless, very few efforts have focused on identification of the very high-risk (vulnerable) individuals with a high burden of asymptomatic atherosclerosis. Since 2003, this critical topic has been the focus of the SHAPE (Screening for Heart Attack Prevention and Education) Task Force and resulted in the establishment of the SHAPE organization (Society for Heart Attack Prevention and Eradication) [5–7]. The SHAPE initiative aims to advance ACVD risk assessment strategies in the asymptomatic population for saving the vulnerable patient, which current strategies have failed to accomplish.

TRADITIONAL PREVENTIVE CARDIOLOGY

Prevention of ACVD is categorized into primary prevention and secondary prevention. Primary prevention can be defined as the prevention of the first heart attack or stroke, while secondary prevention deals with the prevention of the second/recurrent heart attack or stroke. Neither the concept nor the practice of primary prevention existed for ACVD prior to the 1950s when pioneering epidemiologists such as Ancel Key, Jerry and Rose Stamler, William Kannel, Henry Blackburn and others, reported convincing epidemiologic associations between high-fat diet, high serum cholesterol, high blood pressure, smoking, physical inactivity, etc. (termed "risk factors") and ACVD. Despite major accomplishments in reducing the age-adjusted incidence of death from coronary heart disease and stroke (which is partially because of reduced case-fatality rate), the prevalence of ACVD and its associated morbidity, e.g., heart failure, have steadily increased in the past few decades. The incidence and prevalence of most risk factors (except for smoking) have increased or not changed. With the rapidly growing epidemic of obesity, the war against ACVD-prone life style is far from won, if not already lost. It is obvious that our society is facing a serious interruption in the chain of knowledge, attitude, and practice (KAP) to maintain a heart-healthy life (Fig. 1).

Over the past 50 years, great progress has been made in the early detection and management of risk factors as well as the diagnosis and treatment of symptomatic ACVD, particularly ACS. However, very little has been accomplished for asymptomatic ACVD, which accounts for the majority of sudden cardiac death, silent MI, and silent stroke. Unlike most cancers, ACVD remains asymptomatic (subclinical) for decades. Even though the majority of asymptomatic ACVD can be detected and treated, no screening test is currently approved by federal agencies and made available to physicians and patients. Current traditional risk factor-based assessment strategies have clearly proven to be insufficient. A recent report based on the Get with the Guidelines initiative of the American Heart Association which studied 136,905 patients hospitalized with the diagnosis of ACVD, has shockingly revealed the inadequecy of LDL-cholesterol, HDL-cholesterol, and triglyceride in identifying high-risk individuals. The report showed 77, 45.4, and 61.8% of the patients had normal LDL, HDL, and triglyceride, respectively (Fig. 2a–c) [8]. This study has strongly confirmed prior reports suggesting poor predictive value of traditional risk factors, in particular dislipidemia, and clearly highlighted the shortcoming of existing NCEP Guidelines (National Cholesterol Education Program) [9–12].

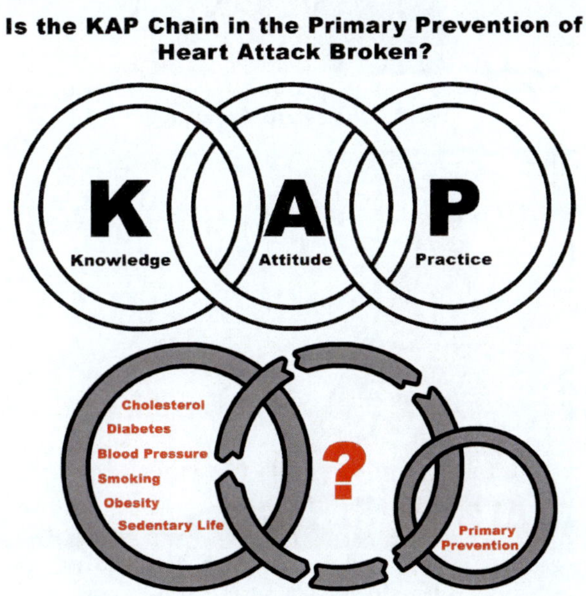

Fig. 1. Most people know that cardiovascular risk factors such as high-fat diet and lack of exercise increase their chance of having a future heart attack, but very few people follow a "heart-healthy" life style. Can heart attacks ever be eradicated by educational campaigns that the American Heart Association has focused on?

In addition to the need for improving risk assessment in asymptomatic individuals, accurate monitoring of the response to therapy in treated patients is essential for success in both primary and secondary prevention of ACVD. In summary, there are two major problems in cardiology; (1) inaccurate individualized assessment of cardiovascular risk as illustrated in Fig. 3 and (2) inadequate

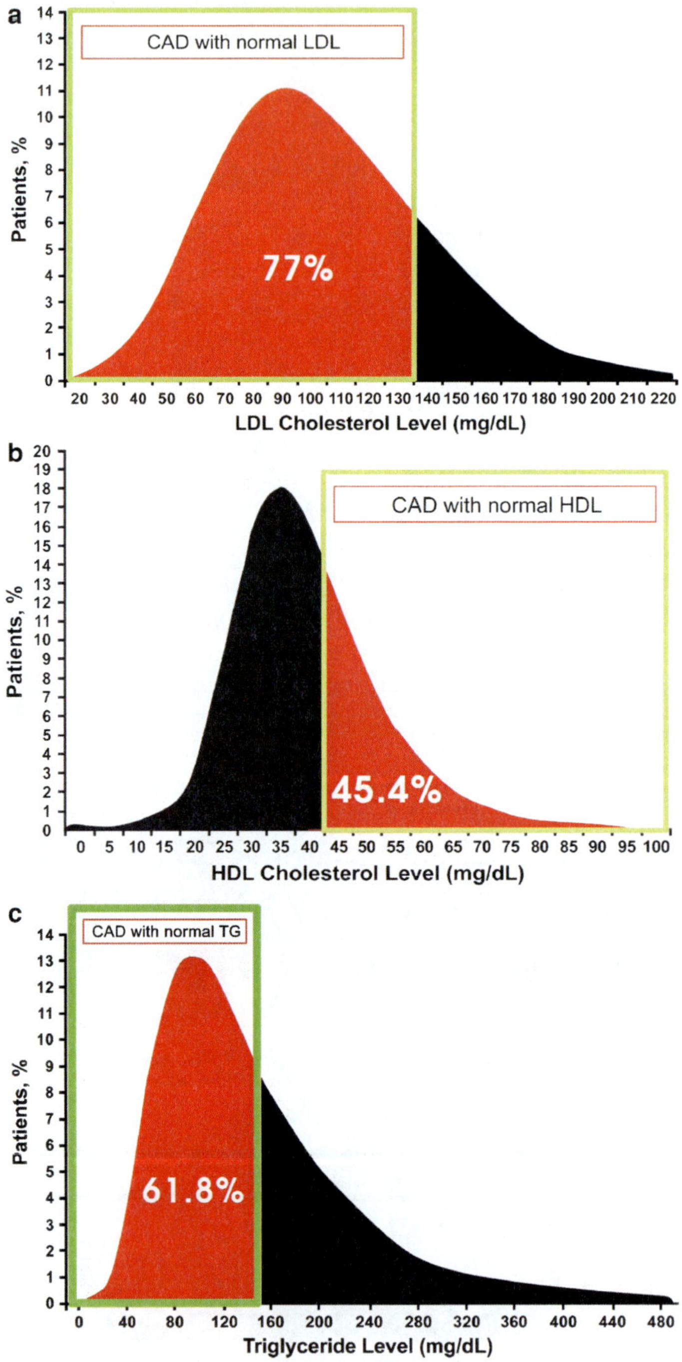

Fig. 1.2 (**a**) Of 136,905 patients hospitalized with CAD, 77% had normal LDL levels below 130 mg/dl. (**b**) Of 136,905 patients hospitalized with CAD, 45.4% had normal HDL levels above 40 mg/dl. (**c**) Of 136,905 patients hospitalized with CAD, 61.8% had normal triglyceride levels below 150 mg/dl.

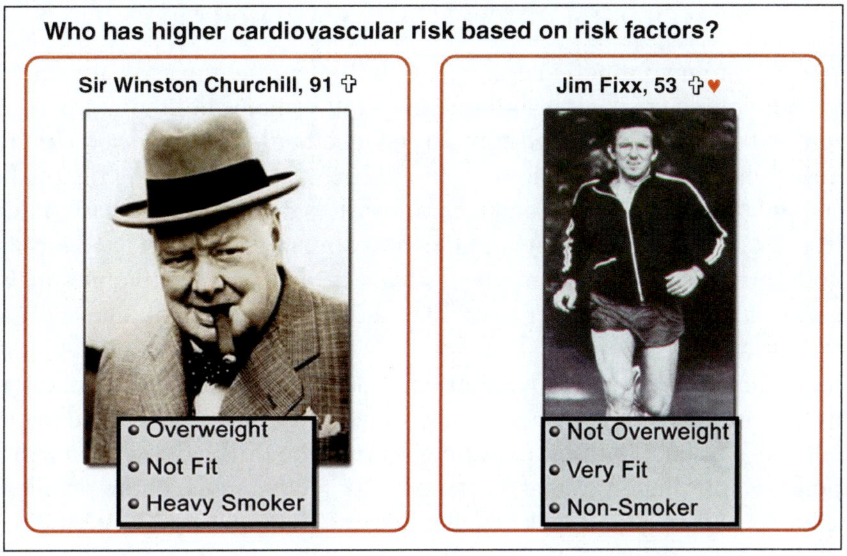
Who has higher cardiovascular risk based on risk factors?
Sir Winston Churchill, 91
Overweight
Not Fit
Heavy Smoker
Jim Fixx, 53
Not Overweight
Very Fit
Non-Smoker

Fig. 3. This figure illustrates the inaccuracy of traditional risk factors for identification of high-risk asymptomatic individuals.

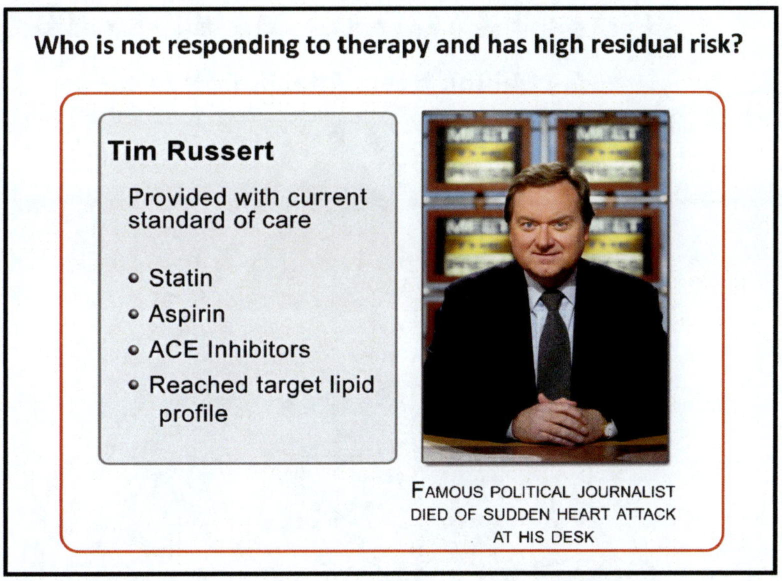

Fig. 4. The sudden death of famous journalist Tim Russert brought to light the problem of inadequate monitoring of response to treatments.

monitoring of the vascular response to treatments as illustrated in Fig. 4. The time has come to adopt new paradigms, beyond traditional ACVD risk factors, to address both these issues.

In this book, leading investigators in the field of ACVD present a new strategy for risk assessment and reduction that is largely based on noninvasive screening for early detection of asymptomatic ACVD itself (subclinical atherosclerosis) rather than for its risk factors. The new strategy stratifies the asymptomatic population based on a screening pyramid in which the intensity of treatment is tailored to the severity of atherosclerosis.

MODERN PREVENTIVE CARDIOLOGY

In the era of Google, remote robotic surgery, sub-millimeter noninvasive imaging, and nanotech-enabled mass proteomic assays, having millions of people (many of whom are indeed health conscious) living with, but unaware of, a huge coronary plaque burden is tragic and simply unacceptable. Physicians and researchers are responsible for taking actions and for helping the medical community to take full advantage of new knowledge and technology to save lives particularly in the very productive segment of the society (<75 years). After all, if investment in seat belts and airbags (low in cost-effectiveness) with proper regulatory provisions can be sold to automobile makers and users, investments for prevention of the number one killer should be successful, and will save many more lives (Fig. 5).

While new tactics aimed at increasing KAP of heart-healthy life styles and reduction of risk factors at the population level are absolutely necessary, new strategies are urgently needed to prevent imminent catastrophic effects. The ultimate preventive strategies must be directed toward the different levels of primary prevention (i.e., prevention of atherosclerosis risk factors in the entire population, mass treatment of atherosclerosis in a smaller at-risk population, and preemptive prevention of events in further smaller presymptomatic population. The first SHAPE guideline is directed at the early detection and

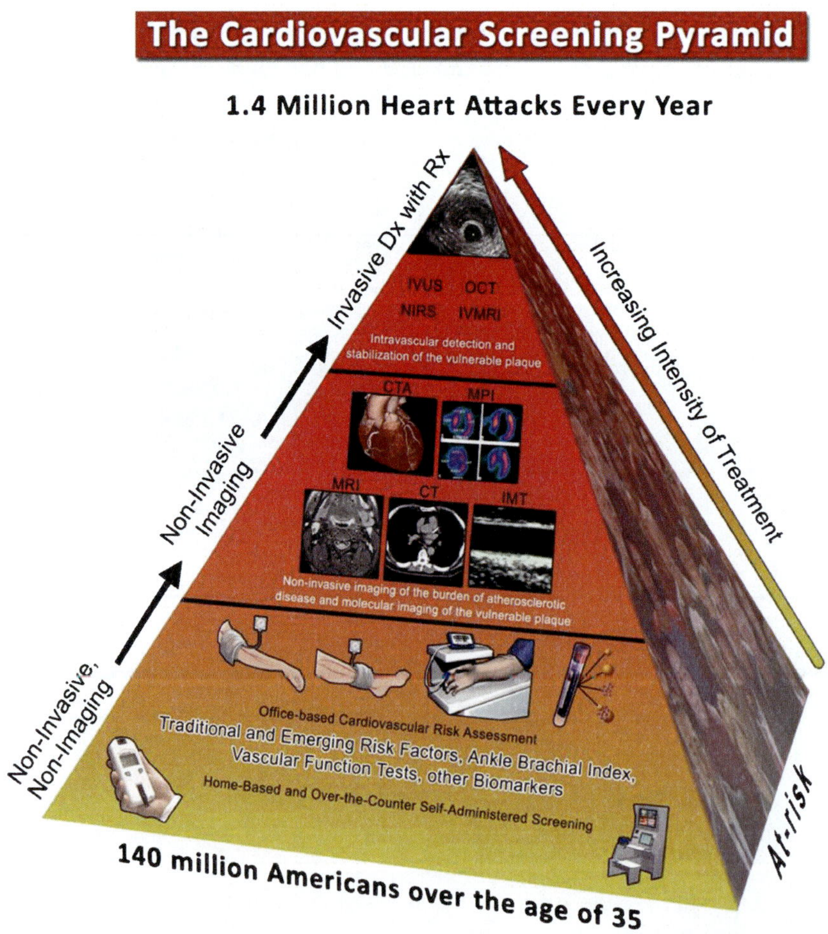

Fig. 5. Screening for asymptomatic atherosclerosis is needed to prevent symptomatic (fatal and or costly) ACVD.

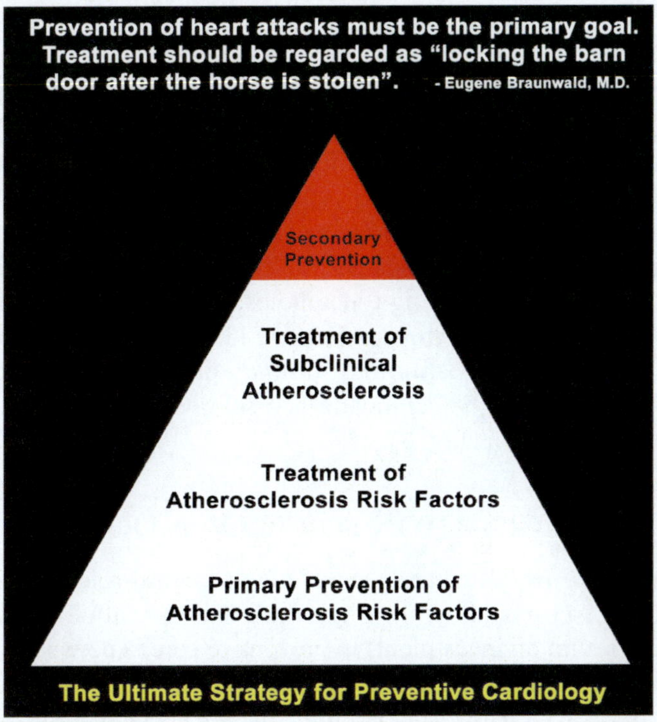

Fig. 6. The ultimate preventive strategies must be directed toward the different levels of primary prevention (i.e., prevention of atherosclerosis risk factors in the entire population, mass treatment of atherosclerosis in a smaller at-risk population, and preemptive prevention of events in further smaller presymptomatic population. The first SHAPE guideline is directed at the early detection and treatment of subclinical atherosclerosis and fills the gap in the existing guidelines.

treatment of subclinical atherosclerosis and fills the gap in the existing guidelines. Implementing such strategies can be visualized in a pyramid approach with the primary prevention of atherosclerosis at the bottom and the primary prevention of events in the presymptomatic population at the top (Fig. 6).

THE BIG PICTURE: HEALTH CARE VS. SICK CARE

The United States "health-care system" is a misnomer, since most of our rapidly rising federal medical care (Medicare) budget is spent on "sick care," i.e., treating existing disease rather than promoting health and preventing disease. In 2007, the USA spent $2.26 trillion on health care, or $7,439 per person, up from $2.1 trillion, or $7,026 per capita, the previous year. This expenditure is forecasted to grow 35% in the next 5 years [13]. Will this be matched by a 35% increase in disease reduction and life expectancy? Obviously no! What, exactly, are Americans paying for? The answer is not clear, but what is clear is that more and more is spent on expensive therapies for the treatment of diseases, most of which are preventable. While this problem remains a hot topic in the media and political arena, little has been done to provide a solution.

PREVENTIVE CARDIOLOGY, POORLY INVESTED

Investment in preventive health care must go far beyond general public recommendations to consume healthy foods, exercise, and avoid smoking. Although issuing educational guidelines and updating the food pyramid are needed, there is much more to be done for preventive health care to reach its full capability. With the growing number of expensive modalities in the tertiary cardiovascular care arena (e.g., drug-eluting stents, cardiac resynchronization therapy, and left ventricular assist devices), the cardiovascular health-care budget is increasingly absorbed into an area with minimum opportunities for adding productive life years. While it is universally agreed that the opportunity for prevention of death and saving quality-adjusted life years (QALY) is far greater in primary than secondary prevention, it is disappointing to see less than 10% of the total cardiovascular care budget routed toward the field of primary prevention. An arsenal of rigorous cost-effectiveness objections and regulatory barriers are exercised against new paradigms in the primary prevention arena. The currently allocated budget for cardiovascular screening (one cholesterol and blood pressure test every 5 years) is woefully inadequate for prevention of the number one killer compared to the preventive screening tests reimbursed for cancer (Fig. 7). In cardiology, primary prevention encompassing decreasing risk factors and screening for and treating subclinical atherosclerosis, is under-invested compared to the less efficacious secondary prevention (Fig. 8).

LEGISLATION FOR PREVENTION

The regulatory bodies and governmental agencies play a central role in this shift. Once the entrepreneurs, businessmen, and, subsequently, the physicians and the entire medical industry realize the opportunity for high ROI (return on investment) in preventive care, a new path will be open to unprecedented progress in our public cardiovascular health care. This strategy, of course, would make sense for other areas of medicine as well. However, given the prevalence and abrupt and fatal nature of heart attack and stroke, such a shift is most needed in the field of preventive cardiology. Currently, preventive cardiovascular health-care strategies are predominantly based on general recommendations and guidelines for heart-healthy life styles. Unlike the treatment of symptomatic ACVD, in which innovative technologies are easily and increasingly adopted, in the primary prevention of ACVD the adoption of new methods and technologies has been extremely slow. This becomes obvious when comparing the number of companies exhibiting at preventive cardiology conferences vs. interventional

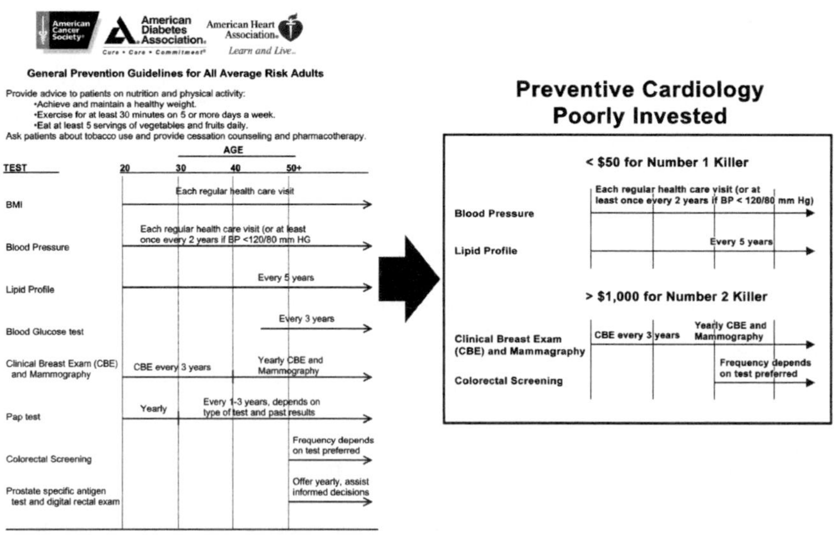

Fig. 7. The current allocation of the US preventive screening budget for the number one killer (CVD) compared to the number two killer (cancer) is very disproportionate.

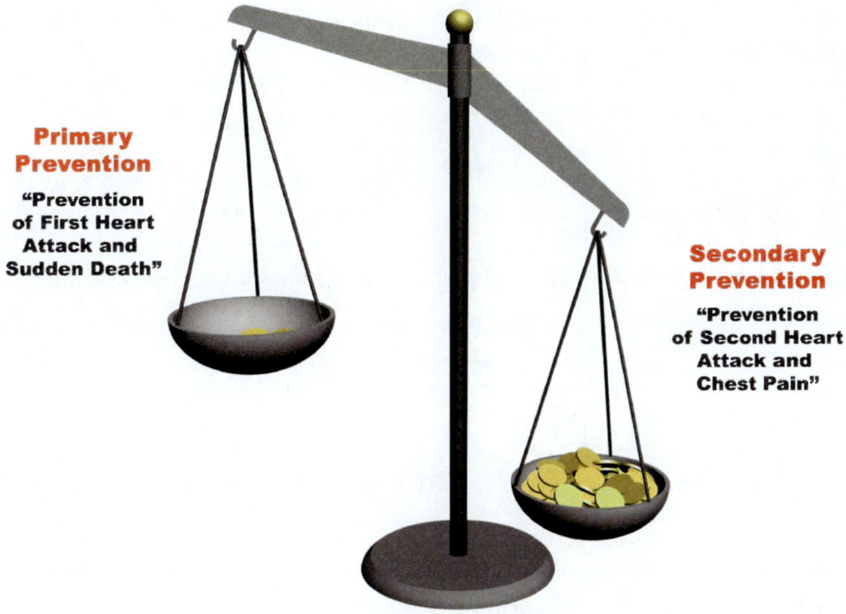
Primary Prevention
"Prevention of First Heart Attack and Sudden Death"
Secondary Prevention
"Prevention of Second Heart Attack and Chest Pain"

Fig. 8. Comparing to the treatment of a heart attack, its prevention is woefully under-invested.

cardiology or cardiovascular surgery meetings. Without creating new opportunities for business developments in the field of primary prevention, it will be hard for the field to grow and fulfill its promises. Attracting investment in free and capitalistic societies can only be successful if ROI is greater than competing business opportunities. Unfortunately, in cardiology practice and business today, ROI in the prevention of the first heart attack and associated sudden death is much lower than ROI in the prevention of chest pain after the first heart attack. Obviously, this investment paradigm is faulty, since primary prevention can save many more lives and results in more productivity by reducing premature death and disability. The SHAPE Task Force helped introduce the first of such legislative initiatives in the United States to Texas legislature. The Texas Heart Attack Preventive Screening Bill (HB1290), which was inspired by the SHAPE guidelines, passed the Senate and became law in Texas effective September 2009. The law mandates insurance coverage for noninvasive imaging of asymptomatic atherosclerosis in the Framingham Intermediate Risk population [14, 15].

Although passing the Texas Heart Attack Preventive Screening law is considered a monumental milestone on the way of shifting cardiovascular health care to primary prevention and has set the stage for other states to follow, it is far from adequate for the ultimate goal of eradicating heart attacks. Additional policy reforms, such as the following, must be seriously considered by the legislative and executive bodies to address the number one killer.

1. Provide more reimbursement incentives for preventive health-care technologies than at present.
2. Empower primary care physicians to utilize state-of-the-art preventive diagnostic technologies.
3. Enforce "pay for benefit" [2] strategy instead of the existing "pay for service" system, and exercise it in all layers of medical care (primary, secondary, and tertiary).
4. Give incentive and funding priorities through NIH, NSF, and other federal research funding agencies to fund proposals with innovative technologies focusing on primary prevention.
5. Empower consumers to take charge of their health by reducing regulatory (FDA) barriers for accessing safe and effective drugs such as statins (over-the-counter access).

6. Give economic incentive (such as tax breaks) to the medical industry for any future products they bring to the market focusing on the primary prevention.
7. Give economic incentive (tax breaks) to at-risk populations to reduce their burden of CVD risk, e.g., weight loss, stop smoking cessation, cholesterol, and blood pressure lowering.
8. Increase the tax on smoking, both consumers and providers.
9. Shift cardiovascular prevention from the hospital and doctors' offices to the home; give incentive to home health monitoring companies and reduce legal barriers for mass adoption of practicing telemedicine and tele-health care.
10. Mandate insurance coverage of screening and treatment of asymptomatic (subclinical) atherosclerosis.

In conclusion, to build the "Field of Dreams" for preventive cardiology and ultimately for the eradication of heart attacks, the government and health-care policy makers need to take the first step to build the ground.

HEART ATTACKS CAN BE ERADICATED

The heart attack epidemic inherited from the twentieth century (over 15million heart attacks every year), makes it difficult for most people to imagine a future in which heart attacks are no longer a threat. Nonetheless, the mission of eradicating heart attacks is no more challenging than the mission of landing humans on Mars. The vision for a heart attack-free future can become a reality in the twenty-first century and can result in a major increase in human life expectancy and socioeconomic development, if the medical community, including academia, industry, and health-care policymakers, shift their investment from the treatment of events that have already occurred to prevention of the first event. Figure 9 illustrates a likely path to arrest the worldwide epidemic of ACVD related mortality and morbidity, particularly heart attacks.

Heart-healthy life style assisted by innovative preventive technologies and personalized medicine will be able to shift the existing in-hospital expensive sick care to the future out-of-hospital inexpensive health care.

1. Era of Screening: Searching for and saving the vulnerable patient: as presented in the SHAPE Task Force report [7], the SHAPE initiative presents the best available strategy to advance the ongoing fight against ACVD, primarily heart attack and stroke [18].
2. Era of "PolyPill": Mass prophylactic therapy of at-risk population using an effective, safe, and inexpensive cocktail of drugs: A future with universal prophylactic therapy for the prevention of ACVD, using a cocktail

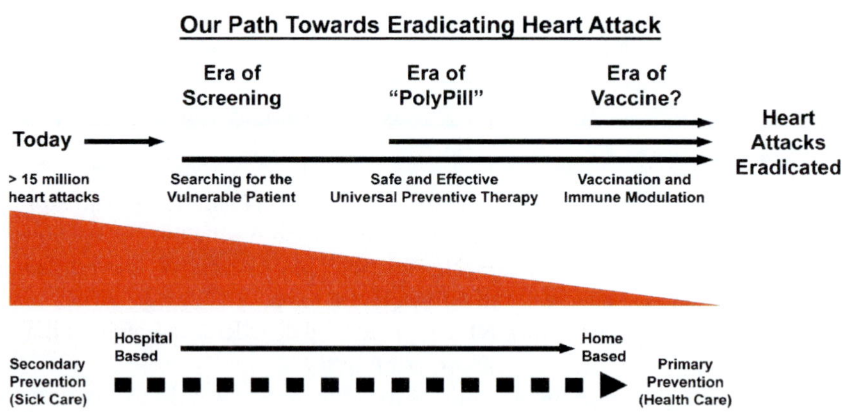

Fig. 9. A likely path to arrest the epidemic of atherosclerotic cardiovascular disease (ACVD) worldwide.

of effective, safe, and inexpensive drugs (packaged compactly) to assure maximum compliance, is on the horizon. Although such a future is most desirable, there are major scientific and regulatory roadblocks that will require time and further investigations [16]. Pending resolution of these issues, the SHAPE strategy remains the best strategy.

3. Era of Vaccine: Primary prevention through immune modulation and vaccination strategies: Vaccination and immune modulation strategies for prevention, regression, and stabilization of atherosclerosis present a most exciting possibility. Atherosclerosis bears many similarities to chronic inflammatory/autoimmune diseases such as rheumatoid arthritis and Alzheimer's disease. Compelling data from experimental models show that such diseases may be challenged by vaccination and immune modulation strategies. Will it be possible to attack ACVD with the same approach? Several studies have shown positive effects of immunization with antigenic LDL preparations. Such ground-breaking approaches may become the panacea for the world's growing epidemic of heart disease [17].

CONCLUSION

Innovation in prevention will shape the future of cardiovascular health care. Heart attacks will be eradicated in the twenty-first century if the medical community, including academia, industry, and health-care policymakers, shift their investment from the treatment of events that have already occurred to prevention of the first event, i.e. "lock the barn door before the horse is stolen."

REFERENCES

1. Yusuf S, Reddy S, Ounpuu S, Anand S. Global burden of cardiovascular diseases: Part II: variations in cardiovascular disease by specific ethnic groups and geographic regions and prevention strategies. Circulation. 2001;104:2855.
2. Lloyd-Jones D, Adams R, Carnethon M, De Simone G, Ferguson TB, Flegal K, Ford E, Furie K, Go A, Greenlund K, Haase N, Hailpern S, Ho M, Howard V, Kissela B, Kittner S, Lackland D, Lisabeth L, Marelli A, McDermott M, Meigs J, Mozaffarian D, Nichol G, O'Donnell C, Roger V, Rosamond W, Sacco R, Sorlie P, Stafford R, Steinberger J, Thom T, Wasserthiel-Smoller S, Wong N, Wylie-Rosett J, Hong Y; American Heart Association Statistics Committee and Stroke Statistics Subcommittee. Heart Disease and Stroke Statistics—2009 Update. A Report From the American Heart Association Statistics Committee and Stroke Statistics Subcommittee. Circulation. 2009;119:e21-e181.
3. Brown MS, Goldstein JLHeart attacks: gone with the century? Science. 1996;272(5262):629.
4. Murabito JM, Evans JC, Larson MG, Levy D. Prognosis after the onset of coronary heart disease. An investigation of differences in outcome between the sexes according to initial coronary disease presentation. Circulation. 1993;88(6):2548-55.
5. Naghavi M, Libby P, Falk E, Casscells SW, Litovsky S, Rumberger J, Badimon JJ, Stefanadis C, Moreno P, Pasterkamp G, Fayad Z, Stone PH, Waxman S, Raggi P, Madjid M, Zarrabi A, Burke A, Yuan C, Fitzgerald PJ, Siscovick DS, de Korte CL, Aikawa M, Juhani Airaksinen KE, Assmann G, Becker CR, Chesebro JH, Farb A, Galis ZS, Jackson C, Jang IK, Koenig W, Lodder RA, March K, Demirovic J, Navab M, Priori SG, Rekhter MD, Bahr R, Grundy SM, Mehran R, Colombo A, Boerwinkle E, Ballantyne C, Insull W Jr, Schwartz RS, Vogel R, Serruys PW, Hansson GK, Faxon DP, Kaul S, Drexler H, Greenland P, Muller JE, Virmani R, Ridker PM, Zipes DP, Shah PK, Willerson JT. From vulnerable plaque to vulnerable patient: a call for new definitions and risk assessment strategies: Part I. Circulation. 2003;108(14):1664-72.
6. Naghavi M, Libby P, Falk E, Casscells SW, Litovsky S, Rumberger J, Badimon JJ, Stefanadis C, Moreno P, Pasterkamp G, Fayad Z, Stone PH, Waxman S, Raggi P, Madjid M, Zarrabi A, Burke A, Yuan C, Fitzgerald PJ, Siscovick DS, de Korte CL, Aikawa M, Juhani Airaksinen KE, Assmann G, Becker CR, Chesebro JH, Farb A, Galis ZS, Jackson C, Jang IK, Koenig W, Lodder RA, March K, Demirovic J, Navab M, Priori SG, Rekhter MD, Bahr R, Grundy SM, Mehran R, Colombo A, Boerwinkle E, Ballantyne C, Insull W Jr, Schwartz RS, Vogel R, Serruys PW, Hansson GK, Faxon DP, Kaul S, Drexler H, Greenland P, Muller JE, Virmani R, Ridker PM, Zipes DP, Shah PK, Willerson JT. From vulnerable plaque to vulnerable patient: a call for new definitions and risk assessment strategies: Part II. Circulation. 2003;108(14):1664-72.
7. Naghavi M, Falk E, Hecht HS, Jamieson MJ, Kaul S, Berman D, Fayad Z, Budoff MJ, Rumberger J, Naqvi TZ, Shaw LJ, Faergeman O, Cohn J, Bahr R, Koenig W, Demirovic J, Arking D, Herrera VL, Badimon J, Goldstein JA, Rudy Y, Airaksinen J, Schwartz RS, Riley WA, Mendes RA, Douglas P, Shah PK. From vulnerable plaque to vulnerable patient -Part III: Executive summary of the Screening for Heart Attack Prevention and Education (SHAPE) Task Force report. Am J Cardiol. 2006;98(2A):2H-15H.
8. Sachdeva et al. Lipid levels in patients hospitalized with coronary artery disease: An analysis of 136,905 hospitalizations in Get With The Guidelines. Am Heart J. 2009;157:111-7.
9. Akosah KO, Schaper A, Cogbill C, Schoenfeld P. Preventing myocardial infarction in the young adult in the first place: how do the National Cholesterol Education Panel III guidelines perform? J Am Coll Cardiol. 2003;41(9):1475-9.

10. Nasir K, Michos ED, Blumenthal RS, Raggi P. Detection of high-risk young adults and women by coronary calcium and National Cholesterol Education Program Panel III guidelines. J Am Coll Cardiol 2005;46:1931-6.
11. Johnson KM, Dowe DA, Brink JA. Traditional Clinical Risk Assessment Tools Do Not Accurately Predict Coronary Atherosclerotic Plaque Burden: A CT Angiography Study. A J Roentgenol 2009;192:235-43.
12. National Health Expenditures, Forecast summary and selected tables. Office of the Actuary in the Centers for Medicare & Medicaid Services, 2008. http://www.cms.hhs.gov/NationalHealthExpendData/Downloads/proj2007.pdf Retrieved Nov 10, 2009.
13. Diamond GA, Denton TA, Matloff JM. Fee-for-benefit: a strategy to improve the quality of health care and control costs through reimbursement incentives. J Am Coll Cardiol. 1993;22(2):343-52.
14. Texas Legislature Online Bill Stages. Bill: HB1290 http://www.legis.state.tx.us/billlookup/BillStages.aspx?LegSess=81R &Bill=HB1290 Retrieved Nov 10, 2009.
15. Falk E, Naghavi M, Shah PK. Legislating screening for atherosclerosis. JAMA. 2008;299(18):2147-8.
16. Jamieson MJ, Naghavi, M. Multi-constituent cardiovascular pills (MCCP)--challenges and promises of population-based prophylactic drug therapy for prevention of heart attack. Curr Pharm Des. 2007;13(10):1069-76.
17. Nilsson J, Hansson GK, Shah PK. Immunomodulation of atherosclerosis: implications for vaccine development. Arterioscler Thromb Vasc Biol. 2005;25(1):18-28.
18. Shah PK. The SHAPE Paradigm: A Commentary Circ Cardiovase Qual Outcomes. 2010;3;106-109.

2 From Vulnerable Plaque to Vulnerable Patient

Morteza Naghavi and Erling Falk

On behalf of the vulrerable patient Consensus writing group*

Contents

Abstract

Atherosclerotic cardiovascular disease results in millions of sudden deaths annually, and coronary artery disease accounts for the majority of this toll. Despite major advances in the treatment of coronary artery disease, a large number of victims of the disease who are apparently healthy die suddenly without prior symptoms. Available screening and diagnostic methods are insufficient to identify the victims before the event occurs. The recognition of the role of the vulnerable plaque has opened new avenues in the field of cardiovascular medicine. This consensus document concludes the following. (1) Rupture-prone plaques are not the only vulnerable plaques. All types of atherosclerotic plaques with high likelihood of thrombotic complications and rapid progression should be considered as vulnerable plaques. We propose a classification for clinical as well as pathological evaluation of vulnerable plaques. (2) Vulnerable plaques are not the only culprit factors for the development of acute coronary syndromes, myocardial infarction,

From: *Asymptomatic Atherosclerosis: Pathophysiology, Detection and Treatment*
Edited by: M. Naghavi (ed.), DOI 10.1007/978-1-60327-179-0_2

and sudden cardiac death. Vulnerable blood (prone to thrombosis) and vulnerable myocardium (prone to fatal arrhythmia) play an important role in the outcome. Therefore, the term "vulnerable patient" may be more appropriate and is proposed now for the identification of subjects with a high likelihood of developing cardiac events in the near future. (3) A quantitative method for cumulative risk assessment of vulnerable patients needs to be developed that may include variables based on plaque, blood, and myocardial vulnerability. This chapter reports the consensus document created among experts on vulnerable plaque, vulnerable blood, and vulnerable myocardium, and provides an outline of the overall risk assessment of the vulnerable patient.

Key words: Atherosclerosis; Vulnerable plaque; Vulnerable blood; Vulnerable myocardium; Vulnerable patient; Plaque rupture

KEY POINTS

- Plaque rupture is the most common type of plaque complication, accounting for ≈70% of fatal acute myocardial infarctions and/or sudden coronary deaths. However, rupture-prone plaques are not the only vulnerable plaques. All types of atherosclerotic plaques with a high likelihood of thrombotic complications and rapid progression should be considered as vulnerable plaques.
- Vulnerable plaques are not the only culprit factors for the development of acute coronary syndromes, myocardial infarction, and sudden cardiac death. Vulnerable blood (prone to thrombosis) and vulnerable myocardium (prone to fatal arrhythmia) play an important role in the outcome.
- A quantitative method for cumulative risk assessment of vulnerable patients needs to be developed that may include variables based on plaque, blood, and myocardial vulnerability.
- The search for the vulnerable patient must follow a pyramid approach, the base of which would start from a comprehensive non-invasive, non-imaging assessment of vascular health along with risk factor measurement. The next step would be non-invasive imaging of atherosclerosis (structure and activity) followed by invasive procedures if risk of an eminent event is expected.
- Longitudinal natural study of vulnerable plaque and vulnerable patients are needed to compare the proposed pyramid-based approach versus the status quo.

INTRODUCTION

Cardiovascular disease has long been the leading cause of death in developed countries, and it is rapidly becoming the number one killer in the developing countries [1]. According to current estimates, 61,800,000 Americans have one or more types of cardiovascular disease [2].

Every year, more than 1 million people in the United States and more than 19 million others worldwide experience a sudden cardiac event (acute coronary syndromes and/or sudden cardiac death). A large portion of this population has no prior symptom [3]. There is considerable demand for diagnosis and treatment of the pathologic conditions that underlie these sudden cardiac events. This consensus document proposes new directions to prevent infarction and sudden cardiac events [4].

UNDERLYING CAUSES OF SUDDEN, FATAL AND NONFATAL CARDIAC EVENTS

Figure 1 delineates the underlying causes of acute cardiac events. The first branch point of the tree indicates patients who lack significant atherosclerosis or related myocardial damage, that is, those who have no ischemic heart disease (see section Nonischemic Vulnerable Myocardium). This leaves the patients with atherosclerosis, some of whom also have a hypercoagulable state (see section Vulnerable (Thrombogenic) Blood).

The next branch point involves the presence or absence of an occlusive or subocclusive thrombus. A thrombus identifies a culprit plaque that may be ruptured or nonruptured.

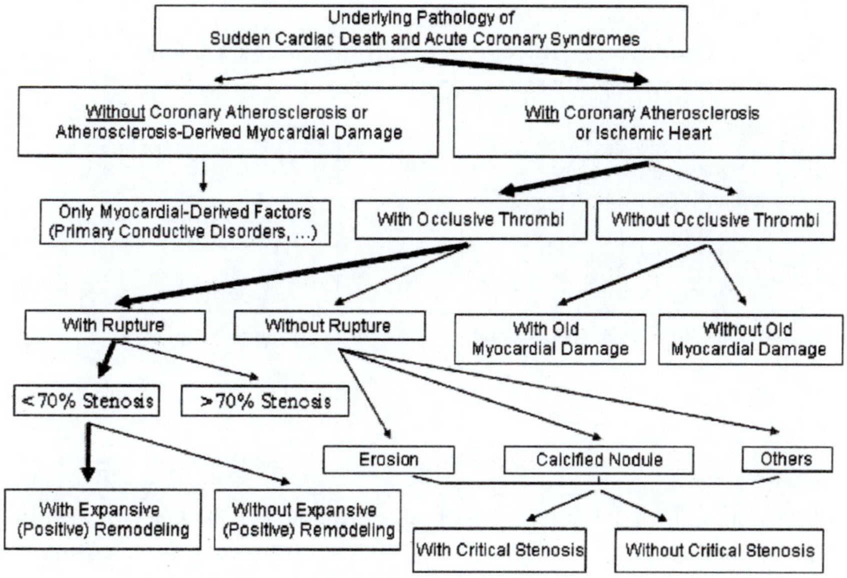

Fig. 1. Proposed diagram of the potential underlying pathology of acute coronary syndrome, (i.e., unstable angina, acute myocardial infarction and sudden cardiac death).

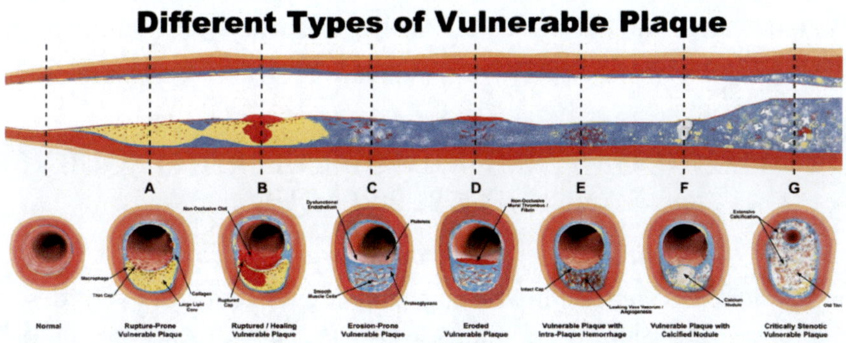

Fig. 2. Different types of vulnerable plaque as underlying cause of acute coronary events (ACS) and sudden cardiac death (SCD). (**a**) Rupture-prone plaque with large lipid core and thin fibrous cap infiltrated by macrophages. (**b**) Ruptured plaque with subocclusive thrombus and early organization. (**c**) Erosion-prone plaque with proteoglycan matrix in a smooth muscle cell-rich plaque. (**d**) Eroded plaque with subocclusive thrombus. (**e**) Intraplaque hemorrhage secondary to leaking vasa vasorum. (**f**) Calcific nodule protruding into the vessel lumen. (**g**) Chronically stenotic plaque with severe calcification, old thrombus, and eccentric lumen.

Plaque rupture is the most common type of plaque complication, accounting for ~70% of fatal acute myocardial infarctions and/or sudden coronary deaths (Fig. 2). Several retrospective autopsy series and a few cross-sectional clinical studies have suggested that thrombotic coronary death and acute coronary syndromes are caused by the plaque features and associated factors presented in Table 1 [5–7]. Most techniques for detecting and treating vulnerable plaque are devoted to rupture-prone plaque. This type of plaque has been termed a "thin-cap fibroatheroma" [8].

In some cases, a deep plaque injury cannot be identified despite a careful search. The thrombus appears to be superimposed on a de-endothelialized, but otherwise intact, plaque. This type of superficial plaque

Table 1
Underlying pathologies of "culprit" coronary lesions

Ruptured plaques (~70%)
Stenotic (20%)
Nonstenotic (50%)
Nonruptured plaques (~30%)
Erosion
Calcified nodule
Others/unknown

Adapted from Falk and associates [6], Davies [7], and Virmani et al. [5]

injury is called "plaque erosion" [9]. Other types of culprit plaques also exist (Fig. 2). In cases involving nonruptured plaques, plaque erosion or nodular calcification usually accompanies the luminal thrombus [5]. Other forms of thrombosis in nonruptured plaques may be described in the future. In all cases that involve a superimposed thrombus, the underlying lesion may be stenotic or nonstenotic. However, nonstenotic lesions are far more frequent than stenotic plaques and account for the majority of culprit ruptured plaques [10].

In cases of sudden cardiac death without thrombosis, we hypothesize that coronary spasm, emboli to the distal intramural vasculature, or myocardial damage related to previous injury may account for a terminal arrhythmic episode.

THE CHALLENGE OF TERMINOLOGY: CULPRIT PLAQUE VERSUS VULNERABLE PLAQUE

Culprit Plaque, a Retrospective Terminology

Interventional cardiologists and cardiovascular pathologists retrospectively describe the plaque responsible for coronary occlusion and death as a *culprit* plaque, regardless of its histopathologic features. For prospective evaluation, clinicians need a similar term for describing such plaques *before* an event occurs. Plaque rupture was reported sporadically by pathologists in the early twentieth century; it became a focus of attention of pioneering scientists in the 1960s (Table 2) and was later documented further by others [11–16].

Since the 1970s, scientists have been seeking the mechanisms responsible for converting chronic coronary atherosclerosis to acute coronary artery disease [11–15, 17]. As insights into this process have evolved, the relevant terminology has been continually updated. In the 1980s, Falk [11] and Davies and Thomas [15] used "plaque disruption" synonymously with "plaque rupture." Later, Muller et al. [18, 19] used "vulnerable" to describe rupture-prone plaques as the underlying cause of most clinical coronary events. When this functional definition was proposed, the plaque considered responsible for acute coronary events (based on retrospective autopsy studies) had a large lipid pool, a thin cap, and macrophage-dense inflammation on or beneath its surface (Fig. 3).

Over the past several years, "vulnerable plaque" has been used sometimes to denote this concept and at other times to denote the specific histopathologic appearance of the above-described plaque. This dual usage is confusing, particularly as plaques can have other histologic features (see Fig. 2) that may also cause acute coronary events [5].

Table 2
Descriptions used by pioneers for culprit plaques [93, 94]

Author	*Year*	*Description used*
Olcott	1931	Plaque rupture
Leary	1934	Rupture of atheromatous abscess
Wartman	1938	Rupture-induced occlusion
Horn	1940	Plaque fissure
Helpern	1957	Plaque erosion
Crawford	1961	Plaque thrombosis
Gore	1963	Plaque ulceration
Byers	1964	Thrombogenic gruel
Chapman	1966	Plaque rupture
Constantinides	1966	Plaque rupture

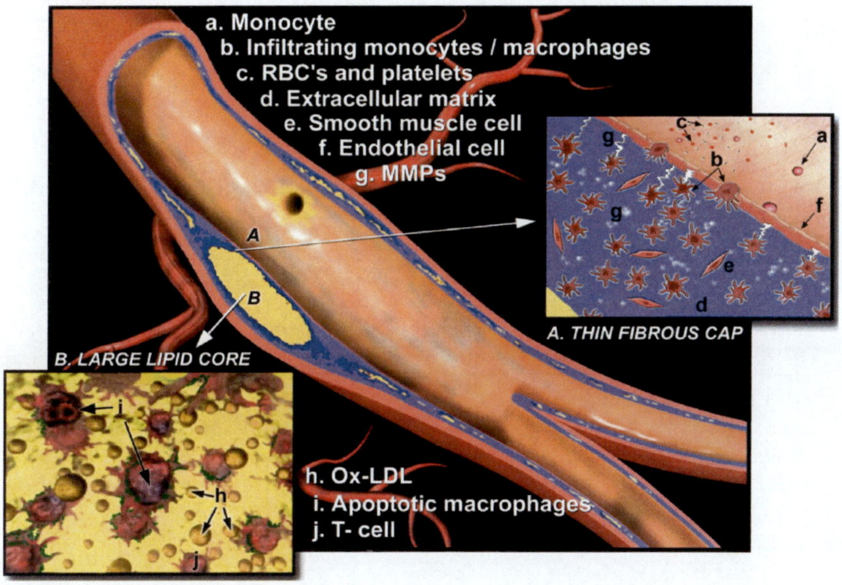

Fig. 3. Schematic figure illustrating the most common type of vulnerable plaque characterized by thin fibrous cap, extensive macrophage infiltration, paucity of smooth muscle cells, and large lipid core, without significant luminal narrowing.

Vulnerable Plaque, a Future Culprit Plaque

The term "vulnerable" is defined by English dictionaries as "susceptible to injury or susceptible to attack," [20] as in "We are vulnerable both by water and land, without either fleet or army" (Alexander Hamilton). It denotes the likelihood of having an event in the future. The term "vulnerable" has been used in various reports in the medical literature, all of which describe conditions susceptible to injury. In this regard, the term "vulnerable plaque" is most suitable to define plaques susceptible to complications. An alternative term, "high-risk plaque," has been proposed [18]. The term "high-risk" is often used to describe the high-risk patient groups with acute coronary syndromes. However, our intention is to provide a terminology to identify apparently healthy subjects at the risk of future events. Therefore, the term vulnerable seems to be more appropriate. Also, because "vulnerable plaque" has already been widely adopted by investigators and clinicians, we recommend that the existing usage of this term be continued. We advise that the underlying morphological features be described broadly enough to include all dangerous plaques that involve a risk of thrombosis and/or rapid progression.

To provide a uniform language to help standardize the terminology, we recommend "vulnerable plaque" to identify all thrombosis-prone plaques and plaques with a high probability of undergoing rapid progression, thus becoming culprit plaques (Table 3). A proposed histopathologic classification for different types of vulnerable plaque is presented in Fig. 2. A list of proposed major and minor criteria for defining vulnerable plaques, based on autopsy studies (culprit plaques), is presented in Table 4.

A large number of vulnerable plaques are relatively uncalcified, relatively nonstenotic, and similar to type IV atherosclerotic lesions described in the American Heart Association classification [21]. However, as depicted in Fig. 3, different types of vulnerable plaques exist. Although Table 1 shows the relative distribution of ruptured and nonruptured culprit plaques, the exact prevalence of each type of vulnerable plaque is unknown and can only be determined in prospective studies.

Table 3
Interchangeable terms used to denote vulnerable plaque

Acceptable but not recommended	*Unacceptable*[a]
High-risk plaque	Soft plaque
Dangerous plaque	Noncalcified plaque
Unstable plaque	AHA type IV plaque

AHA American Heart Association
[a]The term vulnerable plaque refers to all plaques at risk for thrombosis or rapid progression to become culprit lesions. A vulnerable plaque is not necessarily a soft plaque, a non-calcified plaque, an AHA type IV plaque, or a non-stenotic plaque [8, 21]

Table 4
Criteria for defining vulnerable plaque, based on the study of culprit plaques

Major criteria
Active inflammation (monocyte/macrophage and sometimes T-cell infiltration)
Thin cap with large lipid core
Endothelial denudation with superficial platelet aggregation
Fissured plaque
Stenosis >90%
Minor criteria
Superficial calcified nodule
Glistening yellow
Intraplaque hemorrhage
Endothelial dysfunction
Outward (positive) remodeling

Pan-Coronary Vulnerability

Several investigators have noted the presence of more than one vulnerable plaque in patients at risk of cardiovascular events. Mann and Davies [22] and Burke et al. [23] in cardiac autopsy specimens, Goldstein et al. [24] in angiography studies, Nissen [25] and Rioufol et al. [26] with intravascular ultrasound, and Buffon et al. [27] measuring neutrophil myeloperoxidase found multiple rupture-prone or ruptured plaques in a wide range of cardiovascular patient populations. A most recent series of publications on vulnerability reiterated the importance of going beyond a vulnerable plaque and called for evaluating the total arterial tree as a whole [28–30].

Silent-Plaque Rupture

Thrombotic complications that arise from rupture or fissure (small rupture) of a vulnerable plaque may be clinically silent, yet contribute to the natural history of plaque progression and ultimately luminal stenosis [31, 32].

BEYOND THE ATHEROSCLEROTIC PLAQUE

It is important to identify patients in whom disruption of a vulnerable plaque is likely to result in a clinical event. In these patients, other factors beyond plaque (i.e., thrombogenic blood and electrical instability of myocardium) are responsible for the final outcome (Fig. 4). We propose that such patients be referred to as “vulnerable patients.” In fact, plaques with similar characteristics may have different clinical presentations because of blood coagulability (vulnerable blood) or myocardial susceptibility to develop fatal arrhythmia (vulnerable myocardium). The latter may depend on a current or previous ischemic condition and/or a nonischemic electrophysiological abnormality.

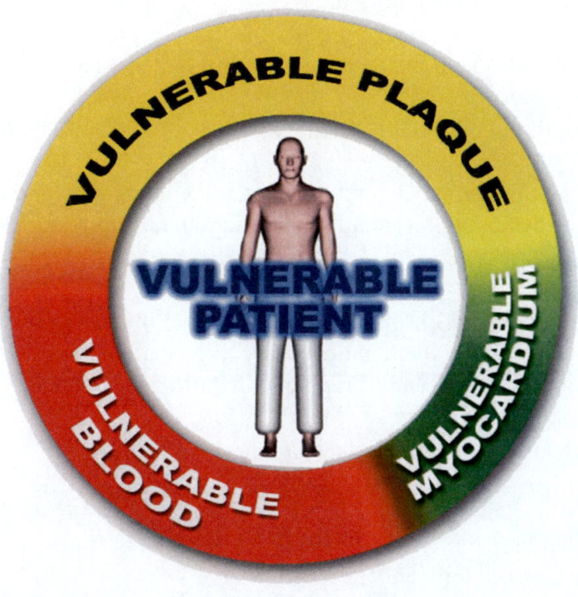

Fig. 4. The risk of a vulnerable patient is affected by vulnerable plaque and/or vulnerable blood and/or vulnerable myocardium. A comprehensive assessment must consider all of the above.

DEFINITION OF A CARDIOVASCULAR VULNERABLE PATIENT

The term "cardiovascular vulnerable patient" is proposed to define subjects susceptible to an acute coronary syndrome or sudden cardiac death based on plaque, blood, or myocardial vulnerability (for example, 1-year risk ≥ 5%). Extensive efforts are needed to quantify an individual's risk of an event according to each component of vulnerability (plaque, blood, and myocardium). Such a comprehensive risk-stratification tool capable of predicting acute coronary syndromes as well as sudden cardiac death would be very useful for preventive cardiology (Fig. 4).

DIAGNOSIS OF VULNERABLE PLAQUE/ARTERY

A number of issues have hampered the establishment of ideal criteria for defining vulnerable plaque: (1) the current body of evidence is largely based on cross-sectional and retrospective studies of culprit plaques; (2) robust prospective outcome studies based on plaque characterization have not been done (because of the lack of a reproducible, validated diagnostic technique); and (3) a lack of a representative animal model of plaque rupture and acute coronary syndrome/sudden death.

On the basis of retrospective evidence, we propose that the criteria listed in Tables 4 and 5 FX be used to define a vulnerable plaque. The sensitivity, specificity, and overall predictive value of each potential diagnostic technique need to be assessed before entering clinical practice.

Table 5
Markers of vulnerability at the plaque/artery level

Markers
Plaque
Morphology/structure
Plaque cap thickness
Plaque lipid core size
Plaque stenosis (luminal narrowing)
Remodeling (expansive vs. constrictive remodeling)
Color (yellow, glistening yellow, red, etc.)
Collagen content versus lipid content, mechanical stability (stiffness and elasticity)
Calcification burden and pattern (nodule vs. scattered, superficial vs. deep, etc.)
Shear stress (flow pattern throughout the coronary artery)
Activity/function
Plaque inflammation (macrophage density, rate of monocyte infiltration and density of activated T cell)
Endothelial denudation or dysfunction (local NO production, anti-/procoagulation properties of the endothelium)
Plaque oxidative stress
Superficial platelet aggregation and fibrin deposition (residual mural thrombus)
Rate of apoptosis (apoptosis protein markers, coronary microsatellite, etc.)
Angiogenesis, leaking vasa vasorum, and intraplaque hemorrhage
Matrix-digesting enzyme activity in the cap (MMPs 2, 3, 9, etc.)
Certain microbial antigens (e.g., HSP60, *C. pneumoniae*)
Pan-arterial
Transcoronary gradient of serum markers of vulnerability
Total coronary calcium burden
Total coronary vasoreactivity (endothelial function)
Total arterial burden of plaque including peripheral (e.g., carotid IMT)

MMP matrix metalloproteinase; *NO* nitric oxide; *IMT* intima-media thickness

Major Criteria

The following are proposed as major criteria for the detection of a vulnerable plaque. The presence of one or a combination of these factors may warrant higher risk of plaque complication. Techniques for detection of vulnerable plaque based on these criteria are briefly summarized here. A detailed discussion of advantages and disadvantages are reviewed elsewhere [33].

Active Inflammation

Plaques with active inflammation may be identified by extensive macrophage accumulation [13]. Possible intravascular diagnostic techniques [34, 35] include thermography (measurement of plaque temperature) [36, 37], contrast-enhanced (CE) MRI [38, 39], fluorodeoxyglucose positron emission tomography [33, 40], and immunoscintigraphy [41]. It has been shown that optical coherence tomography reflects the macrophage content of the fibrous cap [42]. Noninvasive options include MRI with superparamagnetic iron oxide [35, 36] and gadolinium fluorine compounds [43–45].

A Thin Cap With a Large Lipid Core

These plaques have a cap thickness of <100 μm and a lipid core accounting for >40% of the plaque's total volume [8]. Possible intravascular diagnostic techniques include optical coherence tomography (OCT) [46, 47], intravascular ultrasonography (IVUS) [48], high-resolution IVUS [49], elastography (palpography) [50, 51], MRI [52], angioscopy [53], near-infrared (NIR) spectroscopy [54–56], and radiofrequency IVUS analysis [57, 58]. The only noninvasive options are presently MRI and possibly CT [34, 35, 59–62].

Endothelial Denudation with Superficial Platelet Aggregation

These plaques are characterized by superficial erosion and platelet aggregation or fibrin deposition [5]. Possible intravascular diagnostic techniques include angioscopy with dye [63] and matrix-targeted/fibrin-targeted immune scintigraphy and OCT [46, 47]. Noninvasive options include fibrin/matrix-targeted contrast enhanced MRI [64], platelet/fibrin-targeted single photon emission computed tomography [41], and MRI [52].

Fissured/Injured Plaque

Plaques with a fissured cap (most of them involving a recent rupture) that did not result in occlusive thrombi may be prone to subsequent thrombosis, entailing occlusive thrombi or thromboemboli [5]. Possible intravascular diagnostic techniques include OCT [46, 47], IVUS, high-resolution IVUS [49], angioscopy, and MRI [34, 35]. A noninvasive option is fibrin-targeted CE-MRI [64, 65].

Severe Stenosis

On the surface of plaques with severe stenosis, shear stress imposes a significant risk of thrombosis and sudden occlusion. Therefore, a stenotic plaque may be a vulnerable plaque regardless of ischemia. Moreover, a stenotic plaque may indicate the presence of many nonstenotic or less stenotic plaques that can be vulnerable to rupture and thrombosis [24, 66] (Fig. 5). The current standard technique is invasive x-ray angiography [32]. Noninvasive options include multislice CT [67, 68], magnetic resonance angiography with or without a contrast agent, and electron-beam tomography angiography [59, 69–71].

Minor Criteria

For techniques that focus on the plaque level, minor criteria include the following features.

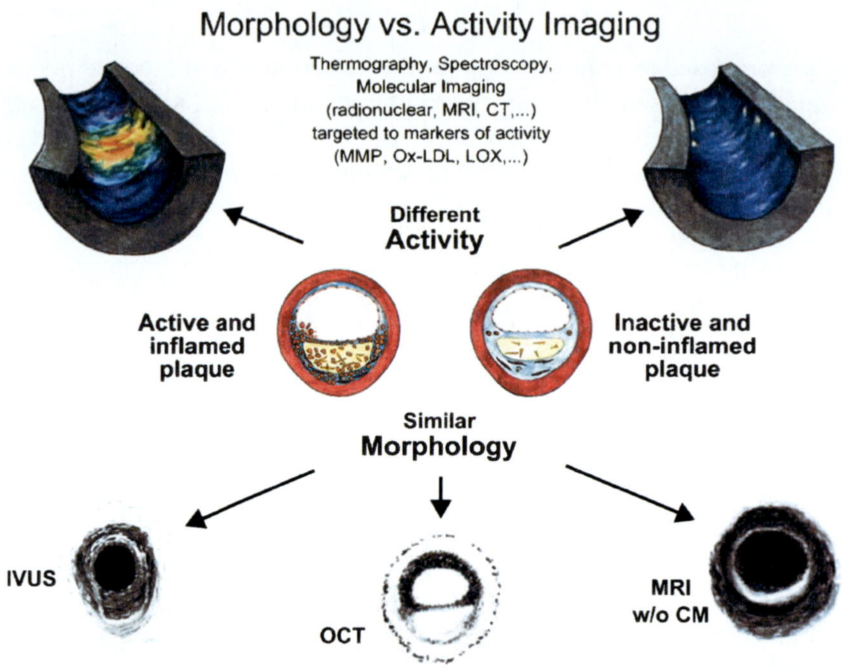

Fig. 5. Plaques with nearly similar morphology in terms of lipid core and fibrous cap (*middle panel*) may look similar with diagnostic imaging aimed at morphology only (*bottom panel*). However, they might look very different using diagnostic methods capable of detecting activity and physiology of the plaques. The *top left* plaque is hot (as evidenced in a thermography image), whereas the *top right* plaque is inactive and detected relatively as a cool plaque.

Superficial Calcified Nodules

These plaques have a calcified nodule within, or very close to, their cap, and this structure protrudes through and can rupture the cap. This event may or may not be associated with severe coronary calcification and a high calcium score [5]. Possible intravascular diagnostic techniques include OCT [46, 47], IVUS and elastography (palpography) [48]. Noninvasive options include electron-beam CT [72], multisection spiral CT [73], and MRI [34, 35].

Yellow Color (on Angioscopy)

Yellow plaques, particularly glistening ones, may indicate a large lipid core and thin fibrous cap, suggesting a high risk of rupture. However, because plaques in different stages can be yellow and because not all lipid-laden plaques are destined to rupture or undergo thrombosis, this criterion may lack sufficient specificity [53, 74]. Possible intravascular diagnostic techniques include angioscopy [73] and transcatheter colorimetry [75]. No diagnostic method has yet been developed for noninvasive angioscopy.

Intraplaque Hemorrhage

Extravasation of red blood cells, or iron accumulation in plaque, may represent plaque instability [76]. Possible intravascular diagnostic techniques include NIR spectroscopy [54, 55], tissue Doppler methods [77], and intravascular MRI. A noninvasive option is MRI [34, 35, 61].

Endothelial Dysfunction

Impaired endothelial vasodilator function occurs in a variety of acute and chronic disease states. Patients with cardiovascular risk factors have endothelial dysfunction. Endothelial dysfunction predicts CHD and stroke [89, 156]. Vulnerable plaques have sites of active inflammation and oxidative stress and are likely to be associated with impaired endothelial function. Possible diagnostic techniques are endothelium-dependent coronary artery dilatation (intravascular) [78] and measurement of flow-mediated dilatation by brachial artery ultrasonography and other emerging techniques (noninvasive) [79].

Expansive (Positive) Remodeling

Many of the nonstenotic lesions undergo "expansive," "positive," or "outward" remodeling, namely compensatory enlargement before impinging significantly on the vascular lumen. This phenomenon was considered as positive remodeling because the luminal area was not affected and stenosis was the only measure of risk. However, with the emphasis on plaque rupture in nonstenotic lesions, the so-called positive remodeling may not be truly positive and beneficial. Several studies have suggested that such remodeling is a potential surrogate marker of plaque vulnerability [80, 81]. In these studies, intravascular ultrasound was used to evaluate remodeling in coronary arteries. A recent study by Kim et al. [82] introduced a noninvasive method for the detection of expansive remodeling in coronary arteries by MRI. CT might also provide a noninvasive method for studying arterial remodeling.

Few of the above techniques have been tested in clinical trials showing ability to predict events. MRI and CT-based approaches are being developed. These technologies and strategies must also be evaluated with regard to their cost-effectiveness.

FUNCTIONAL VERSUS STRUCTURAL ASSESSMENT

A growing body of evidence indicates that different types of vulnerable plaque with various histopathology and biology exist. To evaluate plaque vulnerability, it is evident that a combined approach capable of evaluating structural characteristics (morphology) as well as functional properties (activity) of plaque may be more informative and may provide higher predictive value than a single approach. For instance, a combination of IVUS or OCT with thermography [80, 83] may provide more diagnostic value than each of these techniques alone. Such an arrangement can be useful for both intravascular as well as noninvasive diagnostic methods (Fig. 6). Autopsy [84] and IVUS studies [85] have shown that atherosclerotic lesions are frequently found in young and asymptomatic individuals. It is unclear what percentage of these lesions present morphologies of rupture-prone vulnerable plaques. Moreover, chronic inflammation [86] and macrophage/foam cell formation are an intrinsic part of the natural history of atherosclerosis. These data suggest that screening only based on plaque morphology and/or chronic markers of inflammation may not provide satisfactory predictive value for detection of vulnerable patients.

PAN-ARTERIAL APPROACH

Diagnostic and therapeutic methods may focus on the total burden of coronary artery disease [27]. The coronary calcium score is a good example of using CT for this purpose [72]. The total burden of calcified atherosclerotic plaques in all coronary arteries is identified by ultrafast CT. Extensive efforts are underway to improve image quality, signal processing, and interpretation of detailed components of coronary arteries that lend hope of a new calcium scoring and risk stratification technique based on

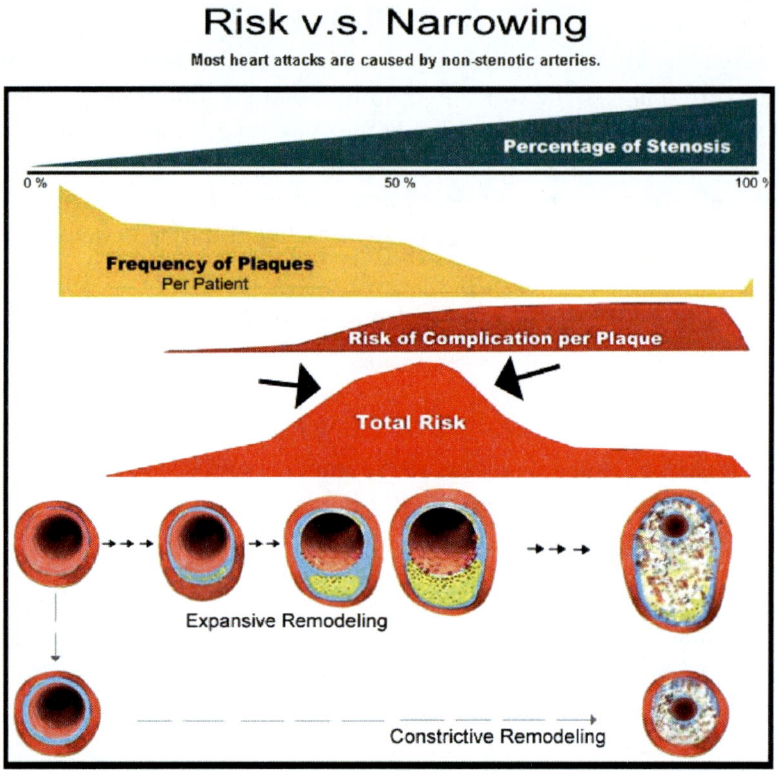

Fig. 6. Correlation between frequency of plaques, degree of stenosis, and risk of complication per plaque as a function of plaque progression. Although the average absolute risk of severely stenotic plaques may be higher than the average absolute risk of mildly stenotic plaques, there are more plaques with mild stenoses than plaques with severe stenoses.

CT information [87]. Like systemic indexes of inflammation (e.g., high sensitive CRP), endothelial dysfunction as measured by impaired flow-mediated vasodilation in the brachial artery can aid in the detection of pan-arterial vulnerability and may serve as a screening tool [88, 89].

Another emerging technique is the measurement of the transcoronary gradient (difference in concentration between coronary ostium and coronary sinus, or between proximal and distal segments of each coronary segment) of various factors, including cytokines [90], adhesion molecules [91], temperature, etc.

It will be important in the future to identify plaques that are on a trajectory of evolution toward a vulnerable state, to find out how long they will stay vulnerable, and to be able to target interventions to those plaques most likely to develop thrombosis. Similarly, factors that protect plaques from becoming vulnerable also need to be identified. It is likely that local hemodynamic factors and three-dimensional morphology may provide insight regarding the temporal course of an evolving plaque.

New studies are unraveling the role of the adventitia and periadventitial connective and adipose tissue in vulnerability of atherosclerotic plaques [92]. Further studies are needed to define the importance of these findings in the detection and treatment of vulnerable plaques.

VULNERABLE (THROMBOGENIC) BLOOD

Serum Markers of Atherosclerosis and Inflammation

Serum markers may predict a patient's risk of acute cardiovascular complications (Table 6). C-reactive protein (CRP) is an independent risk factor and a powerful predictor of future coronary events in the asymptomatic population [154, 155] and in patients with stable and unstable disease. Although CRP is a nonspecific marker of systemic inflammation, it activates endothelium and accumulates in the plaque, suggesting an important role in plaque inflammation [96, 97].

Circulating interleukin-6 levels, which are elevated in patients with acute coronary syndromes, also predict the risk of future coronary events in such patients [98]. Investigators have shown that high plasma concentrations of soluble CD40 ligand may indicate an increased vascular risk in apparently healthy women [99]. Likewise, Hwang et al. [100] showed in a large population-based sample of individuals that circulating levels of soluble intracellular adhesion molecule were predictive of future acute coronary events.

Markers of systemic inflammation, such as soluble adhesion molecules, circulating bacterial endotoxin, soluble human heat-shock protein 60, and antibodies to mycobacterial heat-shock protein 65, may predict an increased risk of atherosclerosis [101]. Pregnancy-associated plasma protein A (PAPP-A) is present in unstable plaques, and its circulating levels are elevated in patients with acute coronary syndromes [102]. Increased serum levels of PAPP-A may reflect instability of atherosclerotic plaques [103].

With major advances in high-throughput genomics and proteomics research, future studies will undoubtedly identify new risk and protective factors and biomarkers that can be used for screening purposes. A recent study suggested an association between several genetic polymorphisms and clinical outcomes, some of which can be possibly related to plaque, blood, and myocardial vulnerability [104]. The tools and knowledge base, made possible by the Human Genome Project, allow the field

Table 6
Serological markers of vulnerability (reflecting metabolic and immune disorders)

Abnormal lipoprotein profile (e.g., high LDL, low HDL, abnormal LDL and HDL size density, lipoprotein [a], etc.)
Nonspecific markers of inflammation (e.g., hsCRP, CD40L, ICAM-1, VCAM-1, P-selectin, leukocytosis, and other serological markers related to the immune system; these markers may not be specific for atherosclerosis or plaque inflammation)
Serum markers of metabolic syndrome (e.g., diabetes or hypertriglyceridemia)
Specific markers of immune activation (e.g., anti-LDL antibody, anti-HSP antibody)
Markers of lipid peroxidation (e.g., ox-LDL and ox-HDL)
Homocysteine
PAPP-A
Circulating apoptosis marker(s) (e.g., Fas/Fas ligand, not specific to plaque)
ADMA/DDAH
Circulating nonesterified fatty acids (e.g., NEFA)

hsCRP high-sensitivity CRP; *CD40L* CD40 ligand; *ICAM* intracellular adhesion molecule; *VCAM* vascular cell adhesion molecule; *MMP* matrix metalloproteinases; *TIMP* tissue inhibitors of MMPs; *LDL* low-density lipoprotein; *HDL* high-density lipoprotein; *HSP* heat shock protein; *ADMA* asymmetric dimethylarginine; *ADMA* dimethylarginine dimethylaminohydrolase; *NEFA* nonesterified fatty acids

to move beyond one or a few single-nucleotide polymorphisms in a priori candidate genes. Genome-wide linkage analyses have been carried out for coronary artery calcification [105], and genome-wide association studies for myocardial infarction are already a reality [106]. Further studies are needed to address the relationship between single-nucleotide polymorphisms in components of each of the plaque, blood, and myocardial vulnerabilities and future outcomes (acute coronary syndromes and sudden cardiac death). However, ongoing proteomic research on serum samples of vulnerable patients collected from prospective studies before the onset of symptoms is most promising.

COAGULATION/ANTICOAGULATION SYSTEM

The importance of the coagulation system in the outcome of plaque complications was reemphasized by Karnicki et al. [107] who in a porcine model demonstrated that the role assigned to lesion-bound tissue factor was not physically realistic and that blood borne factors must have a major role in thrombus propagation. A hematologic disorder is rarely the sole cause of coronary thrombosis and myocardial infarction. Inflammation promotes thrombosis and vice versa [108]. Extensive atherosclerosis may be associated with increased blood thrombogenicity, but the magnitude of thrombogenicity varies from patient to patient, and unstable plaques are much more thrombogenic than stable ones (Table 7).

Some platelet polymorphisms, such as glycoprotein IIIa P1(A2) [109], Ib agene-5T/C Kozak [110], high factor V and factor VII clotting [111], have been reported as independent risk factors for myocardial infarction. Reiner et al. [112] reviewed the associations of known and potential genetic susceptibility markers for intermediate hemostatic phenotypes with arterial thrombotic disease.

Other conditions that lead to a hypercoagulable state are diabetes mellitus, hypercholesterolemia, and cigarette smoking. High levels of circulating tissue factor may be the mechanism of action responsible for the increased thrombotic complications associated with the presence of these cardiovascular risk factors [113]. Acute coronary syndromes are associated with proinflammatory and prothrombotic conditions that involve a prolonged increase in the levels of fibrinogen, CRP, and plasminogen activator inhibitor [114, 115].

Table 7
Blood markers of vulnerability (reflecting hypercoagulability)

Markers of blood hypercoagulability (e.g., fibrinogen, D-dimer, and factor V Leiden)
Increased platelet activation and aggregation (e.g., gene polymorphisms of platelet glycoproteins IIb/IIIa, Ia/IIa, and Ib/IX)
Increased coagulation factors (e.g., clotting of factors V, VII, and VIII; von Willebrand factor; and factor XIII)
Decreased anticoagulation factors (e.g., proteins S and C, thrombomodulin, and antithrombin III)
Decreased endogenous fibrinolysis activity (e.g., reduced t-PA, increased PAI-1, certain PAI-1 polymorphisms)
Prothrombin mutation (e.g., G20210A)
Other thrombogenic factors (e.g., anticardiolipin antibodies, thrombocytosis, sickle cell disease, polycythemia, diabetes mellitus, hypercholesterolemia, hyperhomocysteinemia)
Increased viscosity
Transient hypercoagulability (e.g., smoking, dehydration, infection, adrenergic surge, cocaine, estrogens, postprandial, etc.)

t-PA tissue plasminogen activator; *PAI-1* type 1 plasminogen activator inhibitor

A number of blood abnormalities, including antithrombin III deficiency, protein C or S deficiency, and resistance to activated protein C (also known as factor V Leiden), have been implicated as causes of venous thrombosis. The risk of arterial thrombosis is only modestly increased in these conditions, but these abnormalities are thought to interact with traditional risk factors for arterial thrombosis.

Venous and arterial thromboses are prominent features of the antiphospholipid syndrome. The main antibodies of this syndrome are the anticardiolipin antibody, the lupus anticoagulant, and the IgG antibodies against prothrombin and b_2-glycoprotein [116, 117].

In the nephrotic syndrome, proteinuria results in abnormal concentration and activity of coagulation factors. Moreover, the associated hypoalbuminemia, thrombocytosis, and hypercholesterolemia may induce arterial and venous thrombosis [118].

The importance of the coagulation/fibrinolytic system is highlighted by several autopsy studies that have shown a high prevalence of old plaque disruptions without infarctions. Therefore, an active fibrinolytic system may be able to prevent luminal thrombosis in some cases of plaque disruption [119, 120].

A transient shift in the coagulation and anticoagulation balance is likely to be an important factor in plaque–blood interaction, resulting in an acute event. "Triggers", such as exercise and smoking, which are associated with catecholamine release, may increase the risk of plaque thrombosis [121]. Similarly, metabolic factors, such as postprandial metabolic changes, are associated with increased blood coagulability [122]. Likewise, estrogen replacement therapy can lead to a hypercoagulable state [123].

Finally, plasma viscosity, as well as fibrinogen and white blood cell counts, is positively associated with CHD events as shown by Koenig et al. [124] Furthermore, Junker et al. [125] showed a positive relationship between plasma viscosity and the severity of coronary heart disease (CHD).

VULNERABLE MYOCARDIUM

Ischemic Vulnerable Myocardium Without Prior Atherosclerosis-Derived Myocardial Damage

Abrupt occlusion of a coronary artery is a common cause of sudden death. It often leads to acute myocardial infarction or exacerbation of chest pain [126, 127]. Extensive studies in experimental animals and increasing clinical evidence indicate that autonomic nervous activity has a significant role in modifying the clinical outcome with coronary occlusion [122, 128, 129]. Susceptibility of the myocardium to acute ischemia was reviewed by Airaksinen [130], who emphasized the key role of autonomic tone in the outcome after plaque rupture. Sympathetic hyperactivity favors the genesis of life-threatening ventricular tachyarrhythmias, whereas vagal activation exerts an antifibrillatory effect. Strong afferent stimuli from the ischemic myocardium may impair the arterial baroreflex and lead to hemodynamic instability [131].

There seems to be a wide interindividual variation in the type and severity of autonomic reactions during the early phase of abrupt coronary occlusion, a critical period for out-of-hospital cardiac arrest. The pre-existing severity of a coronary stenosis, adaptation or preconditioning to myocardial ischemia, habitual physical exercise, b-blockade, and gender seem to affect autonomic reactions and the risk of fatal ventricular arrhythmias [130, 132, 133]. Recent studies have documented a hereditary component for autonomic function, and genetic factors may also modify the clinical presentation of acute coronary occlusion [134, 135]. Table 8 depicts conditions and markers associated with myocardial vulnerability.

Table 8
Conditions and markers associated with myocardial vulnerability

- With atherosclerosis-derived myocardial ischemia as shown by
  - ECG abnormalities
    - During rest
    - During stress test
    - Silent ischemia (e.g., ST changes on Holter monitoring)
  - Perfusion and viability disorder
    - PET scan
    - SPECT
  - Wall motion abnormalities
    - Echocardiography
    - MR imaging
    - x-ray ventriculogram
    - MSCT
  - Without atherosclerosis-derived myocardial ischemia
    - Sympathetic hyperactivity
    - Impaired autonomic reactivity
    - Left ventricular hypertrophy
    - Cardiomyopathy (dilated, hypertrophic, or restrictive)
    - Valvular disease (aortic stenosis and mitral valve prolapse)
  - Electrophysiological disorders
    - Long-QT syndrome, Brugada syndrome, Wolff–Parkinson–White syndrome, sinus and atrioventricular conduction disturbances, catecholaminergic polymorphic ventricular tachycardia, T-wave alternans, drug-induced torsades de pointes
    - Commotio cordis
    - Anomalous origination of a coronary artery
    - Myocarditis
    - Myocardial bridging

MSCT multislice computed tomography; *PET* positron emission tomography; *SPECT* single-photon emission computed tomography

Ischemic Vulnerable Myocardium with Prior Atherosclerosis-Derived Myocardial Damage (Chronic Myocardial Damage)

Any type of atherosclerosis-related myocardial injury, such as ischemia, an old or new myocardial infarction, inflammation, and/or fibrosis, potentially increases the patient's vulnerability to arrhythmia and sudden death. In the past few decades, a number of diagnostic methods have been developed for imaging cardiac ischemia and for assessing the risk of developing a life-threatening cardiac arrhythmia. In patients with a history of ischemic heart disease, ischemic cardiomyopathy is the ultimate form of myocardial damage. With the advent of new, effective treatments for hypertension and more efficient management of acute myocardial infarction, deaths resulting from stroke and acute myocardial infarction have steadily decreased [136]. More patients are now surviving acute events, but some develop heart failure or ischemic cardiomyopathy later with the potential for fatal arrhythmias. It is also important to remember that in a significant number of patients sudden cardiac death is the first manifestation of underlying heart disease, and it is still responsible for >450,000 deaths annually in the United States.

Nonischemic Vulnerable Myocardium

A smaller subset of patients experience fatal arrhythmia as a result of diseases other than coronary atherosclerosis. The various forms of cardiomyopathy (dilated, hypertrophic, restrictive, and right ventricular) account for most noncoronary cardiac deaths. Other underlying pathological processes include valvular heart disease, such as aortic stenosis and primary electrical disturbances (long-QT syndromes, Brugada syndrome, Wolff–Parkinson–White syndrome, sinus and atrioventricular conduction disturbances, catecholaminergic polymorphic ventricular tachycardia, and congenital and drug-induced long-QT syndromes with torsades de pointes), and, infrequently, commotio cordis from chest trauma. Less common pathological conditions include anomalous origin of a coronary artery, myocarditis, and myocardial bridging (Table 8). Circulating nonesterified fatty acids are another risk factor for sudden death in middle-aged men, as is elevated serum concentration of CRP; serum measurements may help screening for vulnerable myocardium [137].

The Task Force on Sudden Cardiac Death, organized by the European Society of Cardiology, issued a report that includes detailed diagnostic and therapeutic recommendations for a large number of cardiomyopathic conditions capable of causing sudden cardiac death [138].

Table 9 provides electrophysiological diagnostic criteria and techniques for the detection of myocardial vulnerability.

RISK ASSESSMENT FOR VULNERABLE PATIENTS

Traditional Risk Assessment Strategies

Despite extensive studies and development of several risk prediction models, traditional CHD risk factors fail to predict the development of CHD in a large group of cases (25% [139] to 50% [3, 140, 141]). Risk prediction models developed on the basis of data from long-term population-based follow-up studies may not be able to predict short-term risks for individual persons. The pioneering studies by Ridker et al. [95] who noted a greater impact of an inflammatory marker such as serum CRP than LDL levels, is of interest. Several risk factor assessment models (e.g., Framingham [142], Sheffield [143, 144], New Zealand [145, 146], Canadian [147], British [148], European [149], Dundee [150], Munster [PROCAM] [151], and MONICA [152]) have been developed. However, all of them are based on the traditional risk factors known to contribute to the chronic development of atherosclerosis. Addition of emerging risk factors, particularly those indicative of the activity of the disease (i.e., plaque inflammation), may allow individualized risk assessments to be made.

The traditional risk assessment has been shown to predict long-term outcome in large populations. However, they fall short in predicting near-future events particularly in individual clinical practice. For example, a high Framingham risk score, although capable of forecasting an adverse cardiovascular event in 10 years, clearly falls short in accurately predicting events in individual patients and cannot provide a clear clinical route for cardiologists to identify and treat, to prevent near-future victims of acute coronary syndromes and sudden death. The same is true for coronary evaluations using electrocardiography, myocardial perfusion tests, and coronary angiography. A positive test for coronary stenosis or reversible perfusion defect (ischemia), although considered as a major risk factor, must be coupled in the future with emerging methods of risk assessment for the detection of vulnerable patients to predict more accurately the near-future outcome and prognosis. Those who have no indication of coronary stenosis or myocardial ischemia and who may even lack traditional risk factors may benefit from the techniques now under development that evaluate plaque biology and inflammation.

Table 9
Available techniques for electrophysiological risk stratification of vulnerable myocardium

Diagnostic criteria
Arrhythmia
QT dispersion
QT dynamics
T-wave alternans
Ventricular late potentials
Heart rate variability
Diagnostic techniques
Noninvasive
Resting ECG
Stress ECG
Ambulatory ECG
Signal-averaged ECG
Surface high-resolution ECG
Invasive
Programmed ventricular stimulation
Real-time 3D magnetic-navigated activation map

NEW RISK ASSESSMENT STRATEGIES

We propose a Cumulative Vulnerability Index based on the following:

- Vulnerable plaque/artery
- Vulnerable blood (prone to thrombosis)
- Vulnerable myocardium (prone to life-threatening arrhythmia)

This proposal is by no means intended to disregard the predictive value of traditional risk assessment strategies that have been proven in predicting long-term outcome but instead to strengthen their value in providing higher accuracy, especially for near-term outcomes.

Atherosclerosis is a diffuse and multisystem, chronic inflammatory disorder involving vascular, metabolic, and immune systems with various local and systemic manifestations. Therefore, it is essential to assess total vulnerability burden and not just search for a single, unstable coronary plaque. A composite risk score (e.g., a vulnerability index) that comprises the total burden of atherosclerosis and vulnerable plaque in the coronaries (and aorta and carotid, femoral, etc., arteries) and that includes blood and myocardial vulnerability factors, should be a more accurate method of risk stratification. Such a vulnerability index would indicate the likelihood that a patient with certain factors would have a clinical event in the coming year. Use of the state-of-the-art bioinformatics tools such as neural networks may provide substantial improvement for risk calculations [153].

The information used for developing such risk stratification in the future is likely to come from a combination of smaller prospective studies (e.g., from new imaging techniques) and retrospective cohort studies (e.g., for serum factors) in which the risks for near-future cardiovascular events can be quantitatively calculated. A few such studies have been conducted or are underway [94, 154].

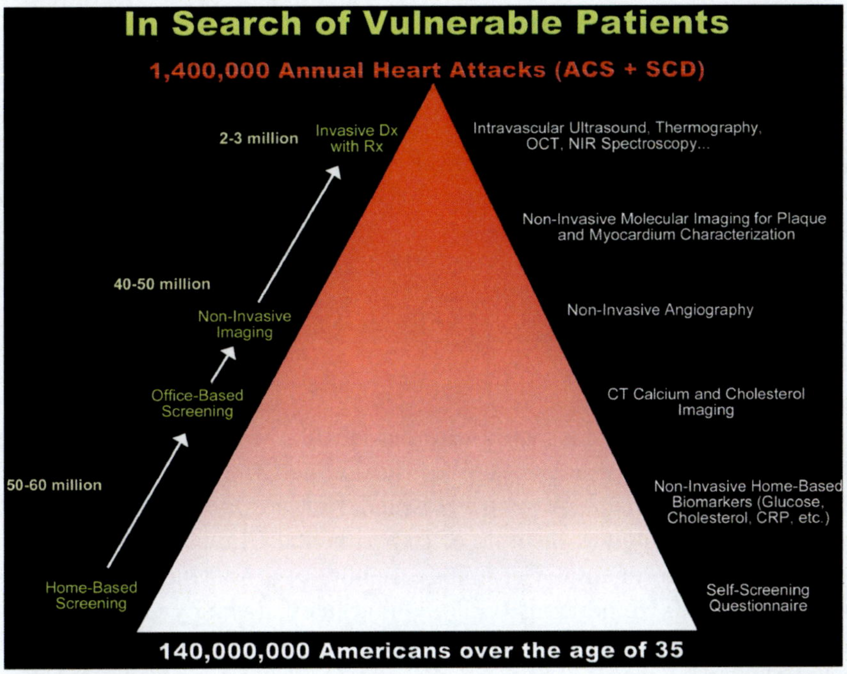

Fig. 7. The Vulnerable Patient Pyramid. This pyramid illustrates a speculative roadmap in search of vulnerable patients (numbers represent population in the United States). The major need is to develop noninvasive, relatively inexpensive, readily available, and accurate screening/diagnostic tools allowing multistep screening of an apparently healthy population and those with known atherosclerosis but whose risks for acute events are uncertain.

In Search of the Vulnerable Patient

The ideal method for screening vulnerable patients should be (1) inexpensive, (2) relatively noninvasive, (3) widely reproducible, (4) readily applicable to an asymptomatic population, and (5) capable of adding predicted value to measurements of established risk factors. Such a method should provide a cost-effective, stepwise approach designed to further stratify risk and provide reliable diagnosis and pathways for monitoring therapy. Obviously, these goals are hard to achieve with today's tools. However, it is well within our reach, if academia and industry in the field of cardiovascular medicine undertake a coordinated effort to embark on developing new screening and diagnostic techniques to identify vulnerable patients (Fig. 7).

The Vulnerable Patient Pyramid This pyramid illustrates a speculative roadmap in search of vulnerable patients (numbers represent population in the United States). The major need is to develop noninvasive, relatively inexpensive, readily available, and accurate screening/diagnostic tools allowing multistep screening of an apparently healthy population and those with known atherosclerosis but whose risks for acute events are uncertain.

*The vulnerable patient consensus writing group:

Morteza Naghavi, MD; Peter Libby, MD; Erling Falk, MD, PhD; S. Ward Casscells, MD; Silvio Litovsky, MD; John Rumberger, MD; Juan Jose Badimon, PhD; Christodoulos Stefanadis, MD; Pedro Moreno, MD; Gerard Pasterkamp, MD, PhD; Zahi Fayad, PhD; Peter H. Stone, MD; Sergio Waxman, MD; Paolo Raggi, MD; Mohammad Madjid, MD; Alireza Zarrabi, MD; Allen Burke, MD; Chun Yuan, PhD; Peter J. Fitzgerald, MD, PhD; David S. Siscovick, MD; Chris L. de Korte, PhD; Masanori

Aikawa, MD, PhD; K. E. Juhani Airaksinen, MD; Gerd Assmann, MD; Christoph R. Becker, MD; James H. Chesebro, MD; Andrew Farb, MD; Zorina S. Galis, PhD; Chris Jackson, PhD; Ik-Kyung Jang, MD, PhD; Wolfgang Koenig, MD, PhD; Robert A. Lodder, PhD; Keith March, MD, PhD; Jasenka Demirovic, MD, PhD; Mohamad Navab, PhD; Silvia G. Priori, MD, PhD; Mark D. Rekhter, PhD; Raymond Bahr, MD; Scott M. Grundy, MD, PhD; Roxana Mehran, MD; Antonio Colombo, MD; Eric Boerwinkle, PhD; Christie Ballantyne, MD; William Insull, Jr, MD; Robert S. Schwartz, MD; Robert Vogel, MD; Patrick W. Serruys, MD, PhD; Goran K. Hansson, MD, PhD; David P. Faxon, MD; Sanjay Kaul, MD; Helmut Drexler, MD; Philip Greenland, MD; James E. Muller, MD; Renu Virmani, MD; Paul M Ridker, MD; Douglas P. Zipes, MD; Prediman K. Shah, MD; James T. Willerson, MD

From The Center for Vulnerable Plaque Research, University of Texas—Houston, The Texas Heart Institute, and President Bush Center for Cardiovascular Health, Memorial Hermann Hospital, Houston (M. Naghavi, S.W.C., S.L., M.M., A.Z., J.T.W.); The Leducq Center for Cardiovascular Research, Department of Medicine, Brigham and Women's Hospital, Harvard Medical School, Boston, Mass (P.L., M.A.); Department of Cardiology and Institute of Experimental Clinical Research, Aarhus University, Aarhus, Denmark (E.F.); Experimental Cardiology Laboratory, Vascular Biology of the University Medical Center in Utrecht, the Netherlands (G.P.); Ohio State University (J.R.); the Zena and Michael A. Wiener Cardiovascular Institute, Mount Sinai Medical Center, New York, NY (Z.F.); Cardiac Catheterization Laboratory at the VA Medical Center, University of Kentucky, Lexington (P.M.); Cardiovascular Division, Department of Medicine, Brigham and Women's Hospital, Harvard Medical School, Boston, Mass (P.H.S.); Division of Cardiology, New England Medical Center, Boston, Mass (S.W.); Department of Medicine, Section of Cardiology, Tulane University School of Medicine, New Orleans, La (P.R.); Department of Cardiovascular Pathology, Armed Forces Institute of Pathology, Washington, DC (A.B., A.F., R.V.); Department of Radiology, University of Washington, Seattle (C.Y.); Stanford University Medical Center Stanford, Calif (P.J.F.); Cardiovascular Health Research Unit, University of Washington, Seattle (D.S.S.); Department of Cardiology, Athens Medical School, Athens, Greece (C.S.); Catheterization Laboratory, Thorax Center, Erasmus University, Rotterdam, the Netherlands (C.L.d.K.); Division of Cardiology, Department of Medicine, University of Turku, Finland (K.E.J.A.); Institute of Arteriosclerosis Research and the Institute of Clinical Chemistry and Laboratory Medicine, Central Laboratory, Hospital of the University of Münster, Munich, Germany (G.A.); Department of Clinical Radiology, University of Münster, Munich, Germany (C.R.B.); Mayo Clinic Medical School, Jacksonville, Fla (J.H.C.); Department of Medicine, Division of Cardiology, Emory University School of Medicine, Atlanta, Ga (Z.S.G.); Bristol Heart Institute, Bristol University, Bristol, United Kingdom (C.J.); Cardiology Division, Massachusetts General Hospital and Harvard Medical School, Boston, Mass (I.-K.J.); Department of Internal Medicine II, Cardiology, University of Ulm, Ulm, Germany (W.K.); University of Kentucky, Lexington, Ky (R.A.L.); R.L. Roudebush VA Medical Center, Indianapolis, Ind (K.M.); School of Public Health, University of Texas—Houston, Houston, Texas (J.D.); Division of Cardiology, University of California Los Angeles, Los Angeles, Calif (M. Navab); Fondazione Salvatore Maugeri, University of Pavia, Pavia, Italy (S.G.P.); Department of Cardiovascular Therapeutics, Pfizer Global Research and Development, Ann Arbor Laboratories, Ann Arbor, Mich (M.D.R.); Paul Dudley White Coronary Care System at St. Agnes HealthCare, Baltimore, Md (R.B.); Center for Human Nutrition, University of Texas Health Science Center, Dallas (S.M.G.); Lenox Hill Hospital, New York, NY (R.M.); Catheterization Laboratories, Ospedale San Raffaele and Emo Centro Cuore Columbus, Milan, Italy (A.C.); Human Genetics Center, Institute of Molecular Medicine, Houston, Tex (E.B.); Department of Medicine, Baylor College of Medicine, Houston, Tex (C.B., W.I.); Minneapolis Heart Institute and Foundation, Minneapolis, Minn (R.S.S.); Division of

Cardiology, University of Maryland School of Medicine, Baltimore, Md (R.V.); Karolinska Institute, Center for Molecular Medicine, Karolinska Hospital, Stockholm, Sweden (G.K.H.); Section of Cardiology, University of Chicago, Ill (D.P.F.); Vascular Physiology and Thrombosis Research Laboratory of the Atherosclerosis Research Center, Cedars-Sinai Medical Center, Los Angeles, California (S.K.); Cardiology Department, Hannover University, Hannover, Germany (H.D.); Department of Medicine, Feinberg School of Medicine, Northwestern University, Chicago, Ill (P.G.); UCLA School of Medicine and Cedars-Sinai Medical Center, Los Angeles, Calif (P.K.S.); Massachusetts General Hospital, Harvard Medical School and CIMIT (Center for Integration of Medicine and Innovative Technology), Boston, Mass (J.E.M.); Cardiovascular Division, Division of Preventive Medicine, Brigham and Women's Hospital, Boston, Mass (P.M.R.); and Indiana University School of Medicine, Krannert Institute of Cardiology, Indianapolis (D.P.Z.).

REFERENCES

1. Yusuf S, Reddy S, Ounpuu S, et al. Global burden of cardiovascular diseases, I: general considerations, the epidemiologic transition, risk factors, and impact of urbanization. *Circulation.* 2001;104:2746–2753.
2. American Heart Association. *2002 Heart and Stroke Statistical Update.* Dallas, TX: American Heart Association; 2002.
3. Myerburg RJ, Interian A Jr, Mitrani RM, et al. Frequency of sudden cardiac death and profiles of risk. *Am J Cardiol.* 1997; 80:10F–19F.
4. Zipes DP, Wellens HJ. Sudden cardiac death. *Circulation.* 1998;98:2334–2351.
5. Virmani R, Kolodgie FD, Burke AP, et al. Lessons from sudden coronary death: a comprehensive morphological classification scheme for atherosclerotic lesions. *Arterioscler Thromb Vasc Biol.* 2000;20:1262–1275.
6. Falk E, Shah PK, Fuster V. Coronary plaque disruption. *Circulation.* 1995;92:657–671.
7. Davies MJ. A macro and micro view of coronary vascular insult in ischemic heart disease. *Circulation.* 1990;82(Suppl II):II-38–II-46.
8. Kolodgie FD, Burke AP, Farb A, et al. The thin-cap fibroatheroma: a type of vulnerable plaque: the major precursor lesion to acute coronary syndromes. *Curr Opin Cardiol.* 2001;16:285–292.
9. Farb A, Burke AP, Tang AL, et al. Coronary plaque erosion without rupture into a lipid core: a frequent cause of coronary thrombosis in sudden coronary death. *Circulation.* 1996;93:1354–1363.
10. Ambrose JA, Tannenbaum MA, Alexopoulos D, et al. Angiographic progression of coronary artery disease and the development of myocardial infarction. *J Am Coll Cardiol.* 1988;12:56–62.
11. Falk E. Plaque rupture with severe pre-existing stenosis precipitating coronary thrombosis: characteristics of coronary atherosclerotic plaques underlying fatal occlusive thrombi. *Br Heart J.* 1983;50:127–134.
12. Friedman M, Van den Bovenkamp GJ. Role of thrombus in plaque formation in the human diseased coronary artery. *Br J Exp Pathol.* 1966;47:550–557.
13. Constantinides P. Pathogenesis of cerebral artery thrombosis in man. *Arch Pathol.* 1967;83:422–428.
14. Chapman I. Relationships of recent coronary artery occlusion and acute myocardial infarction. *J Mt Sinai Hosp N Y.* 1968;35:149–154.
15. Davies MJ, Thomas AC. Plaque fissuring: the cause of acute myocardial infarction, sudden ischaemic death, and crescendo angina. *Br Heart J.* 1985;53:363–373.
16. Thim T, Hagensen MK, Bentzon JF, Falk E. From vulnerable plaque to atherothrombosis. *J Intern Med.* 2008;263(5):506–516.
17. Willerson JT, Campbell WB, Winniford MD, et al. Conversion from chronic to acute coronary artery disease: speculation regarding mechanisms. *Am J Cardiol.* 1984;54:1349–1354.
18. Muller J, Tofler G, Stone P. Circadian variation and triggers of onset of acute cardiovascular disease. *Circulation.* 1989;79:733–743.
19. Muller JE, Abela GS, Nesto RW, et al. Triggers, acute risk factors and vulnerable plaques: the lexicon of a new frontier. *J Am Coll Cardiol.* 1994;23:809–813.
20. Vulnerable. In: *Merriam-Webster's Collegiate Dictionary & Thesaurus.* 11th ed (e-book). Springfield, MA: Merriam-Webster, Inc. 2003.
21. Stary HC, Chandler AB, Dinsmore RE, et al. A definition of advanced types of atherosclerotic lesions and a histological classification of atherosclerosis : a report from the Committee on Vascular Lesions of the Council on Arteriosclerosis, American Heart Association. *Circulation.* 1995;92:1355–1374.
22. Mann J, Davies MJ. Mechanisms of progression in native coronary artery disease: role of healed plaque disruption. *Heart.* 1999;82:265–268.
23. Burke AP, Farb A, Malcom GT, et al. Coronary risk factors and plaque morphology in men with coronary disease who died suddenly. *N Engl J Med.* 1997;336:1276–1282.

24. Goldstein JA, Demetriou D, Grines CL, et al. Multiple complex coronary plaques in patients with acute myocardial infarction. *N Engl J Med*. 2000;343:915–922.
25. Nissen SE. Who is at risk for atherosclerotic disease? Lessons from intravascular ultrasound. *Am J Med*. 2002;112(Suppl 8A):27S–33S
26. Rioufol G, Finet G, Ginon I, et al. Multiple atherosclerotic plaque rupture in acute coronary syndrome. *Circulation*. 2002; 106:804–808.
27. Buffon A, Biasucci LM, Liuzzo G, et al. Widespread coronary inflammation in unstable angina. *N Engl J Med*. 2002; 347:5–12.
28. Casscells W, Naghavi M, Willerson JT. Vulnerable atherosclerotic plaque: a multifocal disease. *Circulation*. 2003;107:2072–2075.
29. Maseri A, Fuster V. Is there a vulnerable plaque? *Circulation*. 2003;107:2068–2071.
30. Kereiakes DJ. The emperor's clothes: in search of the vulnerable plaque. *Circulation*. 2003;107:2076–2077.
31. Davies MJ. Pathology of arterial thrombosis. *Br Med Bull*. 1994;50:789–802.
32. Burke AP, Kolodgie FD, Farb A, et al. Healed plaque ruptures and sudden coronary death: evidence that subclinical rupture has a role in plaque progression. *Circulation*. 2001;103:934–940.
33. Vallabhajosula S, Fuster V. Atherosclerosis: imaging techniques and the evolving role of nuclear medicine. *J Nucl Med*. 1997;38:1788–1796.
34. Fayad ZA, Fuster V. Clinical imaging of the high-risk or vulnerable atherosclerotic plaque. *Circ Res*. 2001;89:305–316.
35. Naghavi M, Madjid M, Khan MR, et al. New developments in the detection of vulnerable plaque. *Curr Atheroscler Rep*. 2001;3:125–135.
36. Stefanadis C, Diamantopoulos L, Vlachopoulos C, et al. Thermal heterogeneity within human atherosclerotic coronary arteries detected in vivo : a new method of detection by application of a special thermography catheter. *Circulation*. 1999;99:1965–1971.
37. Stefanadis C, Toutouzas K, Tsiamis E, et al. Thermal heterogeneity in stable human coronary atherosclerotic plaques is underestimated in vivo: the "cooling effect" of blood flow. *J Am Coll Cardiol*. 2003;41:403–408.
38. Schmitz SA, Coupland SE, Gust R, et al. Superparamagnetic iron oxideenhanced MRI of atherosclerotic plaques in Watanabe hereditable hyperlipidemic rabbits. *Invest Radiol*. 2000;35:460–471.
39. Ruehm SG, Corot C, Vogt P, et al. Magnetic resonance imaging of atherosclerotic plaque with ultrasmall superparamagnetic particles of iron oxide in hyperlipidemic rabbits. *Circulation*. 2001;103:415–422.
40. Lederman RJ, Raylman RR, Fisher SJ, et al. Detection of atherosclerosis using a novel positron-sensitive probe and 18-fluorodeoxyglucose (FDG). *Nucl Med Commun*. 2001;22:747–753.
41. Ciavolella M, Tavolaro R, Taurino M, et al. Immunoscintigraphy of atherosclerotic uncomplicated lesions in vivo with a monoclonal antibody against D-dimers of insoluble fibrin. *Atherosclerosis*. 1999;143:171–175.
42. Tearney GJ, Yabushita H, Houser SL, et al. Quantification of macrophage content in atherosclerotic plaques by optical coherence tomography. *Circulation*. 2003;107:113–119.
43. Krinsky GA, Freedberg R, Lee VS, et al. Innominate artery atheroma: a lesion seen with gadolinium-enhanced MR angiography and often missed by transesophageal echocardiography. *Clin Imaging*. 2001;25:251–257.
44. Bonk RT, Schmiedl UP, Yuan C, et al. Time-of-flight MR angiography with Gd-DTPA hexamethylene diamine co-polymer blood pool contrast agent: comparison of enhanced MRA and conventional angiography for arterial stenosis induced in rabbits. *J Magn Reson Imaging*. 2000;11:638–646.
45. Yuan C, Kerwin WS, Ferguson MS, et al. Contrast-enhanced high resolution MRI for atherosclerotic carotid artery tissue characterization. *J Magn Reson Imaging*. 2002;15:62–67
46. Patwari P, Weissman NJ, Boppart SA, et al. Assessment of coronary plaque with optical coherence tomography and high-frequency ultrasound. *Am J Cardiol*. 2000;85:641–644.
47. Jang I-K, Bouma BE, Kang D-H, et al. Visualization of coronary atherosclerotic plaques in patients using optical coherence tomography: comparison with intravascular ultrasound. *J Am Coll Cardiol*. 2002;39:604–609.
48. Nissen SE. Clinical images from intravascular ultrasound: coronary disease, plaque rupture, and intervention – the inside view. *Am J Cardiol*. 2001;88:16–18.
49. Nissen SE, Yock P. Intravascular ultrasound : novel pathophysiological insights and current clinical applications. *Circulation*. 2001;103:604–616.
50. de Korte CL, Cespedes EI, van der Steen AF, et al. Intravascular ultrasound elastography: assessment and imaging of elastic properties of diseased arteries and vulnerable plaque. *Eur J Ultrasound*. 1998;7:219–224.
51. de Korte CL, Sierevogel MJ, Mastik F, et al. Identification of atherosclerotic plaque components with intravascular ultrasound elastography in vivo: a Yucatan pig study. *Circulation*. 2002;105:1627–1630.
52. Corti R, Osende JI, Fuster V, et al. Artery dissection and arterial thrombus aging: the role of noninvasive magnetic resonance imaging. *Circulation*. 2001;103:2420–2421.
53. Takano M, Mizuno K, Okamatsu K, et al. Mechanical and structural characteristics of vulnerable plaques: analysis by coronary angioscopy and intravascular ultrasound. *J Am Coll Cardiol*. 2001;38:99–104.
54. Cassis LA, Lodder RA. Near-IR imaging of atheromas in living arterial tissue. *Anal Chem*. 1993;65:1247–1256.
55. Moreno PR, Lodder RA, Purushothaman KR, et al. Detection of lipid pool, thin fibrous cap, and inflammatory cells in human aortic atherosclerotic plaques by near-infrared spectroscopy. *Circulation*. 2002;105:923–927.
56. Wang J, Geng YJ, Guo B, et al. Near-infrared spectroscopic characterization of human advanced atherosclerotic plaques. *J Am Coll Cardiol*. 2002;39:1305–1313.

57. Jeremias A, Kolz ML, Ikonen TS, et al. Feasibility of in vivo intravascular ultrasound tissue characterization in the detection of early vascular transplant rejection. *Circulation*. 1999;100:2127–2130.
58. Nair A, Kuban BD, Tuzcu EM, et al. Coronary plaque classification with intravascular ultrasound radiofrequency data analysis. *Circulation*. 2002;106:2200–2206.
59. Helft G, Worthley SG, Fuster V, et al. Progression and regression of atherosclerotic lesions: monitoring with serial noninvasive magnetic resonance imaging. *Circulation*. 2002;105:993–998.
60. Hatsukami TS, Ross R, Polissar NL, et al. Visualization of fibrous cap thickness and rupture in human atherosclerotic carotid plaque in vivo with high-resolution magnetic resonance imaging. *Circulation*. 2000;102:959–964.
61. Yuan C, Mitsumori LM, Ferguson MS, et al. In vivo accuracy of multispectral magnetic resonance imaging for identifying lipid-rich necrotic cores and intraplaque hemorrhage in advanced human carotid plaques. *Circulation*. 2001;104:2051–2056.
62. Yuan C, Zhang S-X, Polissar NL, et al. Identification of fibrous cap rupture with magnetic resonance imaging is highly associated with recent transient ischemic attack or stroke. *Circulation*. 2002;105:181–185.
63. Uchida Y, Nakamura F, Tomaru T, et al. Prediction of acute coronary syndromes by percutaneous coronary angioscopy in patients with stable angina. *Am Heart J*. 1995;130:195–203.
64. Flacke S, Fischer S, Scott MJ, et al. Novel MRI contrast agent for molecular imaging of fibrin: implications for detecting vulnerable plaques. *Circulation*. 2001;104:1280–1285.
65. Corti R, Osende JI, Fayad ZA, et al. In vivo noninvasive detection and age definition of arterial thrombus by MRI. *J Am Coll Cardiol*. 2002;39:1366–1373.
66. Asakura M, Ueda Y, Yamaguchi O, et al. Extensive development of vulnerable plaques as a pan-coronary process in patients with myocardial infarction: an angioscopic study. *J Am Coll Cardiol*. 2001;37:1284–1288.
67. Nieman K, Oudkerk M, Rensing BJ, et al. Coronary angiography with multi-slice computed tomography. *Lancet*. 2001;357: 599–603.
68. Giesler TBU, Ropers D, Ulzheimer S, et al. Noninvasive visualization of coronary arteries using contrast-enhanced multidetector CT: influence of heart rate on image quality and stenosis detection. *AJR Am J Roentgenol*. 2002;179:911–916.
69. Duerinckx AJ. Imaging of coronary artery disease: MR. *J Thorac Imaging*. 2001;16:25–34.
70. Hecht HS. New developments in atherosclerosis imaging: electron beam tomography. *Curr Atheroscler Rep*. 2001;3:417–424.
71. Corti R, Fayad ZA, Fuster V, et al. Effects of lipid-lowering by simvastatin on human atherosclerotic lesions: a longitudinal study by high-resolution, noninvasive magnetic resonance imaging. *Circulation*. 2001;104:249–252.
72. Rumberger JA. Tomographic (plaque) imaging: state of the art. *Am J Cardiol*. 2001;88:66E–69E.
73. Achenbach S, Ropers D, Regenfus M, et al. Noninvasive coronary angiography by magnetic resonance imaging, electron-beam computed tomography, and multislice computed tomography. *Am J Cardiol*. 2001;88:70E–73E.
74. Kodama K, Asakura M, Ueda Y, et al. The role of plaque rupture in the development of acute coronary syndrome evaluated by the coronary angioscope. *Intern Med*. 2000;39:333–335.
75. Lehmann KG, van Suylen RJ, Stibbe J, et al. Composition of human thrombus assessed by quantitative colorimetric angioscopic analysis. *Circulation*. 1997;96:3030–3041.
76. Moulton KS. Plaque angiogenesis and atherosclerosis. *Curr Atheroscler Rep*. 2001;3:225–233.
77. Nasu K, Kawamoto A, Sasaki Y, et al. Measurement of vascular tissue blood flow of the atherosclerotic aorta in Watanabe heritable hypercholesterolemic (WHHL) rabbit by using laser Doppler flowmeter-equipped balloon catheter. *Am J Cardiol*. 1999;84:84P.
78. Drexler H, Zeiher AM, Wollschlager H, et al. Flow-dependent coronary artery dilatation in humans. *Circulation*. 1989;80: 466–474.
79. Vogel RA. Brachial artery ultrasound: a noninvasive tool in the assessment of triglyceride-rich lipoproteins. *Clin Cardiol*. 1999(6 Suppl);22:II34–II39.
80. Varnava AM, Mills PG, Davies MJ. Relationship between coronary artery remodeling and plaque vulnerability. *Circulation*. 2002;105:939–943.
81. Smits PC, Pasterkamp G, Quarles van Ufford MA, et al. Coronary artery disease: arterial remodelling and clinical presentation. *Heart*. 1999;82:461–464.
82. Kim WY, Stuber M, Bornert P, et al. Three-dimensional black-blood cardiac magnetic resonance coronary vessel wall imaging detects positive arterial remodeling in patients with nonsignificant coronary artery disease. *Circulation*. 2002;106:296–299.
83. Naghavi M, Madjid M, Gul K, et al. Thermography basket catheter: in vivo measurement of the temperature of atherosclerotic plaques for detection of vulnerable plaques. *Catheter Cardiovasc Interv*. 2003;59:52–59.
84. Wissler RW, Strong JP. Risk factors and progression of atherosclerosis in youth. PDAY Research Group. Pathological Determinants of Atherosclerosis in Youth. *Am J Pathol*. 1998;153:1023–1033.
85. Tuzcu EM, Kapadia SR, Tutar E, et al. High prevalence of coronary atherosclerosis in asymptomatic teenagers and young adults: evidence from intravascular ultrasound. *Circulation*. 2001;103:2705–2710.
86. Pasterkamp G, Schoneveld AH, van der Wal AC, et al. Relation of arterial geometry to luminal narrowing and histologic markers for plaque vulnerability: the remodeling paradox. *J Am Coll Cardiol*. 1998;32:655–662.
87. Becker CR, Nikolaou K, Muders M, et al. Ex vivo coronary atherosclerotic plaque characterization with multi-detector-row CT. *Eur Radiol*. 2003;12:12.
88. Vogel RA. Heads and hearts: the endothelial connection. *Circulation*. 2003;107:2766–2768.

89. Targonski PV, Bonetti PO, Pumper GM, et al. Coronary endothelial dysfunction is associated with an increased risk of cerebrovascular events. Circulation. 2003;107:2805–2809.
90. Cusack MR, Marber MS, Lambiase PD, et al. Systemic inflammation in unstable angina is the result of myocardial necrosis. J Am Coll Cardiol. 2002;39:1917–1923.
91. Yamamoto H, Uemura S, Tomoda Y, et al. Transcardiac gradient of soluble adhesion molecules predicts progression of coronary artery disease. Int J Cardiol. 2002;84:249–257.
92. Moreno PR, Purushothaman KR, Fuster V, et al. Intimomedial interface damage and adventitial inflammation is increased beneath disrupted atherosclerosis in the aorta: implications for plaque vulnerability. Circulation. 2002;105:2504–2511.
93. Ridker PM, Cushman M, Stampfer MJ, et al. Inflammation, aspirin, and the risk of cardiovascular disease in apparently healthy men. N Engl J Med. 1997;336:973–979.
94. Ridker PM, Hennekens CH, Buring JE, et al. C-reactive protein and other markers of inflammation in the prediction of cardiovascular disease in women. N Engl J Med. 2000;342:836–843.
95. Ridker PM, Rifai N, Rose L, et al. Comparison of C-reactive protein and low-density lipoprotein cholesterol levels in the prediction of first cardiovascular events. N Engl J Med. 2002;347:1557–1565.
96. Pasceri VWJ, Yeh ET. Direct proinflammatory effect of C-reactive protein on human endothelial cells. *Circulation*. 2000;102:2165–2168.
97. Verma SLS, Badiwala MV, Weisel RD, et al. Endothelin antagonism and interleukin-6 inhibition attenuate the proatherogenic effects of C-reactive protein. *Circulation*. 2002;105:1890–1896.
98. Koukkunen H, Penttila K, Kemppainen A, et al. C-reactive protein, fibrinogen, interleukin-6 and tumour necrosis factor-alpha in the prognostic classification of unstable angina pectoris. *Ann Med*. 2001;33:37–47.
99. Schonbeck U, Varo N, Libby P, et al. Soluble CD40L and cardiovascular risk in women. *Circulation*. 2001;104: 2266–2268.
100. Hwang SJ, Ballantyne CM, Sharrett AR, et al. Circulating adhesion molecules VCAM-1, ICAM-1, and E-selectin in carotid atherosclerosis and incident coronary heart disease cases: the Atherosclerosis Risk In Communities (ARIC) study. *Circulation*. 1997;96:4219–4225.
101. Kiechl S, Egger G, Mayr M, et al. Chronic infections and the risk of carotid atherosclerosis : prospective results from a large population study. *Circulation*. 2001;103:10641070.
102. Bayes-Genis A, Conover CA, Overgaard MT, et al. Pregnancy-associated plasma protein A as a marker of acute coronary syndromes. *N Engl J Med*. 2001;345:1022–1029.
103. Beaudeux JL, Burc L, Imbert-Bismut F, et al. Serum plasma pregnancyassociated protein A: a potential marker of echogenic carotid atherosclerotic plaques in asymptomatic hyperlipidemic subjects at high cardiovascular risk. *Arterioscler Thromb Vasc Biol*. 2003;23:e7–e10.
104. Yamada Y, Izawa H, Ichihara S, et al. Prediction of the risk of myocardial infarction from polymorphisms in candidate genes. *N Engl J Med*. 2002;347:1916–1923.
105. Lange LA, Lange EM, Bielak LF, et al. Autosomal genome-wide scan for coronary artery calcification loci in sibships at high risk for hypertension. *Arterioscler Thromb Vasc Biol*. 2002;22:418–423.
106. Ozaki K, Ohnishi Y, Iida A, et al. Functional SNPs in the lymphotoxin-alpha gene that are associated with susceptibility to myocardial infarction. *Nat Genet*. 2002;32:650–654.
107. Karnicki K, Owen WG, Miller RS, et al. Factors contributing to individual propensity for arterial thrombosis. *Arterioscler Thromb Vasc Biol*. 2002;22:1495–1499.
108. Libby P, Simon DI. Inflammation and thrombosis: the clot thickens. *Circulation*. 2001;103:1718–1720.
109. Barakat K, Kennon S, Hitman GA, et al. Interaction between smoking and the glycoprotein IIIa P1(A2) polymorphism in non-ST-elevation acute coronary syndromes. *J Am Coll Cardiol*. 2001;38:1639–1643.
110. Douglas H, Michaelides K, Gorog DA, et al. Platelet membrane glycoprotein Ibα gene –5T/C Kozak sequence polymorphism as an independent risk factor for the occurrence of coronary thrombosis. *Heart*. 2002;87:70–74.
111. Redondo M, Watzke HH, Stucki B, et al. Coagulation factors II, V, VII, and X, prothrombin gene 20210G3A transition, and factor V Leiden in coronary artery disease: high factor V clotting activity is an independent risk factor for myocardial infarction. *Arterioscler Thromb Vasc Biol*. 1999;19:1020–1025.
112. Reiner AP, Siscovick DS, Rosendaal FR. Hemostatic risk factors and arterial thrombotic disease. *Thromb Haemost*. 2001;85:584–595.
113. Sambola A, Osende J, Hathcock J, et al. Role of risk factors in the modulation of tissue factor activity and blood thrombogenicity. *Circulation*. 2003;107:973–977.
114. Passoni F, Morelli B, Seveso G, et al. Comparative short-term prognostic value of hemostatic and inflammatory markers in patients with non-ST elevation acute coronary syndromes. *Ital Heart J*. 2002;3:28–33.
115. Hoffmeister HM, Heller W, Seipel L. Activation markers of coagulation and fibrinolysis: alterations and predictive value in acute coronary syndromes. *Thromb Haemost*. 1999;82:76–79.
116. Vaarala O, Puurunen M, Manttari M, et al. Antibodies to prothrombin imply a risk of myocardial infarction in middle-aged men. *Thromb Haemost*. 1996;75:456–459.
117. Jouhikainen T, Pohjola-Sintonen S, Stephansson E. Lupus anticoagulant and cardiac manifestations in systemic lupus erythematosus. *Lupus*. 1994;3:167–172.

118. Osula S, Bell GM, Hornung RS. Acute myocardial infarction in young adults: causes and management. *Postgrad Med J.* 2002;78:27–30.
119. Burke AP, Kolodgie FD, Farb A, et al. Healed plaque ruptures and sudden coronary death: evidence that subclinical rupture has a role in plaque progression. *Circulation.* 2001;103:934–940.
120. Mann J, Davies MJ. Mechanisms of progression in native coronary artery disease: role of healed plaque disruption. *Heart.* 1999;82:265–268.
121. Servoss SJ, Januzzi JL, Muller JE. Triggers of acute coronary syndromes. *Prog Cardiovasc Dis.* 2002;44:369–380.
122. Silveira A. Postprandial triglycerides and blood coagulation. *Exp Clin Endocrinol Diabetes.* 2001;109:S527–S532.
123. McNagny SE, Wenger NK. Postmenopausal hormone-replacement therapy. *N Engl J Med.* 2002;346:63–65.
124. Koenig W, Sund M, Filipiak B, et al. Plasma viscosity and the risk of coronary heart disease: results from the MONICA-Augsburg Cohort Study, 1984 to 1992. *Arterioscler Thromb Vasc Biol.* 1998;18:768–772.
125. Junker R, Heinrich J, Ulbrich H, et al. Relationship between plasma viscosity and the severity of coronary heart disease. *Arterioscler Thromb Vasc Biol.* 1998;18:870–875.
126. Myerburg RJ, Kessler KM, Castellanos A. Sudden cardiac death: structure, function, and time-dependence of risk. *Circulation.* 1992;85(Suppl I):I-2–I-10.
127. Kannel WB, Doyle JT, McNamara PM, et al. Precursors of sudden coronary death: factors related to the incidence of sudden death. *Circulation.* 1975;51:606–613.
128. Schwartz PJ, Vanoli E, Zaza A, et al. The effect of antiarrhythmic drugs on life-threatening arrhythmias induced by the interaction between acute myocardial ischemia and sympathetic hyperactivity. *Am Heart J.* 1985;109:937–948.
129. Vanoli E, De Ferrari GM, Stramba-Badiale M, et al. Vagal stimulation and prevention of sudden death in conscious dogs with a healed myocardial infarction. *Circ Res.* 1991;68:1471–1481.
130. Airaksinen KE. Autonomic mechanisms and sudden death after abrupt coronary occlusion. *Ann Med.* 1999;31:240–245.
131. Airaksinen KE, Tahvanainen KU, Eckberg DL, et al. Arterial baroreflex impairment in patients during acute coronary occlusion. *J Am Coll Cardiol.* 1998;32:1641–1647.
132. Billman GE, Schwartz PJ, Stone HL. The effects of daily exercise on susceptibility to sudden cardiac death. *Circulation.* 1984;69:1182–1189.
133. Burke AP, Farb A, Malcom GT, et al. Plaque rupture and sudden death related to exertion in men with coronary artery disease. *JAMA.* 1999;281:921–926.
134. Jouven X, Desnos M, Guerot C, et al. Predicting sudden death in the population: the Paris Prospective Study I. *Circulation.* 1999;99:1978–1983.
135. Singh JP, Larson MG, O'Donnell CJ, et al. Heritability of heart rate variability: the Framingham Heart Study. *Circulation.* 1999;99:2251–2254.
136. Claessens C, Claessens P, Claessens M, et al. Changes in mortality of acute myocardial infarction as a function of a changing treatment during the last two decades. *Jpn Heart J.* 2000;41:683–695.
137. Jouven X, Charles MA, Desnos M, et al. Circulating nonesterified fatty acid level as a predictive risk factor for sudden death in the population. *Circulation.* 2001;104:756–761.
138. Priori SG, Aliot E, Blomstrom-Lundqvist C, et al. Task Force on Sudden Cardiac Death of the European Society of Cardiology. *Eur Heart J.* 2001;22:1374–1450.
139. Magnus P, Beaglehole R. The real contribution of the major risk factors to the coronary epidemics: time to end the "only-50%" myth. *Arch Intern Med.* 2001;161:2657–2660.
140. Lefkowitz RJ, Willerson JT. Prospects for cardiovascular research. *JAMA.* 2001;285:581–587.
141. Nieto FJ. Cardiovascular disease and risk factor epidemiology: a look back at the epidemic of the 20th century. *Am J Public Health.* 1999;89:292–294.
142. Anderson KM, Odell PM, Wilson PW, et al. Cardiovascular disease risk profiles. *Am Heart J.* 1991;121:293–298.
143. Ramsay LE, Haq IU, Jackson PR, et al. Targeting lipid-lowering drug therapy for primary prevention of coronary disease: an updated Sheffield table. *Lancet.* 1996;348:387–388.
144. Wallis EJ, Ramsay LE, Ul Haq I, et al. Coronary and cardiovascular risk estimation for primary prevention: validation of a new Sheffield table in the 1995 Scottish health survey population. *BMJ.* 2000;320:671–676.
145. 1996 National Heart Foundation clinical guidelines for the assessment and management of dyslipidaemia. Dyslipidaemia Advisory Group on behalf of the Scientific Committee of the National Heart Foundation of New Zealand. *N Z Med J.* 1996;109:224–231.
146. Jackson R. Updated New Zealand cardiovascular disease risk-benefit prediction guide. *BMJ.* 2000;320:709–710.
147. McCormack JP, Levine M, Rangno RE. Primary prevention of heart disease and stroke: a simplified approach to estimating risk of events and making drug treatment decisions. *CMAJ.* 1997;157:422–428.
148. Joint British recommendations on prevention of coronary heart disease in clinical practice: summary. British Cardiac Society, British Hyperlipidaemia Association, British Hypertension Society, British Diabetic Association. *BMJ.* 2000;320:705–708.
149. Wood D, De Backer G, Faergeman O, et al. Prevention of coronary heart disease in clinical practice: recommendations of the Second Joint Task Force of European and other Societies on Coronary Prevention. *Atherosclerosis.* 1998;140:199–270.
150. Tunstall-Pedoe H. The Dundee coronary risk-disk for management of change in risk factors. *BMJ.* 1991;303:744–747.

151. Assmann G, Cullen P, Schulte H. Simple scoring scheme for calculating the risk of acute coronary events based on the 10-year follow-up of the prospective cardiovascular Munster (PROCAM) study. *Circulation.* 2002;105:310–315.
152. Manhem K, Dotevall A, Wilhelmsen L, et al. Social gradients in cardiovascular risk factors and symptoms of Swedish men and women: the Goteborg MONICA Study 1995. *J Cardiovasc Risk.* 2000;7:359–368.
153. Voss R, Cullen P, Schulte H, et al. Prediction of risk of coronary events in middle-aged men in the Prospective Cardiovascular Münster Study (PROCAM) using neural networks. *Int J Epidemiol.* 2002;31:1253–1264.
154. Arad YSL, Goodman K, Newstein D, et al. Prediction of coronary events with electron beam computed tomography. *J Am Coll Cardiol.* 2000;36:1253–1260
155. Friedman M, Van den Borenkamp G.J. The pathogenesis of a coronary thrombus. *Am J Pathol.* 1966;48:19–44.
156. Friedman M. The pathogenesis of coronary plaques, thromboses, and hemorrhages: an evaluative review. *Circulation.* 1975;52(Suppl III):III34–III40.
157. Halcox JP, Schenke WH, Zalos G, et al. Prognostic value of coronary vascular endothelial function. *Circulation.* 2002;106: 653–658.

3 Pathology of Vulnerability Caused by High-Risk (Vulnerable) Arteries and Plaques

Troels Thim, Mette Kallestrup Hagensen, Jacob Fog Bentzon, and Erling Falk

CONTENTS

ABSTRACT

Atherosclerosis is a slowly progressing systemic (multifocal) arterial disease with focal manifestations caused by one or relatively few stenotic and/or thrombosis-prone (vulnerable) plaques. The coronary arteries, carotid arteries, ilio-femoral arteries, and aorta are especially susceptible to atherosclerosis. The most devastating consequences of atherosclerosis, such as heart attack and stroke, are usually caused by thrombosis precipitated by plaque rupture. Although the morphology of ruptured plaques has been known for decades, it remains poorly understood why a single plaque among many plaques becomes vulnerable and suddenly ruptures. Plaque rupture requires the presence of a lipid-rich (necrotic) core covered by a thin fibrous cap, and the development and detection of "core and cap" are currently explored in basic and clinical research. Other plaque and plaque-related features may be useful markers of vulnerability, including plaque inflammation (macrophage density and activity), neovascularization (angiogenesis), hemorrhage, microcalcification, adventitial inflammation (lymphocytes), and expansive remodeling. Vascular imaging and function testing have the potential to provide a comprehensive assessment of atherosclerosis, including detection of plaque burden, plaque vulnerability, and disease activity. The search for better markers of cardiovascular risk must continue. With the traditional risk-factor-based approach in primary prevention, most individuals

From: *Asymptomatic Atherosclerosis: Pathophysiology, Detection and Treatment*
Edited by: M. Naghavi (ed.), DOI 10.1007/978-1-60327-179-0_3

destined for a near-term heart attack or stroke are misclassified and not identified as being at high risk. Consequently, they are not offered appropriate preventive therapy. Detection of subclinical but high-risk atherosclerosis may change this unfortunate situation.

Key words: Atherosclerosis; Vulnerable plaque; Plaque rupture; Coronary thrombosis; Risk assessment

KEY POINTS OR TOPIC PEARLS

- A "high-risk" or "vulnerable" plaque is a thrombosis-prone plaque
- Plaque rupture is the most common cause of thrombosis in coronary and carotid arteries
- Plaque rupture requires the presence of a lipid-rich (necrotic) core covered by a thin fibrous cap
- In plaque rupture, the tiny fibrous cap is heavily inflamed at the rupture site
- Assessment of subclinical atherosclerosis can improve the prediction of cardiovascular risk

Nearly all of us develop atherosclerosis, but the speed of development and the clinical consequences vary greatly and are difficult to predict. The preclinical incubation period is long, and most people live with atherosclerosis without feeling it or becoming sick from it. Developing the stenotic and/or high-risk (*vulnerable*) plaques responsible for clinical disease takes decades, and by then, atherosclerosis is usually severe and generalized [1, 2]. Furthermore, many first events are fatal, and these can, of course, only be averted by intervention in the disease's preclinical phase. The long incubation period when atherosclerosis is subclinical and harmless offers unique opportunities for the prevention of overt atherosclerotic cardiovascular disease (CVD) by timely detection and treatment of subclinical atherosclerosis. Identification of those in need of preventive therapy remains, however, a major challenge.

Causal risk factors for atherosclerotic CVD are known and constitute important therapeutic targets [3], but their predictive power is limited [4–6]. In fact, most first heart attacks occur in previously asymptomatic individuals with unrecognized atherosclerosis who are misclassified by the Framingham Risk Score as being at low or intermediate risk [7]. Thus, when screening is based on risk factors alone, most individuals destined for an acute atherothrombotic event are not identified and, consequently, not offered adequate preventive treatment. Risk factor exposure is obviously not the only determinant of atherosclerotic CVD, individual susceptibility to the disease must also play an important role. The overall "holistic" effects of exposure to risk factors, known as well as unknown, and susceptibility are captured by the actual amount (burden) and character (activity) of the underlying arterial disease. Therefore, tests for *subclinical atherosclerosis* hold key to reform risk assessment and ensure optimal use of prevention therapy [8].

Atherosclerosis is a systemic arterial disease of multifactorial origin [9]. It begins early in life with multifocal plaque development in medium-sized and large arteries. The coronary arteries, carotid arteries, ilio-femoral arteries, and aorta are particularly susceptible to atherosclerosis. The most devastating consequences of atherosclerosis, such as heart attack and stroke, are caused by superimposed thrombosis [9, 10]. Therefore, the vital question is not why atherosclerosis develops but rather why atherosclerosis, after years of indolent growth, suddenly becomes complicated with luminal thrombosis. If thrombosis-prone plaques could be detected and thrombosis averted, atherosclerosis would be a much more benign disease. The most common type of thrombosis-prone plaques, also known as high-risk or *vulnerable* plaques [11], is the rupture-prone plaque, which constitutes the main focus of this chapter.

PLAQUE RUPTURE

Because of lack of prospective data, we have learned about plaques assumed to be rupture-prone by extrapolating from what we know about ruptured plaques. Plaque rupture is by far the most common cause of arterial thrombosis, and, consequently, the rupture-prone plaque is the most important type of vulnerable plaque and also the best described [11]. Plaque rupture is responsible for approximately 75% of coronary thrombi leading to myocardial infarction and/or death [9, 12] and around 90% of thrombosed carotid plaques causing ischemic stroke [13]. Much less is known about nonrupture related thrombosis and its potential precursor plaques among which the so-called erosion-prone plaque dominates.

The ruptured plaque has been defined as "a plaque with deep injury with a real defect or gap in the fibrous cap that had separated its lipid-rich atheromatous core from the flowing blood, thereby exposing the thrombogenic core of the plaque" [11]. Thus, the presence of a lipid-rich core covered by a fibrous cap is required for plaque rupture [11], and the descriptive term thin-cap fibroatheroma (TCFA) has been suggested for intact plaques at risk of rupture [14]. The exposure of the thrombogenic lipid-rich core in plaque rupture may lead to thrombosis, which covers the rupture site and extends into the lumen [15, 16]. A ruptured plaque with superimposed thrombosis is shown in Fig. 1.

The most extensive and detailed knowledge about ruptured and thus rupture-prone plaques stems from autopsy studies [14–18]. Additional information has been gathered from atherectomy specimen of coronary origin [19, 20] and endarterectomy specimen of carotid origin [13, 21]. Lately, intravascular imaging with optical coherence tomography has provided convincing in vivo evidence of plaque rupture in the coronary arteries of patients with acute myocardial infarction [12]. However, all these techniques have the same limitation: they provide information on the structure and components of ruptured plaques and only by extrapolation do we learn about the features of rupture-prone plaques.

A useful animal model, in which the mechanisms leading to spontaneous plaque rupture could be studied prospectively, would overcome some of these problems, but such a model is not yet available [22].

KEY FEATURES OF RUPTURED PLAQUES: CORE AND CAP

The presence of a lipid-rich (necrotic) core covered by a fibrous cap is a prerequisite for plaque rupture. In the absence of a core there is no fibrous cap, and the plaque cannot rupture. Therefore, the formation of a lipid-rich core is the essential early mechanism in the development of the rupture-prone plaque.

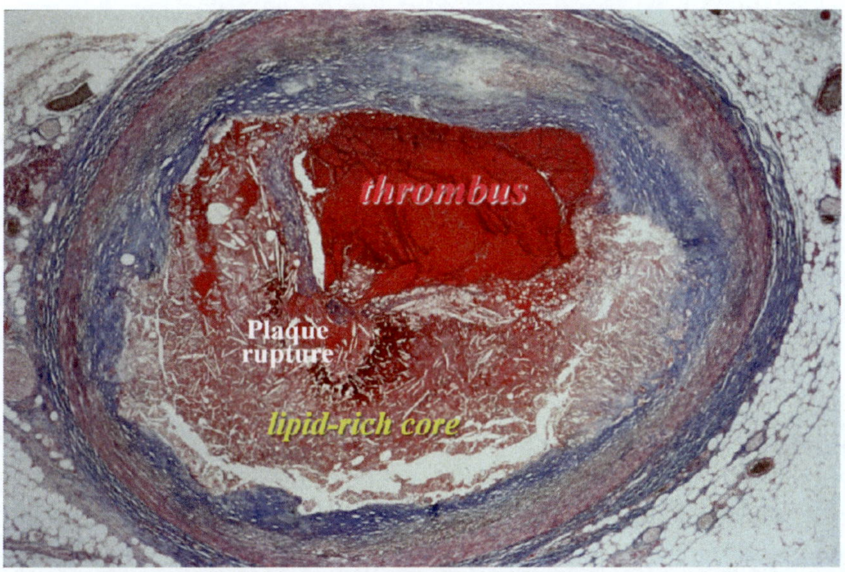

Fig. 1. Fatal coronary thrombosis caused by plaque rupture. There is a defect in the fibrous cap, through which thrombogenic material from the lipid-rich core has been dislodged into the lumen. Plaque hemorrhage is seen beneath the rupture site.

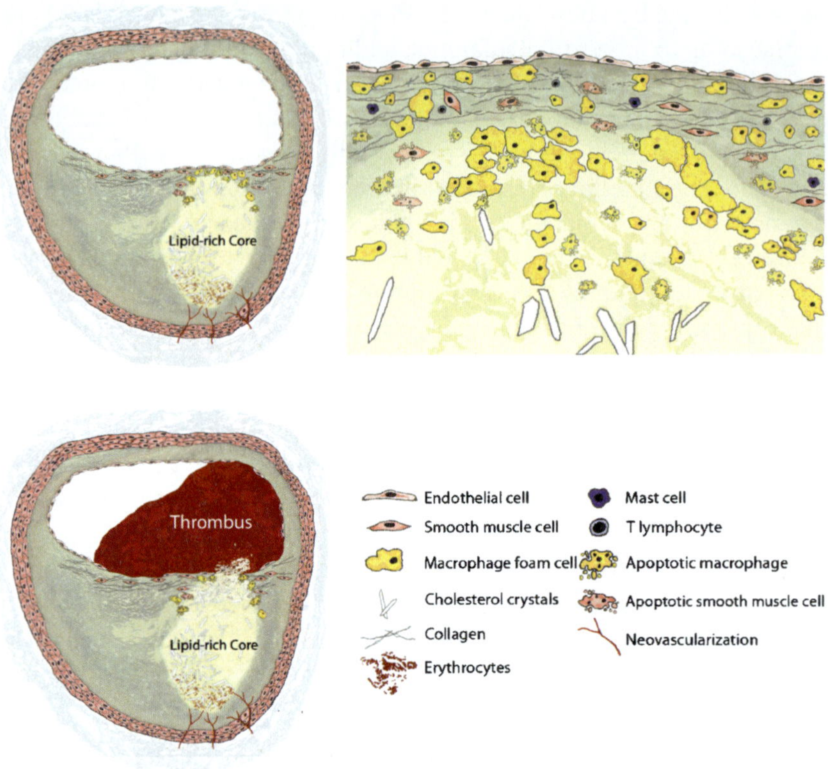

Fig. 2. *Top left panel* illustrates a plaque assumed to be rupture-prone. The lipid-rich core occupies approximately 40% of the plaque area and contains multiple cholesterol crystals. The fibrous cap is thin and inflamed with few smooth muscle cells. Plaque microvessels originating from the adventitia are extending through the media into the base of the plaque. *Top right panel* illustrates the thin and locally weakened fibrous cap. Macrophages are abundantly present whereas smooth muscle cells are scarce. *Bottom left panel* illustrates the corresponding ruptured plaque with consequent thrombus covering the rupture site.

If lipid-rich core formation could be prevented, no plaque ruptures would occur. Later, when the lipid-rich core has formed, the key process is the thinning of the fibrous cap toward its rupture. If fibrous cap thinning could be prevented, no plaque ruptures would occur.

A number of other features are associated with rupture-prone plaques (e.g., angiogenesis, intraplaque hemorrhage, perivascular inflammation, and expansive remodeling). To the extent that these features are causal for plaque rupture, their most likely mode of action is through modulation of the lipid-rich core and the fibrous cap. Figure 2 illustrates the characteristic features of the rupture-prone plaque.

Lipid-Rich Core

A large lipid-rich core is associated with plaque rupture. In human coronary arteries, the lipid-rich cores of ruptured plaques were larger compared to nonruptured plaques and occupied on average 29–34% of plaque area in ruptured plaques [14, 23, 24]. In the carotid artery of symptomatic patients undergoing carotid endarterectomy, a mean lipid-rich core size of 40% of plaque area was found [21]. Similarly in human aortas, ruptured plaques had larger lipid-rich cores than nonruptured plaques, occupying close to 60% of ruptured plaque area [25, 26].

The increase in total plaque lipid content in ruptured compared to intact plaques is predominantly due to increased amounts of free cholesterol and cholesteryl esters, and the ratio of free cholesterol to cholesteryl esters is increased [26–28]. The importance of lipid-rich core size for plaque rupture is comprehensible, because (1) the expansion of the lipid-rich core may erode the fibrous cap from below, and (2) the total lack of supporting collagen in the lipid-rich core confers greater tensile stress to the overlying fibrous cap.

The mechanism of lipid-rich core formation is poorly understood. It has been suggested that smaller pools of accumulated lipid in the basal intima coalesce to a larger pool that due to apoptosis and necrosis of smooth muscle cells and lipid-filled macrophages (foam cells) becomes acellular [14, 29–31]. Cell surface markers on the macrophages in the basal intima of atherosclerotic plaque differ from those in the superficial intima [32]. This may explain a different propensity for apoptosis and necrosis of macrophages in the basal and superficial intima and thereby why lipid-rich cores form in the basal intima [33]. Because cell death is believed to play an important role in the formation of a lipid-rich core, it is also called a necrotic core.

Several sources of lipids contribute to the lipid-rich core and the quantitative importance of these varies between different stages of plaque formation. In atherogenesis in general, the contribution from blood-derived lipoproteins is emphasized [34]. Lipoproteins entering the plaque may be retained and phagocytosed by macrophages which may later die, leaving behind their lipid rich content, and thus contributing to the lipid-rich core [35]. However, lipoproteins may also contribute directly without first passing through foam cells [36]. It has been suggested that intraplaque hemorrhage from neovessels within the plaque may lead to rapid growth of the lipid-rich core and increase its free cholesterol content through the delivery of erythrocyte membranes containing high concentrations of cholesterol [37]. The high free cholesterol content facilitates cholesterol crystal formation, and increased number of cholesterol crystals in the lipid-rich core is associated with plaque rupture [14].

Fibrous Cap

The fibrous cap is simply defined as the connective tissue layer covering the lipid-rich core. It consists of smooth muscle cells and the extracellular matrix they synthesize (mainly collagen and proteoglycans) [14, 29–31]. The cap also contains inflammatory cells, predominantly macrophage foam cells (Fig. 2).

Plaque rupture only occurs when the fibrous cap is extremely thin [17, 38]. In a post mortem series of 41 ruptured coronary plaques, 95% of the fibrous caps were <65 μm thick (mean: 23 μm) [39]. Based on this finding, a thin fibrous cap is usually defined as a cap with a thickness <65 μm [14]. This is in agreement with recent in vivo optical coherence tomography finding of a mean fibrous cap thickness of 49 μm in ruptured coronary plaques in patients with acute myocardial infarction [12]. In carotid endarterectomy specimen with ruptured plaques, the minimal fibrous cap thickness was around 80 μm [40]. In aortas obtained at autopsy, the minimal fibrous cap thickness was around 130 μm in ruptured plaques [26]. These differences in ruptured cap thickness in different vascular territories may reflect differences in vessel wall tension, being lowest in the coronary arteries, intermediate in carotid arteries, and highest in the aorta.

Thinning of the fibrous cap is considered a product of increased matrix degradation by infiltrating macrophages and impaired matrix synthesis due to a decreasing number and/or function of cap smooth muscle cells. Ruptured caps have increased macrophage density and decreased smooth muscle density compared to intact caps [25]. The macrophages possess destabilizing properties through expression of matrix-degrading proteolytic enzymes, e.g., matrix metalloproteinases [41, 42]. Meanwhile, the smooth muscle cells are the principal connective tissue producing cells in the intima, and the matrix they produce is considered to stabilize plaques, protecting against rupture [43].

The reasons for smooth muscle cell loss are poorly understood, but apoptosis has been observed in cap smooth muscle cells in atherosclerotic plaques [44, 45]. Apoptotic loss of smooth muscle cells seems grave taking into account that plaque smooth muscle cells show reduced ability to replicate in vivo and in vitro [14, 46]. Moreover, recent experimental evidence contradicts previous claims that smooth muscle cells in atherosclerotic plaques can be repopulated by circulating progenitor cells [47–49]. Selective apoptosis of smooth muscle cells induced by transgenic techniques in atherosclerotic mice has been reported to induce fibrous cap thinning [50].

Plaque Inflammation

Atherosclerosis is considered a systemic inflammatory disease in which the degree of inflammation within a plaque determines its risk of rupturing [41, 42]. This has led to the misconception that rupture-prone plaques are heavily inflamed. However, the bulk of the rupture-prone plaque is essentially hypocellular with no inflammation. The lipid-rich core is acellular, and large areas of the plaque are dense fibrous or calcified tissue with few or no inflammatory cells (Fig. 3).

In fatal myocardial infarction, advanced coronary plaque contained on average 5–8% inflammatory cells by morphometry [23, 51]. In coronary atherectomy specimens from patients with unstable coronary disease, macrophages occupied approximately 14% of the atherectomized culprit lesion [19], while macrophages only occupied around 1% in carotid endarterectomy specimens from symptomatic patients [21, 52]. These inflammatory infiltrates are not diffusely spread throughout the plaque, but cluster around the lipid-rich core and in the fibrous cap.

However, in contrast to the plaque as a whole, fibrous caps are always heavily inflamed at the site of rupture. In the coronary arteries, a macrophage density of 26% in ruptured fibrous caps has been reported [14]. In the aorta, macrophages take up 14–17% of the cap area in ruptured plaques [25, 26]. At the actual rupture site, only inflammatory cells, predominantly macrophages, are present [17, 53]. Accordingly, it is not diffuse inflammation that characterizes ruptured plaques but rather severe inflammation limited to a tiny plaque component (fibrous cap) or even a small area within this tiny component (site of rupture).

While plaque rupture is always accompanied by local inflammation of the cap, inflammation of morphologically stable plaque types is also a frequent finding [20, 53]. Therefore, inflammation alone is not enough to make a plaque rupture-prone; a core and a thin cap are also required.

Plaque Neovascularization (Angiogenesis)

Rupture-prone plaques are associated with neovascularization extending into the plaque from vasa vasorum in the adventitia (Fig. 2). In rupture-prone and ruptured plaques, the microvessel density is two- to fourfold higher than in stable plaques both in carotid and coronary arteries [54, 55]. Most commonly, the intimal microvessels are present at the base of the plaque and near its shoulder regions, and they may extend well into the plaques surrounding the lipid-rich core which, however, remains avascular [56–58]. These microvessels are fragile and leaky as indicated by the presence of extravasated erythrocytes and plasma proteins [37, 55, 58]. The extent of neovascularization correlates positively with plaque size, lipid content, and the degree of inflammation [54, 55, 58–60].

(Intra)Plaque Hemorrhage

Blood may enter the plaque through a ruptured fibrous cap (plaque hemorrhage) or from fragile neovessels within the plaque (intraplaque hemorrhage). Signs of bleeding from both sources are not uncommon in advanced plaques. Although intraplaque hemorrhage is not directly related to plaque rupture, it may promote rupture by expanding the lipid-rich core and attracting macrophages [37].

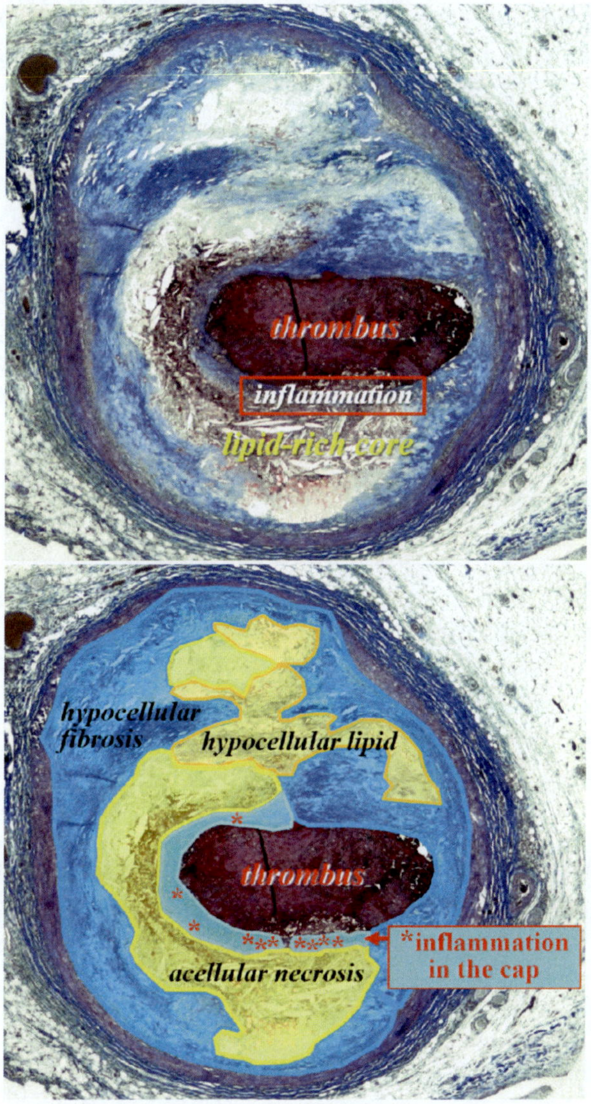

Fig. 3. Ruptured coronary plaque with thrombosis: The thin cap is inflamed whereas the remainder of the plaque is not. Macrophages (*asterisks*) cluster in the cap next to the rupture site. The majority of the plaque consists of acellular lipid-rich core and hypocellular fibrosis and lipid pools.

Expansive Remodeling

The majority of advanced plaques do not cause significant luminal narrowing, because the arterial wall expands as a response to plaque development, known as expansive or positive remodeling [61]. In autopsy studies, expansive remodeling is more pronounced in the proximal portions of the coronary arteries than in the distal portions [62]. Accordingly, plaques that are not detectable on angiography can be observed in the proximal portions of the coronary arteries with intravascular ultrasound [63].

In acute coronary syndromes, 68% of culprit lesions had angiographic stenosis <50% prior to thrombus formation [64]. This is because expansive remodeling is common and makes stenotic plaques relatively rare compared to nonstenotic plaques [64]. Ruptured plaques in particular are associated with expansive remodeling and, consequently, most rupture-prone plaques are asymptomatic and nonstenotic at angiographic examination [53, 62]. This explains, at least in part, why percutaneous coronary intervention added to optimal medical therapy in stable angina may relieve pain without reducing the risk of death, nonfatal myocardial infarction, or other major cardiovascular events [65].

Calcification

The coronary artery calcium content correlates with plaque burden but not with the degree of luminal narrowing [66], and the coronary artery calcium score (CACS) detected by computed tomography is a stronger predictor of cardiovascular events and mortality than conventional risk factors [67, 68].

The calcification pattern seems to differ between different plaque types. Culprit plaques in acute coronary syndromes are less calcified and the calcifications are smaller compared to culprit plaques in stable angina [66, 69, 70]. Therefore, CACS signals coronary atherosclerosis and correlates with risk, although the risk is primarily related to less calcified plaques present along with more calcified and stable plaques.

Rapid Plaque Progression

Plaque rupture in itself does not cause symptoms and the thrombotic response may also remain silent and heal without symptoms [64]. Coronary plaque rupture was identified, as an incidental finding unrelated to the cause of death, in 19 of 129 (15%) persons who died of noncardiac causes [71], and ruptured plaques were also found in carotid endarterectomy specimen from asymptomatic patients [13].

Although clinically silent, nonsymptomatic plaque rupture contributes to stenosis progression [72]. A nonfatal plaque rupture is healed by smooth muscle cells that accumulate at the rupture site and secrete extracellular matrix rich in glycosaminoglycans and collagen [72]. This process heals the plaque defect and organizes residual superimposed thrombus, but it may lead to luminal narrowing [46, 72]. Repeated episodes of rupture and healing are assumed to underlie the rapid but asymptomatic progression of stenoses observed in serial angiography studies [73, 74]. Recent experimental observations indicate that the healing smooth muscle cells originate from the local vessel wall and not from blood-derived progenitor cells [75].

ATHEROTHROMBOSIS

The thrombotic response to plaque rupture consists initially of aggregating platelets, and it may dynamically grow and embolize causing intermittent flow obstruction [76]. In persisting thrombosis, the early platelet-rich thrombus is stabilized by fibrin. If the platelet-rich thrombus is occlusive then blood will stagnate proximal and distal to the occlusion and subsequently coagulate, forming a venous-type thrombus that may propagate proximally and distally [77, 78].

There are three major determinants of the thrombotic response to plaque rupture: the local thrombogenic substrate, local flow disturbances, and the systemic thrombotic propensity [77, 78]. The lipid-rich core exposed by plaque rupture appears to be very thrombogenic [79], probably because of apoptosis-derived microparticles expressing tissue factor [80]. Larger ruptures are likely more thrombogenic than smaller ones. The degree of pre-existing stenosis at the rupture site determines in part the thrombogenic response, probably related to shear-induced platelet activation locally [38, 81, 82]. Systemically, the state of platelet activation, coagulation, and fibrinolysis is critical for the thrombotic response to plaque rupture, documented by the protective effect of antiplatelet agents and anticoagulants in patients at risk of coronary thrombosis. Tissue factor plays an important prothrombotic role not only locally but also in the circulation as blood-borne tissue factor expressed by activated leukocytes and microparticles [83].

THE VULNERABLE PATIENT

The *vulnerable plaque* is upstream in a potentially catastrophic cascade that also includes the thrombotic propensity (*vulnerable blood*), collateral development, and the tendency to ventricular arrhythmias in face of myocardial ischemia (*vulnerable myocardium*) [84, 85]. This chapter deals only with plaque vulnerability, but whether this vulnerability resides in just one, a few, or may plaques (*arterial vulnerability*) remains to be discussed.

Arterial Vulnerability

The presence of more than one vulnerable plaque in a patient with acute coronary syndrome has been debated in relation to different diagnostic and therapeutic strategies. Different definitions of vulnerable plaques have complicated this issue.

As an example, one autopsy study reported that an average of 6.8 vulnerable plaques were present in patients dying from myocardial infarction [86]. However, less than 2 were considered rupture-prone (TCFA), which is by far the most frequent type of vulnerable plaque causing myocardial infarction. This estimate in fact corresponds well with earlier findings of around 2 rupture-prone or ruptured plaques per patient dying from coronary artery disease [24, 38, 39]. Therefore rather than diffuse or multifocal, rupture-prone plaques seem to be oligofocal as highlighted [87].

In the coronary arteries, rupture-prone plaques are predominantly located in the proximal and mid-portions [24] where most coronary occlusions are also observed clinically [88], and where most plaque ruptures and healed plaque ruptures have been observed post mortem [24]. In the carotids, this plaque type is located near the carotid bifurcation [89]. Pioneering studies of ruptured plaques were done on the aorta [25].

Since rupture-prone plaques are located predominantly in the proximal and mid-portions of the coronary arteries, where atherothrombosis has the most devastating consequences and only few of them coexist, there may be a case for local treatment if rupture-prone plaques can be identified.

CONCLUSIONS

Plaque rupture precipitates approximately 75% of all fatal coronary thrombi. The two major determinants of plaque rupture appear to be the size of the lipid-rich core and, in particular, the thickness of the fibrous cap. Only plaques with a very thin cap are at risk of rupture. Plaque rupture is a localized phenomenon in which only a small portion of a tiny fibrous cap needs to be destroyed before the life is at risk. Even in the presence of widespread atherosclerosis, rarely more than a few plaques appear to be at risk of rupture at any given moment.

REFERENCES

1. Roberts WC. Diffuse extent of coronary atherosclerosis in fatal coronary artery disease. Am J Cardiol. 1990;65:2F–6F.
2. Dalager S, Falk E, Kristensen IB, Paaske WP. Plaque in superficial femoral arteries indicates generalized atherosclerosis and vulnerability to coronary death: an autopsy study. J Vasc Surg. 2008;47:296–302.
3. Yusuf S, Hawken S, Ounpuu S, Dans T, Avezum A, Lanas F, McQueen M, Budaj A, Pais P, Varigos J, Lisheng L. Effect of potentially modifiable risk factors associated with myocardial infarction in 52 countries (the INTERHEART study): case-control study. Lancet. 2004;364:937–952.
4. Wald NJ, Hackshaw AK, Frost CD. When can a risk factor be used as a worthwhile screening test? BMJ. 1999;319:1562–1565.
5. Wald NJ, Morris JK, Rish S. The efficacy of combining several risk factors as a screening test. J Med Screen. 2005;12:197–201.
6. Ware JH. The limitations of risk factors as prognostic tools. N Engl J Med. 2006;355:2615–2617.

7. Lauer MS. Primary prevention of atherosclerotic cardiovascular disease: the high public burden of low individual risk. JAMA. 2007;297:1376–1378.
8. Naghavi M, Falk E, Hecht HS, Jamieson MJ, Kaul S, Berman D, Fayad Z, Budoff MJ, Rumberger J, Naqvi TZ, Shaw LJ, Faergeman O, Cohn J, Bahr R, Koenig W, Demirovic J, Arking D, Herrera VL, Badimon J, Goldstein JA, Rudy Y, Airaksinen J, Schwartz RS, Riley WA, Mendes RA, Douglas P, Shah PK. From vulnerable plaque to vulnerable patient – Part III: Executive summary of the Screening for Heart Attack Prevention and Education (SHAPE) Task Force report. Am J Cardiol. 2006;98:2H–15H.
9. Falk E. Pathogenesis of atherosclerosis. J Am Coll Cardiol. 2006;47:C7–12.
10. Thim T, Hagensen MK, Bentzon JF, Falk E. From vulnerable plaque to atherothrombosis. J Intern Med. 2008;263:506–516.
11. Schaar JA, Muller JE, Falk E, Virmani R, Fuster V, Serruys PW, Colombo A, Stefanadis C, Ward CS, Moreno PR, Maseri A, van der Steen AF. Terminology for high-risk and vulnerable coronary artery plaques. Report of a meeting on the vulnerable plaque, June 17 and 18, 2003, Santorini, Greece. Eur Heart J. 2004;25:1077–1082.
12. Kubo T, Imanishi T, Takarada S, Kuroi A, Ueno S, Yamano T, Tanimoto T, Matsuo Y, Masho T, Kitabata H, Tsuda K, Tomobuchi Y, Akasaka T. Assessment of culprit lesion morphology in acute myocardial infarction: ability of optical coherence tomography compared with intravascular ultrasound and coronary angioscopy. J Am Coll Cardiol. 2007;50:933–939.
13. Spagnoli LG, Mauriello A, Sangiorgi G, Fratoni S, Bonanno E, Schwartz RS, Piepgras DG, Pistolese R, Ippoliti A, Holmes DR, Jr. Extracranial thrombotically active carotid plaque as a risk factor for ischemic stroke. JAMA. 2004;292:1845–1852.
14. Virmani R, Kolodgie FD, Burke AP, Farb A, Schwartz SM. Lessons from sudden coronary death: a comprehensive morphological classification scheme for atherosclerotic lesions. Arterioscler Thromb Vasc Biol. 2000;20:1262–1275.
15. Falk E. Stable versus unstable atherosclerosis: clinical aspects. Am Heart J. 1999;138:S421–S425.
16. Davies MJ. The pathophysiology of acute coronary syndromes. Heart. 2000;83:361–366.
17. van der Wal AC, Becker AE, van der Loos CM, Das PK. Site of intimal rupture or erosion of thrombosed coronary atherosclerotic plaques is characterized by an inflammatory process irrespective of the dominant plaque morphology. Circulation. 1994; 89:36–44.
18. Arbustini E, Dal BB, Morbini P, Burke AP, Bocciarelli M, Specchia G, Virmani R. Plaque erosion is a major substrate for coronary thrombosis in acute myocardial infarction. Heart. 1999;82:269–272.
19. Moreno PR, Falk E, Palacios IF, Newell JB, Fuster V, Fallon JT. Macrophage infiltration in acute coronary syndromes. Implications for plaque rupture. Circulation. 1994;90:775–778.
20. van der Wal AC, Becker AE, Koch KT, Piek JJ, Teeling P, van der Loos CM, David GK. Clinically stable angina pectoris is not necessarily associated with histologically stable atherosclerotic plaques. Heart. 1996;76:312–316.
21. Gronholdt ML, Nordestgaard BG, Bentzon J, Wiebe BM, Zhou J, Falk E, Sillesen H. Macrophages are associated with lipid-rich carotid artery plaques, echolucency on B-mode imaging, and elevated plasma lipid levels. J Vasc Surg. 2002;35:137–145.
22. Schwartz SM, Galis ZS, Rosenfeld ME, Falk E. Plaque rupture in humans and mice. Arterioscler Thromb Vasc Biol. 2007; 27:705–713.
23. Kolodgie FD, Burke AP, Skorija KS, Ladich E, Kutys R, Makuria AT, Virmani R. Lipoprotein-associated phospholipase A2 protein expression in the natural progression of human coronary atherosclerosis. Arterioscler Thromb Vasc Biol. 2006;26:2523–2529.
24. Cheruvu PK, Finn AV, Gardner C, Caplan J, Goldstein J, Stone GW, Virmani R, Muller JE. Frequency and distribution of thin-cap fibroatheroma and ruptured plaques in human coronary arteries: a pathologic study. J Am Coll Cardiol. 2007;50:940–949.
25. Davies MJ, Richardson PD, Woolf N, Katz DR, Mann J. Risk of thrombosis in human atherosclerotic plaques: role of extracellular lipid, macrophage, and smooth muscle cell content. Br Heart J. 1993;69:377–381.
26. Felton CV, Crook D, Davies MJ, Oliver MF. Relation of plaque lipid composition and morphology to the stability of human aortic plaques. Arterioscler Thromb Vasc Biol. 1997;17:1337–1345.
27. Katz SS, Shipley GG, Small DM. Physical chemistry of the lipids of human atherosclerotic lesions. Demonstration of a lesion intermediate between fatty streaks and advanced plaques. J Clin Invest. 1976;58:200–211.
28. Lundberg B. Chemical composition and physical state of lipid deposits in atherosclerosis. Atherosclerosis. 1985;56:93–110.
29. Stary HC, Chandler AB, Glagov S, Guyton JR, Insull W, Jr., Rosenfeld ME, Schaffer SA, Schwartz CJ, Wagner WD, Wissler RW. A definition of initial, fatty streak, and intermediate lesions of atherosclerosis. A report from the Committee on Vascular Lesions of the Council on Arteriosclerosis, American Heart Association. Circulation. 1994;89:2462–2478.
30. Stary HC, Chandler AB, Dinsmore RE, Fuster V, Glagov S, Insull W, Jr., Rosenfeld ME, Schwartz CJ, Wagner WD, Wissler RW. A definition of advanced types of atherosclerotic lesions and a histological classification of atherosclerosis. A report from the Committee on Vascular Lesions of the Council on Arteriosclerosis, American Heart Association. Circulation. 1995;92:1355–1374.
31. Stary HC. Natural history and histological classification of atherosclerotic lesions: an update. Arterioscler Thromb Vasc Biol. 2000;20:1177–1178.
32. van der Wal AC, Das PK, Tigges AJ, Becker AE. Macrophage differentiation in atherosclerosis. An in situ immunohistochemical analysis in humans. Am J Pathol. 1992;141:161–168.
33. Tabas I. Consequences and therapeutic implications of macrophage apoptosis in atherosclerosis: the importance of lesion stage and phagocytic efficiency. Arterioscler Thromb Vasc Biol. 2005;25:2255–2264.

34. Tabas I, Williams KJ, Boren J. Subendothelial lipoprotein retention as the initiating process in atherosclerosis: update and therapeutic implications. Circulation. 2007;116:1832–1844.
35. Tedgui A, Mallat Z. Apoptosis as a determinant of atherothrombosis. Thromb Haemost. 2001;86:420–426.
36. Guyton JR. Phospholipid hydrolytic enzymes in a 'cesspool' of arterial intimal lipoproteins: a mechanism for atherogenic lipid accumulation. Arterioscler Thromb Vasc Biol. 2001;21:884–886.
37. Kolodgie FD, Gold HK, Burke AP, Fowler DR, Kruth HS, Weber DK, Farb A, Guerrero LJ, Hayase M, Kutys R, Narula J, Finn AV, Virmani R. Intraplaque hemorrhage and progression of coronary atheroma. N Engl J Med. 2003;349:2316–2325.
38. Falk E. Plaque rupture with severe pre-existing stenosis precipitating coronary thrombosis. Characteristics of coronary atherosclerotic plaques underlying fatal occlusive thrombi. Br Heart J. 1983;50:127–134.
39. Burke AP, Farb A, Malcom GT, Liang YH, Smialek J, Virmani R. Coronary risk factors and plaque morphology in men with coronary disease who died suddenly. N Engl J Med. 1997;336:1276–1282.
40. Trostdorf F, Buchkremer M, Harmjanz A, Kablau M, Jander S, Geiger K, Schmitz-Rixen T, Steinmetz H, Sitzer M. Fibrous cap thickness and smooth muscle cell apoptosis in high-grade carotid artery stenosis. Eur J Vasc Endovasc Surg. 2005;29:528–535
41. Libby P. Inflammation in atherosclerosis. Nature. 2002;420:868–874.
42. Hansson GK. Inflammation, atherosclerosis, and coronary artery disease. N Engl J Med. 2005;352:1685–1695.
43. Schwartz SM, Virmani R, Rosenfeld ME. The good smooth muscle cells in atherosclerosis. Curr Atheroscler Rep. 2000;2:422–429.
44. Bennett MR, Evan GI, Schwartz SM. Apoptosis of human vascular smooth muscle cells derived from normal vessels and coronary atherosclerotic plaques. J Clin Invest. 1995;95:2266–2274.
45. Lutgens E, de Muinck ED, Kitslaar PJ, Tordoir JH, Wellens HJ, Daemen MJ. Biphasic pattern of cell turnover characterizes the progression from fatty streaks to ruptured human atherosclerotic plaques. Cardiovasc Res. 1999;41:473–479.
46. Burke AP, Kolodgie FD, Farb A, Weber DK, Malcom GT, Smialek J, Virmani R. Healed plaque ruptures and sudden coronary death: evidence that subclinical rupture has a role in plaque progression. Circulation. 2001;103:934–940.
47. Bentzon JF, Weile C, Sondergaard CS, Hindkjaer J, Kassem M, Falk E. Smooth muscle cells in atherosclerosis originate from the local vessel wall and not circulating progenitor cells in ApoE knockout mice. Arterioscler Thromb Vasc Biol. 2006;26:2696–2702.
48. Hoofnagle MH, Thomas JA, Wamhoff BR, Owens GK. Origin of neointimal smooth muscle: we've come full circle. Arterioscler Thromb Vasc Biol. 2006;26:2579–2581.
49. Feil S, Hofmann F, Feil R. SM22alpha modulates vascular smooth muscle cell phenotype during atherogenesis. Circ Res. 2004;94:863–865.
50. Clarke MC, Figg N, Maguire JJ, Davenport AP, Goddard M, Littlewood TD, Bennett MR. Apoptosis of vascular smooth muscle cells induces features of plaque vulnerability in atherosclerosis. Nat Med. 2006;12:1075–1080.
51. Kragel AH, Reddy SG, Wittes JT, Roberts WC. Morphometric analysis of the composition of atherosclerotic plaques in the four major epicardial coronary arteries in acute myocardial infarction and in sudden coronary death. Circulation. 1989;80:1747–1756.
52. Verhoeven BA, Moll FL, Koekkoek JA, van der Wal AC, de Kleijn DP, de Vries JP, Verheijen JH, Velema E, Busser E, Schoneveld A, Virmani R, Pasterkamp G. Statin treatment is not associated with consistent alterations in inflammatory status of carotid atherosclerotic plaques: a retrospective study in 378 patients undergoing carotid endarterectomy. Stroke. 2006;37:2054–2060.
53. Pasterkamp G, Schoneveld AH, van der Wal AC, Haudenschild CC, Clarijs RJ, Becker AE, Hillen B, Borst C. Relation of arterial geometry to luminal narrowing and histologic markers for plaque vulnerability: the remodeling paradox. J Am Coll Cardiol. 1998;32:655–662.
54. McCarthy MJ, Loftus IM, Thompson MM, Jones L, London NJ, Bell PR, Naylor AR, Brindle NP. Angiogenesis and the atherosclerotic carotid plaque: an association between symptomatology and plaque morphology. J Vasc Surg. 1999;30:261–268.
55. Virmani R, Kolodgie FD, Burke AP, Finn AV, Gold HK, Tulenko TN, Wrenn SP, Narula J. Atherosclerotic plaque progression and vulnerability to rupture: angiogenesis as a source of intraplaque hemorrhage. Arterioscler Thromb Vasc Biol. 2005;25:2054–2061.
56. Barger AC, Beeuwkes R, III, Lainey LL, Silverman KJ. Hypothesis: vasa vasorum and neovascularization of human coronary arteries. A possible role in the pathophysiology of atherosclerosis. N Engl J Med. 1984;310:175–177.
57. Barger AC, Beeuwkes R, III. Rupture of coronary vasa vasorum as a trigger of acute myocardial infarction. Am J Cardiol. 1990;66:41G–43G.
58. Zhang Y, Cliff WJ, Schoefl GI, Higgins G. Immunohistochemical study of intimal microvessels in coronary atherosclerosis. Am J Pathol. 1993;143:164–172.
59. Kumamoto M, Nakashima Y, Sueishi K. Intimal neovascularization in human coronary atherosclerosis: its origin and pathophysiological significance. Hum Pathol. 1995;26:450–456.
60. Nakano T, Nakashima Y, Yonemitsu Y, Sumiyoshi S, Chen YX, Akishima Y, Ishii T, Iida M, Sueishi K. Angiogenesis and lymphangiogenesis and expression of lymphangiogenic factors in the atherosclerotic intima of human coronary arteries. Hum Pathol. 2005;36:330–340.
61. Glagov S, Weisenberg E, Zarins CK, Stankunavicius R, Kolettis GJ. Compensatory enlargement of human atherosclerotic coronary arteries. N Engl J Med. 1987;316:1371–1375.
62. Burke AP, Kolodgie FD, Farb A, Weber D, Virmani R. Morphological predictors of arterial remodeling in coronary atherosclerosis. Circulation. 2002;105:297–303.

63. Shiran A, Mintz GS, Leiboff B, Kent KM, Pichard AD, Satler LF, Kimura T, Nobuyoshi M, Leon MB. Serial volumetric intravascular ultrasound assessment of arterial remodeling in left main coronary artery disease. Am J Cardiol. 1999;83:1427–1432.
64. Falk E, Shah PK, Fuster V. Coronary plaque disruption. Circulation. 1995;92:657–671.
65. Boden WE, O'Rourke RA, Teo KK, Hartigan PM, Maron DJ, Kostuk WJ, Knudtson M, Dada M, Casperson P, Harris CL, Chaitman BR, Shaw L, Gosselin G, Nawaz S, Title LM, Gau G, Blaustein AS, Booth DC, Bates ER, Spertus JA, Berman DS, Mancini GB, Weintraub WS. Optimal medical therapy with or without PCI for stable coronary disease. N Engl J Med. 2007;356:1503–1516.
66. Sangiorgi G, Rumberger JA, Severson A, Edwards WD, Gregoire J, Fitzpatrick LA, Schwartz RS. Arterial calcification and not lumen stenosis is highly correlated with atherosclerotic plaque burden in humans: a histologic study of 723 coronary artery segments using nondecalcifying methodology. J Am Coll Cardiol. 1998;31:126–133.
67. Budoff MJ, Shaw LJ, Liu ST, Weinstein SR, Mosler TP, Tseng PH, Flores FR, Callister TQ, Raggi P, Berman DS. Long-term prognosis associated with coronary calcification: observations from a registry of 25,253 patients. J Am Coll Cardiol. 2007;49:1860–1870.
68. Greenland P, Bonow RO, Brundage BH, Budoff MJ, Eisenberg MJ, Grundy SM, Lauer MS, Post WS, Raggi P, Redberg RF, Rodgers GP, Shaw LJ, Taylor AJ, Weintraub WS, Harrington RA, Abrams J, Anderson JL, Bates ER, Grines CL, Hlatky MA, Lichtenberg RC, Lindner JR, Pohost GM, Schofield RS, Shubrooks SJ, Jr., Stein JH, Tracy CM, Vogel RA, Wesley DJ. ACCF/AHA 2007 clinical expert consensus document on coronary artery calcium scoring by computed tomography in global cardiovascular risk assessment and in evaluation of patients with chest pain: a report of the American College of Cardiology Foundation Clinical Expert Consensus Task Force (ACCF/AHA Writing Committee to Update the 2000 Expert Consensus Document on Electron Beam Computed Tomography). Circulation. 2007;115:402–426.
69. Ehara S, Kobayashi Y, Yoshiyama M, Shimada K, Shimada Y, Fukuda D, Nakamura Y, Yamashita H, Yamagishi H, Takeuchi K, Naruko T, Haze K, Becker AE, Yoshikawa J, Ueda M. Spotty calcification typifies the culprit plaque in patients with acute myocardial infarction: an intravascular ultrasound study. Circulation. 2004;110:3424–3429.
70. Beckman JA, Ganz J, Creager MA, Ganz P, Kinlay S. Relationship of clinical presentation and calcification of culprit coronary artery stenoses. Arterioscler Thromb Vasc Biol. 2001;21:1618–1622.
71. Davies MJ, Bland JM, Hangartner JR, Angelini A, Thomas AC. Factors influencing the presence or absence of acute coronary artery thrombi in sudden ischaemic death. Eur Heart J. 1989;10:203–208.
72. Mann J, Davies MJ. Mechanisms of progression in native coronary artery disease: role of healed plaque disruption. Heart. 1999;82:265–268.
73. Bruschke AV, Kramer JR, Jr., Bal ET, Haque IU, Detrano RC, Goormastic M. The dynamics of progression of coronary atherosclerosis studied in 168 medically treated patients who underwent coronary arteriography three times. Am Heart J. 1989;117:296–305.
74. Haft JI, Haik BJ, Goldstein JE, Brodyn NE. Development of significant coronary artery lesions in areas of minimal disease. A common mechanism for coronary disease progression. Chest. 1988;94:731–736.
75. Bentzon JF, Sondergaard CS, Kassem M, Falk E. Smooth muscle cells healing atherosclerotic plaque disruptions are of local, not blood, origin in apolipoprotein E knockout mice. Circulation. 2007;116:2053–2061.
76. Falk E. Unstable angina with fatal outcome: dynamic coronary thrombosis leading to infarction and/or sudden death. Autopsy evidence of recurrent mural thrombosis with peripheral embolization culminating in total vascular occlusion. Circulation. 1985; 71:699–708.
77. Falk E. Coronary thrombosis: pathogenesis and clinical manifestations. Am J Cardiol. 1991;68:28B–35B.
78. Falk E, Fernandez-Ortiz A. Role of thrombosis in atherosclerosis and its complications. Am J Cardiol. 1995;75:3B–11B.
79. Fernandez-Ortiz A, Badimon JJ, Falk E, Fuster V, Meyer B, Mailhac A, Weng D, Shah PK, Badimon L. Characterization of the relative thrombogenicity of atherosclerotic plaque components: implications for consequences of plaque rupture. J Am Coll Cardiol. 1994;23:1562–1569.
80. Leroyer AS, Isobe H, Leseche G, Castier Y, Wassef M, Mallat Z, Binder BR, Tedgui A, Boulanger CM. Cellular origins and thrombogenic activity of microparticles isolated from human atherosclerotic plaques. J Am Coll Cardiol. 2007;49:772–777.
81. el Fawal MA, Berg GA, Wheatley DJ, Harland WA. Sudden coronary death in Glasgow: nature and frequency of acute coronary lesions. Br Heart J. 1987;57:329–335.
82. Ruggeri ZM, Mendolicchio GL. Adhesion mechanisms in platelet function. Circ Res. 2007;100:1673–1685.
83. Nemerson Y. A simple experiment and a weakening paradigm: the contribution of blood to propensity for thrombus formation. Arterioscler Thromb Vasc Biol. 2002;22:1369
84. Naghavi M, Libby P, Falk E, Casscells SW, Litovsky S, Rumberger J, Badimon JJ, Stefanadis C, Moreno P, Pasterkamp G, Fayad Z, Stone PH, Waxman S, Raggi P, Madjid M, Zarrabi A, Burke A, Yuan C, Fitzgerald PJ, Siscovick DS, de Korte CL, Aikawa M, Juhani Airaksinen KE, Assmann G, Becker CR, Chesebro JH, Farb A, Galis ZS, Jackson C, Jang IK, Koenig W, Lodder RA, March K, Demirovic J, Navab M, Priori SG, Rekhter MD, Bahr R, Grundy SM, Mehran R, Colombo A, Boerwinkle E, Ballantyne C, Insull W, Jr., Schwartz RS, Vogel R, Serruys PW, Hansson GK, Faxon DP, Kaul S, Drexler H, Greenland P, Muller JE, Virmani R, Ridker PM, Zipes DP, Shah PK, Willerson JT. From vulnerable plaque to vulnerable patient: a call for new definitions and risk assessment strategies: Part I. Circulation. 2003;108:1664–1672.
85. Naghavi M, Libby P, Falk E, Casscells SW, Litovsky S, Rumberger J, Badimon JJ, Stefanadis C, Moreno P, Pasterkamp G, Fayad Z, Stone PH, Waxman S, Raggi P, Madjid M, Zarrabi A, Burke A, Yuan C, Fitzgerald PJ, Siscovick DS, de Korte CL, Aikawa M, Airaksinen KE, Assmann G, Becker CR, Chesebro JH, Farb A, Galis ZS, Jackson C, Jang IK, Koenig W, Lodder RA, March K, Demirovic J, Navab M, Priori SG, Rekhter MD, Bahr R, Grundy SM, Mehran R, Colombo A, Boerwinkle E,

Ballantyne C, Insull W, Jr., Schwartz RS, Vogel R, Serruys PW, Hansson GK, Faxon DP, Kaul S, Drexler H, Greenland P, Muller JE, Virmani R, Ridker PM, Zipes DP, Shah PK, Willerson JT. From vulnerable plaque to vulnerable patient: a call for new definitions and risk assessment strategies: Part II. Circulation. 2003;108:1772–1778.

86. Mauriello A, Sangiorgi G, Fratoni S, Palmieri G, Bonanno E, Anemona L, Schwartz RS, Spagnoli LG. Diffuse and active inflammation occurs in both vulnerable and stable plaques of the entire coronary tree: a histopathologic study of patients dying of acute myocardial infarction. J Am Coll Cardiol. 2005;45:1585–1593.
87. Waxman S, Ishibashi F, Muller JE. Detection and treatment of vulnerable plaques and vulnerable patients: novel approaches to prevention of coronary events. Circulation. 2006;114:2390–2411.
88. Wang JC, Normand SL, Mauri L, Kuntz RE. Coronary artery spatial distribution of acute myocardial infarction occlusions. Circulation. 2004;110:278–284.
89. Dalager S, Paaske WP, Kristensen IB, Laurberg JM, Falk E. Artery-related differences in atherosclerosis expression: implications for atherogenesis and dynamics in intima-media thickness. Stroke. 2007;38:2698–2705.

4 Pathophysiology of Vulnerability Caused by Thrombogenic (Vulnerable) Blood

Giovanni Cimmino, Borja Ibanez, and Juan Jose Badimon

CONTENTS

ABSTRACT

Atherosclerosis constitutes the single most important contributor to the increasing problem of cardiovascular disease. Endothelial dysfunction is considered the early pivotal event in atherogenesis and precedes development of clinically detectable atherosclerotic plaques. The term "vulnerable plaque" identifies an atherosclerotic plaque that is particularly susceptible to disruption, with exposure of tissue factor to the blood flow and subsequent activation of coagulation cascade resulting in lumen occlusion by overlying thrombi. Despite the central role of *vulnerable plaques* in the onset of cardiovascular events, there are still certain situations (e.g. eroded lesions) wherein hyperactive blood (*vulnerable blood*) takes the central role. The magnitude and severity of arterial thrombosis is a complex phenomenon and depends on several factors: arterial vessel wall substrates, local rheologic characteristics of blood flow, and systemic factors in the circulating blood. Biomarker of "vulnerable blood," including blood markers reflecting hypercoagulability, is one tool to identify high-risk individuals for accurate diagnosis and stratification. The importance of the coagulation/fibrinolytic system is highlighted by several autopsic studies that show a high prevalence of old plaque disruptions without infarctions. The imbalance between coagulation and anticoagulation systems is likely to result in an acute event. The prolonged presence of residual thrombus over a disrupted or eroded plaque can induce smooth muscle migration and produce new intima, leading to plaque expansion. Therefore, an active fibrinolytic system may be able to prevent luminal thrombosis in some cases of plaque disruption. Its rapid decline is associated with an increasing plaque burden and

From: *Asymptomatic Atherosclerosis: Pathophysiology, Detection and Treatment*
Edited by: M. Naghavi (ed.), DOI 10.1007/978-1-60327-179-0_4

vulnerability, and it is related to endothelial cell injury. Identification of vulnerable atherosclerotic plaque and improvement of endothelial function represent a primary approach in the management of cardiovascular patients.

Key words: Atherosclerosis; Endothelial dysfunction; Coagulation system; Vulnerable blood; Tissue factor

KEY POINTS

- Acute thrombus formation on disrupted atherosclerotic plaque plays a key role in the onset of ACS. Lesion disruption facilitates the interaction of the circulating blood with the TF from the atherosclerotic lesions.
- Recent evidence has identified two pools of TF. The traditional hypothesis pointed toward apoptotic macrophages as the source of plaque TF. More recent studies have identified a hyperthrombogenic state associated with a circulating TF activity, leading to the concept of "vulnerable blood".
- The circulating TF activity circulates in an "inactive" form and requires to be "activated" to exert its thrombogenic potential.
- Certain pathological conditions such as smoking, hyperlipidemia, and diabetes show a higher incidence of thrombotic complications. These conditions are also characterized by the presence of high levels of circulating TF activity. Recent evidence suggests that circulating TF activity perpetuates the thrombogenic stimulus, leading to the formation of larger and/or more stable thrombus and, thus more severe ACS among those populations with higher levels of circulating TF.
- The new generation of antithrombotic agents are directed toward the inhibition of the TF pathway. The inhibitors of the Factor Xa seem to offer a large therapeutic window, separating the antiplatelet and anticoagulant activities of these therapeutic agents.

INTRODUCTION

Despite significant advances in treating cardiovascular diseases (CVD) over the past 20 years, acute myocardial infarction (AMI), chronic heart failure (CHF), sudden death (SD), and all other manifestations of CVD are still the number one cause of mortality and morbidity in the developing countries [1]. Atherosclerosis and its thrombotic complications are responsible for nearly all cases of CVD [2].

Atherothrombosis is a diffuse immuno-inflammatory process characterized by the deposition of lipid and other blood-borne material within the arterial wall of almost all vascular territories [3]. Atherosclerosis is a diffuse disease that progresses silently until it is clinically manifested. Epidemiological evidence has identified acute thrombus anchored on a ruptured atherosclerotic lesion, in 70–80% of cardiovascular deaths. The major characteristic of atherosclerosis is the deposition of cholesterol in the subendothelial space, leading to the narrowing of the arterial lumen. Lipid accumulation is the result of an imbalance between cholesterol influx and efflux [4]. The magnitude of the thrombotic process, triggered by plaque rupture, is modulated by different elements that determine plaque and blood thrombogenicity. Tissue factor exposure, thrombin formation, fibrin deposition, platelets aggregation, circulating procoagulant microparticles, and soluble tissue factor are key players in thrombus formation and propagation [5–9].

PATHOGENESIS OF ATHEROSCLEROSIS

The deposition of lipid material in the vessel wall starts very early in life. Fatty streaks, the initial macroscopic lesion, have been found in the intima of infants [10]. The normal endothelium is a very active structure that maintains the hemostatic integrity of the arterial tree by creating an antiatherogenic environment [11]. Cardiovascular risk factors, such as high blood pressure, smoking, and high LDL plasma levels, induce endothelial dysfunction, affecting its metabolic activity and generating a proatherogenic environment. Endothelial dysfunction (Fig. 1) is considered the earliest pathological signal of atherosclerosis [12].

The endothelium plays a critical role in the regulation of vascular function through synthesis and release of several vasoactive agents (See Fig. 2). It regulates vascular tone, inhibits platelet and inflammatory cell adhesion, promotes fibrinolysis, and limits vascular proliferation [13]. A central feature of impaired endothelial function, in the presence of cardiac risk factors and under pathological conditions, is impairment in endothelium-derived nitric oxide (NO) bioactivity produced in endothelial cells.

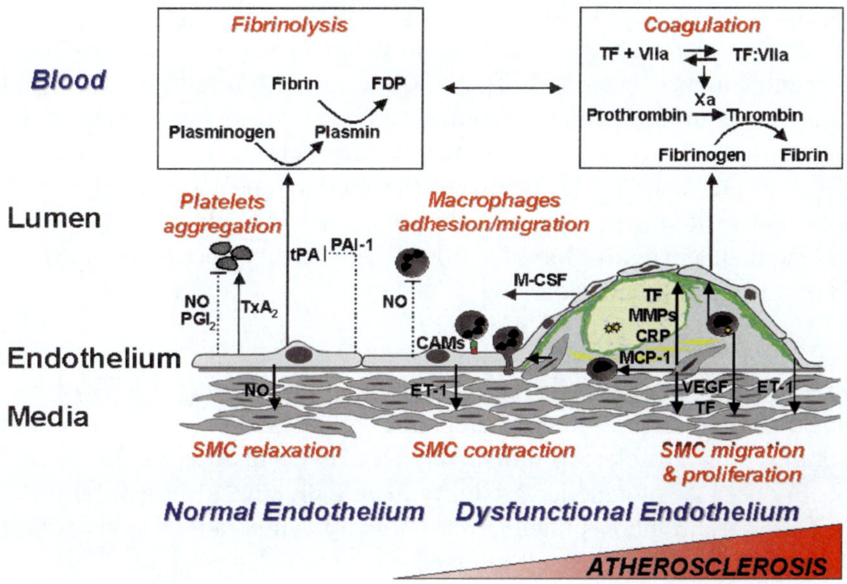

Fig. 1. Atherosclerosis development: from normal endothelium to dysfunctional endothelium.

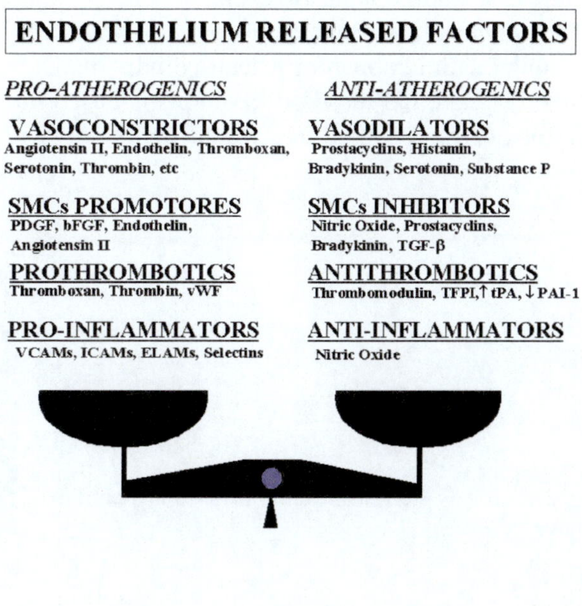

Fig. 2. Factors involved in endothelial function.

NO regulates vascular tone through a dilator action on vascular smooth muscle cells [14]. Additional antiatherogenic functions of NO relate to inhibition of platelet activity, leukocyte adhesion, and vascular smooth muscle cell proliferation. Reduced nitric oxide synthesis or inactivation appears to be a common functional disturbance in the presence of cardiac risk factors and atherothrombosis [15]. Other abnormalities in endothelial function relate, in part, to increased expression of adhesion molecules supporting inflammatory cell recruitment to the vessel wall; enhanced release of constrictor agents such as angiotensin-II that promote vascular growth and alter vascular tone; and loss of antithrombotic function through reduced production of prostacyclin and fibrinolytic factors [16].

Mechanisms underlying impaired endothelial function in various disease states, such as hypertension, diabetes mellitus, hypercholesterolemia, and atherosclerosis, are likely multifactorial. Oxidative stress (defined as an imbalance between endogenous oxidants and antioxidants in favor of the former) also contributes to mechanisms of vascular dysfunction [17–19].

The primary reactive oxygen species produced in the body is superoxide anion (O2-). This anion may inactivate NO and diminish its bioavailability [20]. It can also promote oxidation of the endogenous NO synthase cofactor tetrahydrobiopterin, leading to NO synthase uncoupling, with decreased NO production and increased O2- production from the enzyme [21].

Interaction between O2- and NO leads also to the production of peroxynitrites. They are strong oxidant molecules, able to oxidize proteins, lipids, and nucleic acids, causing vascular cell damage [22]. Finally, O2- facilitates oxidative modification of low-density lipoproteins, which play a key role in the formation of atherosclerotic lesions [23].

Risk Factors, Atherosclerosis progression, Plaque rupture: The Concept of Vulnerability

Despite the advances in imaging and the therapeutic management of cardiovascular risk factors, the clinical manifestations of atherosclerosis remain unpredictable and differ markedly among comparable individuals, probably because of genetic variability in an individual's susceptibility to atherosclerosis and propensity to arterial thrombosis ("*vulnerable blood*"). Vulnerable lesions are often mildy stenotic (less than 50%) and therefore difficult to detect by contrast angiography [24].

Several studies with clinical follow-up have shown that the expected event rate predicted by the population's risk factors may differ several fold from the observed rate [25–32]. Based on these observations, a new concept is born: "vulnerability". It denotes the susceptibility of converting a chronic disease into an acute event.

The only risk factor that seems to have great effect is the individual's age. It is the most discriminatory screening factor in apparently healthy individuals; 96% of deaths from CHD or stroke occur in people aged ≥55 years. On these observations is based the "polypill" strategy in which people with known CVD or over a specified age would be treated with a single daily pill containing 6 components to

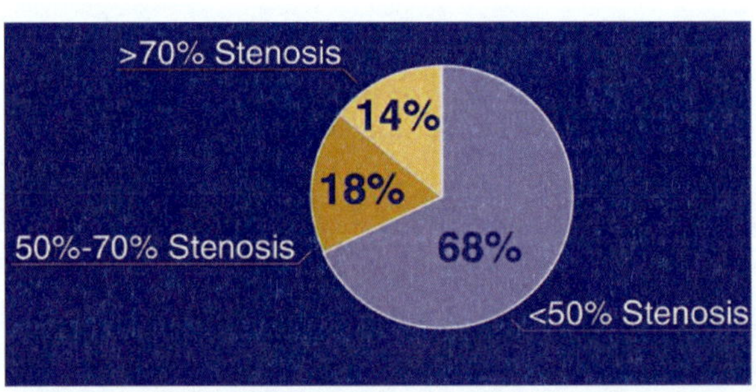

Fig. 3. Coronary stenosis Severity prior to myocardial infarction.

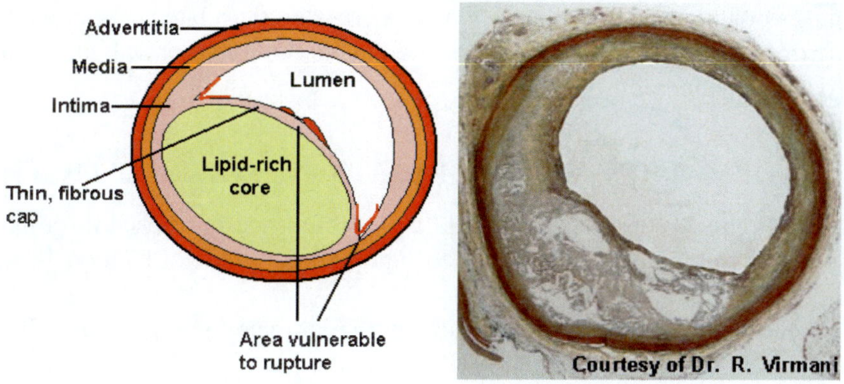

Fig. 4. Vulnerable atherosclerotic plaque.

reduce events and prolong survival, regardless of what current risk assessment algorithms predict [33]. Despite the appeal of such interventions, its effectiveness remains to be proved.

Vulnerable Plaque, a Rupture-Prone Lesion

"Vulnerable plaque" is now used to identify those atherosclerotic lesions prone to disruption (Fig. 4). Certain pathologic features differentiate the so-called stable from the vulnerable lesions. Usually, the vulnerable plaques are mildly stenotic (<50%) with a lipid-rich core that occupies approximately 40% of thc plaque area, and a thin fibrotic core that contains inflammatory cells (macrophages and T-cells) [34]. The rupture or the erosion of the plaque, with the TF exposure to the flow, leads to an intravascular thrombus formation. However, TF exposure alone is not enough for the artery occlusion. It has been shown by Nemerson et al. that after TF exposure, the formation of 1 mm thrombus requires at least 16 h, meaning that there is something more beyond the atherosclerotic plaque.

BEYOND THE ATHEROSCLEROTIC PLAQUE: VULNERABLE MYOCARDIUM AND VULNERABLE BLOOD

The identification of patients in whom disruption of a vulnerable plaque is likely to result in a clinical event is becoming the gold standard in clinical prevention. The presence of plaque is not enough for risk stratification. It has been shown that plaques with similar characteristics may have different clinical presentations because of blood coagulability (vulnerable blood) or myocardial susceptibility, to develop fatal arrhythmia (vulnerable myocardium). Those factors (i.e. thrombogenic blood and electrical instability of myocardium), in addition to pre-existent atherosclerotic plaques, are responsible for the final outcome in patients.

Vulnerable myocardium: Current or the previous ischemic condition and/or a nonischemic electrophysiological abnormality are responsible for malignant or fatal arrhythmias. In patients without prior atherosclerotic-derived injury, abrupt occlusion of a coronary artery leads to SD or AMI. It has been shown that the clinical outcome of these patients correlates with the autonomic nervous activity [35, 36]. Sympathetic hyperactivity favors malignant ventricular tachyarrhythmias, whereas vagal activation has an antifibrillatory effect.

Patients with known atherosclerotic-related damage, such as ischemia, old myocardial infarction, left ventricular dilatation, fibrosis, and inflammation show an increased risk to develop fatal arrhythmia or sudden death.

In a smaller number of cases, various forms of non atherosclerotic-related cardiomyopathy (idiopathic dilatation, hypertrophy, restrictive, and right ventricular disease) and/or valvular heart disease may increase the myocardial vulnerability.

THROMBUS FORMATION AND PROPAGATION: THE ROLE OF THE BLOOD

As described by Virchow more than 100 years ago, occurrence of arterial thrombosis depends on the arterial vessel wall substrates, the local rheologic characteristics of blood flow, and systemic factors in the circulating blood.

Plaque disruption leads to tissue factor and subendothelial material exposure to the blood flow. TF interacts with factor VII and forms the TF-FVII complex, which is converted to TF-FVIIa by FVIIa or already formed TF-FVIIa. The TF-VIIa complex activates factor IX, which in turn activates factor X; alternatively, factor X is directly converted to factor Xa by TF-FVIIa. In combination with factor Va and calcium, Factor Xa catalyzes the conversion of prothrombin to thrombin, thereby leading to fibrin formation, platelet activation, and, ultimately, generation of a thrombus (Fig. 5).

The magnitude of this phenomenon depends on a hyperthrombogenic state triggered by other systemic factors. It has been reported that elevated low HDL cholesterol, cigarette smoking, hyperglycemia are associated with increased blood thrombogenicity [37]. These risk factors seem to share a common biological pathway: increased platelet reactivity and hyper-aggregability, activation of leukocyte-platelet interactions associated with TF release and thrombin activation [38, 39]. However, the real contribution of hemostatic factors is still unknown. Some evidence showed that hypercoagulable states, such as antithrombin deficiency and factor V Leiden generally predispose individuals to venous thrombotic complications, but not to atherosclerosis [40]. The relationship between hemophilic state, such as Factor VIII deficiency and Von Willebrand's disease and atherosclerosis remains to be clarified. Controversial evidence has been reported about those hemophilic diseases [41, 42].

Under physiological conditions, the endogenous fibrinolytic system facilitates the resolution of the thrombi formed at the sites of disrupted atherosclerotic plaques. Impaired plasma fibrinolytic activity has been reported during atherosclerosis, in many prospective studies [43, 44]. Level of fibrinopeptide A,

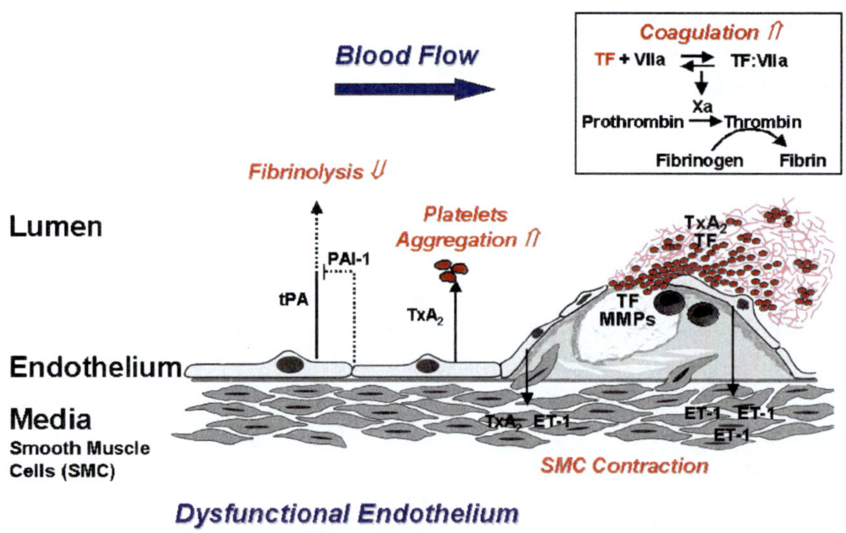

Fig. 5. TF exposure after vessel injury with thrombus formation.

prothrombin activation fragments F1 and F2, and the plasminogen activator inhibitor-1 (PAI-1) are increased in patients with unstable angina and AMI [45, 46]. Fibrinopeptide A fall within a few days of the acute event, while the FI and F2 fragments, a marker of thrombin generation, can persist for up to 6 months [47].

Circulating PAI-1 levels are thought to play an important role in the persistence of microthrombi and a prothrombotic state, resulting in attenuation of thickness of fibrous caps implicated in the vulnerability of atheroma and rupture.

Another crucial role in thrombus formation and propagation comes from microparticles (MPs). MPs are submicron membrane vesicles released by different cell subtypes following cell activation or apoptosis. Even though they are found in the circulating blood of healthy subjects, their levels are increased in many diseases, especially those with a high thrombotic risk. MPs are carriers, at their surface, of phospholipids and proteins specific from the parent cells, which confer them a potential role in many physiological processes, including thrombosis, inflammation, endothelial dysfunction and angiogenesis. Consequently, MPs are being considered as a new key player in atherothrombosis.

Circulating levels of MPs are augmented in cardiac patients as compared with healthy subjects. As circulating MPs increase following AMI, one can wonder whether these MPs are derived from the ruptured plaques [48]. The cellular origin of MPs derived from plaques and from plasma are markedly different [49]. Majority of MPs present in the atherosclerotic plaque originate from macrophages, erythrocytes, and smooth muscle cells, but not from platelets, whereas circulating MPs derived mainly from platelets are not of smooth muscle cell origin. In addition, although MPs are much more abundant in atherosclerotic plaques than in plasma, and account for the procoagulant activity of the lipid core, at least a dozen of the large lesions (such as those found in human carotid arteries) should rupture simultaneously to fully account for circulating levels of MPs in patients with acute coronary syndrome [49]. Circulating MPs bear tissue factor (TF) at their surface and account for the so-called blood-borne TF [50]. They are involved in the formation of TF-platelet hybrids, a critical phenomenon in thrombus propagation, following transfer of TF from leucocyte-MPs to platelet membranes [50]. Platelet-, erythrocyte- and haematopoietic-derived MPs are also involved in in vivo TF-dependent thrombus spreading [51, 52]. In vivo, MPs are captured by thrombus-associated platelets through the interaction of MP-exposed P-selectin glycoprotein ligand-1 with P-selectin from platelets. This leads to an increased concentration of TF which is believed to initiate and accelerate blood coagulation and fibrin formation [53, 54].

But plasma microparticles are not the only source of circulating TF. In 2003, two reports shed more light on the properties of circulating TF. Bogdanov et al demonstrated that circulating TF comprises two distinct proteins: the well known transmembrane "full length" TF (flTF), and an alternatively spliced TF (asTF). asTF is a soluble molecule that, analogously to flTF, requires phospholipids to exhibit its cofactor activity [9]. Concomitantly, Sambola et al demonstrated that the pro-thrombotic state in diabetic, hyperlipidemic, and smoker populations is very likely to be caused by heightened levels of circulating TF activity [55]. The real role of asTF in cardiovascular disease must be elucidated, but due to its characteristics, it may be speculated that it is involved in thrombus propagation.

The activation of coagulation cascade induces proteases that interact not only with coagulation protein zymogens, but also with specific cell receptors that could have proinflammatory effect. Some of these protease activated receptors (PAR-1,-3,-4) can bind thrombin; other receptors (PAR-2) can be activated via TF-FVIIa complex, Factor Xa, or trypsin. It has been shown that PAR-2 activation via TF-FVIIa complex induces release of cytokines, adhesion molecules expression and inflammatory responses in macrophages, while PAR-1 and -4 are involved in cardiac hypertrophy and remodeling on ischemia [56]. Thrombin has a short life in the blood, but it has been shown that it can be sequestered in the atherosclerotic plaque [57]. Its presence in the atherosclerotic lesion could explain the local increased response to thrombin and the perpetuation of arterial thrombosis. Another key player in primary hemostasis is the platelets. In the last few years, they have emerged as crucial cellular determinants of physiologic vascular repair and its pathologic derangement [58]. Platelets that adhere to the vessel wall at sites of endothelial-cell activation contribute to the development of chronic atherosclerotic lesions, and when these lesions rupture, they trigger the acute onset of arterial thrombosis. Some platelet polymorphisms, such as glycoprotein IIIa P1(A2), Ib αgene-5T/C Kozak [59, 60] have been reported as independent risk factors for myocardial infarction.

It has been reported that platelet hyperactivity plays a key role in the progression of diabetic retinopathy and could contribute to the development of nephropathy, especially in patients with a combination of diabetes and arterial hypertension [61, 62]. Serebruany et al. [63] showed that diabetic patients exhibit high platelet activity, and do not respond well to the available combination antiplatelet regimens with aspirin and clopidogrel, when compared with similar patients without diabetes, suggesting a direct interaction between uncontrolled glycemia and platelet activity.

Once activated, platelets release adhesive ligands, as P-selectin, or inflammatory mediators, as CD40 ligand, that mediate the interaction and inflammatory response with endothelium, and stimulate monocytes and macrophages to produce chemoattractants or growth factors [64], perpetuating the inflamed status of the atherosclerotic plaque. Investigators have shown that high plasma concentrations of soluble CD40 ligand may indicate an increased vascular risk in apparently healthy women [65].

The most powerful inflammatory predictor of future coronary events in the asymptomatic population and in patients with stable or unstable disease [66, 67] is the C-reactive protein (CRP). Although CRP is a nonspecific marker of systemic inflammation, it has been shown that it is an independent marker of CVD. It activates endothelium and accumulates in the plaque, suggesting an important role in plaque inflammation [68].

Circulating interleukin-6 levels, which are elevated in patients with ACS, also predict the risk of future coronary events in such patients [69].

These observations suggest the important role that a transient shift in the coagulation and anticoagulation balance is likely to have in the modulation of plaque-blood interaction, leading to an acute cardiac event.

Other metabolic conditions, such as postprandial metabolic changes [70], estrogen replacement therapy [71], plasma viscosity, as well as fibrinogen and white blood cell counts [72] have been also described to be associated with a hypercoagulable.

In the last few years, accumulated evidences suggested the novel role of bone marrow-derived cells in atherosclerosis. It is known that bone marrow-derived macrophages play a critical role in the initiation and propagation of atherosclerosis. The conventional concept that endothelial cells and intimal smooth muscle cells reside within the arterial wall and proliferate, migrate, and secrete what might be needed for expedient healing and repair after injury is changed [73]. With incredible surprise, several experimental studies have suggested that many of the healing smooth muscle cells originated in the bone marrow and were brought to the injured vessel wall with the circulating blood [74]. Some human observations support those studies [75, 76], suggesting their potential involvement in the retardation and stabilization of atherosclerosis in humans. Based on those data, mobilizing atheroprotective cells from the bone marrow and promoting their homing to thrombosis-prone plaques may be a new way to stabilize atherosclerosis against thrombosis and its devastating consequences.

THERAPEUTIC IMPLICATIONS IN THE MODULATION OF TF PATHWAY

The primary function of the coagulation cascade is to promote haemostasis and limit blood loss in response to tissue injury (Fig. 6). This process is greatly regulated to prevent uncontrolled activity.

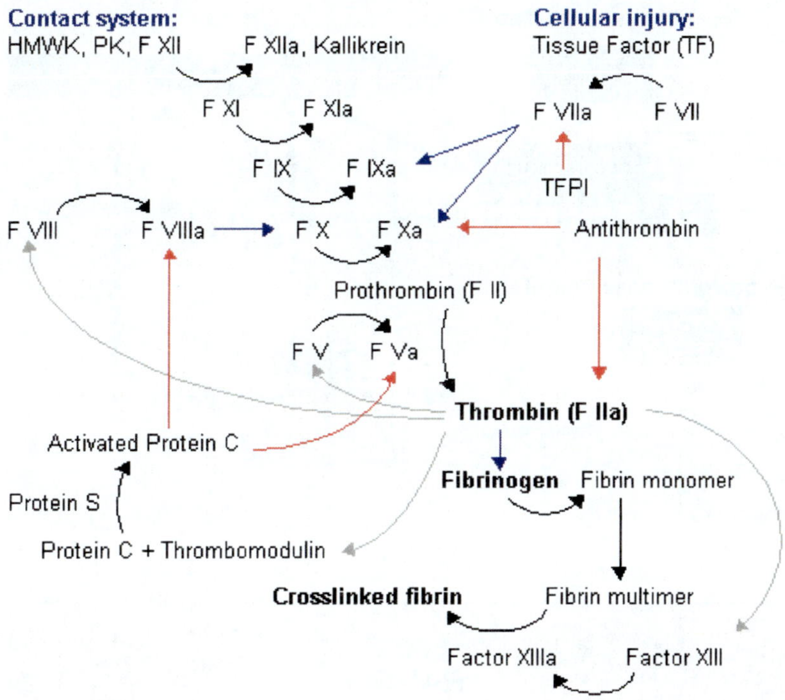

Fig. 6. Coagulation cascade.

However, abnormalities in the coagulation process (initiation, propagation and fibrin formation), with extravascular expression of TF leading to the activation of coagulation proteinases, including FX and prothrombin, contribute to the pathophysiology of several conditions, such as thrombosis, arthritis, cancer, kidney disease, and acute and chronic lung injury.

The role of TF and thrombus formation on disrupted atherosclerotic plaque in acute coronary syndrome has been highly elucidated. However, a autoptic study report on cases of SD due to coronary artery thrombosis has identified frank plaque rupture with thrombus communicated with the lipid core in only 56% of the cases; in the remainder, the thrombi were attached to a superficial erosion that were devoid of endothelial cells [77]. Patients who developed coronary thrombosis on erosions that occurred on non-ruptured, mild to moderate stenotic plaques may have systemic risk factors associated with a hypercoagulable state. As reported by Sambola et al., the increase in blood thrombogenicity observed in the presence of cardiovascular risk factors, such as diabetes, smoking or hyperlipidemia, might be mediated by high levels of circulating TF [55]. The origin of circulating TF (located in blood cells and microparticles and non-cell-bound protein) in plasma is still controversial. However, it has been shown that the elevation of plasma circulating TF is not only the reflection of a heightened TF expression from atherosclerotic lesions but also supports clot formation in vitro [50]. Based on these observations, pharmacological modulation of TF pathway has been explored as a new therapeutic target in the management of thrombotic disorders (Fig. 7).

At the moment different drugs has been developed to manipulate the coagulation cascade. Anticoagulants can inhibit the initiation or propagation of coagulation, or by targeting thrombin, they can attenuate fibrin formation. Drugs that target the tissue factor/factor VIIa complex block the initiation of coagulation, while those that inhibit factor IXa or factor Xa, or their cofactors, factor VIIIa and factor Va, block the propagation of coagulation. Finally, anticoagulants that target thrombin attenuate fibrin generation.

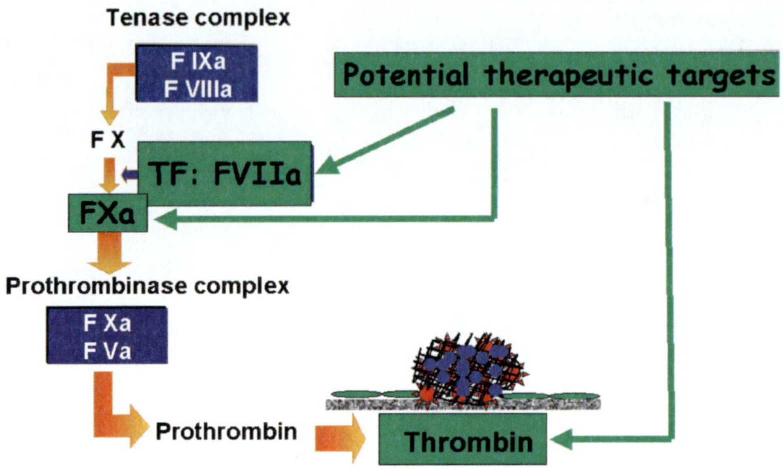

Fig. 7. Therapeutic target in TF pathway.

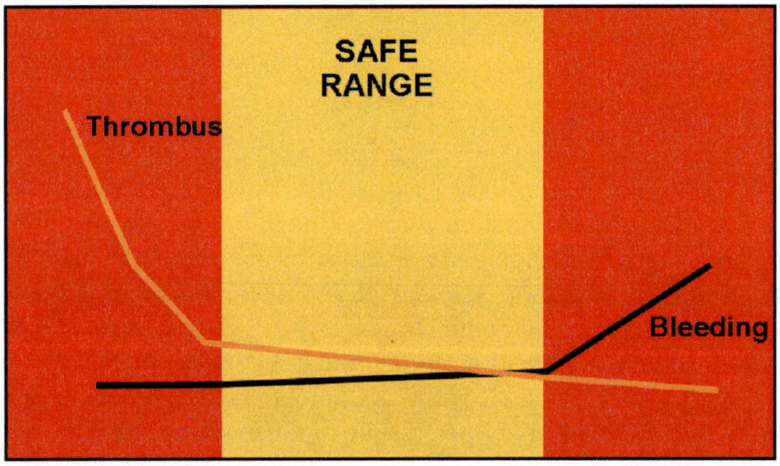

Fig. 8. Best hypothetic anticoagulant.

The best hypothetic anticoagulant should have good bioavailability, no food or drug interactions, rapid onset of action, wide therapeutic window, predictable anticoagulant response, availability of an antidote and no unexpected toxicity (Fig. 8).

Direct and indirect evidence showed that therapeutic approaches based on selective inhibitors of FXa or thrombin rather than traditional, multi-targeted anticoagulants, such as warfarin and unfractionated heparin, are more likely associated with a wider therapeutic window and would therefore be more effective, safer and easier to use [78]. Inhibitors that selectively target the signaling properties of coagulation proteinases without interfering with haemostatic responses would be particularly desirable in the context of conditions associated with extravascular coagulation.

Selective inhibition of FXa is particularly attractive, since FXa is positioned at the convergence point of both the extrinsic and intrinsic coagulation systems. Furthermore, as the levels of serine proteinases are amplified at each step of the coagulation cascade, anticoagulants which target coagulation factors located higher up in the cascade, such as FXa, might be more effective than those directly targeting thrombin [79]. Thrombin is the final effector of blood coagulation. It not only converts fibrinogen to fibrin, but it also renders fibrin resistant to fibrinolysis, by activating FXIII. It is a potent platelet agonist and amplifies its own generation via FVIII and FV activity. Then, inhibition of thrombin may have interesting biological implications.

Factor Xa and thrombin inhibitors include agents with direct and indirect action. Indirect inhibitors act by catalyzing factor Xa inhibition by antithrombin. In contrast, direct factor Xa inhibitors bind directly to the active site of factor Xa, thereby blocking its interaction with its substrates. A prototype of the new indirect factor Xa inhibitors is fondaparinux, a first generation synthetic analog of the antithrombin-binding pentasaccharide found in heparin or LMWH. This drug is FDA approved, licensed for prevention of venous thrombo-embolism (VTE) in patients undergoing high-risk orthopedic surgery and, in some countries, for VTE prevention in general surgical or medical patients. Fondaparinux also is approved as a substitute for heparin or LMWH for initial treatment of VTE.

Direct factor Xa inhibitors are small molecules that reversibly block the active site of factor Xa. Different agents are under investigation in clinical trials. Some of them were stopped prematurely, because of major bleeding. Apixaban and Rivaroxaban are two promising FXa inhibitors.

Indirect thrombin inhibitors act by catalyzing heparin cofactor II. In contrast, direct inhibitors bind to thrombin and block its interaction with substrates.

Direct thrombin inhibitors have properties that give them potential mechanistic advantages over indirect inhibitors. First, because direct thrombin inhibitors do not bind to plasma proteins, they produce a more predictable anticoagulant response. Second, unlike heparin, direct thrombin inhibitors do not bind to PF4. Consequently, the anticoagulant activity of direct thrombin inhibitors is unaffected by the large quantities of PF4 released in the vicinity of platelet-rich thrombi. Finally, direct thrombin inhibitors deactivate fibrin-bound thrombin, as well as fluid-phase thrombin [80].

Three parenteral direct thrombin inhibitors (hirudin, argatroban and bivalirudin) have been licensed in North America for limited indications. The recombinant hirudins, which target thrombin, were the first anticoagulants to be developed that target a specific coagulation factor [81]. Hirudin and argatroban are approved for treatment of patients with heparin-induced thrombocytopenia, whereas bivalirudin is licensed as an alternative to heparin in PCI patients with or without heparin-induced thrombocytopenia. The success of bivaluridin prompted the development of new agents. Two new parenteral direct thrombin inhibitors are currently undergoing phase II evaluation. These are flovagatran and pegmusirudin. There also are three new oral thrombin inhibitors; odiparcil, an indirect inhibitor, and ximelagatran and dabigatran etexilate, which are direct thrombin inhibitors. The first oral, reversible, direct thrombin inhibitor was ximelagatran, a pro-drug of the active-site directed thrombin inhibitor, melagatran. It was a very promising thrombin inhibitor, effective in the prevention of recurrent VTE, primary treatment of VTE and stroke prevention in patients with atrial fibrillation. Unfortunately, because of its potential hepatic toxicity, the drug was withdrawn from the market. A newer oral direct thrombin inhibitor, from the same class of ximelagatran, Dabigatran etexilate is now being evaluated. Preliminary data from the ongoing clinical trials reveals that dabigatran should be safe and effective.

However it remains unclear whether upstream inhibition at the level of factor Xa is safer and/or more effective than downstream inhibition of thrombin. Clinical trials comparing the two classes of anticoagulants are necessary to address this issue.

REFERENCES

1. Yusuf S, Reddy S, Ounpuu S, Anand S. Global burden of cardiovascular diseases: part I: general considerations, the epidemiologic transition, risk factors, and impact of urbanization. Circulation 2001;104(22):2746–2753
2. Viles-Gonzalez JF, Fuster V, Badimon JJ. Atherothrombosis: a widespread disease with unpredictable and life-threatening consequences. Eur Heart J 2004;25:1197–1207

3. Aikawa M, Libby P. The vulnerable atherosclerotic plaque: pathogenesis and therapeutic approach. Cardiovasc Pathol 2004;13:125–138
4. Santos-Gallego CG, Ibanez B, Badimon JJ. HDL-cholesterol: is it really good? Differences between apoA-I and HDL. Biochem Pharmacol 2008;76(4):443–52
5. Toschi V, Gallo R, Lettino M, Fallon JT, Gertz SD, Fernández-Ortiz A, Chesebro JH, Badimon L, Nemerson Y, Fuster V, Badimon JJ. Tissue factor modulates the thrombogenicity of human atherosclerotic plaques. Circulation 1997;95(3):594–599
6. Hutter R, Valdiviezo C, Sauter BV, Savontaus M, Chereshnev I, Carrick FE, Bauriedel G, Lüderitz B, Fallon JT, Fuster V, Badimon JJ. Caspase-3 and tissue factor expression in lipid-rich plaque macrophages: evidence for apoptosis as link between inflammation and atherothrombosis. Circulation 2004;109(16):2001–8. Epub 2004 Apr 12
7. Mallat Z, Tedgui A. Current perspective on the role of apoptosis in atherothrombotic disease. Circ Res 2001;88(10):998–1003
8. Dwyer JH, Allayee H, Dwyer KM, Fan J, Wu H, Mar R, Lusis AJ, Mehrabian M Arachidonate 5-lipoxygenase promoter genotype, dietary arachidonic acid, and atherosclerosis. N Engl J Med 2004;350:29–37
9. Bogdanov VY, Balasubramanian V, Hathcock J, Vele O, Lieb M, Nemerson Y Alternatively spliced human tissue factor: a circulating, soluble, thrombogenic protein. Nat Med 2003;9:458
10. Badimon JJ, Ibanez B, Cimmino G. Genesis and dynamics of atherosclerotic lesions: implications for early detection. Cerebrovasc dis 2009;27(1):38–47
11. Corti R, Fuster V, Badimon JJ. Pathogenetic concepts of acute coronary syndromes. J Am Coll Cardiol 2003;41:7S–14S
12. Chenevard R, Hürlimann D, Béchir M, Enseleit F, Spieker L, Hermann M, Riesen W, Gay S, Gay RE, Neidhart M, Michel B, Lüscher TF, Noll G, Ruschitzka F. Selective COX-2 inhibition improves endothelial function in coronary artery disease. Circulation 2003;107:405–409
13. Ross R. Atherosclerosis- an inflammatory disease. N Engl J Med 1999;340(2):115–126
14. Furchgott RF, Zawadzki JV. The obligatory role of endothelial cells in the relaxation of arterial smooth muscle by acetylcholine. Nature 1980;288:373–376
15. Loscalzo J. Nitric oxide insufficiency, platelet activation, and arterial thrombosis. Circ Res 2001;88:756–762
16. Qian H, Neplioueva V, Shetty GA, et al. Nitric oxide synthase gene therapy rapidly reduces adhesion molecule expression and inflammatory cell infiltration in carotid arteries of cholesterol-fed rabbits. Circulation 1999;99:2979–2982
17. Landmesser U, Harrison DG, Drexler H: Oxidant stress – A major cause of reduced endothelial nitric oxide availability in cardiovascular disease. Eur J Clin Pharmacol 2006;62(suppl 13):13–19
18. Harrison DG. Endothelial control of vasomotion and nitric oxide production: a potential target for risk factor management. Cardiol Clin 1996;14(1):1–15
19. Cai H, Harrison DG. Endothelial dysfunction in cardiovascular diseases: the role of oxidant stress. Circ Res 2000;87:840–844
20. Kojda G, Harrison D. Interactions between NO and reactive oxygen species: pathophysiological importance in atherosclerosis, hypertension, diabetes and heart failure. Cardiovasc Res 1999;43:562–571
21. Vasquez-Vivar J, Kalyanaraman B, Martasek P. The role of tetrahydrobiopterin in superoxide generation from eNOS: enzymology and physiological implications. Free Radic Res 2003;37:121–127
22. Beckman JS, Koppenol WH. Nitric oxide, superoxide, and peroxynitrite: the good, the bad, and ugly. Am J Physiol 1996;5: C1424–C1437
23. Stocker R, Keaney JF Jr. Role of oxidative modifications in atherosclerosis. Physiol Rev 2004;84:1381–1478
24. Virmani R, Kolodgie FD, Burke AP, Farb A, Schwartz SM. Lessons from sudden coronary death: a comprehensive morphological classification scheme for atherosclerotic lesions. Arterioscler Thromb Vasc Biol 2000;20(5):1262–75
25. D'Agostino RB Sr, Grundy S, Sullivan LM, Wilson P; CHD Risk Prediction Group. Validation of the Framingham coronary heart disease prediction scores: results of a multiple ethnic groups investigation. J Am Med Assoc 2001;286(2):180–7
26. Danesh J, Wheeler JG, Hirschfield GM, Eda S, Eiriksdottir G, Rumley A, Lowe GD, Pepys MB, Gudnason V. C-reactive protein and other circulating markers of inflammation in the prediction of coronary heart disease. N Engl J Med 2004;350: 1387–1397
27. Cooper JA, Miller GJ, Humphries SE. A comparison of the PROCAM and Framingham point-scoring systems for estimation of individual risk of coronary heart disease in the second northwick park heart study. Atherosclerosis 2005;181(1):93–100
28. Liu J, Hong Y, D'Agostino RB Sr, Wu Z, Wang W, Sun J, Wilson PW, Kannel WB, Zhao D. Predictive value for the chinese population of the framingham CHD risk assessment tool compared with the chinese multi-provincial cohort study. J Am Med Assoc 2004;291:2591–2599
29. Arad Y, Goodman KJ, Roth M, Newstein D, Guerci AD.Coronary calcification, coronary disease risk factors, C-reactive protein, and atherosclerotic cardiovascular disease events: the St. Francis Heart Study. J Am Coll Cardiol 2005;46:158–165
30. Grundy SM. The changing face of cardiovascular risk. J Am Coll Cardiol 2005;46:173–175
31. Akosah KO, Schaper A, Cogbill C, Schoenfeld P. Preventing myocardial infarction in the young adult in the first place: how do the National Cholesterol Education Panel III guidelines perform? J Am Coll Cardiol 2003;41:1475–1479
32. Brindle P, Emberson J, Lampe F, Walker M, Whincup P, Fahey T, Ebrahim S. Predictive accuracy of the Framingham coronary risk score in British men: prospective cohort study. Br Med J 2003;327(7426):1267
33. Kuller LH. Prevention of coronary heart disease and the national cholesterol education program. Circulation 2006;113:598–600
34. Wald NJ, Law MR. A strategy to reduce cardiovascular disease by more than 80%. Br Med J 2003;326:1419
35. Glagov S, Weisenberg E, Zarins CK, Stankunavicius R, Kolettis GJ. Compensatory enlargement of human atherosclerotic coronary arteries. N Engl J Med 1987;316:1371–1375

36. Schwartz PJ, Vanoli E, Zaza A, Zuanetti G. The effect of antiarrhythmic drugs on life-threatening arrhythmias induced by the interaction between acute myocardial ischemia and sympathetic hyperactivity. Am Heart J 1985;109:937–948
37. Vanoli E, De Ferrari GM, Stramba-Badiale M, Hull SS Jr, Foreman RD, Schwartz PJ. Vagal stimulation and prevention of sudden death in conscious dogs with a healed myocardial infarction. Circ Res 1991;68:1471–81
38. Rauch U, Osende JI, Fuster V, Badimon JJ, Fayad Z, Chesebro JH. Thrombus formation on atherosclerotic plaques: pathogenesis and clinical consequences. Ann Intern Med. 2001;134(3):224–38. Blood 2000;96:170–175
39. Rauch U, Crandall J, Osende JI, Fallon JT, Chesebro JH, Fuster V, Badimon JJ. Increased thrombus formation relates to ambient blood glucose and leukocyte count in diabetes mellitus type 2. Am J Cardiol 2000;86:246–249
40. Dacosta A, Tardy-Poncet B, Isaaz K, Cerisier A, Mismetti P, Simitsidis S, Reynaud J, Tardy B, Piot M, Decousus H, Guyotat D. Prevalence of factor V Leiden (APCR) and other inherited thrombophilias in young patients with myocardial infarction and normal coronary arteries. Heart 1998;80:338–340
41. Srámek A, Reiber JH, Gerrits WB, Rosendaal FR. Decreased coagulability has no clinically relevant effect on atherogenesis: observations in individuals with a hereditary bleeding tendency. Circulation 2001;104:762–67
42. Bilora F, Boccioletti V, Zanon E, Petrobelli F, Girolami A. Hemophilia A, von Willebrand disease, and atherosclerosis of abdominal aorta and leg arteries: factor VIII and von Willebrand factor defects appear to protect abdominal aorta and leg arteries from atherosclerosis. Clin Appl Thromb Hemost 2001;7:311–313
43. Warkentin TE. Hemostasis and atherosclerosis. Can J Cardiol 1995;11(Suppl C):29C–34C
44. Sobel BE, Taatjes DJ, Schneider DJ. Intramural plasminogen activator inhibitor type-1 and coronary atherosclerosis. Arterioscler Thromb Vasc Biol 2003;23(11):1979–1989
45. Douglas JT, Lowe GD, Forbes CD, Prentice CR. Plasma fibrinopeptide A and beta-thromboglobulin in patients with chest pain. Thromb Haemost 1983;50:541–542
46. Alessi MC, Juhan-Vague I. Contribution of PAI-1 in cardiovascular pathology. Arch Mal Coeur Vaiss 2004;97:673–78
47. Merlini PA, Bauer KA, Oltrona L, Ardissino D, Cattaneo M, Belli C, Mannucci PM, Rosenberg RD. Persistent activation of coagulation mechanism in unstable angina and myocardial infarction. Circulation 1994;90:61–68
48. Mallat Z, Hugel B, Ohan J, Lesèche G, Freyssinet JM, Tedgui A. Shed membrane microparticles with procoagulant potential in human atherosclerotic plaques: a role for apoptosis in plaque thrombogenicity. Circulation 1999;99(3):348–353
49. Leroyer AS, Isobe H, Lesèche G, Castier Y, Wassef M, Mallat Z, Binder BR, Tedgui A, Boulanger CM. Cellular origins and thrombogenic activity of microparticles isolated from human atherosclerotic plaques. J Am Coll Cardiol 2007;49:772–7
50. Giesen PL, Rauch U, Bohrmann B, Kling D, Roqué M, Fallon JT, Badimon JJ, Himber J, Riederer MA, Nemerson Y. Blood-borne tissue factor: another view of thrombosis. Proc Natl Acad Sci USA 1999;96:2311–2315
51. Biró E, Sturk-Maquelin KN, Vogel GM, Meuleman DG, Smit MJ, Hack CE, Sturk A, Nieuwland R. Human cell-derived microparticles promote thrombus formation in vivo in a tissue factor-dependent manner. J Thromb Haemost 2003;1:2561–2568
52. Chou J, Mackman N, Merrill-Skoloff G, Pedersen B, Furie BC, Furie B. Hematopoietic cell-derived microparticle tissue factor contributes to fibrin formation during thrombus propagation. Blood 2004;104:3190–3197
53. Furie B, Furie BC. Role of platelet P-selectin and microparticle PSGL-1 in thrombus formation. Trends Mol Med 2004;10:171–8
54. Hrachovinová I, Cambien B, Hafezi-Moghadam A, Kappelmayer J, Camphausen RT, Widom A, Xia L, Kazazian HH Jr, Schaub RG, McEver RP, Wagner DD. Interaction of P-selectin and PSGL-1 generates microparticles that correct hemostasis in a mouse model of hemophilia A. Nat Med 2003;9:1020–1025
55. Sambola A, Osende J, Hathcock J, Degen M, Nemerson Y, Fuster V, Crandall J, Badimon JJ. Role of risk factors in the modulation of tissue factor activity and blood thrombogenicity. Circulation 2003;107(7):973–977
56. Marutsuka K, Hatakeyama K, Sato Y, Yamashita A, Sumiyoshi A, Asada Y. Protease-activated receptor 2 (PAR2) mediates vascular smooth muscle cell migration induced by tissue factor/factor VIIa complex. Thromb Res 2002;107:271–276
57. Bar-Shavit R, Benezra M, Eldor A, Hy-Am E, Fenton JW 2nd, Wilner GD, Vlodavsky I. Thrombin immobilized to extracellular matrix is a potent mitogen for vascular smooth muscle cells: nonenzymatic mode of action. Cell Regul 1990;1(6):453–463
58. Ruggeri ZM. Platelets in atherothrombosis. Nat Med 2002;8:1227–1234
59. Barakat K, Kennon S, Hitman GA, Aganna E, Price CP, Mills PG, Ranjadayalan K, North B, Clarke H, Timmis AD. Interaction between smoking and the glycoprotein IIIa P1(A2) polymorphism in non-ST-elevation acute coronary syndromes. J Am Coll Cardiol 2001;38:1639–1643
60. Douglas H, Michaelides K, Gorog DA, Durante-Mangoni E, Ahmed N, Davies GJ, Tuddenham EG. Platelet membrane glycoprotein Ibalpha gene-5T/C Kozak sequence polymorphism as an independent risk factor for the occurrence of coronary thrombosis. Heart 2002;87(1):70–74
61. Kimura M, Ishizawa M, Miura A, Itaya S, Kanoh Y, Yasuda K, Uno Y, Morita H, Ishizuka T. Platelet protein kinase C isoform content in type 2 diabetes complicated with retinopathy and nephropathy. Platelets 2001;12:138–143
62. Simpson AJ, Booth NA, Moore NR, Lewis SJ, Gray RS. Circulating tissue-type plasminogen activator and plasminogen activator inhibitor type 1 in proliferative diabetic retinopathy: a pilot study. Acta Diabetol 1999;36:155–158
63. Serebruany V, Pokov I, Kuliczkowski W, Chesebro J, Badimon J. Baseline platelet activity and response after clopidogrel in 257 diabetics among 822 patients with coronary artery disease. Thromb Haemost 2008;100:76–82
64. Henn V, Slupsky JR, Gräfe M, Anagnostopoulos I, Förster R, Müller-Berghaus G, Kroczek RA. CD40 ligand on activated platelets triggers an inflammatory reaction of endothelial cells. Nature 1998;391:591–594
65. Schönbeck U, Varo N, Libby P, Buring J, Ridker PM. Soluble CD40L and cardiovascular risk in women. Circulation 2001;104;2266–2268

66. Ridker PM, Cushman M, Stampfer MJ, Tracy RP, Hennekens CH. Inflammation, aspirin, and the risk of cardiovascular disease in apparently healthy men. N Engl J Med 1997;336:973–979
67. Ridker PM, Hennekens CH, Buring JE, Rifai N. C-reactive protein and other markers of inflammation in the prediction of cardiovascular disease in women. N Engl J Med 2000;342:836–843
68. Pasceri V, Willerson JT, Yeh ET. Direct proinflammatory effect of C-reactive protein on human endothelial cells. Circulation 2000;102:2165–2168
69. Koukkunen H, Penttilä K, Kemppainen A, Halinen M, Penttila I, Rantanen T, Pyörälä K. C-reactive protein, fibrinogen, interleukin-6 and tumour necrosis factor-alpha in the prognostic classification of unstable angina pectoris. Ann Med 2001;33:37–47
70. Silveira A. Postprandial triglycerides and blood coagulation. Exp Clin Endocrinol Diabetes 2001;109:S527–S532
71. Davis SR. Postmenopausal hormone-replacement therapy. N Engl J Med 2002;346(1):63–65
72. Koenig W, Sund M, Filipiak B, Döring A, Löwel H, Ernst E. Plasma viscosity and the risk of coronary heart disease: results from the MONICA-Augsburg Cohort Study, 1984 to 1992. Arterioscler Thromb Vasc Biol 1998;18(5):768–772
73. Schwartz SM, Virmani R, Rosenfeld ME. The good smooth muscle cells in atherosclerosis. Curr Atheroscler Rep 2000;2: 422–429
74. Sata M. Circulating vascular progenitor cells contribute to vascular repair, remodeling, and lesion formation. Trends Cardiovasc Med 2003;13:249–253
75. Caplice NM, Bunch TJ, Stalboerger PG, Wang S, Simper D, Miller DV, Russell SJ, Litzow MR, Edwards WD. Smooth muscle cells in human coronary atherosclerosis can originate from cells administered at marrow transplantation. Proc Natl Acad Sci USA 2003;100(8):4754–4759
76. Hill JM, Zalos G, Halcox JP, Schenke WH, Waclawiw MA, Quyyumi AA, Finkel T. Circulating endothelial progenitor cells, vascular function, and cardiovascular risk. N Engl J Med 2003;348:593–600
77. Farb A, Burke AP, Tang AL, Liang TY, Mannan P, Smialek J, Virmani R. Coronary plaque erosion without rupture into a lipid core. A frequent cause of coronary thrombosis in sudden coronary death. Circulation 1996;93:1354–1363
78. Bauer KA. New anticoagulants: anti IIa vs. anti Xa–is one better? J Thromb Thrombolysis 2006;21:67–72
79. Ansell J. Factor Xa or thrombin: is factor Xa a better target? J Thromb Haemost 2007;5(Suppl 1):60–64
80. Weitz JI, Hirsh J, Samama MM; American College of Chest Physicians. New antithrombotic drugs: American College of Chest Physicians Evidence-Based Clinical Practice Guidelines (8th Edition). Chest 2008;133(6 Suppl):234S–256S
81. Weitz J. Factor Xa or thrombin: s thrombin a better target? J Thromb Haemost 2007;5:65–67

5 Vulnerability Caused by Arrhythmogenic Vulnerable Myocardium

Ariel Roguin

CONTENTS

ABSTRACT

Eighty-five percent of those older than 40 years of age dying from cardiac arrest have underlying coronary artery disease on autopsy studies. The most common underlying cause is ventricular fibrillation. Most victims of SCD have severe diffuse multivessel coronary artery disease. Healed myocardial infarctions are present in approximately 50% of victims of SCD. Two conditions appear to be important for the initiation of ventricular fibrillation: an abnormal myocardial substrate (e.g., abnormality of the myocardium, coronary arteries, or cell membrane ion channels) and a transient modulating event (e.g., ischemia). It is the effect of a transient disturbance on a susceptible substrate that is thought to lead to electrical instability.

A number of potential modulating factors have been identified as triggers for SCD, including ischemia, autonomic disturbances, electrolyte and pH derangement, hypoxemia, and drugs.

The most powerful predictor of SCD is poor left ventricular function. Other risk factors for developing SCD mirror those of coronary heart disease and include hypercholesterolemia, hypertension, cigarette smoking, alcohol consumption, physical inactivity, obesity, dietary n-3 polyunsaturated fatty acid intake, diabetes, and left ventricular hypertrophy by electrocardiographic criteria.

This chapter describes methods for identification of vulnerable myocardium and persons at risk, strategies to decrease mortality, and improving event survival.

Early detection of atherosclerosis, which can cause ischemia followed by arrhythmias, is essential for prevention of SCD. Biochemical assays, imaging techniques such as Echocardiography for LV function, CT,

From: *Asymptomatic Atherosclerosis: Pathophysiology, Detection and Treatment*
Edited by: M. Naghavi (ed.), DOI 10.1007/978-1-60327-179-0_5

and MRI for detection of scar, noninvasive electrophysiological tests for vulnerable myocardium, and catheters to localize and characterize vulnerable plaque, in combination with future genomic and proteomic techniques will guide us in the search for vulnerable patients.

Key words: Arrhythmia; Congenital arrhythmias; Coronary artery disease; Primary prevention; Scar; SCD triggers; Sudden death; Treatment

TOPIC PEARLS

1. Eighty-five percent of those older than 40 years of age dying from cardiac arrest have underlying coronary artery disease on autopsy studies.
2. SCD transient modulating factors include ischemia, autonomic disturbances, electrolyte and pH derangement, hypoxemia, and medications.
3. The Vulnerable myocardium can be classified into 3 categories: A. scar (*Ischemic Vulnerable Myocardium With Prior Atherosclerosis-Derived Myocardial Damage*), B. Ischemia (*Ischemic Vulnerable Myocardium Without Prior Atherosclerosis-Derived Myocardial Damage*), and C. Nonischemic (diseases other than coronary atherosclerosis: cardiomyopathy, valvular heart disease, and primary electrical disturbances).
4. Early detection of atherosclerosis, which can cause ischemia followed by arrhythmias, is essential for prevention of SCD.
5. Primary preventive measures in the general population targeting reductions in known cardiovascular risk factors may decrease the mortality from SCD, aimed at both reduction in event rate and improvement in event survival.

A 57-year-old otherwise healthy soccer referee collapsed during a competition after running for 25 minutes. CPR was started immediately and an AED detected a malignant arrhythmia. A DC shock was delivered. The patient was intubated and transferred to the hospital. ST segment depression was observed in AVL V4-6. Angiography revealed mild irregularities in the LAD and RCA and an LCx occlusion which was treated with PCI. The patient was put on hypothermia for 24 hours. The following day all anesthesia agents were stopped and the patient awakened. He gradually returned to full consciousness. During hospitalization and physical examination, as well as ECG recording, he was normal. A treadmill stress test done several days later and an echocardiography were also normal.

Atherosclerotic cardiovascular disease is the leading cause of deaths annually, and coronary heart disease accounts for the majority of this toll. Despite major advances in treatment of coronary heart disease patients, a large number of victims of the disease who are apparently healthy – die suddenly without prior symptoms. Currently, available screening and diagnostic methods are insufficient to identify the victims before the event occurs.

Abnormal heart rhythms, notably atrial and ventricular fibrillation, are leading causes of death and disability. Between 0.5 million and 1 million North Americans and Europeans die each year from sudden cardiac death (SCD), which causes 10–20% of all deaths among adults in the Western world [1]. The most common underlying cause is ventricular fibrillation.

Despite increasing insight into the mechanisms and risk factors of SCD, the populations at high risk for a primary event have not effectively been identified. The population that experiences SCD can broadly be divided into three groups with increasing incidence: (1) primary events in the general population, (2) primary events specifically in persons with known heart disease, and (3) secondary events in individuals with a prior episode of malignant ventricular tachyarrythmia.

The exact mechanism of ventricular fibrillation is poorly understood. There are triggers that act on a vulnerable substrate. Two conditions appear to be important for the initiation of ventricular fibrillation: an abnormal myocardial substrate (e.g., abnormality of the myocardium, coronary arteries, or cell membrane ion channels) and a transient modulating event (e.g., ischemia). It is the effect of a transient disturbance on a susceptible substrate that is thought to lead to electrical instability.

ABNORMAL MYOCARDIAL SUBSTRATE

Eighty-five percent of those older than 40 years of age dying from cardiac arrest have underlying coronary artery disease on autopsy studies. Ten percent have other structural cardiac abnormalities, such as cardiomyopathy and valvular disease, and 5% have no macroscopic structural cardiac abnormality [2,3]. Patients with known molecular abnormalities, such as membrane ion channel defects seen in the monogenic disorders of the long QT and Brugada syndromes, represent a small proportion of the total burden.

Although the link between SCD and coronary artery disease is well established, the anatomic distribution of disease does not help identify those at highest risk. What is notable is that most victims of SCD have severe diffuse multivessel coronary artery disease. Healed myocardial infarctions are present in approximately 50% of victims of SCD [4].

SCD TRIGGERS: TRANSIENT MODULATING FACTORS

A number of potential modulating factors have been identified, including ischemia, autonomic disturbances, electrolyte and pH derangement, hypoxemia, and drugs. Epidemiologic studies regarding these transient factors have furthered our understanding of SCD and guided clinical care in order to prevent an event.

Fifty percent of cardiac arrest survivors develop electrocardiographic changes consistent with acute myocardial infarction, and an additional one-third develop changes consistent with ischemia without infarction. The latter was observed in our patient. Furthermore, on autopsy studies, coronary thrombus has been reported in approximately 75% of SCD victims. Although the exact percentage of patients who experience cardiac arrest secondary to ischemia is unclear, it is evident that in a significant number, ischemia plays an important role. Interventions aimed at reducing the frequency and severity of ischemia, such as thrombolytic therapy and coronary artery bypass grafting, have been associated with decreased incidence of SCD and reduced overall cardiac mortality [1].

The autonomic nervous system in the etiology of SCD, particularly in the setting of ischemia, emotional stress, and vigorous physical exertion, which result in the elevation of circulating catecholamines, may be important triggers for SCD [5–7]. Blocking the adrenergic system with beta-receptor blockade therapy reduces the incidence of SCD.

Electrolyte abnormalities, such as hypokalemia and hypomagnesemia, are often due to diuretic use and may exacerbate the vulnerable myocardium [2].

The Cardiac Arrhythmia Suppression Trial showed that treatment with class Ic antiarrhythmic agents to suppress ventricular arrhythmias post myocardial infarction paradoxically increased mortality from SCD [8]. Subsequent studies came to similar conclusions for Ia, Ib, and pure class III antiarrhythmic drugs [2]. Additionally, a number of noncardiac medications that prolong the QT interval, such as erythromycin and tricyclic antidepressants, also are potentially proarrhythmic. The role that these commonly prescribed medications play in out-of-hospital cardiac arrest has not been well established.

The reasons for SCD are complex and not completely understood. We as clinicians should find who is vulnerable for developing SCD. An expert panel suggested a new definition and proposed risk assessment strategies. They presented a classification for clinical as well as pathological evaluation for SCD. The position paper was called "From Vulnerable Plaque to Vulnerable Patient" [2]. They divided the vulnerable substrate into several parts:

1. *The vulnerable coronary plaque* – Rupture-prone plaques and atherosclerotic plaques with high likelihood of thrombotic complications and rapid progression.
2. *Electrical vulnerability* – Subjects with high likelihood of developing cardiac arrhythmias in the near future. Genetic mutations or variations in gene expression.

3. *Vulnerable blood* – Blood components with more thrombosis risk and an activated coagulation system.
4. *Metabolic vulnerability* – Electrolytes and other chemistry abnormalities.
5. *Vulnerable myocardium* – this can be classified further into 3 categories as describedlater.

Myocardial Scar: Ischemic Vulnerable Myocardium with Prior Atherosclerosis-Derived Myocardial Damage

Any type of atherosclerosis-related myocardial injury, such as ischemia, an old or new myocardial infarction, i.e., scar, inflammation, and/or fibrosis, potentially increases the patient's vulnerability to arrhythmia and sudden death. In patients with a history of ischemic heart disease, ischemic cardiomyopathy with patchy areas of scar is the ultimate form of myocardial damage. The scar can serve as the basis for malignant arrhythmia. Around the scar the electrical conduction might cause re-entry ventricular arrhythmias.

Myocardial Ischemia: Ischemic Vulnerable Myocardium Without Prior Atherosclerosis-Derived Myocardial Damage

Abrupt occlusion of a coronary artery is a common cause of sudden death. It often leads to acute myocardial infarction or exacerbation of chest pain [9]. Extensive studies in experimental animals and increasing clinical evidence indicate that autonomic nervous activity has a significant role in modifying the clinical outcome with coronary occlusion. The autonomic tone has a key role in the outcome after plaque rupture. Sympathetic hyperactivity favors the genesis of life-threatening ventricular tachyarrhythmias. Strong afferent stimuli from the ischemic myocardium may impair the arterial baroreflex and lead to hemodynamic instability [10]·

There seems to be a wide interindividual variation in the type and severity of autonomic reactions during the early phase of abrupt coronary occlusion, a critical period for out-of-hospital cardiac arrest. The pre-existing severity of a coronary stenosis, adaptation or preconditioning to myocardial ischemia, habitual physical exercise, Beta-blockade, and gender seem to affect autonomic reactions and the risk of fatal ventricular arrhythmias [7]. Recent studies have documented a hereditary component for autonomic function, and genetic factors may also modify the clinical presentation of acute coronary occlusion. [11]

In the past few decades, a number of diagnostic methods have been developed for imaging cardiac ischemia and for assessing the risk of developing a life-threatening cardiac arrhythmia. Table 1 depicts conditions and markers associated with myocardial vulnerability.

Nonischemic Vulnerable Myocardium

A subset of patients experience fatal arrhythmia as a result of diseases other than coronary atherosclerosis. The various forms of cardiomyopathy (dilated, hypertrophic, restrictive, and right ventricular) account for most noncoronary cardiac deaths. Other underlying pathological processes include valvular heart disease, such as aortic stenosis and primary electrical disturbances (long-QT syndromes, Brugada syndrome, Wolff–Parkinson–White syndrome, sinus and atrioventricular conduction disturbances, catecholaminergic polymorphic ventricular tachycardia, and congenital and drug-induced long QT syndromes with torsades de pointes). Less common pathological conditions include anomalous origin of a coronary artery, myocarditis, and myocardial bridging.

The Task Force on Sudden Cardiac Death, organized by the European Society of Cardiology, issued a report that includes detailed diagnostic and therapeutic recommendations for a large number of cardiomyopathic conditions capable of causing sudden cardiac death [12] (Table 2).

Table 1
Conditions and markers associated with myocardial vulnerability

With atherosclerosis-derived myocardial ischemia as shown by:
ECG abnormalities:
During rest
During stress test
Silent ischemia (e.g., ST changes on Holter monitoring)
Perfusion and viability disorder:
PET scan
SPECT
Wall motion abnormalities
Echocardiography
MR imaging
Ventriculogram during angiography
MSCT
Without atherosclerosis-derived myocardial ischemia:
Sympathetic hyperactivity
Impaired autonomic reactivity
Left ventricular hypertrophy
Cardiomyopathy (dilated, hypertrophic, or restrictive)
Valvular disease (aortic stenosis and mitral valve prolapse)
Electrophysiological disorders:
Long-QT syndrome, Brugada syndrome, Wolff–Parkinson–White syndrome, sinus and atrioventricular conduction disturbances, catecholaminergic polymorphic ventricular tachycardia, T-wave alternans, and drug-induced torsades de pointes
Commotio cordis
Anomalous origination of a coronary artery
Myocarditis
Myocardial bridging

MSCT indicates multislice computed tomography; PET, positron emission tomography; and SPECT, single-photon emission computed tomography

Table 2
Available techniques for electrophysiological risk stratification of vulnerable myocardium

Diagnostic criteria:
Arrhythmia
QT dispersion
QT dynamics
T-wave alternans
Ventricular late potentials
Heart rate variability
Diagnostic techniques:
Noninvasive
Resting ECG
Stress ECG
Ambulatory ECG
Signal-averaged ECG
Surface high-resolution ECG
Invasive
Programmed ventricular stimulation
Real-time 3D magnetic-navigated activation map

RISK FACTORS

The most powerful predictor of SCD is poor left ventricular function [13]. Other risk factors for developing SCD mirror those of coronary heart disease and include hypercholesterolemia, hypertension, cigarette smoking, alcohol consumption, physical inactivity, obesity, dietary n-3 polyunsaturated fatty acid intake, diabetes, and left ventricular hypertrophy by electrocardiographic criteria [2,12]. Certain risk factors, however, impact the incidence of SCD beyond their effect on coronary heart disease.

Among persons without prior clinically recognized heart disease, dietary intake of long-chain n-3 long polyunsaturated fatty acids (PUFAs) from fatty fish (1 or more servings per week) and higher levels of cell-membrane long-chain n-3 polyunsaturated fatty acids are associated with a lower risk of out-of-hospital cardiac arrest. In contrast, the intake of these fatty acids is not related to the risk of nonfatal myocardial infarction [14] .

Aside from the Mendelian familial syndromes of long QT or Brugada, a hereditary risk for SCD in the general population exists. Those who suffer cardiac arrest are significantly more likely to have had a parent who had SCD [15]. This finding is independent of a familial risk of myocardial infarction.

IDENTIFICATION OF VULNERABLE MYOCARDIUM AND PERSONS AT RISK

Any type of atherosclerosis-related myocardial injury, such as ischemia, an old or new myocardial infarction, inflammation, and/or fibrosis, potentially increases the patient's vulnerability to arrhythmia and sudden death. More patients now survive acute events, and some develop heart failure or ischemic cardiomyopathy later with the potential for fatal arrhythmias. Hence, as the prevalence of the disease increases worldwide, so will the incidence of SCD. Evaluation of patients who are known to have heart disease can identify those at increased risk of SCD, but unfortunately in about more than half of all cases SCD is the initial presenting symptom of heart disease [3].

Although SCD accounts for a significant rate each year, its overall incidence in the general population is low. Predicting SCD in the general population is problematic. In approximately 40–50% of cases of out-of-hospital cardiac arrest due to heart disease, there is no history of clinically recognized heart disease [11]. Efforts to identify high-risk patients using known risk factors in the general population have proved challenging. Combining the risk factors of body mass, cigarette smoking, hypertension, hyperlipidemia, and left ventricular hypertrophy by electrocardiographic criteria, a multivariate model was developed using prospective data on 4,120 middle-aged men from the Albany and Framingham studies to estimate the probability of SCD [16]. While there was a 16-fold increase in risk of SCD from the lowest to the highest risk group, even in the highest risk subgroup of persons without clinically recognized heart disease, the annual incidence of SCD was only 0.7%.

STRATEGIES TO DECREASE MORTALITY

Several strategies must be employed simultaneously to decrease the mortality from SCD, aimed at both reduction in event rate and improvement in event survival. First are primary preventive measures in the general population targeting reductions in known cardiovascular risk factors. Owing to the low incidence of SCD in the general population, these interventions will have to be broad-based, safe, easily administered, acceptable to the general population, and inexpensive. Second is primary prevention of SCD in patients with known heart disease with a focus on pharmacologic therapies. And finally, interventions to improve event survival will be reviewed, with re-evaluation of current emergency medical guidelines and applications of new technologies.

Magnetic-resonance-based visualization of scar morphology would potentially contribute to preprocedural planning for catheter ablation. In catheter ablation of scar-related monomorphic ventricular tachycardia, substrate voltage mapping is used to electrically define the scar during sinus rhythm. However, the electrically defined scar may not accurately reflect the anatomical scar. Magnetic-resonance-based visualization of the scar may elucidate the 3D anatomical correlation between the fine structural details of the scar and scar-related VT circuits [17].

IMPROVING EVENT SURVIVAL

While treatment of critically ill hospitalized patients has improved, the survival rate from cardiac arrest (both in-hospital and out-of-hospital) has remained dismal and essentially unchanged for the last 20 years. Survival to discharge ranges from 1.6 to 20% with congested urban areas and remote suburban areas generally faring the worst [18,19]. To truly improve survival among the victims of SCD will require a paradigm shift in the delivery of emergency care and resuscitation.

OUR PATIENT AND FUTURE DIRECTIONS

Our patient underwent a year before this event a general check-up: the main findings were normal physical examination, a normal ECG and blood tests, and a normal stress test. Unless an AED was present in the scene – he would have to join the SCD statistics. Despite substantial progress in basic, clinical, and epidemiologic research related to life-threatening ventricular arrhythmia, the reduction of mortality from out-of-hospital cardiac arrest due to heart disease remains a challenge for cardiology and is a major public health issue. Clinical and public health efforts to significantly reduce mortality from SCD through the identification of persons at risk face numerous challenges. First, the incidence of SCD in the population is low, even in common high-risk clinical populations. Second, the current risk factors for SCD have a low positive predictive value (most of the patients with the risk factor will not experience sudden death in a particular year) and are not sensitive (many victims of SCD do not have the particular risk factor). Therefore, the use of currently identified risk factors to characterize progressively higher risk groups comes at the cost of decreasing sensitivity, and hence, large numbers of SCD victims have been overlooked.

Recent advances in molecular biology and family studies have contributed important new information related to the mechanisms that provide a substrate for the occurrence of life-threatening ventricular arrhythmias. The study of fundamental mechanisms underlying arrhythmias has led to a marked improvement in treatment for some patients, such as those who can be cured with catheter ablation. Gene delivery and cell-based therapies are also being explored for treating the substrate for re-entry after myocardial infarction or for replacing electronic pacemakers with biological ones. Studies of rare familial syndromes can identify molecules whose dysfunction leads to arrhythmias, ushering in an era of mechanism-based therapeutics. Studies of large populations to identify common genetic variants that predispose individuals to arrhythmias hold similar promise for early detection and intervention in asymptomatic patients at high risk. We are just beginning to understand how new genetic information can be incorporated into diagnosis and therapy.

Table 3 summarizes the recommendations by the ACC/AHA/ESC 2006 guidelines for management of patients with ventricular arrhythmias and the prevention of sudden cardiac death [20]. However, the importance of these findings for clinical care and public health remains limited, since the prevalence of monogenic disorders that increase susceptibility to SCD is low. Real progress in reducing its impact will depend on identification of persons at risk, reduction in those risk factors, and application of techniques – both simple and advanced to improve survival in victims. Ongoing trials in patients with known risk factors will hopefully clarify those interventions that will reduce the incidence of cardiac arrest. Technologies such as AEDs hold promise to improve survival.

Table 3
Recommendations by the ACC/AHA/ESC 2006 guidelines for management of patients with ventricular arrhythmias and the prevention of sudden cardiac death [20]

Test	*To whom, class recommendation and level of evidence*
Resting electrocardiography	Class I Resting 12-lead electrocardiogram (ECG) is indicated in all patients who are evaluated for ventricular arrhythmias. *(Level of Evidence: A)*
Exercise testing	Class I 1. Exercise testing is recommended in adult patients with ventricular arrhythmias who have an intermediate or greater probability of having CHD by age, gender, and symptoms* to provoke ischemic changes or ventricular arrhythmias. *(Level of Evidence: B* 2. Exercise testing, regardless of age, is useful in patients with known or suspected exercise-induced ventricular arrhythmias, including catecholaminergic VT to provoke the arrhythmia, achieve a diagnosis, and determine the patient's response to tachycardia. *(Level of Evidence: B)* Class IIa Exercise testing can be useful in evaluating response to medical or ablation therapy in patients with known exercise-induced ventricular arrhythmias. *(Level of Evidence: B)*
Ambulatory electrocardiography	Class I 1. Ambulatory ECG is indicated when there is a need to clarify the diagnosis by detecting arrhythmias, QT-interval changes, T-wave alternans, or ST changes, to evaluate risk, or to judge therapy. *(Level of Evidence: A)* 2. Event monitors are indicated when symptoms are sporadic to establish whether they are caused by transient arrhythmias. *(Level of Evidence: B)* 3. Implantable recorders are useful in patients with sporadic symptoms suspected to be related to arrhythmias such as syncope when a symptom–rhythm correlation cannot be established by conventional diagnostic techniques. *(Level of Evidence: B*
Electrocardiographic techniques and measurements	Class IIa It is reasonable to use T-wave alternans for improving the diagnosis and risk stratification of patients with ventricular arrhythmias or who are at risk for developing life-threatening ventricular arrhythmias. *(Level of Evidence: A*

Left ventricular function and imaging	Class I 1. Echocardiography is recommended in patients with ventricular arrhythmias who are suspected of having structural heart disease. *(Level of Evidence: B)* 2. Echocardiography is recommended for the subset of patients at high risk for development of serious ventricular arrhythmias or SCD, such as those with dilated, hypertrophic, or RV cardiomyopathies, acute MI survivors, or relatives of patients with inherited disorders associated with SCD. *(Level of Evidence: B)* 3. Exercise testing with an imaging modality (echocardiography or nuclear perfusion (single-photon emission computed tomography [SPECT]) is recommended to detect silent ischemia in patients with ventricular arrhythmias who have an intermediate probability of having CHD by age, symptoms, and gender and in whom ECG assessment is less reliable because of digoxin use, LV hypertrophy, greater than 1-mm ST-segment depression at rest, Wolff-Parkinson-White syndrome, or left bundle-branch block. *(Level of Evidence: B)* 4. Pharmacological stress testing with an imaging modality (echocardiography or myocardial perfusion SPECT) is recommended to detect silent ischemia in patients with ventricular arrhythmias who have an intermediate probability of having CHD by age, symptoms, and gender and are physically unable to perform a symptom-limited exercise test. *(Level of Evidence: B)* Class IIa 1. Magnetic resonance imaging (MRI), cardiac computed tomography (CT), or radionuclide angiography can be useful in patients with ventricular arrhythmias when echocardiography does not provide accurate assessment of LV and RV function and/or evaluation of structural changes. *(Level of Evidence: B)* 2. Coronary angiography can be useful in establishing or excluding the presence of significant obstructive CHD in patients with life-threatening ventricular arrhythmias or in survivors of SCD, who have an intermediate or greater probability of having CHD by age, symptoms, and gender. *(Level of Evidence: C)* 3. LV imaging can be useful in patients undergoing biventricular pacing. *(Level of Evidence: C)*
Electrophysiological Testing in Patients With Coronary Heart Disease.	Class I EP testing is recommended in patients with syncope of unknown cause with impaired LV function or structural heart disease. *(Level of Evidence: B)* Class IIa EP testing can be useful in patients with syncope when bradyarrhythmias or tachyarrhythmias are suspected and in whom noninvasive diagnostic studies are not conclusive. *(Level of Evidence: B)*

Early detection of atherosclerosis which can cause ischemia followed by arrhythmias, as in the case presented, is essential for prevention of SCD. Biochemical assays (e.g., C-reactive protein), imaging techniques as Echocardiography for LV function, CT, and MRI for detection of scar, noninvasive electrophysiological tests for vulnerable myocardium, and emerging catheters to localize and characterize vulnerable plaque, in combination with future genomic and proteomic techniques will guide us in the search for vulnerable patients. This may also lead to the development and deployment of new therapies and ultimately to reduce the incidence of SCD.

REFERENCES

1. Knollmann BC, Roden DM. A genetic framework for improving arrhythmia therapy. Nature 2008; 451:929–936
2. Naghavi M, Libby P, Falk E, et al. From vulnerable plaque to vulnerable patient: a call for new definitions and risk assessment strategies: Part II. Circulation 2003; 108:1772–1778
3. Kannel WB, Thomas HE Jr. Sudden coronary death: the Framingham Study. Ann NY Acad Sci 1982; 382:3–21
4. Reichenbach DD, Moss NS, Meyer E. Pathology of the heart in sudden cardiac death. Am J Cardiol 1977; 39:865–868
5. Leor J, Poole WK, Kloner RA. Sudden cardiac death triggered by an earthquake. New Engl J Med 1996; 334:413–417
6. Empana JP, Jouven X, Lemaitre RN, et al. Clinical depression and risk of out-of-hospital cardiac arrest. Arch Intern Med. 2006; 166:195–200
7. Burke AP, Farb A, Malcom GT, et al. Plaque rupture and sudden death related to exertion in men with coronary artery isease. JAMA 1999; 281:921–926
8. Sotoodehnia N, Zivin A, Bardy GH, Siscovick DS. Reducing mortality from sudden cardiac death in the community: lessons from epidemiology and clinical applications research. Cardiovasc Res 2001; 50:197–209
9. Airaksinen KE. Autonomic mechanisms and sudden death after abrupt coronary occlusion. Ann Med 1999; 31:240–245
10. Airaksinen KE, Tahvanainen KU, Eckberg DL, et al. Arterial baroreflex impairment in patients during acute coronary occlusion. J Am Coll Cardiol 1998; 32:1641–1647
11. Jouven X, Desnos M, Guerot C, et al. Predicting sudden death in the population: the Paris Prospective Study I. Circulation 1999; 99:1978–1983
12. Priori SG, Aliot E, Blomstrom-Lundqvist C, et al. Task Force on Sudden Cardiac Death of the European Society of Cardiology. Eur Heart J 2001; 22:1374–1450
13. Hammermeister KE, DeRouen TA, Dodge HT. Variables predictive of survival in patients with coronary disease. Selection by univariate and multivariate analyses from the clinical, electrocardiographic, exercise, arteriographic, and quantitative angiographic evaluations. Circulation 1979; 59:421–427
14. Lemaitre RN, King IB, Mozaffarian D, Sotoodehnia N, Siscovick DS. Trans-fatty acids and sudden cardiac death. Atheroscler Suppl 2006; 7:13–15
15. Rea TD, Pearce RM, Raghunathan TE, et al. Incidence of out-of-hospital cardiac arrest. Am J Cardiol 2004; 93:1455–1460
16. Kannel WB, Doyle JT, McNamara PM, Quickenton P, Gordon T. Precursors of sudden coronary death. Factors related to the incidence of sudden death. Circulation 1975; 51:606–609
17. Ashikaga H, Sasano T, Dong J, Zviman MM, et al. Magnetic resonance-based anatomical analysis of scar-related ventricular tachycardia: implications for catheter ablation. Circ Res 2007; 101:939–947
18. Mitchell RG, Brady W, Guly UM, Pirrallo RG, Robertson CE. Comparison of two emergency response systems and their effect on survival from out of hospital cardiac arrest. Resuscitation 1997; 35:225–229
19. Markusohn E, Roguin A, Sebbag A et al. Primary percutaneous coronary intervention after out-of-hospital cardiac arrest: patients and outcomes. Isr Med Assoc J 2007; 9:257–259
20. Zipes DP, Camm AJ, Borggrefe M, et al. ACC/AHA/ESC 2006 guidelines for management of patients with ventricular arrhythmias and the prevention of sudden cardiac death – executive summary: a report of the American College of Cardiology/American Heart Association Task Force and the European Society of Cardiology Committee for Practice Guidelines (Writing Committee to Develop Guidelines for Management of Patients With Ventricular Arrhythmias and the Prevention of Sudden Cardiac Death). J Am Coll Cardiol 2006; 48:1064–1108

6 Approach to Atherosclerosis as a Disease: Primary Prevention Based on the Detection and Treatment of Asymptomatic Atherosclerosis

Morteza Naghavi, Erling Falk, Khurram Nasir, Harvey S. Hecht, Matthew J. Budoff, Zahi A. Fayad, Daniel S. Berman, and Prediman K. Shah

CONTENTS

ABSTRACT

Atherosclerosis is a pervasive and malignant disease of the arterial circulation. It is by far the most frequent cause of angina, heart attack (including sudden coronary death), and peripheral arterial disease and is responsible for many cases of stroke. Yet, many individuals, even those with advanced disease, are unaware because they have no symptoms. In 30–50% of these individuals, the first indicator of atherosclerosis is a heart attack, which often is fatal (sudden, unexpected death).

Since there are many pharmacologic and non-pharmacologic therapies to reduce the risk of heart attack and stroke, early detection of atherosclerosis itself, before symptoms occur, can provide a major opportunity to prevent many such events. Since effective screening could confer great public health benefit, it may seem surprising that screening for subclinical atherosclerosis has not yet been incorporated into national and international clinical guidelines. Therapeutic strategies targeted to key at-risk vulnerable patients can reduce the heavy economic burden of symptomatic and end-stage care for cardiovascular disease (CVD).

From: *Asymptomatic Atherosclerosis: Pathophysiology, Detection and Treatment*
Edited by: M. Naghavi (ed.), DOI 10.1007/978-1-60327-179-0_6

There have been two main reasons for this conservative strategy. Firstly, there has been a lack of data convincingly demonstrating that screening for subclinical atherosclerosis improves the assessment of risk beyond that provided by traditional risk factors, such as smoking, hypertension, hypercholesterolemia, and diabetes. Secondly, appropriate instruments for detection of subclinical atherosclerosis have not been widely available to clinicians. The authors of this chapter believe that recent developments have provided us with the requisite data as well as with the necessary methodology. Furthermore, highly effective and safe therapies against atherosclerosis and heart attack are available.

Key words: Atherosclerosis; Asymptomatic Atherosclerosis; Subclinical Atherosclerosis; Non-invasive Screening; Cardiovascular Risk Factors; Framingham Risk Score; Vulnerable Patient; Genetic Susceptibility

KEY POINTS

- Atherosclerosis begins to develop early in life and progresses with time, but the speed of progression is unpredictable and varies markedly among different subjects.
- At every level of risk factor exposure, there is substantial variation in the amount of evolved atherosclerosis, probably because individual susceptibility to atherosclerosis and its risk factors varies greatly, thereby explaining the limited ability to predict clinical outcomes based on risk factor assessment alone.
- Since there are many pharmacologic and non-pharmacologic therapies to reduce the risk of heart attack and stroke, early detection of atherosclerosis itself (regardless of risk factors), before symptoms occur, can provide a major opportunity to prevent many such events.
- It is thought-provoking that cardiovascular disease (CVD) kills more young and middle-aged women than does breast cancer, yet the majority of such women are considered to be at low cardiovascular risk and left untreated based on current risk assessment by using risk factor scoring.
- The time has come to reconsider our traditional, imprecise approach to individual risk assessment using risk factor scoring, and to improve it by a responsible use of novel non-invasive technologies that provide direct assessment of vascular structure and function.

INTRODUCTION

BURDEN OF DISEASES CAUSED BY ATHEROSCLEROSIS

Cardiovascular disease (CVD) is the leading cause of death in the United States and most developed countries (Fig. 1a). Atherosclerotic CVD is responsible for the majority of CVD. Nearly all coronary heart disease (CHD), intermittent claudication and critical limb ischemia, and most strokes, result from atherosclerotic vascular changes (Fig. 1b). CHD alone is the single largest killer of American males and females (>500,000 annually), causing more than 1 of every 5 deaths [1]. The lifetime risk of developing CHD after age 40 is 49% for men and 32% for women [1]. This year an estimated 700,000 Americans will have a first heart attack, and approximately 500,000 will have a recurrent attack [1]. Because the risk of CHD increases markedly with age, and women live longer than men, almost as many women ultimately die of CHD as do men [1].

Although heart attack treatment has improved markedly in recent years, myocardial infarction with severe heart muscle damage or sudden unexpected death remains an all too common first manifestation of coronary atherosclerosis (see Fig. 2). These attacks usually occur in patients who are not receiving the benefits of preventive therapies of proven efficacy because their arterial disease was unrecognized (asymptomatic), and/or they had been misclassified by conventional risk factors into a treatment goal not in line with their individual burden of atherosclerosis (see Fig. 3).

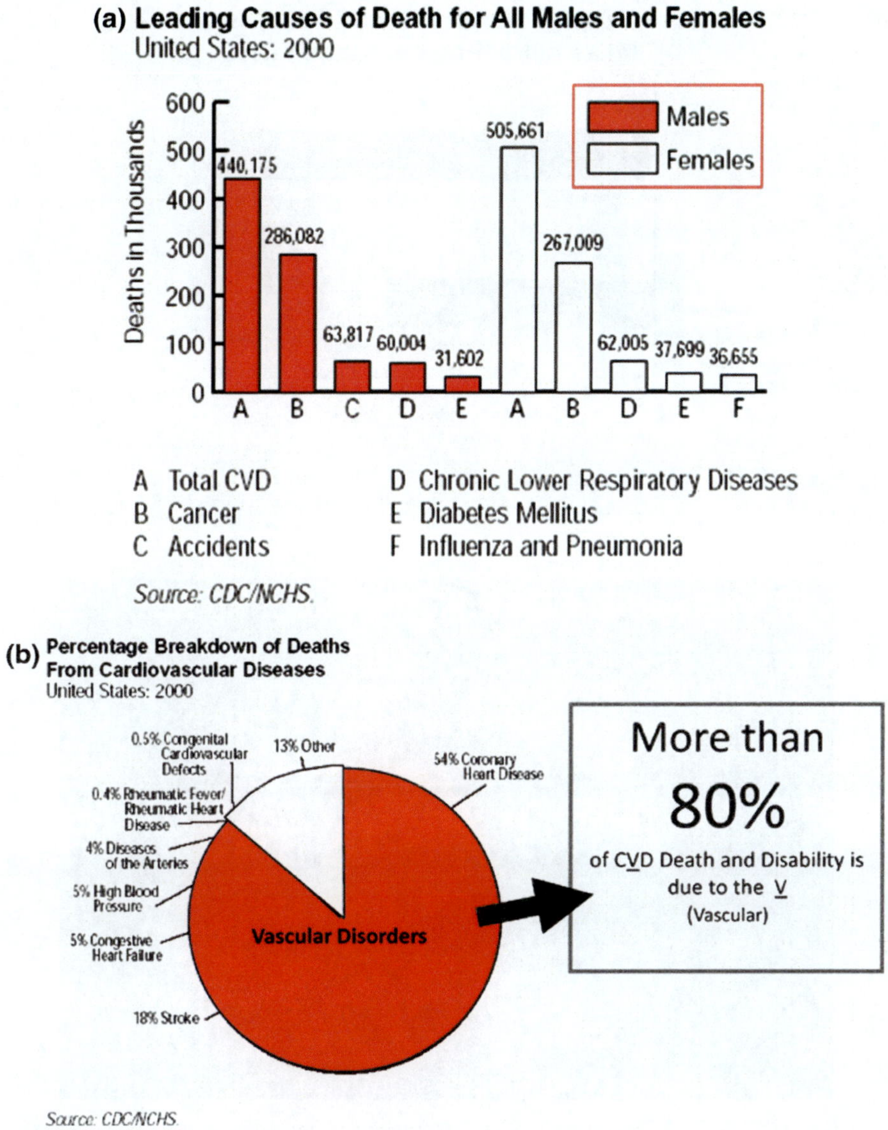

Fig. 1. (**a**) Cardiovascular disease (CVD) leads the cause of death in the United States both for men and women. (**b**) the majority of CVD death and disability is caused by the vascular (V) component of CVD.

RISK FACTORS VS SUSCEPTIBILITY VS VULNERABILITY

Most heart attacks and many cases of ischemic stroke are caused by disruption of an atherosclerotic plaque with superimposed thrombosis. Atherosclerosis begins to develop early in life and progresses with time, but the speed of progression is unpredictable and varies markedly among different subjects. At every level of risk factor exposure, there is substantial variation in the amount of evolved atherosclerosis, probably because the individual susceptibility to atherosclerosis and its risk factors varies greatly, thereby explaining the limited ability to predict clinical outcomes based on risk factor assessment alone.

A newer understanding of the natural history of atherosclerosis, from endothelial dysfunction and activation, to intimal accumulation of lipids, inflammatory cells, and growth of smooth muscle cells,

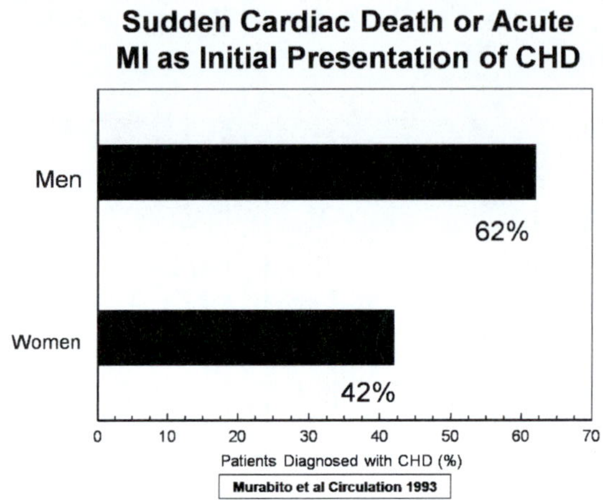

Fig. 2. Leading causes of death for all males and females.

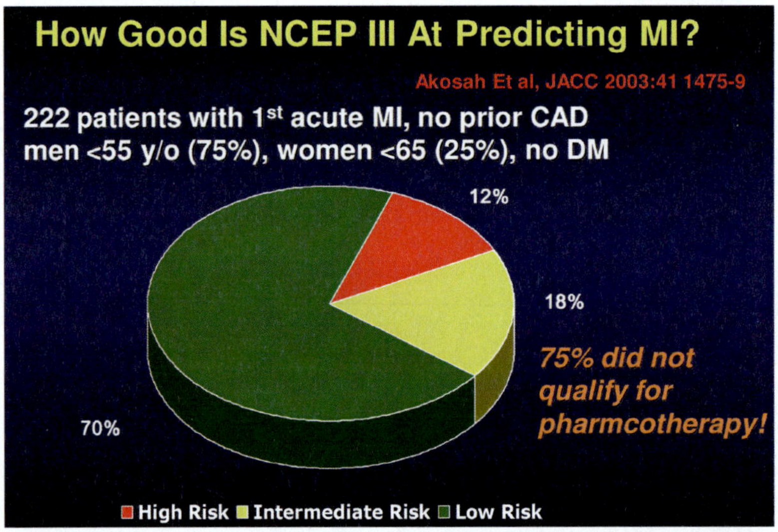

Fig. 3. Risk Assessment based solely on risk factors misclassifies patients at immediate risk of coronary events.

to plaque formation, disruption, and thrombosis, provides the opportunity to identify the high-risk or vulnerable patient at various stages of the process. Refinement of diagnostic methods should greatly enhance our ability to identify individuals with early-onset atherosclerosis that is likely to progress, thereby offering the opportunity for preventive intervention.

The prevalence of 1 or more major risk factors (beyond age) is very high among Americans aged 40 years and above who develop CHD (Table 1). However, it is also high among those who do not develop CHD, illustrating that when risk factors are almost universally present in a population they do not predict the development of disease in individuals [2–5]. Instead, individual susceptibility to atherosclerosis and vulnerability to acute events determine individual risk. In the present context, vulnerability to clinical manifestations of atherosclerosis can be considered to reside in a host of unmeasured factors, including genetic variation, but, more prag-

Table 1
Risk factors are ubiquitous among Americans aged 40–59 years, also among those not dying from coronary heart disease

	CHA, death		*MRFIT, death*	
RiskFartor	CHD	Non-CHD	CHD	Non-CHD
Men, n	1068	8026	17416	*257996*
Cholesterol ≥ 200 mg/dL (≥5.18 mmol/L)	72%	62%	77%	*65%*
DBP > 80 mm Hg or SBP > 120 mm Hg	91%	83%	89%	78%
Current smoking	*52%*	40%	49%	*35%*
Diabetes	7.1%	3.0%	*5.6%*	1.5%
Cholesterol ≥ 240 mg/dL (≥6.22 mmol/L)	30%	21%	37%	24%
DBP ≥ 90 mm Hg or SBP ≥ 140 mm Hg	73%	60%	*56%*	36%
Women, n	*465*	*7188*	NA	NA
Cholesterol ≥ 200 mg/dL (≥5.18 mmol/L)	77%	67%	NA	NA
DBP > 80 mm Hg or SBP > 120 mm Hg	87%	72%	NA	NA
Current smoking	*52%*	*35%*	NA	NA
Diabetes	*5.6%*	2.1%	NA	NA
Cholesterol ≥ 240 mg/dL (≥6.22 mmol/L)	39%	27%	NA	NA
DBP ≥ 90 mm Hg or SBP ≥ 140 mm Hg	71%	47%	NA	NA

Abbreviations: CHA, Chicago Heart Association Detection Project in Industry; CHD, coronary heart disease; DSP, diastolic blood pressure; MRFIT, Multiple Risk Factor Intervention Trial; NA, not applicable; SBP, systolic blood pressure. Adapted from Greenland et al. [6]

matically, can also be considered to be the presence or absence of the underlying subclinical atherosclerosis, and the susceptibility to thrombotic (vulnerable blood) and arrhythmic (vulnerable myocardium) complications.

The poor predictive power of major traditional risk factors was clearly demonstrated by Weissler [7] who calculated a weak likelihood ratio of 1.03 to 1.42 for prediction of coronary events in men and women (See Table 2). Despite the high frequency of this risk profile in the population with CHD events. This apparent paradox is attributable to the presence of 1 or more risk factors in a great many individuals with no CHD [7].

The inability of the traditional risk factors to identify the at-risk population is the basis of the "Polypill" strategy, in which people with known CVD or over 55 without known disease , are treated with a single daily pill containing 6 components to reduce the risk factor level, regardless of what current risk assessment algorithms predict [8]; 96% of deaths from CHD or stroke occur in people aged 55 and over [8].

CURRENT GUIDELINES IN PRIMARY PREVENTION

The current primary prevention guidelines recommend initial risk assessment and then risk classification based on risk factors (e.g. the Framingham Risk Score in the United States and the SCORE in Europe), followed by risk reducing goal-directed therapy when necessary [9–12]. Although this approach may identify persons at very low or very high risk of a heart attack or stroke within the next 10 years, the majority of the population belongs to an intermediate risk group, in which the predictive power of risk factors is low. Since most heart attacks occur in this group (high population attributable risk), many individuals at risk are likely to be not properly identified and, thus, not treated

Table 2
Predictive power for CHD death, or CHD or nonfatal myocardial infarction, in men and women aged 18–59 Years (From Weissler [7])

Sex	% Sensitivity	Specificity	Complement of specificity (100-specificity)	Positive likelihood ratio (95% cl)
CHD Death				
Men	87.5	33.0	67.0	1.31 (1.30–1.32)
Women	93.1	33.1	66.9	1.39 (1.35–1.42)
CHD Death or nonfatal myocardial infarction				
Men	90.4	25.9	84.1	1.07 (1.03–1.11)
Women	87.9	27.6	72.4	1.21 (1.14–1.28)

Abbreviations: CHD, coronary heart disease; CI, confidence interval

to more appropriate "individualized" goals, whereas others are misclassified as being at high risk and are unnecessarily treated with pharmacologic therapy, perhaps for the rest of their lives. This strategy is not cost-effective, and, more importantly, is not good medicine.

The serious limitations of current guidelines are recognized by the American Heart Association (AHA), the National Cholesterol Education Program (NCEP) expert panel, and by the European Third Joint Task Force [9–11]. Therefore, the use of non-invasive screening tests that identify abnormal arterial structure and function for risk prediction in a given individual can be an option for advanced risk assessment in appropriately selected persons, particularly in those with multiple risk ww who are judged to be at intermediate (~indeterminate) risk [9–11]. Such tests include carotid intima-media thickness (IMT) measured by ultrasound, coronary artery calcification determined by computed tomography (CT), endothelial vasomotor dysfunction evaluated by ultrasound, ankle/brachial blood pressure ratio (ABI), and magnetic resonance imaging (MRI) techniques [9–11].

CHD Risk Equivalents

Patients who already have developed clinical atherosclerotic disease have declared themselves to be at continued high risk (vulnerable) [13]. Current American and European guidelines also recognize groups of patients who are at similar high risk [9–11], including those with diabetes, severe hyperlipidemia or hypertension, as well as patients in whom atherosclerosis and/or its consequences have been demonstrated by non-invasive testing. For example, the presence of myocardial ischemia appropriately identified by stress testing qualifies as a diagnosis of CHD. Moreover, the identification of obstructive atherosclerosis in carotid or ilio-femoral arteries is considered a CHD risk equivalent and should be treated aggressively; atherosclerosis in one vascular bed predicts atherosclerosis in other vascular beds.

CHD risk equivalents include peripheral arterial disease (whether diagnosed by ABI, lower limb blood flow studies, or clinical symptoms), carotid artery disease (transient ischemic attack or stroke of carotid origin, or > 50% stenosis on angiography or ultrasound), abdominal aortic aneurysms, as well as 2 or more risk factors with a10-year CHD risk of greater than 20% [9,12]. However, existing guidelines do not recognize severe nonobstructive coronary atherosclerosis as a CHD risk equivalent, a view which demands reconsideration, since most heart attacks originate from nonobstructive coronary plaques.

SCREENING FOR SILENT DISEASE TO PREVENT DEADLY DISEASE

In a recent scientific statement, the American Cancer Society (ACS), the AHA, and the American Diabetes Association announced a new collaborative initiative to create a national commitment to the prevention and early detection of cancer, cardiovascular disease, and diabetes [14].

The ACS recommends that screening for (1) breast cancer begins at age 20 and includes mammography from age 40 (at least annually), (2) cervical cancer begins no later than age 21 (Pap test), (3) colorectal cancer begins at age 50 (several options), and (4) prostate cancer begins at age 50 (prostate-specific antigen test and digital rectal examination annually) (Table 3).

The AHA recommends that assessment of cardiovascular risk begins at age 20 and is repeated at regular intervals, preferentially by calculating the Framingham Risk Score (Table 3) [14]. In contrast to cancer, early detection of CVD by screening with the best available technology is not mentioned, although CVD kills more individuals than all cancers combined. In the United States in the year 2001, 56,887 died from colorectoanal cancer, 41,809 from breast cancer, 30,719 from prostate

Table 3
General prevention guidelines for all average-risk adults (From [14])

American Cancer Society · American Diabetes Association. Cure • Care • Commitment® · American Heart Association. Learn and Live.

General Prevention Guidelines for All Average Risk Adults

Provide advice to patients on nutrition and physical activity:
- •Achieve and maintain a healthy weight.
- •Exercise for at least 30 minutes on 5 or more days a week.
- •Eat at least 5 servings of vegetables and fruits daily.

Ask patients about tobacco use and provide cessation counseling and pharmacotherapy.

TEST	AGE 20	30	40	50+
BMI	Each regular health care visit →			
Blood Pressure	Each regular health care visit (or at least once every 2 years if BP <120/80 mm HG →			
Lipid Profile	Every 5 years →			
Blood Glucose test			Every 3 years →	
Clinical Breast Exam (CBE) and Mammography	CBE every 3 years		Yearly CBE and Mammography →	
Pap test	Yearly	Every 1-3 years, depends on type of test and past results →		
Colorectal Screening				Frequency depends on test preferred →
Prostate specific antigen test and digital rectal exam				Offer yearly, assist informed decisions →

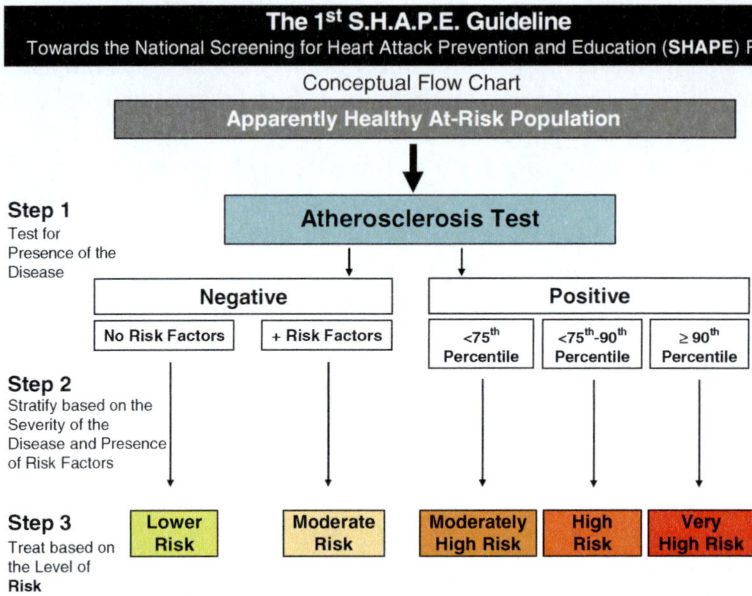

Fig. 4. Conceptual flow chart illustrating the principles of the new algorithm underlying the proposed screening for heart attack prevention and education (SHAPE) guidelines described in the executive summary of this report.

cancer and more than 500,000 from atherosclerosis [1]. It is thought-provoking that CVD kills more young and middle-aged women than breast cancer, yet the majority of such women are considered to be at low cardiovascular risk and left untreated based on current risk assessment by risk factor scoring [15]. It seems plausible that early detection of asymptomatic (preclinical) atherosclerosis by screening followed by appropriate treatment could prevent the devastating consequences of this disease.

THE TIME HAS COME

The time has come to reconsider our traditional, imprecise approach to individual risk assessment in primary prevention. In this book we propose a formal strategy for assessment of the risk of clinical CVD that is largely based on non-invasive screening for the disease itself (subclinical atherosclerosis) rather than its risk factors (Fig. 4). The purpose is to identify those who are susceptible to atherosclerosis and its thrombotic and arrhythmogenic complications (vulnerable patients) and initiate appropriate care to prevent heart attack, and to avoid treatment of those who don't need it.

REFERENCES

1. American Heart Association. Heart Disease and Stroke Statistics – 2004 Update. Dallas, TX, AHA 2003. Available at: http://www.americanheart.org/downloadable/heart/1079736729696HDSStats2004UpdateREV3-19-04.pdf

2. Wald NJ, Law M, Watt HC, Wu T, Bailey A, Johnson AM, Craig WY, Ledue TB, Haddow JE. Apolipoproteins and ischaemic heart disease: implications for screening. Lancet 1994;343:75–79.
3. Wald NJ, Hackshaw AK, Frost CD. When can a risk factor be used as a worthwhile screening test? BMJ 1999;319:1562–5.
4. Law MR, Wald NJ. Risk factor thresholds: their existence under scrutiny. BMJ 2002;324:1570–1576.
5. Law MR, Wald NJ, Morris JK. The performance of blood pressure and other cardiovascular risk factors as screening tests for ischaemic heart disease and stroke. J Med Screen 2004;11:3–7.
6. Greenland P, Knoll MD, Stamler J, Neaton JD, Dyer AR, Garside DB, Wilson PW. Major risk factors as antecedents of fatal and nonfatal coronary heart disease events. JAMA 2003;290:891–897.
7. Weissler AM. Traditional risk factors for coronary heart disease. JAMA 2004;291:299–300. Letter.
8. Wald NJ, Law MR. A strategy to reduce cardiovascular disease by more than 80%. BMJ 2003;326:1419
9. National Cholesterol Education Program (NCEP) Expert Panel on Detection, Evaluation, and Treatment of High Blood Cholesterol in Adults (Adult Treatment Panel III). Third Report of the National Cholesterol Education Program (NCEP) Expert Panel on Detection, Evaluation, and Treatment of High Blood Cholesterol in Adults (Adult Treatment Panel III) final report. Circulation 2002;106:3143–421. (http://circ.ahajournals.org/cgi/reprint/106/25/3143)
10. Smith SC Jr, Greenland P, Grundy SM. AHA Conference Proceedings. Prevention conference V: Beyond secondary prevention: Identifying the high-risk patient for primary prevention: executive summary. Circulation 2000;101:111–116.
11. De Backer G, Ambrosioni E, Borch-Johnsen K, Brotons C, Cifkova R, Dallongeville J, Ebrahim S, Faergeman O, Graham I, Mancia G, Manger Cats V, Orth-Gomer K, Perk J, Pyorala K, Rodicio JL, Sans S, Sansoy V, Sechtem U, Silber S, Thomsen T, Wood D; Third Joint Task Force of European and Other Societies on Cardiovascular Disease Prevention in Clinical Practice. European guidelines on cardiovascular disease prevention in clinical practice. Third Joint Task Force of European and Other Societies on Cardiovascular Disease Prevention in Clinical Practice. Eur Heart J 2003;24:1601–1610. (Full text available at: http://www.escardio.org/NR/rdonlyres/A0EF5CA5-421B-45EF-A65C-19B9EC411261/0/CVD_Prevention_03_full.pdf)
12. Grundy SM, Cleeman JI, Merz CN, Brewer HB Jr, Clark LT, Hunninghake DB, Pasternak RC, Smith SC Jr, Stone NJ. Implications of recent clinical trials for the National Cholesterol Education Program Adult Treatment Panel III guidelines. Circulation 2004;110:227–39.
13. Law MR, Watt HC, Wald NJ. The underlying risk of death after myocardial infarction in the absence of treatment. Arch Intern Med 2002;162:2405–10.
14. Preventing Cancer, Cardiovascular Disease, and Diabetes. A Common Agenda for the American Cancer Society, the American Diabetes Association, and the American Heart Association. Harmon Eyre, MD, Chief Medical Officer, American Cancer Society; Richard Kahn, PhD, Chief Scientific and Medical Officer, American Diabetes Association;Rose Marie Robertson, MD, FAHA, Chief Science Officer, American Heart Association; the ACS/ADA/AHA Collaborative Writing Committee *Circulation*. 2004;109:3244–3255.
15. Nasir K, Michos ED, Blumenthal RS, Raggi P. Detection of high-risk young adults and women by coronary calcium and National Cholesterol Education Program Panel III guidelines. J Am Coll Cardiol. 2005 Nov 15;46(10):1931–1936. Epub 2005 Oct 20.

I

Risk Factors and Circulating Markers of Asymptomatic Atherosclerotic Cardiovascular Disease

7 History of the Evolution of Cardiovascular Risk Factors and the Predictive Value of Traditional Risk-Factor-Based Risk Assessment

Amit Khera

Contents

Abstract

The near epidemic rise in cardiovascular disease deaths in the early and middle twentieth century necessitated a more complete understanding of the risk factors for these illnesses. Through histologic examinations, animal studies, clinical and geographical observations and, ultimately, through large, prospective epidemiologic studies, the major traditional risk factors for cardiovascular disease were discovered, which paved the way for successful public health programs and interventions over the past few decades. However, cardiovascular disease remains a formidable global health challenge, especially in developing countries, and the utility of traditional risk factors as targets of therapy does not equate to accuracy for disease prediction. As up to 20% of those affected by coronary heart disease have no traditional risk factors, and since risk factor levels between those with and without cardiovascular disease overlap significantly, individual risk factors are poor predictors of cardiovascular events. Global risk assessment in the form of multivariable equations, such as the Framingham Risk Score that incorporate multiple traditional risk factors, have improved accuracy and are well suited for population screening through office-based practices. Recently, many limitations of current risk assessment with modified Framingham algorithms have emerged, including poor calibration in various ethnic groups, misclassification of risk in young people and women, and potential missed opportunities for preventive efforts by focusing solely on short-term risk. While traditional risk factors will certainly form the cornerstone of future cardiovascular

From: *Asymptomatic Atherosclerosis: Pathophysiology, Detection and Treatment*
Edited by: M. Naghavi (ed.), DOI 10.1007/978-1-60327-179-0_7

risk assessment strategies, their utility will be enhanced by newly developed algorithms or paradigms for their use, or by incorporating novel risk factors and emerging risk assessment technologies into risk assessment.

Key words: Blood pressure; Cardiovascular disease; Cholesterol; Framingham risk score; Risk assessment; Risk factors

KEY POINTS

- Several lines of evidence have implicated traditional risk factors such as elevated cholesterol, high blood pressure, diabetes, and smoking in the development and complications of atherosclerotic disease.
- The cornerstone of the "high-risk" strategy of disease prevention is the ability to identify those at highest risk who warrant the most intensive treatment.
- The utility of traditional risk factors as targets of therapy does not equate to accuracy for disease prediction, and individual risk factors are poor predictors of cardiovascular disease.
- Global risk assessment in the form of multivariable equations that incorporate multiple traditional risk factors, such as the Framingham Risk Score, is currently the standard of care for risk assessment.
- Recently, many limitations of the Framingham Risk Score have emerged, including poor calibration in various ethnic groups, misclassification of risk in young people and women, and potential missed opportunities for preventive efforts by focusing solely on short-term risk.
- The use of newly developed algorithms involving traditional risk factors, incorporating novel risk factors in these algorithms, and the use of emerging risk assessment technologies will most likely enhance cardiovascular risk assessment strategies in the future.

CLINICAL CASE

KC is a 61-year-old Caucasian woman who presents for evaluation of her cardiovascular risk. Her 68-year-old sister was recently diagnosed with coronary artery disease, and she had to undergo coronary artery bypass surgery. KC has a history of hypertension that is reasonably controlled with diuretic therapy and a distant history of tobacco use, as well as a borderline elevated low-density lipoprotein cholesterol and low HDL cholesterol. How should she be evaluated and counseled about her risk for cardiovascular disease (CVD), including the need for pharmacologic therapy?

HISTORICAL PERSPECTIVE ON CARDIOVASCULAR RISK FACTORS

In the early part of the 1900s, several changes in U.S. society led to significant increases in CVD death rates, which reached their peak soon after WWII (Fig. 1) [1]. Similar trends were seen in Western European countries, and contributing factors included the transition to an urban, industrialized economy with accompanying changes in diet, and reductions in physical activity [2]. The impact of these social changes was accentuated by the concomitant decline in death rates from infectious diseases. Surprisingly, little was known at that time about the risk factors for coronary heart disease (CHD), the principal illness associated with the near epidemic rise in CVD death rates. It was anticipated that the identification of these factors could result in new strategies for the prevention of CVD. The use of epidemiologic methods had previously been implemented primarily in the study of infectious illness, but had not been applied to any significant degree for the study of CVD. In light of the significant public health impact of CVD, the U.S. Preventive Health Service initiated the development of an epidemiologic study of CVD in 1947 [3]. The town of Framingham, Massachusetts, a predominantly white, middle-class industrial and trading center 21 miles west of Boston was selected, and enrollment

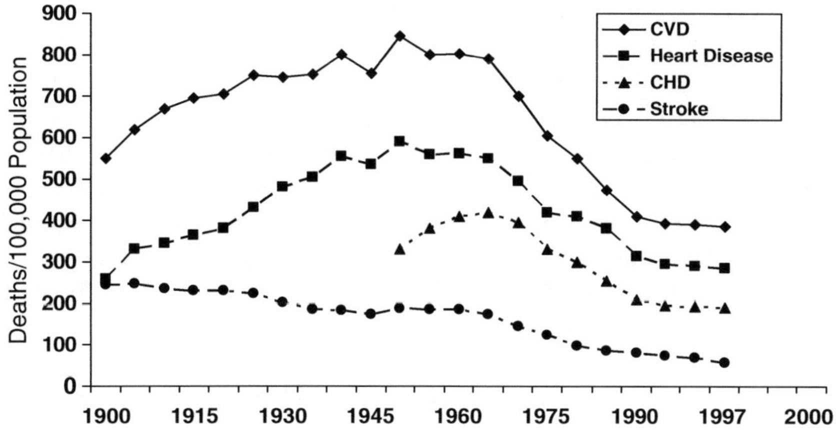

Fig. 1. Age-adjusted mortality rates from cardiovascular diseases in the U.S. 1900–1997. CVD indicates cardiovascular disease; CHD, coronary heart disease (from [1]).

of the 5,209 men and women began in 1948. Not long afterward in 1957, Ancel Keyes and colleagues embarked upon a large international collaborative effort known as the Seven Countries Study to evaluate inter- and intracountry determinants of heart disease [4].

Identifying Cardiovascular Disease Risk Factors

As the prototypical risk factor, serum cholesterol is now unequivocally linked to the development of atherosclerosis. The evolution of the acceptance of this risk factor has spanned almost two centuries and has encompassed many different sources of evidence. Early evidence came from Virchow's microscopic characterizations of atherosclerosis in the midnineteenth century, which included a description of the characteristic cholesterol crystals evident inside the plaques. In the early twentieth century, Anitschkow and colleagues revealed that atheroma could be experimentally induced in animals fed diets enriched with cholesterol [5]. The links between cholesterol and dietary fat levels with atherosclerosis were bolstered by numerous additional animal studies and observational reports in the first few decades of the twentieth century [6]. Around the same time, observations emerged about crosscountry differences in dietary cholesterol and fat consumption and the risk for atherosclerosis, with lower CVD prevalence in populations in Africa, Asia, and Latin America compared with those in Europe. The methods of ultracentrifugation also emerged soon after WWII and permitted characterization and quantification of lipoprotein subclasses. The early Framingham experience and the pooled experience from several smaller studies reported as the Cooperative Lipoprotein Study in the 1950s confirmed the association between serum cholesterol levels and incident CHD [7,8]. Yet, definitive evidence for a causal role of serum cholesterol came from the Lipid Research Clinics Coronary Primary Prevention Trial, which demonstrated reduced CHD events with lipid-lowering therapy [9].

Although awareness of hypertension dates back to at least 2,600 BC in ancient China, a reliable noninvasive measure of blood pressure was not developed until 1896 with the advent of the first mercury sphygmomanometer [10]. While early observations suggested that high blood pressure was associated with adverse cardiovascular consequences, others felt that hypertension was "essential" and in the words of Paul Dudley White, an "important compensation mechanism" [11]. Indeed, despite knowledge of longstanding high blood pressure, Franklin D. Roosevelt's physician proclaimed that his death from cerebral hemorrhage in 1945 "came out of the clear sky" [12]. However, findings from epidemiologic studies reported in the 1950s as well as the advent of effective medications to lower blood pressure around this time increased the acceptance of high blood pressure as a modifiable risk factor for CVD. Ultimate validation of high blood pressure as a CVD risk factor came from the Veterans Administration trials in the late 1960s and early 1970s that reported improved CVD outcomes in hypertensive patients treated with antihypertensive drugs [13].

In addition to cholesterol levels and high blood pressure, epidemiologic studies in the 1950s implicated smoking and obesity as correlates with CVD risk, and described the joint effects of these factors on the predisposition for CVD (Fig. 2) [8,14,15]. In 1959, the first public statement on CVD prevention and risk factors was presented, including mention of hypercholesterolemia, elevated blood pressure, smoking, obesity, and family history [16]. The original term "risk factor" was coined by Framingham Heart Study investigators in one of their initial manuscripts published in 1961 [14]. Subsequently, several large epidemiologic studies have evaluated the relationship between these traditional risk factors and CVD. The Seven Countries Study demonstrated that crosscountry differences in CVD rates were related to dietary consumption of saturated fats, while within population rates corresponded with serum cholesterol, blood pressure, and cigarette smoking [4]. In the U.S., the enormous (Multiple Risk Factor Intervention Trial) MRFIT program comprising 347,978 men followed from the late 1970s also demonstrated an association between serum cholesterol concentration, cigarette consumption, and blood pressure with CV events [17]. Several ongoing population-based cohort studies such as the Atherosclerosis Risk in Communities Study (ARIC) in the U.S. and MONICA (Multinational MONItoring of trends and determinants in CArdiovascular disease) studies in Europe have revealed similar findings and continue to contribute to our understanding of risk factors for CVD.

Cumulatively, these myriad investigations involving the laboratory, animal studies, clinical observations, and epidemiologic cohorts have laid the framework for what are now considered major

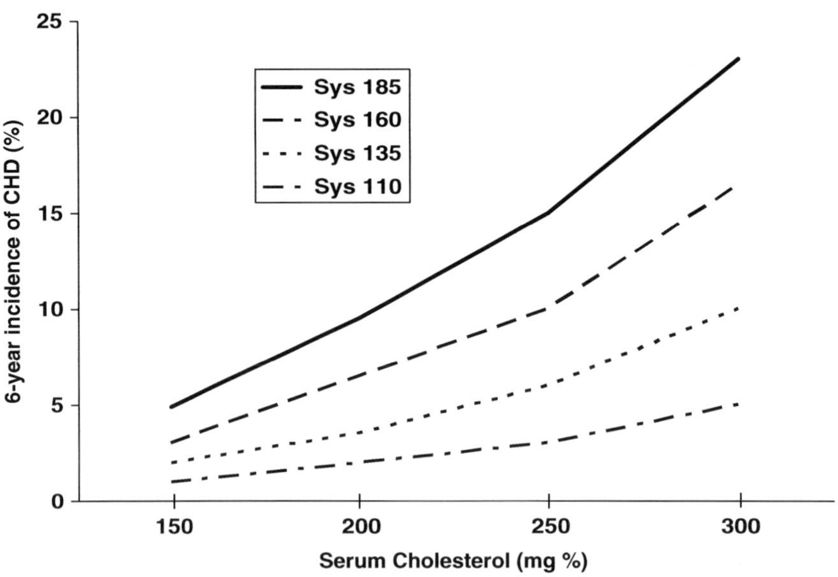

Fig. 2. Joint effects of serum cholesterol and systolic blood pressure on coronary heart disease rates in the Framingham Heart Study. Data are for men aged 44–62 years. CHD indicates coronary heart disease; Sys, systolic blood pressure. (from [14]).

Table 1
Risk factors for cardiovascular disease

Major risk factors	*Other risk factors*
Cigarette smoking	Obesity
Elevated blood pressure	Physical inactivity
Elevated serum total (and LDL) cholesterol	Dietary habits
Low serum HDL cholesterol	Family history of premature CHD
Diabetes mellitus	
Advancing age	

LDL Low-density lipoprotein, *HDL* High-density lipoprotein, *CHD* Coronary heart disease. (adapted from [37])

traditional risk factors for CVD (Table 1). Currently, more than 250 putative risk factors for CVD have been described, but most are markers of disease rather than having any causal relationship and lack the extensive evidence supporting a link to atherosclerosis as with the major traditional risk factors [18]. The identification of these major risk factors paved the way for preventive efforts to impact rates of CVD. The landmark Surgeon General report on adverse effects of smoking in 1964 hastened the significant decline in smoking rates in the 1960s and 1970s [19]. In addition, campaigns to reduce dietary fat intake in the 1960s and 1970s [20], to treat hypertension in the 1970s and 1980s [21], and to reduce blood lipid levels in the 1980s and 1990s [22] have made major contributions to the dramatic reduction of CVD death rates in the past half century.

The identification and the modification of traditional CV risk factors have been a tremendous public health success in the twentieth century. However, CVD remains the leading cause of death in economically developed nations and is emerging as a serious health epidemic in developing nations. As additional CVD prevention strategies are developed, it is important to note the distinction between the utility of traditional risk factors as targets of preventive strategies versus their utility as predictors of those who will be afflicted by CVD.

STRATEGIES FOR PREVENTION OF CARDIOVASCULAR DISEASE

Population-Based Strategy

Two different, but complementary approaches have been utilized for the prevention of CVD (Fig. 3) [23]. The *population-based* strategy attempts to shift the distribution of risk factors in the entire population to a lower average level (i.e., shifting the mean blood pressure), often utilizing public health measures, and has made a considerable impact upon the CVD death rates in the twentieth century. In support of this strategy, several studies have demonstrated that achieving optimal levels of multiple risk factors results in markedly lower rates of CVD [24–26]. Stamler et al. examined over 360,000 subjects from the MRFIT and Chicago Heart Association Detection Project in Industry studies and determined long-term outcomes in those with a low risk factor burden (serum cholesterol <200 mb/dl, blood pressure ≤120/80 mmHg, no current smoking, no diabetes, no myocardial infarction, normal ECG) [25]. Subjects with optimal levels of these risk factors had a 77–92% reduction in CHD death and an increase in life expectancy of 6–10 years compared with those without such profiles. The results of this and other similar studies suggest that shifting the distribution of risk factors in the

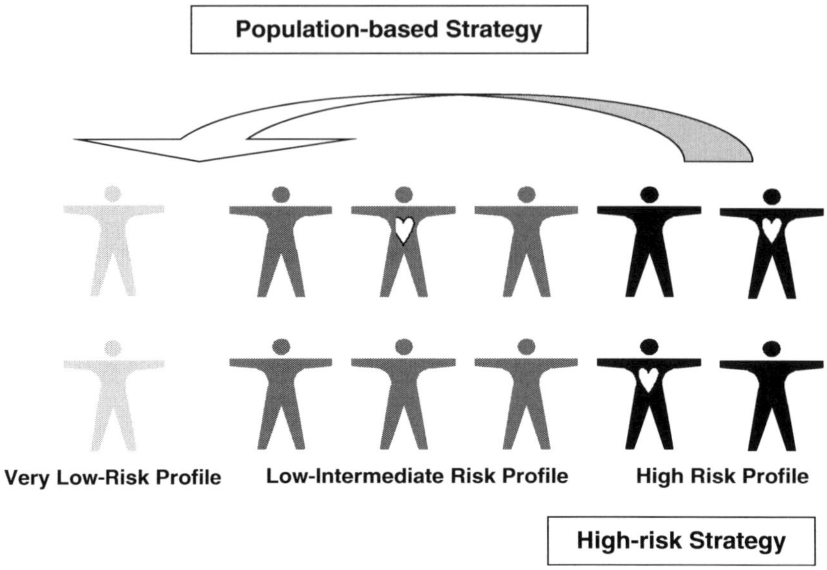

Fig. 3. Strategies for cardiovascular disease prevention. Population-based strategies shift the overall distribution of risk factors. High-risk strategies target those with high-risk profile.

population to optimal levels could have a major impact on CVD and should be the cornerstone of public health efforts for CVD prevention.

High-Risk Strategy

The population-based strategy also has many shortcomings. While the entire population is impacted by the preventive measures, only a small fraction would have actually been affected by disease, resulting in overtreatment of the majority of individuals. Such considerations are most relevant when pharmacologic therapies or other more aggressive measures are required to treat risk factors, resulting in an unfavorable risk-benefit ratio. An alternative preventive strategy for CVD is termed the *high-risk* strategy [23]. This approach involves setting a threshold of risk, and focusing treatment strategies on individuals who exceed this risk, such as treating blood pressure in a patient once they are considered hypertensive.

Traditional medical practice centers on this approach, which identifies patients with "illness" (or risk), thereby requiring treatment. There are several advantages to this strategy such as providing intervention that are appropriate to the individual, thereby creating a more favorable risk-benefit ratio. Importantly, this strategy also improves cost effectiveness of various therapies. For example, the cost per quality-adjusted life-year gained using HMG-CoA reductase inhibitors (statins) in primary prevention populations is estimated as $54,000–$1.4 million compared with $1800–$40,000 for secondary prevention populations that are at higher risk [27]. In addition, knowledge of underlying CV risk can enhance physician and patient motivation toward adopting preventive measures [28]. One major application of the high-risk strategy in CVD prevention is to determine appropriate candidates for pharmacologic lipid-lowering therapy use, where the intensity of treatment is matched to the level of risk [29]. However, the utility of the high-risk strategy in CVD prevention is predicated upon widely available, reliable measures of CV risk on which to base treatment decisions.

PREDICTIVE VALUE OF TRADITIONAL RISK FACTORS FOR CARDIOVASCULAR DISEASE

Individual Risk Factors and Risk Factor Counting

Although individual traditional risk factors may be associated with the development of CVD, they are generally poor discriminators of CV risk when used alone. One explanation for this observation is that the distribution of individual risk factors between those with and without CVD overlaps substantially (Fig. 4) [30]. In the Women's Health Study, although LDL cholesterol levels were associated with incident CV events, 46% of these events occurred in women with LDL levels below 130 mg/dl [31]. Similarly, approximately 32% of the excess coronary deaths related to blood pressure are related to values found within the "normal" range (<120/80 mmHg) [32].

One routinely used technique to evaluate the utility of risk assessment strategies is the receiver operating characteristic curve analysis (ROC). The area under the ROC curve (AUC) estimates the probability that the risk function will assign a higher value to those who will develop an event compared to those who will not [33]. Essentially, it assesses how well the risk factor or factors can *discriminate* between affected and unaffected persons with a value of 0.5 (or 50%) being no better than chance and a value of 1.0 being perfect discrimination. An analogous term for AUC is the c-statistic, and values in the range of 0.7–0.9 are considered good while values greater than 0.9 are considered excellent for discrimination. The c-statistic for individual risk factors such as lipid values and blood pressure generally ranges between 0.6 and 0.7 when used alone [34], which is suboptimal for clinical purposes.

An alternative strategy used by clinicians is to rely on the number of risk factors, or risk factor counting, to quantify risk and to determine the appropriateness of therapy. The hazards of this approach were demonstrated in analysis of more than 122,000 patients enrolled in clinical trials of CHD, including myocardial infarction, unstable angina, and percutaneous coronary intervention [35]. In this study, 15% of women and almost 20% of men had none of the four conventional CHD risk factors (hypercholesterolemia, hypertension, smoking, and diabetes) upon diagnosis of CHD at trial entry (Fig. 5). In addition, more than 50% of women and 60% of men had only 0 or 1 of these risk factors. In addition, there is considerable overlap in the risk factor prevalence between those with and without CHD death, as demonstrated in the Framingham Heart Study cohort. While approximately 90% of middle-aged subjects who died of CHD had ≥1 major risk factor, 75–85% of those free of CHD death also had at least one risk factor [36]. Thus, individual risk factors appear to have poor specificity for the prediction of CVD. Risk factor interactions are complex involving joint effects,

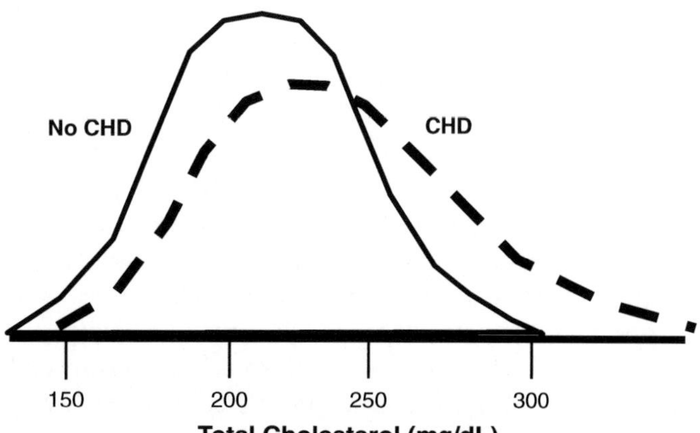

Fig. 4. Total cholesterol levels overlap significantly between those with and without coronary heart disease. Data are from 26-year follow-up of the Framingham Heart Study. CHD indicates coronary heart disease (adapted from [30]).

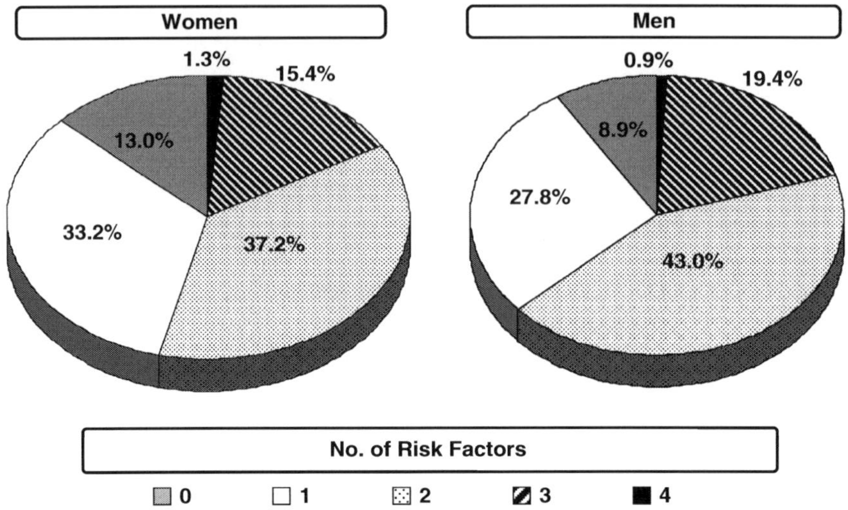

Fig. 5. Number of cardiovascular risk factors in patients with coronary heart disease. In an analysis of 122,458 patients enrolled in randomized clinical trials of coronary heart disease, 15.4% of women and 19.4% of men had none of the four major risk factors (hypertension, hypercholesterolemia, diabetes mellitus, current smoking) [35].

threshold levels, and multiplicative interactions that magnify CHD risk, requiring a more comprehensive approach to risk assessment.

Global Risk Assessment Equations

The limitations of individual risk factors for evaluation of CV risk have led to the concept of global risk assessment in the form of predictive equations [37]. These algorithms are mathematical functions derived from multivariable modeling of various weighted well-established risk factors, which provide a probability estimate of developing CVD in a given time period. The currently recommended standard for assessing CHD risk in the U.S. is the Framingham Risk Score (FRS) (Fig. 6a and b) [29,38]. It was derived from the Framingham Heart Study population and initially consisted of a point scoring system based on categories of age, total cholesterol (or LDL cholesterol), HDL cholesterol, systolic blood pressure, diabetes, and smoking status, with separate algorithms for men and women. The point total is converted into an estimate of the 10-year (short-term) risk of "soft" coronary events including angina pectoris, coronary insufficiency, myocardial infarction, and coronary death [38]. A modified version of this algorithm which does not incorporate diabetes status and which predicts 10-year risk of "hard" CHD endpoints (CHD death or myocardial infarction) was endorsed by the National Cholesterol Education Program Adult Treatment Panel III (NCEP-ATP III) report, and is the version predominantly used in clinical practice in the U.S. [29].

Other versions of the FRS have been developed for the prediction of stroke, peripheral vascular disease, and congestive heart failure [39–41]. More recently, the Framingham investigators have created a multivariable risk function for the assessment of composite CVD risk, including CHD and all these other components [42]. Several other risk functions have been developed for countries in Europe and Asia. In 2003, the European Society of Cardiology guidelines on CVD prevention presented a new global risk assessment algorithm called SCORE [43,44]. This risk function was developed from 12 European cohort studies and provides two separate scoring systems for countries with a lower and higher prevalence of CVD. While this algorithm incorporates the same traditional

a

Step 1: Age

Years	Points
20-34	-9
35-39	-4
40-44	0
45-49	3
50-54	6
55-59	8
60-64	10
65-69	11
70-74	12
75-79	13

Step 2: Total Cholesterol

TC (mg/dL)	Points at Age 20-39	Points at Age 40-49	Points at Age 50-59	Points at Age 60-69	Points at Age 70-79
<160	0	0	0	0	0
160-199	4	3	2	1	0
200-239	7	5	3	1	0
240-279	9	6	4	2	1
^{3}280	11	8	5	3	1

Step 3: HDL-Cholesterol

HDL-C (mg/dL)	Points
≥60	-1
50-59	0
40-49	1
<40	2

Step 4: Systolic Blood Pressure

Systolic BP (mm Hg)	Points if Untreated	Points if Treated
<120	0	0
120-129	0	1
130-139	1	2
140-159	1	2
≥160	2	3

Step 5: Smoking Status

	Points at Age 20-39	Points at Age 40-49	Points at Age 50-59	Points at Age 60-69	Points at Age 70-79
Nonsmoker	0	0	0	0	0
Smoker	8	5	3	1	1

Step 6: Adding Up the Points

Age	—
Total cholesterol	—
HDL-cholesterol	—
Systolic blood pressure	—
Smoking status	—
Point total	

Step 7: CHD Risk

Point Total	10-Year Risk
<0	<1%
0	1%
1	1%
2	1%
3	1%
4	1%
5	2%
6	2%
7	3%
8	4%
9	5%
10	6%
11	8%
12	10%
13	12%
14	16%
15	20%
16	25%
≥17	≥30%

Absolute 10-year risk of CHD death or MI

Fig. 6. (**a**) Framingham Risk Score algorithm for men. NCEP-ATPIII version of the Framingham Risk Score [29]. Ten-year risk of coronary heart disease death or myocardial infarction is calculated by adding points for age, total cholesterol, HDL-cholesterol, systolic blood pressure, and smoking status and comparing the summed point total to the 10-year risk percent. CHD indicates coronary heart disease; MI, myocardial infarction.

b

Step 1: Age

Years	Points
20-34	-7
35-39	-3
40-44	0
45-49	3
50-54	6
55-59	8
60-64	10
65-69	12
70-74	14
75-79	16

Step 2: Total Cholesterol

TC (mg/dL)	Points at Age 20-39	Points at Age 40-49	Points at Age 50-59	Points at Age 60-69	Points at Age 70-79
<160	0	0	0	0	0
160-199	4	3	2	1	1
200-239	8	6	4	1	1
240-279	11	8	5	3	2
^{3}280	13	10	7	4	2

Step 3: HDL-Cholesterol

HDL-C (mg/dL)	Points
≥60	-1
50-59	0
40-49	1
<40	2

Step 4: Systolic Blood Pressure

Systolic BP (mm Hg)	Points if Untreated	Points if Treated
<120	0	0
120-129	1	3
130-139	2	4
140-159	3	5
≥160	4	6

Step 5: Smoking Status

	Points at Age 20-39	Points at Age 40-49	Points at Age 50-59	Points at Age 60-69	Points at Age 70-79
Nonsmoker	0	0	0	0	0
Smoker	9	7	4	2	1

Step 6: Adding Up the Points

Age	—
Total cholesterol	—
HDL-cholesterol	—
Systolic blood pressure	—
Smoking status	—
Point total	

Step 7: CHD Risk

Point Total	10-Year Risk
<9	<1%
9	1%
10	1%
11	1%
12	1%
13	2%
14	2%
15	3%
16	4%
17	5%
18	6%
19	8%
20	11%
21	14%
22	17%
23	22%
24	27%
≥25	≥30%

Absolute 10-year risk of CHD death or MI

Fig. 6. (continued) (**b**) Framingham Risk Score algorithm for women.

risk factors as the FRS, it is calibrated more accurately for European populations and predicts 10-year risk of composite CVD death, thus expanding the focus from CHD but excluding nonfatal events.

The FRS has several desirable properties that led to its broad endorsement as the primary method for CV risk assessment in the U.S. and other countries [29,45]. This algorithm yields an overall c-statistic of approximately 0.75–0.80, which suggests reasonable ability to discriminate risk from a population perspective [38]. Its components are inexpensive to measure and it can be easily applied in an office-based setting with both paper and computer-based tools to facilitate its use [29]. The low cost and the ease of use of this tool by primary care providers are critical factors for any risk assessment strategy that is applied broadly to the general population. Also, the components of this score, except for age, are largely modifiable risk factors which are thought to be causal in the etiology of atherosclerosis.

Limitations of Traditional Risk Assessment Strategies

Despite the many advantages of the FRS, it also has several shortcomings as a method of assessing CV risk. While discrimination ability of 80% may be suitable from a population perspective, it may be suboptimal on an individual level. Also, the c-statistic may not adequately measure the true utility of this tool [46], or encompass its functionality in clinical practice. In addition, the currently used Framingham risk function was derived from the homogenous, predominantly white, middle-class population of Framingham, Massachusetts, which limits its generalizability to other populations including ethnic minorities. Other subgroups for which the FRS appears to have suboptimal performance include women and younger individuals. Finally, the focus on short-term risk may result in undertreatment and false reassurance of those with lower short-term, but high long-term risk.

Racial/Ethnic Groups

The FRS has been extensively evaluated in several different racial and ethnic groups. A comprehensive analysis by D'Agostino and colleagues examined its utility in 6 prospective, ethnically diverse cohorts consisting of over 23,000 participants and demonstrated reasonable consistency in performance between blacks and whites, although the c-statistics were slightly lower in blacks (Table 2) [47]. However, the FRS was poorly calibrated for risk assessment in Japanese Americans, Hispanics, and Native Americans, with significant overestimation of cardiovascular risk in these groups. Reports from Chinese and other

Table 2
Discrimination and calibration of Framingham risk score in ethnically diverse cohorts

	White				*Black*	*Japanese American*	*Hispanic*	*Native American*
	FHS	ARIC	PHS	CHS	ARIC	HHP	PR	SHS
Men								
c-statistic	0.79	0.75	0.63	0.63	0.67	0.72	0.69	0.69
χ^2 statistic		13.8		13.2	6.2	66.0	142.0	10.6
Women								
c-statistic	0.83	0.83		0.66	0.79			0.75
χ^2 statistic	3.7	5.3		10.4	5.0			22.7

Data represent unadjusted performance characteristics of the Framingham risk function in large cohort studies of different ethnic groups. Increasing values for the χ-statistic represent improved discrimination, while higher values for the χ^2 statistic signify worse calibration (>20=poor calibration)
FHS indicates Framingham Heart Study; ARIC, Atherosclerosis Risk in Communities Study; PHS, Physicians' Health Study; CHS, Cardiovascular Health Study; PR, Puerto Rico Heart Health Program; SHS, Strong Heart Study. (adapted from [47])

Asian populations have also described an overestimation of CHD risk using the FRS [48,49], although only limited assessments are available in those of South Asian descent [50]. Finally, studies of several European cohorts have similarly revealed overestimation of risk when applying the Framingham risk function to those populations, leading to the adoption of the SCORE algorithm [51,52].

Importantly, the FRS appears to have adequate discrimination in the aforementioned populations as measured by the c-statistic, in that it can order those with higher and lower risk appropriately. However, it is poorly calibrated in quantifying absolute risk in these groups as they vary widely in their average baseline risks for CVD, which greatly impacts the precision of short term risk estimation [47]. From a quantitative standpoint, simple statistical adjustments to recalibrate the Framingham function have improved its performance in most [49,51,53], but not in all the cohorts studied [54]. However, recalibrated algorithms for different demographic groups are not widely available for routine clinical practice, and the appropriateness of recalibration for different ethnic groups currently residing inside the U.S. is unknown. As such, the use of the FRS in patients of certain ethnic groups, such as those of Asian and Hispanic descent, must be viewed with caution for clinical decision making.

Young Individuals

Despite meeting statistical measures of utility, a study by Akosah et al. demonstrated the limitations of the FRS in a real-world setting as it pertains to younger adults [55]. The authors performed a retrospective study of 222 young men (≤55 years) and women (≤65 years) hospitalized in their institution with an acute myocardial infarction. After calculating 10-year risk based upon the FRS, only 12% of this cohort would have been considered high risk prior to their event, with 18% categorized as intermediate risk and 70% lower risk (Fig. 7). Furthermore, only 25% of men and 18% of women would have been eligible for statin therapy prior to their events based upon their risk categories and application of the NCEP ATPIII guidelines. These findings were supported by those of Nasir et al. demonstrating that greater than 76 and 61% of young individuals with moderate and high-risk levels of coronary artery calcium, respectively, would not qualify for lipid-lowering therapy based upon NCEP ATPIII and traditional risk assessment algorithms [56]. The discrepancy between CV risk implied by this marker and therapeutic recommendations in young individuals was of significantly greater magnitude than the discrepancy seen in older individuals.

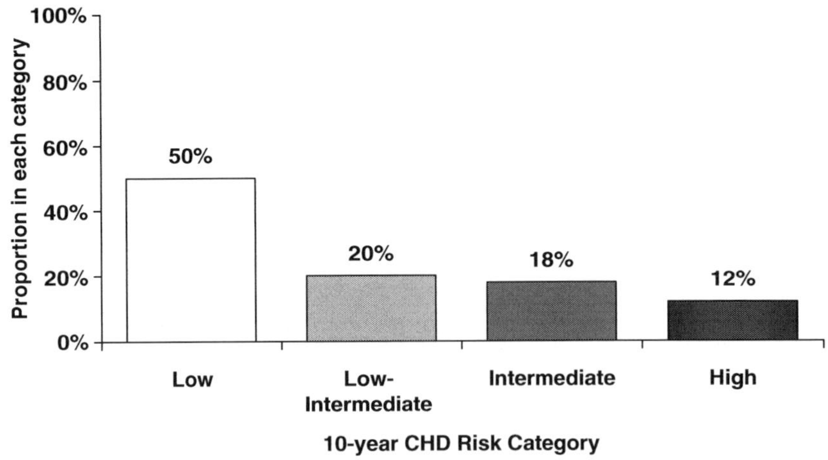

Fig. 7. Current cardiovascular risk assessment strategies underestimate risk in younger individuals. An analysis of 222 young men (age ≤55) and women (≤65) admitted with a myocardial infarction showed that 70% would have been categorized as lower risk and only 12% as high risk based upon the NCEP-ATP III risk assessment algorithm [55]. CHD indicates coronary heart disease.

While increasing age is the strongest risk factor for CVD, the heavy weighting of age in the Framingham algorithm can lead to misclassification of risk in younger individuals with a large risk factor burden. Indeed, Berry et al. demonstrated that in over 10,000 male subjects aged 30–39, the calculated FRS only exceeded the treatment threshold of >10% 10-year risk in those in the top decile of risk factor burden, despite substantial risk factor burden in those of lower deciles [57]. Certain young subjects, such as those with a strong family history of myocardial infarction, may also have risk that exceeds FRS estimates [58], but family history information is not incorporated in the Framingham algorithm.

Women

According to an analysis from the NHANES study, approximately 95% of women aged 20–79 without CHD or CHD equivalents are classified as low risk by the FRS algorithm compared with just 74% of similar age men (Fig. 8) [59]. While women generally develop CVD at later ages than men, this classification of risk by the FRS most likely underestimates the short-term risk of CVD in many women. In one study examining102 sisters of patients with premature CHD, 98% of these women were categorized as low risk by the FRS, although 12% had moderate risk coronary artery calcium scores (>100) and 6% had high-risk scores (>400) [56]. In addition, in the previously mentioned study by Nasir et al., 78 and 64% of women with intermediate and high-risk coronary artery calcium scores, respectively, would be ineligible for lipid-lowering therapy based on NCEP ATPIII guidelines, which rely on risk categorization by the FRS [56].

Due to these limitations, a novel risk score termed the Reynolds Risk Score was recently developed to enhance CV risk prediction in women [60]. This algorithm included traditional as well as emerging risk factors and improved measures of global fit and calibration compared with traditional Framingham algorithms, and demonstrated modest improvements in discrimination of CV events as measured by the c-statistic. In addition, this new model reclassified 40–50% of women categorized into the 5- <20% 10-year risk groups by FRS into higher or lower risk categories. Nevertheless, only a small proportion of all women (~10%) are within this 5–20% FRS range, and validation of this algorithm in women from other cohorts has not been performed [61].

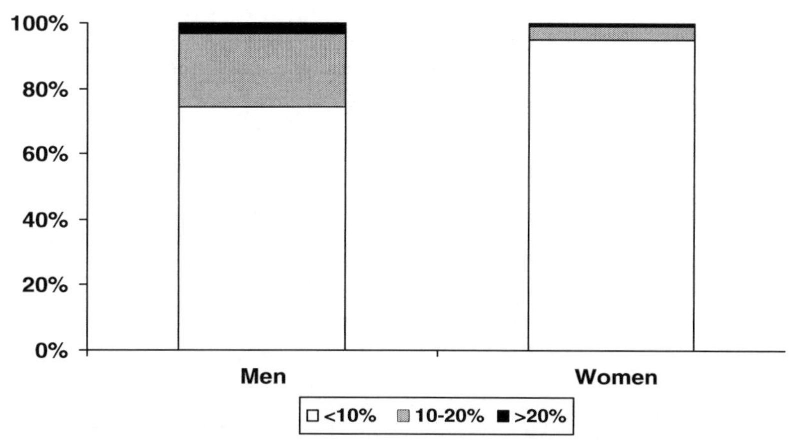

Fig. 8. Distribution of 10-year risk categories in men and women from NHANES 1999–2002. Ten-year risk of coronary heart disease events in men and women based upon the modified Framingham algorithm. Approximately 95% of women without coronary heart disease or coronary heart disease equivalents are categorized as low risk [59]. NHANES indicates National Health and Nutrition Examination Survey.

Short-Term Risk vs. Lifetime Risk

Most current CV risk assessment strategies including the FRS, SCORE algorithm, and others assess for near-term (i.e. 10-year) risk, which facilitates cost effectiveness and risk-benefit analyses of preventive strategies. While there are certain benefits to shorter-term estimates, solely focusing on the next decade may hinder opportunities for long-term risk reduction and foster a false sense of reassurance in those with low short-term, but high long-term risks.

Estimates from the Framingham Heart Study suggest that approximately 50% of men and 33% of women will develop CHD over their lifetimes starting from age 40 [62]. Most of those who eventually suffer from this illness will have been categorized as low short-term risk by the current FRS algorithm when applied at a younger age. Importantly, the traditional risk factors can be used to stratify long-term CV risks in both men and women (Fig. 9), and optimal levels of all major risk factors result in markedly low lifetime CVD risk (approximately 5% in men and 8% in women from age 50) [63]. Thus, assessment of lifetime risk using traditional risk factors may be a valuable adjunct to short-term CV risk assessment, especially since risk factor modification that begins earlier in life has been shown to magnify the long-term benefits [64].

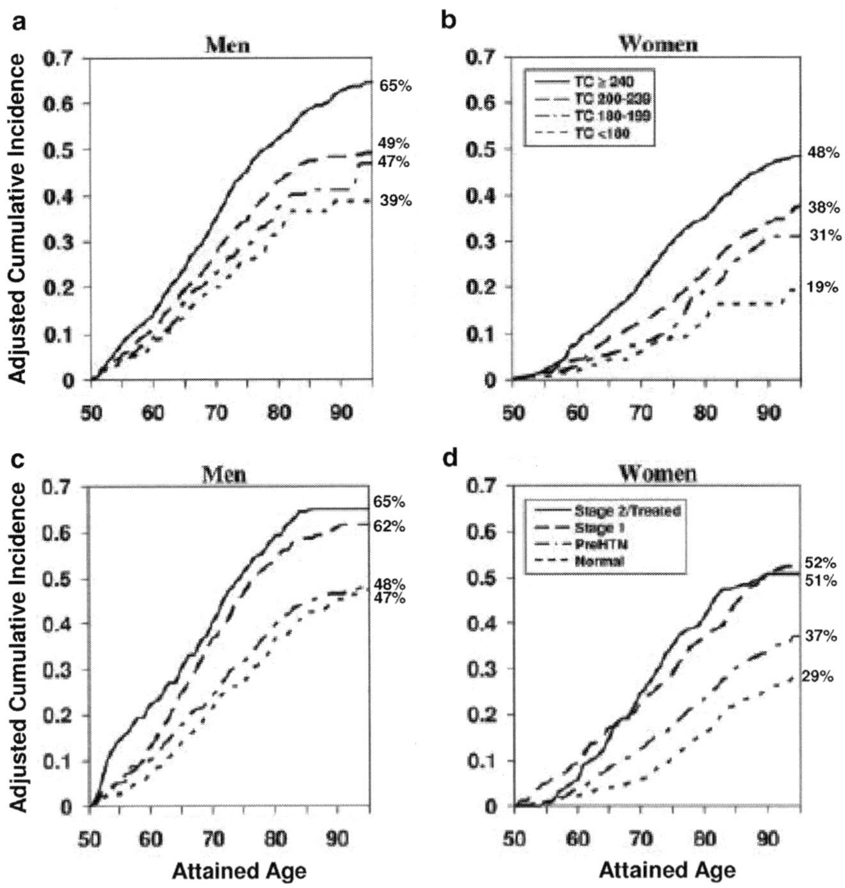

Fig. 9. Lifetime risk of cardiovascular disease is dependent upon traditional risk factor levels. The cumulative lifetime risk of cardiovascular disease in men and women from age 50 until 95 years in men and women is related to total cholesterol levels (**a** and **b**) and blood pressure category (**c** and **d**). TC indicates total cholesterol; HTN, hypertension (adapted from [63]).

CONCLUSIONS

Contributions from a range of investigative studies have culminated in the identification of the major traditional risk factors for CV disease over the past several decades. Interventions targeting these risk factors have yielded dramatic reductions in CV disease death rates, yet CV disease remains the leading cause of death in economically developed countries and is poised to become a major health epidemic in developing nations. Identifying those at highest risk for CV events will permit selectively targeting those in greatest need of risk reduction therapies, particularly pharmacologic agents. Global risk assessment using multiple risk factor equations such as the Framingham Risk Score have overcome some of the limitations of individual risk factors for CV risk assessment and have become the mainstay for risk assessment on the population level. However, a growing appreciation for the many shortcomings of traditional risk-factor-based risk assessment coupled with the identification of novel risk factors, emerging risk assessment technologies, and new concepts regarding earlier intervention, and lifelong risk evaluation are rapidly changing the landscape of cardiovascular risk prediction.

REFERENCES

1. Cooper R, Cutler J, Desvigne-Nickens P, et al. Trends and disparities in coronary heart disease, stroke, and other cardiovascular diseases in the United States: findings of the national conference on cardiovascular disease prevention. Circulation 2000;102(25):3137–47.
2. Gaziano JM. Global burden of cardiovascular disease. In: Zipes D, Libby P, Bonow R, Brauwnwald E, eds. Braunwald's Heart Disease. 7th ed. Philadelphia, PA: Elsevier; 2005:1–19.
3. Dawber TR, Meadors GF, Moore FE, Jr. Epidemiological approaches to heart disease: the Framingham Study. Am J Public Health 1951;41(3):279–81.
4. Keyes A, Aravanis C, Blackburn H, et al. Seven Countries. A Multivariate Analysis of Death and Coronary Heart Disease. Cambridge, MA: Harvard University Press; 1980.
5. Anitschkow N. Experimental arteriosclerosis in animals. In: Cowdry EV, ed. Arteriosclerosis. New York: Macmillan; 1933:271–322.
6. Stamler J. Established major coronary risk factors. In: Marmot M, Elliot P, eds. Coronary Heart Disease Epidemiology. Oxford: Oxford University Press; 1992:35–66.
7. Evaluation of serum lipoprotein and cholesterol measurements as predictors of clinical complications of atherosclerosis; report of a cooperative study of lipoproteins and atherosclerosis. Circulation 1956;14(4 Part 2):691–742.
8. Dawber TR, Moore FE, Mann GV. Coronary heart disease in the Framingham study. Am J Public Health 1957;47(4 Part 2):4–24.
9. The Lipid Research Clinics Coronary Primary Prevention Trial results. I. Reduction in incidence of coronary heart disease. JAMA 1984;251(3):351–64.
10. Basile JN, Ventura H. A historical look at hypertension: celebrating 100 years with the Southern Medical Association. South Med J 2006;99(12):1412–3.
11. White P. In: Heart disease. 2nd ed. New York: Mcmillan; 1937:326.
12. Messerli FH. This day 50 years ago. N Engl J Med 1995;332(15):1038–9.
13. Effects of treatment on morbidity in hypertension. Results in patients with diastolic blood pressures averaging 115 through 129 mm Hg. JAMA 1967;202(11):1028–34.
14. Kannel WB, Dawber TR, Kagan A, Revotskie N, Stokes J, 3rd. Factors of risk in the development of coronary heart disease – six year follow-up experience. The Framingham Study. Ann Intern Med 1961;55:33–50.
15. Hammond EC, Horn D. The relationship between human smoking habits and death rates: a follow-up study of 187,766 men. J Am Med Assoc 1954;155(15):1316–28.
16. White P, Sprague H, Stamler J, et al. A Statement on Arteriosclerosis, Main Cause of Heart Attacks and Strokes. New York: National Health Education Council; 1959.
17. Neaton JD, Kuller LH, Wentworth D, Borhani NO. Total and cardiovascular mortality in relation to cigarette smoking, serum cholesterol concentration, and diastolic blood pressure among black and white males followed up for five years. Am Heart J 1984;108(3 Pt 2):759–69.
18. Hopkins PN, Williams RR. A survey of 246 suggested coronary risk factors. Atherosclerosis 1981;40(1):1–52.
19. US Department of Health Education and Welfare PHSP. Smoking and Health: Report of the Advisory Committee to the Surgeon General of the Public Health Service. Washington, DC: US Government Printing Office; 1964.

20. American Heart Association, Central Committee for Medical and Community Programs. Dietary Fat and its Relation to Heart Attacks and Stroke. New York: American Heart Association; 1961.
21. National Conference on High Blood Pressure Education, National Heart and Lung Institute. DHEW Publication (NIH) 73–486. Washington, DC: US Government Printing Office; 1973.
22. National Cholesterol Education Program. High blood cholesterol in adults: report of the expert panel on detection, evaluation, and treatment. NIH Pub. No. 88–2925. Bethesda, MD: National Heart, Lung, and Blood Institute; 1988.
23. Rose G. Sick individuals and sick populations. Int J Epidemiol 1985;14(1):32–8.
24. Daviglus ML, Stamler J, Pirzada A, et al. Favorable cardiovascular risk profile in young women and long-term risk of cardiovascular and all-cause mortality. JAMA 2004;292(13):1588–92.
25. Stamler J, Stamler R, Neaton JD, et al. Low risk-factor profile and long-term cardiovascular and noncardiovascular mortality and life expectancy: findings for 5 large cohorts of young adult and middle-aged men and women. JAMA 1999;282(21):2012–8.
26. Stampfer MJ, Hu FB, Manson JE, Rimm EB, Willett WC. Primary prevention of coronary heart disease in women through diet and lifestyle. N Engl J Med 2000;343(1):16–22.
27. Prosser LA, Stinnett AA, Goldman PA, et al. Cost-effectiveness of cholesterol-lowering therapies according to selected patient characteristics. Ann Intern Med 2000;132(10):769–79.
28. Kalia NK, Miller LG, Nasir K, Blumenthal RS, Agrawal N, Budoff MJ. Visualizing coronary calcium is associated with improvements in adherence to statin therapy. Atherosclerosis 2006;185(2):394–9.
29. Executive summary of the third report of The National Cholesterol Education Program (NCEP) Expert panel on detection, evaluation, and treatment of high blood cholesterol in Adults (Adult Treatment Panel III). JAMA 2001;285(19):2486–97.
30. Castelli WP. Lipids, risk factors and ischaemic heart disease. Atherosclerosis 1996;124 Suppl:S1–9.
31. Ridker PM, Rifai N, Rose L, Buring JE, Cook NR. Comparison of C-reactive protein and low-density lipoprotein cholesterol levels in the prediction of first cardiovascular events. N Engl J Med 2002;347(20):1557–65.
32. Stamler J, Stamler R, Neaton JD. Blood pressure, systolic and diastolic, and cardiovascular risks. US population data. Arch Intern Med 1993;153(5):598–615.
33. Hanley JA, McNeil BJ. The meaning and use of the area under a receiver operating characteristic (ROC) curve. Radiology 1982;143(1):29–36.
34. Danesh J, Wheeler JG, Hirschfield GM, et al. C-reactive protein and other circulating markers of inflammation in the prediction of coronary heart disease. N Engl J Med 2004;350(14):1387–97.
35. Khot UN, Khot MB, Bajzer CT, et al. Prevalence of conventional risk factors in patients with coronary heart disease. JAMA 2003;290(7):898–904.
36. Greenland P, Knoll MD, Stamler J, et al. Major risk factors as antecedents of fatal and nonfatal coronary heart disease events. JAMA 2003;290(7):891–7.
37. Grundy SM, Pasternak R, Greenland P, Smith S, Jr., Fuster V. Assessment of cardiovascular risk by use of multiple-risk-factor assessment equations: a statement for healthcare professionals from the American Heart Association and the American College of Cardiology. Circulation 1999;100(13):1481–92.
38. Wilson PW, D'Agostino RB, Levy D, Belanger AM, Silbershatz H, Kannel WB. Prediction of coronary heart disease using risk factor categories. Circulation 1998;97(18):1837–47.
39. Kannel WB, D'Agostino RB, Silbershatz H, Belanger AJ, Wilson PW, Levy D. Profile for estimating risk of heart failure. Arch Intern Med 1999;159(11):1197–204.
40. Murabito JM, D'Agostino RB, Silbershatz H, Wilson WF. Intermittent claudication. A risk profile from The Framingham Heart Study. Circulation 1997;96(1):44–9.
41. Wolf PA, D'Agostino RB, Belanger AJ, Kannel WB. Probability of stroke: a risk profile from the Framingham Study. Stroke 1991;22(3):312–8.
42. D'Agostino RB, Sr., Vasan RS, Pencina MJ, et al. General cardiovascular risk profile for use in primary care: the Framingham Heart Study. Circulation 2008;117:743–53.
43. De Backer G, Ambrosioni E, Borch-Johnsen K, et al. European guidelines on cardiovascular disease prevention in clinical practice. Third Joint Task Force of European and other societies on Cardiovascular Disease Prevention in Clinical Practice. Eur Heart J 2003;24(17):1601–10.
44. Graham I, Atar D, Borch-Johnsen K, et al. European guidelines on cardiovascular disease prevention in clinical practice: full text Fourth Joint Task Force of the European Society of Cardiology and other societies on cardiovascular disease prevention in clinical practice (constituted by representatives of nine societies and by invited experts). Eur J Cardiovasc Prev Rehabil 2007;14(Suppl 2):S1–113.
45. Pearson TA, Blair SN, Daniels SR, et al. AHA guidelines for primary prevention of cardiovascular disease and stroke: 2002 Update: consensus panel guide to comprehensive risk reduction for adult patients without coronary or other atherosclerotic vascular diseases. American Heart Association Science Advisory and Coordinating Committee. Circulation 2002;106(3):388–91.
46. Cook NR. Use and misuse of the receiver operating characteristic curve in risk prediction. Circulation 2007;115(7):928–35.
47. D'Agostino RB, Sr., Grundy S, Sullivan LM, Wilson P. Validation of the Framingham coronary heart disease prediction scores: results of a multiple ethnic groups investigation. JAMA 2001;286(2):180–7.

48. Barzi F, Patel A, Gu D, et al. Cardiovascular risk prediction tools for populations in Asia. J Epidemiol Community Health 2007;61(2):115–21.
49. Liu J, Hong Y, D'Agostino RB, Sr., et al. Predictive value for the Chinese population of the Framingham CHD risk assessment tool compared with the Chinese Multi-Provincial Cohort Study. JAMA 2004;291(21):2591–9.
50. Bhopal R, Fischbacher C, Vartiainen E, Unwin N, White M, Alberti G. Predicted and observed cardiovascular disease in South Asians: application of FINRISK, Framingham and SCORE models to Newcastle Heart Project data. J Public Health (Oxf) 2005;27(1):93–100.
51. Brindle P, Emberson J, Lampe F, et al. Predictive accuracy of the Framingham coronary risk score in British men: prospective cohort study. BMJ 2003;327(7426):1267.
52. Hense HW, Schulte H, Lowel H, Assmann G, Keil U. Framingham risk function overestimates risk of coronary heart disease in men and women from Germany – results from the MONICA Augsburg and the PROCAM cohorts. Eur Heart J 2003;24(10):937–45.
53. Marrugat J, Subirana I, Comin E, et al. Validity of an adaptation of the Framingham cardiovascular risk function: the VERIFICA Study. J Epidemiol Community Health 2007;61(1):40–7.
54. Wu Y, Liu X, Li X, et al. Estimation of 10-year risk of fatal and nonfatal ischemic cardiovascular diseases in Chinese adults. Circulation 2006;114(21):2217–25.
55. Akosah KO, Schaper A, Cogbill C, Schoenfeld P. Preventing myocardial infarction in the young adult in the first place: how do the National Cholesterol Education Panel III guidelines perform? J Am Coll Cardiol 2003;41(9):1475–9.
56. Nasir K, Michos ED, Blumenthal RS, Raggi P. Detection of high-risk young adults and women by coronary calcium and National Cholesterol Education Program Panel III guidelines. J Am Coll Cardiol 2005;46(10):1931–6.
57. Berry JD, Lloyd-Jones DM, Garside DB, Greenland P. Framingham risk score and prediction of coronary heart disease death in young men. Am Heart J 2007;154(1):80–6.
58. Philips B, de Lemos JA, Patel MJ, McGuire DK, Khera A. Relation of family history of myocardial infarction and the presence of coronary arterial calcium in various age and risk factor groups. Am J Cardiol 2007;99(6):825–9.
59. Ajani UA, Ford ES. Has the risk for coronary heart disease changed among U.S. adults? J Am Coll Cardiol 2006;48(6):1177–82.
60. Ridker PM, Buring JE, Rifai N, Cook NR. Development and validation of improved algorithms for the assessment of global cardiovascular risk in women: the Reynolds Risk Score. JAMA 2007;297(6):611–9.
61. Ford ES, Giles WH, Mokdad AH, Myers GL. Distribution and correlates of C-reactive protein concentrations among adult US women. Clin Chem 2004;50(3):574–81.
62. Lloyd-Jones DM, Larson MG, Beiser A, Levy D. Lifetime risk of developing coronary heart disease. Lancet 1999;353(9147):89–92.
63. Lloyd-Jones DM, Liu K, Tian L, Greenland P. Narrative review: assessment of C-reactive protein in risk prediction for cardiovascular disease. Ann Intern Med 2006;145(1):35–42.
64. Cohen JC, Boerwinkle E, Mosley TH, Jr., Hobbs HH. Sequence variations in PCSK9, low LDL, and protection against coronary heart disease. N Engl J Med 2006;354(12):1264–72.

8 Comprehensive Lipid Profiling Beyond LDL

Benoit J. Arsenault, S. Matthijs Boekholdt, John J.P. Kastelein, and Jean-Pierre Després

CONTENTS

ABSTRACT

Although many trials have documented the benefits of lowering plasma LDL cholesterol levels for the primary and secondary prevention of cardiovascular disease (CVD), about two thirds of CVD cases cannot be prevented. As CVD morbidity and mortality rates continue to increase in developed and developing societies, despite several improvements in CVD management, this observation suggests that other risk factors beyond LDL cholesterol and other traditional CVD risk factors may yield new insights into the assessment and management of CVD risk. It is now well-recognized that abdominally obese and insulin-resistant individuals have a strong tendency to develop a typical dyslipidemia that is independent of LDL cholesterol levels. This typical dyslipidemia has been called "atherogenic" dyslipidemia in the ATP-III guidelines, which is in fact a misnomer because it implies that other dyslipidemias are not atherogenic. This atherogenic dyslipidemia usually accompanies a high intra-abdominal or visceral adipose tissue (VAT) accumulation and is often associated with elevated plasma levels of triglycerides and apolipoprotein B

From: *Asymptomatic Atherosclerosis: Pathophysiology, Detection and Treatment*
Edited by: M. Naghavi (ed.), DOI 10.1007/978-1-60327-179-0_8

and with decreased HDL cholesterol and apolipoprotein A-I concentrations. It is also associated with an increased preponderance of small, dense LDL particles which have a stronger tendency to undergo oxidation, even among individuals with plasma LDL cholesterol levels in the normal range. Altogether, these observations suggest that currently available algorithms might not necessarily identify these abdominally obese and dyslipidemic individuals at increased CVD risk. The so-called "hypertriglyceridemic waist" phenotype, on the basis of a simple measurement of waist circumference in combination with plasma triglyceride levels, is a simple tool that can be easily used by general practitioners to identify people carrying atherogenic metabolic abnormalities which put them at increased CVD risk.

Key words: LDL-cholesterol; LDL-size; Apolipoprotein B; Abdominal obesity; Metabolic syndrome; Dyslipidemia

KEY POINTS

- Intra-abdominal adipose tissue accumulation is the most prevalent cause of the metabolic syndrome and is commonly associated with the high-triglyceride, low-HDL atherogenic dyslipidemia
- Even in the presence of LDL cholesterol levels in the normal range, individuals with abnormal LDL physicochemical properties are at increased CVD risk
- The apoB/apoAI ratio represents a marker of lipid abnormalities that may provide information on CVD risk beyond traditional lipid variables
- The hypertriglyceridemic waist phenotype represents a simple and useful tool in clinical practice for the initial screening of individuals likely to have features of the metabolic syndrome, an often under-diagnosed and puzzling CVD risk factor.

INTRODUCTION

Two patients are in the waiting room of a primary care center. They both have their annual appointments with their family doctor. The first patient is 42 years old; is a construction worker; does not smoke and exercises on a regular basis. He has a body-mass index (BMI) of 27 kg/m^2, a waist circumference of 94 cm, plasma LDL cholesterol concentrations in the normal range, and a negative family history for CVD. His physician calculates his Framingham risk score and estimates that he has a 10-year risk of 4%, putting him in the low-risk category. After having congratulated his patient for his low Framingham risk score and for his relatively healthy lifestyle, the doctor invites the second patient into his office. This man is also in his early forties and has a BMI comparable to that of the first patient with a slightly elevated waist circumference (100 cm). The second patient is a businessman; is under a lot of stress;and he spends an average of 60 h per week at the office. He does not have time to exercise and has no other choice but to eat rapidly available, energy-dense, fast food. His LDL cholesterol concentration is similar to that of the first patient and his systolic blood pressure is slightly elevated. The table charts suggest that this patient has a Framingham risk score of 6%, also putting him in the low risk category. However, despite this low Framingham score, this patient complains of sporadic chest pain on exercise, chronic thirst and vision problems, and the physician also notices that his patient was completely out of breath after having finished tying his shoelaces. This patient presented clear signs of coronary artery disease and of insulin resistance; clinical manifestations that the Framingham risk score completely failed to identify. Looking back at his two previous patients, this family physician had several questions in mind: How can two middle-aged individuals with comparable BMIs and essentially similar Framingham risk scores show such disparate clinical manifestations? Can body composition or lifestyle habits affect this relationship to such an extent? Can other CVD risk factors/markers explain this discrepancy? Can I, as a family physician with a limited budget, obtain information about CVD risk factors to better identify people at cardiovascular risk?

In the next section we will address these questions by discussing the lipid and other metabolic abnormalities that promote atherogenesis in an LDL-independent manner.

Throughout the next sections, it should become obvious to the reader that patients who arrive at the clinic with an elevated waist circumference and insulin resistance are at increased risk because they have an increased accumulation of visceral adipose tissue (VAT), the most prevalent cause of the metabolic syndrome and of the "LDL-independent" dyslipidemia.

PATHOPHYSIOLOGICAL EVIDENCE CONNECTING INTRA-ABDOMINAL ADIPOCYTES, INSULIN RESISTANCE, ECTOPIC FAT DEPOSITION AND THE ATHEROGENIC DYSLIPIDEMIA

There is now considerable pathophysiological evidence indicating that adipocytes located in the intra-abdominal cavity (omental, mesenteric, perirenal, etc.) have different metabolic properties compared to adipocytes located in subcutaneous depots (truncal, gluteal, femoral, etc.) [1]. Obese pre-menopausal women generally store excess energy in subcutaneous depots. These "healthy," small-sized and insulin sensitive adipocytes are known to be highly competent in storing circulating triglycerides and are therefore associated with a normal metabolic profile, even in the presence of a positive daily energy balance [2]. On the other hand, men and post-menopausal women have a greater genetic and hormonal predisposition for storing excess energy in intra-abdominal depots. This body fat distribution is associated with an increased risk of developing type 2 diabetes and CVD, even in the presence of a "normal" BMI.

As the role of adipose tissue as an endocrine organ is increasingly recognized, the distinctive patterns of adipokine secretion of visceral and subcutaneous depots have been studied extensively. Dysfunctional adipose tissue, as localized in VAT, secretes a number of inflammatory markers such as tumor necrosis factor-α (TNF-α) and interleukin-6 (IL-6), which in turn promote the hepatic secretion of C-reactive protein (CRP), an acute phase inflammation marker that is strongly associated with CVD risk [3]. It is now also well-recognized that the pro-inflammatory state observed in individuals with an increased VAT accumulation is a direct cause of macrophage infiltration of VAT, a phenomenon associated with adipose tissue hypoxia and impaired blood flow through adipose tissue that is not observed in subcutaneous obesity [4]. Among other adipose tissue-derived hormones, plasma levels of adiponectin are decreased in visceral obesity. This adipokine, which is by far the most abundant of all adipose-tissue derived circulating hormones, improves endothelial function by decreasing monocyte adhesion, foam cell formation and smooth muscle cell migration and proliferation, and by increasing nitric oxide production in the vessel wall. Many prospective studies have shown that adiponectin, together with low plasma HDL cholesterol levels are predictive of increased CVD risk [5]. As adiponectin decreases glucose production in the liver and increases β-oxidation of fatty acids and glucose transport in the skeletal muscle, hypoadiponectinemia is frequently observed in insulin-resistant individuals. Adiponectin promotes the proliferation of small and insulin-sensitive adipocytes, a process known as adipogenesis, through the activation of the nuclear receptor peroxisome-proliferator activated receptor-γ (PPAR-γ). This process is decreased by inflammatory markers such as TNF-α which directly inhibit the expression of the adiponectin gene. As opposed to TNF-α, adiponectin decreases IL-6 expression and reduces apoptosis in adipose tissue, a process likely to prevent the enlargement of adipocytes. As enlarged adipocytes show poor insulin sensitivity and enhanced lipolysis, adiponectin plays important paracrine and autocrine roles in adipose tissue [6]. As insulin is essential for triglyceride storage in adipose tissue, insulin resistance in intra-abdominal adipocytes reduces lipoprotein lipase (LPL) activity, a crucial regulator of chylomicron and very low-density lipoproteins (VLDL) catabolism. This decreased LPL activity is largely responsible for the exaggerated postprandial hypertriglyceridemia observed in abdominally obese, insulin-resistant people. The cardiovascular complications associated with obesity are therefore thought to be exacerbated during the postprandial state, which is present during the majority of the day among people in developed societies [7]. The acylation-stimulating protein (ASP) is another enzyme that enhances postprandial triglyceride clearance and facilitates glucose uptake in adipocytes [8]. ASP also efficiently reduces catecholamine-stimulated non-esterified fatty acids (NEFA) release from adipocytes. Although ASP activity or concentration has not clearly been investigated in the context of VAT, it is reasonable to believe that VAT might be associated with a defect in ASP action. Adipose tissue insulin resistance also increases hormone sensitive lipase (HSL) activity, which enhances lipolysis in adipocytes, a process that increases the flux of NEFA to the liver via the portal vein [9]. This "portal theory" is the common denominator between VAT accumulation and hepatic, intramyocellular and epicardial fat deposition, a phenomenon also known as ectopic fat deposition [10]. A fatty liver is associated with many pathophysiological abnormalities, such as increased triglyceride synthesis and their secretion in large, triglyceride-enriched VLDL particles as well as increased production of glucose, CRP and apolipoprotein B (apoB). Degradation of apoB and insulin are also reduced in the fatty liver, leading to increased plasma levels of apoB and insulin [11]. The increased plasma levels of triglyceride, apoB, NEFAs, insulin, glucose and CRP observed in abdominally obese subjects could therefore be the consequences of the increased portal flux of NEFAs from the expanded visceral fat depot to the liver.

The hepatic nuclear receptor PPAR-α is a key regulator of the lipoprotein–lipid metabolism [12]. Its activation by either fatty acids or fibric acid derivatives increases the expression of a cluster of genes including apolipoprotein AI (apoAI), apolipoprotein AII (apoAII) and LPL and reduces the expression of apolipoprotein CIII (apoCIII), a potent inhibitor of LPL. Activation of PPAR-α in the liver also increases cellular NEFA oxidation and inhibits VLDL secretion. In macrophages, fibric acid derivatives have been shown to increase the expression of SR-B1/CLA-1, increasing HDL-receptor activity and stimulating reverse cholesterol transport to the liver. Thus, PPAR-α activation merits further consideration, as its role in counteracting the high triglyceride, low-HDL dyslipidemia might represent an interesting pathway to decrease CVD risk in subjects with "on target" LDL cholesterol levels.

BEYOND LDL CHOLESTEROL: THE IMPORTANCE OF PHYSICOCHEMICAL PROPERTIES OF LDL PARTICLES IN THE DEVELOPMENT OF ATHEROSCLEROSIS

It is now well-recognized that early phases of atherosclerosis are characterized by endothelial dysfunction, a condition highly correlated with increased blood pressure and metabolic syndrome [13]. This clinical phenotype is thought to create an attractive environment for lipid-loaded macrophages and for naturally or enzymatically-modified, atherogenic LDL particles. Epidemiological evidence tells us that the risk of developing CVD is strongly and positively associated with LDL levels. However, in reality, not every patient with elevated LDL cholesterol levels develops CVD, nor does every patient with on-target plasma LDL levels remain free of CVD. Part of this inconsistency may be explained by heterogeneity of LDL particles. Over the last 15 years, many investigations have established the notion that small, dense LDL particles are an important risk factor for atherosclerosis [14]. Small, dense LDL particles, also known as LDL pattern B (LDL size <255 Å) are observed in the context of hypertriglyceridemia and low HDL cholesterol concentration. The enhanced hepatic VLDL production observed in the context of VAT and ectopic fat deposition, along with the decreased LPL activity observed under these circumstances contribute to the elevation of circulating triglycerides during both the fasting and the postprandial state. Triglyceride concentrations are by far the best correlate of LDL particle size [15]; in fact, individuals with triglyceride levels below 1.7 mmol/l are almost invariably characterized by the absence of small dense LDL in the circulation. Hypertriglyceridemia increases plasma concentrations of remnant-like particles, which also promote endothelial dysfunction and an increase in circulating small, dense LDL particles [16]. Moreover, hepatic lipase (HL) is another enzyme that may contribute to the small, dense LDL phenotype. HL, which activity is also increased in abdominal obesity, hydrolyzes triglycerides and phospholipids in LDL and HDL particles, thereby reducing mean LDL particle size and reducing HDL2 cholesterol levels, the most anti-atherogenic fraction of HDL particles [17]. In addition, hypertriglyceridemia facilitates cholesteryl-ester transfer protein (CETP) mediated exchange of cholesteryl ester against triglycerides between HDL and apoB-containing particles, a process than does not require energy [18]. As a result, LDL and HDL particles become enriched in triglycerides and as a consequence, good substrates for HL activity, which results in the formation of small and dense LDL and HDL particles. Biological consequences of small, dense LDL are summarized below. As small, dense HDL particles are likely to be excreted by the kidney (contributing to reduced plasma HDL cholesterol levels), these altered HDL particles cannot exert their anti-atherogenic effects (which are summarized in the next section). Although LDL particle size is influenced by various environmental factors as described above, it is of great interest to mention that heritability studies and other methods applied in genetic epidemiology have suggested that at least 30% of LDL particle size is genetically influenced [19].

Small, dense LDL particles have a reduced affinity for the LDL receptor [20]. As a consequence, their plasma half-life becomes longer, which makes these particles more susceptible to oxidation. In addition, small dense LDL particles undergo oxidation more easily than normal LDL particles. It has already been shown that VAT accumulation and the secretory phospholipase A2-IIA, which is thought to hydrolyze phospholipids at the surface of LDL particles, are strongly associated with the presence of both small dense LDL and oxidized LDL (oxLDL). Oxidation of LDL particles increases their atherogenic potential because they are more readily incorporated into macrophages, leading to foam cell formation, which in turn enhances various pro-atherogenic and chronic inflammatory pathways in the vessel wall [21]. In patients with an acute coronary syndrome or coronary artery disease, dysfunctional endothelium contains not only oxLDL, but also antibodies against the oxidized form of LDL particles, as opposed to normal arteries [22].

OxLDLs are toxic to endothelial cells and together with reactive oxygen species (ROS) may initiate an inflammatory response through the activation of the nuclear factor-κB pathway. The balance between "normal" and oxLDL is determined by many factors such as the scavenging capacity of the antioxidant defense system, and the balance between pro-oxidant agents such as myeloperoxidase, lipoxygenase and ROS and anti-oxidants like flavonoids, Co enzyme Q10 and β-carotene [23]. In people with either hyperglycemia and/or insulin resistance, LDL particles are also likely to be glycated by advanced glycation ends (AGEs), which slows LDL catabolism in a similar manner as observed for small dense LDLs and oxLDLs. Glycoxidation of LDL particles can also occur when glycation and oxidation act synergistically to irreversibly modify LDL particles [24]. Figure 1 summarizes the relationship between LDL particle size, particle concentration, apoB and the biological consequences of the small, dense LDL phenotype. Such phenomena could explain some of the differences in CVD between our two patients discussed above.

Many studies have shown that modified LDL particles are associated with CVD risk. For instance, in the Québec Cardiovascular Study, LDL peak particle size determined by gradient gel electrophoresis was found to be a predictor of ischemic heart disease (IHD) independently from triglyceride and HDL cholesterol levels [25]. In another analysis among participants of this cohort, cholesterol levels within small LDL particles were also predictive of an increased IHD risk [26], a finding that was confirmed in the EPIC-Norfolk prospective population study [27]. In the latter, however, the relationship between cholesterol levels in small LDL particles and coronary heart disease risk was not found to be totally independent from triglyceride and HDL cholesterol levels, highlighting the close relationship between

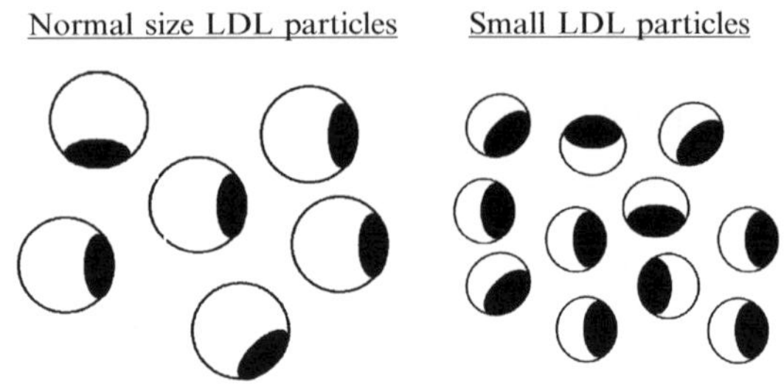

Patient	#1	#2
[LDL cholesterol]	LOW	LOW
[apoB]	LOW	INCREASED
Density	LOW	INCREASED
Affinity for LDL receptor	GOOD	DECREASED
Susceptibility to oxidation/glycation	LOW	INCREASED
Plasma half-life	LOW	INCREASED
Atherogenic potential	LOW	INCREASED

Fig. 1. Schematic representations of physicochemical properties and pathophysiology of LDL particles upon homeostatic conditions (*left*) and in metabolic syndrome and related disorders (*right*).

hypertriglyceridemia, low HDL cholesterol levels and small, dense LDL, a finding that has been observed in several previous investigations [14]. Because at any given LDL level, small LDL size needs to be compensated by an increased number of lipoproteins, measurement of the LDL particle concentration is another approach to quantifying this atherogenic metabolic dyslipidemia. The number of circulating LDL particles can be measured by nuclear magnetic resonance spectroscopy, or, crudely, by measuring the plasma concentration of apoB, because each LDL particle contains one apoB molecule. An elevated number of LDL particles is associated with increased cardiovascular risk [28]. The role of apoB in estimating cardiovascular risk is discussed below.

BEYOND LDL QUANTITY AND QUALITY: HDL CHOLESTEROL AND RESIDUAL CVD RISK

The benefits of carrying elevated plasma HDL have been recognized for decades. The Framingham Heart Study identified HDL cholesterol as an important CVD risk factor in 1977 [29]. The investigators reported that subjects with the highest LDL and lowest HDL cholesterol levels had the highest CHD risk. Even in subjects with low LDL cholesterol, a decrease in HDL cholesterol concentrations has been associated with an increased CHD risk. However, an important finding in that early publication was the fact that among subjects with the highest plasma LDL cholesterol levels, participants with the highest HDL cholesterol levels were not at increased CHD risk, suggesting that the risk associated with LDL levels could be counteracted by elevated HDL cholesterol levels, whereas the opposite did not appear to be true. In the Helsinki Heart Study, a rise of 8% in HDL cholesterol levels obtained with the PPAR-α agonist gemfibrozil was associated with a 24% decrease in CVD events, independently from obtained plasma triglyceride and LDL cholesterol levels [30]. Similar finding were observed in the Veterans Affairs High-Density Lipoprotein Cholesterol Intervention Trial (VA-HIT), in which coronary events were reduced by 22% in the gemfibrozil treatment arm, compared with placebo [31].

Plasma HDL cholesterol levels are low in many pathophysiological conditions such as in abdominal obesity, metabolic syndrome (low-HDL cholesterol is a feature of the metabolic syndrome), in smoking individuals, in individuals with a poor diet and in sedentary individuals. Lifestyle therapy is therefore thought to be an excellent way of increasing plasma HDL cholesterol. Mutations or polymorphisms in several genes implicated in HDL metabolism such as, lecithin cholesteryl acetyl-transferase (LCAT), CETP, ATP-binding cassette A1 (ABCA1), LPL and HL also might explain altered plasma HDL levels observed in some individuals [32].

The main "anti-atherogenic" role of HDL particles is believed to be the stimulation of reverse cholesterol transport, an important physiological process in which excess cholesterol is removed from the peripheral organs, brought back to the liver and excreted as bile salts via the intestine [33]. Nascent HDL particles come from the liver and the small intestine. These small particles contain one apoAI molecule on their surface and virtually no lipids in the hydrophobic core. These nascent HDL particles interact with peripheral cells such as macrophages and acquire free cholesterol and phospholipids via either the ABCA1, the scavenger receptor class B type 1 (SR-B1) or by passive diffusion. At this point, these nascent HDL particles are discoidal. Upon activation by apoAI, LCAT esterifies free cholesterol within HDL particles and increases the lipid content of HDL particles. At this stage, these HDL particles are part of the HDL3 sub fraction and their metabolic purposes will not be fulfilled until they accept and "esterify" more cholesterol to become larger (±80–85 Å). These HDL2 particles are thought to represent the most cardio protective sub fraction of HDL particles, as they have many anti-atherogenic functions [34]. Another important function of HDL particles is undoubtedly their anti-oxidant property. HDL particles directly inhibit oxidation of LDL particles and inhibit the infiltration of oxLDL in the vessel wall [35]. However, in abdominally obese men, this anti-oxidant activity has been shown to be reduced substantially [36, 37]. The anti-oxidant properties are likely to be attributable to apoAI and other proteins carried by HDL such as paraoxonase-1 and glutathione. Vice versa, oxidation of apoAI has been shown to result in dysfunctional HDL particles [38]. It is now well-recognized that chronic inflammation is associated with the development of atherosclerosis and that this pathological state also contributes to the elevated plasma levels of a large number of circulating cytokines, creating a vicious circle between inflammation and atherosclerosis. HDL particles exert a certain number of anti-inflammatory actions such as inhibiting monocyte infiltration into the vessel wall mainly through the down regulation of a number of circulating inflammatory markers such as mediators of monocyte adhesion and proliferation (E-selectin, MCP-1, ICAM-1 and VCAM-1). HDL also has certain antithrombotic effects such as the reduction of platelet activation and aggregation, an observation that might help explain the fact that patients with either high HDL or apoAI levels also have a reduced risk of recurrent venous thromboembolism [39]. In addition, HDL also suppresses apoptosis of endothelial cells, preserving endothelial function, and HDL particles have other beneficial effects on endothelial cells such as the expression of endothelial nitric oxide synthase (eNOS) and prostacyclin, two key enzymes involved in endothelium function and vasodilatation. Furthermore, HDL particles inhibit the vasoconstrictor endothelin-1.

Upon certain biological circumstances, these anti-inflammatory and anti-oxidant properties of HDL particles can be altered, suggesting that, similarly to LDL particles, a closer look at HDL physico-chemical properties could perhaps provide insight into the cardio protective effects of HDL particles. In abdominally obese individuals, HDL particles have been shown to be smaller and denser, and to correlate well with certain features of the metabolic syndrome [40]. Such small HDL particles may have reduced capacity of exerting reverse cholesterol transport and anti-atherogenic properties. In a cross-sectional study of 347 patients with first myocardial infarction (MI), cholesteryl ester transfer rates (from HDL toward endogenous apoB-containing lipoproteins) were highest in patients with small HDL particles and increased non-HDL cholesterol levels [41]. Of interest, this group of patients had a younger age at first MI compared to patients with large HDL particles and low non-HDL cholesterol levels, suggesting that these patients might have been characterized by other metabolic disorders that accompany the small HDL phenotype, such as an increased CETP activity and other features of the metabolic syndrome. As conventional lipid risk factors explain the reductions in CHD events in VA-HIT only partially, Otvos and colleagues showed that beyond the benefits attributable to increased HDL cholesterol and decreased triglyceride levels, the number of circulating HDL and LDL particles provided further information about the prevention of CHD events in that trial [42]. These results suggest that on top of conventional lipid risk factors, the physicochemical properties of lipoproteins may provide additional information for cardiovascular risk prediction.

CLINICAL UTILITY OF APOLIPOPROTEINS VERSUS TRADITIONAL LIPIDS IN ASSESSING CVD RISK

In the INTERHEART study, nine potentially modifiable risk factors accounted for 90 and 94% of the population attributable risk of MI in men and women, respectively [43]. Among these risk factors, abnormal lipids, described by the apoB/apoAI ratio had the strongest association with risk of MI. The large-scale AMORIS (Apolipoprotein-related MOrtality RIsk Study) observed a similar association between apoB/apoAI ratio and MI risk in more than 175,000 participants. This relationship was even found to be independent of the total to HDL cholesterol ratio [44]. A recent sub study, in the Treating to New Targets (TNT) and Incremental Decrease in End Points Through Aggressive Lipid Lowering (IDEAL) trials, suggests that apoB levels predict cardiovascular risk even at very low LDL-C levels [45]. Over the past decade, there have been several findings favoring the use of the apoB/apoAI ratio as opposed to traditional lipid levels or ratios. First, from a pathophysiological standpoint apoB is the major apolipoprotein carried by virtually all atherogenic lipoproteins (VLDL, IDL and LDL), suggesting that on top of estimating plasma LDL cholesterol (90% of circulating apoB is carried by LDL), apoB may be a better reflection of the total burden of atherogenic particles. Moreover, since each LDL particle contains one apoB molecule, measurement of apoB may be an appropriate tool to identify people with a high LDL particle concentration, which corresponds to the small dense LDL phenotype. Although the evidence highlighting the benefits of carrying elevated HDL cholesterol levels are irrefutable, paying closer attention to apoAI levels may also be relevant in clinical practice as the anti-inflammatory and anti-oxidant properties of HDL particles are thought to be attributable to apoAI rather than to the overall number of HDL particles or their cholesterol content.

Finally, it is important to highlight the numerous methodological advantages of measuring the apoB/apoAI ratio as opposed to standard cholesterol levels or ratios. First, the methodology for the measurement of apoB and apoAI has been standardized by the International Federation of Clinical Chemistry [46] and the measurement errors are usually less than 5%. More importantly, a reliable measurement of the apoB/apoAI ratio does not require the participant to be at the fasting state. The predictive value of the apoB/apoAI ratio has been confirmed in several studies, but further large-scale studies are still needed. In this context, another important question remains: Can a simple, inexpensive and practical clinical tool improve the identification of the LDL-independent dyslipidemia and improve CHD risk prediction in the context of global cardio metabolic risk?

THE HYPERTRIGLYCERIDEMIC WAIST: A HANDY TOOL FOR CLINICIANS

As mentioned above, increased VAT accumulation contributes to the small, dense LDL phenotype, low levels of HDL cholesterol and an increased apoB/apoAI ratio, independently from age, sex, blood pressure, LDL cholesterol levels and other traditional CVD risk factors [2]. However, computed tomography is not a feasible tool for cardiovascular risk prediction. In order to avoid this caveat and to estimate VAT, we have previously recommended the measurement of waist circumference in primary care settings [47]. Although waist circumference represents a crude estimate of VAT accumulation, an important limitation of waist is that this measurement also captures the amount of "cardio protective" subcutaneous abdominal fat, especially in pre-menopausal women [48]. Recent evidence from the EPIC-Norfolk study has also suggested that an increased hip circumference, a crude marker of subcutaneous adipose tissue accumulation, might be associated with a decreased CHD risk [49]. On the basis of these observations, it has been suggested that the measurement of waist-to-hip ratio might represent an excellent marker of the cardiovascular risk associated with body composition. We have proposed that the simultaneous measurement of plasma triglyceride levels, a marker of dysfunctional adipose tissue, lipid overflow and altered NEFA metabolism may provide a better estimate of VAT than the measurement of waist alone (Fig. 2). The concept of "hypertriglyceridemic waist" was first introduced in the literature by Lemieux et al. [50] in 2000 as an attempt to identify, at low cost, patients carrying specific features of the metabolic syndrome (hyperinsulinemia, hyperbetaapolipoproteinemia and small LDL particles) that had been found to increase risk of IHD more than 20-fold [51]. The association of the combination of increased waist circumference and elevated triglyceride levels with the atherogenic metabolic risk profile was investigated in men and women who participated in the third National Health and Nutrition Examination Survey (NHANES III). In this cross-sectional report of 9,183 adults, this phenotype was associated with higher plasma levels of insulin, fasting glucose and uric acid and with lower plasma levels of HDL cholesterol. Subjects with the hypertriglyceridemic waist phenotype were also more likely to have diabetes, underlining the association of this clinical phenotype to the "lipotoxic" nature of VAT [52].

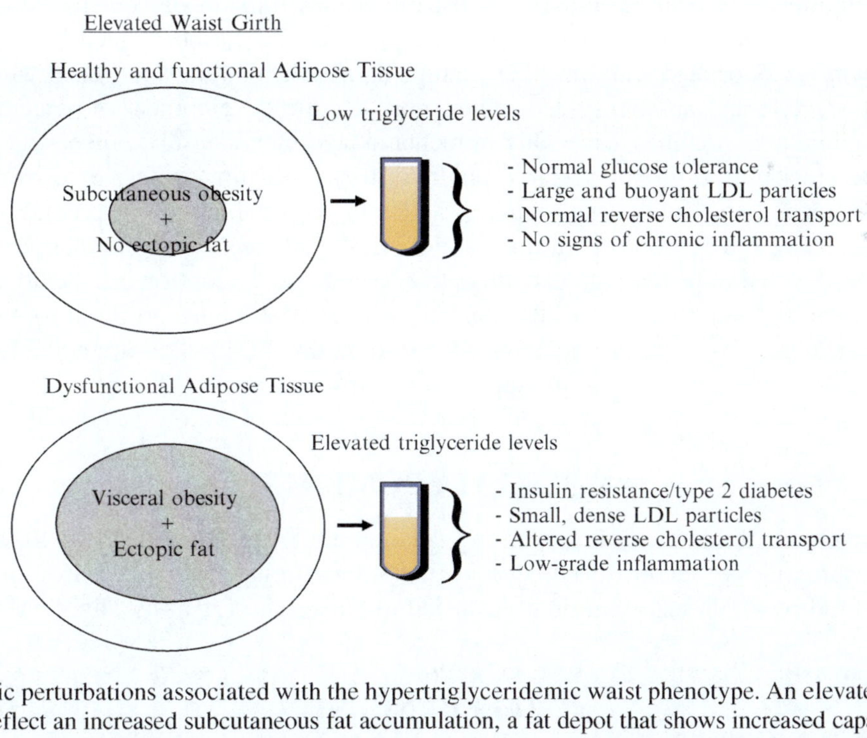

Fig. 2. Metabolic perturbations associated with the hypertriglyceridemic waist phenotype. An elevated waist circumference might reflect an increased subcutaneous fat accumulation, a fat depot that shows increased capacity for triglyceride storage (*top*). Despite an elevated waist circumference, this phenotype is associated with low plasma triglyceride levels, with normal glucose tolerance and with no specific features of the metabolic syndrome. In combination with elevated triglyceride levels (*bottom*), an elevated waistline is likely to be associated with ectopic fat deposition, insulin resistance and many other features of the metabolic syndrome that considerably increase CVD and diabetes risk.

So far, the association between the hypertriglyceridemic waist phenotype and CVD risk has been investigated in a number of studies. In a sample of 557 postmenopausal women who were followed for an average of 8.5 years, the combined presence of elevated waist circumference and triglyceride levels was found to be the best indicator of cardiovascular risk, independently from the other components of the metabolic syndrome [53]. In a cohort composed of 3,430 French men, those with the hypertriglyceridemic waist phenotype were twice as likely to encounter a CVD event during the 7.5 years follow-up compared to men with both low waist circumference and triglyceride levels [54]. Thus, hypertriglyceridemic waist phenotype may be an excellent and cheap screening tool in primary care practice to identify people with atherogenic dyslipidemia who are at increased cardiovascular risk.

CONCLUSION

Individuals with VAT accumulation are likely to show other features of the metabolic syndrome such as an increased preponderance of small, dense and often oxidized LDL particles, hypertriglyceridemia, increased plasma apoB and fasting insulin levels as well as decreased in HDL cholesterol and apoAI levels. The presence of the typical high triglyceride, low HDL atherogenic dyslipidemia, is associated with an increased CVD risk, beyond LDL cholesterol and other traditional CVD risk factors. Furthermore, there is now increasing evidence that the hypertriglyceridemic waist phenotype may represent a simple and inexpensive clinical tool that could help health professionals, general practitioners, internists, cardiologists and even diabetologists in diagnosing such features of the metabolic syndrome in clinical practice. This emerging clinical phenotype should be used, together with the Framingham risk score, to identify and predict global cardiovascular risk in preventive cardiology. To this date, the best treatment for this atherogenic dyslipidemia associated with excess visceral obesity remains lifestyle modification. Indeed, an active lifestyle, characterized by increased daily energy expenditure, (independently from the intensity of physical activity) is associated with low VAT accumulation, whereas a positive energy balance caused by a sedentary lifestyle and an energy-dense diet promotes the development of visceral obesity and associated metabolic abnormalities, especially in men and post-menopausal women.

Although we are facing a global obesity epidemic, today's health professionals often neglect to encourage and reinforce the notion that regular practice of physical activity is crucial in maintaining a healthy "waist" and to stay away from this "silent" LDL-independent dyslipidemia. Considerable efforts should be devoted in primary care settings to encourage the adoption of a healthy lifestyle and this should be achieved via regular consultations with other health care professionals, with specific training in physical activity science and/or nutrition, to annihilate the "obesogenic" lifestyle habits that have been adopted by too many individuals in our Westernized world.

ACKNOWLEDGMENTS

Benoit J. Arsenault is recipient of a training scholarship from Hôpital Laval Research Centre. Jean-Pierre Després is the Scientific Director of the International Chair on Cardiometabolic Risk which is supported by an unrestricted grant awarded to Université Laval by Sanofi Aventis.

REFERENCES

1. Mauriège P, Galitzky J, Berlan M, et al. Heterogeneous distribution of beta and alpha-2 adrenoceptor binding sites in human fat cells from various fat deposits: functional consequences. Eur J Clin Invest 1987;17:156–65.
2. Després JP, Lemieux I. Abdominal obesity and metabolic syndrome. Nature 2006;444:881–7.
3. Lemieux I, Pascot A, Prud'homme D, et al. Elevated C-reactive protein: another component of the atherothrombotic profile of abdominal obesity. Arterioscler Thromb Vasc Biol 2001;21:961–7.

4. Goossens GH. The role of adipose tissue dysfunction in the pathogenesis of obesity-related insulin resistance. Physiol Behav 2008;94(2):206–18.
5. Okamoto Y, Kihara S, Funahashi T, et al. Adiponectin: a key adipocytokine in metabolic syndrome. Clin Sci (Lond) 2006;110: 267–78.
6. Hammarstedt A, Andersson CX, Rotter Sopasakis V, et al. The effect of PPARgamma ligands on the adipose tissue in insulin resistance. Prostaglandins Leukot Essent Fatty Acids 2005;73:65–75.
7. Blackburn P, Lamarche B, Couillard C, et al. Postprandial hyperlipidemia: another correlate of the "hypertriglyceridemic waist" phenotype in men. Atherosclerosis 2003;171:327–36.
8. Cianflone K, Zakarian R, Couillard C, et al. Fasting acylation-stimulating protein is predictive of postprandial triglyceride clearance. J Lipid Res 2004;45:124–31.
9. Després JP. Is visceral obesity the cause of the metabolic syndrome? Ann Med 2006;38:52–63.
10. Kantartzis K, Rittig K, Balletshofer B, et al. The relationships of plasma adiponectin with a favorable lipid profile, decreased inflammation, and less ectopic fat accumulation depend on adiposity. Clin Chem 2006;52:1934–42.
11. Kotronen A, Yki-Jarvinen H. Fatty liver: a novel component of the metabolic syndrome. Arterioscler Thromb Vasc Biol 2008;28:27–38.
12. Fruchart JC, Staels B, Duriez P. PPARS, metabolic disease and atherosclerosis. Pharmacol Res 2001;44:345–52.
13. Jonk AM, Houben AJ, de Jongh RT, et al. Microvascular dysfunction in obesity: a potential mechanism in the pathogenesis of obesity-associated insulin resistance and hypertension. Physiology (Bethesda) 2007;22:252–60.
14. Rizzo M, Berneis K. Low-density lipoprotein size and cardiovascular risk assessment. QJM 2006;99:1–14.
15. McNamara JR, Jenner JL, Li Z, et al. Change in LDL particle size is associated with change in plasma triglyceride concentration. Arterioscler Thromb 1992;12:1284–90.
16. Heine RJ, Dekker JM. Beyond postprandial hyperglycaemia: metabolic factors associated with cardiovascular disease. Diabetologia 2002;45:461–75.
17. Carr MC, Hokanson JE, Zambon A, et al. The contribution of intraabdominal fat to gender differences in hepatic lipase activity and low/high density lipoprotein heterogeneity. J Clin Endocrinol Metab 2001;86:2831–7.
18. de Grooth GJ, Klerkx AH, Stroes ES, et al. A review of CETP and its relation to atherosclerosis. J Lipid Res 2004;45: 1967–74.
19. Bossé Y, Pérusse L, Vohl MC. Genetics of LDL particle heterogeneity: from genetic epidemiology to DNA-based variations. J Lipid Res 2004;45:1008–26.
20. Marcel YL, Hogue M, Weech PK, et al. Expression of apolipoprotein B epitopes in lipoproteins. Relationship to conformation and function. Arteriosclerosis 1988;8:832–44.
21. Boullier A, Bird DA, Chang MK, et al. Scavenger receptors, oxidized LDL, and atherosclerosis. Ann N Y Acad Sci 2001;947:214–22; discussion 22–3.
22. Holvoet P, Vanhaecke J, Janssens S, et al. Oxidized LDL and malondialdehyde-modified LDL in patients with acute coronary syndromes and stable coronary artery disease. Circulation 1998;98:1487–94.
23. Scheffer PG, Teerlink T, Heine RJ. Clinical significance of the physicochemical properties of LDL in type 2 diabetes. Diabetologia 2005;48:808–16.
24. Lyons TJ. Glycation and oxidation: a role in the pathogenesis of atherosclerosis. Am J Cardiol 1993;71:26B-31B.
25. Lamarche B, Tchernof A, Moorjani S, et al. Small, dense low-density lipoprotein particles as a predictor of the risk of ischemic heart disease in men. Prospective results from the Québec Cardiovascular Study. Circulation 1997;95:69–75.
26. St-Pierre AC, Cantin B, Dagenais GR, et al. Low-density lipoprotein subfractions and the long-term risk of ischemic heart disease in men: 13-year follow-up data from the Québec Cardiovascular Study. Arterioscler Thromb Vasc Biol 2005;25:553–9.
27. Arsenault BJ, Lemieux I, Després JP, et al. Cholesterol levels in small LDL particles predict the risk of coronary heart disease in the EPIC-Norfolk prospective population study. Eur Heart J 2007;28:2770–7.
28. Kathiresan S, Otvos JD, Sullivan LM, et al. Increased small low-density lipoprotein particle number: a prominent feature of the metabolic syndrome in the Framingham Heart Study. Circulation 2006;113:20–9.
29. Gordon T, Castelli WP, Hjortland MC, et al. High density lipoprotein as a protective factor against coronary heart disease. The Framingham Study. Am J Med 1977;62:707–14.
30. Frick MH, Elo O, Haapa K, et al. Helsinki Heart Study: primary-prevention trial with gemfibrozil in middle-aged men with dyslipidemia. Safety of treatment, changes in risk factors, and incidence of coronary heart disease. N Engl J Med 1987;317:1237–45.
31. Robins SJ, Collins D, Wittes JT, et al. Relation of gemfibrozil treatment and lipid levels with major coronary events: VA-HIT: a randomized controlled trial. JAMA 2001;285:1585–91.
32. Boekholdt SM, Souverein OW, Tanck MW, et al. Common variants of multiple genes that control reverse cholesterol transport together explain only a minor part of the variation of HDL cholesterol levels. Clin Genet 2006;69:263–70.
33. Link JJ, Rohatgi A, de Lemos JA. HDL cholesterol: physiology, pathophysiology, and management. Curr Probl Cardiol 2007;32:268–314.
34. Cannon CP. High-density lipoprotein cholesterol and residual cardiometabolic risk in metabolic syndrome. Clin Cornerstone 2007;8 Suppl 6:S14–23.
35. Zhang B, Bai H, Liu R, et al. Serum high-density lipoprotein-cholesterol levels modify the association between plasma levels of oxidatively modified low-density lipoprotein and coronary artery disease in men. Metabolism 2004;53:423–9.
36. Perségol L, Verges B, Gambert P, et al. Inability of HDL from abdominally obese subjects to counteract the inhibitory effect of oxidized LDL on vasorelaxation. J Lipid Res 2007;48:1396–401.

37. Perségol L, Foissac M, Lagrost L, et al. HDL particles from type 1 diabetic patients are unable to reverse the inhibitory effect of oxidised LDL on endothelium-dependent vasorelaxation. Diabetologia 2007;50:2384–7.
38. Zheng L, Nukuna B, Brennan ML, et al. Apolipoprotein A-I is a selective target for myeloperoxidase-catalyzed oxidation and functional impairment in subjects with cardiovascular disease. J Clin Invest 2004;114:529–41.
39. Eichinger S, Pecheniuk NM, Hron G, et al. High-density lipoprotein and the risk of recurrent venous thromboembolism. Circulation 2007;115:1609–14.
40. Pascot A, Lemieux I, Prud'homme D, et al. Reduced HDL particle size as an additional feature of the atherogenic dyslipidemia of abdominal obesity. J Lipid Res 2001;42:2007–14.
41. Zeller M, Masson D, Farnier M, et al. High serum cholesteryl ester transfer rates and small high-density lipoproteins are associated with young age in patients with acute myocardial infarction. J Am Coll Cardiol 2007;50:1948–55.
42. Otvos JD, Collins D, Freedman DS, et al. Low-density lipoprotein and high-density lipoprotein particle subclasses predict coronary events and are favorably changed by gemfibrozil therapy in the Veterans Affairs High-Density Lipoprotein Intervention Trial. Circulation 2006;113:1556–63.
43. Yusuf S, Hawken S, Ounpuu S, et al. Effect of potentially modifiable risk factors associated with myocardial infarction in 52 countries (the INTERHEART study): case-control study. Lancet 2004;364:937–52.
44. Walldius G, Jungner I, Aastveit AH, et al. The apoB/apoA-I ratio is better than the cholesterol ratios to estimate the balance between plasma proatherogenic and antiatherogenic lipoproteins and to predict coronary risk. Clin Chem Lab Med 2004;42: 1355–63.
45. Kastelein JJP, van der Steeg, WA, Holme, I, Gaffney, M, Cater, NB, Barter, P, Deedwania, P, Olsson, AG, Boekholdt, SM, Demicco, DA, Szarek, M, LaRosa, JC, Pedersen, TR, Grundy, SM, for the TNT and IDEAL study groups. Lipids, apolipoproteins and their ratios in relation to cardiovascular events on statin treatment. Pooled analyses of the TNT and IDEAL Trials. Circulation 2008;117(23):3002–9.
46. Marcovina SM, Albers JJ, Kennedy H, et al. International Federation of Clinical Chemistry standardization project for measurements of apolipoproteins A-I and B. IV. Comparability of apolipoprotein B values by use of International Reference Material. Clin Chem 1994;40:586–92.
47. Pouliot MC, Després JP, Lemieux S, et al. Waist circumference and abdominal sagittal diameter: best simple anthropometric indexes of abdominal visceral adipose tissue accumulation and related cardiovascular risk in men and women. Am J Cardiol 1994;73:460–8.
48. Lemieux I, Drapeau V, Richard D, et al. Waist girth does not predict metabolic complications in severely obese men. Diabetes Care 2006;29:1417–9.
49. Canoy D, Boekholdt SM, Wareham N, et al. Body fat distribution and risk of coronary heart disease in men and women in the European Prospective Investigation Into Cancer and Nutrition in Norfolk cohort: a population-based prospective study. Circulation 2007;116:2933–43.
50. Lemieux I, Pascot A, Couillard C, et al. Hypertriglyceridemic waist: a marker of the atherogenic metabolic triad (hyperinsulinemia; hyperapolipoprotein B; small, dense LDL) in men? Circulation 2000;102:179–84.
51. Lamarche B, Tchernof A, Mauriège P, et al. Fasting insulin and apolipoprotein B levels and low-density lipoprotein particle size as risk factors for ischemic heart disease. JAMA 1998;279:1955–61.
52. Kahn HS, Valdez R. Metabolic risks identified by the combination of enlarged waist and elevated triacylglycerol concentration. Am J Clin Nutr 2003;78:928–34.
53. Tanko LB, Bagger YZ, Qin G, et al. Enlarged waist combined with –elevated triglycerides is a strong predictor of accelerated atherogenesis and related cardiovascular mortality in postmenopausal women. Circulation 2005;111:1883–90.
54. Czernichow S, Bruckert E, Bertrais S, et al. Hypertriglyceridemic waist and 7.5-year prospective risk of cardiovascular disease in asymptomatic middle-aged men. Int J Obes (Lond) 2007;31(5):791–6.

9 New Blood Biomarkers of Inflammation and Atherosclerosis

Natalie Khuseyinova and Wolfgang Koenig

CONTENTS

ABSTRACT

During the past decade, compelling experimental and clinical evidence has demonstrated that both systemic and local inflammation might play a prominent role in the pathogenesis of atherosclerosis and its clinical complications. Since inflammatory processes accompany all stages of atherosclerosis,

From: *Asymptomatic Atherosclerosis: Pathophysiology, Detection and Treatment*
Edited by: M. Naghavi (ed.), DOI 10.1007/978-1-60327-179-0_9

measurement of plasma/serum concentrations of circulating inflammatory biomarkers might aid in identifying individuals at high risk for cardiovascular disease (CVD). In particular, such biomarkers might add to the predictive value of the atherogenic lipoprotein phenotype to further improve assessment of future global cardiovascular (CV) risk, since many of these molecules can be measured systemically by sensitive assays, and elevated concentrations in the circulation have been shown to be associated with future CV events. Determination of several of these molecules carries important prognostic information, independent of traditional risk factors, and may turn out to be useful in improving risk stratification. However, for most of these biomarkers, the clinical utility has not yet been firmly established.

Key words: Biomarkers; Atherosclerosis; Inflammation; Pathophysiology; Risk prediction

KEY POINTS

- The inflammatory response represents an important contributor of atherothrombosis. Screening for low-grade inflammation, using several novel biomarkers might provide an important tool for identifying individuals at increased risk, who would benefit most from targeted preventive interventions.
- To be implemented into clinical practice, these markers, however, should fulfill certain requirements, such as providing independent information on risk prediction in addition to global risk assessment, being reliable and easily reproducible, and showing high sensitivity and specificity. Finally, simple and robust assays should be commercially available.
- In the future, simultaneous assessment of several biomarkers, a so-called "multi-marker approach," might allow to reveal in more detail the complex and multi-factorial origin of atherothrombosis, thereby opening a new avenue to combat this still widespread disease.

INTRODUCTION

In the era of "global risk assessment," risk stratification in primary prevention is usually done on the basis of one of the available risk scores like the Framingham risk score, the PROCAM Score or the European Society of Cardiology SCORE. On the basis of the result of these scores, which, however, take into account only a limited number of cardiovascular (CV) risk factors, subjects are stratified into those at high (10-year risk >20%), low (10-year risk <10%), or intermediate risk (10-year risk of 10–20%). There are clear recommendations in the guidelines as to what to do with subjects at high risk (life-style changes or prescription of a statin) or low risk (re-evaluation 3–5 years later). However, for those at intermediate risk, whose group comprises a relatively large group of approximately 25–40% of the population [1], no clear recommendations exist. Therefore, they might be candidates for additional testing, to increase or decrease their actual risk. This has prompted the search for novel blood biomarkers, relevant to the pathophysiology of atherosclerosis, e.g., representing inflammatory pathways, coagulation, platelet aggregation, lipoproteins or lipid-related variables. To date, a number of blood biomarkers are available for this purpose, but most of them are not yet applicable in the clinical routine for various reasons [2]. This chapter summarizes our current knowledge based on observations from experimental and clinical studies with emphasis on potential mechanisms of action and on clinical utility of inflammatory biomarkers as predictors of cardiovascular risk.

C-REACTIVE PROTEIN

This classical acute phase reactant, which is mainly produced by hepatocytes under transcriptional control of several cytokines, mainly interleukin-6 (IL-6), represents the most extensively studied pro-inflammatory molecule. Indeed, data from more than 25 prospective studies indicate that elevated C-reactive protein (CRP) is strongly associated with future CV risk in apparently healthy men and women, patients with stable angina pectoris (AP), those with acute coronary syndrome (ACS), after myocardial infarction (MI), and in patients with the metabolic syndrome (MetS). Based on such compelling evidence, the recent AHA/CDC consensus report [3] recommends the measurement of CRP as the only biomarker among all available candidates, albeit only in asymptomatic subjects at intermediate risk for future coronary heart disease (CHD) events (10-year risk of 10–20%) and in selected patients after an ACS. However, more recent studies have demonstrated only a modest prognostic power of CRP by showing a 50% increased risk associated with elevated concentrations, while earlier meta-analysis had reported a twofold increased risk [4]. In addition, there is an ongoing discussion whether or not CRP is simply an innocent bystander in the atherosclerotic process or is causally involved in atherogenesis [5]. Nonetheless, to date, of all emerging biomarkers investigated with respect to CV disease risk prediction, the most extensive and robust database exists for CRP. Still, its incremental predictive value above and beyond traditional risk factors, as well as its causal involvement in atherogenesis have not been definitely proven. Eventually, these issues might be solved on the basis of individual subject data in a meta-analysis currently prepared by the Emerging Risk Factors Collaboration Group [6], and further genetic studies and appropriate animal models.

SERUM AMYLOID P

Serum amyloid P (SAP) represents, like CRP, another member of the pentraxin family, a highly conserved group of molecules that may play a role in innate immunity [7]. SAP is synthesized and secreted only in hepatocytes and has a half-life of approximately 24 h. SAP, however, in contrast to CRP, is only mildly affected during acute or chronic inflammation and serum concentrations remain close to the normal range (10–50 mg/L) [7]. Physiological functions of SAP are not entirely elucidated. SAP probably is best known as a universal constituent of amyloid deposits that are characteristic of systemic amyloidosis, including cerebral amyloid in Alzheimer's disease and in type 2 diabetes mellitus (T2DM). In addition, SAP has also been found in atherosclerotic plaque [8], which has generated interest to consider it as a marker for the future CVD risk prediction. Jenny et al. [9] reported for the first time on the association of SAP and CVD outcomes. In multivariable adjusted analyses in elderly subjects from the prospective Cardiovascular Health Study (CHS), using a case-cohort design, they found a 66% increased risk for angina, and a 39% increased risk for combined CVD, across extreme quartiles of SAP distribution. However, no significant association was found for stroke and CVD death, and the association with MI was also non-significant in quartile analysis, but was significant when the risk was computed for a one standard deviation increase. The next important step, obviously, is the need to replicate such results in diverse populations. However, and most critically, basic research has to provide convincing arguments regarding the potential underlying pathophysiology of SAP in CVD.

FIBRINOGEN

Fibrinogen is another acute phase reactant and plays a central role in the coagulation cascade. Elevated fibrinogen levels lead to formation of tight and rigid network structures, decrease the deformability of the clot and render it less amenable to endogenous fibrinolysis [10]. There is also evidence of other potential mechanisms, involving fibrinogen in both the early and the later stages of the atherothrombotic process, such as modulation of endothelial cell (EC) permeability, and further promotion of EC migration [10]. It provides an adsorptive surface for the extracellular accumulation of low density lipoprotein (LDL) and further facilitates cholesterol transfer from platelet to monocytes/macrophages, thereby playing a role in foam cell formation [10]. The clinical and epidemiologic evidence demonstrating an association between elevated fibrinogen levels and future CHD are unequivocal [11]. The published data are remarkably strong and consistent, despite the diversity of populations studied, the variable length of follow-up (FU), different definitions of endpoints, and the various analytical methods applied in the absence of an International Standard at the time most of these studies were done. Moreover, in a recent publication from the Fibrinogen Studies Collaboration (FSC) [12], a comprehensive meta-analysis of individual data on 154,211 subjects without known CVD at baseline, coming from 31 prospective studies with information on plasma fibrinogen and major disease outcomes has shown a significant and independent association of elevated fibrinogen levels and CV morbidity and mortality: An increase in fibrinogen level by 1 g/L was associated with approximately a twofold increase in risk for CHD. Thus, fibrinogen undoubtedly represents a strong and independent risk factor for future CV events. However, despite this well-established association, the proof of a causal involvement of fibrinogen in atherogenesis is still pending. In addition, lack of adequate standardization of fibrinogen assays limits its clinical utility.

PLASMINOGEN ACTIVATOR INHIBITOR-1

Plasminogen activator inhibitor (PAI)-1, belonging to the super-family of serpins (i.e., α1-protease inhibitor class of *ser*ine *p*rotease *in*hibitors), is an important component of the plasminogen/plasmin system with a half-life of approximately 6 min. By suppression of tissue-type and urokinase-type plasminogen activator, PAI-1 represents a pivotal inhibitor of fibrinolysis [13]. Under physiological conditions PAI-1 favors the stabilization of fibrin, thereby protecting the organism from increased risk of bleeding. However, even a light excess in PAI-1 levels could cause impaired fibrinolytic function, thus contributing to a prothrombotic state and to atherogenesis. Indeed, large amounts of PAI-1 were found in advanced human atheromatous plaque [14]. Furthermore, in the acute clinical setting, PAI-1 is released during the first hours of ST-elevation MI and predicted 30-day mortality [15]. In addition, higher levels of PAI-1 activity were associated with increased risk for re-infarctions in MI-survivors during a 3-year FU [13]. However, the vast majority of primary and secondary prevention studies found an association between increased PAI-1 levels and subsequent incident CHD only in univariate analysis, and such association disappeared after controlling for traditional CV risk factors [13]. These findings were further reflected in a subsequent meta-analysis [16], which revealed an odds ratio (OR) of 0.98 (95 % confidence interval (CI), 0.53–1.81) across extreme tertiles of baseline PAI-1 concentrations. Thus, the independence of the prognostic ability of PAI-1 seems to be questionable. In contrast to clinical and epidemiological studies, experimental data seem to be much more convincing. Genetic deficiency of PAI-1 prolongs the time to occlusive thrombosis following photochemical injury of the carotid atherosclerotic plaque in apoE-deficient (apoE$^{-/-}$) mice [13]. Conversely, transgenic mice that over-express PAI-1 demonstrated development of coronary arterial thrombosis and sub-endothelial infarction [13]. Thus, further research is needed to elucidate a real role of increased PAI-1 concentrations in cardiometabolic disorders.

D-DIMER

Fibrin D-dimer has been suggested as a global marker for direct measurement of the ongoing turnover of cross-linked fibrin and for an activation of the hemostatic system without reflecting changes in fibrinogen and fibrin status [17]. In addition, D-dimer assays are more stable, and more practical to detect even small amounts of intravascular clot. Therefore, D-dimer plays an important role in the detection of hypercoagulable states such as acute symptomatic deep vein thrombosis, pulmonary embolism or disseminated intravascular coagulation, showing a high negative predictive value [17].

Assuming that thrombogenesis represents one of the fundamental parts of complicated atherosclerotic disease, measurement of D-dimer might be useful to identify patients at high risk for future coronary events. Efforts to introduce D-dimer as a strong and independent prognostic marker of future CVD have been summarized in meta-analyses with a total of 1,535 incident CHD events and found an approximately 70% increased risk for incident CHD associated with being in the top tertile (T) of the D-dimer distribution [17]. Further studies supported the magnitude of such an association. In the Atherosclerosis Risk in Communities (ARIC) study [17], including 326 incident CHD cases and a referent cohort of 720 individuals, D-dimers showed the most powerful predictive value for incident CHD among various markers of fibrinolysis and coagulation, with a relative risk (RR) of 4.21 (95% CI 1.9–9.6; for top vs. bottom quintile). Finally, in WOSCOPS [18], and the Womens Health Initiative (WHI) observational study [19], the strength of the association between elevated levels of D-dimer and CV events was similar to those found in meta-analysis, revealing multivariate-adjusted risk estimates of 1.86 (95% CI, 1.24–2.8) and 1.7 (95% CI, 1.0–2.9), respectively.

INTERLEUKIN-6

IL-6 is a 26 kDa single chain glycoprotein, produced by many cell types including activated monocytes/macrophages and endothelial cells, as well as by adipose tissue [5]. The most important function of this cytokine represents the amplification of the inflammatory cascade. During an acute phase response, IL-6, acting on hepatocytes, promotes synthesis of several acute phase reactants, such as CRP, serum amyloid A, and fibrinogen [5]. Moreover, IL-6 might exert a direct pro-atherogenic role e.g., by stimulation of macrophages to secrete monocyte chemoattractant protein-1 (MCP-1), by activation of platelets, or by increasing plasma concentrations of fibrinogen and PAI-1 [5]. The vast majority of clinical and epidemiological studies are in support of its pro-atherogenic properties. For instance, elevated IL-6 levels in patients with unstable AP, who participated in the FRISC II trial ($n=3{,}269$), were independently associated with a twofold increased mortality in both the conservative arm of the trial at 6 months and the interventional arm at 12 months [20]. In the primary prevention setting, IL-6 also possessed strong predictive ability for future CVD risk assessment, as has been documented in several large studies [2]. Thus, IL-6 might play an important direct pathogenic role in atherogenesis in addition to its role in the amplification of the inflammatory cascade, by initiating an acute phase response. Moreover, circulating or locally produced IL-6 may favor the onset of a prothrombotic state, which could increase the risk of atherosclerotic complications, especially during later stages of atheroma development.

INTERLEUKIN-18

The pleiotropic proinflammatory cytokine interleukin-18 (IL-18) has been considered as a crucial and potent mediator of atherosclerotic plaque destabilization and vulnerability, due to its ability to induce interferon (INF)-γ and to enhance the expression of matrix metalloproteinases (MMPs). IL-18 is widely expressed in cells of hemopoietic and non-hemopoietic lineages and is synthesized as a 23 kDa biologically inert precursor, which is further cleaved by caspase 1 (or IL-1β-converting enzyme) to yield the mature and active 18.3 kDa glycoprotein [21]. Increased IL-18 expression in human atherosclerotic plaque has been shown in lesions prone to rupture [22]. In animal models, inhibition of IL-18 or knockout of the IL-18 gene led to the reduction of atherosclerotic plaque development and progression [22]. Conversely, direct administration of IL-18, enhanced atherogenesis in an INF-γ-dependent manner, even in the absence of T-cells, and promoted a switch to a vulnerable plaque phenotype by decreasing intimal collagen content and cap-to-core ratio [22].

Whereas experimental studies on the role of IL-18 in atherogenesis are relatively consistent and promising, the clinical relevance for this biomarker yet needs to be established. Within the Athero*Gene* study, conducted in 1,229 CHD patients, increased IL-18 levels at baseline were independently associated with future CV death during a 3.9-year FU [23]. However, at 5.9 years, IL-18 concentrations were no longer predictive of outcome [24]. In the PRIME Study, a cohort of apparently healthy subjects from France and Northern Ireland, elevated IL-18 concentrations were associated with an increased risk for subsequent CHD events, but such an association was only seen when data from both populations were pooled for analysis [25]. In a large case-cohort study in initially healthy, middle-aged men and women from the MONICA/KORA Augsburg populations with a mean FU of 11 years, concentrations of IL-18 were measured in 382 case subjects with incident CHD and in 1,980 non-case subjects. In multivariable analyses there was no statistically significant association, neither in men nor in women [26]. This large population-based case-cohort study therefore suggests that IL-18 might only serve as a marker of future CV events in men with manifest CHD and/or in areas of high absolute risk of CHD, and thus, further studies are needed to evaluate its true clinical value.

NEOPTERIN

Neopterin might represent another marker of increased monocytes/macrophages activity – a pyrazino-pyrimidine derivative and a by-product of the guanosine triphosphate-biopterin pathway. Neopterin is synthesized and released in increased amounts by human monocytes/macrophages only upon stimulation by INF-γ during Th1-type immune response [27]. Thus, it serves as a soluble marker of cell-mediated immune activation and therefore might, at least partially, reflect an increased inflammatory response during atherosclerotic plaque rupture [28]. Experimental evidence has demonstrated that neopterin may act pro-oxidatively under certain environmental conditions, and it was found to support LDL oxidation. Moreover, neopterin induces the expression of inducible nitric oxide (NO) synthase in vascular smooth muscle cells (SMCs) and stimulates cellular adhesion molecules and tissue factor expression in coronary endothelial cells. These in vitro observations seem to be confirmed by further clinical studies [28], which nicely showed that increased circulating levels of neopterin were independently associated with rapid angiographic coronary artery stenosis progression, in patients with chronic stable angina. Elevated concentrations of neopterin were found in patients with ACS compared to patients with stable forms of CHD, which also correlated with the presence of both angiographically complex lesions and increased CV risk [28]. The predictive ability of elevated neopterin levels to identify patients at long-term risk of death or recurrent coronary events after ACS was further confirmed among participants of the PROVE-IT-TIMI 22 trial [29]. Taken together, these findings suggest that increased neopterin concentrations might reflect disease activity and predispose to vulnerability in ACS.

MATRIX METALLOPROTEINASES

MMPs belong to a family of multi-domain zinc-dependent endopeptidases that promote degradation of all protein and proteoglycan-core-protein components of the extracellular matrix (ECM) [30]. MMPs are involved in the embryonic development and morphogenesis, wound healing, and tissue resorption. On the other hand, MMPs might be implicated in vascular and cardiac remodeling as a result of dysregulated activation of these enzymes [30]. In addition, MMPs are highly expressed in macrophage-rich areas of the atherosclerotic plaque, especially at the shoulder region of the cap, which might promote weakening of the fibrous cap and subsequent destabilization of atherosclerotic lesions [30].

Several cross-sectional studies have demonstrated significantly increased concentrations of MMPs in patients with ACS compared to healthy controls or in patients with more advanced CHD [30]. However, to date, only one prospective study conducted in 1,227 patients with angiographically confirmed CHD, showed that increased concentrations of MMP-9 at baseline were associated with future CV death [31]. Surprisingly, high concentrations of the endogenous tissue inhibitors of metalloproteinase-1 (TIMP-1) were also predictive of future CV death in this study [32], which has been confirmed by others [33]. Thus, undoubtedly, MMPs play an important role in plaque destabilization, but further studies are needed to prove or disprove their clinical usefulness for risk assessment.

PREGNANCY-ASSOCIATED PLASMA PROTEIN A

Pregnancy-associated plasma protein A (PAPP-A) is a high-molecular mass, zinc binding metalloproteinase which may be produced by different activated cells in unstable plaques and released into the extracellular matrix. Using specific monoclonal antibodies, PAPP-A was found to be abundantly expressed in both eroded and ruptured coronary and carotid plaques, mainly in monocyte/macrophages present in the cap and shoulder region, but was only minimally expressed in stable plaque [34]. PAPP-A is a specific activator of insulin-like growth factor-1 (IGF-1) and acts by degrading IGF binding proteins-4 and -5, thus allowing active IGF-1 to bind to cell-surface type 1 IGF receptors [35]. IGF-1 induces cell proliferation, differentiation, migration, inflammatory cell activation, LDL-cholesterol uptake, and release of inflammatory cytokines, thereby contributing to plaque progression and destabilization. Whether PAPP-A directly degrades extracellular matrix remains unclear. Several studies in patients with ACS, but also with stable CHD have investigated PAPP-A as a potential marker of risk for clinical complications [34]. In a cohort of 200 patients with troponin negative ACS, PAPP-A levels independently predicted ischemic cardiac events and need for revascularization during 6-month FU [34]. Within the CAPTURE trial, PAPP-A levels indicated increased risk of death and MI in both troponin negative and troponin positive patients [34]. In multivariable analysis, PAPP-A, soluble CD40 ligand, IL-10 and vascular endothelial growth factor (VEGF) were independent predictors of the outcome. Similarly, in patients with ST-elevation MI (STEMI), PAPP-A levels were increased, and predicted 12-month risk of death and recurrent non-fatal MI [34]. It has also been suggested that PAPP-A may be a suppressor rather than a mediator of inflammation and tissue damage [36]. Also, there is recent evidence for the presence of an ACS-related isoform of PAPP-A, which is not complexed with the proform of the eosinophilic major basic protein (proMBP), that should result in the development of more specific assays [37]. Thus, further mechanistic and clinical studies are needed to assess the potential utility of PAPP-A for risk stratification in the ACS.

MYELOPEROXIDASE

Myeloperoxidase (MPO), a member of the heme peroxidase super-family, is a leukocyte-derived enzyme, which is stored within the azurophilic granules of polymorphonuclear neutrophils and monocytes and is secreted upon leukocyte activation and degranulation [38]. The molecular mass of this hemoprotein is approximately 120–140 kDa. Initially, it was assumed that the physiological role of this enzyme could be considered as part of the innate immune system and therefore is in the host defense against infection, taking into account very potent bactericidal and viricidal properties of MPO. Indeed, generation of free radicals and diffusible oxidants by catalyzation of chloride and hydrogen peroxide (H_2O_2) to hypochlorous acid (HOCl) – represents a major source of its antimicrobial activity, presumably by oxidizing key functional components of ingested microorganisms [39]. However, the fact that under certain circumstances, MPO-derived reactive oxidizing and chlorinating species can overwhelm local antioxidant defenses, and therefore might lead to oxidative damage of the arterial wall have highlighted their possible pro-atherogenic role. Indeed, MPO and its oxidation products were found to be markedly enriched in human atherosclerotic lesions compared to control vessels, where they co-localize with macrophages [38]. MPO could be also involved in the development of endothelial dysfunction, since it utilizes the atheroprotective endothelial-derived NO as a substrate. Nonetheless, a most pivotal characteristic of MPO remains its ability to activate MMPs and deactivate inhibitors of MMPs, that promote the weakening of the fibrous cap and lead to the destabilized atherosclerotic plaque.

In line with these findings are the results of two prospective studies in patients with ACS. MPO concentrations have been measured in the CAPTURE trial in 1,090 patients with ACS [40]. Baseline MPO levels predicted an increased risk for adverse CV events, and this effect was even more pronounced in patients without myocardial necrosis. In a large cohort of patients with chest pain, a single measurement of MPO on admission, independently predicted acute MI [41]. Thus, MPO might be a promising prognostic marker for CV events, especially in the ACS. However, further studies are needed to replicate these findings and to establish a potential role for MPO as a predictor of incident CHD in initially healthy subjects. In particular pre-analytical issues need to be critically evaluated.

OXIDIZED LDL

The oxidative modification hypothesis of atherogenesis suggests that the most significant event in early lesion formation is lipid oxidation, placing oxLDL in a central role for the development of this disease [42]. OxLDL has a large number of biological actions and consequences, including injuring ECs, expressing adhesion molecules, recruiting leukocytes and retaining them, as well as the formation of foam cells [42]. Furthermore, elevated oxLDL could play a role in the transition from stable to vulnerable, unstable plaque, and this assumption is supported by recent studies showing that oxLDL stimulates MMP-1 and -9 expressions in human vascular EC and in monocyte-derived macrophages, as well as up-regulates the expression of MMP-1 and -3 in human coronary ECs through its endothelial receptor LOX-1 [2] (Fig. 1).

Salonen et al. [43] were the first to conduct a prospective, population-based, nested case-control study in which the titer of auto antibodies to malondialdehyde-modified LDL and native LDL was associated with accelerated progression of carotid atherosclerosis. More recently, data of a first prospective nested case-control study from two population-based MONICA/KORA Augsburg surveys showed that plasma oxLDL was the strongest predictor of CHD events compared to a conventional lipoprotein profile, and other traditional risk factors for CHD [44]. Further studies are warranted to establish the clinical relevance of oxLDL measurement in various stages of the atherosclerotic process and identify the specific pathophysiological mechanisms by which oxLDL exerts it deleterious effects.

GLUTATHIONE PEROXIDASE

Although antioxidant studies in four different animal models of atherosclerosis (rabbit, mouse, hamster and monkey) mainly showed positive results, several large-scale, double-blind, placebo-controlled trials evaluating the effects of different antioxidant compounds on cardiovascular outcome were inconsistent and rather disappointing [45]. Nonetheless, it seems justified to assume that oxLDL may indeed play a key role in the generation of inflammatory processes in atherosclerotic lesions and that anti-oxidative mechanisms still may be important in the pathophysiology of the disease. Therefore, the role of glutathione peroxidase (GPx), a selenium-containing enzyme with potent antioxidant properties, could be important in this context. GPx utilizes glutathione to reduce hydrogen peroxide

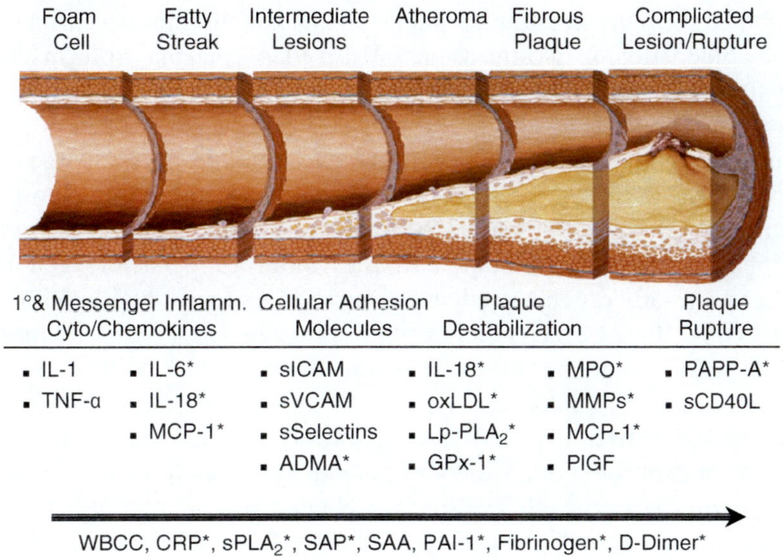

Fig. 1. Markers of inflammation and plaque instability: from foam cell to plaque rupture (modified after Ref. [2]) * biomarkers, which are covered in this review. *IL* interleukin, *TNF-α* tumor necrosis factor-α; *MCP-1* monocyte chemoattractant protein-1; *sICAM* soluble intercellular adhesion molecule-1; *sVCAM* soluble vascular cell adhesion molecule; *ADMA* asymmetric dimethylarginine; *oxLDL* oxidized low density lipoprotein; *Lp-PLA$_2$* lipoprotein associated phospholipase A$_2$; *GPx-1* glutathione peroxidase; *MPO* myeloperoxidase; *MMPs* matrix metalloproteinases; *PlGF* placental growth factor; *PAPP-A* pregnancy-associated plasma protein-A; *sCD40L* soluble CD40 ligand; *CRP* C-reactive protein; *sPLA$_2$* secretory type II phospholipase A$_2$; *SAP* serum amyloid P; *SAA* serum amyloid A; *PAI-1* plasminogen activator inhibitor; *WBCC* white blood cell count.

and lipid peroxides to water and lipid alcohols, respectively [46]. To date, four isoforms of GPx have been identified, with GPx-1, as an intracellular molecule, being more intensively studied. Experimental studies in GPx-1 knock-out mice have demonstrated an increased oxidation of LDL or have developed endothelial dysfunction due to deficiency in bioactive nitric oxide as compared to wild-type mice [47]. This enzyme might also inhibit transcription of 5-lipoxygenase as well as leukotriene and prostanoid synthesis in mononuclear cells and macrophages, EC, platelets, and leukocytes [47]. In one prospective study, risk of future fatal and non-fatal CV events associated with baseline activity of erythrocyte GPx-1 and superoxide dismutase activity was investigated in 636 patients with angiographically confirmed CHD and was found to be inversely associated with increasing GPx-1 activity [48]. Decreased concentrations of GPx were significantly associated with increased CV risk according to the extent of atherosclerosis. However, there is no data so far on the clinical utility of this enzyme in the primary prevention setting. Clearly, such studies need to be done as well as the replication of already existing findings in further studies, before any sound conclusions can be drawn on the potential value of this biomarker in CV risk assessment.

LIPOPROTEIN-ASSOCIATED PHOSPHOLIPASE A$_2$

Lipoprotein-associated phospholipase A$_2$ (Lp-PLA$_2$) represents another emerging biomarker for atherosclerotic disease and is presently under intensive investigation [49]. Lp-PLA$_2$, a 45.4 kDa protein, is a calcium-independent member of the phospholipase A$_2$ family. It is produced mainly by monocytes, macrophages, T-lymphocytes, and mast cells and has been found to be up-regulated in atherosclerotic lesions, especially in complex plaque, as well as in thin cap coronary lesions prone to rupture [50]. In the bloodstream, two-thirds of the Lp-PLA$_2$ plasma isoform circulates primarily bound to low-density lipoproteins (LDL), the other third is distributed between HDL and very low-density lipoproteins (VLDL).

Lp-PLA$_2$ may promote oxidation of LDL and recent investigations have stressed the pro-atherogenic properties of this enzyme. After LDL oxidation within the arterial wall, a short acyl group at the *sn*-2 position of phospholipids becomes susceptible to the hydrolytic action of Lp-PLA$_2$ that cleaves an oxidized phosphatidylcholine component of the lipoprotein particle generating two potent pro-inflammatory and pro-atherogenic mediators, namely lysophosphatidyl-choline (LysoPC) and oxidized fatty acid (oxFA). LysoPC is a potent chemo-attractant for T-cells and monocytes, promotes endothelial cell dysfunction, stimulates macrophage proliferation, and induces apoptosis in SMCs and macrophages. Several studies in initially healthy subjects but also in those with manifest atherosclerosis have found an association between increased concentrations of Lp-PLA$_2$ and future coronary and cerebrovascular events, independent of a variety of potential confounders [49]. However, measurement of Lp-PLA$_2$ in the early phase of the ACS was not associated with increased risk for recurrent events. Apart from an important role of Lp-PLA$_2$ in the prediction of future CV disease, this enzyme could also represent an attractive, novel therapeutic target, since initial studies have demonstrated a significant clinical benefit by inhibiting this enzyme through azetidinones, a new class of compounds acting as acylating inhibitors of the enzymatic activity of Lp-PLA$_2$ or by pyromidones [51]. However, no clear recommendation on its clinical usefulness can be given until further data document its incremental value, in addition to traditional risk factors.

TYPE II SECRETORY PHOSPHOLIPASE A$_2$

Type II secretory phospholipase (sPLA$_2$-II), another well studied member of the phospholipase A$_2$ family, is a Ca^{2+}-dependent, 14 kDa enzyme [52]. SPLA$_2$ is an acute phase reactant, circulating levels of which greatly increase during systemic inflammatory conditions and is under regulatory control of various pro-inflammatory compounds such as IL-1β, IL-6, TNF-α or INF-γ [52]. The catalytic function of this enzyme is related to the hydrolysis of the *sn*-2 acyl group of glycerophospholipids, with further liberation of fatty acids and lysophospholipids. However, in contrast to Lp-PLA$_2$, sPLA$_2$-II can also hydrolyze unmodified phospholipids. Possible atherogenic mechanisms of sPLA$_2$-II consist in the release of various lipid mediators at the site of lipoprotein retention in the arterial wall that, in turn, may trigger local inflammatory cellular responses [52]. Furthermore, in arterial tissue, sPLA$_2$-II may also directly modify LDL particles to become more atherogenic, thereby making sPLA$_2$-II-treated lipoproteins more susceptible to further lipid oxidation and enzymatic modification [53]. In vivo studies of transgenic mice overexpressing human sPLA$_2$-II showed an enhanced formation of bioactive oxidized phospholipids, as well as an increased formation of atherosclerotic lesions [52]. Furthermore, circulating sPLA$_2$-II in blood has been demonstrated to predict coronary events in initially healthy subjects, in patients with manifest CHD as well as in patients with unstable angina, including patients with severe ACS. In the EPIC Norfolk study [54], comprising 3,314 apparently healthy subjects, elevated levels of sPLA$_2$ at baseline were associated with an increased risk of future CHD events. We also investigated whether sPLA$_2$ is associated with prognosis in a large cohort of patients with clinically overt CHD, and found sPLA$_2$ mass to be associated with an increased risk of future cardiovascular events during a FU of 4.1 years (HR 1.92 (95% CI, 1.05–3.51) for T3 vs. T1) [55]. Although consistent, most of the above studies in CHD patients were relatively small and results in healthy subjects have to be replicated in other cohorts until the clinical usefulness of sPLA$_2$-II in the prediction of CHD may be established.

ASYMMETRIC DIMETHYLARGININE

Asymmetric dimethylarginine (ADMA), being an endogenous competitive inhibitor of all major isoforms of NO synthase and thereby playing a pivotal role in vascular function [56], has been suggested to be a novel marker of endothelial dysfunction and increased risk of CVD [28]. Indeed, reduced bioavailability of the major endothelium-derived vasoactive mediator NO, due to inhibitory action of ADMA, might lead to the promotion of atherosclerosis through impaired endothelium-dependent vasodilation, increased platelet and leukocyte aggregation and adhesion to endothelium, enhanced SMCs proliferation and extracellular matrix production [56]. In addition, ADMA also exerts pro-apoptotic effects and suppresses progenitor cell mobilization, differentiation and function.

Increased ADMA concentrations in peripheral blood are found in various clinical situations such as acute coronary and intensive care settings, as well as in patients with hypertension, hyperlipidemia, hyperhomocysteinemia, peripheral arterial occlusive disease, congestive heart failure, stroke, pulmonary hypertension, and end-stage renal disease [28]. Moreover, in several cross-sectional and prospective studies, elevated ADMA concentrations independently predicted CHD outcome in certain populations at increased CV risk, such as hemo-dialysis patients or diabetic patients. Within the Athero*Gene* study [57], a secondary prevention study including patients with angiographically confirmed CHD, it has been demonstrated that increased concentrations of ADMA at baseline were associated with future CV death during a 2.6-year FU. Maas et al. [58] conducted a first prospective study and investigated the association between ADMA concentrations and risk of future CHD in a nested case-control design in a large cohort of initially healthy subjects. The major finding clearly showed that increase of ADMA was independently associated with increased risk for future fatal and nonfatal coronary events in non-smoking men but not in smoking men, thereby pointing to a significant interaction of smoking and ADMA-associated CV risk.

CYSTATIN C

Cystatin C has been proposed to represent a superior marker for detection of chronic kidney disease (CKD), which seems very sensitive to small changes in glomerular filtration rate (GFR) [59]. Cystatin C is a 13 kDa protein and is being a housekeeping gene, produced at a constant rate by all nucleated cells. It has multiple biological functions, including controlling extracellular proteolysis due to its inhibitory effects on cysteine peptidase, such as e.g., cathepsins [59]. It also exerts antibacterial activities and might be considered as a modulator of the immune system. So far, several prospective studies have highlighted the prognostic significance of cystatin C for CVD, chronic heart failure (CHF), and CKD in various settings [59]. In subjects without overt CKD it also seems to be a much stronger predictor of death, CVD, and incident CKD among the elderly, compared to creatinine and estimated GFR. For instance, Jernberg et al. [60] showed that elevated cystatin C was associated with mortality among persons hospitalized with ACS. We could also demonstrate that elevated cystatin C predicted secondary cardiovascular events within a cohort of post-MI patients ($n = 1{,}033$) participating in an in-hospital rehabilitation program after acute MI or coronary revascularization [61]. Patients in the top quintile of the cystatin C distribution had a more than twofold increased risk for a secondary CVD event compared to those in the bottom quintile, even after controlling for a large variety of potential confounders, including markers of inflammation and traditional markers of impaired renal function. Furthermore, the independency of the association between cystatin C and CVD events from creatinine and creatinine clearance strongly suggests that cystatin C may represent more than just a marker of glomerular filtration. Data from the Heart and Soul Study [62] clearly showed that elevated cystatin C concentrations were able to predict all-cause mortality, future CV events, and incident CHF among ambulatory subjects with stable CHD, and even among persons without microalbuminuria or low estimated GFR. Therefore, cystatin C seems to be a promising and clinically useful marker, which provides complementary information to the so far known risk determinants in patients with CHD. However, evidence that cystatin C concentrations may be altered by age, gender, BMI, cigarette smoking, CRP, and thyroid dysfunction, might unfortunately limit the utility of this emerging marker in routine clinical practice.

MONOCYTE CHEMOATTRACTANT PROTEIN-1

MCP-1 (CCL2) is the most important chemokine that regulates migration and infiltration of monocytes/macrophages [63]. Its effects are mainly mediated through the CC chemokine receptor 2 (CCR2). ECs, monocytes, and/or SMC express MCP-1 in response to various cytokines, growth factors, oxLDL, and CD40 L and thus MCP-1 expression is increased in atherosclerotic lesions, in particular in macrophage-rich areas. MCP-1 causes chronic vascular inflammation, induces proliferation and migration of SMCs, migration of ECs, neovascularization in plaque, oxidative stress, and thrombosis [63]. Activation of the MCP-1/CCR2 pathway has also been shown to induce expression of MMPs, thus suggesting its involvement in plaque destabilization. In animal models, the expression of MCP-1 was directly related to the extent of atherosclerosis and macrophage infiltration into the atherosclerotic lesion, and anti-monocyte MCP-1 gene therapy limited the progression and destabilization of established atherosclerosis in apolipoprotein E-knockout mice [63]. Based on these findings, MCP-1 could present an interesting, novel target for intervention to reduce atherosclerotic complications. Consistent with such experimental data, in the Orbofiban in Patients with Unstable coronary Syndromes (OPUS)-TIMI 16 trial, elevated levels of MCP-1 were associated with risk of death or MI after 10 months, independent of a variety of CV risk factors, clinical and ECG characteristics, renal function, and markers of necrosis and inflammation [64]. However, although in a large case-cohort study from the MONICA/KORA Augsburg database, elevated levels of MCP-1 preceded CHD events, they were not independent predictors of risk, once traditional risk factors were also considered [65]. Thus, further studies in various populations are needed to potentially establish MCP-1 as a clinically useful biomarker.

SUMMARY AND CONCLUSION

The rapidly increasing literature on biomarkers in CVD has provided us with valuable new information regarding the pathophysiology of this complex disorder. However, before such information can be translated into the clinical setting, a number of criteria have to be fulfilled before any biomarker can be used routinely. It is not sufficient to simply demonstrate a more or less strong association between a biomarker and CV outcome. Morrow [66] has put together an extensive list of requirements that cover pre-analytical issues, assay methods, costs involved, strength of the association found in various studies, and the potential incremental value over and above existing routinely measured traditional risk factors. Unless such information has been convincingly shown, widespread clinical use of biomarkers to refine risk predication cannot be recommended. Thus, there is still some way to go before we may have an ideal reliable diagnostic tool in our hands that enables us to identify atherosclerosis at its earliest still asymptomatic stage, with economically acceptable costs.

REFERENCES

1. Greenland P, Smith SC Jr, Grundy SM. Improving coronary heart disease risk assessment in asymptomatic people: role of traditional risk factors and noninvasive cardiovascular tests. Circulation. 2001;104:1863–1867.
2. Koenig W, Khuseyinova N. Biomarkers of atherosclerotic plaque instability and rupture. Arterioscler Thromb Vasc Biol. 2007;27:15–26.

3. Pearson TA, Mensah GA, Alexander RW, Anderson JL, Cannon RO 3rd, Criqui M, Fadl YY, Fortmann SP, Hong Y, Myers GL, Rifai N, Smith SC Jr, Taubert K, Tracy RP, Vinicor F; Centers for Disease Control and Prevention; American Heart Association. Markers of inflammation and cardiovascular disease: application to clinical and public health practice: a statement for healthcare professionals from the Centers for Disease Control and Prevention and the American Heart Association. Circulation. 2003;107:499–511.
4. Danesh J, Wheeler JG, Hirschfield GM, Eda S, Eiriksdottir G, Rumley A, Lowe GD, Pepys MB, Gudnason V. C-reactive protein and other circulating markers of inflammation in the prediction of coronary heart disease. N Engl J Med. 2004;350: 1387–1397.
5. Rattazzi M, Puato M, Faggin E, Bertipaglia B, Zambon A, Pauletto P. C-reactive protein and interleukin-6 in vascular disease: culprits or passive bystanders? J Hypertens. 2003;21:1787–1803.
6. The Emerging Risk Factors Collaboration. The Emerging Risk Factors Collaboration: analysis of individual data on lipid, inflammatory and other markers in over 1.1 million participants in 104 prospective studies of cardiovascular diseases. Eur J Epidemiol. 2007;22:839–869.
7. Pepys MB, Booth DR, Hutchinson WL, Gallimore JR, Collins PM, Hohenester E. Amyloid P component. A critical review. Amyloid. 1997;4:274–295.
8. Li XA, Hatanaka K, Ishibashi-Ueda H, Yutani C, Yamamoto A. Characterization of serum amyloid P component from human aortic atherosclerotic lesions. Arterioscler Thromb Vasc Biol. 1995;15:252–257.
9. Jenny NS, Arnold AM, Kuller LH, Tracy RP, Psaty BM. Serum amyloid P and cardiovascular disease in older men: results from the Cardiovascular Health Study. Arterioscler Thromb Vasc Biol. 2007;27:352–358.
10. Kamath S, Lip GYH. Fibrinogen: biochemistry, epidemiology and determinants. Q J Med 2003;96:711–729.
11. Koenig W. Fibrin(ogen) in cardiovascular disease: an update. Thromb Haemost. 2003;89:601–609.
12. Fibrinogen Studies Collaboration. Plasma fibrinogen level and the risk of major cardiovascular diseases and nonvascular mortality: an individual participant meta-analysis. JAMA. 2005;294:1799–1809.
13. Vaughan DE. PAI-1 and atherothrombosis. J Thromb Haemost. 2005;3:1879–1883.
14. Falkenberg M, Tjarnstrom J, Ortenwall P, Olausson M, Risberg B. Localization of fibrinolytic activators and inhibitors in normal and atherosclerotic vessels. Thromb Haemost. 1996;75:933–938.
15. Collet JP, Montalescot G, Vicaut E, Ankri A, Walylo F, Lesty C, Choussat R, Beygui F, Borentain M, Vignolles N, Thomas D. Acute release of plasminogen activator inhibitor-1 in ST-segment elevation myocardial infarction predicts mortality. Circulation. 2003;108:391–394
16. Lowe GD, Danesh J, Lewington S, Walker M, Lennon L, Thomson A, Rumley A, Whincup PH. Tissue plasminogen activator antigen and coronary heart disease. Prospective study and meta-analysis. Eur Heart J. 2004;25:252–259.
17. Lowe GD. Fibrin D-dimer and cardiovascular risk. Semin Vasc Med. 2005;5:387–398.
18. Lowe GD, Rumley A, McMahon AD, Ford I, O'Reilly DS, Packard CJ; West of Scotland Coronary Prevention Study Group. Interleukin-6, fibrin D-dimer, and coagulation factors VII and XIIa in prediction of coronary heart disease. Arterioscler Thromb Vasc Biol. 2004;24:1529–1534.
19. Pradhan AD, LaCroix AZ, Langer RD, Trevisan M, Lewis CE, Hsia JA, Oberman A, Kotchen JM, Ridker PM. Tissue plasminogen activator antigen and D-dimer as markers for atherothrombotic risk among healthy postmenopausal women. Circulation. 2004;110:292–300.
20. Lindmark E, Diderholm E, Wallentin L, Siegbahn A. Relationship between interleukin 6 and mortality in patients with unstable coronary artery disease: effects of an early invasive or noninvasive strategy. JAMA. 2001;286:2107–2113.
21. Gracie JA, Robertson SE, McInnes IB. Interleukin-18. J Leukoc Biol. 2003;73:213–224
22. Caligiuri G, Kaveri S, Nicoletti A. When interleukin-18 conducts, the Preludio sounds the same no matter who plays. Arterioscler Thromb Vasc Biol. 2005;25:655–657.
23. Blankenberg S, Tiret L, Bickel C, Peetz D, Cambien F, Meyer J, Rupprecht HJ; Athero*Gene* Investigators. Interleukin-18 is a strong predictor of cardiovascular death in stable and unstable angina. Circulation. 2002;106:24–30.
24. Tiret L, Godefroy T, Lubos E, Nicaud V, Tregouet DA, Barbaux S, Schnabel R, Bickel C, Espinola-Klein C, Poirier O, Perret C, Munzel T, Rupprecht HJ, Lackner K, Cambien F, Blankenberg S; Athero*Gene* Investigators. Genetic analysis of the interleukin-18 system highlights the role of the interleukin-18 gene in cardiovascular disease. Circulation. 2005; 112:643–650.
25. Blankenberg S, Luc G, Ducimetiere P, Arveiler D, Ferrieres J, Amouyel P, Evans A, Cambien F, Tiret L; PRIME Study Group Interleukin-18 and the risk of coronary heart disease in European men: the Prospective Epidemiological Study of Myocardial Infarction (PRIME). Circulation. 2003;108:2453–2459.
26. Koenig W, Khuseyinova N, Baumert J, Thorand B, Loewel H, Chambless L, Meisinger C, Schneider A, Martin S, Kolb H, Herder C. Increased concentrations of C-reactive protein and IL-6 but not IL-18 are independently associated with incident coronary events in middle-aged men and women: results from the MONICA/KORA Augsburg case-cohort study, 1984–2002. Arterioscler Thromb Vasc Biol. 2006;26:2745–2751.
27. Murr C, Widner B, Wirleitner B, Fuchs D. Neopterin as a marker for immune system activation. Curr Drug Metab. 2002;3:175–187.
28. Pacileo M, Cirillo P, De Rosa S, Ucci G, Petrillo G, D'Amore SM, Sasso L, Maietta P, Spagnuolo R, Chiariello M. The role of neopterin in cardiovascular disease. Monaldi Arch Chest Dis. 2007;68:68–73.
29. Ray KK, Morrow DA, Sabatine MS, Shui A, Rifai N, Cannon CP, Braunwald E. Long-term prognostic value of neopterin: a novel marker of monocyte activation in patients with acute coronary syndrome. Circulation. 2007;115:3071–3078.

30. Jones CB, Sane DC, Herrington DM. Matrix metalloproteinases: a review of their structure and role in acute coronary syndrome. Cardiovasc Res. 2003;59:812–823.
31. Blankenberg S, Rupprecht HJ, Poirier O, Bickel C, Smieja M, Hafner G, Meyer J, Cambien F, Tiret L; Athero*Gene* Investigators. Plasma concentrations and genetic variation of matrix metalloproteinase 9 and prognosis of patients with cardiovascular disease. Circulation. 2003;107:1579–1585.
32. Lubos E, Schnabel R, Rupprecht HJ, Bickel C, Messow CM, Prigge S, Cambien F, Tiret L, Munzel T, Blankenberg S. Prognostic value of tissue inhibitor of metalloproteinase-1 for cardiovascular death among patients with cardiovascular disease: results from the Athero*Gene* study. Eur Heart J. 2006;27:150–156.
33. Cavusoglu E, Ruwende C, Chopra V, Yanamadala S, Eng C, Clark LT, Pinsky DJ, Marmur JD. Tissue inhibitor of metalloproteinase-1 (TIMP-1) is an independent predictor of all-cause mortality, cardiac mortality, and myocardial infarction. Am Heart J. 2006;151:1101.e1–1101.e8.
34. Thorn EM, Khan IA. Pregnancy-associated plasma protein-A: an emerging cardiac biomarker. Int J Cardiol. 2007;117:370–372.
35. Bunn RC, Fowlkes JL. Insulin-like growth factor binding protein proteolysis. Trends Endocrinol Metab. 2003;14:176–181.
36. Conti E, Andreotti F, Zuppi C. Pregnancy-associated plasma protein a as predictor of outcome in patients with suspected acute coronary syndromes. Circulation. 2004;109:e211–212.
37. Qin QP, Kokkala S, Lund J, Tamm N, Qin X, Lepantalo M, Pettersson K. Immunoassays developed for pregnancy-associated plasma protein-A (PAPP-A) in pregnancy may not recognize PAPP-A in acute coronary syndromes. Clin Chem. 2006;52:398–404.
38. Nicholls SJ, Hazen SL. Myeloperoxidase and cardiovascular disease. Arterioscler Thromb Vasc Biol. 2005;25:1102–1111.
39. Eiserich JP, Baldus S, Brennan ML, Ma W, Zhang C, Tousson A, Castro L, Lusis AJ, Nauseef WM, White CR, Freeman BA. Myeloperoxidase, a leukocyte-derived vascular NO oxidase. Science. 2002;296:2391–2394.
40. Baldus S, Heeschen C, Meinertz T, Zeiher AM, Eiserich JP, Munzel T, Simoons ML, Hamm CW; CAPTURE Investigators. Myeloperoxidase serum levels predict risk in patients with acute coronary syndromes. Circulation. 2003;108:1440–1445.
41. Brennan ML, Penn MS, Van Lente F, Nambi V, Shishehbor MH, Aviles RJ, Goormastic M, Pepoy ML, McErlean ES, Topol EJ, Nissen SE, Hazen SL. Prognostic value of myeloperoxidase in patients with chest pain. N Engl J Med. 2003; 349:1595–1604.
42. Jessup W, Kritharides L, Stocker R. Lipid oxidation in atherogenesis: an overview. Biochem Soc Trans. 2004;32:134–138.
43. Salonen JT, Yla-Herttuala S, Yamamoto R, Butler S, Korpela H, Salonen R, Nyyssonen K, Palinski W, Witztum JL. Autoantibody against oxidised LDL and progression of carotid atherosclerosis. Lancet. 1992;339:883–887.
44. Meisinger C, Baumert J, Khuseyinova N, Loewel H, Koenig W. Plasma oxidized low-density lipoprotein, a strong predictor for acute coronary heart disease events in apparently healthy, middle-aged men from the general population. Circulation. 2005;112:651–657.
45. Vivekananthan DP, Penn MS, Sapp SK, Hsu A, Topol EJ. Use of antioxidant vitamins for the prevention of cardiovascular disease: metaanalysis of randomised trials. Lancet. 2003:361:2017–2023.
46. Ursini F, Maiorino M, Roveri A. Phospholipid hydroperoxide glutathione peroxidase (PHGPx): more than an antioxidant enzyme? Biomed Environ Sci. 1997;10:327–332.
47. Lackner KJ, Blankenberg S. Atherosclerosis, oxidative stress and glutathione peroxidase-1: a new kid on the block. Ital Heart J. 2004;5:169–172.
48. Blankenberg S, Rupprecht HJ, Bickel C, Torzewski M, Hafner G, Tiret L, Smieja M, Cambien F, Meyer J, Lackner KJ; Athero*Gene* Investigators. Glutathione peroxidase 1 activity and cardiovascular events in patients with coronary artery disease. N Engl J Med. 2003;349:1605–1613.
49. Khuseyinova N, Koenig W. Predicting the risk of cardiovascular disease: where does lipoprotein-associated phospholipase A(2) fit in? Mol Diagn Ther. 2007;11:203–217.
50. Kolodgie FD, Burke AP, Skorija KS, Ladich E, Kutys R, Makuria AT, Virmani R. Lipoprotein-associated phospholipase A2 protein expression in the natural progression of human coronary atherosclerosis. Arterioscler Thromb Vasc Biol. 2006; 26:2523–2529.
51. Zalewski A, Macphee C. Role of lipoprotein-associated phospholipase A2 in atherosclerosis: biology, epidemiology, and possible therapeutic target. Arterioscler Thromb Vasc Biol. 2005;25:923–931.
52. Hurt-Camejo E, Camejo G, Peilot H, Oorni K, Kovanen P. Phospholipase A(2) in vascular disease. Circ Res. 2001;89:298–304.
53. Sartipy P, Camejo G, Svensson L, Hurt-Camejo E. Phospholipase A(2) modification of low density lipoproteins forms small high density particles with increased affinity for proteoglycans and glycosaminoglycans. J Biol Chem. 1999;274: 25913–25920.
54. Boekholdt SM, Keller TT, Wareham NJ, Luben R, Bingham SA, Day NE, Sandhu MS, Jukema JW, Kastelein JJ, Hack CE, Khaw KT. Serum levels of type II secretory phospholipase A2 and the risk of future coronary artery disease in apparently healthy men and women: the EPIC-Norfolk Prospective Population Study. Arterioscler Thromb Vasc Biol. 2005;25:839–846.
55. Koenig W, Vossen CY, Brenner H, Rothenbacher D. Type II secretory phospolipase A_2 plasma concentrations predict cardiovascular events in patients with coronary heart disease. Circulation. 2007;116:II_841 (Abstract).
56. Böger RH. Asymmetric dimethylarginine (ADMA): a novel risk marker in cardiovascular medicine and beyond. Ann Med. 2006;38:126–136.

57. Schnabel R, Blankenberg S, Lubos E, Lackner KJ, Rupprecht HJ, Espinola-Klein C, Jachmann N, Post F, Peetz D, Bickel C, Cambien F, Tiret L, Münzel T. Asymmetric dimethylarginine and the risk of cardiovascular events and death in patients with coronary artery disease: results from the Athero*Gene* Study. Circ Res. 2005;97:e53-e59.
58. Maas R, Schulze F, Baumert J, Löwel H, Hamraz K, Schwedhelm E, Koenig W, Böger RH. Asymmetric dimethylarginine, smoking, and risk of coronary heart disease in apparently healthy men: prospective analysis from the population-based Monitoring of Trends and Determinants in Cardiovascular Disease/Kooperative Gesundheitsforschung in der Region Augsburg study and experimental data. Clin Chem. 2007;53:693–701.
59. Madero M, Sarnak MJ, Stevens LA. Serum cystatin C as a marker of glomerular filtration rate. Curr Opin Nephrol Hypertens. 2006;15:610–616.
60. Jernberg T, Lindahl B, James S, Larsson A, Hansson LO, Wallentin L. Cystatin C: a novel predictor of outcome in suspected or confirmed non-ST-elevation acute coronary syndrome. Circulation. 2004;110:2342–2348.
61. Koenig W, Twardella D, Brenner H, Rothenbacher D. Plasma concentrations of cystatin C in patients with coronary heart disease and risk for secondary cardiovascular events: more than simply a marker of glomerular filtration rate. Clin Chem. 2005;51:321–327.
62. Ix JH, Shlipak MG, Chertow GM, Whooley MA. Association of cystatin C with mortality, cardiovascular events, and incident heart failure among persons with coronary heart disease: data from the Heart and Soul Study. Circulation. 2007;115:173–179.
63. Coll B, Alonso-Villaverde C, Joven J. Monocyte chemoattractant protein-1 and atherosclerosis: is there room for an additional biomarker? Clin Chim Acta. 2007;383:21–29.
64. De Lemos JA, Morrow DA, Sabatine MS, Murphy SA, Gibson CM, Antman EM, McCabe CH, Cannon CP, Braunwald E. Association between plasma levels of monocyte chemoattractant protein-1 and long-term clinical outcomes in patients with acute coronary syndromes. Circulation. 2003;107:690–695.
65. Herder C, Baumert J, Thorand B, Martin S, Lowel H, Kolb H, Koenig W. Chemokines and incident coronary heart disease: results from the MONICA/KORA Augsburg case-cohort study, 1984–2002. Arterioscler Thromb Vasc Biol. 2006;26:2147–2152.
66. Morrow DA, de Lemos JA. Benchmarks for the assessment of novel cardiovascular biomarkers. Circulation. 2007;115:949–952.

10 Genomics and Proteomics: The Role of Contemporary Biomolecular Analysis in Advancing the Knowledge of Atherosclerotic Coronary Artery Disease

Gary P. Foster and Naser Ahmadi

CONTENTS

ABSTRACT

Despite major advances in the treatment of coronary heart disease (CHD), a large number of individuals die suddenly without prior symptoms. The currently available screening and diagnostic methods are insufficient to identify vulnerable patients before an event occurs. Genomic and proteomic studies of atherosclerosis promise to bridge epidemiology and basic biology, and advance our understanding of the basic biomolecular mechanisms of this disease processes. Proteins from vascular cells or atherosclerotic plaques that are present in plasma are modified along the different steps of atherosclerotic development, and they constitute additional candidates for vascular research, particularly in the search for novel biological markers of cardiovascular risk. Opportunities to translate genomic and proteomic information into cardiovascular clinical practice have never been greater, but their fruition requires validation in large independent cohorts that will be achieved only through collaborative efforts. In this chapter, we summarize genomic and proteomic techniques and the most recent results obtained by application of these high-throughput strategies to cardiovascular disease.

From: *Asymptomatic Atherosclerosis: Pathophysiology, Detection and Treatment*
Edited by: M. Naghavi (ed.), DOI 10.1007/978-1-60327-179-0_10

Key words: Coronary heart disease; Genomics; Proteomics

It is estimated that between 20 and 33% of individuals with significant coronary artery disease are misclassified by the Framingham Risk Assessment [1, 2]. These findings suggest the presence of important undiscovered patho-physiologic mechanisms. Recent advances in genomic and proteomic technologies hold great promise for transforming the practice of medicine through a more comprehensive understanding of the biomolecular mechanisms responsible for a wide variety of diseases.

The actual term "genomics" is thought to have been originally coined by Dr. Tom Roderick, a geneticist at the Jackson Laboratory (Bar Harbor, ME), over beer at a meeting held in Maryland on the mapping of the human genome in 1986 (Wikipedia, *Genomics*). Genomics refers to the study of an organism's entire genome or the sum total of the genes. Following the same logic, proteomics refers to the study of an organism's entire proteome.

It is anticipated that genomic approaches applied to atherosclerosis will identify associated genes and biomolecular pathways, whereas proteomic studies should provide verification of genomic findings and identify a more refined family of clinically relevant biomarkers. The coupling of information gained through these new methodologies to our traditional tools should significantly sharpen our ability to assess and modify the management of cardiovascular disease. Realizing the potential to translate genomic and proteomic information into cardiovascular clinical practice will necessitate a detailed pathway to discovery, followed by validation in large independent cohorts. These efforts will only be achieved through collaborative efforts between diverse specialties within the cardiovascular research community.

Despite steady progress in some portions of the developed world, atherosclerotic cardiovascular disease remains a growing public health burden throughout the world [3–5]. Although population statistics provide helpful guidelines, meaningful advances in cardiovascular research cannot be fully realized unless translated to care of individual patients [6].

Combining a refined set of biomarkers with currently available screening tools promises to promote this translational process. Before a personalized medicine approach to atherosclerosis can become reality, researchers must validate novel markers across different cohorts and in relation to various environmental modifiers. The operation of intricate networks of genes, environmental factors, and gene-by-environment interactions further complicates the understanding of the genetic components of atherosclerosis [7, 8]. To address these concerns, combined genomic approaches, often called *genomic convergence*, are necessary [9].

The human genome project (HGP) and International HapMap project (IHMP) provide a massive library of DNA-based information that can be searched for meaningful associations with data gained from genomic studies. Differential expressions of thousands of genes can now be assessed in a variety of biological samples under different conditions. The HGP and IHMP laid the groundwork for studies of genetic susceptibility to disease, and expression databases that assist with the definition of disease subtypes and variants, related to environmental interactions.

Although less mature, proteomic libraries are under construction and hold great promise in complementing the information cataloged through the efforts of the HGP and IHMP (Table 1).

GENETIC STUDIES OF ATHEROSCLEROTIC CARDIOVASCULAR DISEASE

Knowledge of the human genome sequence and the advent of technologies that enable rapid surveillance of entire genomes and proteomes have fundamentally changed the study of disease patho-physiology. These high-throughput technologies and concomitant advances in bioinformatics methodologies have paved the way for the genetic dissection of chronic disease, and for the accelerated coupling of data to the definition of the molecular pathways linking specific gene variants

Table 1
Comparison of current methods of genetic and proteomic research

Method	*Strength*	*Limitations*	*Findings*
Genetic linkage	Evaluates individual genes with large effect	Low resolution and power for complex diseases (requires fine mapping/gene study)Family-based study only (may not explain gene expression of general population)	LDL and HMG-CoA reductase inhibitor, chromosomal locus and CAD, , MEF2A and ALOX5AP with MI and stroke risk
Genetic association	More resolution and statistical power for complex diseases as compared to linkage analysisFamily-based or unrelated subjects gene study	Need large sample size for replication (~2,000 cases + 2,000 controls) to detect genetic markers with small effect	clinical phenotype, such as MI, differing levels of a biomarker such as C-reactive protein and cholesterol
Candidate gene	Lower cost than genome-wide study-Customized choice of SNPs	Evaluated only the genes chosen for analysis	*CRP* SNPs, *ALOX5AP*
Whole genome	Surveys entire genome, and evaluates maximum amount of information per assayIdentifies variants with relatively small effect	Very expensive due to SNP volumeRequires comprehensive Bioinformatics Requires good coverage (avoid missing a region of interest) and multiple rounds of replication	Genetic variants within CRP to cardiovascular disease
Gene expression	Real-time Dynamic information about pathophysiological changesCustomized chips for panels of genes related to a process (e.g., inflammation) Microarray analysis that covers genes within the human genome (20–38.5 K)	Susceptible to experimental and pathphysiologic variabilityPossible bias in types of discovered genes discovered based on the selected chips mRNA expression and ultimate protein expression may not be closely associated	Transcriptional profiling of peripheral blood leukocytes, Expression profiling of atheromata in human aortic tissue, gene expression associated with atherosclerotic lesion progression (*H2-Eb1* and *H2-Ab1, Runx2*, an *Spp1*etc)
Proteomic	Protein expression	Post-translational modificationsSusceptible to experimental and pathphysiologic variability	HSP27, LDL-associated apolipoproteins, and *many* others
Complementary genomic and proteomic	Real-time Dynamic information about pathophysiological changesCustomized chips for panels of genes related to a process (e.g., inflammation) High resolution and power for protein and genomic profiling	Requires comprehensive BioinformaticsSusceptible to experimental and pathphysiologic variability	Cardiovascular disease-related proteins in human plasma

SNP single nucleotide polymorphism, *MEF2A* myocyte enhancer factor-2, *MI* myocardial infarction, *ALOX5AP* arachidonate 5-lipoxygenase activating protein gene

to cell dysfunction. These approaches have led to the identification of gene loci of rheumatoid arthritis (RA) [10], systemic lupus erythematosus (SLE) [11], and numerous other autoimmune diseases [12]. These successes indicate the enormous potential for high-throughput technologies to generate the molecular knowledge needed for radical improvement in the quality of health care delivery (Table 2).

Table 2
Prior contemporary genomic and proteomic studies in CAD

Authors	*Studied cohort*	*Technique*	*Findings*
Prior Genomic studies in CAD			
Seo et al. [28]	Atherosclerotic aortic tissue from heart donors	Gene expression patterns using microarray analysis	208 genes were identified whose expression patterns provided the power to correctly classify mild and severe atherosclerotic disease in 29 out of 31 samples (93.5%)
Patino et al. [29]	Carotid atherosclerosis were compared with controls	Gene expression signatures	PMC gene expression profiling might have utility in the detection of atherosclerosis. A number of regulatory genes and transcription factors that were significantly altered in the disease group were found
Tabibiazar et al. [30]	Mouse genetic model (apoE-deficient, C57B1/6J, CH3) that induces atherosclerosis with diet (normal vs. high fat diet) and age	Gene expression was performed by microarray analysis	Gene classifier groups with the ability to correctly distinguish between temporal stages of aortic atherosclerosis were isolated. Atherosclerosis related mouse genes were matched to human orthologs and accurately classified disease and control groups
Ma et al. [31]	PMCs from four individuals with CAD in comparison with three healthy male controls	Gene expression was performed by microarray analysis (using 10,378 cDNA clones chosen form a library using an Affymetrix arrayer)	108 differentially expressed genes (>2 fold) were found (65 upregulated and 43 downregulated). Genes for 3 secreted proteins were chosen from the differentially expressed list (pro-platelet basic protein, platelet factor 4, coagulation factor XIII A1) and reverse transcriptase polymerase chain reaction (RT-PCR) was performed which confirmed up-regulation of the three secreted proteins
Prior proteomic studies in CAD			
Tabibiazar et al. [32]	Proteomic signature of atherosclerosis in diseased and controlled groups of Mouse model	Protein expression was performed by microarray analysis	After applying several algorithms, an expression pattern of 7 proteins (Ccl21, Ccl9, Csf3, Tnfsf11, Vegfa, Ccl11, Ccl2) were found to distinguish disease from control group with up to 100% accuracy

(continued)

Table 2 (continued)

Authors	*Studied cohort*	*Technique*	*Findings*
Duran et al. [33]	Proteomic analysis on proteins secreted from human carotid atherosclerotic plaques	2 dimensional electrophoretic gels was performed	42 spots in the normal group compared with 154 spots in the diseased group were identified and showed the different expression of proteins between the disease and control groups
You et al. [34]	Proteomic analysis on ten diseased and seven normal coronary arteries from patients undergoing heart transplantation or from autopsy specimens	Two dimensional gel electrophoresis was performed. Protein identification was performed with LC-tandem mass spectroscopy ion trap and a protein identification program	Analysis of the 2D gel maps identified one protein spot that which showed a consistently higher level of expression in the diseased arteries. Mass spectrometry identified this protein spot as ferritin light chain (1.9x control expression)
Donahue et al. [35]	Plasma samples from 53 males with CAD and 53 age, race and disease matched controls	Albumin and immunoglobulins were removed from plasma samples. Samples were then separated into 12,960 fractions by cation exchange and two reversed-phase chromatography steps. Proteins were then analyzed by liquid chromatography–electrospray ionization tandem mass spectrometry	95 differentially expressed proteins in a variety of broad categories were found. In addition, 17 differentially expressed genes were identified based on a formula of peak size and percent of fractions of expressed proteins
Zimmerli et al. [36]	Urine samples from 88 individuals with CAD and 282 controls	Spot urine samples were analyzed using ESI–TOF–MS	15 proteins were differentially expressed with patterns that distinguished the disease and control groups with 98% sensitivity and 83% specificity

Among the myriad of genomic technologies now available, the methods used to screen for disease-conferring gene variants, and to assess entire genome or proteome expression levels have particular potential for medical benefit.

Such knowledge will allow for definition of the molecular determinants of disease expression and persistence, and thereby identify both biomarkers for use in diagnosis and risk prediction and targets on which to focus prevention and treatment.

Of particular relevance to the prevention and management of disease are technologies such as high-throughput DNA genotyping, microarray-based gene-expression profiling, and mass spectrometry-facilitated protein profiling platforms that collectively support the comprehensive analysis of DNA sequence variants across the genome and the global gene and protein expression changes that distinguish health from disease. Now used extensively in all facets of biomedical investigation, genomic and proteomic tools are already beginning to pinpoint molecular variants that influence risk and outcome in common diseases, and to thereby inform and direct development of novel molecular biomarkers and drug targets. As evidenced by recent advances in DNA sequencing methods, continued improvements in the scope, power, and cost efficiency of genomic and proteomic technologies should ensure their capacity to provide the scale and depth of knowledge required for translating genome sequence information into major medical impact.

TECHNIQUES USED IN THE GENOMIC AND PROTEOMIC STUDIES

Bioinformatics. Includes three components (1) the development and implementation of tools that enable efficient retrieval, access, and management of different types of information; (2) the development of new algorithms and statistics with which to assess relations among members of large data sets; (3) the analysis and interpretation of various types of data (from genomic and proteomic analyses) [13].

Basic local alignment search tool (BLAST). "Software program from NCBI for searching public databases for homologous DNA sequences or proteins." [13]

Hierarchical clustering. An unsupervised clustering approach used to determine patterns in gene expression data with an output that resembles a tree-like structure. [13]

Self-organizing map (SOM). An algorithm that organizes the clusters of gene expression data or multidimensional data in a two-dimensional grid, such that clusters that are close together in the grid are more similar than those further apart [13].

Expressed sequence tags (EST). A unique short DNA sequence (100–300 base pairs) derived from a cDNA library that can be mapped to a unique locus in the genome and serves to identify that gene locus [13].

Mass spectrometry (MS). A technique for measuring and analyzing molecules that involves introducing enough energy into a target molecule to cause its disintegration. The resulting fragments are then analyzed, based on their mass:charge ratios, to produce a molecular fingerprint. The resulting mass spectrum is a graph (often a histogram) of ion intensity as a function of mass:charge ratio [13].

Microarray technology. Hybridization-based tool used to analyze how large numbers of genes interact with each other and how a cell's regulatory network controls a vast battery of genes simultaneously; used for genotyping, mapping, sequencing, and sequence detection. Microarrays are constructed by applying biomolecules with a robot in an orderly fashion, on a rectangular grid of spots on a slide or chip (that serves as matrix), labeled with a fluorescent probe and scanned with a microscope or specialized imaging equipment. The rows represent genes, and the columns represent different samples. First, an array of gene-specific probes is embedded on a matrix. Nucleic acids (mRNA or cDNA) are then isolated from test samples and converted into labeled targets. The labeled targets are then incubated with the solid state probes, allowing targets to hybridize with probes. The hybridization of probes and targets is measured (after the incubation, nonhybridized samples are washed away) with dye fluorescence or radioactivity [13].

Molecular profiling (MP). "A global view of mRNA, protein patterns, and DNA alterations in various cell types and disease processes" [13].

Single-nucleotide polymorphism (SNP). "A SNP is a location in the gene where certain individuals have one DNA base (e.g., A), and others have a different base (e.g., C). SNPs and point mutations are structurally identical, differing only in their frequency. Variations that occur in 1% or less of a population are considered point mutations, and those occurring in more than 1% are SNPs. This distinction is practical and reflects the fact that low frequency mutations cannot be used effectively in genetic studies as genetic markers, while more common ones can" [13].

NCBI: National Center for Biotechnology Information.

GENETIC LINKAGE STUDIES

Using families and anonymous DNA markers, genetic linkage studies correlate inherited genomic regions with inherited familial characteristics (Figs. 1–3). Although the many genes and environmental factors influencing atherosclerosis make direct linkage difficult, numerous examples link phenotypes with atherosclerotic cardiovascular disease. A recent linkage analysis has successfully identified specific genes that may contribute to cardiovascular event risk, for example, myocyte enhancer factor-2 (MEF2A) with myocardial infarction (MI) risk [14], and arachidonate 5-lipoxygenase activating protein gene (ALOX5AP) with MI and stroke risk [15]. Helgadottir et al. [15] showed linkage between the ALOX5AP gene region and MI in 296 Icelandic families, including 713 subjects. The ALOX5AP gene encodes the enzyme 5-lipoxygenase activating protein (FLAP), which participates in leukotriene synthesis. Such leukotrienes, especially leukotriene B4 (LTB4), mediate inflammation within the vasculature and participate in murine atherosclerosis [16]. The clinical utility of these

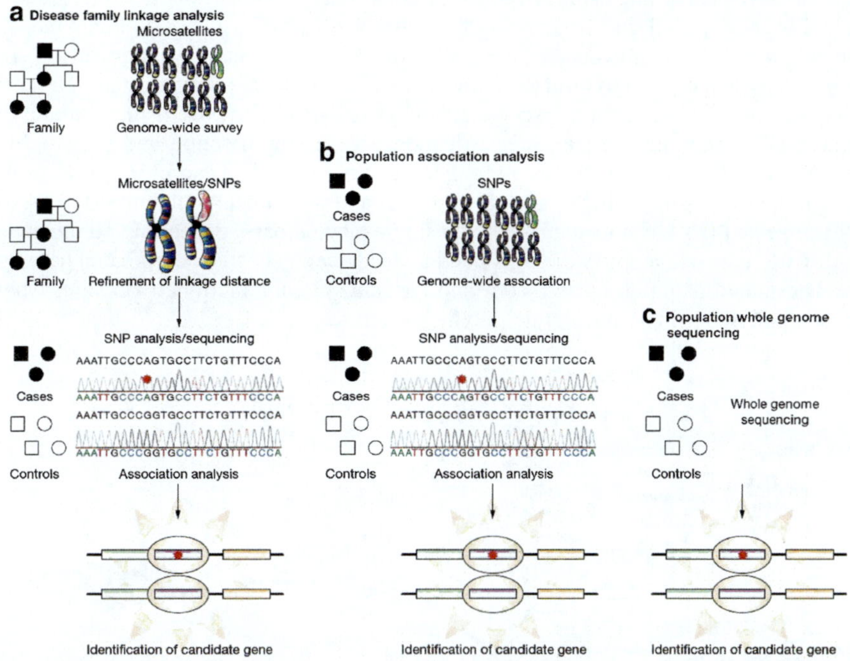

Fig. 1. Strategies for disease gene mapping. A number of genomic tools are used to screen for disease susceptibility genes. (**a**) Genome-wide screens using microsatellite markers spaced at approximately 10 cM intervals across the genome can be used to survey multicase families and identify marker loci that cosegregate (are linked) with disease. If significant linkage is detected, the linkage interval can be refined by further genotyping using microsatellite markers and/or SNPs to evaluate marker-disease linkage in multicase families or marker-disease associations in families or cases and controls. Sequencing is then used to search for disease-associated variants in selected candidate genes. (**b**) Genome-wide screens using SNP markers spaced at 5–10 kb intervals can be used to genotype cases and controls to search for marker loci associated with disease. Loci showing significant associations are then reanalyzed using additional SNPs or sequencing to identify the disease-causing mutations. (**c**) It may soon be possible to directly screen for disease-associated variants using high-throughput sequencing technologies to directly sequence cases and controls. Abbreviation: *SNP* single nucleotide polymorphism.

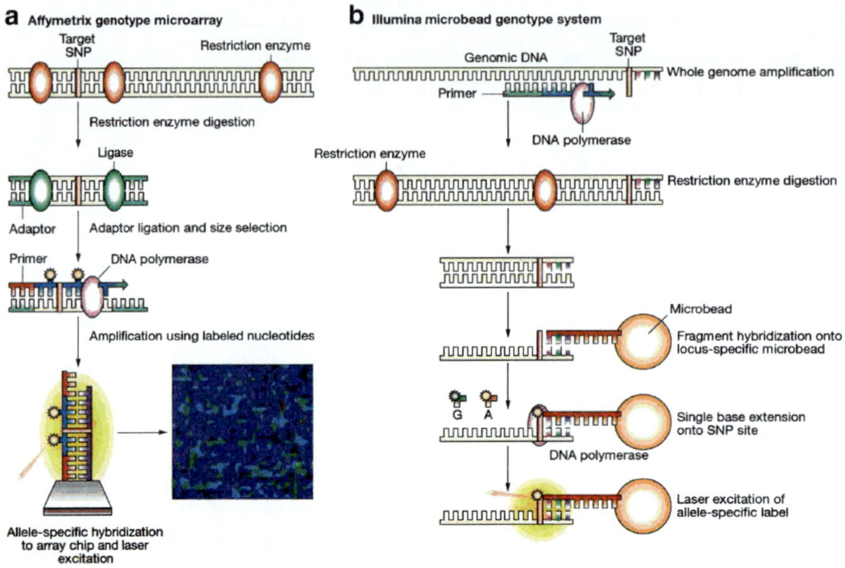

Fig. 2. Two ultra-high-throughput single nucleotide polymorphism genotyping platforms for use in genome-wide association analyses. (**a**) SNP genotyping using Affymetrix (Santa Clara, CA) high-density oligonucleotide microarrays. Genomic DNA samples are digested into fragments of random sizes using a restriction enzyme. Adaptors are then ligated to the fragment ends to create universal priming sites for PCR amplification. Fragments of sizes 250–1,000 bp are amplified, fluorescently labeled and hybridized to the array. The arrays are scanned and SNP genotypes are determined using specialized software following laser detection. (**b**) SNP genotyping using Illumina bead arrays (San Diego, CA). Genomic DNA samples are subjected to genome-wide amplification and the amplified DNA is then fragmented by enzyme digestion. Fragments are hybridized to SNP-specific bead chips, each of which carries two probes that enable simultaneous genotyping of both SNP alleles and that anneal with template DNA at a site one base before the SNP. The annealed DNA is now extended by a single labeled base, depending on the genotype at the SNP. The extended samples are stained to amplify the signal and allow detection of the incorporated base by laser excitation, and genotypes are determined using an array reader and specialized computational software. Abbreviations: PCR, polymerase chain reaction; SNP, single nucleotide polymorphism

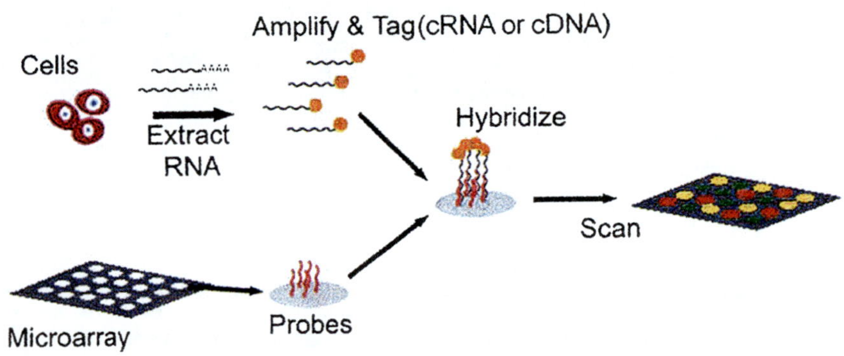

Fig. 3. Microarrays. Cells are processed for mRNA extraction, tagged with a fluorescent marker, and then hybridized onto a microarray with probes. If a complementary strand is present on the microarray, mRNA will bind to microarray and level of fluorescence will indicate level of expression.

findings remains unclear as the selection criteria allow for a significant percentage of individuals with potentially dangerous coronary disease to be included in the control groups and do not exclude the possibility of false positives in the disease groups.

GENETIC ASSOCIATION STUDIES

Genetic association studies seek to identify differences in the inheritance of particular single nucleotide polymorphism (SNP) alleles among subjects with a differing clinical phenotype, such as myocardial infarction (cases vs. control subjects) or differing levels of a biomarker such as C-reactive protein (CRP) or cholesterol (high vs. low levels) [17].

CANDIDATE GENE ASSOCIATION STUDIES

Association studies may utilize a candidate gene or genome-wide approach. Such studies are often based on a selection of candidate genes on assumptions about biologically relevant genes. Thus, candidate gene studies are biased against identification of novel genes.

Combining different genetic methodologies facilitates discovery. Genetic association studies help refine regions identified by linkage studies. After identifying linkage between MI and the region containing ALOX5AP [18], a focused candidate gene sequence the entire gene in 93 affected individuals and 93 control subjects to identify a panel of 48 common SNPs in ALOX5AP and determine differences in the inheritance of a particular pattern of SNPs, or haplotype, between subjects with MI ($n=779$) and control subjects ($n=624$). As in the above investigations, the clinical utility of these findings remains unclear as the selection criteria allow for a significant percentage of individuals with potentially dangerous coronary disease to be included in the control groups and do not exclude the possibility of false positives in the disease groups.

GENOME-WIDE ASSOCIATION STUDIES

Genome-wide association studies examine hundreds of thousands of SNPs throughout the genome. Such studies, although not hypothesis-driven, are ideally suited to discovering previously unrecognized pathways for particular diseases.

The most significant disadvantage of genome-wide association studies involves the statistical conundrum of multiple comparisons inherent in simultaneously performing association tests on thousands of markers. A study of 500,000 SNPs with a false-positive rate of 0.1% would generate 500 false-positive results, a very large number that necessitates multiple rounds of replication to confirm an association. Thus, thoroughly replicated results from genome-wide association studies applied to cardiovascular disease and related phenotypes have just now begun to appear [9]. Another limitation of SNP association studies is their inability to determine which SNPs may affect gene expression or function. The SNPs may influence gene expression (e.g., by altering a transcriptional activator binding site in the promoter), or gene function (e.g., by causing an amino acid change). Transcriptional activators (TA), repressors (TR), and mRNA turnover influence mRNA levels independent of SNP genotypes; these mechanisms would only be detectable by expression profiling. Although mRNA levels may vary within and among cells, regulation of protein trafficking, turnover, or structure could affect a protein level or function independently from genotype or mRNA regulation. SNPs represent static information (the genome), expression profiles are dynamic (the transcriptome) and may show physiological fluctuations.

A recent study, performed following a genome-wide microsatellite marker scan on 42 French Canadian families with 284 individuals, provided evidence for a CHD susceptibility locus on chromosome 8 with an NPL score of 3.14 ($P=0.001$) at D8S1106. Linkage to this locus was verified by fine mapping, in an enlarged sample of 50 families with 320 individuals [19].

In similar fashion, a genome-wide scan performed on 236 nuclear families of the Quebec Family Study (QFS) revealed a quantitative trait locus (QTL) for LDL peak-particle size (LDL-PPD) on the

17q21 region that encodes the myeloperoxidase (MPO) gene, which, by its reactive intermediates, can oxidize LDL. They found no significant differences between the MPO gene variants and LDL-PPD and concluded that they are unlikely to be responsible for the quantitative trait locus reported on 17q21. However, the c.-653G > A is associated with plasma LDL-C and LDL-apoB concentrations [20].

The clinical utility of these findings remains unclear as the selection criteria allows for a significant percentage of individuals with potentially dangerous coronary disease to be included in the control groups and the possibility of false positives in the disease groups.

GENE EXPRESSION PROFILING IN CARDIOVASCULAR DISEASE

Microarray technology [8] provides a method to rapidly analyze biologic specimens for gene expression patterns of 20,000–38,500 genes that comprise the human genome.

Gene expression or transcriptional profiling is especially advantageous in genomic studies designed to detect an environmental stimulus. This extension of the concept to cell culture has permitted investigation of the influence of vascular dynamics on transcripts related to atherosclerosis.

Detection of transcripts in circulating cells offers convenient clinical application of transcriptional profiling; however it may not reflect gene expression in atherosclerotic lesions.

Transcriptional profiling of platelets in patients with acute coronary syndromes showed changes in gene transcription of megakaryocytesand myeloid-related protein-14, 2 weeks before the onset of symptoms [9].

Previous studies [21] showed augmented expression of 72 genes including HMG-CoA reductase in macrophage-rich tissue of human atherosclerotic lesions as compared with expression profiles of normal intimal tissue and THP-1 macrophage-like cells. In addition, studies on the transcriptional effect of statin therapy on peripheral monocytes [22] demonstrated that statins inhibit expression of inflammatory cytokine interleukin-1b, which are normally present at high levels in subjects with CAD [23]. Such findings show that the potential clinical utility of genomic techniques to identify associated genes also provides incremental values to detect additional drug targets and their effects.

PROTEOMIC PROFILING IN ATHEROSCLEROSIS

Gene association or transcriptional profiling studies cannot assess potentially important post-transcriptional variables including alternative splicing of mRNA, control subjects on protein translation, and post-translational processing of proteins. Protein markers may provide more accurate real-time information about patho-physiology than stable germ-line markers such as SNPs. As with genomics, potential benefits to the clinical community include better tools for diagnosis, cardiac biomarkers, and identification of therapeutic targets. Proteomic assessment of cardiovascular disease starts with the selection of tissue samples. For example, a study on sampled endarterectomy sections containing atherosclerotic plaque showed decreased expression of heat shock protein-27 (HSP27) in plaque compared with healthy tissue, and confirmed these results by showing a similar trend for the amount of soluble HSP27 in plasma of subjects with atherosclerotic cardiovascular disease [24].

Similar to genomic markers, proteomic studies require rigorous validation of technology platforms and experimental results. The pilot phase of the plasma proteome project identified 345 cardiovascular disease-related proteins in human plasma [25, 26]. These catalogs were developed to identify additional novel proteins that might be associated with cardiovascular disease in future proteomic discovery experiments. Such databases accelerate the identification of unknown markers present in atherosclerotic cardiovascular disease.

Identifying relevant proteomic markers will benefit from comparison with genetic and genomic data. Future experiments should compare fluctuations of cardiovascular biomarkers with other epidemiologic factors such as age, gender, ethnicity, and a variety of environmental exposures already recognized to influence disease risk and outcome.

COMPLEMENTARY GENOMIC AND PROTEOMIC APPROACHES

Analysis of plasma to identify real-time markers of CAD is highly desirable since plasma is easily collected and provides a practical method to test for reproducibility [27]. Contemporary proteomic analysis allows evaluation of the proteome through mass spectrometry, microarray analysis and electrophoresis technology. Characteristic protein expression patterns have been established for a variety of cancers, infectious diseases and inflammatory disorders [28–36].

As noted above, contemporary genomic analysis allows evaluation of the entire genome through microarray technology. This technology has the ability to identify the expression levels of 38,500 individual genes within a sample of peripheral blood monocytes [37]. In a number of studies, complementary genomic and proteomic results have demonstrated a robust method to distinguish disease and control groups [30, 32]. Likewise, the use of novel pattern recognition algorithms has the potential to provide unique and robust patterns that are both sensitive and specific to CAD. These signature patterns will provide the basis for prospective validation testing to determine diagnostic strength and possible clinical utility.

The ability of mass spectrometry to generate highly accurate mass-to-charge ratio (*m/z*) of various protein components in a complex mixture (such as blood plasma), and the subsequent spectra of very high resolution has made it a powerful protein profiling tool. Accurate analysis of huge volumes of resulting data requires mathematical expertise and sophisticated software tools to facilitate pattern recognition. The ability to detect patterns of differential protein expression between control and diseased samples forms the basis for proteomic pattern diagnostics [38]. These diagnostic patterns are highly dependent on the algorithms used to preprocess the raw data to remove background noise, to identify and compare peaks from various spectra, and training algorithms used to recognize common components of patterns [39, 40].

Prior studies using elegant animal models have been instrumental in establishing experimental design and in narrowing our focus to specific regions of interest within the genome and proteome [41]. However, human data will ultimately be necessary to define characteristic gene and protein expression patterns for CAD.

Although analyses of atherosclerotic tissue samples have revealed new insights, coronary tissue sampling will never be an acceptable method to screen for disease. Evaluation of individuals with atherosclerotic disease elsewhere in the vascular system (e.g., carotid arterial intimal medial thickness) may also be of limited value where the experimental concern is CAD. The patchy distribution of atherosclerotic disease argues against a paradigm that assumes uniform distribution of disease. Other important limitations of prior studies are poorly defined disease and control groups. Use of secondary evidence through clinical events alone has the risk of including individuals without CAD in the disease group (false positives). Of equal importance is that the absence of secondary evidence of CAD, such as an absence of events or coronary stenosis thresholds on arteriography, does not assure the absence of CAD within the control group (false negatives). Contamination of both disease and control groups markedly limits the ability to understand the implications of the study results. Although many of the human studies mentioned previously are to be commended for their bimolecular methods, each have questionable methods in establishing disease and control groups.

CLINICAL APPLICATIONS OF GENOMICS TO CARDIOVASCULAR MEDICINE

Genomic-Based Cardiovascular Risk Prediction Models

In atherosclerosis, many factors influence disease predisposition and therapeutic response, providing an appropriate testing ground for a personalized medicine approach based on convergence of information. Future risk assessment models will likely incorporate a patient's genomic, proteomic, and environmental information, using statistical models to identify marker-disease associations and correct for confounders such as gene–environment interactions.

Screening for early detection of high-risk (vulnerable) patients with asymptomatic atherosclerosis and monitoring their response to treatments in order to reduce sudden cardiovascular events remain a major challenge in preventive cardiology [3–5].

Pathologic studies of autopsy specimens have attempted to establish stages of CAD within the vessel wall [42]. These stages suggest progressive vessel enlargement (positive remodeling) with the collection of plaque within the vessel wall until luminal stenosis and occlusion occur. Positive, negative and intermediate remodeling have been demonstrated by intravascular ultrasound (IVUS) and CCT [43], where the various forms of remodeling that fall within the disease process are the subject of current investigation [44–48] (Fig. 4).

The association between angiographic stenosis severity and acute coronary events (myocardial infarction or unstable angina) is poor. Indeed, the majority of acute coronary syndromes are the result of rupture of plaques that cause <50% luminal stenosis [49–54]. Studies concerning the diagnostic accuracy of CTA have demonstrated a good agreement with conventional coronary angiography resulting in a sensitivity and specificity of approximately 88% and 98% [55]. The high negative predictive value of 97–100% renders CCT a particularly useful tool to rule out the presence of CAD in patients with an intermediate pretest likelihood. Moreover, comparative studies have demonstrated that anatomic imaging with CCT may provide information complementary to the traditionally used techniques for functional assessment [56].

An essential step in identifying markers specific to CAD is to establish pure disease and control groups. Several methods are available to measure the coronary vessel wall, each of which has their relative strengths and weaknesses (Table 3). Optical coherence tomography and intravascular ultrasound provide very high resolution of the vessel wall from within the vessel lumen. By their nature, these studies are very invasive and impractical for stratifying patients into disease groups. Magnetic resonance imaging and echocardiography are both noninvasive methods that have the ability to image coronary arteries; however, each has significant limitations in comprehensive analysis and spatial resolution making them poor modalities for stratifying patients into disease groups. CCT provides the best method to stratify patients into disease groups as it is noninvasive and provides high spatial resolution images of the entire coronary artery tree.

Our group has attempted to improve on the shortcomings of prior studies by combining contemporary coronary imaging with genomic microarray analysis, proteomic mass spectrometry analysis,

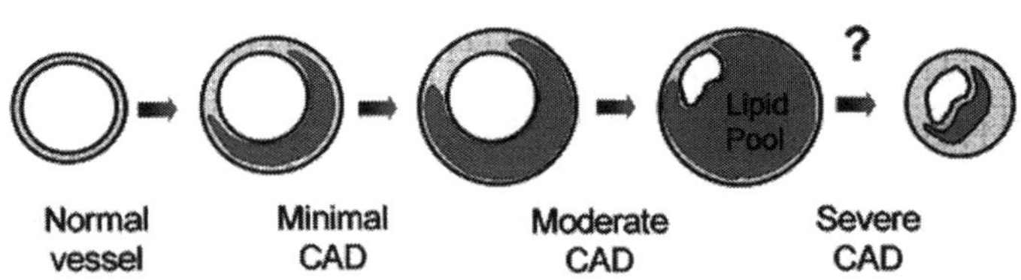

Fig. 4. Diagram demonstrating the various forms of coronary atherosclerotic remodeling

Table 3

	Invasiveness	*Spatial resolution*	*Ability to image all coronaries*	*Ability to include or exclude CAD in an individual patient*	*Ease of use*
OCT	++++	++++	+	+	+
IVUS	++++	+++	+	+	+
MRI	+	+	+++	+	++
TTE	+	+++	+	+	++
CCT	+	++	++++	+++	++++

OCT optical coherence tomography, *IVUS* intravascular ultrasound, *CCT* multidetector cardiac computed tomographic angiography, *MRI* magnetic resonance imaging, *TTE* transthoracic echocardiography

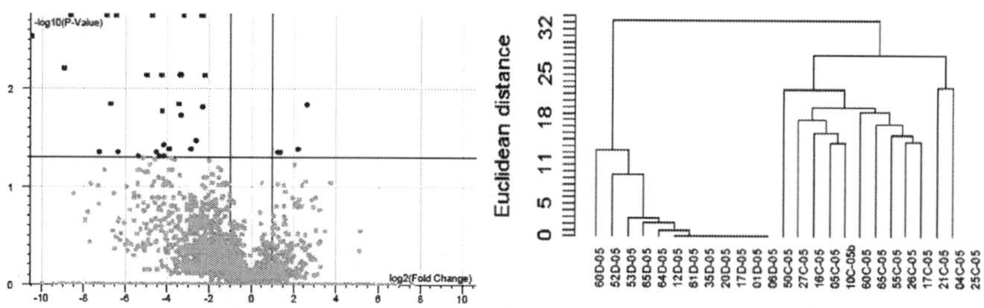

Fig. 5. *Left* Volcano plot: Different expression of peptide mass profile between CAC (*black*) and control (*gray*) cohorts. *Right* Hierachical clustering analysis: Distinct clinical relevant classes between CAD (D) and control (C) cohorts

novel pattern recognition algorithms and bioinformatics approaches. Our study evaluated the proteome of low risk patients, with normal coronary arteries on CTA, and vulnerable patients with noncalcified and mixed coronary plaques (<50% luminal stenosis) on CTA, using electron spray ionization mass spectrometry (ESI–MS) and Surface-enhanced laser desorption/ionization (SELDI). Contemporary proteomic analysis demonstrated distinct protein expression patterns in vulnerable patients as compared with patients with normal coronaries (Fig. 5).

SUMMARY

- Rapid advances in genomic and proteomic technology have the potential to provide a novel understanding of the underlying mechanisms responsible for atherosclerotic cardiovascular disease.
- Genetic and proteomic markers will add to the diagnostic accuracy of traditional tools with the potential to predict the onset, severity, vulnerability and activity of atherosclerotic plaques.
- Early results from several genomic and proteomic studies provide proof of concept for consistent and reproducible markers.
- Clinical translation of these bimolecular findings will require validation in prospective studies that encompass large, ethnically diverse cohorts.
- Despite test sophistication, high-throughput automation will allow clinical laboratories to offer testing at costs similar to most diagnostic imaging studies. Interpreting such test results will truly provide a challenge. Indeed, prospective validation of new risk markers will likely limit the rate of progress more than any technical or experimental factors.

REFERENCES

1. Akosah KO, McHugh VL, Barnhart SI, Schaper AM, Mathiason MA, et al. Carotid ultrasound for risk clarification in young to middle-aged adults undergoing elective coronary angiography. Am J Hypertens 2006;19(12):1256–61
2. Ahmadi N, Choe D, Khandhar S. Foster GP Outcomes of individuals with discordance between the Framingham risk score and the coronary artery calcification score. Circulation 2008;118:S-994
3. Naghavi M, Libby P, Falk E, Casscells SW, Litovsky S, et al. From vulnerable plaque to vulnerable patient: a call for new definitions and risk assessment strategies: Part I. Circulation 2003;108(14):1664–72.
4. Naghavi M, Libby P, Falk E, Casscells SW, Litovsky S, et al. From vulnerable plaque to vulnerable patient: a call for new definitions and risk assessment strategies: Part II. Circulation. 2003;108(15):1772–8
5. Naghavi M, Falk E, Hecht HS, Jamieson MJ, Kaul S, et al. SHAPE Task Force. From vulnerable plaque to vulnerable patient – Part III: Executive summary of the Screening for Heart Attack Prevention and Education (SHAPE) Task Force report. Am J Cardiol. 2006 Jul 17;98(2A):2H–15H. Epub 2006 Jun 12.
6. Rosamond WD, Chambless LE, Folsom AR, et al. Trends in the incidence of myocardial infarction and in mortality due to coronary heart disease, 1987 to 1994. N Engl J Med 1998;339:861–7
7. Boerwinkle E, Ellsworth DL, Hallman DM, Biddinger A. Genetic analysis of atherosclerosis: a research paradigm for the common chronic diseases. Hum Mol Genet 1996;5:1405–10.
8. Hunter DJ. Gene–environment interactions in human diseases. Nat Rev Genet 2005;6:287–98.
9. Tuomisto TT, Binder BR, Yla-Herttuala S. Genetics, genomics and proteomics in atherosclerosis research. Ann Med 2005;37:323–32.
10. Begovich AB, et al. A missense single-nucleotide polymorphism in a gene encoding a protein tyrosine phosphatase (PTPN22) is associated with rheumatoid arthritis. Am J Hum Genet 2004;75:330–7
11. Prokunina L, et al. A regulatory polymorphism in PDCD1 is associated with susceptibility to systemic lupus erythematosus in humans. Nat Genet 2002;32:666–9
12. Cargill M, et al. A large-scale genetic association study confirms IL12B and leads to the identification of IL23R as psoriasis-risk genes. Am J Hum Genet 2007;80:273–90
13. Vasan RS. Biomarkers of cardiovascular disease: molecular basis and practical considerations. Circulation 2006;113(19):2335–62. Review
14. Topol EJ. The genomic basis of myocardial infarction. J Am Coll Cardiol 2005;46:1456–65.
15. Helgadottir A, Manolescu A, Thorleifsson G, et al. The gene encoding 5-lipoxygenase activating protein confers risk of myocardial infarction and stroke. Nat Genet 2004;36:233–9.
16. Mehrabian M, Allayee H, Wong J, et al. Identification of 5-lipoxygenase as a major gene contributing to atherosclerosis susceptibility in mice. Circ Res 2002;91:120–6.
17. Shiffman D, Ellis SG, Rowland CM, et al. Identification of four gene variants associated with myocardial infarction. Am J Hum Genet 2005;77:596–605.
18. Bijnens AP, Lutgens E, Ayoubi T, Kuiper J, Horrevoets AJ, Daemen MJ. Genome-wide expression studies of atherosclerosis: critical issues in methodology, analysis, interpretation of transcriptomics data. Arterioscler Thromb Vasc Biol 2006;26:1226–35
19. Engert JC, Lemire M, Faith J, Brisson D, Fujiwara TM, Roslin NM, Brewer CG, Montpetit A, Darmond-Zwaig C, Renaud Y, Doré C, Bailey SD, Verner A, Tremblay G, St-Pierre J, Bétard C, Platko J, Rioux JD, Morgan K, Hudson TJ, Gaudet D. Identification of a chromosome 8p locus for early-onset coronary heart disease in a French Canadian population. Eur J Hum Genet 2008;16(1):105–14.
20. Dolley G, Lamarche B, Després JP, Bouchard C, Pérusse L, Vohl MC. Myeloperoxidase gene sequence variations are associated with low-density-lipoprotein characteristics. J Hum Genet 2008;53(5):439–46.
21. Goldstein JL, Brown MS. The LDL receptor defect in familial hypercholesterolemia. Implications for pathogenesis and therapy. Med Clin North Am 1982;66:335–62.
22. Breslow JL. Genetic differences in endothelial cells may determine atherosclerosis susceptibility. Circulation 2000;102:5–6.
23. Pajukanta P, Cargill M, Viitanen L, et al. Two loci on chromosomes 2 and X for premature coronary heart disease identified in early- and late-settlement populations of Finland. Am J Hum Genet 2000; 67:1481–93.
24. Francke S, Manraj M, Lacquemant C, et al. A genome-wide scan for coronary heart disease suggests in Indo-Mauritians a susceptibility locus on chromosome 16p13 and replicates linkage with the metabolic syndrome on 3q27. Hum Mol Genet 2001;10:2751–65.
25. Harrap SB, Zammit KS, Wong ZY, et al. Genome-wide linkage analysis of the acute coronary syndrome suggests a locus on chromosome 2. Arterioscler Thromb Vasc Biol 2002;22:874–8.
26. Broeckel U, Hengstenberg C, Mayer B, et al. A comprehensive linkage analysis for myocardial infarction and its related risk factors. Nat Genet 2002;30:210–4.
27. Barnea E, Sorkin R, Ziv T, Beer I, Admon A. Evaluation of prefractionation methods as a preparatory step for multidimensional based chromatography of serum proteins. Proteomics 2005;5:3367–75.
28. Seo D, Wang T, Dressman H, et al. Gene expression phenotypes of atherosclerosis. Arterioscler Thromb Vasc Biol 2004;24:1922–7
29. Patino WD, Mian OY, Kang JG, et al. Circulating transcriptome reveals markers of atherosclerosis. Proc Natl Acad Sci U S A 2005;102:3423–8

30. Tabibiazar R, Wagner RA, Ashley EA, et al. Signature patterns of gene expression in mouse atherosclerosis and their correlation to human coronary disease. Physiol Genomics 2005;22:213–26
31. Ma J, Liew CC. Gene profiling identifies secreted protein transcripts from peripheral blood cells in coronary artery disease. J Mol Cell Cardiol 2003;35:993–8
32. Tabibiazar R, Wagner RA, Deng A, Tsao PS, Quertermous T. Proteomic profiles of serum inflammatory markers accurately predict atherosclerosis in mice. Physiol Genomics 2006;25:194–202.
33. Duran MC, Mas S, Martin-Ventura JL, et al. Proteomic analysis of human vessels: application to atherosclerotic plaques. Proteomics 2003;3:973–8.
34. You SA, Archacki SR, Angheloiu G, et al. Proteomic approach to coronary atherosclerosis shows ferritin light chain as a significant marker: evidence consistent with iron hypothesis in atherosclerosis. Physiol Genomics 2003;13:25–30.
35. Donahue MP, Rose K, Hochstrasser D, et al. Discovery of proteins related to coronary artery disease using industrial-scale proteomics analysis of pooled plasma. Am Heart J 2006;152:478–85.
36. Zimmerli LU, Schiffer E, Zurbig P, Good DM, Kellmann M, Mouls L, Pitt AR, Coon JJ, Schmeider RE, Peter KH, Mischak H, Kolch W, Delles C, Dominiczak AF. Urinary proteomic biomarkers in coronary artery disease. Mol Cell Proteomics 2008;7:290–298.
37. Damani SB Topol EJ. Future use of genomics in coronary artery disease. J Am Coll Cardiol 2007;50:1933–40.
38. Rodland KD. Proteomics and cancer diagnosis: the potential of mass spectrometry. Clin Biochem 2004;37:579–83.
39. Diamandis EP. Analysis of serum proteomic patterns for early cancer diagnosis: drawing attention to potential problems. J Natl Cancer Inst 2004;96:353–6.
40. Diamandis EP. Mass spectrometry as a diagnostic and a cancer biomarker discovery tool: opportunities and potential limitations. Mol Cell Proteomics 2004;3:367–78.
41. Arab S, Gramolini AO, Ping P, Kislinger T, Stanley B, van Eyk J, Ouzounian M, MacLennan DH, Emili A, Liu PP.Cardiovascular proteomics: tools to develop novel biomarkers and potential applications. J Am Coll Cardiol. 2006;48(9):1733–41. Epub 2006 Oct 17. Review.
42. Glagov S, Weisenberg E, Zarins CK, Stankunavicius R, Kolettis GJ. Compensatory enlargement of human atherosclerotic coronary arteries. N Engl J Med 1987;316:1371–5.
43. Hirose M, Kobayashi Y, Mintz GS, et al. Correlation of coronary arterial remodeling determined by intravascular ultrasound with angiographic diameter reduction of 20% to 60%. Am J Cardiol 2003;92:141–5.
44. Nicholls SJ, Tuzcu EM, Sipahi I, et al. Relationship between atheroma regression and change in lumen size after infusion of apolipoprotein A-I Milano. J Am Coll Cardiol 2006;47:992–7.
45. Schoenhagen P, Tuzcu EM, Apperson-Hansen C, et al. Determinants of arterial wall remodeling during lipid-lowering therapy: serial intravascular ultrasound observations from the reversal of atherosclerosis with aggressive lipid lowering therapy (REVERSAL) trial. Circulation 2006;113:2826–34.
46. Schoenhagen P, Tuzcu EM, Stillman AE, et al. Non-invasive assessment of plaque morphology and remodeling in mildly stenotic coronary segments: comparison of 16-slice computed tomography and intravascular ultrasound. Coron Artery Dis 2003;14:459–62.
47. Sipahi I, Tuzcu EM, Moon KW, et al. Does the extent and direction of arterial remodeling predict subsequent progression of coronary atherosclerosis? A serial intravascular ultrasound study. Heart 2007.
48. Sipahi I, Tuzcu EM, Schoenhagen P, et al. Static and serial assessments of coronary arterial remodeling are discordant: an intravascular ultrasound analysis from the reversal of atherosclerosis with aggressive lipid lowering (REVERSAL) trial. Am Heart J 2006;152:544–50.
49. Bruschke AV, Kramer JR Jr, Bal ET, Haque IU, Detranto RC, Goormastic M. The dynamics of progression of coronary atherosclerosis studied in 168 medically treated patients who underwent coronary arteriography three times. Am Heart J 1989;117:296–305.
50. Hackett D, Davies G, Maseri A. Pre-existing coronary stenosis in patients with first myocardial infarction are not necessarily severe. Eur Heart J 1988;9:1317–23.
51. Haft JI, Haik BJ, Goldstein JE, Brodyn NE. Development of significant coronary artery lesions in areas of minimal disease: a common mechanism for coronary disease progression. Chest 1988;94:731–736.
52. Lichtlen PR, Nikutta P, Jost S, Deckers J, Wiese B, Rafflenbeul W. INTACT Study Group. Anatomical progression of coronary artery disease in humans as seen by prospective, repeated, quantitated coronary angiography. Circulation 1992;86:828–838.
53. Loree HM, Kamm RD, Stringfrellow RG, Lee RT. Effects of fibrous cap thickness on peak circumferential stress in model atherosclerotic vessels. Circ Res 1992;71:850–8.
54. Mann JM, Davies MJ. Vulnerable plaque: relation of characteristics to degree of stenosis in human coronary arteries. Circulation 1996;94:928–931
55. Stein PD, Yaekoub AY, Matta F, Sostman HD, 64-Slice CT for diagnosis of coronary artery disease: a systemic review. Am J Med 2008;121:715–25.
56. Budoff MJ, Rasouli ML, Shavelle DM, Gopal A, Gul KM, Mao SS, Liu SH, McKay CR. Cardiac CT angiography (CTA) and nuclear myocardial perfusion imaging (MPI)-a comparison in detecting significant coronary artery disease. Acad Radiol. 2007;14(3):252–7.

11 Circulating Endothelial Progenitor Cells: Mechanisms and Measurements

Jonathan R. Murrow and Arshed A. Quyyumi

CONTENTS

From: *Asymptomatic Atherosclerosis: Pathophysiology, Detection and Treatment*
Edited by: M. Naghavi (ed.), DOI 10.1007/978-1-60327-179-0_11

Abstract

Endothelial progenitor cells (EPC) are defined as a population of bone marrow-derived monocytes that migrate to sites of vascular injury and participate in new blood vessel formation, either by proliferation or by paracrine mechanisms. In circulation, these cells are thought to bear certain cell surface markers such as CD34, CD133, and VEGFR2 that permit enumeration by flow cytometry. While the capacity to grow in culture is another defining feature of EPC, methodology of culture assays and the constituents of the resultant EPC colonies remain a subject of controversy. In vivo, mobilization of EPC from bone marrow is mediated by matrix metalloproteinases and nitric oxide. Homing to sites of vascular injury is achieved in part via binding of cell surface receptors on EPC to tissue-derived factors up-regulated in ischemic tissues. Levels of EPC assessed by flow cytometry and by cell culture correlate with the presence of cardiac risk factors or overt atherosclerosis, where subjects with increasing levels of vascular injury (defined by the presence of cardiac risk factors or of known vascular disease) tend to have lower levels of circulating EPC. These observations prompt further study into the mechanisms of vascular injury and repair while offering a prospect for novel therapeutic strategies.

Key words: Endothelial progenitor cell; Vascular repair; Angiogenesis

KEY POINTS

- Endothelial progenitor cells (EPC) are generally defined as a population of bone marrow derived monocytes that migrate to sites of vascular injury and participate in new blood vessel formation.
- EPCs are currently measured by flow cytometric analysis of unique cell surface markers as well as by colony forming units in cell culture.
- Although mechanisms continue to be defined, levels of circulating EPCs generally correlate with vascular health, where lower numbers are associated with the presence of risk factors for atherosclerosis as well as overt cardiovascular disease.
- The regenerative properties of EPCs challenge past concepts of atherosclerosis as purely a manifestation of an unmitigated accumulation of vascular injury.

INTRODUCTION

The pathobiology of atherosclerosis has been largely attributed to processes of repeated vascular injury leading to plaque development and expansion, subsequent tissue ischemia, and ultimately infarction [1]. Risk factors including advanced age, tobacco smoking, hypertension, high cholesterol, and diabetes mellitus have been identified as the root causes of this injury; accordingly, the last half-century's cardiovascular therapeutics have sought to mitigate the effects of these exposures. This concept of unchecked vascular injury has been revised in the light of the discovery of a population of endogenous mononuclear cells that reside in the bone marrow, mobilize in response to tissue injury, and repair injured vascular tissue. These so-called endothelial progenitor cells (EPC) and their regenerative properties have challenged the classic Ross hypothesis, offering the possibility of another mode of treating atherosclerotic vascular disease. The precise identity of the EPC remains elusive. EPC have thus necessarily been defined by their functions – that they originate in the bone marrow, circulate in peripheral blood, home to sites of vascular injury, and participate in new blood vessel formation [2]. Ever since the notion was first entertained that blood vessels could be formed de novo from circulating blood components, researchers have sought to define the true identity of these EPC, to understand their role in vascular homeostasis and pathology, and to relate their functions to common clinical syndromes.

HISTORICAL PERSPECTIVE

The identification of EPC began with observations, was advanced by animal models, and has been refined by modern molecular and cellular techniques. In 1893 Renault first theorized that leukocytes might give rise to tissue structure [3]. In the 1920s, Alexis Carrel and others leant support to this notion by observing that mononuclear leukocytes cultured from the blood of adult chickens differentiated into cells which resembled fibroblasts and organized into tubules [3, 4]. In experimenting with a variety of cell culture conditions in the Carrel Laboratory at the Rockefeller Institute, Parker found that "isolated blood cells, in a plasma substratum, are capable of constructing highly organized channels that are analogous to the capillaries of the organism." [5] The idea that these angiogenic cells might arise from the bone marrow became clear in 1950, when White and co-workers described the formation of blood vessels from the cultured bone marrow cells of adult chickens [3].

Feigl and co-workers in 1985 created an animal model of vascular injury by implanting pledgets in sheep aorta, upon which activated monocytes from the peripheral circulation participated in the formation of new endothelium over organized thrombus [6]. These spindle-shaped layers of "pre-endothelium" that had derived from the blood pool evinced immuno-histochemical properties of mature endothelial cells while retaining primitive ultra structural features of undifferentiated mesenchymal cells [7, 8]. Implicating the bone marrow as the repository for angiogenic cells, bone marrow-derived cells implanted on synthetic vascular prostheses yielded complete endothelialization relative to uncoated control grafts [9].

Asahara and colleagues in 1997 provided the strongest evidence that new blood vessel formation is partly attributable to a population of bone marrow-derived monocytes. CD34-positive mononuclear cells isolated from humans demonstrated an endothelial phenotype in vitro. Moreover, these cells participated in neo-angiogenesis in a mouse hind limb ischemia model [10], thus defining a cell population that exhibited key features of an endothelial progenitor – a bone marrow heritage, an ability to mobilize and to home to sites of injury, and a role in regenerating new blood vessels.

BONE MARROW ORIGINS

Evidence supporting the bone-marrow origins of angiogenic cells, as opposed to lineage of these cells from progenitors resident in the vessel wall, comes from experimental and clinical chimerism – settings where gender-mismatched cardiac or vascular tissue is engrafted in a host animal or patient [11]. In allograft chimeric mouse models of cardiac transplant, bone marrow precursors of the host mediate the development of transplant coronary vasculopathy, mimicking the injury to microvessels seen in transplant graft arteriosclerosis in humans [12]. Autopsy and endomyocardial biopsy specimens from gender-mismatched cardiac transplant patients reveal endothelial cells in the coronary arteries of cardiac grafts that are comprised in large part from extra-cardiac sources, which is thought to include bone marrow niches [13]. These bone marrow derived new endothelial cells predominate in the microcirculation, can be noted as early as 1 month after cardiac transplant, and may serve as a major contributor to transplant arteriopathy [14, 15].

Additional support for the notion that circulating EPC arise from the bone marrow comes from the discovery of EPC precursors that reside within the marrow. This population of multipotent adult progenitor cells (MAPC) co-purifies with mesenchymal stem cells and gives rise to circulating EPC. Lacking cell surface markers of EPC or mature endothelial cells, these MAPCs differentiate into an endothelial progenitor phenotype with key features of EPC (including angiogenic potential) when cultured [16, 17].

EPC IN THE CIRCULATION: CELL SURFACE MARKERS AS MARKERS OF LINEAGE

In addition to their bone marrow origins, EPC are identified by their presence – albeit infrequent – in the peripheral circulation. Flow cytometry using fluorescently-labeled antibodies to key cell surface markers (most notably CD34, CD133, and vascular endothelial growth factor receptor 2 (VEGFR-2)), is one method of quantifying populations of circulating endothelial progenitors [18, 19] (see Fig. 1).

All hematopoietic stem cells express CD34, and EPC (and thus endothelial cells) are thought to arise from differentiation from this common precursor. While this marker is lost by hematopoietic cells as they differentiate into blood components, it is retained by a population of cells that have phenotypic characteristics of an endothelial progenitor [20–22]. As these EPC differentiate into mature endothelial cells, the CD34 surface marker is not uniformly expressed, with less expression in larger vessels and heterogeneous expression in capillary beds [23]. Thus, the CD34 marker helps to identify in the peripheral circulation, a population of cells enriched for EPC but not mature endothelial cells. The function of the CD34 surface protein is not known. Messenger RNA expression patterns suggest that while CD34 protein is involved in post-natal blood vessel development, it has no clear role as an adhesion molecule or in signal transduction on either endothelial cells or hematopoietic progenitors [23, 24]. CD34-positive cells cultured in the presence of VEGF take on properties of endothelial cells in forming cobblestone monolayers, in staining for von Willebrand factor, and in incorporating acetylated low-density lipoprotein. Moreover, when CD34-positive cells are injected into a canine bone marrow transplant model, they localize and colonize implanted Dacron aortic grafts, contributing to neo-endothelialization [25]. Purified CD34-positive cells from peripheral human blood allow faster restoration of flow in a rodent model of hind limb ischemia [26]. As they differentiate into endothelial cells in culture and take on the structure and function of endothelial cells in vivo, cells bearing the CD34 marker appear to be a population of cells enriched for immature cells with true angiogenic potential.

CD133 (or AC133) is a 5-transmembrane antigen identifying a population of cells which demonstrate the EPC phenotype when cultured with VEGF and stem cell growth factor [27, 28]. The neointima that lines implanted left ventricular assist devices in heart failure patients consists of CD133-positive cells. Since mature endothelial cells do not express CD133, cells bearing this marker likely represent a true progenitor subset of mononuclear cells [29]. The function of the CD133 protein is unknown. Although reverse-transcriptase PCR demonstrates CD133 mRNA in most adult human tissues and cell type, expression of the CD133 antigen is largely restricted to CD34-positive cells, and thus serves as a unique identifier of cells bearing angiogenic potential [30].

The vascular endothelial growth factor receptor (VEGFR-2) – also identified as the kinase-domain receptor (KDR) – is another endothelial-specific marker of EPCs expressed on mature endothelial cells as well as on cell populations enriched for EPC [29, 31]. The VEGFR-2 marker defines peripheral mononuclear cells that contribute to neo-endothelialization, and its co-expression with CD133 has been used to identify a population enriched for EPC [29]. [32] Of note, these double positive cells are quite rare, representing between 0.01 and 0.0001% of the circulating mononuclear population [19].

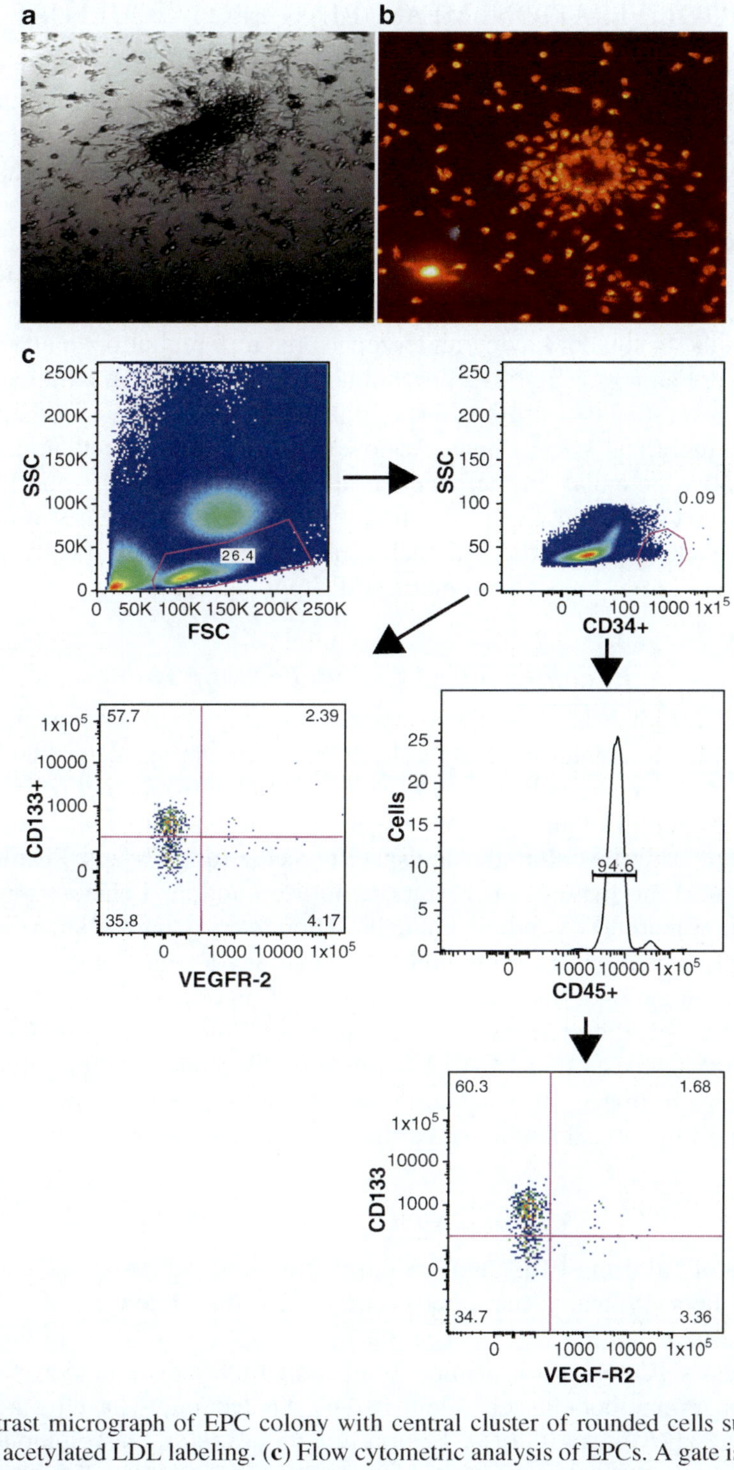

Fig. 1. (**a**) Phase contrast micrograph of EPC colony with central cluster of rounded cells surrounded by radiating thin, flat cells. (**b**) DiI acetylated LDL labeling. (**c**) Flow cytometric analysis of EPCs. A gate is defined for the mononuclear cells. A subpopulation is identified for cells labeled with fluorescence-labeled anti-CD34 antibody. Counts may be obtained for dual positive cells expressing CD133 and VEGFR-2 surface markers or further refined selecting for CD45 medium subpopulations.

PROLIFERATION: MEASURING EPC IN CULTURE

The capacity to grow in culture is another defining feature of EPC, and colony counts have been used as a surrogate for measuring the functional robustness of circulating progenitor populations. Controversy arises from the fact that differing culture techniques yield colonies with differing phenotypes – raising questions about the most appropriate method of isolating cell colonies enriched for EPC [33]. Presently, three techniques have emerged as principal ways of culturing EPC, each bearing unique colonies.

Controversy exists as well over the cellular composition of EPC colonies (by whatever method of cultivation), though there is consensus that these colonies are not merely cultures of circulating mature endothelial cells. In spite of having undergone some differentiation to an endothelial cell phenotype (including expression of VEGFR-2), mononuclear cells grown in culture retain properties of immature cells with reparative capabilities [34]. Unlike cultured mature endothelial cells (i.e., those isolated from human umbilical vein or bone marrow tissue), cultured circulating EPC are unique in their higher proliferative potential, in their increased sensitivity to angiogenic factors, and in their ability to form new blood vessels in vivo [34]. Culture techniques have focused on isolating this population of cells while excluding hematopoietic cells and mature endothelial cells, in order to obtain a true quantitative measure of a subject's circulating EPC population.

Endothelial Cell Colony Forming Unit

The method adapted from Asahara's and co-workers' work isolates angiogenic mononuclear cells while seeking to avoid contamination of the culture from circulating mature endothelial cells [10]. From peripheral blood, the mononuclear layer of cells is isolated from other peripheral blood components by centrifugation in a Ficol gradient. After plating on fibronectin (which binds mature endothelial cells), non-adherent cells are cultured using specific media for 4–7 days. Resultant spindle shaped colonies form, which exhibit features of migration, proliferation, and elaboration of growth factors, while sharing structural features of endothelial cells. Though a standard nomenclature is lacking, the Asahara technique has been dubbed the endothelial cell colony forming unit (EC-CFU) method [35]. Subsequent work has sought to define the cellular composition of colonies, finding that in addition to staining for endothelial specific markers, colonies contain CD14-positive and CD45-positive monocytes [36]. Other work suggests that EC-CFUs are primarily composed of cells of the monocyte–macrophage lineage, with limited intrinsic angiogenic capacity [36, 37]. Nonetheless, this technique is the most widely used in clinical studies of cardiovascular disease.

Circulating Angiogenic Cells

A second method of culturing EPC involves cultivating both adherent and non-adherent cells in growth media for 4 days. Typically, these cells do not form the same type of colonies as EC-CFU. However, they are similar in their cell surface marker expression, in their in vitro function, and in their capacity for neo-vascularization in models of hind limb ischemia [35, 38, 39]. As they are highly angiogenic in animal models, cells identified by this technique have been dubbed circulating angiogenic cells (CAC) [35]. As with EC-CFUs, cellular analysis suggests a monocyte–macrophage lineage for CACs in culture, even while exhibiting phenotypic characteristics of endothelial cells (i.e., endothelial nitric oxide synthase up-regulation and endothelial specific marker expression) [35, 40].

Endothelial Cell Forming Colonies

A third technique isolates peripheral blood mononuclear cells that adhere to collagen and are subsequently cultivated for 5–22 days after plating. Termed endothelial cell forming colonies (ECFC), this approach has been described as a "late-outgrowth" or "outgrowth endothelial cell" (OEC) assay as it identifies cells beyond the time period at which either EC-CFUs or CACs are typically evaluated. Early outgrowth cells (4–7 days) appear spindle-shaped and have higher angiogenic cytokine secretion [37]. Meanwhile, late outgrowth cell colonies (greater than 21 days) form a cobblestone layer, have higher expression of mature endothelial cell markers, produce more nitric oxide, and may possess a greater capacity to form capillaries in vitro and in vivo [37, 41–43]. ECFCs isolated from this method do not express hematopoietic antigens, or have features of a monocyte–macrophage lineage, but do have robust proliferative potential and form blood vessels in vivo [44]. While in vitro and in vivo studies support their characterization as a more refined population of EPC, clinical studies of how these cells impact vascular health and disease are limited.

CONTROVERSIES

As noted, the composition of cell colonies by each of the above culture techniques is heterogeneous – containing cells with a variety of lineages and phenotypes. Angiogenic cells have been shown to arise from CD34-negative mononuclear precursors [45]. In addition, the cellular composition of EPC colonies includes non-monocytic cell types, including T lymphocytes that secrete high levels of angiogenic cytokines that contribute to adhesion, migration and tubule formation via a SDF-1 signaling pathway. These T cell subtypes correlate inversely with age and cardiac risk factors, suggesting their role as a biomarker for vascular disease [46]. Moreover, cells in these colonies do not typically express the same surface markers as circulating progenitor populations measured by flow cytometry. EC-CFU, CAC, and ECFC express monocyte/macrophage markers (CD14, Mac-1 and CD11c) but do not ubiquitously express CD34 or CD133. Whatever their identity, cells within colonies contribute to experimental angiogenesis [10, 37, 39]. These cell populations, however, likely represent different cell subtypes than those measured by flow cytometry [40]. Thus, measuring progenitor cell levels by both culture and by flow cytometry likely identifies populations enriched for, but not exclusively composed of, true EPC.

MECHANISMS: MOBILIZATION, HOMING, PATHOGENESIS

Mobilization

Quantitative measure of EPC measured by flow cytometry and by culture demonstrates an ability of this cell population to mobilize in response to a variety of homeostatic and pathologic stimuli. This mobilization from the bone marrow to sites of vascular injury is thought to be mediated by matrix metalloproteinases (MMP) in a nitric oxide-dependent process [47]. MMP-2 and MMP-9 are proteolytic enzymes that contribute to hematopoietic cell migration and tissue localization in both normal health and in response to injury. Stromal derived factor (SDF)-1 induces the secretion of MMP-2 and MMP-9 from circulating CD34-positive cells. In vitro, CD34-positive cells from cord blood incubated with MMP-2 and MMP-9 rich media increases cell migration [47].

Endothelial nitric oxide synthase (eNOS)-deficient mice demonstrate the importance of NO in neo-vascularization by its effect on EPC mobility. VEGF-induced mobilization of EPCs is reduced in eNOS knock-out mice [48]. Infusion of wild type EPCs, but not bone marrow transplantation, rescues mice and suggests a defect in progenitor cell mobilization (mediated by MMP-9) – as the mechanism of impaired neo-vascularization to hind limb ischemia in this mouse model [49].

Circulating endogenous cytokines may also contribute to EPC mobilization. Increased VEGF levels are associated with angiogenesis, and exogenously administered VEGF increases EPC counts in peripheral blood as well as post-natal angiogenesis in vivo [50]. Erythropoietin (EPO), when administered exogenously enhances EPC mobilization from the bone marrow. Moreover, serum EPO and VEGF levels are associated with bone marrow derived progenitor cells as well as with the number and function of circulating EPCs [51].

Homing

Once mobilized from the bone marrow, circulating EPC home to sites of vascular injury via the binding of ischemic tissue-derived factors to cell surface receptors on EPC [52]. At the site of injury, an endogenous integrin-linked kinase (ILK) responds to hypoxia in endothelial cells by up-regulating intracellular adhesion molecule (ICAM)-1 and SDF-1 [53–55]. SDF-1 binds to its receptor CXCR-4 which is expressed on circulating CD34-positive mononuclear cells [56].

Other mechanisms of EPC localization include $\alpha_4\beta_1$ integrins homing to integrin ligands vascular–cellular adhesion molecules (VCAM) and cellular fibronectin [57]. CCN1, a cysteine-rich heparin-binding protein, is expressed by vascular cells in response to atherosclerotic plaque formation and mechanical stress. CCN1 stimulates migration of CD34-positive cells, release of MMP-9, and expression of integrins [58]. Finally, c-kit and its membrane-bound ligand is involved in EPC recruitment by microvascular endothelial cells [59].

Pathogenesis

Circulating levels of EPC-enriched populations are depressed in subjects with atherosclerosis or cardiac risk factors [60, 61]. Whether this represents a primary deficiency in vascular repair potential or a suppression of circulating reparative cells in response to risk factors (i.e., tobacco smoke, diabetes, etc.) remains to be elucidated. Pre-clinical work has identified several mechanisms by which EPC function is impaired. C-reactive protein (HsCRP), a biomarker associated with increased cardiovascular risk [62], is associated with increased CFUs within a healthy cohort, but when cultured in the presence of CRP (≥15 mcg/mL), isolated EPCs from peripheral blood demonstrated reduced CFU number, with inhibited expression of endothelial markers (Tie-2, lectin, and VE-cadherin) [63, 64]. CRP exposure was associated with a decrease in endotheli63al NO synthase mRNA expression by EC-CFU [64]. Additionally, plasma concentrations of asymmetric dimethylarginine (ADMA) in subjects with stable angina inversely correlate with the number of circulating CD34-positive/CD133-positive cells and EC-CFU. Ex vivo studies show that incubation with ADMA results in decreased EC-CFU counts, decreased differentiation, and attenuated tubule formation. Endothelial NO synthase activity was decreased in EPC incubated in ADMA, suggesting a possible mechanism of effect. Notably, co-incubation of EPC with rosuvastastin abolished these deleterious effects of ADMA [65].

CLINICAL CORRELATIONS

While the identity of the true EPC and its precise mechanism of effect remains to be fully elucidated, several studies have identified clear association between various measurements of progenitor cell number and activity in the circulation and the presence of cardiac risk factors or overt atherosclerosis. In this way, the estimation of EPC by flow cytometry and by cell culture serves as a biomarker of the underlying health or disease state of an individual. A biomarker is a biologic measure which may be employed to identify normal or abnormal processes at the level of pre-disease (at risk), pre-clinical (screening), diagnosis (overt disease), disease severity, staging, response to therapy, or prognosis [66]. Measures of EPC have been studied as putative biomarkers for cardiovascular disease in this context.

RISK FACTORS

In an at-risk cohort of middle-aged men, the level of EC-CFU was inversely associated with the calculated Framingham Risk Score and directly related to vascular health (assessed by endothelial function studies) [60]. In a similar at-risk population, a likewise negative association has been shown between EPC counts by flow cytometry and an increasing number of cardiac risk factors (male gender, advancing age, sedentary lifestyle, hypertension, hyperlipidemia and diabetes) [61]. Moreover, independent of overt risk factors, CD34-positive cell counts inversely correlate with the presence of the metabolic syndrome [67]. Finally, subjects with asymptomatic peripheral atherosclerotic disease (identified by ultrasound in the carotid arteries, the abdominal aorta, or femoral arteries) have decreased circulating EPCs measured by flow cytometry [68, 69].

MALE SEX

EC-CFU counts and migratory function are increased in women versus men, with differences likely mediated by estrogen [70]. Estrogen-deficiency is associated with significantly decreased EPC in the periphery and bone marrow in animal models of ovariectomy, an effect restored by estrogen therapy. The mechanism is mediated via a caspase-8-dependent pathway, suggesting modulation of apoptosis. Women with increased plasma estrogen concentrations displayed significantly increased level of circulating EPC [71]. Interestingly, circulating CAC increases with gestational age in pregnancy, correlating with serum estradiol levels [72].

AGING

Aging is associated generally with modestly lower EPC counts by flow cytometry, while EC-CFU counts have been less consistently depressed in studies of elderly subjects relative to young individuals [73, 74]. However, functional measures such as survival, migration, and proliferation are markedly decreased with advancing age [75].

PHYSICAL ACTIVITY

Moderate exercise for 28 days in subjects with stable coronary artery disease resulted in a significant increase in circulating CACs. This phenomenon appears to be NO-dependent because the increase in EPCs with exercise was attenuated in eNOS knock-out mice and in wild-type mice treated with an NO blocker [76]. Additionally, acute dynamic exercise in healthy subjects is associated with a nearly fourfold increase in circulating EPCs (CD133-positive cells). Cultured angiogenic cells isolated before and after exercise demonstrated similar patterns of secreted angiogenic growth factors [77].

HYPERTENSION

Subjects with essential hypertension have lower circulating CD34-positive/KDR-positive cells in comparison to normotensive controls [78]. By culture, however, no difference was observed in counts of progenitor cells cultivated by a late outgrowth of CACs [79]. Ex vivo studies of peripheral mononuclear cells cultured from hypertensive patients demonstrate accelerated senescence and reduced telemorase activity in comparison to cells from healthy controls [80].

SMOKING

EPC identified by culture and by flow cytometry are significantly decreased in smokers, with a dose dependent effect [61, 81, 82]. EPC growth, migration, adherence, and tube formation are all impaired in smokers versus non-smoking controls [82]. Treatment of cultured peripheral mononuclear cells with benzo(a)pyrene – a polycyclic aromatic hydrocarbon component of tobacco smoke – results in impaired EPC number and colonies in a dose-dependent manner, suggesting a mechanism by which smoking affects EPC count and influences vascular disease [83]. Smoking cessation was associated with a rapid increase in CD34-positive/CD133-positive mononuclear cells, with a greater effect in "light smokers" (<20 cigarettes per day) than in "heavy smokers" (>20 cigarettes per day) [81]. For those who continue to smoke, green tea consumption may improve EPC levels and endothelial function [84].

DIABETES

In diabetics, quantitative and qualitative differences have been observed in EPC isolated from peripheral blood. Generally, circulating CAC and EC-CFU in diabetics are fewer in number, and have decreased mobilization, adhesion, migration, and proliferation. [85–87] These abnormalities are mediated by NO deficiency and reactive oxygen species and may account for increased susceptibility of diabetics to vascular injury and cardiovascular disease. EC-CFU counts from type 1 diabetics were 44% lower than in matched non-diabetic controls, a reduction that inversely correlated with levels of glycosylated hemoglobin [88]. Similar findings were noted in type 2 diabetics with coronary disease, where CD34-positive cell counts were fewer [89].

EPC from type 2 diabetics demonstrated reduced adhesion, migration, and proliferation in response to hypoxia (as a model for issue ischemia) compared with non-diabetic controls [85]. Mobilization of EPC from the bone marrow in response to injury is attenuated in diabetic mice, a deficit not fully restored when resident bone marrow cells are replaced with progenitors from non-diabetic animals [85]. EPC from diabetic subjects were less likely to participate in tubule formation when compared to controls [86].

Hyperglycemia may mediate these abnormalities, as exposure of mononuclear cells from healthy subjects to high glucose reduces the colony number and proliferative capacity, while increasing senescence, impairing migration, and decreasing tube formation [90]. Nitric oxide bioavailability, which is reduced in diabetic subjects, may be another mechanism of abnormal EPC function. In EPC exposed to high glucose media, the functional abnormalities improve with co-incubation with exogenous NO sources such as sodium nitroprusside [90]. Moreover, CD34-positive cells isolated from diabetic subjects demonstrate reduced migration, which corrects with co-incubation with NO donors [87]. Additionally, excess free radicals from the generation of reactive oxygen species have been implicated in EPC dysfunction in diabetics as it has been in measures of endothelial vasomotor dysfunction in these subjects [91]. EPCs cultured from diabetic patients produce excess superoxide that impairs neo-endothelialization [92, 93].

Among anti-diabetic therapies, thiazolidenediones have been associated with improvements in quantitative and qualitative measures of EPC. Rosiglitazone exposure in vitro is associated with a sixfold increase in CFU counts while promoting differentiation of EPC to mature endothelial cells [94]. Pioglitazone therapy is associated with an increase of circulating EPC counts (as defined by

EC-CFU assays) and improvements in migration, adhesion, proliferation, and survival. Notably, these effects may be independent of glycemic control, as study participants all had hemoglobin A1c values less than 7% [95].

ATHEROSCLEROTIC CORONARY ARTERY DISEASE: STABLE ANGINA

CD34-positive and CD133-positive/KDR-positive monocytes measured by flow cytometry are decreased in subjects with stable coronary artery disease in comparison to healthy controls. [89, 96] Trends in EPC colony counts, however, vary based on the culture technique. In subjects referred for coronary angiography, the level of EC-CFU inversely correlated with the likelihood of multi-vessel coronary artery disease [97]. By contrast, subjects referred for coronary angiography had CAC levels that directly correlate with the presence of angiographically significant coronary artery disease, with the highest levels in those subjects referred for revascularization [98].

Among patients with stable coronary artery disease, circulating EPC levels may serve as a marker for the potential to form collateral coronary vessels. Among subjects with isolated left anterior descending coronary artery disease undergoing percutaneous coronary intervention, adequate collateral flow index (defined as ≥0.25) is strongly associated with counts of circulating CD34-positive/CD133-positive precursor cells. In subjects with inadequate collateral flow indices, counts of EPCs in circulation and in culture are significantly reduced [99].

ATHEROSCLEROTIC CORONARY ARTERY DISEASE: UNSTABLE ANGINA AND MYOCARDIAL INFARCTION

In contrast to subjects with stable angina, those with unstable coronary syndromes show markedly increased levels of EPC by flow cytometry. Although this relationship is less reproducible when considering cell counts by culture, CD34-positive and CD34-positive/VEGFR-2-positive mononuclear cells increase in the setting of acute infarction, can remain elevated for several months, and may serve as a prognostic marker for recovery. Cell culture of peripheral blood mononuclear cells showed greater proliferation at day 7 versus day 1 after infarct [100, 101]. Moreover, in the setting of ST-segment elevation myocardial infarction (STEMI), expression of the EPC homing marker CXCR4 is elevated. EPC maturation is promoted as endothelial cells, early cardiac, muscle and endothelial markers (assessed by RT-PCR of mRNA) are expressed at higher levels by mononuclear cells in the setting of acute infarct [102].

Measures of EPC by flow cytometry carry prognostic value. In quantitative and qualitative measures, EPC predict prognosis in coronary artery disease and appear to be markers of reparative potential. CD34-positive/KDR-positive cell counts from peripheral blood inversely correlate with a higher incidence of adverse cardiovascular events (over a 10 month follow up period) [103]. In patients with coronary artery disease, increased levels of CD34-positive/KDR-positive cells was associated with a reduced risk of cardiovascular death, ischemia, revascularization, and hospitalization [104]. Ex vivo studies of EPCs collected 1 week after acute myocardial infarction show that cells' capability to differentiate predict infarct size regression as assessed by myocardial perfusion imaging [105].

In subjects with cardiomyopathy as a consequence of coronary artery disease, EPC counts are reduced. In addition, proliferation, migration, and angiogenic potential are impaired. [106–108] These measures correlate inversely with worsening New York Heart Association functional class and all cause mortality [107–109].

Among therapies for coronary artery disease, 3-hydroxy-3-methylglutaryl coenzyme A (HMG-CoA) reductase inhibitor (statin) use has been shown to augment levels of circulating progenitor cells.

Treatment of patients with stable coronary artery disease with atorvastatin 40 mg daily resulted in a 1.5-fold increase in the number of circulating CD34-positive/KDR-positive cells observed 1 week after starting therapy, followed by a threefold increase in EPC counts at the end of the study period [38]. Notably, this effect is not observed with improved cholesterol levels after ezetimibe therapy [110].

In addition to increases in circulating EPC counts, EPC function (such as proliferation, migration, adhesion, and survival) improves with statin therapy, correlating to improvements in neo-endothelialization seen in statin treated animals [38, 111, 112].

CARDIAC SURGERY

Vascular injury and exposure to cardiopulmonary bypass (CPB) during cardiac surgery results in increases in EPC counts. Coronary artery bypass surgery was associated with a rapid increase in circulating EPC levels (both by flow cytometry and EC-CFU) measured 6 h postoperatively [113, 114]. This EPC surge is less robust in elderly patients, suggesting that reparative capacity may be limited with advanced age [113, 115]. Coronary artery bypass grafting with CPB was associated with impaired EPC migratory function and viability in comparison to patients subjected to off-pump surgery [116]. However, homing signals may be increased after CPB exposure, as circulating CD34-positive/CXCR4-positive cells are increased in this setting [117].

STROKE

A strong inverse correlation is observed between the numbers of circulating CD34-positive and CD133-positive cells and a history of stroke [118, 119]. In the setting of patients with chronic hypoperfused areas, cerebral blood flow measures correlated directly with circulating CD34-positive levels [119]. In acute stroke, EPC counts by FACS and EC-CFU counts positively correlated with prognosis and reduced infarct growth, suggesting increased reparative potential after cerebral infarct enhances recovery [120, 121]. Levels of CD34-positive/KDR-positive cells inversely correlate with the burden of carotid atherosclerosis in stroke patients [122].

PERIPHERAL VASCULAR DISEASE

Subjects with peripheral arterial disease, both diabetic and non-diabetic, have lower levels of circulating EPC (measured by flow cytometry), with impaired proliferation and adhesion ex vivo [123, 124]. Acute and chronic exercise increases EPC levels in subjects with ischemic PAD, which may be associated with increases in plasma VEGF levels [125, 126].

SUMMARY

A population of bone-marrow derived mononuclear cells has been identified that contributes to maintenance of vascular health and to repair of atherosclerotic vascular disease. These EPC are rare in the periphery, and understanding of their identity as a unique population of cells continues to evolve. Whether measures of this cell population serves as an index of the regenerative potential of an individual or a measure of vascular injury remains to be defined. Nevertheless, these concepts challenge past understanding of the pathogenesis of vascular disease and offer novel therapeutic strategies for the future.

REFERENCES

1. Ross R. The pathogenesis of atherosclerosis: a perspective for the 1990s. Nature 1993;362(6423):801–9.
2. Ingram DA, Caplice NM, Yoder MC. Unresolved questions, changing definitions, and novel paradigms for defining endothelial progenitor cells. Blood 2005;106(5):1525–31.
3. Ribatti D. The discovery of endothelial progenitor cells: an historical review. Leuk Res 2007;31(4):439–44.
4. Carrel A, Ebeling AH. Pure cultures of large mononuclear leucocytes. J Exp Med 1922;36(4):365–77.
5. Parker RC. The development of organized vessels in cultures of blood cells. Science 1933;77(2005):544–6.
6. Feigl W, Susani M, Ulrich W, et al. Organisation of experimental thrombosis by blood cells. Evidence of the transformation of mononuclear cells into myofibroblasts and endothelial cells. Virchows Arch A Pathol Anat Histopathol 1985;406(2):133–48.
7. Leu HJ, Feigl W, Susani M. Angiogenesis from mononuclear cells in thrombi. Virchows Arch A Pathol Anat Histopathol 1987;411(1):5–14.
8. Scott SM, Barth MG, Gaddy LR, et al. The role of circulating cells in the healing of vascular prostheses. J Vasc Surg 1994;19(4):585–93.
9. Noishiki Y, Tomizawa Y, Yamane Y, et al. Autocrine angiogenic vascular prosthesis with bone marrow transplantation. Nat Med 1996;2(1):90–3.
10. Asahara T, Murohara T, Sullivan A, et al. Isolation of putative progenitor endothelial cells for angiogenesis. Science 1997;275(5302):964–6.
11. Hillebrands J-L, Klatter FA, van den Hurk BMH, et al. Origin of neointimal endothelium and {{alpha}}-actin-positive smooth muscle cells in transplant arteriosclerosis. J Clin Invest 2001;107(11):1411–22.
12. Hu Y, Davison F, Zhang Z, et al. Endothelial replacement and angiogenesis in arteriosclerotic lesions of allografts are contributed by circulating progenitor cells. Circulation 2003;108(25):3122–7.
13. Simper D, Wang S, Deb A, et al. Endothelial progenitor cells are decreased in blood of cardiac allograft patients with vasculopathy and endothelial cells of noncardiac origin are enriched in transplant atherosclerosis. Circulation 2003;108(2):143–9.
14. Minami E, Laflamme MA, Saffitz JE, et al. Extracardiac progenitor cells repopulate most major cell types in the transplanted human heart. Circulation 2005;112(19):2951–8.
15. Ii M, Losordo DW. Transplant graft vasculopathy: a dark side of bone marrow stem cells? Circulation 2003;108(25):3056–8.
16. Reyes M, Dudek A, Jahagirdar B, et al. Origin of endothelial progenitors in human postnatal bone marrow. J Clin Invest 2002;109(3):337–46.
17. Moore MAS. Putting the neo into neoangiogenesis. J Clin Invest 2002;109(3):313–5.
18. Rustemeyer P, Wittkowski W, Greve B, et al. Flow-cytometric identification, enumeration, purification, and expansion of CD133+ and VEGF-R2+ endothelial progenitor cells from peripheral blood. J Immunoassay Immunochem 2007;28(1):13–23.
19. Khan SS, Solomon MA, McCoy JP, Jr. Detection of circulating endothelial cells and endothelial progenitor cells by flow cytometry. Cytometry B Clin Cytom 2005;64(1):1–8.
20. Civin CI, Strauss LC, Brovall C, et al. Antigenic analysis of hematopoiesis. III. A hematopoietic progenitor cell surface antigen defined by a monoclonal antibody raised against KG-1a cells. J Immunol 1984;133(1):157–65.
21. Katz FE, Tindle R, Sutherland DR, et al. Identification of a membrane glycoprotein associated with haemopoietic progenitor cells. Leuk Res 1985;9(2):191–8.
22. Andrews RG, Singer JW, Bernstein ID. Monoclonal antibody 12–8 recognizes a 115-kd molecule present on both unipotent and multipotent hematopoietic colony-forming cells and their precursors. Blood 1986;67(3):842–5.
23. Fina L, Molgaard HV, Robertson D, et al. Expression of the CD34 gene in vascular endothelial cells. Blood 1990;75(12):2417–26.
24. Ito A, Nomura S, Hirota S, et al. Enhanced expression of CD34 messenger RNA by developing endothelial cells of mice. Lab Invest 1995;72(5):532–8.
25. Shi Q, Rafii S, Wu MH-D, et al. Evidence for circulating bone marrow-derived endothelial cells. Blood 1998;92(2):362–7.
26. Schatteman GC, Hanlon HD, Jiao C, et al. Blood-derived angioblasts accelerate blood-flow restoration in diabetic mice. J Clin Invest 2000;106(4):571–8.
27. Gehling UM, Ergun S, Schumacher U, et al. In vitro differentiation of endothelial cells from AC133-positive progenitor cells. Blood 2000;95(10):3106–12.
28. Yin AH, Miraglia S, Zanjani ED, et al. AC133, a novel marker for human hematopoietic stem and progenitor cells. Blood 1997;90(12):5002–12.
29. Peichev M, Naiyer AJ, Pereira D, et al. Expression of VEGFR-2 and AC133 by circulating human CD34(+) cells identifies a population of functional endothelial precursors. Blood 2000;95(3):952–8.
30. Shmelkov SV, Jun L, St Clair R, et al. Alternative promoters regulate transcription of the gene that encodes stem cell surface protein AC133. Blood 2004;103(6):2055–61.
31. Terman BI, Dougher-Vermazen M, Carrion ME, et al. Identification of the KDR tyrosine kinase as a receptor for vascular endothelial cell growth factor. Biochem Biophys Res Commun 1992;187(3):1579–86.
32. Nowak G, Karrar A, Holmen C, et al. Expression of vascular endothelial growth factor receptor-2 or Tie-2 on peripheral blood cells defines functionally competent cell populations capable of reendothelialization. Circulation 2004;110(24):3699–707.
33. Shantsila E, Watson T, Tse HF, et al. New insights on endothelial progenitor cell subpopulations and their angiogenic properties. J Am Coll Cardiol 2008;51(6):669–71.

34. Bompais H, Chagraoui J, Canron X, et al. Human endothelial cells derived from circulating progenitors display specific functional properties compared with mature vessel wall endothelial cells. Blood 2004;103(7):2577–84.
35. Prater DN, Case J, Ingram DA, et al. Working hypothesis to redefine endothelial progenitor cells. Leukemia 2007;21(6):1141–9.
36. Ingram DA, Mead LE, Tanaka H, et al. Identification of a novel hierarchy of endothelial progenitor cells using human peripheral and umbilical cord blood. Blood 2004;104(9):2752–60.
37. Sieveking DP, Buckle A, Celermajer DS, et al. Strikingly different angiogenic properties of endothelial progenitor cell subpopulations: insights from a novel human angiogenesis assay. J Am Coll Cardiol 2008;51(6):660–8.
38. Dimmeler S, Aicher A, Vasa M, et al. HMG-CoA reductase inhibitors (statins) increase endothelial progenitor cells via the PI 3-kinase/Akt pathway. J Clin Invest 2001;108(3):391–7.
39. Kalka C, Masuda H, Takahashi T, et al. Transplantation of ex vivo expanded endothelial progenitor cells for therapeutic neovascularization. Proc Natl Acad Sci USA 2000;97(7):3422–7.
40. Rehman J, Li J, Orschell CM, et al. Peripheral blood "endothelial progenitor cells" are derived from monocyte/macrophages and secrete angiogenic growth factors. Circulation 2003;107(8):1164–9.
41. Lin Y, Weisdorf DJ, Solovey A, et al. Origins of circulating endothelial cells and endothelial outgrowth from blood. J Clin Invest 2000;105(1):71–7.
42. Gulati R, Jevremovic D, Peterson TE, et al. Diverse origin and function of cells with endothelial phenotype obtained from adult human blood. Circ Res 2003;93(11):1023–5.
43. Hur J, Yoon C-H, Kim H-S, et al. Characterization of two types of endothelial progenitor cells and their different contributions to neovasculogenesis. Arterioscler Thromb Vasc Biol 2004;24(2):288–93.
44. Yoder MC, Mead LE, Prater D, et al. Redefining endothelial progenitor cells via clonal analysis and hematopoietic stem/progenitor cell principals. Blood 2007;109(5):1801–9.
45. Rookmaaker MB, Vergeer M, van Zonneveld AJ, et al. Endothelial progenitor cells: mainly derived from the monocyte/macrophage-containing CD34- mononuclear cell population and only in part from the hematopoietic stem cell-containing CD34+ mononuclear cell population. Circulation 2003;108(21):e150; author reply e150.
46. Hur J, Yang HM, Yoon CH, et al. Identification of a novel role of T cells in postnatal vasculogenesis: characterization of endothelial progenitor cell colonies. Circulation 2007;116(15):1671–82.
47. Lapidot T, Dar A, Kollet O. How do stem cells find their way home? Blood 2005;106(6):1901–10.
48. Goichberg P, Kalinkovich A, Borodovsky N, et al. cAMP-induced PKCzeta activation increases functional CXCR4 expression on human CD34+ hematopoietic progenitors. Blood 2006;107(3):870–9.
49. Aicher A, Heeschen C, Mildner-Rihm C, et al. Essential role of endothelial nitric oxide synthase for mobilization of stem and progenitor cells. Nat Med 2003;9(11):1370–6.
50. Asahara T, Takahashi T, Masuda H, et al. VEGF contributes to postnatal neovascularization by mobilizing bone marrow-derived endothelial progenitor cells. EMBO J 1999;18(14):3964–72.
51. Heeschen C, Aicher A, Lehmann R, et al. Erythropoietin is a potent physiologic stimulus for endothelial progenitor cell mobilization. Blood 2003;102(4):1340–6.
52. Askari AT, Unzek S, Popovic ZB, et al. Effect of stromal-cell-derived factor 1 on stem-cell homing and tissue regeneration in ischaemic cardiomyopathy. Lancet 2003;362(9385):697–703.
53. Lee SP, Youn SW, Cho HJ, et al. Integrin-linked kinase, a hypoxia-responsive molecule, controls postnatal vasculogenesis by recruitment of endothelial progenitor cells to ischemic tissue. Circulation 2006;114(2):150–9.
54. Yamaguchi J-i, Kusano KF, Masuo O, et al. Stromal cell-derived factor-1 effects on ex vivo expanded endothelial progenitor cell recruitment for ischemic neovascularization. Circulation 2003;107(9):1322–8.
55. Ceradini DJ, Kulkarni AR, Callaghan MJ, et al. Progenitor cell trafficking is regulated by hypoxic gradients through HIF-1 induction of SDF-1. Nat Med 2004;10(8):858–64.
56. Mohle R, Bautz F, Rafii S, et al. The chemokine receptor CXCR-4 is expressed on CD34+ hematopoietic progenitors and leukemic cells and mediates transendothelial migration induced by stromal cell-derived factor-1. Blood 1998;91(12):4523–30.
57. Jin H, Aiyer A, Su J, et al. A homing mechanism for bone marrow-derived progenitor cell recruitment to the neovasculature. J Clin Invest 2006;116(3):652–62.
58. Grote K, Salguero G, Ballmaier M, et al. The angiogenic factor CCN1 promotes adhesion and migration of circulating CD34+ progenitor cells: potential role in angiogenesis and endothelial regeneration. Blood 2007;110(3):877–85.
59. Dentelli P, Rosso A, Balsamo A, et al. C-KIT, by interacting with the membrane-bound ligand, recruits endothelial progenitor cells to inflamed endothelium. Blood 2007;109(10):4264–71.
60. Hill JM, Zalos G, Halcox JPJ, et al. Circulating endothelial progenitor cells, vascular function, and cardiovascular risk. N Engl J Med 2003;348(7):593–600.
61. Vasa M, Fichtlscherer S, Aicher A, et al. Number and migratory activity of circulating endothelial progenitor cells inversely correlate with risk factors for coronary artery disease. Circ Res 2001;89(1):E1–7.
62. Pearson TA, Mensah GA, Alexander RW, et al. Markers of inflammation and cardiovascular disease: application to clinical and public health practice: a statement for healthcare professionals from the Centers for Disease Control and Prevention and the American Heart Association. Circulation 2003;107(3):499–511.

63. Ciulla MM, Giorgetti A, Silvestris I, et al. Endothelial colony forming capacity is related to C-reactive protein levels in healthy subjects. Curr Neurovasc Res 2006;3(2):99–106.
64. Verma S, Kuliszewski MA, Li SH, et al. C-reactive protein attenuates endothelial progenitor cell survival, differentiation, and function: further evidence of a mechanistic link between C-reactive protein and cardiovascular disease. Circulation 2004;109(17):2058–67.
65. Thum T, Tsikas D, Stein S, et al. Suppression of endothelial progenitor cells in human coronary artery disease by the endogenous nitric oxide synthase inhibitor asymmetric dimethylarginine. J Am Coll Cardiol 2005;46(9):1693–701.
66. Vasan RS. Biomarkers of cardiovascular disease: molecular basis and practical considerations. Circulation 2006;113(19):2335–62.
67. Fadini GP, de Kreutzenberg SV, Coracina A, et al. Circulating CD34+ cells, metabolic syndrome, and cardiovascular risk. Eur Heart J 2006;27(18):2247–55.
68. Chironi G, Walch L, Pernollet MG, et al. Decreased number of circulating CD34+KDR+ cells in asymptomatic subjects with preclinical atherosclerosis. Atherosclerosis 2007;191(1):115–20.
69. Hughes AD, Coady E, Raynor S, et al. Reduced endothelial progenitor cells in European and South Asian men with atherosclerosis. Eur J Clin Invest 2007;37(1):35–41.
70. Hoetzer GL, MacEneaney OJ, Irmiger HM, et al. Gender differences in circulating endothelial progenitor cell colony-forming capacity and migratory activity in middle-aged adults. Am J Cardiol 2007;99(1):46–8.
71. Strehlow K, Werner N, Berweiler J, et al. Estrogen increases bone marrow-derived endothelial progenitor cell production and diminishes neointima formation. Circulation 2003;107(24):3059–65.
72. Sugawara J, Mitsui-Saito M, Hoshiai T, et al. Circulating endothelial progenitor cells during human pregnancy. J Clin Endocrinol Metab 2005;90(3):1845–8.
73. Aznaouridis K, Ozkor M, Murrow J, Mavromatis K, Sher S, Jorgensen J, Sutcliffe D, Hameed D, Harris W, Taylor WR, Alexander RW, Quyyumi A. Association of endothelial progenitor cell colonies with cardiovascular risk factors. J Am Coll Cardiol 2008;51:A98–177.
74. Hoetzer GL, Van Guilder GP, Irmiger HM, et al. Aging, exercise, and endothelial progenitor cell clonogenic and migratory capacity in men. J Appl Physiol 2007;102(3):847–52.
75. Heiss C, Keymel S, Niesler U, et al. Impaired progenitor cell activity in age-related endothelial dysfunction. J Am Coll Cardiol 2005;45(9):1441–8.
76. Laufs U, Werner N, Link A, et al. Physical training increases endothelial progenitor cells, inhibits neointima formation, and enhances angiogenesis. Circulation 2004;109(2):220–6.
77. Rehman J, Li J, Parvathaneni L, et al. Exercise acutely increases circulating endothelial progenitor cells and monocyte-/macrophage-derived angiogenic cells. J Am Coll Cardiol 2004;43(12):2314–8.
78. Pirro M, Schillaci G, Menecali C, et al. Reduced number of circulating endothelial progenitors and HOXA9 expression in CD34+ cells of hypertensive patients. J Hypertens 2007;25(10):2093–9.
79. Delva P, Degan M, Vallerio P, et al. Endothelial progenitor cells in patients with essential hypertension. J Hypertens 2007;25(1):127–32.
80. Imanishi T, Moriwaki C, Hano T, et al. Endothelial progenitor cell senescence is accelerated in both experimental hypertensive rats and patients with essential hypertension. J Hypertens 2005;23(10):1831–7.
81. Kondo T, Hayashi M, Takeshita K, et al. Smoking cessation rapidly increases circulating progenitor cells in peripheral blood in chronic smokers. Arterioscler Thromb Vasc Biol 2004;24(8):1442–7.
82. Michaud SE, Dussault S, Haddad P, et al. Circulating endothelial progenitor cells from healthy smokers exhibit impaired functional activities. Atherosclerosis 2006;187(2):423–32.
83. van Grevenynghe J, Monteiro P, Gilot D, et al. Human endothelial progenitors constitute targets for environmental atherogenic polycyclic aromatic hydrocarbons. Biochem Biophys Res Commun 2006;341(3):763–9.
84. Kim W, Jeong MH, Cho SH, et al. Effect of green tea consumption on endothelial function and circulating endothelial progenitor cells in chronic smokers. Circ J 2006;70(8):1052–7.
85. Capla JM, Grogan RH, Callaghan MJ, et al. Diabetes impairs endothelial progenitor cell-mediated blood vessel formation in response to hypoxia. Plast Reconstr Surg 2007;119(1):59–70.
86. Tepper OM, Galiano RD, Capla JM, et al. Human endothelial progenitor cells from type II diabetics exhibit impaired proliferation, adhesion, and incorporation into vascular structures. Circulation 2002;106(22):2781–6.
87. Segal MS, Shah R, Afzal A, et al. Nitric oxide cytoskeletal-induced alterations reverse the endothelial progenitor cell migratory defect associated with diabetes. Diabetes 2006;55(1):102–9.
88. Loomans CJ, de Koning EJ, Staal FJ, et al. Endothelial progenitor cell dysfunction: a novel concept in the pathogenesis of vascular complications of type 1 diabetes. Diabetes 2004;53(1):195–9.
89. Eizawa T, Ikeda U, Murakami Y, et al. Decrease in circulating endothelial progenitor cells in patients with stable coronary artery disease. Heart 2004;90(6):685–6.
90. Chen YH, Lin SJ, Lin FY, et al. High glucose impairs early and late endothelial progenitor cells by modifying nitric oxide-related but not oxidative stress-mediated mechanisms. Diabetes 2007;56(6):1559–68.
91. Goldin A, Beckman JA, Schmidt AM, et al. Advanced glycation end products: sparking the development of diabetic vascular injury. Circulation 2006;114(6):597–605.

92. Thum T, Fraccarollo D, Schultheiss M, et al. Endothelial nitric oxide synthase uncoupling impairs endothelial progenitor cell mobilization and function in diabetes. Diabetes 2007;56(3):666–74.
93. Sorrentino SA, Bahlmann FH, Besler C, et al. Oxidant stress impairs in vivo reendothelialization capacity of endothelial progenitor cells from patients with type 2 diabetes mellitus: restoration by the peroxisome proliferator-activated receptor-gamma agonist rosiglitazone. Circulation 2007;116(2):163–73.
94. Wang CH, Ciliberti N, Li SH, et al. Rosiglitazone facilitates angiogenic progenitor cell differentiation toward endothelial lineage: a new paradigm in glitazone pleiotropy. Circulation 2004;109(11):1392–400.
95. Wang CH, Ting MK, Verma S, et al. Pioglitazone increases the numbers and improves the functional capacity of endothelial progenitor cells in patients with diabetes mellitus. Am Heart J 2006;152(6):1051.e1–8.
96. Wang HY, Gao PJ, Ji KD, et al. Circulating endothelial progenitor cells, C-reactive protein and severity of coronary stenosis in Chinese patients with coronary artery disease. Hypertens Res 2007;30(2):133–41.
97. Kunz GA, Liang G, Cuculi F, et al. Circulating endothelial progenitor cells predict coronary artery disease severity. Am Heart J 2006;152(1):190–5.
98. Guven H, Shepherd RM, Bach RG, et al. The number of endothelial progenitor cell colonies in the blood is increased in patients with angiographically significant coronary artery disease. J Am Coll Cardiol 2006;48(8):1579–87.
99. Lambiase PD, Edwards RJ, Anthopoulos P, et al. Circulating humoral factors and endothelial progenitor cells in patients with differing coronary collateral support. Circulation 2004;109(24):2986–92.
100. Shintani S, Murohara T, Ikeda H, et al. Mobilization of endothelial progenitor cells in patients with acute myocardial infarction. Circulation 2001;103(23):2776–9.
101. Massa M, Rosti V, Ferrario M, et al. Increased circulating hematopoietic and endothelial progenitor cells in the early phase of acute myocardial infarction. Blood 2005;105(1):199–206.
102. Wojakowski W, Tendera M, Michalowska A, et al. Mobilization of CD34/CXCR4+, CD34/CD117+, c-met+ stem cells, and mononuclear cells expressing early cardiac, muscle, and endothelial markers into peripheral blood in patients with acute myocardial infarction. Circulation 2004;110(20):3213–20.
103. Schmidt-Lucke C, Rossig L, Fichtlscherer S, et al. Reduced number of circulating endothelial progenitor cells predicts future cardiovascular events: proof of concept for the clinical importance of endogenous vascular repair. Circulation 2005;111(22):2981–7.
104. Werner N, Kosiol S, Schiegl T, et al. Circulating endothelial progenitor cells and cardiovascular outcomes. N Engl J Med 2005;353(10):999–1007.
105. Numaguchi Y, Sone T, Okumura K, et al. The impact of the capability of circulating progenitor cell to differentiate on myocardial salvage in patients with primary acute myocardial infarction. Circulation 2006;114(1 Suppl):I114–9.
106. Heeschen C, Lehmann R, Honold J, et al. Profoundly reduced neovascularization capacity of bone marrow mononuclear cells derived from patients with chronic ischemic heart disease. Circulation 2004;109(13):1615–22.
107. Valgimigli M, Rigolin GM, Fucili A, et al. CD34+ and endothelial progenitor cells in patients with various degrees of congestive heart failure. Circulation 2004;110(10):1209–12.
108. Kissel CK, Lehmann R, Assmus B, et al. Selective functional exhaustion of hematopoietic progenitor cells in the bone marrow of patients with postinfarction heart failure. J Am Coll Cardiol 2007;49(24):2341–9.
109. Michowitz Y, Goldstein E, Wexler D, et al. Circulating endothelial progenitor cells and clinical outcome in patients with congestive heart failure. Heart 2007;93(9):1046–50.
110. Landmesser U, Bahlmann F, Mueller M, et al. Simvastatin versus ezetimibe: pleiotropic and lipid-lowering effects on endothelial function in humans. Circulation 2005;111(18):2356–63.
111. Llevadot J, Murasawa S, Kureishi Y, et al. HMG-CoA reductase inhibitor mobilizes bone marrow-derived endothelial progenitor cells. J Clin Invest 2001;108(3):399–405.
112. Walter DH, Rittig K, Bahlmann FH, et al. Statin therapy accelerates reendothelialization: a novel effect involving mobilization and incorporation of bone marrow-derived endothelial progenitor cells. Circulation 2002;105(25):3017–24.
113. Scheubel RJ, Zorn H, Silber RE, et al. Age-dependent depression in circulating endothelial progenitor cells in patients undergoing coronary artery bypass grafting. J Am Coll Cardiol 2003;42(12):2073–80.
114. Roberts N, Xiao Q, Weir G, et al. Endothelial progenitor cells are mobilized after cardiac surgery. Ann Thorac Surg 2007;83(2):598–605.
115. Dimmeler S, Vasa-Nicotera M. Aging of progenitor cells: limitation for regenerative capacity? J Am Coll Cardiol 2003;42(12):2081–2.
116. Ruel M, Suuronen EJ, Song J, et al. Effects of off-pump versus on-pump coronary artery bypass grafting on function and viability of circulating endothelial progenitor cells. J Thorac Cardiovasc Surg 2005;130(3):633–9.
117. Mieno S, Ramlawi B, Boodhwani M, et al. Role of stromal-derived factor-1alpha in the induction of circulating CD34+CXCR4+ progenitor cells after cardiac surgery. Circulation 2006;114(1 Suppl):I186–92.

118. Ghani U, Shuaib A, Salam A, et al. Endothelial progenitor cells during cerebrovascular disease. Stroke 2005;36(1):151–3.
119. Taguchi A, Matsuyama T, Moriwaki H, et al. Circulating CD34-positive cells provide an index of cerebrovascular function. Circulation 2004;109(24):2972–5.
120. Yip HK, Chang LT, Chang WN, et al. Level and value of circulating endothelial progenitor cells in patients after acute ischemic stroke. Stroke 2008;39(1):69–74.
121. Sobrino T, Hurtado O, Moro MA, et al. The increase of circulating endothelial progenitor cells after acute ischemic stroke is associated with good outcome. Stroke 2007;38(10):2759–64.
122. Lau KK, Chan YH, Yiu KH, et al. Burden of carotid atherosclerosis in patients with stroke: relationships with circulating endothelial progenitor cells and hypertension. J Hum Hypertens 2007;21(6):445–51.
123. Fadini GP, Sartore S, Albiero M, et al. Number and function of endothelial progenitor cells as a marker of severity for diabetic vasculopathy. Arterioscler Thromb Vasc Biol 2006;26(9):2140–6.
124. Shaffer RG, Greene S, Arshi A, et al. Flow cytometric measurement of circulating endothelial cells: the effect of age and peripheral arterial disease on baseline levels of mature and progenitor populations. Cytometry B Clin Cytom 2006;70(2):56–62.
125. Sandri M, Adams V, Gielen S, et al. Effects of exercise and ischemia on mobilization and functional activation of blood-derived progenitor cells in patients with ischemic syndromes: results of 3 randomized studies. Circulation 2005;111(25):3391–9.
126. Shaffer RG, Greene S, Arshi A, et al. Effect of acute exercise on endothelial progenitor cells in patients with peripheral arterial disease. Vasc Med 2006;11(4):219–26.

12 Family History: An Index of Genetic and Environmental Predisposition to Coronary Artery Disease

Shivda Pandey and Khurram Nasir

Contents

Abstract

It is well known that family history of coronary heart disease reflects genetic predisposition to develop atherosclerosis. Individuals with a family history of premature CHD are at a significantly increased risk for CHD events. They form a potential target population for early, aggressive primary prevention strategies. However, the conventional cardiovascular risk factors (age, total cholesterol, smoking, HDL cholesterol, and systolic blood pressure) are precisely characterized and incorporated in the Framingham Risk evaluation algorithm. They do not include family history information as a criterion to guide primary prevention endeavors. Emerging evidence indicates that subjects with positive family history are unequivocally a high-risk group and candidates for prompt primary prevention efforts. In this chapter, we have highlighted overwhelming evidence indicating positive family history of CHD to be associated with an independent predictor of subclinical CHD markers, such as assessed CAC, Carotid-IMT, flow-mediated dilatation, among various others. On the basis of these facts, we propose following modifications in the risk

From: *Asymptomatic Atherosclerosis: Pathophysiology, Detection and Treatment*
Edited by: M. Naghavi (ed.), DOI 10.1007/978-1-60327-179-0_12

prediction algorithm currently being used. Individuals in the Framingham low risk category, (estimated 10-year coronary mortality <10%) with family history, can be considered as intermediate risk and be targets for further risk stratification using CAC testing. On the other hand, those within the "intermediate-risk" range should be considered as high risk and treated aggressively as CHD equivalent with LDL goals of less than 70 mg/dl, and lipid lowering therapy be initiated, if LDL≥100 mg/dl. We believe that this will be a cost effective approach in utilizing appropriate therapies and advance risk stratifying tools, such as CAC testing, in this vulnerable population.

Key words: Carotid IMT; Coronary artery calcification; Family history of heart disease; Framingham risk score

KEY POINTS

- Family history of premature CHD is an independent predictor of future CHD events.
- Extensive evidence exists, demonstrating strong relationship between markers of subclinical atherosclerosis and family history of premature CHD, explaining in part, high risk associated with this trait.
- Individuals in the Framingham low risk category (estimated 10-year coronary mortality <10%) with family history can be considered as intermediate risk and be targets for further risk stratification using CAC testing.
- On the other hand, those within the "intermediate-risk" range, should be considered as high risk and treated aggressively as CHD equivalent with LDL goals less than 70 mg/dl, and lipid lowering therapy be initiated, if LDL≥100 mg/dl.

Ms. TP is an asymptomatic 51-year-old mildly obese woman who presented herself for a routine health maintenance examination. She smokes a pack a day for the past 7 years. Her blood pressure is 134/90, controlled on antihypertensive medication. LDL and HDL-cholesterol levels are 135 and 47 mg/dl, respectively. She is not a diabetic and is not on any other medication besides the antihypertensives. Further questioning revealed a history of myocardial infarction in her father and brother at ages 46 and 49, respectively. After computing the Framingham Risk Score, she belonged to the low risk category (10-year risk of hard cardiovascular events <10%).

The above case scenario has been cited to underscore the importance of certain risk factors that have been demonstrated to independently predict coronary heart disease, but are unfortunately not adequately represented in the currently followed risk prediction algorithms [1, 2]. The role of family history of premature coronary heart disease as an independent risk factor for subclinical atherosclerosis cannot be overemphasized [3–7]. Similarly, obesity is an independent predictor of coronary events [8–11], both alone and as a part of the entire constellation of the metabolic syndrome [12–15]. Also, there is abundant literature to support the fact that the Framingham risk equation underestimates the cardiovascular risk in women [16–18]. Therefore, we realize that these three risk factors determine a sizable vulnerable population that deserves more aggressive preventive efforts than what it is currently receiving. We will subsequently discuss in detail the family history component of susceptibility to coronary heart disease.

FAMILY HISTORY: AN INDEX OF GENETIC AND ENVIRONMENTAL PREDISPOSITION TO CAD

It is not hard to conceptualize that individuals with family members developing premature coronary heart disease will have a greater propensity of developing the same. The pathogenesis of coronary heart disease involves a complex interplay of numerous intricate biochemical processes namely lipid metabolism, inflammatory response, endothelial function, platelet function, thrombosis, fibrinolysis, homocysteine metabolism, insulin sensitivity, and blood pressure regulation [19]. Although each process is affected by extrinsic environmental variables, it entails systematic function of several receptors, chemical messengers, and signaling pathways, the expression in which is governed by the genetic constitution. Topol et al. [20] have used genomics research to delineate 4 discrete biological pathways contributing to CAD and specifically MI – altered lipoprotein handling, disruption of endothelial integrity, arterial inflammation, and thrombosis. They have also presented a brief overview, highlighting the key genes implicated in each pathway.

At the same time, the environmental component is also very important and it is reasonable to state that members of a family are more likely to demonstrate similar lifestyle patterns that might lead to the development of CAD if they are unhealthy and predisposed to the same. To summarize, family members share the genetic, environmental, social and behavioral determinants of coronary heart disease, and this forms the rationale for family-centered approaches to cardiovascular disease prevention.

ROLE OF FAMILY HISTORY IN PREDICTING CARDIOVASCULAR RISK

Although family history of premature coronary heart disease has been positively correlated with various traditional cardiovascular risk factors [21, 22], there are several studies to demonstrate that it is an independent predictor of cardiovascular morbidity and mortality [23–35]. In 1979, Thelle et al. [32] used the case-control design to show that there were no significant differences in conventional cardiovascular risk factors between those who had family history compared to those without. Therefore, they postulated that the contribution of family history to cardiovascular risk is independent of traditional risk factors. A few years later, Shea et al. [25] reported that odds ratios (ORs) for overall, stratified and matched comparisons of cardiovascular events in relatives of patients with documented CAD, and control subjects ranged between 2.0 and 3.9 (*P* less than 0.01 for all comparisons), once again indicating the significant and independent risk posed by family history. They further pointed out that this risk might be of greater magnitude in those otherwise classified as low-risk. In yet another case-control study as a part of the Stockholm Heart Epidemiology program (SHEEP), Leander et al. [24] demonstrated that the adjusted OR of myocardial infarction was 2.0 (95% confidence interval [CI] = 1.6–2.6) for men reporting ≥1 affected parent or sibling, compared with men with no family history of coronary heart disease, and 3.4 (95% CI = 2.1–5.9) for those reporting ≥2 affected parents or siblings. The corresponding ORs for women were 2.1 (95% CI = 1.5–3.0) and 4.4 (95% CI = 2.4–8.1). They also reported synergistic interactions between family history and traditional risk factors like smoking, high LDL-cholesterol and low HDL-cholesterol in women and a similar relationship between family history and diabetes mellitus in men.

There are numerous prospective studies to corroborate the above stated results. Colditz et al. [33] computed relative risk ratios for angina pectoris, fatal and non-fatal myocardial infarction separately in women, with premature and non-premature parental history of myocardial infarction compared to those with no family history in the overall cohort of 117,156 women initially free of CAD. The relative risk ratios for angina, fatal and non-fatal MI in women with premature (<60 years) parental history of MI were 3.4 (95% CL 2.2, 5.2), 5.0 (95% CL 2.7, 9.2) and 2.8 (95% CL 1.8, 4.3) respectively. The respective values in women with non-premature (>60 years) parental history of MI were 1.9 (95% CL 1.2, 3.2), 2.6 (95% CL 1.1, 5.8) and 1.0 (95% CL 0.5, 1.8). They further demonstrated that these values were only mildly attenuated after multivariate adjustment with conventional risk factors, thus indicating that family history of myocardial infarction is an independent predictor of impending coronary events. In a similar study with men, Colditz et al. [34] reported that individuals with positive family history had a greater likelihood of developing CAD (relative risk = 2.2, 95% confidence interval,

1.2–3.8 for maternal history; relative risk = 1.7, 95% confidence interval 1.2–2.3 for paternal history). The risk of MI increased with decreasing age at parental MI. And again, the associations were not sizably affected by controlling for diet or established risk factors. In yet another prospective study, Myers et al. [27] established that parental history of CAD death increased the risk of CAD by 29% and that it was as important a predictor of hard events as any other traditional risk factor. They also pointed out that family history in an otherwise low-risk individual is especially a major determinant of future CAD.

The third category of studies to establish the role of family history in predicting CAD risk is prospective with validated family history information. Family history data could be accurately ascertained for the Framingham offspring cohort where both parents belonged to the original Framingham cohort. Lloyd et al. [30] utilized the advantage of this study design to demonstrate that the ORs for greater risk of coronary events in men and women with premature parental cardiovascular disease compared to those without were 2.6 (95% CI 1.7–4.1) and 2.3 (95% CI 1.3–4.3) respectively. After multivariate adjustment, the resultant ORs were 2.0 (95% CI 1.2–3.1) for men and 1.7 (95% CI 0.9–3.1) for women. They also reported that premature parental CVD was associated with a significantly higher coronary risk in intermediate multivariable risk quintile, as compared to the low and high risk. Thus, the authors suggested that family history data might be especially valuable to guide primary prevention plan in individuals classified as intermediate risk, according to conventional cardiovascular risk factors. Murabito et al. [35] used a similar setting to evaluate the role of sibling history as a risk determinant for cardiovascular disease in middle-aged adults. They reported a significant association between sibling CVD and incident coronary events, the age- and sex-adjusted OR being 1.55; 95% CI 1.19–2.03. Adjustment with multiple risk factors did not appreciably weaken the relationship, the adjusted OR being 1.45; 95% CI 1.10–1.91. They further demonstrated that multivariable-adjusted OR for sibling CVD (1.99; 95% CI, 1.32–3.00) exceeded that for parental CVD (1.45; 95% CI, 1.02–2.05).

After evaluating 122,155 Utah families, Williams et al. [36] further underscored the relevance of family history data by showing that the families with positive family risk scores (FRS≥0.5) were only 14% of the general population but accounted for 72% of patients with early CHD and 48% of CHD at all ages. These findings clearly point out that the relatively small proportion of "at-risk families" bears the major brunt of coronary heart disease and deserves aggressive and specifically targeted prevention measures. The authors also suggested that lifestyle and behavior modifications could be specifically tailored for and effectively implemented in families.

FAMILY HISTORY AND SUBCLINICAL ATHEROSCLEROSIS

The degree of subclinical atherosclerosis can be quantified by using a number of tools namely coronary artery calcium, carotid intima-media thickness, inflammatory markers, indicators of endothelial function and so on. Several studies have evaluated the relationship between family history of coronary artery disease and the burden of subclinical atherosclerosis [4–6, 37–40]. This association assumes particular importance because it delineates the population with an existing burden of asymptomatic disease that is most likely to benefit from timely prevention endeavors. We will now briefly discuss a few salient findings of these studies.

Coronary artery calcium and carotid-IMT were the markers of subclinical atherosclerosis to demonstrate maximum strength of association with FH in terms of the magnitude of OR (approximately 2–3). The results of three large prospective studies, evaluating the association between family history and CAC, namely MESA [4], Framingham Heart Study [6] and Dallas Heart Study [5], clearly demonstrated that it is an independent and significant predictor of the burden of atherosclerosis.

Nasir et al. [41] demonstrated that sibling history is more reflective of familial susceptibility of atherosclerosis as compared to parental history of CHD. They reported that ORs (95% CI) for presence of CAC in men with FH of premature CHD in parents only, in siblings only and combined FH were 1.3(1.1–1.6), 2.3(1.7–3.6) and 2.5(1.8–3.3) respectively. A similar trend was observed among women. Michos et al. [42] and later Philips et al. [43] showed a synergistic interaction between family history and metabolic risk factors as determinants of prevalent CAC. However, Philips et al. [43] reported that FH was not significantly associated with CAC in older individuals. Nevertheless, they also suggested that their results could have possibly been adulterated by survivor bias and competing risk.

Similarly, most of the studies focused on the relationship between family history and carotid IMT, reported a significant and independent association. Wang et al. [39] used validated family history information from the Framingham Offspring cohort to establish that age-adjusted mean internal carotid IMT in subjects with family history of premature CHD compared to those without were 1.13, versus 1.04 mm in men, $P<0.01$ and 0.92, versus 0.85 mm in women, $P=0.03$. Jounala et al. [40] reported that subjects with family history of CHD had higher carotid IMT compared to those without (0.600 ± 0.109 vs. 0.578 ± 0.089 mm; age- and sex-adjusted P value 0.003). They also demonstrated that in subjects with positive family history, carotid IMT was more strongly associated with cardiovascular risk factors (P for interaction$=0.007$). Zureik et al. [44], however, denied any statistically significant association between parental death from MI and carotid-IMT. They mentioned that the results could have been seriously hampered by survivor and self-selection bias, in addition to possible misclassification of subjects according to parental history of premature death from MI.

Other studies using miscellaneous markers of subclinical coronary artery disease (inflammatory mediators [38] such as CRP, fibrinogen, D-dimer etc; flow-mediated dilatation as an index of endothelial function [37]; perfusion defects on PET [45] and measures of artery elasticity [46]) further corroborated the association between family history of CAD and subclinical atherosclerosis.

RELEVANCE OF FAMILY HISTORY DATA IN THE GENOMIC ERA

Guttmacher et al. [47] eloquently describe the perception of the current and exponentially progressive "genomic world" as "space-age images of microarray chips, bioinformatics, and designer drugs". It appears attractive to discard the archaic family history information for far more sophisticated genetic tools, but as the authors suggest, novel advancements supplement instead of replacing the established method. Family history is a cost-effective, well-recognized, individualized genomic means that encompasses all the complex genetic and ecologic interactions that lead to the development of coronary heart disease.

Although classic teaching emphasizes the role of family history in Mendelian disorders, it is unfair to overlook its importance in the pathogenesis of the far more common multi-factorial disorders [47]. However, unlike the other multi-factorial disorders such as Age-related macular degeneration, and Type 2 Diabetes Mellitus, wherein precise genomic delineations exist, we have still not been able to distinctly characterize the precise genetic markers for CHD [20]. Damani et al. [20] also added that "we are just now entering an age where rapid genomic delineation of the susceptibility for MI is becoming possible". It is important to realize that the exorbitant cost associated with this project might pose a major logistic challenge [20]. Therefore, in the current scenario it certainly doesn't appear prudent to disregard family history information, which is an invaluable parameter to assess genetic and environmental susceptibility to CAD.

OBSTACLES PRECLUDING THE INCORPORATION OF FAMILY HISTORY IN RISK ALGORITHMS

Family history is undoubtedly an independent risk factor for CAD development; several challenges have however prohibited its inclusion in the commonly followed risk prediction algorithms [48]. The most frequently raised concern is regarding the validity and recall bias of self-reported family history information. Different studies have critically evaluated and compared the validated and self reported methods [49, 50]. In a unique validation study [49] using objective clinical assessments in a two-generation population-based sample, the authors reported that positive predictive value (PPV), positive likelihood ratio, negative predictive value, and negative predictive ratio for reports of premature parental heart attack were 28% (CI, 22–34%), 8.6(CI, 6.8–10.9), 99(98–100) and 0.28(0.22–0.36), respectively. They added that the low PPV is probably reflective of low prevalence rather than low predictive value per se, as suggested by the high likelihood ratios. On the whole, there is sufficiently strong evidence to substantiate the validity and accuracy of self-reported family history.

Most primary care physicians also find it extremely cumbersome to collect, organize and interpret family history information. The technically sound Family Risk Score (FRS) method [36] was developed to address the issue of heterogeneity among different families. However, it appears logistically challenging to practice it in the primary care setting on a regular basis. This has proven to be an invincible challenge, discouraging the physicians to utilize the wealth of family history data. Moreover, it is unfortunate that most primary care physicians elicit this information in order to support an already existing diagnosis of CHD [51].

Obtaining detailed medical histories of the patient's relatives inevitably puts forth ethical and legal concerns. However, Kardia et al. [52] distinctly point out that "physicians obtaining family histories in the course of practice, outside the research context, are not required by the Office of Human Research Protections to obtain consent from third parties; rather, the ethics involved in the physician-patient relationship apply". They further discuss the importance of enhancing "genetic awareness" among patients and identifying risk prone families to help the susceptible members accordingly.

AN ALTERNATIVE RISK PREDICTION ALGORITHM

We realize that individuals with positive family history are unequivocally a high-risk group and deserve prompt primary prevention efforts. Ironically, if we place them in the currently followed risk prediction algorithm [48], they fall in the least-risk category and receive cholesterol-lowering therapy only when LDL levels exceed 190 mg/dl. In the light of this observation, we propose to suggest the following modifications (see Figs. 1 and 2) in the existing risk stratification and primary prevention guidelines. Individuals in the Framingham low risk category (estimated 10-year coronary mortality <10%) with family history can be considered as intermediate risk and be targets for further risk stratification using coronary artery calcium scores. Similarly, individuals with family history already in the Framingham intermediate risk category (estimated 10-year coronary mortality 10–20%) can be promoted to the high risk group and receive aggressive risk factor lowering therapy. This provides a feasible way to meaningfully incorporate valuable family history information to guide primary preventive efforts in individuals who are very likely to benefit from them.

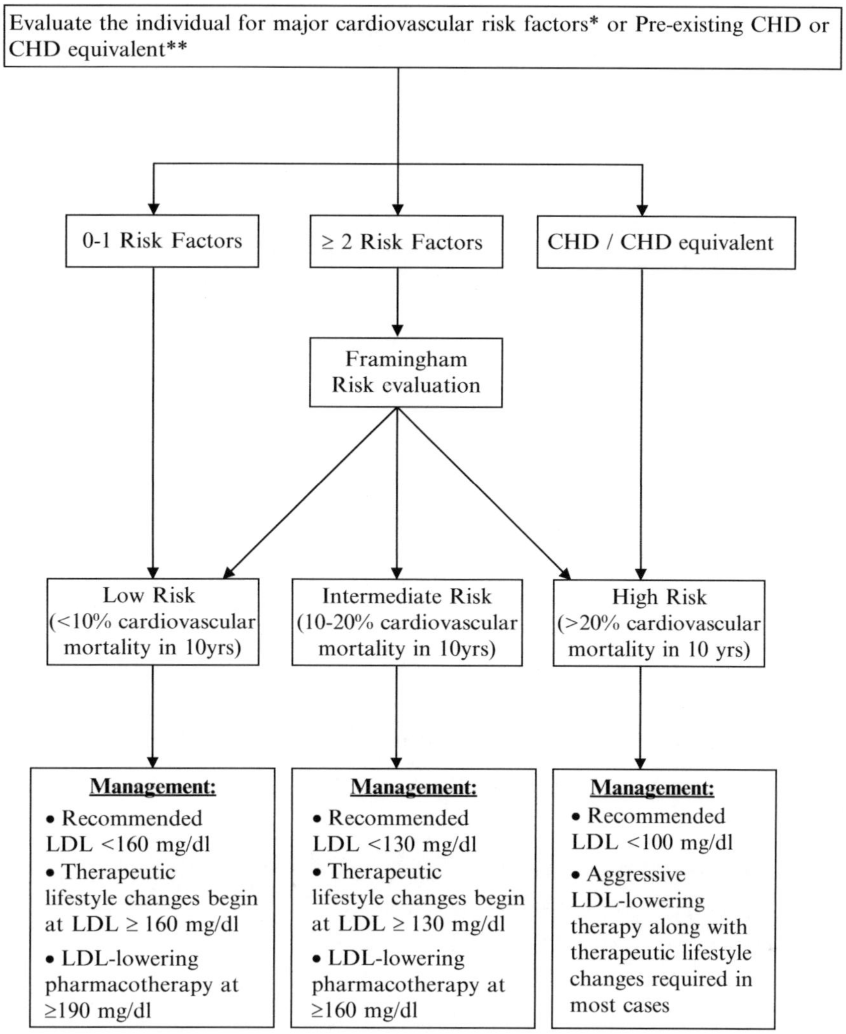

*Major cardiovascular risk factors are smoking, age, HDL-cholesterol, systolic blood pressure and family history of premature coronary heart disease.

**Conditions that are considered as CHD equivalents include diabetes mellitus ;other clinical forms of atherosclerotic disease such as peripheral vascular disease, abdominal aortic aneurysm and symptomatic carotid artery disease.

Fig. 1. Current ATP III cardiovascular risk evaluation algorithm.

WHAT THE FUTURE HOLDS FOR THE FAMILY HISTORY COMPONENT OF CARDIOVASCULAR RISK

In one of the previous sections, we discussed that detailed family history data is inconvenient and cumbersome to utilize in clinical practice. We also mentioned the conspicuous lack of "genetic literacy" in both patients and physicians. Innovative software techniques and nation-wide awareness campaigns to overcome these obstacles are already on their way [47].

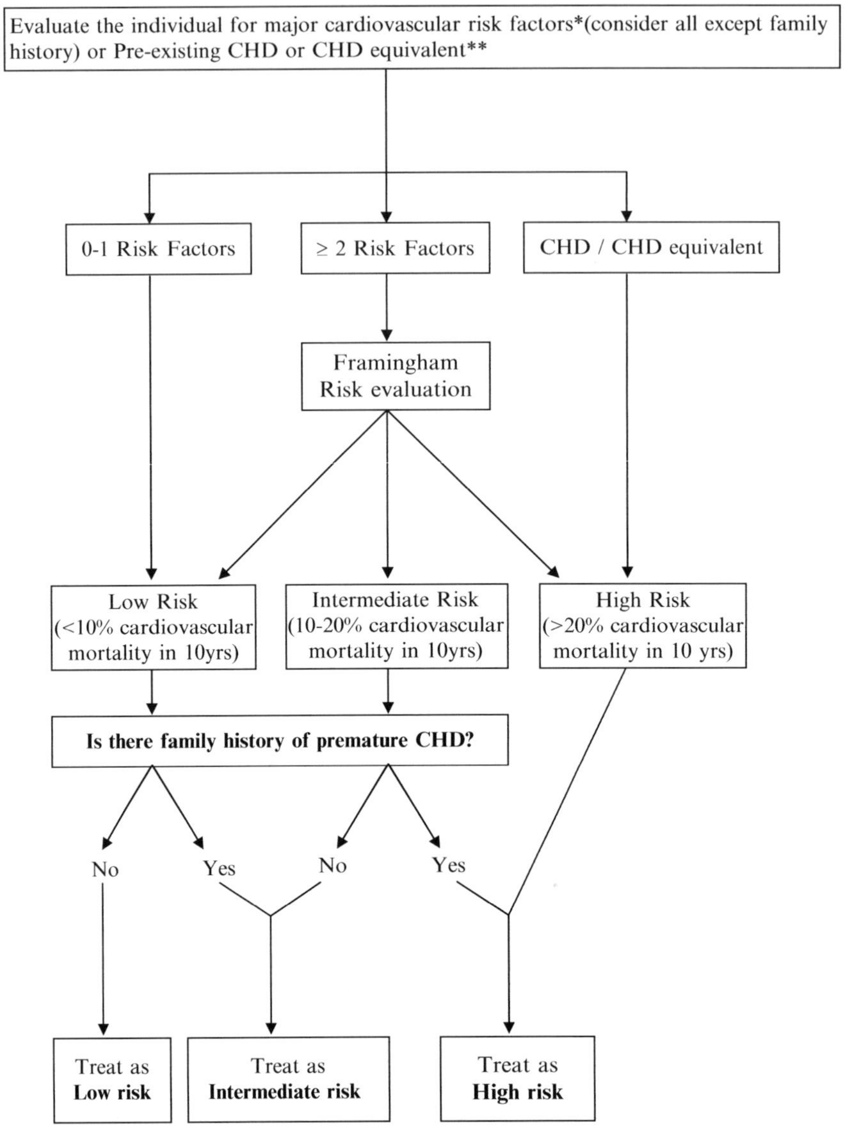

Fig. 2. Suggested cardiovascular risk evaluation algorithm.

Although we have a lucid picture of the relevance of family history in primary prevention of CAD, there is compelling need towards future research endeavors working out the logistics of using this information. We still need to establish the feasibility, usefulness and therapeutic impact of incorporating family history information in CAD prevention guidelines, through meticulously structured clinical studies.

REFERENCES

1. Nasir K, Michos ED, Blumenthal RS, Raggi P. Detection of high-risk young adults and women by coronary calcium and National Cholesterol Education Program Panel III guidelines. J Am Coll Cardiol. 2005;46:1931–6.
2. Akosah KO, Schaper A, Cogbill C, Schoenfeld P. Preventing myocardial infarction in the young adult in the first place: how do the National Cholesterol Education Panel III guidelines perform? J Am Coll Cardiol. 2003;41:1475–9.

3. Scheuner MT, Whitworth WC, McGruder H, Yoon PW, Khoury MJ. Familial risk assessment for early-onset coronary heart disease. Genet Med. 2006;8:525–31.
4. Nasir K, Budoff MJ, Wong ND, Scheuner MT, Herrington D, Arnett DK, Szklo M, Greenland P, Blumenthal RS. Family history of premature coronary heart disease and coronary artery calcification: Multi-Ethnic Study of Atherosclerosis (MESA). Circulation. 2007;116:619–26.
5. Patel MJ, de Lemos JA, Philips B, Murphy SA, Vaeth PC, McGuire DK, Khera A. Implications of family history of myocardial infarction in young women. Am Heart J. 2007;154:454-60
6. Parikh NI, Hwang SJ, Larson MG, Cupples LA, Fox CS, Manders ES, Murabito JM, Massaro JM, Hoffmann U, O'Donnell CJ. Parental occurrence of premature cardiovascular disease predicts increased coronary artery and abdominal aortic calcification in the Framingham Offspring and Third Generation cohorts. Circulation. 2007;116:1473–81.
7. Lloyd-Jones DM, Nam BH, D'Agostino RB, Levy D, Murabito JM, Wang TJ, Wilson PWF, O'Donnell CJ. Parental cardiovascular disease as a risk factor for cardiovascular disease in middle-aged adults: a prospective study of parents and offspring. JAMA. 2004;291:2204–11.
8. Bogers RP, Bemelmans WJ, Hoogenveen RT, Boshuizen HC et al. Association of overweight with increased risk of coronary heart disease partly independent of blood pressure and cholesterol levels: a meta-analysis of 21 cohort studies including more than 300 000 persons. Arch Intern Med. 2007;167:1720–8.
9. Perez Perez A, Ybarra Munoz J, Blay Cortes V, de Pablos Velasco P. Obesity and cardiovascular disease. Public Health Nutr. 2007;10:1156–63.
10. Poirier P, Giles TD, Bray GA, Hong Y, Stern JS, Pi-Sunyer FX, Eckel RH. Obesity and cardiovascular disease: pathophysiology, evaluation, and effect of weight loss: an update of the 1997 American Heart Association Scientific Statement on Obesity and Heart Disease from the Obesity Committee of the Council on Nutrition, Physical Activity, and Metabolism. Circulation. 2006;113:898–918.
11. Hubert HB, Feinleib M, McNamara PM, Castelli WP. Obesity as an independent risk factor for cardiovascular disease: a 26-year follow-up of participants in the Framingham Heart Study. Circulation. 1983;67:968–77.
12. Haffner SM. Relationship of metabolic risk factors and development of cardiovascular disease and diabetes. Obesity (Silver Spring). 2006;14:121S–7S.
13. Grundy SM. Metabolic syndrome: connecting and reconciling cardiovascular and diabetes worlds. J Am Coll Cardiol. 2006;47:1093–100.
14. Bonora E. The metabolic syndrome and cardiovascular disease. Ann Med. 2006;38:64–80.
15. Wong ND. Metabolic syndrome: cardiovascular risk assessment and management. Am J Cardiovasc Drugs. 2007;7:259–72.
16. Hecht HS, Superko HR. Electron beam tomography and National Cholesterol Education Program guidelines in asymptomatic women. J Am Coll Cardiol. 2001;37:1506–11.
17. Michos ED, Vasamreddy CR, Becker DM, Yanek LR, Moy TF, Fishman EK, Becker LC, Blumenthal RS. Women with a low Framingham risk score and a family history of premature coronary heart disease have a high prevalence of subclinical coronary atherosclerosis. Am Heart J. 2005;150:1276–81.
18. Michos ED, Nasir K, Braunstein JB, Rumberger JA, Budoff MJ, Post WS, Blumenthal RS. Framingham risk equation underestimates subclinical atherosclerosis risk in asymptomatic women. Atherosclerosis. 2006;184:201–6.
19. Scheuner MT. Genetic predisposition to coronary artery disease. Curr Opin Cardiol. 2001;16:251–60.
20. Damani SB, Topol EJ. Future use of genomics in coronary artery disease. J Am Coll Cardiol. 2007;50:1933–40.
21. Becker DM, Yook RM, Moy TF, Blumenthal RS. Markedly high prevalence of coronary risk factors in apparently healthy African-American and white siblings of persons with premature coronary heart disease. Am J Cardiol. 1998;82:1046–51.
22. Rissanen AM, Nikkila EA. Aggregation of coronary risk factors in families of men with fatal and non-fatal coronary heart disease. Br Heart J. 1979;42:373–80.
23. Friedlander Y, Siscovick DS, Weinmann S, et al. Family history as a risk factor for primary cardiac arrest. Circulation. 1998;97:155–160.
24. Leander K, Hallqvist J, Reuterwall C, Ahlbom A, de Faire U. Family history of coronary heart disease, a strong risk factor for myocardial infarction interacting with other cardiovascular risk factors: results from the Stockholm Heart Epidemiology Program (SHEEP). Epidemiology. 2001;12:215–21.
25. Shea S, Ottman R, Gabrieli C, Stein Z, Nichols A. Family history as an independent risk factor for coronary artery disease. J Am Coll Cardiol. 1984;4:793–801.
26. Friedlander Y, Kark JD, Stein Y. Family history of myocardial infarction as an independent risk factor for coronary heart disease. Br Heart J. 1985;53:382–7.
27. Myers RH, Kiely D, Cupples LA, Kannel WB. Parental history is an independent risk factor for coronary artery disease: the Framingham Study. Am Heart J. 1990;120:963–69.
28. Jousilahti P, Puska P, Vartiainen E, Pekkanen J, Tuomilehto J. Parental history of premature coronary heart disease: an independent risk factor of myocardial infarction. J Clin Epidemiol. 1996;49:497–503.
29. Pohjola-Sintonen S, Rissanen A, Liskola P, Luomanmaki K. Family history as a risk factor of coronary heart disease in patients under 60 years of age. Eur Heart J. 1998;19:235–9.
30. Lloyd-Jones DM, Nam BH, D'Agostino RB, Levy D, Murabito JM, Wang TJ, Wilson PW, O'Donnell CJ. Parental cardiovascular disease as a risk factor for cardiovascular disease in middle-aged adults: a prospective study of parents and offspring. JAMA. 2004;291:2204–11.

31. Castro-Bieras A, Muniz J, Fernandes-Fuertes I, Lado-Canosa A et al. Family history as an independent risk factor for ischaemic heart disease in a low incidence area (Galicia, Spain). Eur Heart J. 1993;14:1445–50.
32. Thelle DS, Forde OH. The cardiovascular study in Finnmark county: coronary risk factors and the occurrence of myocardial infarction in first degree relatives and in subjects of different ethnic origin. Am J Epidemiol. 1979;110:708–15.
33. Colditz GA, Stampfer MJ, Willett WC, Rosner B, Speizer FE, Hennekens CH. A prospective study of parental history of myocardial infarction and coronary heart disease in women. Am J Epidemiol. 1986;123:48–58.
34. Colditz GA, Rimm EB, Giovannucci E, Stampfer MJ, Rosner B, Willett WC. A prospective study of parental history of myocardial infarction and coronary artery disease in men. Am J Cardiol. 1991;67:933–8.
35. Murabito JM, Pencina MJ, Nam BH, D'Agostino RB, Wang TJ, Lloyd-Jones DM, Wilson PWF, O'Donnell CJ. Sibling cardiovascular disease as a risk factor for cardiovascular disease in middle-aged adults. JAMA. 2005;294:3117–23.
36. Williams RR, Hunt SC, Heiss G, Province MA, Bensen JT, Higgins M, Chamberlain RM, Ware J, Hopkins PN. Usefulness of cardiovascular family history data for population-based preventive medicine and medical research (the Health Family Tree Study and the NHLBI Family Heart Study). Am J Cardiol. 2001;87:129–35.
37. Clarkson P, Celermajer DS, Powe AJ, Donald AE, Henry RMA, Deanfield JE. Endothelium-dependent dilatation is impaired in young healthy subjects with a family history of premature coronary disease. Circulation. 1997;96:3378–83.
38. Margaglione M, Cappucci G, Colaizzo D, Vecchione G, Grandone E, Di Minno G. C-reactive protein in offspring is associated with the occurrence of myocardial infarction in first-degree relatives. Arterioscler Thromb Vasc Biol. 2000;20:198–203.
39. Wang TJ, Nam BH, D'Agostino RB, Wolf PA, Lloyd-Jones DM, Mac Rae CA, Wilson PW, Polak JF, O'Donnell CJ. Carotid intima-media thickness is associated with premature parental coronary heart disease: the Framingham Heart Study. Circulation. 2003;108:572–6.
40. Juonala M, Viikari JSA, Räsänen L, Helenius H, Pietikäinen M, Raitakari OT. Young adults with family history of coronary heart disease have increased arterial vulnerability to metabolic risk factors: the Cardiovascular Risk in Young Finns Study. Arterioscler Thromb Vasc Biol. 2006;26:1376–82.
41. Nasir K, Michos ED, Rumberger JA, Braunstein JB, Post WS, Budoff MJ, Blumenthal RS. Coronary artery calcification and family history of premature coronary heart disease: sibling history is more strongly associated than parental history. Circulation. 2004;110:2150–6.
42. Michos ED, Nasir K, Rumberger JA, Vasamreddy CR, Braunstein JB, Budoff MJ, Blumenthal RS. Relation of family history of premature coronary heart disease and metabolic risk factors to risk of coronary arterial calcium in asymptomatic subjects. Am J Cardiol. 2005;95:655–7.
43. Philips B, de Lemos J, Patel M, McGuire DK, Khera A. Relation of family history of myocardial infarction and the presence of coronary arterial calcium in various age and risk factor groups. Am J Cardiol. 2007;99:825–9.
44. Zureik M, Touboul PJ, Bonithon-Kopp C, Courbon D, Ruelland I, Ducimetière P. Differential association of common carotid intima-media thickness and carotid atherosclerotic plaques with parental history of premature death from coronary heart disease: the EVA study. Arterioscler Thromb Vasc Biol. 1999;19:366–71.
45. Sdringola S, Patel D, Gould KL. High prevalence of myocardial perfusion abnormalities on positron emission tomography in asymptomatic persons with a parent or sibling with coronary artery disease. Circulation. 2001;103:496–501.
46. Riley WA, Freedman DS, Higgs NA, Barnes RW, Zinkgraf SA, Berenson GS. Decreased arterial elasticity associated with cardiovascular disease risk factors in the young. Bogalusa Heart Study. Arteriosclerosis. 1986;6:378–86.
47. Guttmacher AE, Collins FS, Carmona RH. The family history–more important than ever. N Engl J Med. 2004;351:2333–6.
48. Expert panel on detection, evaluation, and treatment of high blood cholesterol in adults. Executive summary of the third report of the National Cholesterol Education Program (NCEP) Expert panel on detection, evaluation, and treatment of high blood cholesterol in adults (Adult Treatment Panel III). JAMA. 2001;285:2486–97.
49. Murabito JM, Nam BH, D'Agostino RB, Lloyd-Jones DM, O'Donnell CJ, Wilson PWF. Accuracy of offspring reports of parental cardiovascular disease history: the Framingham Offspring Study. Ann Intern Med. 2004;140:434–40.
50. Bensen JT, Liese AD, Rushing JT et al. Accuracy of proband reported family history: the NHLBI Family Heart Study (FHS). Genet Epidemiol. 1999;17:141–50.
51. Scheuner MT, Wang SJ, Raffel LJ, Larabell SK, Rotter JI. Family history: a comprehensive genetic risk assessment method for the chronic conditions of adulthood. Am J Med Genet. 1997;71:315–24.
52. Kardia SL, Modell SM, Peyser PA. Family-centered approaches to understanding and preventing coronary heart disease. Am J Prev Med. 2003;24:143–51.
53. Guttmacher AE, Collins FS, Carmona RH. The family history–more important than ever. N Engl J Med. 2004;351:2333–6.
54. O'Donnell CJ. Family history, subclinical atherosclerosis, and coronary heart disease risk: barriers and opportunities for the use of family history information in risk prediction and prevention. Circulation. 2004;110:2074–6.

13 Endothelial Activation Markers in Sub-clinical Atherosclerosis: Insights from Mechanism-Based Paradigms

Victoria L.M. Herrera and Joseph A. Vita

CONTENTS

ABSTRACT

Endothelial cell (EC) activation mediates inflammation and involves several effectors such as E-selectin, P-selectin, ICAM-1, and VCAM-1. These EC activation markers are detected to be significantly increased in clinical coronary artery disease (CAD), and mildly increased in subclinical CAD compared with non-disease reference groups. Because inflammation is implicated in all stages of CAD and thought to underlie plaque destabilization and rupture, monitoring the increase in EC activation markers could be a surrogate endpoint in the monitoring of subclinical coronary artery disease (subCAD) progression,

From: *Asymptomatic Atherosclerosis: Pathophysiology, Detection and Treatment*
Edited by: M. Naghavi (ed.), DOI 10.1007/978-1-60327-179-0_13

and/or response to prevention/intervention strategies. While CAD progression is complex, and requires the contemporaneous analysis of multi-pathway markers, monitoring EC activation markers could provide insight into subCAD progression, especially when levels approach those detected in acute coronary syndromes (ACS). Clearly, mechanism-based deductions provide compelling evidence that EC activation markers should be integrated into the management of subCAD; however, much study remains to be done.

Key words: Endothelial activation biomarkers; E-selectin; P-selectin; VCAM-1; ICAM-1

TOPIC PEARLS

- *An unequivocal mandate.* "The need to identify individuals at risk for concerted intervention before problems manifest" [1] underlies the mandate for advancing the management of subclinical atherosclerosis.
- *Integrating Endothelial cell (EC) activation markers in real-time coronary artery disease (CAD) management – beyond predicting risk 1–2 or even 10 years later.* Since EC activation is implicated in plaque progression and destabilization, monitoring of EC activation provides a mechanism-based approach that, coupled to emerging plaque-biology diagnostic tools, could provide real-time insight into plaque progression and destabilization.
- *Re-establishing endothelial health.* Targeting the pharmacological modulation of pathological EC activation in order to reestablish endothelial health and integrity provides a management benchmark that is mechanism-based. Clinical research needs to be done to validate this mechanism-based hypothesis and determine best diagnostic and treatment strategies.
- *A balancing act.* Since EC activation is required in a normal physiological response to common triggers (e.g., wounds, infections, and remodeling), long-term inhibition of increased EC activation in CAD will not be physiological. Therapy directed at limiting EC activation "spikes" would have to permit physiological responses, while avoiding pathological responses that contribute to atherosclerosis.
- *Limitations of systemic EC markers.* Current analysis modalities of systemic EC activation markers is limited by non-information on the site of EC activation. This limitation requires integration with other emerging diagnostic tools, such as plaque molecular imaging, and/or a vascular bed-specific marker.

CASE PRESENTATION

A 52 year old man presents himself to his physician, for an annual examination. He is well without symptoms of cardiovascular disease. He is a nonsmoker and has no history of hypertension or diabetes mellitus. A recent screening colonoscopy was normal. There is no family history of premature CAD. Blood pressure is 130/80 mmHg, and physical examination is normal. A lipid profile demonstrates a total cholesterol of 183, HDL cholesterol 53, triglycerides 70, and LDL cholesterol of 116 mg/dL. C-reactive protein is 0.52 mg/L. His coronary calcium score by computed tomography scanning of the heart is 100 and is in the intermediate range for age and gender.

The patient is concerned about his risk for coronary heart disease and currently exercises regularly and maintains a low-fat diet. He asks whether he should start treatment with a statin to lower his cholesterol levels. Current guidelines suggest that this patient has low risk for cardiovascular events and that there is no indication for drug therapy [2].

MANAGEMENT QUESTIONS

- How best to monitor the patient's subclinical coronary artery disease (subCAD), prevent CAD progression, and intervene effectively before a cardiac event?
- Will analysis of a panel of biomarkers, including EC activation markers, help in monitoring subclinical atherosclerosis and guide management in order to prevent CAD progression?

INTRODUCTION: A PERSPECTIVE OF OPPORTUNITY AND CHALLENGES

EC activation plays a pivotal role in all stages of CAD – not just plaque initiation, but plaque progression and destabilization as well [1]. Intuitively, therefore, EC activation markers could provide monitoring parameters, as well as mechanism-based treatment benchmarks for management of all stages of the disease. Emerging non-invasive structural and functional imaging technologies (*see Chaps. 19–27*) now make it possible to identify individuals with subCAD, but important questions remain about optimal management of early disease. A review of the current information on EC activation markers in acute coronary syndromes (ACS) provides a rationale for integration of EC activation markers in the management of individuals with subclinical atherosclerosis. At the same time, however, the said review also highlights the complexities and challenges that require sorting out. Nevertheless, with improving technologies to better detect asymptomatic or subCAD, integrating EC activation markers into subclinical atherosclerosis management may become feasible, and help meet the mandate to "identify individuals at risk for concerted intervention before problems manifest" [1].

As a requirement for the accumulation of inflammatory cells, endothelial activation seems rather straightforward. However, endothelial activation is complex rather than stereotyped, since the specific stimulus/i, mediator/s of, responders to, and biological context of endothelial activation affect downstream outcomes differentially, as well as synergistically. Nevertheless, dissection of this complexity is important in the elucidation of mechanisms of CAD plaque progression and destabilization, in order to decipher the functional implications of elevated markers of endothelial activation, hence elucidating prognostic parameters that could underlie mechanism-based intervention and/or prevention strategies.

The well-recognized role of local inflammation as a predecessor for plaque rupture suggests potential utility of EC activation as biomarkers for plaque progression or even as intervention-targets themselves. However, emerging data speak about a more complex role for EC activation in coronary atherosclerosis, since key effectors of EC activation are reported to also recruit endothelial progenitor cells (EPCs), as they do leukocytes (Table 1). This dual role is not surprising, given that wound healing would

Table 1
Causal roles of EC activation in atherosclerosis demonstrated in mouse knockout (null deficiency by gene-targeting) models

EC activation effectors	*Counter ligand*	*Double knockout with ApoE$^{-/-}$*	*Function*
E-selectin	ESL-1, PSGL-1, CD43, CD44,	Decreased plaque	WBC capture, tethering and rolling Platelet rolling EPC homing
P-selectin	PSGL-1	Decreased plaque	WBC capture, tethering and rolling Platelet rolling
	PSGL		EPC homing
ICAM-1	LFA-1 or CD11a/CD18	Decreased plaque	WBC adhesion
	LFA-1		T-cell transendothelial passage
	LFA-1		EPC homing
VCAM-1	VLA-4 or CD49d/CD29	Embryonic lethal VCAM1$^{D4D/D4D}$Ldlr$^{-/-}$ mice: decreased plaque	WBC adhesion

(continued)

Table 1
(continued)

EC activation effectors	*Counter ligand*	*Double knockout with ApoE$^{-/-}$*	*Function*
	SPARC		Transendothelial migration
	VLA-4		EPC homing
PECAM-1	PECAM-1, CD177	Decreased plaque	WBC transendothelial migration
			Mechanoresponsive
			Maintenance of vascular permeability barrier

ApoE$^{-/-}$; ApoE-deficient knockout mouse; EPC, endothelial progenitor cell; ESL-1, E-selecting ligand-1; LFA-1, lymphocyte function-associated antigen-1; PSGL-1, P-selectin glycoprotein ligand; SPARC, secreted protein acidic and rich in cysteine; VCAM1$^{D4D/D4D}$Ldlr$^{-/-}$, double knockout of LDL receptor-deficiency and mutant VCAM-1 with immunoglobulin-like domain #4 deleted; VLA-4, very late antigen-4; WBC, white blood cells (monocytes, neutrophils, lymphocytes); references: [10–12, 18–19, 21–24, 54–58].

require both inflammatory cells and progenitor cells. More complexly, EC activation also participates in platelet rolling, and as seen with PECAM-1, in some anti-inflammatory events (Table 1).

CONCEPTS

Definition of EC Activation

There is no uniform agreement on the definition of endothelial activation, thus reflecting its complexity.

- Endothelial activation is involved in a spectrum of physiological and pathogenic events. On the one hand it is a regulated life-saving physiologic response to fight infections or participate in wound healing, and on the other, a dysregulated "life-threatening" response seen in pathologic conditions, such as adult-respiratory distress syndrome, sepsis, vasculitides, disseminated intravascular coagulation (DIC).
- A general definition of endothelial activation is a change in phenotype or function, in response to stimuli from the environment, such as cytokines, thrombin, bacterial endotoxin, microbial products, hemodynamic perturbations, oxidants, hypoxia, radiation [3, 4], leading to the expression of molecules that mediate adhesion and/or recruitment of leukocytes [3–6].
- Notably, only the activated endothelium participates in the inflammatory response [7].
- Since inflammation is involved in all forms of plaque ([8]; *reviews*, [1, 9]), it follows that endothelial activation is present in all forms of plaque.

Components of EC activation: VCAM-1, ICAM-1, E-selectin, P-selectin

The adhesion and transmigration of leukocytes from the blood into the arterial wall in inflammation occurs via a multi-step paradigm, through selectins and adhesion molecules expressed by the "activated" endothelium [10, 11]. The established view was that selectins (E-selectin and P-selectin) underlie the 1st step of weak *rolling* interaction that allows leukocytes to roll along the endothelium, until a 2nd step of *tethering* or tighter adhesion occurs with the expression of adhesion molecules (intercellular adhesion molecule-1 or ICAM-1, and vascular cell adhesion molecule-1 or VCAM-1 on ECs, followed by a 3rd step of *transmigration* across the endothelium via platelet and EC adhesion molecule-1 (PECAM-1) and other cellular adhesion molecules [10, 11]. However, functional redundancy among the different EC activation players is evident [12], akin to a fail-safe system with back-up contingencies.

Roles of Endothelial Activation in CAD

EC activation is involved in CAD plaque initiation, progression and destabilization via its central role in inflammation, and emerging roles in platelet rolling and EPC recruitment.

EC activation-mediated inflammation is implicated in plaque initiation, progression, destabilization and disruption, leading to both the "clinically silent" discontinuous plaque growth, and the "clinically overt" event or ACS [1, 9]. Direct evidence for this role lies in the detection of expression of adhesion molecules and selectins, which is increased in the atherosclerotic plaque compared to normal endothelium in humans [13, 14]. The presence of EC activation effectors on plaques per se is concordant with observed inflammatory-based (T-cells, monocytes, and neutrophils) mechanisms of plaque progression and destabilization. Causal evidence for roles of EC activation effectors in atherosclerotic plaque initiation and growth in size, are obtained from studies using gene-targeted null-deficiency (knockout) mouse models (Table 1), albeit limited to aortic root plaques. Knockout mice lacking ICAM-1 or P-selectin exhibited marked delay in atherosclerotic lesion formation in double knockout models: ICAM-$1^{-/-}$/Apo$E^{-/-}$ mice and P-selectin$^{-/-}$/Apo$E^{-/-}$ mice [15, 16]. VCAM-1 null deficiency is embryonic lethal [17]. E-selectin$^{-/-}$ null mice do not elicit decreased atherosclerotic lesions due to redundancy with P-selectin, but with the combined triple knockout model, E-selectin$^{-/-}$, P-selectin$^{-/-}$, and Apo$E^{-/-}$ null mice, atherosclerotic lesions are decreased in size (*a review*, [18]).

Studies in mouse knockout models also implicate EC activation effectors, E-selectin and P-selectin, in platelet rolling ([19]; Table 1), which can thus contribute to inflammation-mediated increase in plaque thrombogenicity [20].

More recently, emerging reports implicate E-selectin, ICAM-1 and VCAM-1 in the recruitment of EPCs to ischemic areas or pathogenically inflamed tissues – with neovascularization as the common targeted outcome.

- E-selectin: E-selectin knockout mice reveal that just as E-selectin participates in tethering leukocytes, E-selectin participates in EPC homing to ischemic areas [21]. More specifically, E-selectin stimulated not only ECs to express ICAM-1, but also EPCs to secrete interleukin-8 (IL-8), leading to enhanced migration and incorporation in to EC capillary formation [21]. We note however, that E-selectin null-deficiency is not embryonic lethal, and such mice display normal embryonic vasculogenesis and angiogenesis.
- ICAM-1: ICAM-1 is also involved in recruitment of EPCs to ischemic areas. In-vitro data show that EPCs are recruited to ECs through ICAM-1/beta-2 integrin interaction [22]. In vivo mouse model data show that inhibition of ICAM-1 via anti-ICAM-1 antibody decreased EPC recruitment to ischemic areas, concordant with in-vitro data [22].
- VCAM-1: Not surprisingly, Duan et al. [23] have also observed VCAM-1 participating in EPC recruitment to ischemic areas. This is corroborated by the detection of selective recruitment of EPCs to inflamed joint tissue in rheumatoid arthritis, via the VCAM-1/very late activation antigen-4 adhesive system [24]. Together, these findings provide evidence of VCAM-1's role in EPC recruitment in pathogenic states typified by inflammation and neovascularization.
- P-selectin: EPCs express PSGL-1, the interacting partner for P-selectin. Expression of P-selectin on activated endothelium can therefore participate in EPC recruitment.

Altogether, demonstrated roles of EC activation effectors in proatherogenic-proinflammatory recruitment of leukocytes and in pro-repair recruitment of EPCs is not surprising given that both are involved in wound healing. This dual role could underlie the variation in association of EC activation markers and prognosis risk stratification after ACS (Table 1). In the context of CAD, EC activation triggers leukocyte recruitment as inflammatory response to lipid-influx, as well as EPC recruitment to participate in repair of sites of endothelial injury, and/or in the maintenance of endothelial integrity. On the other hand, EPCs could also contribute to neovascularization of plaques, thus allowing plaque growth, as well as providing an avenue for plaque instability through pathologic angiogenesis in plaque.

Increased Soluble EC Activation Markers Represent Increased Endothelial Expression of Said Markers

In-vitro data show that increased expression of cell adhesion molecules on activated EC surface is associated with increased levels of soluble adhesion molecules [25]. Increased cell adhesion molecules have been detected in different stages of CAD (see Tables 2 and 3), concordant with observations in other pathological conditions associated with EC activation, such as: infectious diseases, cancer, chronic inflammatory disease [26]. Likewise, circulating P-selectin has been shown to be shed from activated endothelium and platelets [19].

Table 2
Review of multi-marker clinical studies of EC activation markers

Overview of Multi-marker Clinical Studies of EC Activation Markers

	Stable Angina	Unstable Angina	Acute Myocardial Infarction	Predict Future Risk	
	↑	↑	↑	Cardiac event post MI	Extent of atherosclerosis
VCAM-1	❶❷❸④	❶❷❸④	❶❷	❼❽❾❿⑩	❾⑩
ICAM-1	❶❷❸④	❶❷❸④	❶❷	❼❽❾❿⑩	❾⑩
E-selectin	❶❷❸④❺	❶❷❸④❺	❶❷	❼❽❾❿⑩	⑩
P-selectin	①②❸❹❺❻	①❷❸❹❺❻	①	❼❽❾❿⑩	⑩

Legend: ↑, significantly increased from disease-free reference group; EC, endothelial cell; ICAM-1, intercellular adhesion molecule; MI, myocardial infarction; VCAM-1, vascular cell adhesion molecule

❶–❿, studies demonstrate increased levels of EC activation marker

①–⑩, studies report no significant change in EC activation marker

References: ❶ and ①: Soeki et al. [53]; ❷: Guray et al. [32]; ❸: Turhan et al. [54]; ❹ and ④: Parker et al. [55]; ❺: Atalar et al. 2001 [56]; ❻: Draz et al. [57]; ❼: Mulvihill et al. [28]; ❽: Ray et al. [29]; ❾: Peter et al. [58]; ❿: Blankenberg et al. [27]; ⑩: Hope and Meredith [30]

Table 3
Relative levels of EC activation markers in subclinical and clinical atherosclerosis

	Hwang et al. [33]			*Guray et al. [32]*			
n	240	224	166	29	34	45	43
	Ref. grp (ng/ml)	subCAA (% incr)	subCAD (% incr)	Ref. grp (ng/ml)	SA (% incr)	UA (% incr)	AMI (% incr)
VCAM-1	461	–0.7	3.91	110	94.81	138.6	196.22
ICAM-1	244	16.1	18.22	237	56.04	65.0	73.60
E-selectin	33	26.5	17.07	29	8.79	38.8	53.75

AMI, acute myocardial infarction; ref. grp, disease-free reference group; SA, stable angina; subCAA, subclinical carotid artery atherosclerosis; subCAD, subclinical coronary artery disease; UA, unstable angina

% increase = [test – reference]/reference × 100

CURRENT INFORMATION

Key Insights and Lessons from Clinical Studies of EC Activation Markers

The pivotal role of inflammation in the pathogenesis of atherosclerosis suggests that anti-inflammatory therapy might be useful for primary and secondary prevention. Indeed, it has been suggested that therapy that targets the effectors of inflammation may provide benefits above and beyond currently available risk reduction therapy [1]. A number of observational studies have shown that plasma levels of markers of EC activation have predictive values in patients with ACS, while some report non-informativeness of EC activation markers to discriminate stable angina (SA) from ACS, or to predict future risk of cardiac events or extent of atherosclerosis (Table 2).

While most studies detect increased levels of EC activation markers with symptomatic CAD, and delineate SA, unstable angina (UA) and acute myocardial infarction (AMI) from each other by level of increase in one or more EC activation markers (Table 2), a few report on predictive risk of a cardiac event after AMI [27–29]. However, negative predictive ability is also reported for all four EC activation markers [30]. The predictive values reported are quite encouraging given that systemic EC activation markers do not discriminate site of EC activation – plaque surface, plaque neo-vessels, plaque-subjacent adventitial vaso vasorum, other-site vascular endothelium – or the stimulus for EC activation.

In the study by Hope and Meredith [30], the failure of all four EC activation markers (VCAM-1, ICAM-1, P-selectin) to predict CAD progression reiterates that monitoring EC activation alone might not be sufficient, and that the simultaneous determination of biomarkers that reflect different pathophysiological processesimproves risk stratification in patients with ACS [31]. More importantly, the variable results of studies relating EC activation markers to ACS speaks for the complexity of CAD, the complexity of EC activation marker expression, release and clearance, as well as reflect methodological and analytical challenges.

HOW BEST TO INTEGRATE EMERGING INFORMATION INTO CLINICAL PRACTICE IN ORDER TO IMPROVE THE MANAGEMENT OF SUB-CLINICAL CORONARY ARTERY DISEASE (SubCAD)

Monitoring Increase of EC Activation Markers as a Way to Monitor risk for Progression of Subclinical CAD

Beyond analysis of classical risk factors, changes in EC activation markers could provide a personalized and mechanism-based risk-stratification. Abnormal results might trigger more aggressive monitoring and/or facilitate specific interventions.

Since actual values of EC activation markers span a broad range as seen in the group means of levels in normals (29–33 ng/ml for E-selectin, 237–244 ng/ml for ICAM-1, and 110–461 ng/ml for VCAM-1, Table 3), inter-marker comparative analyses require an informative and valid numerical transformation. To do this, comparative analysis of levels reported in the literature of EC activation markers were converted to a % increase of mean marker levels attained in a particular CAD-stage group of patients (subclinical coronary atherosclerosis, SA, UA, AMI) compared to levels detected in disease-free reference subjects within the same research dataset. Comparative analysis (Table 3) was limited to studies reporting similar group mean levels detected in disease-free reference groups [32, 33]. Having a common metric allows inter-marker analysis and analysis for trends across different studies conducted with different protocols. Utilizing % increase from disease-free reference levels has been reported by Murphy et al. [34], wherein they detected 41.8% increase in sICAM-1 levels in ACS patients compared to healthy controls ($P<0.01$) [34]

As shown in Table 3, the levels of VCAM-1 and ICAM-1 markers are slightly elevated compared to disease-free reference groups in subclinical atherosclerosis represented by subclinical carotid artery atherosclerosis (subCAA) and subclinical coronary atherosclerosis (subCAD) [33]. Patients with SA, UA, and AMI display higher levels [32]. This elevation provides a rationale for the use of EC activation markers in the management of subclinical CAD. Since EC activation underlies inflammation, and since inflammation underlies plaque progression and destabilization, the detection of marked increases in EC activation in patients with subCAD that approach levels detected in patients with SA and/or ACS denotes likely increasing inflammation-mediated plaque progression. This hypothesis needs to be tested, and if proven, should prompt further clinical investigation, if not intervention.

It should be noted however, that not all studies have shown a correlation between EC activation markers and subclinical disease. Observations by Hulthe et al. [35] in 391 healthy men detected association of sICAM-1 with subclinical carotid and femoral artery atherosclerosis, but not VCAM-1, or E-selectin. Furthermore, EC activation markers cannot distinguish different sites of subclinical atherosclerosis, carotid vs coronary artery atherosclerosis [33], as well as carotid vs femoral artery atherosclerosis [35].

Upon graphing the % increase values for VCAM-1, ICAM-1 and E-selectin obtained from data reported in Hwang et al. [33] and Guray et al. [32] (Table 3, Fig. 1), a larger delta-increase is detected from the sum of markers rather than when individually analyzed, thus suggesting that considering the sum of two or more EC activation markers could be more robust in distinguishing progression of subCAD to SA or ACS. This observation makes sense since collectively they all contribute to different steps in leukocyte recruitment with some functional redundancy (*a review*, [18]).

A mechanism-based perspective would state that examining the sum % increase in EC activation markers compared with disease-free reference levels (Fig. 1) might be useful, since EC activation markers have redundant and overlapping functions. For example, leukocyte rolling is decreased but not eliminated in ICAM-1 knockout mice, an observation that is likely explained by a compensatory increase in VCAM-1 expression [36]. Clinical studies would be required to validate this idea.

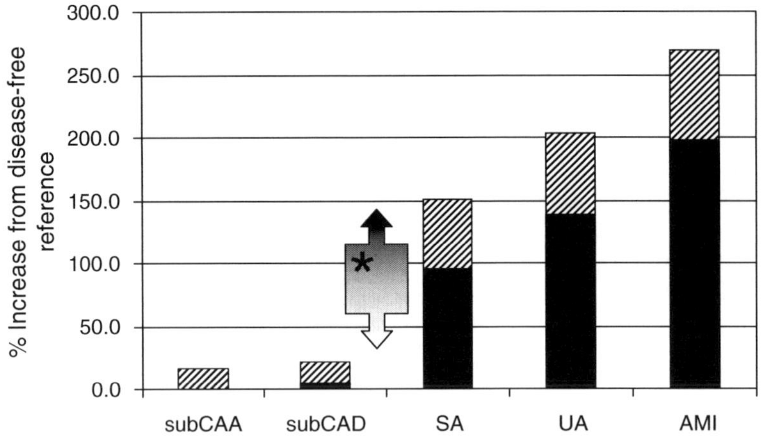

Fig. 1. Additive % increase from disease-free reference of ICAM-1 and VCAM-1 levels in different stages of CAD (data from Table 3, Hwang et al. [33] and Guray et al. [32]). Additive % increase from disease-free reference of ICAM-1 levels (hatched bar), and VCAM-1 levels (solid bar); subCAA, subclinical carotid artery atherosclerosis; subCAD, subclinical coronary atherosclerosis; SA, stable angina; UA, unstable angina; AMI, acute myocardial infarction; * within arrow-box: pictorially depicts gap between asymptomatic atherosclerosis (subCAA, subCAD) from symptomatic atherosclerosis (SA, UA, or AMI). Gap represents putative interval that could be monitored prospectively in patients with asymptomatic atherosclerosis, in order to identify patients approaching levels associated with symptomatic atherosclerosis (SA, UA, or AMI).

It should be noted however, that monitoring EC activation markers should not be done in isolation, but rather as part of a multi-marker panel that includes "cognate partners" that interact with EC activation effectors [37], such as ICAM-1 and cd11b+ monocytes [34]. The analysis of cognate partners could be more informative as elevation of both would imply a mechanism for a self-sustaining interactive process through reciprocal activation of said "cognate partners." Additionally, the analysis of EC activation markers should be done along with other plaque progression events such as constitutive activation of inflammatory cells, endothelial injury, and thrombogenicity, as this mechanism-based multi-marker panel could be expected to provide a more robust testing scheme for plaque progression in patients with subCAD [37]. This paradigm is illustrated in Fig. 2. This theoretical framework for integrating EC activation markers into the management of subCAD needs to be tested.

Monitoring Decrease of EC Activation Levels as Potential Treatment Benchmarks for Subclinical Atherosclerosis

We posit that, while the use of EC activation biomarkers for diagnosis of specific plaque-stages, especially imminent destabilization and/or rupture, is complicated and requires evaluation of partners and downstream effects [37], the value of EC activation as a treatment-benchmark in the management of subclinical CAD could be more attainable. Since inflammation is involved in all stages of plaque progression [1], detection of decreasing trends upon serial analysis of EC activation markers, rather than increase, could be a surrogate endpoint indicating attenuation or reversal of plaque progression, in lieu of imaging plaque regression. Reports, albeit not universal, of elevated EC activation distinguishing SA from control, or AMI from UA, SA and healthy controls (Tables 2 and 3), and reports on the predictive value of EC activation biomarkers in several studies for future cardiac events, albeit not all, after ACS (Table 2), support the concept for integrating EC activation biomarkers in monitoring treatment response. In support of this paradigm using EC activation marker levels as therapy-response functional-benchmarks, Marschang et al. [38] reported that statin therapy reduced P-selectin levels which correlated with the progression of CAD.

We note however, that as with monitoring plaque progression, monitoring treatment response and reversal or attenuation of plaque progression would also necessitate investigation of inflammation, endothelial integrity and thrombogenicity (Fig. 2). We note however, that since inflammation occurs earlier, monitoring EC activation markers could be more informative in subCAD than monitoring thrombogenicity in early plaque stages. Clinical studies are needed to test this paradigm.

DEDUCED MECHANISM-BASED POTENTIAL PARADIGMS FOR INTEGRATING EC ACTIVATION MARKERS

While EC activation cannot stand as sole biomarkers for plaque progression, or impending plaque destabilization, EC activation does stand as a logical, potential intervention target that awaits clinical study. Basis for this potential is inferred from experimental in-vitro, animal model, and plaque-based studies. Briefly, the following deductions can be made, which formulate rational hypotheses for consideration in clinical studies.

1. Since EC activation mediates inflammatory cell influx into plaques, and since monocytes, T-cells and neutrophils are implicated in plaque progression and destabilization [1], it is logical to hypothesize that treatments aimed at controlling increased EC activation could prevent progression of plaque.
2. Since reciprocal activation of ECs and inflammatory cells occurs in ACS, and thus, provides a mechanism for sustained plaque inflammation [34], normalization of EC activation could provide a break in the inflammation cascade, which likely underlies plaque progression and destabilization.

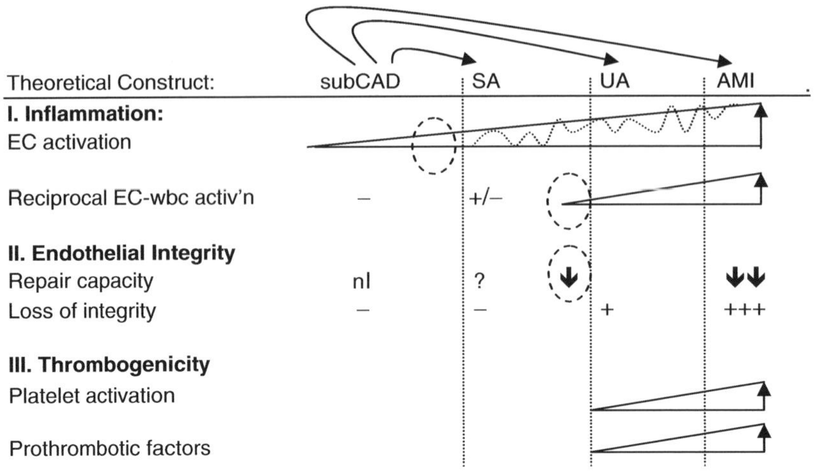

Fig. 2. Scheme depicting increasing trend of EC activation (Figure 1, Table 3) in the context of other key pathogenic pathways of plaque progression. This theoretical construct depicts the rationale for monitoring EC activation in patients with asymptomatic or subclinical atherosclerosis, and the rationale for monitoring multiple pathogenic pathways associated with plaque progression in clinical CAD. EC, endothelial cell; wbc, white blood cell; subCAD, subclinical coronary artery disease; SA, stable angina; UA, unstable angina; AMI, acute myocardial infarction. (–), no change; nl, normal levels; (ê), decrease; r, denotes reported increasing trend in levels; wavy dotted line, depicts putative temporal or diurnal variation in levels of EC activation markers which could confound analysis unless accounted for via serial analysis. Multiple curved arrows from subCAD depicts the notion that subCAD can progress clinically and present as SA or UA or AMI.

3. Since EC activation can contribute to thrombogenicity via increased endothelial expression of tissue factor (TF), a key initiator of coagulation cascade [39], and release of endothelial microparticles with TF [40], targeting the modulation of EC activation, could contribute to the attenuation of pro-thrombogenic changes, thus decreasing risk for plaque progression and atherothrombosis.
4. Since inflammation (EC activation and activated leukocyte recruitment) causes various forms of plaque disruption via contribution to EC apoptosis and matrix degradation [1], regulating increased EC activation levels to normal would allow EC repair capacity to "catch-up" and attenuate risk for plaque disruption.
5. Since EC activation and inflammation are implicated in endothelial apoptosis-mediated plaque denudation [41], regulating EC activation-mediated apoptosis could attenuate plaque endothelial erosion, and hence decrease risk for plaque progression.

Observations reporting that 50% of CHD cases do not have elevated LDL cholesterol levels, and 20% of major adverse events occur in patients with no accepted risk factors [42], albeit controversial, support the contention made by the analysis of inflammation in atherosclerosis [1] that addressing proinflammatory pathways of atherosclerosis pathogenesis is a compelling treatment goal. In plaque progression, stimuli for EC activation can arise from activated macrophages and T-cells within the plaque [1], from aging-associated pro-inflammation mechanisms (*a review*, [43]), from advanced glycation end products associated with aging and oxidative stress [44], and from senescent ECs per se [45].

EVIDENT LIMITATIONS AND CHALLENGES

Limitations

1. The lack of consensus in observations of EC activation markers in different clinical studies suggest a complexity that has not been satisfactorily dealt with. This complexity could be due to the lack of protocolized

measurements of EC activation markers, missing EC activation markers, and the need to simultaneously evaluate EC activation state along with its "partners," especially those with feedback loop connections to EC activation.
2. With the lack of consensus, currently, there is neither any definition of normal, nor established clinical thresholds for action.
3. Diurnal variation of soluble E- and P-selectin and sICAM-1 could confound analysis of predictive value of adhesion molecules.

As reported by Osmancik et al. [46], diurnal variation of sP-selectin in patients with CAD is observed. Evening levels represent the shed forms of the morning membrane-bound P-selectin [46]. In contrast, levels of E-selectin and sICAM-1 did not exhibit diurnal variation.

Challenges

1. Integration of EC activation markers into a monitoring scheme.

   While mechanism-based studies provide compelling evidence for the projected utility of EC activation markers when used in proper analytical context, effective integration of EC activation markers still needs to be delineated and tested clinically following frameworks put forward by Mosca [48], Keeney [47], Vasan [49]. The integration strategy will most likely require contemporaneous assessment of plaque-specific biology and status of reciprocal activation markers affecting endothelial integrity, inflammation and thrombogenicity. Currently, technological developments need to occur to address these.

2. Finding effective therapies that modulate endothelial activation or facilitate endothelial health.

   Effective therapy should control pathological increases in EC activation-mediated inflammation and subsequent inflammation-mediated plaque progression or destabilization, while allowing EPC-mediated endothelial repair. Finding effective therapies other than lipid-lowering is imperative, since lipid-lowering therapy, while effective, is not enough. Analysis by Marschang et al. [38] showed that treatment with statin therapies did not alter levels of several EC activation markers, such as E-selectin, VCAM-1, ICAM-1, PECAM-1, after 6 months, even if coronary calcium scores decreased. Interestingly, observed decrease in P-selectin levels correlated with the reduction in coronary calcium scores as measured by electron beam computed tomography ($r^2=0.393$, $P<0.0001$). Notably however, 43% (20/47 patients) in the treated group required intervention (stents, angioplasties) within the 6 month observation period despite the statin therapy [38]. This suggests that (1) statin therapy was not sufficient to alter plaque progression in 20/47 patients who required intervention, and that (2) persistence of increased levels of EC activation markers (VCAM-1, E-selectin, ICAM-1, PECAM-1) most likely represents ongoing plaque progression despite lipid lowering therapy. The reported decrease in hsCRP levels and P-selectin levels in the treated group suggests a decrease to some extent with statin therapy, but clearly not enough in at least 20/47 patients who progressed to a cardiac event requiring intervention, as reported by Marschang et al. [38].

MECHANISM-BASED PRIORITIES FOR FUTURE DIRECTIONS TO DETERMINE CLINICAL UTILITY OF EC ACTIVATION MARKERS

Three key issues need to be addressed for the determination of clinical utility of EC activation markers. Addressing these will also facilitate the subsequent integration of said EC activation markers in the management of subclinical CAD.

1. *Need for development of standardized protocols for measurement of EC activation markers, along with other biomarkers of CAD.* Currently, gender-specific and age-specific "normal levels" have not been delineated due to the lack of standardized protocols. Determination of "normal" is important to decipher physiological variation from pathological increases.

2. *Need to identify plaque stage-specific and site-specific discrimination of EC activation through molecular imaging or vascular bed-specific markers.* Molecular imaging of the plaque is a critical emerging field [50]. Molecular imaging targeting VCAM-1 has been successful in identifying inflammatory changes in atherosclerosis using magnetic resonance, non-invasive imaging of a VCAM-1 internalizing nano particle [51]. Dual-targeted micro particles of iron oxide increased capacity to detect the activated endothelium in aortic root plaques of ApoE-deficient mice via MRI-based molecular imaging of VCAM-1 and P-selectin, expressed on activated endothelium [52].
3. *Need for serial cross-talk analysis.* Since CAD is complex, identification of an informative panel for analysis of reciprocal activation affecting endothelial integrity, inflammation, thrombogenicity, needs to be done [37]. This analysis will be strongly aided by the development of functional-imaging modalities to analyze plaque biology.

"REPORT CARD" FOR INTEGRATING EC ACTIVATION MARKERS IN THE MANAGEMENT OF SUBCAD

Analysis of EC activation markers within the context of the "Ten Questions to Consider before Using Novel Risk Factors in Clinical Practice" [48] reveals that the current state of information illustrates some answers, but more importantly highlights questions remaining to be answered (Table 4).

While it is clear the much remains to be done, mechanism-based projections of the importance of inflammation in plaque progression and destabilization, and the role of EC activation in inflammation, provide compelling basis to advance new clinical paradigms that accomplish the monitoring of subCAD and subsequent prevention of plaque progression, as proposed [1]. This to-be-established paradigm follows the precedence set by the established paradigm of early cancer diagnosis and treatment.

SUMMARY

Key Points

- *An unequivocal mandate.* "The need to identify individuals at risk for concerted intervention before problems manifest" [1] underlies the mandate for advancing the management of subclinical atherosclerosis. This mandate parallels the cancer treatment mandate – microscopic cancers are monitored, aggressively eliminated when detected, and metastatic tumorigenesis prevented with cytotoxic therapy, which by themselves impose life-threatening health risks to patients.
- *Harnessing the information in monitoring changes in EC activation markers in real-time CAD management – beyond predicting risk 1–2 or even 10 years later.* Since EC activation is implicated in plaque progression and destabilization, monitoring of EC activation provides a mechanism-based approach which, coupled to emerging plaque-biology diagnostic tools, could provide real-time insight into plaque progression and destabilization.
- *Regulating EC activation state that effectively prevents cardiac events.* Targeting the pharmacological modulation of pathological EC activation in order to reestablish endothelial health and integrity provides a management benchmark that is mechanism-based. Clinical research needs to be done to validate this mechanism-based hypothesis and determine best diagnostic and treatment strategies.

Practical Tips

- Lessons from monitoring EC activation markers in ACS prognosis are *a priori* applicable concepts for the monitoring and management of subclinical atherosclerosis. Intuitively, as measures of inflammation, EC activation marker levels that approach levels described in ACS or SA provide mechanism-based rationale for further investigation.
- Analysis of sum % increase of different EC activation markers (VCAM-1, ICAM-1) could be more informative than analyzing markers individually, since it will be a common unit of measure for EC activation markers which

Table 4
2008 "Report Card" on Steps to Clinical Application of EC Activation Markers

Key Points Raised in "Ten Questions to Consider before using Novel Risk Factors in Clinical Practice" [48]	*2008 "report card" on EC activation markers*	*Future steps*
1. Convenient, standardized valid test	Not available	1. Establish standardized testing protocols • Consensus on kit used, timing of bleed, processing, storage, testing of sample
2. Population norms to guide interpretation results	Not established	2. Conduct coordinated, multicenter studies • Disease free "reference" values • Alternatively, patient-specific baseline values for serial analysis
3. Additional clinical significant prognosis above traditional risk factors	Emerging	3. Study after standardized test protocols agreed upon
4. Change in clinical management on the basis of EC activation marker levels	Not established	4. Study how to treat the disease and not just the risk factors (lipid lowering) • Mechanism-based rationale provides validation for said study
5. Risk factor specific for the condition targeted for intervention or prevention	Not possible with current EC activation markers	5. Since current EC activation markers are not specific for CAD-associated inflammation: • Study combinatorial analysis which could provide insight into CAD-specific inflammation • Explore CAD-specific EC activation markers • Study association of increased EC activation by other causes (e.g., diabetes) and increased CAD-risk
6. Direct and indirect risks of screening (false positive, false negative results)	Not known	6. Clinical studies testing whether: • Serial testing of EC activation marker coupled with other biomarker and imaging technologies could decrease false positive results in subCAD • Multi-marker additive analysis could eliminate false-negative results
7. Intervention which alters risk factor leads to clinical benefit	Not available	7. Clinical studies to determine predictive value of EC activation markers, and whether they comprise surrogate endpoints for various prevention or intervention strategies – other than a cardiac event
8. Clinical benefit for risk factors that are not causal	Not applicable	8. Not applicable
9. Traditional risk factors evaluated and appropriately treated	A given in subclinical CAD	9. Complex pathogenesis of CAD requires evaluation and treatment strategies of multiple risk factors when present
10. Overall benefit of new risk factor outweighs adverse consequences and costs with screening and follow-up	Unknown	10. Clinical studies to assess overall benefit • Evaluating markers of a key pathway for plaque progression (i.e., EC-mediated inflammation) allows for monitoring the disease, and not just 10 year risk for coronary heart disease as would be accomplished with the Framingham risk score

have different disease-free reference levels. This could better elicit trends in EC activation marker levels. Owing to the complexity of CAD, a one-marker "gold standard" is unlikely.

- At a minimum, EC activation should be analyzed in the context of endothelial repair/injury mismatch, reciprocal endothelial-leukocyte-platelet activation, and plaque biology.

Potential Pitfalls

- Since EC activation is required in normal physiological response to common triggers (e.g., wounds, infections, remodeling), long-term inhibition of increased EC activation in CAD will not be physiological. Therapy directed at limiting EC activation "spikes" would have to permit physiological responses, while avoiding pathological responses that contribute to atherosclerosis. Achieving this goal is a more difficult treatment paradigm compared to simple suppression of EC activation.
- Current analysis modalities of systemic EC activation markers is limited by non-information on the site of EC activation – plaque surface vs plaque microvessels, plaque *vs* systemic vascular beds. This limitation requires integration with other emerging diagnostic tools such as plaque molecular imaging, and/or a vascular bed-specific marker.

REFERENCES

1. Libby P. Inflammation in atherosclerosis. Nature 2002;420:868–874.
2. ATP III Final Report PDF. Third report of the National Cholesterol Education Program (NCEP) expert panel on detection, evaluation, and treatment of high blood cholesterol in adults (Adult Treatment Panel III) final report. Circulation 2002;106:3143–3421.
3. Cines DB, Pollak ES, Buck CA, et al. Endothelial cells in physiology and in the pathophysiology of vascular disorders. Blood 1998;91:3527–2561.
4. Zimmerman GA, Albertine KH, Carveth HJ, et al. Endothelial activation in ARDS. Chest 1999;116:18S–24S.
5. Luscinskas FW, Gimbrone MA. Endothelial-dependent mechanisms in chronic inflammatory leukocyte recruitment. Annu Rev Med 1996;47:413–421.
6. Pober JS, Cotran RS. The role of endothelial cells in inflammation. Transplantation 1990;50:537–544.
7. Ward PA, Hunninghake GW. Lung inflammation and fibrosis. Am J Respir Crit Care Med 1998;157:S123–S129.
8. Ross R. Atherosclerosis – an inflammatory disease. N Engl J Med 1999;340:115–126.
9. Spagnoli LG, Bonanno E, Sangiorgi G, et al. Role of inflammation in atherosclerosis. J Nucl Med 2007;48:1800–1815.
10. Bevilacqua MP. Endothelial-leukocyte adhesion molecules. Annu Rev Immunol 1993;11:767–804.
11. Springer TA. Traffic signals for lymphocyte recirculation and leukocyte emigration: the multistep paradigm. Cell 1993;76:301–314.
12. Labow MA, Norton CR, Rumberger JM, et al. Characterization of E-selectin-deficient mice: demonstration of overlapping function of the endothelial selectins. Immunity 1994;1:709–720.
13. Poston RN, Haskard DO, Coucher JR, et al. Expression of intercellular adhesion molecule-1 in atherosclerotic plaques. Am J Pathol 1992;140:665–673.
14. Wood KM, Cadogan MD, Ramshaw AL, et al. The distribution of adhesion molecules in human atherosclerosis. Histopathology 1993;22:437–444.
15. Collins RG, Velji R, Guevara NV, et al. P-selectin or intercellular adhesion molecule (ICAM-1) deficiency substantially protects against atherosclerosis in apoE deficient mice. J Exp Med 2000;191:189–194.
16. Johnson RC, Chapman SM, Dong ZM, et al. Absence of P-selectin delays fatty streak formation in mice. J Clin Invest 1997;99:1037–1043.
17. Gurtner GC, Davis V, Li H, et al. Targeted disruption of the murine VCAM1 gene: essential role of VCAM-1 in chorioallantoic fusion and placentation. Genes Dev 1994;9:1–14.
18. Galkina E, Ley K. Vascular adhesion molecules in atherosclerosis. Arterioscler Thromb Vasc Biol 2007;27:2292–2301.
19. Hartwell DW, Wagner DD. New discoveries with mice mutant in endothelial and platelet selectins. Thromb Haemost 1999;82:850–857.
20. Shah PK. Molecular mechanisms of plaque instability. Curr Opin Lipidol 2007;18:492–499.
21. Oh IY, Yoon CH, Hur J, et al. Involvement of E-selectin in recruitment of endothelial progenitor cells and angiogenesis in ischemic muscle. Blood 2007;110:3891–3899.
22. Yoon CH, Hur J, Oh IY, et al. Intercellular adhesion molecule-1 is upregulated in ischemic muscle, which mediates trafficking of endothelial progenitor cells. Arterioscler Thromb Vasc Biol 2006;26:1066–1072.

23. Duan H, Cheng L, Sun X, et al. LFA-1 and VLA-4 involved in human high proliferative potential-endothelial progenitor cells homing to ischemic tissue. Thromb Haemost 2006;96:807–815.
24. Silverman MD, Haas CS, Rad AM, et al. The role of vascular cell adhesion molecule 1/very late activation antigen 4 in endothelial progenitor cell recruitment to rheumatoid arthritis synovium. Arthritis Rheum 2007;56:1817–1826.
25. Leeuwenberg JF, Smeets EF, Neefjes JJ, et al. E-selectin and intercellular adhesion molecule-1 are released by activated human endothelial cells in vitro. Immunology 1992;77:543–549.
26. Gearing AJ, Newman W. Circulating adhesion molecules in disease. Immunol Today 1993;14:506–512.
27. Blankenberg S, Rupprecht HJ, Bickel C, et al. for the AtheroGene Investigators. Circulating cell adhesion molecules and death in patients with coronary artery disease. Circulation 2001;104:1336–1342.
28. Mulvihill NT, Foley JB, Murphy RT, et al. Risk stratification in unstable angina and non-Q wave myocardial infarction using soluble cell adhesion molecules. Heart 2001;85:623–627.
29. Ray KK, Morrow DA, Shui A, et al. Relation between soluble intercellular adhesion molecule-1, statin therapy, and long-term risk of clinical cardiovascular events inpatients with previous acute coronary syndrome (from PROVE IT-TIMI 22). Am J Cardiol 2006;98:861–865.
30. Hope SA, Meredith IT. Cellular adhesion molecules and cardiovascular disease. Part II. Their association with conventional and emerging risk factors, acute coronary events and cardiovascular risk prediction. Int Med J 2003;33:450–462.
31. Heeschen C, Dimmeler S, Hamm CW, et al. Pregnancy-associated plasma protein-A levels in patients with acute coronary syndromes. J Am Coll Cardiol 2005;45:229–237.
32. Guray U, Erbay AR, Guray Y, et al. Levels of soluble adhesion molecules in various clinical presentations of coronary atherosclerosis. Int J Cardiol 2004;96:235–240.
33. Hwang SJ, Ballantyne CM, Sharrett AR, et al. Circulating adhesion molecules VCAM-1, ICAM-1, and E-selectin in carotid atherosclerosis and incident coronary heart disease cases: the Atherosclerosis Risk in Communities (ARIC) study. Circulation 1997;96:4219–4225.
34. Murphy RT, Foley JB, Crean P, et al. Reciprocal activation of leukocyte-endothelial adhesion molecules in acute coronary syndromes. Int J Cardiol 2003;90:247–252.
35. Hulthe J, Wikstrand J, Mattsson-Hulten L, et al. Circulating ICAM-1 (intercellular cell-adhesion molecule 1) is associated with early stages of atherosclerosis development and with inflammatory cytokines in healthy 58-year-old men: the Atherosclerosis and Insulin Resistance (AIR) study. Clin Sci (Lond) 2002;103(2):123–129.
36. Sumagin R, Sarelius IH. A role for ICAM-1 in maintenance of leukocyte-endothelial cell rolling interactions in inflamed arterioles. Am J Physiol Heart Circ Physiol 2007;293:H2786–2798.
37. Herrera VLM. Endothelial biomarkers of vulnerable plaque progression. *In* Waksman R, Serruys PW, Schaar J (eds) The vulnerable plaque, 2nd edn. Informa UK Ltd., Colchester, UK, 2007.
38. Marschang P, Griedrich GJ, Ditlbacher H, et al. Reduction of soluble P-selectin by statins is inversely correlated with the progression of coronary artery disease. Int J Cardiol 2006;6:183–190.
39. Moons AH, Levi M, Peters RJ. Tissue factor and coronary artery disease. Cardiovasc Res 2002;53:313–325.
40. Morel O, Toti F, Hugel B, et al. Procoagulant microparticles: disrupting the vascular homeostasis equation. Arterioscler Thromb Vasc Biol 2006;26:2594–2604.
41. Valgimigli M, Merli E, Malagutti P, et al. Endothelial dysfunction in acute and chronic coronary syndromes: evidence for a pathogenetic role of oxidative stress. Arch Biochem Biophys 2003;420:255–261.
42. Tsimikas S, Willerson JT, Ridker PM. C-reactive protein and other emerging blood biomarkers to optimize risk stratification of vulnerable patients. J Am Coll Cardiol 2006;47:C19–C31.
43. Sarkar D, Fisher PB. Molecular mechanisms of aging-associated inflammation. Cancer Lett 2006;236:13–23.
44. Yan SF, D'Agati V, Schmidt AM, et al. Receptor for Advanced Glycation Endproducts (RAGE): a formidable force in the pathogenesis of the cardiovascular complications of diabetes & aging. Curr Mol Med 2007;7:699–710.
45. Kletsas D, Pratsinis H, Mariatos G, et al. The proinflammatory phenotype of senescent cells: the p53-mediated ICAM-1 expression. Ann NY Acad Sci 2004;1019:330–332.
46. Osmancik P, Kvasnicka J, Widimsky P, et al. Diurnal variation of soluble E- and P-selectin, and intercellular adhesion molecule-1 inpatients with and without coronary artery disease. Cardiology 2004;102:194–199.
47. Keeney JF Jr. Circulating biomarkers in acute coronary syndromes. Something different or more of the same? Circulation 2005;112:778–780.
48. Mosca L. Editorial. N Engl J Med. 2002;347:1615–1617.
49. Vasan R. Biomarkers of cardiovascular disease. Molecular basis and practical considerations. Circulation 2006;113:2335–2362.
50. Choudhury RP, Fuster V, Fayad ZA. Molecular, cellular and functional imaging of atherothrombosis. Nat Rev Drug Discov 2005;18–30.
51. Nahrendorf M, Jaffer FA, Kelly KA, et al. Noninvasive vascular cell adhesion molecule-1 imaging identifies inflammatory activation of cells in atherosclerosis. Circulation 2006;114:1504–1511.
52. McAteer MA, Schneider JE, Ali ZA, et al. Magnetic resonance imaging of endothelial adhesion molecules in mouse atherosclerosis using dual-targeted microparticles of iron oxide. Arterioscler Thromb Vasc Biol 2008;28:77–83.
53. Soeki T, Tamura Y, Shinohara H, et al. Increased soluble platelet/endothelial cell adhesion molecule-1 in the early stages of acute coronary syndromes. Int J Cardiol 2003;90:261–268.

54. Turhan H, Erbay AR, Yasar AS, et al. Plasma soluble adhesion molecules; intercellular adhesion molecule-1, vascular cell adhesion molecule-1 and E-selectin levels in patients with isolated coronary artery ectasia. Coron Artery Dis 2005;16:45–50.
55. Parker C, Vita JA, Freedman JE. Soluble adhesion molecules and unstable coronary artery disease. Atherosclerosis 2001;156: 417–424.
56. Atalar E, Aytemir K, Haznedaroglu I, et al. Increased plasma levels of soluble selectins in patients with unstable angina. Int J Cardiol 2001;78:69–73.
57. Draz N, Hamdy MS, Gomaa Y, et al. Soluble P-selectin is a marker of plaque destabilization in unstable angina. Egyp J Immuno 2003;10:83–87.
58. Peter K, Nawroth P, Conradt C, et al. Circulating vascular cell adhesion molecule-1 correlates with the extent of human atherosclerosis in contrast to circulating intercellular adhesion molecule-1, E-selectin, P-selectin, and thrombomodulin. Arterioscler Thromb Vasc Biol 1997;17:505–512.

II

Non Invasive, Non Imaging, Assessment of Asymptomatic Atherosclerotic Cardiovascular Disease

14 Exercise Stress Testing in Asymptomatic Individuals and Its Relation to Subclinical Atherosclerotic Cardiovascular Disease

Kevin S. Heffernan

CONTENTS

ABSTRACT

Exercise testing is one of the most widely used modalities for the initial evaluation of coronary artery disease (CAD) and its severity. Although primarily used in the evaluation of myocardial ischemia, the exercise test provides additional clinical information that has become only recently appreciated. The initial part of this chapter reviews the diagnostic and prognostic power of the traditional exercise test in asymptomatic patients. The latter part of the chapter examines nontraditional (i.e., nonelectrogardiographic) variables as a means of refining the prognostic capabilities of the exercise test. Particular emphasis is placed on the capability of exercise test variables to provide novel insight into underlying atherosclerotic cardiovascular disease burden in asymptomatic patients.

Key words: Exercise test; ST-segment; Chronotropic incompetence; Heart rate recovery

THE TRADITIONAL EXERCISE TEST: RELIANCE ON ST-SEGMENT

The exercise test remains a safe diagnostic tool with an event rate of approximately 0.8–1.2 per 10,000 tests [1, 2]. The use of exercise testing for screening purposes in asymptomatic patients has been a topic of debate [3, 4]. Although several studies have successfully used the exercise test to refine risk

From: *Asymptomatic Atherosclerosis: Pathophysiology, Detection and Treatment*
Edited by: M. Naghavi (ed.), DOI 10.1007/978-1-60327-179-0_14

stratification and predict extent of coronary artery disease (CAD) in intermediate-risk asymptomatic patients [5–8], the American Heart Association, American College of Cardiology, and the US Preventive Services Task Force do not currently recommend the exercise test as a screening tool [4, 9, 10]. This is due, in large part, to the pervasive findings of poor diagnostic and prognostic capability of the traditional exercise test in low-risk populations.

The traditional exercise test relies on changes in ST-segment as a means of detecting obstructive coronary CAD. A positive or abnormal exercise test is traditionally defined as horizontal or downsloping ST-segment depression ≥ 0.1 mV for 80 ms [11]. This is related to a generalized subendocardial ischemia from coronary obstruction and is proportional to myocardial oxygen demand [11]. Sensitivity of a test refers to percentage of times a test gives a positive result in patients with CAD. Specificity is the percentage of times a test gives a negative result in those without CAD. The traditional exercise test has a sensitivity and specificity for obstructive CAD of 68% (range 23–100%) and 77% (range 17–100%), respectively [11, 12]. These values appear to be lower in women compared with men [13]. Thus, exercise testing that relies on ST-segment for diagnosis does not detect all patients with obstructive CAD, and as many as 25% of patients with a positive exercise test may not have obstructive CAD on coronary angiography. This is problematic because false positive testing may lead to further invasive and costly testing and concomitantly increased physical/psychological risk to the patient.

Most arguments against exercise testing for screening purposes are founded on Bayes theorem, which states that the probability of a patient having disease is dependent on the disease probability before the test and on the probability that the test will provide a true positive [4, 14]. Given the low specificity and sensitivity of the exercise test for detecting asymptomatic patients with CAD, the predictive value (i.e., how accurately the test result identifies the presence or absence of CAD in patients) will be low in those with low risk.

It has been suggested that several factors hamper the diagnostic value of ST-segment changes in asymptomatic patients including referral bias, verification bias, failure of ST-segment changes to reflect workload and degree of myocardial ischemia, and use of coronary angiography as the gold standard [4]. Indeed, coronary angiography performed in the resting state does not provide a complete picture of vascular function in response to stress as it fails to provide insight into atherosclerotic cardiovascular disease (ACVD) burden, endothelial dysfunction, and autonomic dysfunction (i.e., stress-induced vasoconstriction causing ischemia in the absence of obstructive CAD) [14].

Methods have been devised in an attempt to improve the diagnostic capabilities of ST-segment changes. The duke treadmill score (DTS) is considered by many to be one of the most significant advances in exercise testing in recent years [11]. The DTS has been shown to improve risk stratification in symptomatic patients [15], and almost all current major guidelines advocate inclusion of this score when exercise testing [10]. The DTS is calculated as (exercise time − (5 × maximum ST-segment depression in mm) − (4 × angina index)), where exercise time is measured in minutes during the Bruce protocol and angina index as 0 = none, 1 = nonlimiting, and 2 = exercise-limiting. Although the DTS is an independent predictor of overall mortality and cardiac mortality in asymptomatic women, it does not appear to be a better predictor than exercise capacity alone and does not provide additional prognostic information [16]. The prognostic capability of the DTS in asymptomatic men is not known.

Heart rate (HR) adjustment of ST-segment may also substantially improve the sensitivity and specificity of exercise testing [17–19]. Increases in HR with exercise are linearly related to changes in myocardial oxygen demand [14]. ST-segment depression during exercise testing is dependent not only on coronary artery obstruction but also on excess myocardial oxygen demand. Thus, HR adjustment of ST-segment depression is physiologically logical [14]. Two methods have been devised to correct ST-segment for HR. The ST/HR slope is a linear regression-based method calculated from the maximal rate of change of ST-segment depression relative to HR during the period of active ischemia that accompanies end-exercise. HR is used as the independent variable while ST-segment depression as the dependent variable and the greatest slope with a statistically significant correlation coefficient amongst all leads is taken as the final test value. The ST/HR index represents the average change in ST-segment depression relative to HR change over the entire course of exercise (maximum ST-segment depression/HRpeak – HRrest). The ST/HR index has been shown to improve risk stratification by more than threefold in low-risk asymptomatic men and women and by fivefold in high-risk asymptomatic men. In the multiple risk factor intervention trial, an ST/HR index > 1.6 mV/bpm identified a group of men in whom therapy aimed at reducing coronary heart disease (CHD) risk factors decreased the 7-year relative risk of CHD death by 61% [20]. Authors from this study suggested that exercise ECG using HR-adjusted indexes of ST-segment depression may be used in the screening of asymptomatic subjects at increased risk of CHD for more accurate identification of those who will benefit most from risk factor-reduction programs [20].

The association between coronary and carotid atherosclerosis is well established. Thus, it is not surprising that a positive exercise test is also associated with ACVD. A significant independent association between carotid intima-media thickness (IMT) and ischemic ST-segment depression has been reported in asymptomatic older adults, and the increase in IMT appears to increase in parallel with the increase in risk of myocardial ischemia [21]. The likelihood of CAD increases 2.39-fold for each 0.1 mm increase in IMT [21]. Moreover, IMT is an independent predictor for CAD, increasing the risk by almost twofold for each 0.1 mm increase in IMT [21]. Similarly, ST/HR slope is also associated with carotid hypertrophy (measured as carotid cross-sectional area index and carotid wall thickness) in asymptomatic patients independently of traditional cardiac risk factors [22]. Hence, evidence exists to suggest that asymptomatic patients with a positive exercise test have a greater prevalence and severity of ACVD.

NONELECTROCARDIOGRAPHIC MEASURES OBTAINED FROM THE EXERCISE TEST

Given findings that the ST-segment is a poor prognostic and diagnostic marker in asymptomatic patients and the presence or absence of symptoms is a relatively poor predictor of risk, it has been proposed that measures other than those associated with myocardial ischemia be examined in asymptomatic patients [4, 14]. Even in the absence of angina or ST-segment depression, the exercise test can provide useful information about cardiovascular risk and ACVD burden.

Blood Pressure Response to Exercise Testing and Recovery

During an incremental exercise test, systolic blood pressure (SBP) rises with exercise intensity as a result of increasing cardiac output, whereas diastolic blood pressure (DBP) remains relatively stable. The blood pressure response to exercise testing provides important prognostic information. Exercise-induced hypotension (i.e., a fall in SBP below resting levels) or an attenuated rise in SBP (i.e., an increase in SBP < 10 mmHg) has been associated with poor prognosis [23]. Exertional hypotension has been attributed to left ventricular dysfunction, ischemia, papillary muscle dysfunction, and mitral regurgitation [11]. Although associated with severe CAD and mortality in symptomatic patients [23], exercise-induced hypotension is not predictive of mortality risk in individuals with a normal ST-segment response to exercise testing [11]. SBP recovery following exercise testing (measured as peak SBP during exercise/SBP at 3 min of recovery) has also been shown to be related to severity of CAD and to independently predict mortality [24, 25]. However, slow SBP recovery is not a predictor of mortality in lower-risk asymptomatic patients [26].

An exaggerated rise in SBP during exercise, often defined as an absolute pressure>210 mmHg in men and >190 mmHg in women, is a predictor of future sustained hypertension, CV events, and mortality [27–30], although this is not a universal finding [31]. While the mechanisms for an exaggerated SBP response to exercise are unknown, several have been purported including autonomic dysfunction secondary to carotid atherosclerosis, inflammation, reduced nitric oxide bioavailability, and concomitant endothelial dysfunction. An exaggerated SBP response has been shown to be associated with numerous correlates of atherosclerotic disease burden such as left ventricular hypertrophy, stroke, albumineria, white blood cell count, heightened sympathetic nervous activity, insulin resistance, and hypercholesterolemia [32, 33].

An exaggerated SBP response to exercise testing may provide novel insight into subclinical atherosclerotic disease burden. In healthy normotensive and prehypertensive men and women with no ECG abnormalities during exercise and no history of CAD, those with an exaggerated SBP response to exercise testing demonstrate impaired endothelial function as measured by flow-mediated dilation of the brachial artery [34–36]. Aortic distensibility is also reduced in patients with an exaggerated SBP response to exercise testing [37]. Jae et al. examined the exercise BP response to exercise testing as it relates to carotid atherosclerosis [38]. Patients used in this investigation consisted of apparently men undergoing an exercise stress test for screening purposes. Carotid atherosclerosis was defined as stenosis greater than 25% or carotid IMT greater than 1.2 mm. Results revealed that those individuals with an exaggerated SBP response were almost three times more likely to have carotid atherosclerosis compared with individuals with a normal SBP response (Fig. 1). This association remained after adjusting for potential confounders such as lipid profile, body mass index, glucose, hemoglobin A1c, fibrinogen, and peak oxygen uptake.

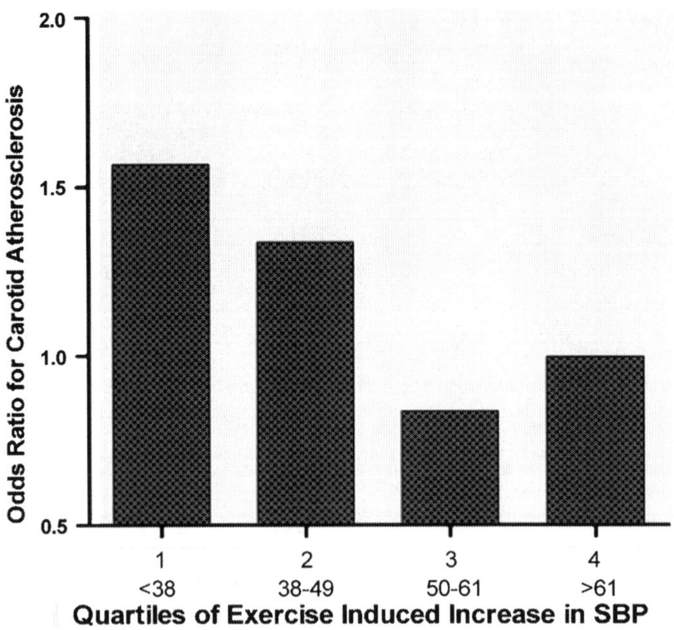

Fig. 1. Odds ratio for carotid atherosclerosis according to exercise-induced systolic blood pressure (*SBP*) increases in quartiles after adjusting for age, smoking, body mass index, total cholesterol, low-density lipoprotein cholesterol, high-density lipoprotein cholesterol, triglycerides, resting systolic blood pressure/diastolic blood pressure, resting heart rate, glucose, hemoglobin A1c, fibrinogen, white blood cell count, maximal heart rate, and peak oxygen uptake.

Chronotropic Response to Exercise Testing and Recovery

With increasing exercise intensity, HR increases due to a combination of vagal withdrawal followed by sympathoexcitation. During exercise recovery, HR decreases because of parasympathetic reactivation and sympathetic withdrawal. The clinical utility of the rapid initial increase in HR is currently questionable. While one study notes that a rapid increase in HR predicts better survival in a clinical population [39], another study notes the opposite [40]. At the present time, HR measured during the first minute of exercise testing should not be used for clinical decision making [39].

Chronotropic incompetence (CI) may be defined as an attenuated HR response to exercise relative to metabolic demand. The most commonly reported methods of defining CI are as follows:

1. Failure to achieve 85% of age-predicted maximal HR (220-age), or
2. Failure to achieve 80% of HR reserve (maximal exercise HR – resting HR)/(age-predicted maximal HR-resting HR) × 100%, or
3. Low chronotropic response index (i.e., value < 0.8) that requires either an estimate or the direct measurement of functional capacity (% of HR reserve achieved/% metabolic reserve achieved)

CI has been attributed to autonomic dysfunction and is an independent predictor of CAD events and mortality in healthy patients [41, 42]. In 1975, Ellestad and Wan examined the HR response to exercise testing in 2,700 patients and discovered that patients with CI devoid of ST-segment alterations had a four times greater incidence of CAD than those without CI during a 4-year follow-up [43]. Since this initial discovery, numerous studies in large cohorts such as the Framingham Heart Study have confirmed the notion that CI is a strong and independent predictor of death, even after accounting for ST-segment changes, physical activity, and traditional cardiovascular risk factors (i.e., Framingham risk score) in asymptomatic patients [6, 44].

CI may also provide novel insight into subclinical atherosclerotic disease burden. In symptomatic patients referred for exercise testing due to chest pain, CI has been shown to be associated with impaired endothelial function as assessed by brachial artery flow-mediated dilation [45]. These patients also have elevated vascular inflammatory biomarkers associated with atherosclerotic disease burden such as C-reactive protein, monocyte chemoattractant protein-1, and N-terminal probrain natriuretic peptide [45]. The relationship between CI and carotid atherosclerosis has also been examined in apparently healthy asymptomatic patients undergoing an exercise stress test for screening purposes [46]. Individuals with CI were almost two times more likely to have carotid atherosclerosis, defined as stenosis greater than 25% or carotid IMT greater than 1.2 mm, compared with individuals with a normal HR response (Fig. 2). This finding remained after adjusting for potential confounders such as age, SBP, lipid profile, body mass index, glucose, hemoglobin A1c, and peak oxygen uptake.

Heart rate recovery (HRR) after exercise testing results from concerted sympathetic withdrawal and vagal reactivation. HRR is calculated as maximal HR during the exercise test – HR at 1 min of recovery or at 2 min of recovery. Slow HRR may be defined as a recovery value:

1. <12 bpm at 1-min recovery if the recovery protocol consists of a cool-down period
2. <18 bpm at 1-min recovery if the recovery period consists of supine rest
3. <22 bpm at 2-min recovery if the recovery period consists of seated rest
4. <42 bpm at 2 min if submaximal exercise testing is employed

Slow HRR is an independent predictor of mortality and has prognostic value in asymptomatic men and women even after accounting for Framingham and European Risk Scores [8, 47–50]. A recent observational study also noted that in patients with imaging evidence of myocardial ischemia, an abnormal HRR was associated with a trend toward attenuating the survival improvement associated

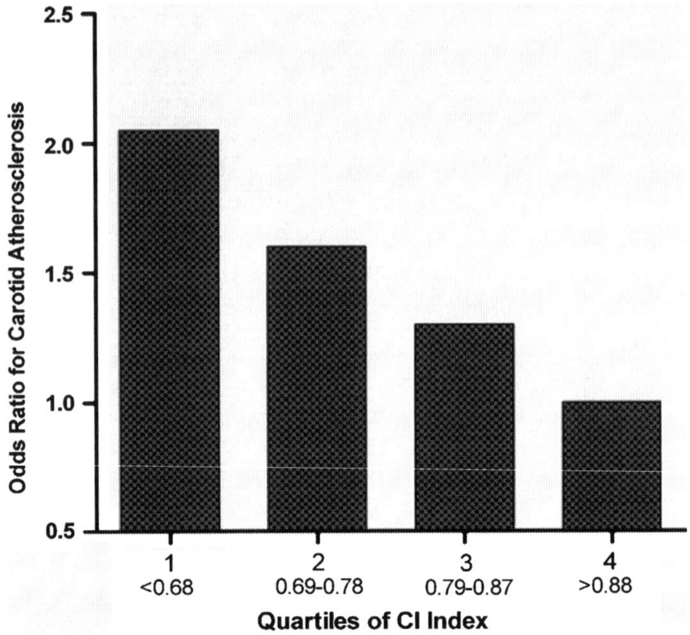

Fig. 2. Unadjusted odds ratio for carotid atherosclerosis by quartiles of chronotropic incompetence (CI) index.

with early revascularization [51]. Thus, HRR has potential for identification of patients who might benefit from intervention and advanced treatment.

Slow HRR in apparently healthy men is related to several biomarkers of atherosclerotic disease burden such as C-reactive protein, white blood cell count, plasminogen activator inhibitor 1, tissue plasminogen activator, and fibrinogen [52, 53]. In symptomatic patients referred for exercise testing due to chest pain, slow HRR has been shown to be associated with impaired endothelial function as assessed by brachial artery flow-mediated dilation [54]. In apparently healthy young men, slow HRR is also associated with aortic stiffness as assessed by pulse wave velocity [55] and impaired nitroglycerin-mediated dilation of the brachial artery [56], a measure of endothelial-independent vascular dysfunction. However, slow HRR in young adulthood does not appear to be predictive of future coronary artery calcification [57]. A relationship between HRR and carotid atherosclerosis has also been noted. In apparently healthy asymptomatic men undergoing an exercise stress test for screening purposes, those with slow HRR were almost four times more likely to have carotid atherosclerosis, defined as stenosis greater than 25% or carotid IMT greater than 1.2 mm, compared with individuals with a normal HR response (Fig. 3) [58]. This finding remained after adjusting for potential confounders such as age, SBP, lipid profile, body mass index, glucose, fibrinogen, and peak oxygen uptake.

Exercise Capacity

Measures of exercise capacity, or the amount of work completed before exhaustion, reflect the functional limits of the cardiovascular system during the exercise test. The most accurate assessment of exercise capacity is by direct measurement of peak oxygen uptake with metabolic/ventilatory gas analysis. Oxygen uptake is often expressed in multiples of metabolic equivalents (METs). One MET is equivalent to approximately 3.5 mL oxygen/kg bodyweight/minute and reflects the basal oxygen requirement to maintain life in the resting state. Given practicality of use, metabolic gas analysis may not be feasible in select clinical settings. Exercise capacity may be estimated from exercise test dura-

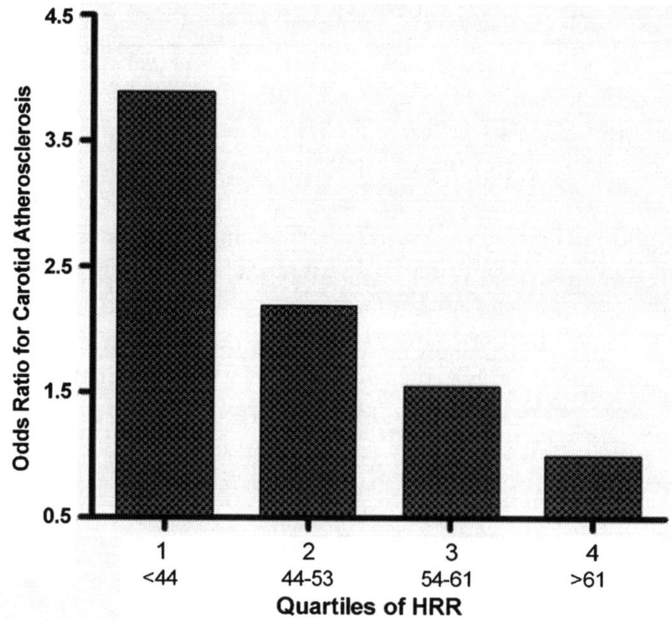

Fig. 3. Unadjusted odds ratio for carotid atherosclerosis by quartiles of heart rate recovery (*HRR*).

tion using validated equations and nomograms. Estimates of exercise capacity have been found to provide reasonably accurate estimates of directly measured capacity [59, 60].

Numerous population studies have now examined the relationship between exercise capacity and cardiovascular risk [61, 62]. Results unequivocally demonstrate that impaired exercise capacity is predictive of increased risk/mortality even after controlling for standard risk factors (Framingham and European Risk Scores) [5, 6, 8, 47, 60, 63]. In a recent study, it was shown that the combination of low exercise capacity and high systematic coronary risk evaluation (SCORE) values was associated with more than fivefold increased risk for CVD death in asymptomatic men after adjusting for potential confounders such as CRP, blood lipids, family history of CAD, and exercise-induced ST-segment change [64]. When adjusting for age and other risk factors, each MET increase in exercise capacity results in a 10–25% improvement in survival [11]. It has been suggested that functional capacity is the most important variable obtained from a standard exercise test [4, 14]; one issue that has yet to be resolved is an accurate definition of "abnormal" functional capacity. While some studies advocate clear cut-points (<7 METs in men and <5 METs in women), others have defined abnormal as simply the lowest quartile within a specific cohort.

Low exercise capacity/low peak oxygen uptake is associated with a greater inflammatory state (i.e., elevated C-reactive protein and white blood cell count) and greater levels of fibrinogen [65–67]. Asymptomatic men with low exercise capacity (<10 METS) also have greater coronary artery calcium (CAC) than men with high exercise capacity [68]. LaMonte et al. found that exercise capacity adds prognostic information to CAC scores in asymptomatic men [68]. Exercise tolerance > 10 METs is associated with lower risk for CAD events, independent of traditional risk factors, abnormal exercise ECG responses, and CAC scores [68]. Interestingly, the cardioprotective effects of having exercise tolerance > 10 METs carried over to those men with significant subclinical ACVD (CAC scores >400) [68]. Numerous studies acknowledge that high peak oxygen uptake (a measure of cardiorespiratory fitness) is associated with reduced arterial stiffness, reduced wave reflection, and greater flow-mediated dilation of the brachial artery (see Chap. 54). Several studies also note an inverse association between peak oxygen uptake and carotid IMT [69–71].

Combining Exercise Test Measures to Improve Prognosis: The Quest for Global Risk Scores

Several studies have begun combining exercise test variables in an attempt to improve prognostic capability (Table 1). Myers et al. examined whether cardiovascular risk may be more powerfully predicted when both CI and HRR are considered together [72]. Patients having a normal chronotropic response to exercise and recovery had a mortality rate of only 0.25–0.5% [72]. Having both abnormal CI and HRR increased the risk of CV mortality more than fourfold [72].

Mora et al. found that asymptomatic men that have both low HRR and low exercise capacity have a relative risk of CV death 3.5 times higher than those with high HRR and high exercise capacity (20-year follow-up) (Fig. 4) [5]. Women that have both low HRR and low exercise capacity have a relative risk of CV death 8.5 times higher than those with high HRR and high exercise capacity (20-year follow-up) (Fig. 5) [5]. The most interesting finding of this study was that in low-intermediate risk men and women, half of the women and just under half of the men with Framingham Risk Score 10–19% and half of the women with FRS 6–9% would be reclassified as high risk on the

Table 1
Relation of exercise test variables to markers of subclinical atherosclerotic disease in asymptomatic patients

Exercise test variable	*Definition/description*	*Relation to subclinical atherosclerotic disease*
ST-segment	Horizontal or down-sloping ST-segment depression ^{3}0.1 mV for 80 ms	Risk of CAD (defined by exercise-induced ischemia) ↑ 2.39-fold for each 0.1 mm ↑ in IMT
HR/ST slope	HR plotted against ST-segment depression via linear regression; the greatest statistically significant slope between all leads taken as final value	ST/HR slope > 3.47 μV/bpm associated with 50% greater prevalence of carotid plaque
Exaggerated SBP	SBP > 210 mmHg in men and >190 mmHg in women	Exaggerated SBP in men associated with greater risk of carotid atherosclerosis, LV hypertrophy, reduced aortic distensibility and reduced brachial FMD
Chronotropic incompetence	<85% of age-predicted HR_{max} or <80% of $HR_{reserve}$ or Low chronotropic response index; % of HR reserve achieved/% metabolic reserve achieved	CI associated with greater prevalence of carotid atherosclerosis, reduced brachial FMD and higher levels of C-reactive protein, monocyte chemoattractant protein-1, and N-terminal probrain natriuretic peptide
Heart rate recovery	$HR_{peak} - HR_{@1\text{-min recovery}}$ or $HR_{peak} - HR_{@2\text{-min recovery}}$	Slow HRR associated with greater prevalence of carotid atherosclerosis, higher arterial stiffness and reduced brachial FMD
Exercise capacity	Direct measurement via metabolic gas exchange analysis Estimated in men: 14.7–0.11 × Age Estimated in women: 14.7–0.13 × Age	Inverse association between peak oxygen uptake and carotid atherosclerosis

HR heart rate, *SBP* systolic blood pressure, *IMT* intima-media thickness, *FMD* flow-mediated dilation

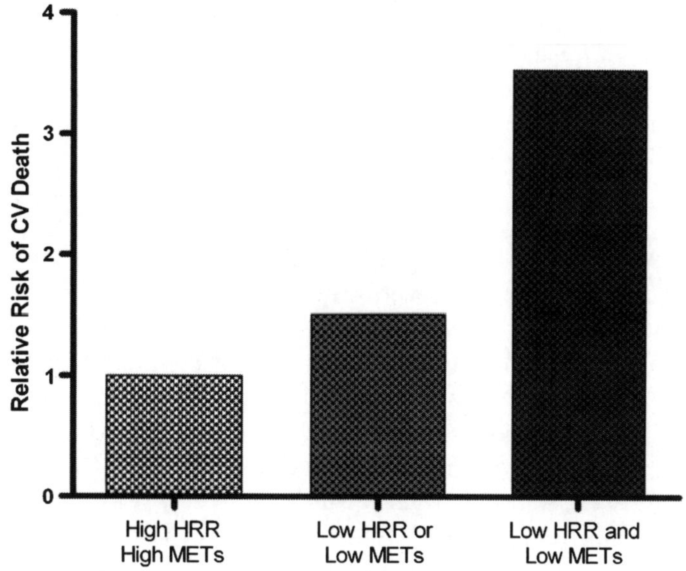

Fig. 4. Relative risk of cardiovascular death at 20-year follow-up by HRR/METs in men.

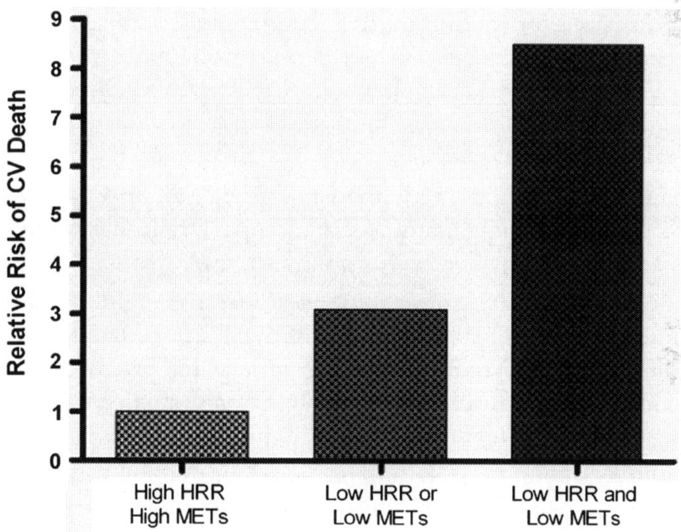

Fig. 5. Relative risk of cardiovascular death at 20-year follow-up by HRR/METs in women.

basis of having low HRR and low exercise capacity [5]. Similar results were reported by Aktas et al. in a group of asymptomatic patients undergoing exercise tests for screening purposes [8]. When matched for the European SCORE, those with slow HRR and/or low exercise capacity had higher mortality rates than those with normal HRR and exercise capacity [8]. The addition of HRR and exercise capacity to SCORE values increased the c-index, a measure of predictive accuracy ranging from 0.5 (no discriminating ability) to 1.0 (perfect discrimination), from 0.73 to 0.76 [8].

The most recent advance in the field of exercise testing is the development of a nomogram for predicting all-cause mortality from several traditional and nontraditional exercise test variables such as ST-segment depression, angina, abnormal HRR, METs achieved, and ventricular ectopy during recovery [73]. This model, validated in 30,000 patients with suspected CAD and a normal resting ECG, performed better than the DTS and further assisted with risk reclassification [73]. Sixty four percent of patients initially classified as high risk by the DTS were reclassified as low-intermediate risk with the use of this nomogram [73]. Overall, the nomogram reclassified 21% of patients [73]. Global risk scores that include traditional ECG-based measures (i.e., ST-segment depression), anginal symptoms, and non-ECG measures offer promise as a means of improving utility of the exercise test.

FUTURE DIRECTIONS AND CONCLUDING REMARKS

Recent studies have argued that combining exercise testing with measures of ACVD may increase prognostic/diagnostic power for the detection of significant obstructive CAD. For example, in symptomatic patients, electron beam tomography-derived CAC scores combined with exercise ECG responses improve diagnostic accuracy for the identification of significant obstructive CAD [74, 75]. Similar results have been attained when combining carotid IMT and exercise testing [76]. Future research is needed to examine the clinical utility of combining measures of ACVD with exercise testing for improving specificity and sensitivity for CAD detection in asymptomatic patients.

The exercise test may also be used as a stressor to aid in revealing abnormal vascular responses that are not apparent at rest. Heffernan et al. has shown that PWV measured during exercise recovery can be vastly different in different clinical cohorts despite similar resting values, suggesting an exercise stress-induced vascular dysfunction [77]. Finger pulse-wave amplitude (a measure of peripheral microvascular function) obtained during exercise testing reveals patients with CAD manifest progressive arterial vasoconstriction during incremental exercise intensity while healthy individuals exhibit vasodilation [78]. Measures of arterial wave reflection from radial tonometry during exercise testing and recovery have been shown to unearth abnormal vascular responses with aging and disease that are not apparent at rest [79]. Brachial artery flow-mediated dilation applied to the exercise recovery period may also hold promise as a means of expounding on ACVD burden [80]. Future research is warranted to examine the predictive significance of arterial responsiveness to acute exercise testing.

There are currently no large-scale, randomized trials that demonstrate the clinical utility of the exercise test for screening purposes in asymptomatic individuals. Ultimately, a randomized clinical outcome trial is required whereby patients are randomized to either a traditional exercise test or an exercise test incorporating non-ECG variables. Would reclassification and subsequent treatment improve outcome?

In conclusion, the traditional exercise test and its reliance on ST-segment depression has poor diagnostic and prognostic capabilities in asymptomatic patients. It is speculated that the ST-segment as a measure of myocardial ischemia does not provide insight into underlying ACVD burden, endothelial dysfunction, inflammation, and autonomic dysfunction, subsequently limiting its predictive usefulness. Measuring the initial HR response or SBP recovery currently lacks clinical utility in asymptomatic patients and requires more research. Combining measures such as exercise BP response, CI, HRR, and exercise capacity with standard risk scores (Framingham/European Risk Score) and standard exercise test measures (DTS) may improve prognostic capabilities of the exercise test in asymptomatic patients while at the same time providing novel insight into ACVD burden and potentially vascular endothelial dysfunction, inflammation, and autonomic dysfunction.

TOPIC PEARLS

- Exercise testing is currently not recommended by AHA/ACC/US Preventive Services Task Force for screening purposes in low-risk asymptomatic patients due to low specificity and sensitivity for detecting CAD.
- Exercise testing may be of value for asymptomatic patients categorized as intermediate risk (one or more risk factor defined as hypercholesterolemia, hypertension, diabetes, smoking, or family history of premature CAD) and asymptomatic patients initiating a regular exercise training program.

- Addition of non-ECG-derived measures such as exercise BP response, CI, HRR, and exercise capacity greatly improves the prognostic capability of the exercise test and may aid in risk restratification of asymptomatic patients.
- Even in the absence of ST-segment changes and angina, non-ECG results obtained from the exercise test (i.e., exercise BP response, CI, HRR, and exercise capacity) provide novel insight into underlying ACVD burden, inflammatory state, and autonomic dysfunction.

CASE STUDY

A 56-year old man wishes to start a regular exercise program and is referred for exercise testing (standard treadmill Bruce protocol). The patient is a nonsmoking, nondiabetic apparently healthy man with a family history of CHD and a body mass index of 26.6 kg/m^2. His total cholesterol is 216 mg/dl, HDL is 41 mg/dl, and blood pressure (BP) is 135/85 mmHg. He is not taking BP medication. According to his Framingham Risk Score, this patient has a 10-year risk of 12%. The patient attained an exercise capacity of nine METs with no angina or ST-segment depression. The test was terminated because of volitional fatigue (rating of perceived exertion of 19 on the Borg Scale of 6–20). According to the DTS (score of 7), this patient is at low risk. The patient had a resting HR of 68 bpm and achieved a peak exercise HR of 154 bpm. His HR during an active recovery was 142 bpm 1 min after the test and 124 bpm 2 min after the test. BP during the last stage of exercise was 218/90 mmHg.

According to the Framingham Risk Score and the DTS, this patient is low-intermediate risk. This patient had a normal chronotropic response but an exaggerated BP response, slow HRR, and fairly low exercise capacity. According to the work of Mora et al [5], this patient may be reclassified as high risk. Moreover, the abnormal HR and BP response suggest that this patient may be three to four times more likely to have carotid atherosclerosis, endothelial dysfunction, and a heightened inflammatory state. Follow-up blood work and ultrasound imaging revealed this patient to have carotid stenosis>25%, IMT>1.2 mm, and a CRP level of 2.6 mg/L.

REFERENCES

1. Gibbons L, Blair SN, Kohl HW, Cooper K. The safety of maximal exercise testing. Circulation 1989;80:846–52.
2. Myers J, Voodi L, Umann T, Froelicher VF. A survey of exercise testing: methods, utilization, interpretation, and safety in the VAHCS. J Cardiopulm Rehabil 2000;20:251–8.
3. Greenland P, Smith SC, Jr., Grundy SM. Improving coronary heart disease risk assessment in asymptomatic people: role of traditional risk factors and noninvasive cardiovascular tests. Circulation 2001;104:1863–7.
4. Lauer M, Froelicher ES, Williams M, Kligfield P. Exercise testing in asymptomatic adults: a statement for professionals from the American Heart Association Council on Clinical Cardiology, Subcommittee on Exercise, Cardiac Rehabilitation, and Prevention. Circulation 2005;112:771–6.
5. Mora S, Redberg RF, Sharrett AR, Blumenthal RS. Enhanced risk assessment in asymptomatic individuals with exercise testing and Framingham risk scores. Circulation 2005;112:1566–72.
6. Balady GJ, Larson MG, Vasan RS, Leip EP, O'Donnell CJ, Levy D. Usefulness of exercise testing in the prediction of coronary disease risk among asymptomatic persons as a function of the Framingham risk score. Circulation 2004;110:1920–5.
7. Gibbons LW, Mitchell TL, Wei M, Blair SN, Cooper KH. Maximal exercise test as a predictor of risk for mortality from coronary heart disease in asymptomatic men. Am J Cardiol 2000;86:53–8.
8. Aktas MK, Ozduran V, Pothier CE, Lang R, Lauer MS. Global risk scores and exercise testing for predicting all-cause mortality in a preventive medicine program. JAMA 2004;292:1462–8.
9. Fowler-Brown A, Pignone M, Pletcher M, Tice JA, Sutton SF, Lohr KN. Exercise tolerance testing to screen for coronary heart disease: a systematic review for the technical support for the U.S. Preventive Services Task Force. Ann Intern Med 2004;140:W9–24.
10. Gibbons RJ, Balady GJ, Bricker JT, et al. ACC/AHA 2002 guideline update for exercise testing: summary article: a report of the American College of Cardiology/American Heart Association Task Force on Practice Guidelines (Committee to Update the 1997 Exercise Testing Guidelines). Circulation 2002;106:1883–92.
11. Froelicher VF, Myers JN. Manual of Exercise Testing, 3rd ed. Philadelphia: Mosby; 2007.

12. Gianrossi R, Detrano R, Mulvihill D, et al. Exercise-induced ST depression in the diagnosis of coronary artery disease. A meta-analysis. Circulation 1989;80:87–98.
13. Nasir K, Redberg RF, Budoff MJ, Hui E, Post WS, Blumenthal RS. Utility of stress testing and coronary calcification measurement for detection of coronary artery disease in women. Arch Intern Med 2004;164:1610–20.
14. Kligfield P, Lauer MS. Exercise electrocardiogram testing: beyond the ST segment. Circulation 2006;114:2070–82.
15. Shaw LJ, Peterson ED, Shaw LK, et al. Use of a prognostic treadmill score in identifying diagnostic coronary disease subgroups. Circulation 1998;98:1622–30.
16. Gulati M, Arnsdorf MF, Shaw LJ, et al. Prognostic value of the duke treadmill score in asymptomatic women. Am J Cardiol 2005;96:369–75.
17. Okin PM, Anderson KM, Levy D, Kligfield P. Heart rate adjustment of exercise-induced ST segment depression. Improved risk stratification in the Framingham Offspring Study. Circulation 1991;83:866–74.
18. Okin PM, Grandits G, Rautaharju PM, et al. Prognostic value of heart rate adjustment of exercise-induced ST segment depression in the multiple risk factor intervention trial. J Am Coll Cardiol 1996;27:1437–43.
19. Okin PM, Lauer MS, Kligfield P. Chronotropic response to exercise. Improved performance of ST-segment depression criteria after adjustment for heart rate reserve. Circulation 1996;94:3226–31.
20. Okin PM, Prineas RJ, Grandits G, et al. Heart rate adjustment of exercise-induced ST-segment depression identifies men who benefit from a risk factor reduction program. Circulation 1997;96:2899–904.
21. Nagai Y, Metter EJ, Earley CJ, et al. Increased carotid artery intimal-medial thickness in asymptomatic older subjects with exercise-induced myocardial ischemia. Circulation 1998;98:1504–9.
22. Okin PM, Roman MJ, Schwartz JE, Pickering TG, Devereux RB. Relation of exercise-induced myocardial ischemia to cardiac and carotid structure. Hypertension 1997;30:1382–8.
23. Dubach P, Froelicher VF, Klein J, Oakes D, Grover-McKay M, Friis R. Exercise-induced hypotension in a male population. Criteria, causes, and prognosis. Circulation 1988;78:1380–7.
24. Laukkanen JA, Kurl S, Salonen R, Lakka TA, Rauramaa R, Salonen JT. Systolic blood pressure during recovery from exercise and the risk of acute myocardial infarction in middle-aged men. Hypertension 2004;44:820–5.
25. McHam SA, Marwick TH, Pashkow FJ, Lauer MS. Delayed systolic blood pressure recovery after graded exercise: an independent correlate of angiographic coronary disease. J Am Coll Cardiol 1999;34:754–9.
26. Ellis K, Pothier CE, Blackstone EH, Lauer MS. Is systolic blood pressure recovery after exercise a predictor of mortality? Am Heart J 2004;147:287–92.
27. Laukkanen JA, Kurl S, Rauramaa R, Lakka TA, Venalainen JM, Salonen JT. Systolic blood pressure response to exercise testing is related to the risk of acute myocardial infarction in middle-aged men. Eur J Cardiovasc Prev Rehabil 2006;13:421–8.
28. Sharabi Y, Ben-Cnaan R, Hanin A, Martonovitch G, Grossman E. The significance of hypertensive response to exercise as a predictor of hypertension and cardiovascular disease. J Hum Hypertens 2001;15:353–6.
29. Matthews CE, Pate RR, Jackson KL, et al. Exaggerated blood pressure response to dynamic exercise and risk of future hypertension. J Clin Epidemiol 1998;51:29–35.
30. Allison TG, Cordeiro MA, Miller TD, Daida H, Squires RW, Gau GT. Prognostic significance of exercise-induced systemic hypertension in healthy subjects. Am J Cardiol 1999;83:371–5.
31. Lauer MS, Pashkow FJ, Harvey SA, Marwick TH, Thomas JD. Angiographic and prognostic implications of an exaggerated exercise systolic blood pressure response and rest systolic blood pressure in adults undergoing evaluation for suspected coronary artery disease. J Am Coll Cardiol 1995;26:1630–6.
32. Miyai N, Arita M, Morioka I, Takeda S, Miyashita K. Ambulatory blood pressure, sympathetic activity, and left ventricular structure and function in middle-aged normotensive men with exaggerated blood pressure response to exercise. Med Sci Monit 2005;11:CR478–84.
33. Jae SY, Fernhall B, Lee M, et al. Exaggerated blood pressure response to exercise is associated with inflammatory markers. J Cardiopulm Rehabil 2006;26:145–9.
34. Stewart KJ, Sung J, Silber HA, et al. Exaggerated exercise blood pressure is related to impaired endothelial vasodilator function. Am J Hypertens 2004;17:314–20.
35. Chang HJ, Chung J, Choi SY, et al. Endothelial dysfunction in patients with exaggerated blood pressure response during treadmill test. Clin Cardiol 2004;27:421–5.
36. Chang HJ, Chung JH, Choi BJ, et al. Endothelial dysfunction and alteration of nitric oxide/cyclic GMP pathway in patients with exercise-induced hypertension. Yonsei Med J 2003;44:1014–20.
37. Bitigen A, Turkyilmaz E, Barutcu I, et al. Aortic elastic properties in patients with hypertensive response to exercise. Circ J 2007;71:727–30.
38. Jae SY, Fernhall B, Heffernan KS, et al. Exaggerated blood pressure response to exercise is associated with carotid atherosclerosis in apparently healthy men. J Hypertens 2006;24:881–7.
39. Leeper NJ, Dewey FE, Ashley EA, et al. Prognostic value of heart rate increase at onset of exercise testing. Circulation 2007;115:468–74.
40. Falcone C, Buzzi MP, Klersy C, Schwartz PJ. Rapid heart rate increase at onset of exercise predicts adverse cardiac events in patients with coronary artery disease. Circulation 2005;112:1959–64.
41. Lauer MS, Francis GS, Okin PM, Pashkow FJ, Snader CE, Marwick TH. Impaired chronotropic response to exercise stress testing as a predictor of mortality. JAMA 1999;281:524–9.

42. Lauer MS, Mehta R, Pashkow FJ, Okin PM, Lee K, Marwick TH. Association of chronotropic incompetence with echocardiographic ischemia and prognosis. J Am Coll Cardiol 1998;32:1280–6.
43. Ellestad MH, Wan MK. Predictive implications of stress testing. Follow-up of 2700 subjects after maximum treadmill stress testing. Circulation 1975;51:363–9.
44. Lauer MS, Okin PM, Larson MG, Evans JC, Levy D. Impaired heart rate response to graded exercise. Prognostic implications of chronotropic incompetence in the Framingham Heart Study. Circulation 1996;93:1520–6.
45. Huang PH, Leu HB, Chen JW, et al. Comparison of endothelial vasodilator function, inflammatory markers, and N-terminal pro-brain natriuretic peptide in patients with or without chronotropic incompetence to exercise test. Heart 2006;92:609–14.
46. Jae SY, Fernhall B, Heffernan KS, et al. Chronotropic response to exercise testing is associated with carotid atherosclerosis in healthy middle-aged men. Eur Heart J 2006;27:954–9.
47. Mora S, Redberg RF, Cui Y, et al. Ability of exercise testing to predict cardiovascular and all-cause death in asymptomatic women: a 20-year follow-up of the lipid research clinics prevalence study. JAMA 2003;290:1600–7.
48. Cole CR, Foody JM, Blackstone EH, Lauer MS. Heart rate recovery after submaximal exercise testing as a predictor of mortality in a cardiovascularly healthy cohort. Ann Intern Med 2000;132:552–5.
49. Nishime EO, Cole CR, Blackstone EH, Pashkow FJ, Lauer MS. Heart rate recovery and treadmill exercise score as predictors of mortality in patients referred for exercise ECG. JAMA 2000;284:1392–8.
50. Morshedi-Meibodi A, Larson MG, Levy D, O'Donnell CJ, Vasan RS. Heart rate recovery after treadmill exercise testing and risk of cardiovascular disease events (The Framingham Heart Study). Am J Cardiol 2002;90:848–52.
51. Chen MS, Blackstone EH, Pothier CE, Lauer MS. Heart rate recovery and impact of myocardial revascularization on long-term mortality. Circulation 2004;110:2851–7.
52. Jae SY, Ahn ES, Heffernan KS, et al. Relation of heart rate recovery after exercise to C-reactive protein and white blood cell count. Am J Cardiol 2007;99:707–10.
53. Jae SY, Carnethon MR, Ahn ES, et al. Association between heart rate recovery after exercise testing and plasminogen activator inhibitor 1, tissue plasminogen activator, and fibrinogen in apparently healthy men. Atherosclerosis 2008;197:415–9.
54. Huang PH, Leu HB, Chen JW, et al. Usefulness of attenuated heart rate recovery immediately after exercise to predict endothelial dysfunction in patients with suspected coronary artery disease. Am J Cardiol 2004;93:10–3.
55. Fei DY, Arena R, Arrowood JA, Kraft KA. Relationship between arterial stiffness and heart rate recovery in apparently healthy adults. Vasc Health Risk Manag 2005;1:85–9.
56. Girod JP, Garcia MJ, Saunders S, Drinko J, Brotman DJ. Relation of brachial artery reactivity to nitroglycerin and heart rate recovery following exercise in healthy male volunteers. Am J Cardiol 2005;96:447–9.
57. Kizilbash MA, Carnethon MR, Chan C, et al. The association of heart rate recovery immediately after exercise with coronary artery calcium: the coronary artery risk development in young adults study. Clin Auton Res 2007;17:46–9.
58. Jae SY, Carnethon MR, Heffernan KS, et al. Slow heart rate recovery after exercise is associated with carotid atherosclerosis. Atherosclerosis 2008;196:256–61.
59. Morris CK, Myers J, Froelicher VF, Kawaguchi T, Ueshima K, Hideg A. Nomogram based on metabolic equivalents and age for assessing aerobic exercise capacity in men. J Am Coll Cardiol 1993;22:175–82.
60. Gulati M, Black HR, Shaw LJ, et al. The prognostic value of a nomogram for exercise capacity in women. N Engl J Med 2005;353:468–75.
61. Laukkanen JA, Kurl S, Salonen R, Rauramaa R, Salonen JT. The predictive value of cardiorespiratory fitness for cardiovascular events in men with various risk profiles: a prospective population-based cohort study. Eur Heart J 2004;25:1428–37.
62. Laukkanen JA, Lakka TA, Rauramaa R, et al. Cardiovascular fitness as a predictor of mortality in men. Arch Intern Med 2001;161:825–31.
63. Wei M, Kampert JB, Barlow CE, et al. Relationship between low cardiorespiratory fitness and mortality in normal-weight, overweight, and obese men. JAMA 1999;282:1547–53.
64. Laukkanen JA, Rauramaa R, Salonen JT, Kurl S. The predictive value of cardiorespiratory fitness combined with coronary risk evaluation and the risk of cardiovascular and all-cause death. J Intern Med 2007;262:263–72.
65. Aronson D, Sheikh-Ahmad M, Avizohar O, et al. C-Reactive protein is inversely related to physical fitness in middle-aged subjects. Atherosclerosis 2004;176:173–9.
66. Church TS, Barlow CE, Earnest CP, Kampert JB, Priest EL, Blair SN. Associations between cardiorespiratory fitness and C-reactive protein in men. Arterioscler Thromb Vasc Biol 2002;22:1869–76.
67. Church TS, Finley CE, Earnest CP, Kampert JB, Gibbons LW, Blair SN. Relative associations of fitness and fatness to fibrinogen, white blood cell count, uric acid and metabolic syndrome. Int J Obes Relat Metab Disord 2002;26:805–13.
68. LaMonte MJ, Fitzgerald SJ, Levine BD, et al. Coronary artery calcium, exercise tolerance, and CHD events in asymptomatic men. Atherosclerosis 2006;189:157–62.
69. Rauramaa R, Rankinen T, Tuomainen P, Vaisanen S, Mercuri M. Inverse relationship between cardiorespiratory fitness and carotid atherosclerosis. Atherosclerosis 1995;112:213–21.
70. Lakka TA, Laukkanen JA, Rauramaa R, et al. Cardiorespiratory fitness and the progression of carotid atherosclerosis in middle-aged men. Ann Intern Med 2001;134:12–20.
71. Jae SY, Carnethon MR, Heffernan KS, Choi YH, Lee MK, Fernhall B. Association between cardiorespiratory fitness and prevalence of carotid atherosclerosis among men with hypertension. Am Heart J 2007;153:1001–5.
72. Myers J, Tan SY, Abella J, Aleti V, Froelicher VF. Comparison of the chronotropic response to exercise and heart rate recovery in predicting cardiovascular mortality. Eur J Cardiovasc Prev Rehabil 2007;14:215–21.

73. Lauer MS, Pothier CE, Magid DJ, Smith SS, Kattan MW. An externally validated model for predicting long-term survival after exercise treadmill testing in patients with suspected coronary artery disease and a normal electrocardiogram. Ann Intern Med 2007;147:821–8.
74. Lamont DH, Budoff MJ, Shavelle DM, Shavelle R, Brundage BH, Hagar JM. Coronary calcium scanning adds incremental value to patients with positive stress tests. Am Heart J 2002;143:861–7.
75. Schmermund A, Baumgart D, Sack S, et al. Assessment of coronary calcification by electron-beam computed tomography in symptomatic patients with normal, abnormal or equivocal exercise stress test. Eur Heart J 2000;21:1674–82.
76. Akosah KO, McHugh VL, Barnhart SI, et al. Carotid ultrasound for risk clarification in young to middle-aged adults undergoing elective coronary angiography. Am J Hypertens 2006;19:1256–61.
77. Heffernan KS, Jae SY, Fernhall B. Racial differences in arterial stiffness after exercise in young men. Am J Hypertens 2007;20:840–5.
78. Rozanski A, Qureshi E, Bauman M, Reed G, Pillar G, Diamond GA. Peripheral arterial responses to treadmill exercise among healthy subjects and atherosclerotic patients. Circulation 2001;103:2084–9.
79. Sharman JE, McEniery CM, Dhakam ZR, Coombes JS, Wilkinson IB, Cockcroft JR. Pulse pressure amplification during exercise is significantly reduced with age and hypercholesterolemia. J Hypertens 2007;25:1249–54.
80. Padilla J, Harris RA, Wallace JP. Can the measurement of brachial artery flow-mediated dilation be applied to the acute exercise model? Cardiovasc Ultrasound 2007;5:45.

15 The Ankle Brachial Index

Matthew A. Allison and Mary M. McDermott

Contents

Abstract

The ankle brachial index (ABI) is defined as the ratio of systolic blood pressures in the ankles to that in the arms. The arteries typically interrogated for calculating the ABI include the brachial arteries in the arms and the posterior tibial and/or dorsalis pedis arteries in the legs. Owing to physiologic considerations, the ratio of the pressures in the ankles to that in the legs is normally greater than 1.00. Values lower than this usually indicate significant flow-limiting atheroocclusive disease in the lower extremities. Previous studies have demonstrated the ABI to be a valid and reproducible method for detecting asymptomatic peripheral arterial disease (PAD) or confirming the presence of significant lower extremity atherosclerotic disease in those with symptoms consistent with intermittent claudication. Since it is simple, inexpensive, and non-invasive, the ABI is suitable for screening asymptomatic individuals and in community-based studies. As the measurement is typically highly reproducible, this technique can also be used in the clinical setting, including the vascular laboratory. In this chapter, we review the epidemiology of PAD with a focus on the use of the ABI for detecting this disease. The measurement techniques, methods of calculating, and interpretation of the ABI are discussed. We also describe the associations between the ABI and both prevalent and incident cardiovascular disease, as well as functional limitations. Finally, clinical considerations are provided.

Key words: Ankle brachial index; Atherosclerosis; Lower extremities; Peripheral arterial disease; Subclinical cardiovascular disease

From: *Asymptomatic Atherosclerosis: Pathophysiology, Detection and Treatment*
Edited by: M. Naghavi (ed.), DOI 10.1007/978-1-60327-179-0_15

KEY POINTS

- The ankle brachial index (ABI) is a valid and reproducible measure of significant lower extremity atheroocclusive disease.
- There are several methods for calculating the ABI that may result in different estimates for peripheral arterial disease and magnitudes of associations with cardiovascular disease (CVD) risk factors.
- An abnormally low ABI is significantly associated with higher risks for prevalent and incident fatal and nonfatal CVD, as well as functional limitations.

CASE SCENARIO

A 64-year-old male with a history of hypertension presents at his physician's office with results of a screening test for lower extremity peripheral arterial disease (PAD) that was performed at his local shopping mall. The patient paid a fee to have several screening tests performed, including testing for lower extremity PAD by the ankle brachial index (ABI), which, he was told, required additional follow-up with his physician. His ABI was 0.90 in his right leg and 0.75 in his left leg. He smoked one pack of cigarettes daily for 40 years but quit nearly 10 years ago. His current medications include atenolol 50 mg daily, amlodipine 10 mg daily, and 81 mg of aspirin daily. He has no history of coronary artery disease, kidney disease, or cerebrovascular disease. He reports no pain in his legs with walking. He has no complaints of chest pain or shortness of breath. He describes a fairly sedentary lifestyle. The patient asks about the significance of the results of the screening test for PAD and whether any treatments are indicated.

SYSTEMIC NATURE OF ATHEROSCLEROSIS

Atherosclerosis is a chronic inflammatory process that proceeds through a relatively standard sequence of pathophysiologic steps and is the result of injurious stimuli to the endothelium of the arterial wall [1]. Left unabated, this process can result in the development of atheromatous plaques that impinge on or occlude the arterial lumen, leading to downstream tissue ischemia and necrosis. Arterial branch points and vascular areas with increased shear stress or increased turbulence of blood flow are sites where there is a tendency for atherosclerosis to initiate and progress. As such, atherosclerotic plaques can be found throughout the vasculature. Indeed, previous angiographic and computed tomography studies have demonstrated the highest prevalence of atherosclerosis in the distal abdominal aorta and bilateral iliac/femoral arteries [2,3].

The excess accumulation of atherosclerosis in the arteries of the lower extremities can result in flow-limiting stenosis and a pressure drop distal to the stenosis that can be detected by standard blood pressure (BP) measurement techniques utilizing a Doppler probe. The obstruction of blood flow may also result in a reduction of oxygen supply to the musculature distal to the obstruction during exercise. If significant, the reduced oxygen supply may result in symptoms associated with tissue ischemia. Intermittent claudication (IC) is the most classic clinical manifestation of tissue ischemia in the lower extremities and is one of the conditions in the disease category of PAD.

PERIPHERAL ARTERIAL DISEASE

PAD is atherosclerosis in the arterial system of the lower extremities. This disease classification is distinct from peripheral vascular disease, which may include disorders of both the venous and the arterial systems. Representative conditions of PAD include IC and gangrene of the feet or toes. Both are typically due to the extensive accumulation of atherosclerotic plaques that lead to tissue ischemia and, in the case of gangrene, necrosis. In some cases, arterial revascularization is performed to restore adequate oxygen supply distal to the obstruction. Owing to the underlying cause of the arterial obstruction, these revascularization cases are also classified as PAD.

As stated previously, the atherosclerosis associated flow-limiting stenoses in the arterial system of the lower extremities result in not only tissue ischemia, but also a pressure drop distal to the luminal obstruction. Sans a diagnosis of subclavian stenosis, this pressure drop results in a lower systolic BP in the lower extremity relative to the systolic BP in the upper extremity. Calculation of the ratio of lower extremity to upper extremity systolic BP results in a value called the ABI. As it is indicative of significant atherosclerotic disease in the lower extremity [or extremities], an abnormal ABI is indicative of lower extremity PAD. Importantly, an abnormal ABI may be present in the absence of associated symptomatology while approximately 30% of those with IC have an abnormal ABI [4, 5]. In this way, the ABI may be viewed as a measure of subclinical cardiovascular disease (CVD).

Community-based studies in the United States have estimated the prevalence of PAD to be between 5 and 8 million individuals [6]. PAD is rare in those under age 50 but the prevalence increases rapidly by doubling with every decade increase in age [6]. Beyond the morbidity associated with lower extremity ischemia, a diagnosis of PAD is important since individuals with this condition have an increased risk for incident total and cardiovascular mortality when compared to those without PAD (see later). This, coupled with the relatively high prevalence, makes PAD a significant public health problem. Accordingly, the ABI may be an appropriate candidate for screening of subclinical atherosclerosis in an effort to reduce the burden of not only PAD, but also other CVD morbidity and mortality.

THE ANKLE BRACHIAL INDEX

ABI is the ratio of Doppler-recorded systolic pressures in the lower to upper extremities. In persons without lower extremity atherosclerosis, arterial pressures increase with greater distance from the heart, because of increasing impedance with increasing arterial taper [7]. This phenomenon results in higher systolic pressures at the ankle compared to the brachial arteries in persons without PAD. Thus, persons without significant lower extremity atherosclerosis have an ABI > 1.00.

The ABI is a simple, noninvasive tool to assess the presence and extent of atherosclerosis in the lower extremities. The methodology for obtaining the systolic BPs necessary to calculate the ABI is standard but there are variations in how many measurements are obtained in each extremity and which artery is used in the ankles.

Measurement Technique (Fig. 1)

The examination should be conducted in a quiet, warm, and comfortable room. Have the participant lie supine on an examination table. The head and heels must be at the same level. The entire head and both feet must be on the table and not overhanging as having the feet even slightly lower than the rest of the body will produce an invalid ABI measurement.

Have the participant rest quietly for at least 5 min before beginning the measurement. Place an appropriately sized BP cuff around both arms, based on arm circumference at the midpoint. The cuff width must be at least 40% of the arm circumference. The three cuff sizes should be employed as follows:

1. Adult (12 cm width) cuff for an arm circumference of <32 cm
2. Large adult (16 cm width) cuff for an arm circumference of 32–42 cm
3. Thigh (20 cm width) cuff for an arm circumference of ^{3}43 cm

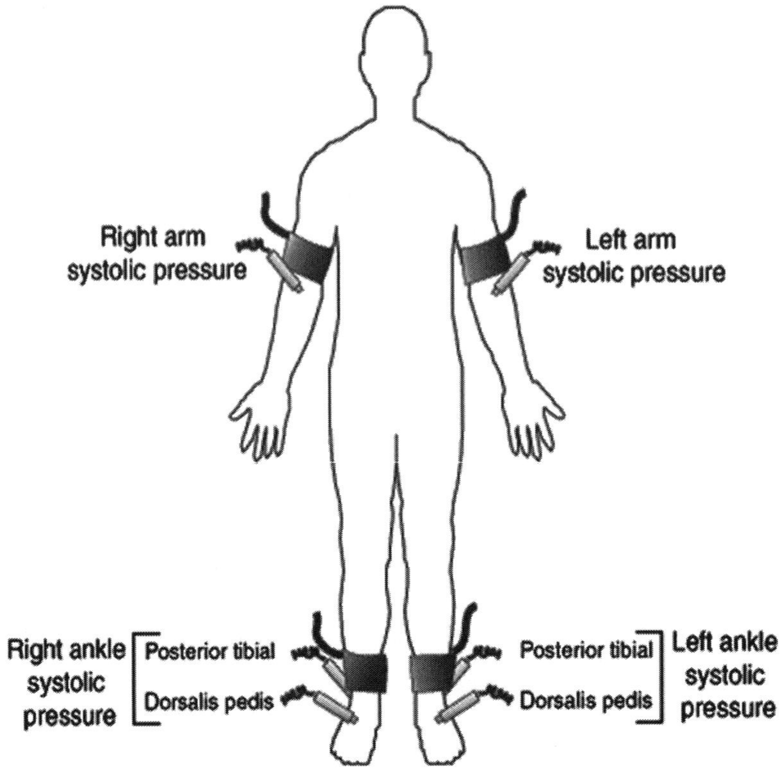

Fig. 1. Measurement of the ankle brachial index.

Place an adult (12 cm) cuff size on each ankle. Place the cuff so that the lower portion rests 3 cm above the greatest protuberance of the medial malleolus. All four cuffs should be in place before the first systolic BP is taken.

By palpation, locate the brachial artery on both arms as well as the dorsalis pedis and posterior tibial arteries on both legs. Mark the location of each artery with a marker. Sometimes an ankle pulse will not be palpable but can be found with the Doppler. Place ultrasound conducting gel over the end of the Doppler. After palpating the location of the pulse, turn on the Doppler and place the probe over the artery. Place the probe in line with the artery and move it from side to side until the strongest pulse is heard. Inflate the cuff to 20 mmHg above the last audible pulse sound. If the pulse cannot be obliterated, raise the pressure to a maximum of 300 mmHg. If not obliterated at this point, the artery is considered "noncompressible." Deflate the cuff slowly allowing the pressure to drop at a rate of 2 mmHg/s. Record the pressure at which the first sustained (more than one beat) pulse reappears. This is the systolic pressure at this location. Deflate the cuff completely. Using the procedure just described, systolic BPs are obtained in the following locations:

1. Right and left brachial arteries
2. Right and left posterior tibial arteries
3. Right and left dorsalis pedis arteries

It is important to record if the pressure in an artery is not detectable or noncompressible as these values will need to be considered when computing the ABI value.

Different Ways of Calculating the Ankle Brachial Index

ABI can be calculated for each lower extremity artery by dividing the systolic pressure measured in the dorsalis pedis and posterior tibial arteries in each limb by the brachial artery pressure. The traditional method of ABI calculation is to use the highest arterial pressure in each limb to calculate the ABI [8]. However, a recent study shows that the sensitivity of the ABI for diagnosing PAD varies according to how lower extremity arterial pressures are used to calculate the ABI. In one study in which 107 patients (208 limbs) underwent angiographic evaluation using digital subtraction angiography, investigators found that the sensitivity of the ABI for PAD (defined as ABI<0.90) varied from 69% when the highest arterial pressure in the ankle was used to 84% when the lowest arterial pressure in the ankle was used to calculate the ABI [9]. The specificity of the ABI for a diagnosis of PAD varied from 83% when the highest arterial pressure at the ankle was used to 64% when the lowest arterial pressure at the ankle was used to calculate the ABI. In a separate study of 216 individuals who underwent arterial duplex ultrasonography, the sensitivity and the specificity of the ABI for PAD (defined as ABI<0.90) were 89 and 63%, respectively, when the lowest arterial pressure was used to calculate the ABI [10]. The sensitivity and specificity of the ABI for PAD were 68 and 99%, respectively, when the highest arterial pressure was used to calculate the ABI [10].

Interpretation of the ABI

In individuals without manifest CVD (to include PAD), the mean ABI is on or about 1.13 [11]. Traditionally, an ABI cut-point of 0.90 or less has been considered evidence of significant atherosclerosis in the lower extremities and therefore, PAD. Moreover, an ABI of 0.90 or less has been consistently shown to be associated with prevalent and incident CVD morbidity and mortality (see below). There is also evidence that as the ABI value decreases below this cut-point, the more severe the atherosclerosis and the more sensitive the ABI is for detecting CVD. However, recent studies have challenged the use of the 0.90 cut-point as the best discriminator of abnormal from normal. [11–14] These studies suggest that it may be more appropriate to consider the entire range of the ABI values. For example, several studies have now demonstrated that those with an ABI between 0.90 and 1.00 have higher levels of several CVD risk factors and greater subclinical atherosclerosis in other vascular beds compared to those with an ABI above 1.00 [12–14]. There is also limited evidence that those with an ABI between 1.0 and 1.1 have higher levels of carotid intimal medial thickness [14]. Finally, when the ABI is analyzed as a continuous variable, those individuals with no CVD risk factors had values closest to 1.13 [11].

To further substantiate the use of the entire range of ABI values, recent research has revealed that higher (>1.30 or 1.40) values may be clinically relevant. An ABI value greater than 1.30 is significantly associated with higher levels of coronary artery calcium, diabetes, and higher body mass index [14, 15] An ABI>1.40 is associated with a significantly worse quality of life on several scales, higher rates of CVD comorbidities, and a higher risk for incident CVD [15–17]. These "high ABI" values represent "stiff" arteries in the lower extremities that may be due to medial calcification. Importantly, there is a nonperfect overlap between arterial stiffness and atherosclerosis, which begs the question of whether these high ABI values should be classified as PAD or not.

Age-Associated Progression of Ankle Brachial Index

An important clinical consideration in patients who have a previous ABI measurement is the change of the ABI value over time. Unfortunately, there have been limited studies conducted on this topic. In a study of 508 Veteran's Affairs patients, the mean change in ABI over 4.6 years was 0.06

with 42% of patients demonstrating a decrease in both legs, 33% an increase in both legs, and 25% had an increase in one leg and a decrease in the other. Similarly, in subjects over the age of 65 from the Cardiovascular Health Study, 9.5% had significant progression of the ABI defined as a decrease of 0.15 over 6 years and converting to a value<0.90. The mean ABI decrease in this group was 0.33 [18]. In terms of clinical symptoms, there is a significant association between ABI progression and both leg symptoms at rest and the presence of symptomatic PAD in either limb [19].

Cardiovascular Risk Factors for an Abnormal Ankle Brachial Index

There is a consistent association between several of the traditional CVD risk factors and an ABI<0.90 ("low ABI"). In the Framingham Offspring Study, every 10 year increase in age was associated with more than a 2.5 times higher risk for a low ABI after adjustment for the standard risk factors [20]. Compared to non-Hispanic Whites, African Americans have approximately twice the odds for a low ABI while Hispanic and Chinese Americans have been found to have a 50% lower odds of an ABI<0.90. These associations been reported to be independent of traditional and novel CVD risk factors [21, 22].

Of the major risk factors for CVD, diabetes and cigarette smoking have the largest magnitude of associations with a low ABI. Individuals with diabetes have two to four times the prevalence [23] and risk [24] while an impaired fasting glucose has been associated with a 20% increase in risk after adjustment for other CVD risk factors [25]. The risk associated with cigarette smoking ranges from 2.0 to 4.5 [20]. High LDL cholesterol is also associated with an increased risk, but these associations have not always been statistically significant. However, individuals with familial hypercholesterolemia have a substantially higher prevalence of a low ABI than controls.[26] Of the inflammatory or "novel" risk factors, interleukin-6, CRP, and fibrinogen have been found to be significantly associated with PAD; although the magnitude of the association after adjustment for the traditional CVD risk factors is modest [22]. The risk of a low ABI in those with documented coronary heart disease (CHD) is over twofold than for those without this condition [20].

Importantly, the relationship between the ABI and cardiovascular risk factors is nonlinear, and may be described as a backward J or U-shape [15]. That is, the prevalence and/or mean values of risk factors such as cigarette smoking, fasting plasma glucose, and waist circumference are highest in those with an ABI<0.9, lowest for those with an ABI 1.0–1.39, and intermediate in those above 1.4. This "stiff artery" high ABI group is also characterized by a high prevalence of individuals with type-2 diabetes as well as markers for this condition, such as fasting serum insulin levels and body mass index.

The Association Between the Ankle Brachial Index and Cardiovascular Disease

Concomitant Prevalent Cardiovascular Disease

Individuals with an ABI<0.9 have higher prevalence rates of several cardiovascular comorbidities. For instance, male subjects in the Atherosclerosis Risk in Communities (ARIC) Study who had an ABI<0.90 had a two- to threefold higher odds for prevalent CHD (depending on ethnic group) and over a fourfold higher odds for cerebrovascular disease (i.e., stroke or transient ischemic attack). Similarly, in unselected primary care patients over the age of 65 from Germany, those with an ABI<0.90 were found to have significantly higher rates of diabetes [adjusted odds ratio (AOR): 1.8], hypertension (AOR: 2.2), lipid disorders (AOR: 1.3), and other coexisting atherothrombotic diseases (any cerebrovascular event: AOR: 1.8; any cardiovascular event: AOR: 1.5) [27]. In another study of primary care patients, over half of those with lower extremity PAD had coexisting CVD [28]. Of note, the association between PAD and other CVD morbidities is not limited to those without manifest CVD. Among patients with coronary artery and other vascular morbidities, the prevalence of cardiovascular risk factors, including the metabolic syndrome, is higher in those with a low ABI [29]. The low ABI is also significantly associated with coronary atherosclerosis as measured by angiography [30, 31].

Incident Total Mortality

Compared with those with no evidence of lower extremity PAD, individuals with an ABI<0.80 have been shown to have an increased risk of dying that was 3.1 for deaths from all causes, 5.9 for all deaths from CVD and 6.6 for deaths from CHD (Fig. 2) [32]. Results from the Cardiovascular Health Study confirm the increased mortality rates among those with an ABI<0.90 but also indicate that the association may be stronger in those without CVD at baseline [33]. The increased mortality rates are not limited to those with an ABI<0.90. In an elegant study by O'Hare and colleagues, and compared to those with an ABI between 1.1 and 1.2, individuals with an ABI between 0.90 and 1.00 had a significantly higher risk of death (HR: 1.40, 95% CI: 1.20–1.63) while those with an ABI>1.40 had a 57% higher risk of mortality (95% CI: 1.07–2.31). There are reports of increased rates of mortality for a low or high ABI among other ethnic groups to include Native Americans [15].

Incident Fatal and Nonfatal Cardiovascular Disease

An abnormally low ABI predicts an increased risk for future coronary and cerebrovascular events. In subjects between the age of 55 and 74 enrolled in the Edinburgh Artery Study, an ABI<0.90 was significantly predictive of an increased risk of fatal myocardial infarction (relative risk: 1.69, $p<0.05$), even after further adjustment for prevalent CVD, diabetes, and conventional risk factors [34]. The Cardiovascular Health Study also found a significantly higher risk for fatal MI after 6 years among those with an ABI<0.90. However, the relative risk was higher in those without CVD at baseline (RR: 2.03) than among those with CVD at baseline (RR: 1.52) [33].

An ABI<0.90 has been found to be significantly associated with incident nonfatal cardiovascular events and revascularization procedures. Compared to an ABI in the highest quartile, the Rotterdam study found a 55 and 59% increase in risk for nonfatal MI in those with an ABI<1.10 and 0.97, respectively [35]. Results from the ARIC Study suggest a significant trend for incident stroke over 7 years when using the spectrum of the ABI (<0.80, 0.80–0.90, etc.) [36]. Despite an elevated risk for

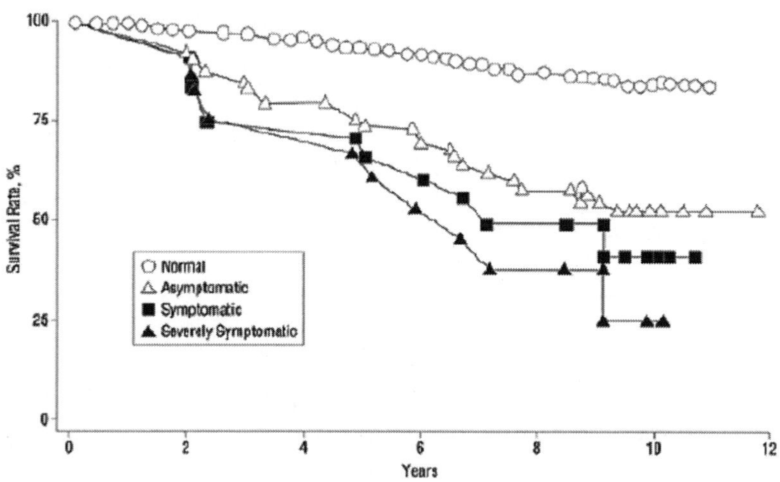

Fig. 2. Associations of peripheral arterial disease and total mortality [32].

mortality among those with a high ABI, additional results from ARIC do not suggest an increased risk for incident CVD in those with an ABI above 1.3 or 1.4 [37]. In a population of patients referred for angiography, the estimated cumulative rate free of cardiovascular events was 90% for ABI>0.90 and 73% for ABI<0.90 ($p = 0.02$) which remained significant after adjustment for age, low-density lipoprotein cholesterol, carotid and femoral intima-media thickness, and degree of coronary stenosis (Gensini score) [31]. In addition, a low ABI in those with CHD has been associated with a 2.5 times higher risk for CVD morbidity [38].

Doobay and colleagues conducted a meta-analysis of nine PAD studies that recorded incident CVD. In this analysis, the authors reported the sensitivity and the specificity of an ABI<0.90 in predicting incident CHDs to be 16.5 and 92.7%, while for incident stroke, these values were 16.0 and 92.2%, and for incident cardiovascular mortality, the sensitivity and specificity were 41.0 and 87.9%, respectively. These results indicate a high specificity, but a relatively low sensitivity, of an ABI<0.90 for future cardiovascular outcomes and suggest that the ABI may be a rational component of the vascular risk assessment among selected individuals [39].

The Association Between the Ankle Brachial Index and Functional Limitations

A range of functional limitations have been described in persons with lower extremity PAD, even among those with asymptomatic disease [40–42]. The Walking and Leg Circulation Study (WALCS) cohort is an observational, longitudinal study of persons with PAD. Among 740 WALCS participants with and without PAD, lower ABI values were associated with greater impairment in functional performance, independent of the presence or type of exertional leg symptoms, suggesting that lower extremity ischemia may influence lower extremity functional performance regardless of the presence or absence of exertional leg symptoms. In separate analyses, 40% of WALCS participants with PAD who reported no exertional leg symptoms developed leg symptoms during a 6-min walk test, suggesting that some persons with PAD have severely restricted their activity level in order to avoid leg symptoms [40]. Among WALCS participants, those who were both asymptomatic and inactive had significantly poorer performance on some measures of lower extremity functioning than PAD participants in WALCS who had classical symptoms of IC [40]. At 2-years of follow-up, PAD participants who reported no exertional leg symptoms at baseline were at particularly high risk for becoming unable to walk for 6-min continuously at 2 year follow-up compared to participants without PAD [43].

The Women's Health and Aging Study (WHAS) also demonstrated that asymptomatic PAD is significantly associated with impaired lower extremity performance compared to persons without PAD. The WHAS cohort included 933 community dwelling disabled women age 65 and older with a valid ABI measurement. Although only about 7% of these WHAS participants reported being told by their physician that they had PAD, 35% had an ABI less than 0.90. Of the 327 participants with PAD, 61% reported no exertional leg symptoms. Among 574 participants with and without PAD who reported no exertional leg symptoms, lower ABI values were associated with greater limitations in measures of lower extremity performance that included slower walking speed at usual and fastest pace over 4 m, fewer blocks walked during the past week, and a higher prevalence of inability to walk ¼ mile and walk up and down stairs without assistance. However, lower ABI values in the WHAS were not associated with greater limitations in any of four measures of upper extremity functioning. These findings suggest that lower extremity ischemia may have a direct negative effect on lower extremity functional performance among persons without exertional leg symptoms.

Use of the Ankle Brachial Index in Clinical Practice

The 34th Bethesda Conference on the prevention of CVDs focused on the use of subclinical measures of atherosclerosis as tools for enhancing screening and prediction of incident CHD. The detection gap between those who endure a CHD event and those who are actually identified as at risk by traditional risk stratification techniques was the impetus for recommendations advocating further examination of the utility of subclinical measures. The ABI was one of the subclinical measures deemed potentially useful for CHD risk stratification [44].

Since that conference, there have been many reports in this area. In 2005 and based on the available evidence, the United States Preventive Services Task Force (USPSTF) issued the following recommendations: "The USPSTF found fair evidence that screening with [the] ankle brachial index can detect adults with asymptomatic PAD. The evidence is also fair that screening for PAD among asymptomatic adults in the general population would have few or no benefits because the prevalence of PAD in this group is low and because there is little evidence that treatment of PAD at this asymptomatic stage of disease, beyond treatment based on standard cardiovascular risk assessment, improves health outcomes. The USPSTF also found fair evidence that screening asymptomatic adults with the ankle brachial index could lead to some small degree of harm, including false-positive results and unnecessary work-ups. Thus, the USPSTF concludes that, for asymptomatic adults, harms of routine screening for PAD exceed benefits" [45].

This recommendation has been challenged on the basis that "most patients with PAD have neither classic symptoms of leg claudication nor threatened limbs but have an extraordinarily high rate of adverse cardiovascular events, such as myocardial infarction, stroke, and death – events that should serve as a key rationale for screening. Medical therapy, including risk factor modification and antiplatelet medications, is known to reduce cardiovascular morbidity and mortality rates in these patients. [Therefore], the Task Force's recommendation against PAD detection may itself adversely result in inadequate recognition and treatment of PAD, with adverse public health consequences" [46]. Accordingly, there have been requests for the USPSTF to re-evaluate its current recommendation for screening with the ABI, while other organizations have recommended the use of the ABI in screening asymptomatic adults as well as adults at higher risk for CVD, such as patients with diabetes [8, 47]. The American Diabetes Association currently recommends annual screening for PAD in people with diabetes that includes obtaining a history of claudication, palpation of pedal pulses, and consideration of obtaining an ABI [45].

A different question is the use of the ABI in symptomatic patients; that is, in those with IC or leg symptoms that may be due to occlusive atherosclerotic disease. In these cases, it seems reasonable to consider performing the ABI as part of the diagnostic evaluation. In this regard, the American Heart Association and the Trans-Atlantic Inter-Society Consensus (TASC) Panel recommend performing an ABI in those patients who present with IC [8, 47].

Treatment Considerations for those with a low Abnormal Ankle Brachial Index

The initial consideration for treatment of an abnormally low ABI is whether the patient has symptoms of lower extremity arterial occlusive disease. If no symptoms are present, due to the strong association between a low ABI and other CVD, the treatment plan should focus on optimization of risk factors for CVD such as BP and both serum glucose and lipid levels as well as smoking cessation. If lower extremity symptoms are present, the treatment plan should also include therapies aimed at relief of symptoms. Moreover, in the context of a normal ABI in an asymptomatic patient, the clinician should consider the presence of and treatment for functional limitations.

The American Heart Association and the American College of Cardiology have published guidelines for treatment of CVD risk factors in patients with PAD [8]. To summarize, LDL cholesterol should be reduced to less than 100 mg/dL using hydroxymethyl glutaryl coenzyme-A reductase inhibitors. However, based on clinical trials demonstrating greater benefit from more intensive LDL lowering, more recent commentaries suggest that lowering LDL to <70 mg/dL is a therapeutic option for patients with PAD. In the case when there are elevated triglyceride and normal LDL cholesterol levels, a fibric acid derivative may be considered. In nondiabetic PAD patients with hypertension, therapy should be administered to achieve a goal of <140 mmHg systolic and 90 mmHg diastolic, while in PAD patients with hypertension and either diabetes or chronic renal disease, the goal is to reduce the systolic to <130 mmHg and the diastolic to <80 mmHg. Of note, beta-adrenergic blocking drugs are not contraindicated in patients with PAD. The aim in diabetic patients with PAD is to reduce the fasting blood sugar to <126 mg/dL and have regular preventive care of the feet. There is some evidence that reduction of the hemoglobin A1C levels to <7% can reduce the microvascular complications of diabetes. Finally, smoking cessation should be strongly encouraged for all PAD patients who are current smokers.

In patients with PAD, treatment with cyclo-oxygenase inhibitors (aspirin) is recommended as a means of reducing the risk for myocardial infarction and stroke [8]. In those cases when aspirin is contraindicated, ADP inhibitors (i.e., clopridogrel) are considered an effective alternative. Oral anticoagulation with warfarin is not recommended as a means of reducing CVD risk.

Treatment of Functional Impairment in Patients with PAD

In 2008, only two medications were FDA approved for treating walking impairment because of symptoms of IC. Pentoxifylline was approved in 1984 for treatment of walking limitation due to IC symptoms. However, more recent studies suggest that pentoxifylline is no better than placebo for improving walking symptoms related to PAD. Cilostazol, a phosphodiesterase type III inhibitor, was FDA approved in 1999 for improving walking limitation related to PAD. Among persons with IC, cilostazol is associated with an approximately 40 to 50% improvement in walking performance as compared to placebo [48]. In comparison, supervised treadmill walking exercise is associated with more than 100% improvement in walking performance among persons with PAD and IC [49]. The most effective supervised walking programs include walking exercise at least three times weekly, last at least 6 months, and include walking exercise to maximal discomfort. However, many patients with IC do not have access to supervised treadmill exercise programs because of lack of insurance coverage. Although asymptomatic PAD is associated with significant functional impairment, currently there are no FDA-approved medications for treating functional limitations associated with PAD. Similarly, exercise programs have not been tested in a large cohort of patients with asymptomatic PAD.

CASE SCENARIO (REVISITED)

The individual presented at the beginning of this chapter fulfills the ABI criteria for PAD and is typical of those at risk for PAD – the presence of several major CVD risk factors (i.e., age, hypertension, and smoking). As described earlier, individuals with a low ABI are at increased risk for incident CVD morbidity and mortality independent of other CVD risk factors. As such, these patients should be counseled about their increased risk for CVD and encouraged to consider lifestyle changes to reduce this risk. Concomitantly, the clinician should consider intensive risk factor reduction to lower the LDL cholesterol below 70 mg/dL. The patient should also be treated with antiplatelet therapy and encouraged to walk for exercise. Given the presence of PAD, a screening treadmill test to rule out ischemia is appropriate before prescribing exercise for this patient.

REFERENCES

1. Stary HC, Chandler AB, Dinsmore RE, Fuster V, Glagov S, Insull W, Jr., Rosenfeld ME, Schwartz CJ, Wagner WD, Wissler RW. A definition of advanced types of atherosclerotic lesions and a histological classification of atherosclerosis. A report from the Committee on Vascular Lesions of the Council on Arteriosclerosis, American Heart Association. Arterioscler Thromb Vasc Biol 1995; 15(9): 1512–31
2. Allison MA, Criqui MH, Wright CM. Patterns and risk factors for systemic calcified atherosclerosis. Arterioscler Thromb Vasc Biol 2004; 24(2): 331–6
3. DeBakey ME, Lawrie GM, Glaeser DH. Patterns of atherosclerosis and their surgical significance. Ann Surg 1985; 201(2): 115–31
4. Criqui MH, Denenberg JO, Bird CE, Fronek A, Klauber MR, Langer RD. The correlation between symptoms and non-invasive test results in patients referred for peripheral arterial disease testing. Vasc Med 1996; 1(1): 65–71
5. Criqui MH, Fronek A, Barrett-Connor E, Klauber MR, Gabriel S, Goodman D. The prevalence of peripheral arterial disease in a defined population. Circulation 1985; 71(3): 510–5
6. Allison MA, Ho E, Denenberg JO, Langer RD, Newman AB, Fabsitz RR, Criqui MH. Ethnic-specific prevalence of peripheral arterial disease in the United States. Am J Prev Med 2007; 32(4): 328–33
7. Yuan-Cheng CF. Blood flow in arteries: pressure and velocity waves in large arteries and the effects of geometric nonuniformity. In: Biodynamics – circulation. New York: Springer-Verlag; 1984; pp 133–6
8. Hirsch AT, Haskal ZJ, Hertzer NR, Bakal CW, Creager MA, Halperin JL, Hiratzka LF, Murphy WR, Olin JW, Puschett JB, Rosenfield KA, Sacks D, Stanley JC, Taylor LM, Jr., White CJ, White J, White RA, Antman EM, Smith SC, Jr., Adams CD, Anderson JL, Faxon DP, Fuster V, Gibbons RJ, Hunt SA, Jacobs AK, Nishimura R, Ornato JP, Page RL, Riegel B. ACC/AHA 2005 Practice Guidelines for the management of patients with peripheral arterial disease (lower extremity, renal, mesenteric, and abdominal aortic): a collaborative report from the American Association for Vascular Surgery/Society for Vascular Surgery, Society for Cardiovascular Angiography and Interventions, Society for Vascular Medicine and Biology, Society of Interventional Radiology, and the ACC/AHA Task Force on Practice Guidelines (Writing Committee to Develop Guidelines for the Management of Patients With Peripheral Arterial Disease): endorsed by the American Association of Cardiovascular and Pulmonary Rehabilitation; National Heart, Lung, and Blood Institute; Society for Vascular Nursing; TransAtlantic Inter-Society Consensus; and Vascular Disease Foundation. Circulation 2006; 113(11): e463–654
9. Niazi K, Khan TH, Easley KA. Diagnostic utility of the two methods of ankle brachial index in the detection of peripheral arterial disease of lower extremities. Catheter Cardiovasc Interv 2006; 68(5): 788–92
10. Schroder F, Diehm N, Kareem S, Ames M, Pira A, Zwettler U, Lawall H, Diehm C. A modified calculation of ankle-brachial pressure index is far more sensitive in the detection of peripheral arterial disease. J Vasc Surg 2006; 44(3): 531–6
11. Aboyans V, Criqui MH, McClelland RL, Allison MA, McDermott MM, Goff DC, Jr., Manolio TA. Intrinsic contribution of gender and ethnicity to normal ankle-brachial index values: the Multi-Ethnic Study of Atherosclerosis (MESA). J Vasc Surg 2007; 45(2): 319–27
12. Allison MA, Laughlin GA, Barrett-Connor E. Association between the ankle-brachial index and carotid intimal medial thickness in the Rancho Bernardo Study. Am J Cardiol 2006; 98(8): 1105.
13. Allison MA, Laughlin GA, Barrett-Connor E, Langer R. Association between the ankle-brachial index and future coronary calcium (the Rancho Bernardo Study). Am J Cardiol 2006; 97(2): 181–6
14. McDermott MM, Liu K, Criqui MH, Ruth K, Goff D, Saad MF, Wu C, Homma S, Sharrett AR. Ankle-brachial index and subclinical cardiac and carotid disease: the multi-ethnic study of atherosclerosis. Am J Epidemiol 2005; 162(1): 33–41
15. Resnick HE, Lindsay RS, McDermott MM, Devereux RB, Jones KL, Fabsitz RR, Howard BV. Relationship of high and low ankle brachial index to all-cause and cardiovascular disease mortality: the Strong Heart Study. Circulation 2004; 109(6): 733–9
16. Allison M, Criqui M, Hiatt W, Hirsch A. A high ankle brachial index is associated with increased cardiovascular disease morbidity and worse quality of life. Circulation 2007; 115(8): e283
17. O'Hare AM, Katz R, Shlipak MG, Cushman M, Newman AB. Mortality and cardiovascular risk across the ankle-arm index spectrum: results from the Cardiovascular Health Study. Circulation 2006; 113(3): 388–93
18. Kennedy M, Solomon C, Manolio TA, Criqui MH, Newman AB, Polak JF, Burke GL, Enright P, Cushman M. Risk factors for declining ankle-brachial index in men and women 65 years or older: the Cardiovascular Health Study. Arch Intern Med 2005; 165(16): 1896–902
19. Bird CE, Criqui MH, Fronek A, Denenberg JO, Klauber MR, Langer RD. Quantitative and qualitative progression of peripheral arterial disease by non-invasive testing. Vasc Med 1999; 4(1): 15–21

20. Murabito JM, Evans JC, Nieto K, Larson MG, Levy D, Wilson PW. Prevalence and clinical correlates of peripheral arterial disease in the Framingham Offspring Study. Am Heart J 2002; 143(6): 961–5
21. Criqui M, Vargas V, Ho E, Koppel D, Denenberg J, Fronek A, Langer R. Ethnicity and peripheral arterial disease: the San Diego Population Study. Circulation 2002; 105: e113
22. Allison MA, Criqui MH, McClelland RL, Scott JM, McDermott MM, Liu K, Folsom AR, Bertoni AG, Sharrett AR, Homma S, Kori S. The effect of novel cardiovascular risk factors on the ethnic-specific odds for peripheral arterial disease in the Multi-Ethnic Study of Atherosclerosis (MESA). J Am Coll Cardiol 2006; 48(6): 1190–7
23. Gregg EW, Sorlie P, Paulose-Ram R, Gu Q, Eberhardt MS, Wolz M, Burt V, Curtin L, Engelgau M, Geiss L. Prevalence of lower-extremity disease in the U.S. adult population >=40 years of age with and without diabetes: 1999–2000 National Health and Nutrition Examination Survey. Diabetes Care 2004; 27(7): 1591–7
24. Newman AB, Siscovick DS, Manolio TA, Polak J, Fried LP, Borhani NO, Wolfson SK. Ankle-arm index as a marker of atherosclerosis in the Cardiovascular Health Study. Cardiovascular Heart Study Collaborative Research Group. Circulation 1993; 88(3): 837–45
25. Beks PJ, Mackaay AJ, de Neeling JN, de Vries H, Bouter LM, Heine RJ. Peripheral arterial disease in relation to glycaemic level in an elderly Caucasian population: the Hoorn study. Diabetologia 1995; 38(1): 86–96
26. Kroon A, Ajubi N, van Asten W, Stalenhoef A. The prevalence of peripheral vascular disease in familial hypercholesterolaemia. J Intern Med 1995; 238(5): 451–9
27. Diehm C, Schuster A, Allenberg JR, Darius H, Haberl R, Lange S, Pittrow D, von Stritzky B, Tepohl G, Trampisch HJ. High prevalence of peripheral arterial disease and co-morbidity in 6880 primary care patients: cross-sectional study. Atherosclerosis 2004; 172(1): 95–105
28. Hirsch AT, Criqui MH, Treat-Jacobson D, Regensteiner JG, Creager MA, Olin JW, Krook SH, Hunninghake DB, Comerota AJ, Walsh ME, McDermott MM, Hiatt WR. Peripheral arterial disease detection, awareness, and treatment in primary care. JAMA 2001; 286(11): 1317–24
29. Gorter PM, Olijhoek JK, van der Graaf Y, Algra A, Rabelink TJ, Visseren FL. Prevalence of the metabolic syndrome in patients with coronary heart disease, cerebrovascular disease, peripheral arterial disease or abdominal aortic aneurysm. Atherosclerosis 2004; 173(2): 363–9
30. Otah KE, Madan A, Otah E, Badero O, Clark LT, Salifu MO. Usefulness of an abnormal ankle-brachial index to predict presence of coronary artery disease in African-Americans. Am J Cardiol 2004; 93(4): 481–3
31. Papamichael CM, Lekakis JP, Stamatelopoulos KS, Papaioannou TG, Alevizaki MK, Cimponeriu AT, Kanakakis JE, Papapanagiotou A, Kalofoutis AT, Stamatelopoulos SF. Ankle-brachial index as a predictor of the extent of coronary atherosclerosis and cardiovascular events in patients with coronary artery disease. Am J Cardiol 2000; 86(6): 615–8
32. Criqui MH, Langer RD, Fronek A, Feigelson HS, Klauber MR, McCann TJ, Browner D. Mortality over a period of 10 years in patients with peripheral arterial disease. N Engl J Med 1992; 326(6): 381–6
33. Newman AB, Shemanski L, Manolio TA, Cushman M, Mittelmark M, Polak JF, Powe NR, Siscovick D. Ankle-arm index as a predictor of cardiovascular disease and mortality in the Cardiovascular Health Study The Cardiovascular Health Study Group. Arterioscler Thromb Vasc Biol 1999; 19(3): 538–45
34. Lee AJ, Price JF, Russell MJ, Smith FB, van Wijk MCW, Fowkes FGR. Improved prediction of fatal myocardial infarction using the ankle brachial index in addition to conventional risk factors: the Edinburgh Artery Study. Circulation 2004; 110(19): 3075–80
35. van der Meer IM, Bots ML, Hofman A, del Sol AI, van der Kuip DA, Witteman JC. Predictive value of noninvasive measures of atherosclerosis for incident myocardial infarction: the Rotterdam Study. Circulation 2004; 109(9): 1089–94
36. Tsai AW, Folsom AR, Rosamond WD, Jones DW. Ankle-brachial index and 7-year ischemic stroke incidence: the ARIC study. Stroke 2001; 32(8): 1721–4
37. Wattanakit K, Folsom AR, Duprez DA, Weatherley BD, Hirsch AT. Clinical significance of a high ankle-brachial index: insights from the Atherosclerosis Risk in Communities (ARIC) Study. Atherosclerosis 2006; Epub ahead of print
38. Criqui MH, Denenberg JO. The generalized nature of atherosclerosis: how peripheral arterial disease may predict adverse events from coronary artery disease. Vasc Med 1998; 3(3): 241–5
39. Doobay AV, Anand SS. Sensitivity and specificity of the ankle-brachial index to predict future cardiovascular outcomes: a systematic review. Arterioscler Thromb Vasc Biol 2005; 25(7): 1463–9
40. McDermott MM, Greenland P, Liu K, Guralnik JM, Criqui MH, Dolan NC, Chan C, Celic L, Pearce WH, Schneider JR, Sharma L, Clark E, Gibson D, Martin GJ. Leg symptoms in peripheral arterial disease: associated clinical characteristics and functional impairment. JAMA 2001; 286(13): 1599–606
41. McDermott MM, Fried L, Simonsick E, Ling S, Guralnik JM. Asymptomatic peripheral arterial disease is independently associated with impaired lower extremity functioning: the Women's Health And Aging Study. Circulation 2000; 101(9): 1007–12
42. McDermott MM, Greenland P, Liu K, Guralnik JM, Celic L, Criqui MH, Chan C, Martin GJ, Schneider J, Pearce WH, Taylor LM, Clark E. The ankle brachial index is associated with leg function and physical activity: the Walking and Leg Circulation Study. Ann Intern Med 2002; 136(12): 873–83
43. McDermott MM, Guralnik JM, Ferrucci L, Criqui MH, Greenland P, Tian L, Liu K, Tan J. Functional decline in lower-extremity peripheral arterial disease: associations with comorbidity, gender, and race. J Vasc Surg 2005; 42(6): 1131–7
44. Taylor AJ, Merz CN, Udelson JE. 34th Bethesda Conference: executive summary – can atherosclerosis imaging techniques improve the detection of patients at risk for ischemic heart disease? J Am Coll Cardiol 2003; 41(11): 1860–2

45. U.S. Preventive Services Task Force. Screening for peripheral arterial disease, topic page. In: Ned Calonge (ed) Guide to clinical preventive services. Rockville: Agency for Healthcare Research and Quality; 2005
46. Beckman JA, Jaff MR, Creager MA. The United States preventive services task force recommendation statement on screening for peripheral arterial disease: more harm than benefit? Circulation 2006; 114(8): 861–6
47. Norgren L, Hiatt WR, Dormandy JA, Nehler MR, Harris KA, Fowkes FG. Inter-society consensus for the management of peripheral arterial disease (TASC II). J Vasc Surg 2007; 45 Suppl S: S5–67
48. Beebe HG, Dawson DL, Cutler BS, Herd JA, Strandness DE, Jr., Bortey EB, Forbes WP. A new pharmacological treatment for intermittent claudication: results of a randomized, multicenter trial. Arch Intern Med 1999; 159(17): 2041–50
49. Gardner AW, Poehlman ET. Exercise rehabilitation programs for the treatment of claudication pain. A meta-analysis. JAMA 1995; 274(12): 975–80

16 Arterial Elasticity/Stiffness

Daniel A. Duprez and Jay N. Cohn

CONTENTS

ABSTRACT

The major pathophysiologic process initiating atherosclerotic cardiovascular disease is the deficiency of arterial endothelial function. The rate of progression of cardiovascular disease is highly variable. Changes in small arterial elasticity/stiffness are the first signs of cardiovascular disease in asymptomatic subjects as an expression of endothelial dysfunction. Measurement of arterial stiffness with different noninvasive techniques provides information about the functional and structural vascular changes at the level of the aorta, the muscular conduit arteries, the peripheral branches, and the microvascular components. Arterial stiffness has been related to the coronary heart disease risk scores. Now, there is evidence that arterial stiffness is a predictor for cardiovascular events in the general population, in patients with hypertension, end-stage renal disease, and impaired glucose intolerance. Future studies are warranted to demonstrate the value of follow-up of arterial elasticity/stiffness as a marker of improvement in arterial wall health during antihypertensive, antidiabetic, and lipid-lowering therapy. Promising study results show that measurement of arterial stiffness can become an important part of the routine assessment of patients in daily practice.

Key words: Arterial stiffness; Cardiovascular disease prevention; Cardiovascular events; Coronary heart disease risk score; Hypertension; Large and small artery elasticity; Pulse contour analysis; Pulse wave velocity

From: *Asymptomatic Atherosclerosis: Pathophysiology, Detection and Treatment*
Edited by: M. Naghavi (ed.), DOI 10.1007/978-1-60327-179-0_16

KEY POINTS

- Endothelial dysfunction results in stiffening of the small arteries
- Structural changes in the large conduit arteries decrease their elasticity and increase stiffness
- Risk factors and effective preventive therapy alter prognosis by functional and structural effects on the arteries
- A focus on arterial elasticity can improve the diagnostic and therapeutic approach to cardiovascular disease

The earliest changes in the vasculature that lead to advancing vascular disease occur in the endothelium. Small artery elasticity can be considered as a surrogate marker for endothelial dysfunction.

The arterial vasculature is the target organ of aging and atherosclerosis that precipitates morbid cardiovascular events. Functional and structural changes in the arterial vasculature lead to a rise in blood pressure as a consequence of a reduced cross-sectional area of the resistance vessels, as well as to thrombotic and hemorrhagic events that affect primarily the myocardium and brain [1–3]. Blood pressure has become a major identifier of vascular disease in clinical practice, because epidemiologic data have demonstrated a close relationship between the resting blood pressure and the risk for subsequent cardiovascular events [4].

The earliest changes in the vasculature that presage advancing vascular disease occur in the endothelium, which is the primary source of nitric oxide to protect the artery and maintain its low vascular smooth muscle tone [5]. When nitric oxide bioactivity is deficient the small arteries will constrict and the large conduit arteries may be infiltrated by lipids that can result in atherosclerotic plaques [6]. Consequently, small arterial elasticity or stiffness may be an early marker for the patient who is developing functional or structural vascular disease and is in need of aggressive intervention. This early vascular disease is not always accompanied by a pressure above the threshold currently defined as hypertension [7]. The term prehypertension is currently in use and ideally would be confined to those patients whose high-normal pressure is a consequence of endothelial dysfunction.

Although atherosclerotic plaques and morbid events are classic manifestations of conduit artery disease, which may be visualized by ultrasound or angiographic studies, the function of small arteries in the microcirculation is uniquely stiffened by endothelial dysfunction.

These considerations have raised the possibility of utilizing arterial elasticity measurements as a guide to the diagnosis of early vascular disease and as a means of monitoring the response to therapy in patients who have begun treatment.

ARTERIAL STIFFNESS AND MEASUREMENTS

Noninvasive measurement of arterial elasticity entails measurement of surrogate parameters that are intrinsically associated with arterial elasticity/stiffness. A number of computerized devices are now available that enable quantification of global indices of arterial stiffness, as well as regional and local abnormalities.

Pulse pressure is the difference between systolic and diastolic blood pressure and has been in the past considered as one of the simplest measures of arterial stiffness. However, pulse pressure alone is inadequate to assess arterial stiffness accurately. Problems include the influence of stroke volume and the "normal" amplification of the pressure wave as it travels from the aorta to the periphery. The arterial pressure wave has two principal components, the wave generated by the heart, which travels away from the heart, and the reflected wave, which returns to the heart from peripheral sites, predominantly in the lower part of the body. Thus pulse pressure measured at any peripheral arterial site cannot serve as a satisfactory assessment of arterial stiffness.

Table 1
Different techniques to estimate arterial elasticity/stiffness

Technique	*Device (Manufacturer)*	*Measurements*
Pulsewave velocity (PWV)	Complior (Artech)	Carotid-femoral PWV Carotid-radial PWV
Pulse contour analysis (systole)	Sphygmocor (Atcor)	Aortic pressure Augmentation Index
Pulse contour analysis (diastole)	CV Profilor (HDI)	Small artery elasticity (C_2) Large artery elasticity (C_1)
Ultrasound	Multiple	Cross-sectional compliance and distensibility

Noninvasive measurement of arterial stiffness entails measurement of surrogate parameters that are intrinsically associated with stiffness (Table 1). This involves three main methodologies: (1) pulse transit time, (2) analysis of the arterial pressure pulse and its wave contour, and (3) direct stiffness estimation using measurements of diameter and distending pressure [8–11]. These surrogate parameters are related to the functional effects of arterial stiffness and as such can be used to quantify changes. A number of computerized devices are now available that enable quantification of global, regional, and local indices of stiffness. This availability has raised the possibility of utilizing arterial stiffness measurements as a guide to the diagnosis of early vascular disease and as a means of monitoring the response to therapy.

The velocity of the arterial pulse wave or pulse wave velocity can be assessed by measuring an arterial wave form, usually recorded with an ultrasonic transducer, at a proximal and a more distal vascular site. The sites usually selected for assessment in clinical practice are the carotid artery and the femoral artery. The time delay between the carotid and the femoral divided by the distance between these two sites, usually estimated on the surface with a ruler or tape measure, is used to calculate the velocity of the pulse wave between these two sites in the conduit artery system. The pulse wave velocity is sensitive to blood pressure because of the nonlinear pressure-volume relationship of vascular tissue. Therefore, the higher the pressure, the more rapid the pulse wave velocity. The pulse wave velocity is also dependent upon local changes in the structure of the arterial system, so that the thicker and less distensible aorta with aging results in a more rapid pulse wave velocity.

Another frequently used technique is pulse contour analysis (Fig. 1). An arterial waveform can be recorded over any accessible peripheral artery, including the radial artery, the brachial artery, the femoral artery, and the carotid artery. The technique of pulse contour analysis requires an independent method to quantitate the pressure, and this is usually obtained from an arm cuff. Waveform analysis can involve assessment of both the systolic and the diastolic portions. A critical component of pulse contour analysis is the influence of reflected waves or oscillations arising from more distal vascular sites and branch points where the forward arterial wave is reflected backward [12]. These oscillations can be detected in the waveform and are analyzed in systole as an augmentation of late systolic pressure and in diastole as an oscillation superimposed on the diastolic pressure decay. Systolic pressure analysis has the advantage of being visually detectable merely by examining the systolic wave form and calculating the ratio of the late systolic to early systolic pressure [13]. The late systolic peak can usually be recognized, often interrupting a plateau that defines the early peak. Sometimes, however, the pressures merge and no augmentation can be defined. The approach used by one instrument is to utilize a computer program that attempts to recreate from the radial waveform a pressure waveform representing a carotid pressure wave [14]. This exercise involves use of a "transfer function" to

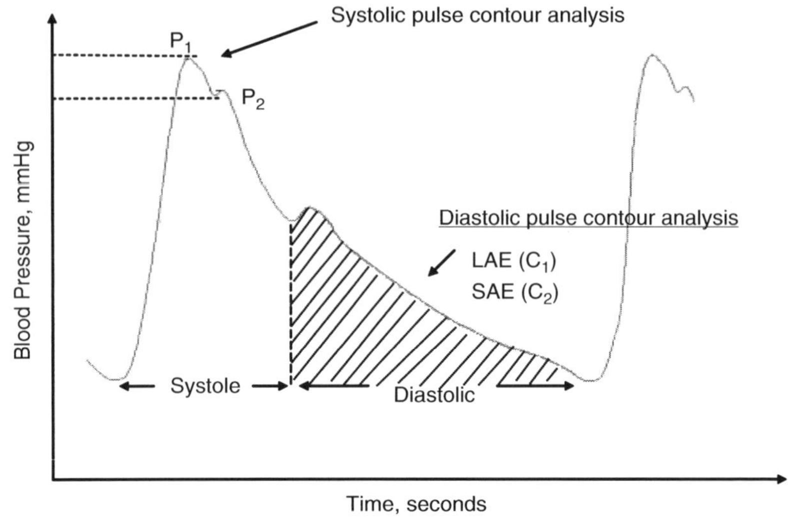

Fig. 1. Systolic and diastolic pulse contour analysis. P_1, first peak; P_2, second peak; LAE: large artery elasticity; SAE: small artery elasticity.

accomplish the reconstruction. Since this "transfer function" would be expected to vary with age, disease, and treatment, some investigators have discouraged its use and encouraged use of the peripheral waveform for analyzing augmentation [15]. Since wave reflection is induced by stiffening of the small arteries, whereas wave transit time is influenced by stiffening of the large arteries, and since the augmentation index is dependent on both the reflected wave and its rapid transit back to the root of the aorta, an increase in augmentation index is a function of both small and large artery stiffness (nonspecific).

Small artery elasticity is reduced in the presence of endothelial dysfunction and also as a consequence of structural changes in the smaller vascular segments. Small artery effects can be separated from large artery effects by computer analysis of the diastolic decay of the arterial wave form. This analysis is dependent on modeling the circulation as a modified Windkessel in which compliance and resistance are in parallel [11]. Despite the assumptions required for this model-dependent analysis, small artery elasticity (C_2 in the model) can be separated from large artery elasticity (C_1 in the model).

Conduit arteries can be visualized with appropriate ultrasound techniques to evaluate the thickness of the wall, which usually is defined as intima-medial thickness (IMT) and diameter. This technique has been applied particularly to the carotid artery, where visualization in the neck is easily feasible and the IMT of the proximal and distal wall of the carotid artery can be measured. Cross-sectional compliance and distensibility are calculated from the arterial wall movements and the blood pressure, unfortunately usually obtained from the arm rather from the artery being studied [16].

ARTERIAL STIFFNESS AS PREDICTOR FOR HYPERTENSION

Changes in arterial elasticity/stiffness are detectable before blood pressure rises to a level diagnostic of hypertension. The goal for identifying and managing hypertension should be broadened from simply initiating treatment once an arbitrary "high" level of blood pressure elevation has been reached and should be focused on maintaining vascular health.

Hypertension is a major risk factor for atherosclerotic events, but some normotensive persons are clearly at greater risk for cardiovascular events than are hypertensive individuals. In fact, a hypothetical analysis of the Framingham epidemiologic studies showed that more normotensive than hypertensive persons experience cardiovascular events [17]. Damage to the endothelium – whether caused by a gene, hypertension, diabetes, elevated cholesterol, smoking, or aging, or (as is most commonly the case) a combination of two or more of these risk factors – appears to be the key in the progression to atherosclerosis and cardiovascular events [18]. Therefore, the goal for identifying and managing hypertension should be broadened from simply initiating treatment once an arbitrary "high" level of BP elevation has been reached and should be focused on maintaining vascular health, in which endothelial function plays a key role [19]. Consequently therapeutic decision making should use a model that brings together several factors that might serve to better define the at-risk individual. This new model centers around the health of the vascular wall and especially the endothelium. Such an approach evolves from a recent proposed redefinition of hypertension, which would define the condition as "a state of abnormal arterial function and structure associated with endothelial dysfunction, vascular smooth muscle constriction or remodeling, increased impedance to left ventricular ejection, and propensity for atherosclerosis, often but not always manifested by an elevated blood pressure" [20].

The conventional wisdom, as presented, is that arterial stiffness is the result of hypertension rather than its cause, but there is now evidence that the relationship between hypertension and arterial stiffness may be bidirectional. In the ARIC Study (Atherosclerosis Risk in Communities), using high-resolution B-mode ultrasound examination of the left common carotid artery, Liao et al. [21] found that one standard deviation increase in arterial stiffness was associated with a 15% greater risk of future hypertension, independent of established risk factors and level of blood pressure. Another study by Dernellis and Panaretou [22] provided evidence that increased aortic stiffness precedes hypertension. Aortic stiffness was determined by M-Mode echocardiography which involved calculating aortic systolic and diastolic diameters and using standard equations to calculate aortic strain, distensibility, and stiffness index. They found that aortic stiffness in normotensive individuals was a predictor of future hypertension after correcting for risk factors that included systolic blood pressure, age, sex, body mass index, heart rate, total cholesterol, diabetes, smoking, alcohol consumption, and physical activity. On the other hand, the relationship between blood pressure and arterial properties is reciprocal; it has been shown in the Bogalusa Heart Study that childhood blood pressure predicted arterial stiffness assessed an average of 26.5 years later by brachial – ankle pulse wave velocity [23]. Those who had higher blood pressure levels in childhood had stiffer arteries 26 years later, which suggests that blood pressure even in early childhood plays a role in the process of arterial stiffening. Mechanistically, arterial stiffness may be the consequence of repetitive cycles of stress and strain and the attendant induction of vascular smooth muscle cell growth and synthesis of matrix components dependent on endothelial dysfunction. These processes influence vascular stiffness, which may further increase blood pressure and initiate a positive feedback loop. The observed predictability of childhood blood pressure for arterial stiffness in young adulthood is at variance with the situation in middle-aged and older adults in whom impaired elasticity or compliance of the artery is considered an antecedent factor for systolic hypertension and widened pulse pressure [21, 24].

Abnormalities of the arterial vasculature that precede cardiovascular morbid events are likely to occur in a temporal sequence (Fig. 2). The initial abnormalities appear to be functional, in large part related to endothelial dysfunction associated with decreased bioavailability of NO [25]. A decrease in constitutive release of NO, which maintains low small artery tone, may be the initial abnormality, but it is soon accompanied by a decrease in stimulated release of endothelial vasodilators, as manifested by a reduction in flow-mediated dilation of conduit arteries [26, 27]. These functional abnormalities of the vasculature should precede and are mechanistic precursors of the structural alterations that are responsible for thickening of the conduit artery wall [28], increases in pulse pressure, and atherosclerotic plaque development. These structural changes may also result in additional functional abnormalities. But cross-sectional studies suggest that this sequence of vascular

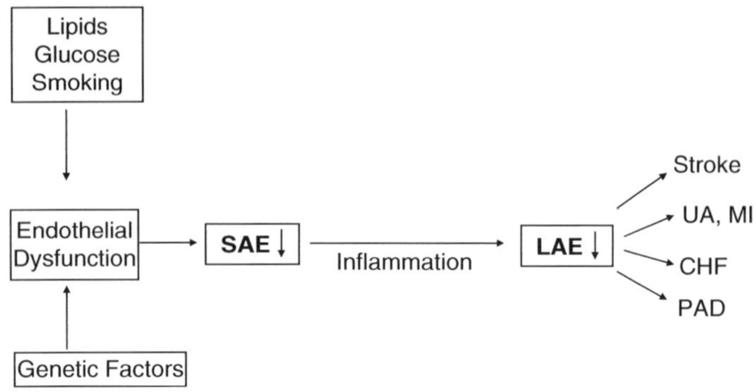

Fig. 2. Temporal sequence of the development of cardiovascular events. (*SAE* Small artery elasticity, *LAE* Large artery elasticity, *UA* Unstable angina, *MI* Myocardial infarction, *CHF* Congestive heart failure, *PAD* Peripheral arterial disease).

manifestations of vascular disease is not always present. Sometimes the structural changes present without obvious functional changes, and these structural changes are not necessarily expressed throughout the entire vasculature.

ARTERIAL ELASTICITY/STIFFNESS AND CHD RISK SCORE

The classical coronary heart disease risk score is a biostatistical risk approach and does not provide information about personalized cardiovascular disease. Changes in arterial elasticity can be considered as an early marker for cardiovascular disease.

The Framingham risk score indicates the individual's 10-year absolute risk for developing coronary heart disease and is the most frequently applied score in daily practice. This approach needs to be considered as a biostatistical risk and does not provide information about personalized cardiovascular disease. Changes in arterial elasticity can be considered as early markers for cardiovascular disease [29]. There is need for more information regarding the relationship between CHD risk score and arterial stiffness.

The Prospective Study of the Vasculature in Uppsala Seniors (PIVUS) study aimed to evaluate the feasibility and the relation to the Framingham risk score of three techniques to assess arterial stiffness in an elderly population with a mean age of 70 years [30]. These three parameters for arterial stiffness were the following: (1) arterial distensibility of the carotid artery by ultrasonography; (2) augmentation index by pulse wave analysis; and (3) the stroke volume to pulse pressure ratio by echocardiography. All three indices of arterial stiffness were inter-related. Although all the techniques were correlated to Framingham risk score, only carotid artery distensibility and the stroke volume to pulse pressure ratio were independently related to coronary risk, suggesting complementary use of these two indices of arterial stiffness in the future.

In order to investigate a possible association between augmentation index and cardiovascular risk, augmentation index was related to the level of cardiovascular risk in 216 subjects with or without cardiovascular disease [31]. Each individual's cardiovascular risk was evaluated using three different risk scores; the "coronary risk chart" of the European Society of Cardiology that is based on the Framingham study [32]. Since all Framingham risk scores were originally developed to predict cardiovascular risk in patients without a previous history of cardiovascular disease, the investigators additionally used two risk scores that allowed us to classify patients with pre-existing cardiovascular disease. The SMART (Second Manifestations of ARTerial disease) risk score was developed in a cross-sectional study of patients who experienced their first cardiovascular events. The EPOZ (Epidemiological Prevention study of Zoetermeer) risk score was derived in a follow-up study which included subjects at relatively high risks, and all-cause mortality was used as the primary outcome parameter [33]. Augmentation index was derived by pulse wave analysis using carotid applanation tonometry. Augmentation index significantly increased with increasing risk scores and was significantly correlated to the three cardiovascular risk scores. These findings suggest that augmentation index may be a useful marker of cardiovascular risk.

We studied indices from systolic and diastolic pulse contour analysis from the radial pressure waveform and correlated these indices with traditional risk factors in asymptomatic individuals screened for cardiovascular disease [13]. The systolic indices were augmentation pressure, augmentation index, and systolic reflective index and the diastolic indices were large and small artery elasticity. These indices were then correlated to each other as well as to individual traditional risk factors and the Framingham risk score. All indices were significantly correlated to the Framingham risk score, which was stronger in women than men, but when adjusted for age only diastolic indices remained significant in women.

PREDICTIVE VALUE OF ARTERIAL ELASTICITY/STIFFNESS FOR CARDIOVASCULAR EVENTS

Cross-sectional studies show that arterial stiffness is correlated with atherosclerotic lesions. Longitudinal studies have demonstrated independent predictive value of arterial stiffness, assessed by pulse wave velocity, large and small artery elasticity, augmentation index, and central pulse pressure for cardiovascular events.

Indirect evidence for the influence of arterial stiffness on cardiovascular events comes from cross-sectional studies showing that arterial stiffness and cardiovascular risk factors for atherosclerotic lesions are correlated. A major limitation of these studies is their cross-sectional nature. Although these studies show a clear association between aortic stiffness and other markers of cardiovascular risk or atherosclerosis, it is not possible to conclude that arterial stiffness is predictive of cardiovascular events because patients were not followed prospectively.

Table 2 reports the longitudinal studies, which have demonstrated the independent predictive value of arterial stiffness, assessed by pulse wave velocity, large and small artery elasticity, augmentation index, and central pulse pressure for cardiovascular events. The largest amount of evidence has been given for aortic stiffness, measured through carotid-femoral pulse wave velocity. Aortic stiffness has independent predictive value for all-cause and cardiovascular mortalities, fatal and nonfatal coronary events, and fatal strokes in the general population [34, 35], the elderly [36–38], patients with uncomplicated essential hypertension [39–42], impaired glucose intolerance [43], end-stage renal disease [44–47]. We demonstrated that in an asymptomatic population, small artery elasticity was predictive of cardiovascular morbid events, thus confirming the temporal sequence of atherosclerotic disease described earlier [48].

Although measures of stiffness provide useful prognostic information concerning the occurrence of cardiovascular events, the value of changes in arterial stiffness as a guide to the reduction in cardiovascular events with treatment is yet to be unequivocally demonstrated. Arterial stiffness attenuation may reflect the true reduction of arterial wall damage, whereas blood pressure, blood glucose, and lipids can be normalized in a few weeks by using antihypertensive, antidiabetic, and lipid-lowering drugs, leading to a strong reduction in cardiovascular risk scores, but without yet any improvement of atherosclerotic lesions and arterial stiffness, which requires a long-lasting correction of abnormalities. A temporal dissociation is thus expected between the improvement of cardiovascular risk factors and a reduced arterial stiffness.

Table 2
Predictive value of arterial elasticity/stiffness on cardiovascular morbidity and mortality in different patient populations

Type of patient	*N*	*Parameter*	*Events*	*Follow-up (years)*	*Authors (Ref.)*
General population	1,678	Aortic PWV	CV mortality	9.4	Willum-Hansen et al. [34]
General population	492	Aortic PWV	CV mortality	10.0	Shokawa et al. [35]
General population	419	Large and small artery elasticity	CV events	6.0	Grey et al. [48]
Elderly	2,835	Aortic PWV	CV mortality	4.1	Mattace-Raso et al. [36]
Elderly	2,488	Aortic PWV	CV mortality and events	4.6	Sutton-Tyrrel et al. [37]
Elderly	141	Aortic PWV	CV mortality	2.5	Meaume et al. [38]
Hypertension	1,980	Aortic PWV	CV mortality	9.3	Laurent et al. [39]
Hypertension	1,045	Aortic PWV	CHD events	5.7	Boutouyrie et al. [40]
Hypertension	1,715	Aortic PWV	Fatal strokes	7.9	Laurent et al. [41]
Hypertension	2,073	Central pulse pressure and carotid AIx	CV events	3.4	Williams et al. [42]
Impaired glucose tolerance	571	Aortic PWV	All cause mortality	10.7	Cruickshank et al. [43]
ESRD	241	Aortic PWV	CV mortality	6.0	Blacher et al. [44]
ESRD	265	Aortic PWV	CV mortality	5.2	Shoij et al. [45]
ESRD	180	Central pulse pressure	All cause mortality	4.3	Safar et al. [46]
ESRD	180	Carotid AIx	All cause and CV mortality	4.3	London et al. [47]

PWV Pulse wave velocity, *AIx* Augmentation index, *CHD* Coronary Heart Disease, *ESRD* End-stage renal disease, *N* Number of patients

PREVENTIVE TREATMENT

There is now evidence that preventive therapies can improve arterial elasticity/stiffness in asymptomatic subjects to slow progression of early cardiovascular disease. Surrogate markers such as arterial elasticity for the biological process in the arteries and heart that progress to morbid events should serve as an attractive means of identifying those at risk and demonstrating their response to therapy.

Most cardiovascular events are a consequence of a progressive atherosclerotic process that can be detected long before symptoms develop. Dysfunction of the vascular endothelium seems to be a key in the progression to atherosclerosis and cardiovascular events. Identifying individuals with early markers for this vascular disease process raises the possibility for pharmacotherapy to slow the progression and delay or prevent future morbid events.

As the underlying mechanisms of vascular disease and the effects of renin-angiotensin system inhibition on these processes have been further defined, the therapeutic focus has begun to shift toward prevention of disease progression at earlier stages. Noninvasive diagnostic tests are now available to assess otherwise healthy individuals for subclinical CV disease. We performed the DETECTIV pilot study, which allowed evaluation of the efficacy of the angiotensin II receptor blocker, valsartan versus placebo on the severity of vascular and cardiac function and structural alterations. These abnormalities were quantitated by ten tests of vascular and cardiac health (Rasmussen Disease Score) in high-risk asymptomatic individuals with either prehypertension or controlled blood pressure <140/90 mm Hg [49]. During 6 months of valsartan therapy, vascular function benefits included improved small artery elasticity and a reduction in systolic and diastolic blood pressure within the normotensive range. A further increase in small artery elasticity and a reduction in left ventricular mass after 12 months of therapy are consistent with a slowly developing structural effect superimposed on the early functional benefit. These data on delayed cardiac and vascular effects suggest that longer-term therapy might display more dramatic benefits on structure of the vasculature and heart. As a pilot study DETECTIV was not designed to assess morbid events. Indeed, the population eligible for participation in DETECTIV had no evidence for overt disease that would place them at high immediate risk. The goal in this population is to slow disease progression from its earliest detection to hopefully delay or prevent morbid events during the patients' productive years. Demonstration of this morbid event prevention would require a long study in a very large population. In the meantime, however, surrogate markers such as arterial elasticity should serve as an attractive means of identifying those at risk and documenting efficacy of therapy.

CONCLUSIONS

Endothelial dysfunction is the primary target in the pathogenesis of cardiovascular disease. Several techniques are available to measure arterial stiffness. Each of these provides different and perhaps complementary data that may offer unique insights into vascular health. Surrogate markers, especially small artery elasticity, may offer the most sensitive guide to early vascular disease likely to progress and to the functional response of the vasculature to therapy.

REFERENCES

1. Cohn JN. Arterial stiffness, vascular disease and risk of cardiovascular events. Circulation. 2006;113:601–3.
2. Folkow B. Hypertensive structural changes in systemic precapillary resistance vessels: how important are they for in vivo haemodynamics? J Hypertens. 1995;13(12 Pt 2):1546–59.
3. Lip GY, Blann AD, Edmunds E, Beevers DG. Baseline abnormalities of endothelial function and thrombogenesis in relation to prognosis in essential hypertension. Blood Coagul Fibrinolysis. 2002;13:35–41.
4. Menotti A, Lanti M, Kafatos A, et al. Seven Countries Study. The role of a baseline casual blood pressure measurement and of blood pressure changes in middle age in prediction of cardiovascular and all-cause mortality occurring late in life: a cross-cultural comparison among the European cohorts of the Seven Countries Study. J Hypertens. 2004;22:1683–90.
5. Widlansky ME, Gokce N, Keaney JF, Vita JA. The clinical implications of endothelial dysfunction. J Am Coll Cardiol. 2003;42:1149–60.
6. Gilani M, Kaiser DR, Bratteli CW, et al. Role of nitric oxide deficiency and its detection as a risk factor in pre-hypertension. JASH. 2007;1:45–55.
7. Duprez D, Cohn JN. Monitoring vascular health beyond blood pressure. Curr Hypertens Rep. 2006;8:287–91.
8. Davies JI, Struthers AD. Pulse wave analysis and pulse wave velocity: a critical review of their strengths and weaknesses. J Hypertens. 2003;21:463–72.
9. McVeigh GE. Pulse waveform analysis and arterial wall properties. Hypertension. 2003;41:1010–11.
10. O'Rourke MF, Staessen JA, Vlachopoulos C, Duprez D, Plante GE. Clinical applications of arterial stiffness; definitions and reference values. Am J Hypertens. 2002;15:426–44.
11. Finkelstein SM, Cohn JN. First- and third-order models for determining arterial compliance. J Hypertens. 1992;10 Suppl:S11–4.
12. Cohn JN. Pathophysiologic and prognostic implications of measuring arterial compliance in hypertensive disease. Prog Cardiovasc Dis. 1999;41:441–50.
13. Duprez DA, Kaiser DR, Whitwam W, et al. Determinants of radial artery pulse wave analysis in asymptomatic individuals. Am J Hypertens. 2004;17:647–53.
14. Karamanoglu M, O'Rourke MF, Avolio AP, Kelly RP. An analysis of the relationship between central aortic and peripheral upper limb pressure waves in man. Eur Heart J. 1993;14:160–7.

15. Millasseau SC, Patel SJ, Redwood SR, Ritter JM, Chowienczyk PJ. Pressure wave reflection assessed from the peripheral pulse: is a transfer function necessary? Hypertension. 2003;41:1016–20.
16. Duprez DA, De Buyzere ML, Verloove HH, et al. Influence of the arterial blood pressure and nonhemodynamic factors on regional arterial wall properties in moderate essential hypertension. J Hum Hypertens. 1996;10:251–6.
17. Atilla K, Vasan RS. Prehypertension and risk of cardiovascular disease. Expert Rev Cardiovasc Ther. 2006;1:111–7.
18. Brunner H, Cockcroft JR, Deanfield J, et al. Working Group on Endothelins and Endothelial Factors of the European Society of Hypertension. Endothelial function and dysfunction. Part II: Association with cardiovascular risk factors and diseases. A statement by the Working Group on Endothelins and Endothelial Factors of the European Society of Hypertension. J Hypertens. 2005;23:233–46.
19. Duprez DA, Cohn JN. Small artery elasticity index, endothelial function and cardiovascular risk. In: Safar ME, O'Rourke MF (ed) Handbook of Hypertension: Arterial Stiffness in Hypertension, vol.23. Elsevier, The Netherlands, 2006, 16:257–65.
20. Giles TD, Berk BC, Black HR, et al. Expanding the definition and classification of hypertension. J Clin Hypertens. 2005;7:505–12.
21. Liao D, Arnett DK, Tyroler HA, et al. Arterial stiffness and the development of hypertension. The ARIC study. Hypertension. 1999;34:201–6.
22. Dernellis J, Panaretou M. Aortic stiffness is an independent predictor of progression to hypertension in nonhypertensive subjects. Hypertension. 2005;45:426–31.
23. Li S, Chen W, Srinivasan SR, Berenson GS. Childhood BP as a predictor of arterial stiffness in young adults the Bogalusa heart study. Hypertension. 2004;43:541–6.
24. Arnett DK, Glasser SP, McVeigh G, et al. Blood pressure and arterial compliance in young adults: the Minnesota Children's Blood Pressure Study. Am J Hypertens. 2001;14:200–5.
25. McVeigh GE, Allen PB, Morgan DR, Hanratty CG, Silke B. Nitric oxide modulation of blood vessel tone identified by arterial waveform analysis. Clin Sci (Lond). 2001;100:387–93.
26. Clarkson P, Celermajer DS, Powe AJ, Donald AE, Henry RM, Deanfield JE. Endothelium-dependent dilatation is impaired in young healthy subjects with a family history of premature coronary disease. Circulation. 1997;96:3378–83.
27. Anderson TJ, Uehata A, Gerhard MD, et al. Close relation of endothelial function in the human coronary and peripheral circulation. J Am Coll Cardiol. 1995;26:1235–41.
28. Barenbrock M, Hausberg M, Kosch M, Golubev SA, Kisters K, Rahn KH. Flow-mediated vasodilation and distensibility in relation to intima-media thickness of large arteries in mild essential hypertension. Am J Hypertens. 1999;12:973–9.
29. Cohn JN, Duprez DA, Grandits GA. Arterial elasticity as part of a comprehensive assessment of cardiovascular risk and drug treatment. Hypertension. 2005;46:217–20.
30. Lind L, Fors N, Hall J, Marttala K, Stenborg A. A comparison of three different methods to determine arterial compliance in the elderly: the Prospective Investigation of the Vasculature in Uppsala Seniors (PIVUS) study. J Hypertension. 2006;24:1083–8.
31. Nurnberger J, Keflioglu-Scheiber A, Opazo Saez AM, Wenzel RR, Philipp T, Schafers RF. Augmentation index is associated with cardiovascular risk. J Hypertension. 2002;20:2407–14.
32. Fourth Joint Task Force of the European Society of Cardiology and Other Societies on Cardiovascular Disease Prevention in Clinical Practice. European guidelines on cardiovascular disease prevention in clinical practice: executive summary. Eur Heart J. 2007;28:2375–414.
33. Simons PC, Algra A, Bots ML, Grobbee DE, van der Graaf Y. Common carotid intima – media thickness and arterial stiffness: indicators of cardiovascular risk in high-risk patients. The SMART Study (Second Manifestations of ARTerial disease). Circulation. 1999;100:951–57.
34. Willum-Hansen T, Staessen JA, Torp-Pedersen C, et al. Prognostic value of aortic pulse wave velocity as index of arterial stiffness in the general population. Circulation. 2006;113:664–70.
35. Shokawa T, Imazu M, Yamamoto H, et al. Pulse wave velocity predicts cardiovascular mortality: findings from the Hawaii-Los Angeles-Hiroshima study. Circ J. 2005;69:259–64.
36. Mattace-Raso FUS, van der Cammen TJM, Hofman A et al. Arterial stiffness and risk of coronary heart disease and stroke. The Rotterdam Study. Circulation. 2006;113:657–63.
37. Sutton-Tyrrell K, Najjar SS, Boudreau RM, et al. Elevated aortic pulse wave velocity, a marker of arterial stiffness, predicts cardiovascular events in well-functioning older adults. Circulation. 2005;111:3384–90.
38. Meaume S, Benetos A, Henry OF, Rudnichi A, Safar ME. Aortic pulse wave velocity predicts cardiovascular mortality in subjects >70 years of age. Arterioscler Thromb Vasc Biol. 2001;21:2046–50.
39. Laurent S, Boutouyrie P, Asmar R, et al. Aortic stiffness is an independent predictor of all-cause and cardiovascular mortality in hypertensive patients. Hypertension. 2001; 37:1236–41.
40. Boutouyrie P, Tropeano AI, Asmar R, et al. Aortic stiffness is an independent predictor of primary coronary events in hypertensive patients: a longitudinal study. Hypertension. 2002;39:10–5.
41. Laurent S, Katsahian S, Fassot C, et al. Aortic stiffness is an independent predictor of fatal stroke in essential hypertension. Stroke. 2003;34:1203–6.
42. Williams B, Lacy PS, Thom SM, et al. Differential impact of blood pressure-lowering drugs on central aortic pressure and clinical outcomes: principal results of the Conduit Artery Function Evaluation (CAFE) study. Circulation. 2006;113:1213–25.

43. Cruickshank K, Riste L, Anderson SG, Wright JS, Dunn G, Gosling RG. Aortic pulse-wave velocity and its relationship to mortality in diabetes and glucose intolerance: an integrated index of vascular function? Circulation. 2002;106:2085–90.
44. Blacher J, Guerin AP, Pannier B, Marchais SJ, Safar ME, London GM. Impact of aortic stiffness on survival in end-stage renal disease. Circulation. 1999;99:2434–9.
45. Shoji T, Emoto M, Shinohara K, et al. Diabetes mellitus, aortic stiffness, and cardiovascular mortality in end-stage renal disease. J Am Soc Nephrol. 2001;12:2117–24.
46. Safar ME, Blacher J, Pannier B, et al. Central pulse pressure and mortality in end-stage renal disease. Hypertension. 2002;39:735–8.
47. London GM, Blacher J, Pannier B, Guerin AP, Marchais SJ, Safar ME. Arterial wave reflections and survival in end-stage renal failure. Hypertension. 2001;38:434–8.
48. Grey E, Bratteli C, Glasser SP, et al. Reduced small artery but not large artery elasticity is an independent risk marker for cardiovascular events. Am J Hypertension. 2003;16:265–9.
49. Duprez DA, Florea ND, Jones K, Cohn JN. Beneficial effects of valsartan in asymptomatic individuals with vascular or cardiac abnormalities: the DETECTIV Pilot Study. J Am Coll Cardiol. 2007;50:835–9.

17 Assessment of Endothelial Function in Clinical Practice

Jeffrey T. Kuvin

Contents

Abstract

Endothelial cell function represents an important marker of vascular health. The clinical evaluation of vascular function has become an important tool to assess cardiovascular risk and prognosis. Vasorelaxation, a measure of endothelial function, can be measured by assessing the response to pharmacological or other stressors in the vasculature. Coronary artery endothelial testing assesses the vascular bed of most clinical interest; however, peripheral vascular testing offers a more practical approach to testing a variety of patient populations and clinical scenarios. Recently, clinical applications have been developed to allow for real-time assessment of vascular function. Tools that are portable and can be used in the ambulatory setting to assess endothelial function testing are now available. Knowledge regarding a patient's endothelial health appears to be useful for identifying patient subgroups at risk for future cardiovascular events, determining response to treatments, and perhaps evaluating individuals who should receive medical therapy, but do not qualify according to present guidelines. The true clinical utility of vascular function testing has not yet been determined; however, physiologic testing provides unique information about the health on an individuals' vasculature. The search for reliable, robust markers of endothelial function and their potential use in clinical practice are discussed further in this chapter.

Key words: Endothelium; Vascular function; Vasorelaxation; Brachial artery reactivity; Peripheral arterial tonometry; Plethysmography; Hyperemia

From: *Asymptomatic Atherosclerosis: Pathophysiology, Detection and Treatment*
Edited by: M. Naghavi (ed.), DOI 10.1007/978-1-60327-179-0_17

KEY POINTS

- Endothelial function represents a barometer of vascular health.
- Testing for endothelial function is feasible and provides important information regarding cardiovascular risk.
- Vasomotor function may be measured by assessing the response to pharmacological and other stressors in the coronary and peripheral vasculature.
- There are a variety of patient populations and clinical scenarios, which most likely derive benefit from more information regarding vascular health.
- There are many attractive features for performing ambulatory physiologic testing of vascular function, and the methodology is evolving toward user-friendly applications.

INTRODUCTION

For years, the basic and clinical sciences have focused on blood vessel reactivity and the functional role of the endothelium. The vascular endothelium comprises complex physiology, and disturbances in cellular function may be an early marker of atherosclerosis. These multipurpose cells act in an autocrine, paracrine, and endocrine fashion. One major function of endothelial cells is to regulate vascular tone, which occurs through a balance between specific vasoactive substances, most notably, nitric oxide. Endothelial cells also perform important functions related to platelet activation, leukocyte adhesion, and thrombosis. If disturbed, the delicate balance maintained by the endothelium may be disrupted, thus allowing for the development of vascular dysfunction, and ultimately, atherosclerosis (Fig. 1).

Endothelial function represents a barometer of vascular health, and subtle changes in the vasculature may have profound effects on atherosclerosis-related morbidity and mortality. Recently, clinical applications have been developed to allow for real-time assessment of vascular reactivity. The search for reliable, robust markers of endothelial function, and their potential use in clinical practice will be discussed in this chapter.

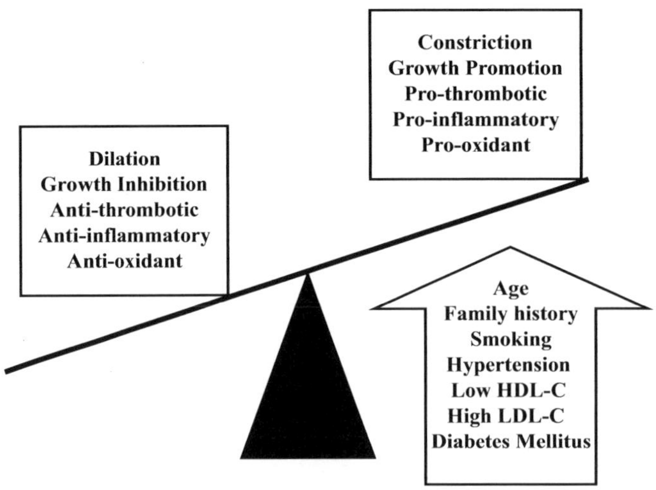

Fig. 1. Endothelial dysfunction. Healthy endothelial cells provide a balance between beneficial and detrimental functions of the vasculature. In the presence of cardiovascular risk factors, the scale tips toward endothelial dysfunction, and ultimately, increased cardiovascular events.

CLINICAL TOOLS TO ASSESS ENDOTHELIAL FUNCTION

Vascular relaxation may be measured by assessing the response to pharmacological and other stressors in the coronary and peripheral vasculature [1,2]. Intracoronary infusion of acetylcholine in the coronary vasculature results in muscarinic receptor activation on endothelial cells, thereby releasing nitric oxide. Typically, the release of excess vasodilators results in dilation of the blood vessels and hyperemia. This process, however, is disturbed in patients with endothelial cell dysfunction, even in the absence of atherosclerotic plaque. Dysfunctional endothelium result in decreased vasodilation and, in some individuals, paradoxical vasoconstriction ensues [1].

Coronary artery endothelial testing assesses the arterial bed of most clinical interest, but carries risks of coronary ischemia, as well as the inherent potential complications of cardiac catheterization, including cost. Often considered the gold standard for endothelial function testing, the limitations of coronary artery testing do not allow for its widespread use, thus limiting its clinical utility. Nevertheless, this technique has been helpful in defining the clinical utility of endothelial function testing and has been instrumental in the development of an in vivo model to evaluate vascular function. Numerous interventions known to decrease cardiovascular risk, such as cholesterol-lowering therapies and smoking cessation, have been linked to early improvements in coronary endothelial function. Robust data now exist suggesting impaired coronary artery endothelial function portends adverse long-term cardiovascular risk [3, 4]. Halcox et al. followed patients over 4 years and measured changes in coronary vascular resistance and epicardial artery diameter following administration of intracoronary acetylcholine [5]. In this study, endothelial function predicted cardiovascular events in patients with coronary artery disease as well as in subjects with no angiographic evidence of atherosclerosis.

Endothelial dysfunction and atherosclerosis are diffuse disease processes; thus, there is a physiologic basis for assessing the endothelium-dependent vasomotion in the peripheral vasculature. Numerous methods to evaluate the peripheral arterial system have emerged as alternatives to coronary endothelial function testing. Testing the peripheral circulation has inherent benefits, such as the ability to utilize noninvasive tools due to the superficial location of many of peripheral vascular beds as well as cost advantages.

The most commonly used technique for assessing peripheral endothelial function testing is brachial artery reactivity testing (BART). This tool utilizes high-resolution vascular ultrasound before and during a period of reactive hyperemia induced by brachial artery occlusion [6]. Vasodilation results from the release of nitric oxide due to shear stress and changes in hydrostatic pressure; thus, a lack of vasodilation suggests a decreased level of endogenous vasodilators and endothelial dysfunction. Although less commonly used to test vascular function, the carotid, superficial femoral, and radial arteries may also be evaluated by similar techniques [7, 8].

Testing peripheral arterial endothelial function with BART can provide information regarding future cardiovascular risk. Our group has shown that normal brachial artery reactivity predicts the absence of coronary artery disease and the amount of vasodilation correlates well with exercise treadmill tolerance [9]. It has also been shown that patients with diminished brachial artery function have an increased risk for future cardiovascular events and the need for revascularization [10]. Abnormal brachial artery vasomotion tested in high-cardiovascular risk patients undergoing vascular surgery is an independent risk factor for short- and long-term adverse events [11, 12], even after correcting for traditional cardiovascular risk factors. Impaired peripheral endothelial function independently predicts adverse outcome in specific patient cohorts, such as those with heart failure [13]. Finally, improved flow-mediated dilation of the brachial artery over a period of time appears to portend better cardiovascular outcomes [14].

Gender-based differences in peripheral arterial vasomotion have been identified, and flow-mediated dilation in women correlates well with cardiovascular risk, especially in postmenopausal women [15].

Interestingly, flow-mediated dilation is not necessarily similar among the sexes, and a higher cut-point for flow-mediated dilation is likely required to optimize the sensitivity of BART for identifying women who have significant coronary atherosclerosis, compared with similarly aged men [16]. Modena and colleagues have prospectively shown, in a cohort of >2,000 postmenopausal women, that FMD provides incremental prognostic information for future cardiovascular risk [17]. BART has also been tested in a prospective fashion in postmenopausal women with hypertension and impaired brachial artery vasomotion [18]. Following 6 months of treatment with optimal blood pressure therapy, brachial artery vasoreactivity remained abnormal in 150 patients, and improved in the remaining 250 patients. After approximately 5 years, patients whose flow-mediated dilation remained impaired had significantly more cardiovascular events than did those patients whose endothelial function improved with treatment, thus suggesting that endothelial function testing might provide information about which patients derive benefit from a specific intervention.

Venous occlusion plethysmography is an additional peripheral vascular technology for evaluating peripheral vasomotor function. This modality involves measuring volume changes by mercury strain gages during hyperemia in the forearm. Infusion of vasoactive agents, including drugs to release nitric oxide or inhibitors of endothelial nitric oxide synthase, allows for the evaluation of specific mechanisms of vascular function and dysfunction. This tool has been used to evaluate vascular function in a variety of patient populations. Measuring the vasoactive response to brachial artery infusion of acetylcholine in patients with known coronary artery disease has been shown to be a prognostic marker for future cardiovascular events [19]. Assessment of forearm endothelial function is also a marker of long-term cardiovascular events in patients with hypertension [20].

Abnormalities in pulse wave amplitude have long been described in the peripheral circulation in patients with atherosclerosis [21] and may be an early independent marker of future cardiac events [22]. Newer technologies, such as peripheral arterial tonometry (PAT), allow for the noninvasive evaluation of pulse wave amplitude and have been linked to endothelial function, cardiovascular risk, and the presence or absence of coronary artery disease. PAT digitally records arterial pulse waves before and during reactive hyperemia, and the derived ratio is labeled PAT hyperemia. PAT hyperemia correlates with brachial artery as well as coronary artery endothelial function testing [23, 24] and seems to capture a nitric-oxide-mediated pathway related to flow-mediated vasodilation [25]. PAT hyperemia has been shown to be an adequate surrogate marker to assess for changes in vascular function over time [26] and has been closely linked with cardiovascular risk factors in the Framingham cohort [27]. It has been shown that interventions known to induce vasodilation via activation of the nitric oxide system, such as flavanol-rich foods, improve pulse wave amplitude measurements [28]. The true prognostic importance of this test, up to this point, remains untested.

There are several other devices for measuring indices related to pulse wave and pulse volume, thereby allowing for mathematical models to provide data regarding central arterial tone. These data reveal diastolic wave forms, elasticity, vascular resistance as well as an augmentation index, and many of these indices have been associated with cardiovascular risk factors [29, 30] and have been utilized as surrogate markers in drug intervention studies [31]. Digital thermal monitoring of the fingers and hands during reactive hyperemia has also been associated with cardiovascular risk, coronary artery calcium scores, and other markers of atherosclerosis.

In addition to vascular imaging techniques, blood testing might provide a sense of endothelial health and disease. Cellular adhesion molecules play an important role in vascular function and are expressed on the surface of damaged endothelial cells. Cellular adhesion molecules are released into the circulation, and increased levels have been linked to cardiovascular risk and atherosclerosis [32]. C-reactive protein, urine levels of nitric oxide metabolites, and vascular extracellular superoxide dismutase may also be reflective of endothelial function [33, 34]. Finally, endothelial progenitor cells derived from bone marrow have a role in ongoing endothelial repair and might represent a surrogate biologic marker for vascular function and cardiovascular risk. A decrease in circulating number of endothelial progenitor cells contributes to endothelial dysfunction and cardiovascular disease progression. In healthy men, a decreased level of circulating endothelial progenitor cells correlates with increased Framingham risk factor score as well as abnormal flow-mediated brachial-artery reactivity [35]. Strategies to increase circulating endothelial progenitor cells are similar to traditional risk factor modification. In addition, targets aimed at increasing bone marrow production of these cells, with erythropoietin, granulocyte-macrophage colony-stimulating factor, and vascular endothelial growth factor, might prove beneficial for vascular health.

ENDOTHELIAL FUNCTION TESTING IN CLINICAL PRACTICE

There are a variety of patient populations and clinical scenarios for which the practitioner and patient would likely derive benefit from more information regarding vascular health [36]. Knowledge regarding the health of the endothelium in a given patient would likely be useful to identify patient subgroups at higher risk for cardiovascular events, yet who might not qualify for medical therapy according to present guidelines (Fig. 2). For example, given inherent insufficiencies in risk factor assessment, real-time physiologic assessment of endothelial function might be a welcome addition to the physicians' diagnostic armamentarium, allowing for determination of subjects who represent higher than expected cardiovascular risk and should be considered for initiation or intensification of therapy. By identifying patients with decreased endothelial function despite having "normal" standard testing, such as a low Framingham risk score or an unremarkable stress test, one might be able to define a subgroup of patients who would likely benefit from aggressive medical or lifestyle interventions [37]. Thus, in this era of early and aggressive risk factor assessment and modification, physiologic tools addressing arterial function make sense and are likely to have a role.

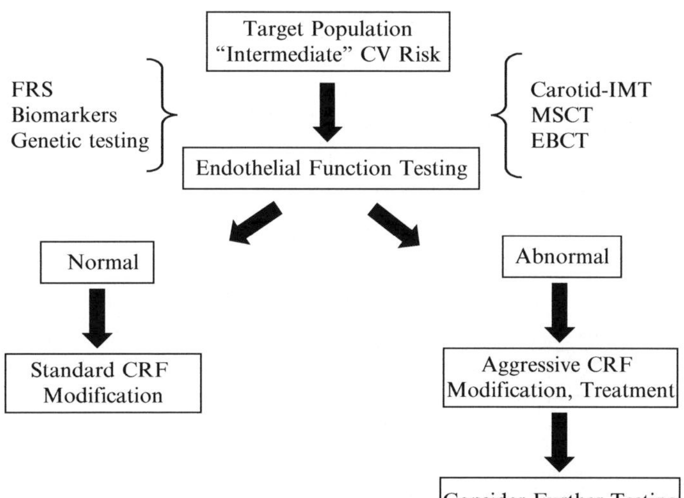

Fig. 2. Potential algorithm for endothelial function testing in clinical practice. For intermediate risk cardiovascular patients, endothelial function testing might be employed in the clinical setting to further determine risk and need for aggressive risk factor control or further cardiovascular testing. *CV* cardiovascular; *FRS* Framingham risk score; *IMT* intima media thickness; *MSCT* multislice computed tomography; *EBCT* electron beam computed tomography; *CRF* cardiovascular risk factor.

Thus far, the methods presently being utilized to evaluate vascular function are primarily used in specialized center involved in clinical research, performed by highly trained technical staff. This presents numerous barriers to incorporating these tests in clinical practice. The lack of standardization of these techniques remains a significant limitation. While manuscripts describing the methodology are common, standardization of the technical aspects of endothelial function testing is lacking [38], which limits the ability to provide comparisons of data between various groups and understanding of what constitutes "normal" vs. "abnormal." Depending on the technique employed, there is often significant variability in data regarding endothelial function. For example, BART is performed with upper arm cuff or forearm occlusion. The amount of ischemia is different with these two techniques and results in varying levels of brachial reactivity and vasodilation. Thus, within this one technique for assessing endothelial function, there are different strategies for achieving reactive hyperemia with significantly different, and uncomparable, results.

In addition to inherent issues with the various techniques, there is physiologic variability in endothelial function testing. Similar to blood pressure and heart rate measurements, the practitioner needs to take issues such as timing, environment, emotions, and other factors, into consideration when analyzing the data. Most of the tests for endothelial function, therefore, are used for their strong negative predictive values. The inconsistency regarding financial reimbursement and the lack of understanding of billing codes for vascular function testing also limit its clinical use and applicability. Societies and professional organizations will need to address these issues, which underscores the potential benefits and utility of routinely testing vascular function.

Other important potential barriers to routine clinical use of endothelial function testing are related to the notion of whether or not it is important to address abnormal endothelial function. While it seems that coronary endothelial function is a predictor of future cardiovascular events, further prognostic data with some of the peripheral vascular techniques, suggesting strong correlations between abnormal endothelial function with increased cardiovascular events, are needed. In addition, while repeat testing of the endothelium might prove valuable in monitoring a patient's response to therapy or intervention, the link between certain therapies and improved cardiovascular endpoints is not always clear. On the one hand, for example, various antioxidant preparations have been linked to enhanced endothelial function; however, large clinical trials have necessarily been able to demonstrate improved clinical outcomes [39, 40]. On the other hand, for example, there is little doubt about the long-term beneficial effects of statin therapy in select patients; however, the effect of this class of medications on endothelial function remains mixed [41]. Thus, there is a complex relationship between endothelial function and cardiovascular outcomes.

Feasibility of performing endothelial function testing is a significant issue when considering these tests for clinical practice. Certainly, given the invasive nature of coronary artery testing as well as infusion of vasoactive medications in the peripheral circulation, these techniques have limited applicability in large populations and will likely not play a major role in routine practice. Thus far, even noninvasive techniques have been performed in research laboratories under highly controlled conditions, in part, due to large equipment size and lack of portability. Thus, with newer technology, some of these barriers seem to be decreasing, thereby perhaps increasing their potential use in clinical practice. Devices that are small and portable enough to be used in the ambulatory clinic setting and might improve the feasibility of endothelial function testing in the ambulatory population are now available. In addition, due to labile changes in endothelial function, in part related to diet, timing of the test, medications, and environmental factors, assessment of vascular endothelial function in a busy outpatient clinic has not seemed appropriate. Some of these perceived barriers, indeed, should not be a hindrance to performing ambulatory testing. For example, the chronic use of vasoactive medications,

Table 1
Peripheral vascular endothelial function testing is feasible in the ambulatory setting

	Non-CAD subjects (n = 28)	*CAD subjects (n = 32)*	*p Value*
Flow-mediated dilation (FMD) of the brachial artery (%)	11.5 ± 0.8	6.8 ± 1.1	0.001
Peripheral arterial tonometry (PAT) hyperemia	2.4 ± 0.1	2.0 ± 0.1	0.02

Relationship between FMD and PAT hyperemia ($p < 0.05$)
FMD Sensitivity for coronary artery disease 83%, negative predictive value 74%
PAT Sensitivity for coronary artery disease 92%, negative predictive value 78%

particularly non-nitrates, has been shown to have no significant effect on brachial artery function, suggesting that it is not necessary to withhold most cardiac medications prior to endothelial function testing [42] (Table 1).

Our group has performed a study to evaluate the role of noninvasive vascular testing in the large and small vessels of the upper extremity in the ambulatory clinic population. We determined that both BART and PAT hyperemia, tested in the clinic, correlated with the extent of cardiovascular risk and the presence or absence of coronary artery disease [43]. In addition, we noted that ambulatory flow-mediated dilation of the brachial artery as well as PAT hyperemia correlated with each other. None of the clinic patients had prior knowledge they were going to undergo vascular function testing prior to their arrival in clinic; thus, they did not hold their cardioactive medications or limit their food intake. Thus, studies such as this support the potential use of noninvasive vascular endothelial function testing in ambulatory populations.

ENDOTHELIAL FUNCTION TESTING IN THE CLINIC: ARE WE THERE YET?

It is well accepted that coronary and peripheral endothelial function testing represent a gage of vascular health, and impaired vasomotion is important to the pathogenesis and prognosis of cardiovascular disease. There are many attractive features for performing ambulatory physiologic testing of vascular function, and the methodology is evolving toward user-friendly applications. Endothelial function testing must compete with other noninvasive tests, such as quantification of coronary calcification by electron-beam computed tomography [44] and measurement of carotid artery intima-media thickness [45], which focus more on vascular anatomy than physiology. As the technology advances and data evolve linking changes in endothelial function to clinical improvement and better cardiovascular outcomes, it is likely that endothelial function testing will gain in popularity for the identification of cardiovascular risk, especially asymptomatic individuals yet who do not qualify for medical therapy according to present guidelines [46, 47].

ACKNOWLEDGMENTS

Dr. Kuvin has received research grants from SonoSite, Inc. and Itamar-Medical, Inc. manufacturers of noninvasive monitoring devices to assess endothelial function.

REFERENCES

1. Ludmer P, Selwyn A, Shook T, et al. Paradoxical vasoconstriction induced by acetylcholine in atherosclerotic coronary arteries. N Engl J Med. 1986;315:1046–1051.
2. Neunteufl T, Katzenschlager R, Hassan A, et al. Systemic endothelial dysfunction is related to the extent and severity of coronary artery disease. Atherosclerosis. 1997;129:111–118.
3. Suwaidi J, Hamasaki S, Higano S, et al. Long-term follow-up of patients with mild coronary artery disease and endothelial dysfunction. Circulation. 2000;101:948–954.
4. Schachinger V, Britten M, Zeiher A. Prognostic impact of coronary vasodilator dysfunction on adverse long-term outcome of coronary heart disease. Circulation. 2000;101:1899–1906.
5. Halcox J, Schenke W, Zalos G, et al. Prognostic value of coronary vascular endothelial dysfunction. Circulation. 2002;106:653–658.
6. Corretti M, Anderson T, Benjamin E, et al. Guidelines for the ultrasound assessment of endothelial-dependent flow-mediated vasodilation of the brachial artery. J Am Coll Cardiol. 2002;39:257–265.
7. Rubenfire M. Rajagopalan S. Mosca L. Carotid artery vasoreactivity in response to sympathetic stress correlates with coronary disease risk and is independent of wall thickness. J Am Coll Cardiol. 2000;36:2192–2197.
8. Celermajer DS, Sorensen KE, Gooch VM, et al. Non-invasive detection of endothelial dysfunction in children and adults at risk of atherosclerosis. Lancet. 1992;340:1111–1115.
9. Kuvin J, Patel R, Sliney K, et al. Peripheral vascular endothelial function testing as a non-invasive indicator of coronary artery disease. J Am Coll Cardiol. 2001;38;1843–1849.
10. Neunteufl T, Heher S, Katzenschlager R, et al. Long-term prognostic value of flow-mediated dilation in the brachial artery of patients with chest pain. Am J Cardiol. 2000;86:207–210.
11. Gokce N, Keaney J, Hunter L, et al. Risk stratification for postoperative cardiovascular events via noninvasive assessment of endothelial function. Circulation. 2002;105:1567–1572.
12. Gokce N, Keaney JF Jr, Hunter LM, et al. Predictive value of noninvasively determined endothelial dysfunction for long-term cardiovascular events in patients with peripheral vascular disease. J Am Coll Cardiol. 2003;41:1769–1775.
13. Heitzer T, Baldus S, von Kodolitsch Y, Rudolph V, Meinertz T. Systemic endothelial dysfunction as an early predictor of adverse outcome in heart failure. Arterioscler Thromb Vasc Biol. 2005;25:1174–1179.
14. Suessenbacher A, Frick M, Alber HF, Barbieri V, Pachinger O, Weidinger F. Association of improvement of brachial artery flow-mediated vasodilation with cardiovascular events. Vasc Med. 2006;11:239–244.
15. Gatto NM, Hodis HN, Liu CR, Liu CH, Mack WJ. Brachial artery vasoreactivity is associated with cross-sectional and longitudinal anatomical measures of atherosclerosis in postmenopausal women with coronary artery disease. Atherosclerosis. 2008;196:674–681.
16. Patel AR, Kuvin JT, Sliney KA, et al. Gender-based differences in brachial artery flow-mediated vasodilation as an indicator of significant coronary artery disease. Am J Cardiol. 2005;96:1223–1236.
17. Rossi R, Nuzzo A, Origliani G, Modena MG. Prognostic role of flow-mediated dilation and cardiac risk factors in post-menopausal women. J Am Coll Cariol. 2008;51:997–1002.
18. Modena M, Bonetti L, Coppi F, et al. Prognostic role of reversible endothelial dysfunction in hypertensive postmenopausal women. J Am Coll Cardiol. 2002;40:505–510.
19. Heitzer T, Schlinzig T, Krohn K, et al. Endothelial dysfunction, oxidative stress, and risk of cardiovascular events in patients with coronary artery disease. Circulation. 2001;104:2673–2678.
20. Perticone F, Ceravolo R, Pujia A, et al. Prognostic significance of endothelial dysfunction in hypertensive patients. Circulation. 2001;104:191–196.
21. Carter, S. Indirect systolic pressures and pulse waves in arterial occlusive diseases in the lower extremities. Circulation. 1968;37:624–638.
22. Hedblad, B, Ogren, M, Isacsson, S-O, et al. Low pulse wave amplitude during reactive leg hyperemia: an independent early marker for ischaemic heart disease and death. Results from the 21-year follow-up of the prospective cohort study 'Men born in 1914', Malmo, Sweden. J Int Med. 1994;236:161–168.
23. Kuvin J, Patel A, Sliney K, et al. Assessment of peripheral vascular endothelial function with finger arterial pulse wave amplitude. Am Heart J. 2003;146:168–174.
24. Bonetti PO, Pumper GM, Higano ST, Holmes DR, Kuvin JT, Lerman A. Noninvasive identification of patients with early coronary atherosclerosis by assessment of digital reactive hyperemia. J Am Coll Cardiol. 2004;44:2137–2141.
25. Nohria A, Gerhard-Herman M, Creager MA, Hurley S, Mitra D, Ganz P. The role of nitric oxide in the regulation of digital pulse volume amplitude in humans. J Appl Physiol. 2006;101:545–548.
26. Bonetti P, Barsness G, Keelan P, et al. Enhanced external counterpulsation improves endothelial function in patients with symptomatic coronary artery disease. J Am Coll Cardiol. 2003;41:1761–1768.
27. Hamburg N, Keyes M, Larson MG, et al. Digital microvascular function is related to cardiovascular risk factors in the community: The Framingham Heart Study. Circulation. 2007;116:II–846.
28. Fisher ND, Hughes M, Gerhard-Herman M, Hollenberg NK. Flavanol-rich cocoa induces nitric-oxide-dependent vasodilation in healthy humans. J Hypertens. 2003;21:2281–2286.

29. Nurnberger J, Keflioglu-Scheiber A, Opazo Saez AM, Wenzel RR, Philipp T, Schafers RF. Augmentation index is associated with cardiovascular risk. J Hypertens. 2002;20:2407–2414.
30. Covic A, Goldsmith DJ, Panaghiu L, Covic M, Sedor J. Analysis of the effect of hemodialysis on peripheral and central arterial pressure waveforms. Kidney Int. 2000;57:2634–2643.
31. The CAFÉ Investigators. Differential impact of blood pressure-lowering drugs on central aortic pressure and clinical outcomes: principal results from the Conduit Artery Function Evaluation (CAFÉ) study. Circulation. 2006;113:1213–1225.
32. Parker C, Vita JA, Freedman JE. Soluble adhesion molecules and unstable coronary artery disease. Atherosclerosis. 2001;156:417–424.
33. Ridker PM, Rifai N, Rose L, Burning JE, Cook NR. Comparison of C-reactive protein and low-density lipoprotein cholesterol levels in the prediction of first cardiovascular events. N Engl J Med. 2002;347:1557–1565.
34. Rodriguez-Plaza LG, Alfieri AB, Cubeddu LX. Urinary excretion of nitric oxide metabolites in runners, sedentary individuals and patients with coronary artery disease: effects of 42 km marathon, 15 km racc and a cardiac rehabilitation program. J Cardiovasc Risk. 1997;4:367–372.
35. Hill JM, Zalos G, Halcox JP, et al. Circulating endothelial progenitor cells, vascular function, and cardiovascular risk. N Engl J Med. 2003;348:593–600.
36. Kuvin J, Karas R. The clinical utility of vascular endothelial function testing: ready for prime-time? Circulation. 2003;107:3243–3247.
37. Soman P, Dave DM, Udelson JE, et al.Vascular endothelial dysfunction is associated with reversible myocardial perfusion defects in the absence of obstructive coronary artery disease. J Nucl Cardiol. 2006;13:756–760.
38. Kuvin J, Patel A, Karas R. Need for standardization of non-invasive assessment of vascular endothelial function. Am Heart J. 2001;141:327–328.
39. Chauhan A, More RS, Mullins PA, et al. Aging-associated endothelial dysfunction in humans is reversed by l-arginine. J Am Coll Cardiol. 1996;28:1796–1804.
40. Quyyumi AA. Does acute improvement of endothelial dysfunction in coronary artery disease improve myocardial ischemia? A double-blind comparison of parenteral d- and l-arginine. J Am Coll Cardiol. 1998;32:904–911.
41. Vita JA, Yeung AC, Winniford M, et al. Effect of cholesterol-lowering therapy on coronary endothelial vasomotor function in patients with coronary artery disease. Circulation. 2000;102:846–851.
42. Gokce N, Holbrook M, Hunter LM, et al. Acute effects of vasoactive drug treatment on brachial artery reactivity. J Am Coll Cardiol. 2002;40:761–765.
43. Kuvin JT, Mammen A, Mooney P, Alsheikh-Ali AA, Karas RH. Assessment of peripheral vascular endothelial function in the ambulatory setting. Vasc Med. 2007;12:13–16.
44. Keelan P, Bielak L, Ashai K, et al. Long-term prognostic value of coronary calcification detected by electron-beam computed tomography in patients undergoing coronary angiography. Circulation. 2001;104:412–417.
45. O'Leary D, Polak J, Kronmal R, et al. Carotid-artery intima and media thickness as a risk factor for myocardial infarction and stroke in older adults. N Engl J Med. 1999;340:12–22.
46. Naghavi M, Falk E, Hecht HS, et al. SHAPE Task Force. From vulnerable plaque to vulnerable patient – Part III: Executive summary of the Screening for Heart Attack Prevention and Education (SHAPE) Task Force report. Am J Cardiol. 2006;98:2H–15H.
47. Napoli C, Lerman LO, de Nigris F, Gossl M, Balestrieri ML, Lerman A. Rethinking primary prevention of atherosclerosis-related diseases. Circulation. 2006;114:2517–2527.

18 Digital (Fingertip) Thermal Monitoring of Vascular Function: A Novel, Noninvasive, Nonimaging Test to Improve Traditional Cardiovascular Risk Assessment and Monitoring of Response to Treatments

Matthew Budoff, Naser Ahmadi, Stanley Kleis, Wasy Akhtar, Gary McQuilkin, Khawar Gul, Timothy O'Brien, Craig Jamieson, Haider Hassan, David Panthagani, Albert Yen, Ralph Metcalfe, and Morteza Naghavi

CONTENTS

From: *Asymptomatic Atherosclerosis: Pathophysiology, Detection and Treatment*
Edited by: M. Naghavi (ed.), DOI 10.1007/978-1-60327-179-0_18

Abstract

Digital thermal monitoring (DTM) is a noninvasive, inexpensive, easily performed, operator-independent vascular function test designed to complement the existing, risk-factor based assessment of vascular health and to monitor the vascular response to therapies. It is similar to a blood pressure device, with the addition of adhesive temperature probes on the right and left index fingertips that measure fingertip temperature fall and rebound during a brief (2–5 min), arm-cuff occlusion, and release procedure (reactive hyperemia). The higher the temperature rebound, the better the vascular reactivity. In our studies, we have found that DTM indices of vascular reactivity correlate strongly with the number of cardiovascular risk factors, measured by the Framingham Risk Score (FRS), and with the burden of asymptomatic (subclinical) coronary atherosclerosis, measured by coronary calcium score and CT angiography, as well as with myocardial perfusion defects on nuclear stress testing in symptomatic subjects. Moreover, our studies have shown that DTM provides incremental predictive value over risk factor assessment for the identification of high-risk patients with both subclinical atherosclerosis (Coronary Artery Calcium Score ≥100) and coronary artery stenosis (CT angiography showing ≥50% stenosis). Finally, DTM indices of vascular function have shown reproducibility comparable to blood pressure measurements. These very promising findings will require corroboration, particularly in long-term, prospective studies and clinical trials. It is important to emphasize that DTM is not intended to replace measurement of risk factors or advanced imaging tests. Rather, its purpose is to complement them by providing a powerful, noninvasive vascular function assessment of coronary health.

Key words: Digital (fingertip) thermal monitoring (DTM); Framingham risk score; Coronary calcium score; Vascular function; Endothelial dysfunction; Reactive hyperemia; Vascular reactivity

KEY POINTS

- DTM is a new, noninvasive, nonimaging vascular function test based on monitoring fingertip temperature during an arm-cuff induced reactive hyperemia test.
- Fingertip temperature drops during cuff occlusion and rebounds after releasing the cuff. The higher the temperature rebound (TR), the better the vascular function.
- Lower fingertip temperature rebound is associated with higher burden of cardiovascular risk factors measured by Framingham Risk Score (FRS).
- Lower fingertip temperature rebound is associated with higher burden of atherosclerotic plaques measured by coronary artery calcium score.
- The combination of low fingertip temperature rebound and high Framingham risk score (FRS) provides a larger area under the ROC curve compared with either TR or FRS alone for detection of both nonobstructive and obstructive coronary artery disease.
- These findings are promising and require corroboration by other cardiovascular researchers.

RISK ASSESSMENT FOR PRIMARY PREVENTION OF CVD

The majority of people with cardiovascular disease have no symptoms; however, it is well known that the cardiovascular disease epidemic will result in 30% of *all* global deaths [1]. It is vital to determine those who are on the path to cardiovascular disease, *before* their symptoms present themselves. In addition, these asymptomatic patients are not receiving pharmacological therapies as part of a preventative regimen.

RISK FACTOR MEASUREMENT – FRAMINGHAM RISK SCORE

All major advisory bodies, including the American Heart Association and European Society of Cardiology, advocate traditional risk factor approaches in identifying asymptomatic individuals at high risk of developing CHD, as well as determining the aggressiveness of treatment in these individuals. These approaches incorporate traditional risk factors, such as the patient's age, sex, and the presence and extent of established, modifiable coronary risk factors – hypertension, hyperlipidemia, diabetes mellitus, cigarette smoking – in the prediction and reduction of coronary risk. A 10-year risk of myocardial infarction/CHD death can be predicted for a given patient based on these major risk factors. Asymptomatic patients are generally categorized as low (<10%), intermediate (10–20%), or high risk (>20%), based upon their respective scores [3]. According to these guidelines, low-risk patients can be reassured and educated about therapeutic lifestyle changes. Intermediate-risk patients may require further risk stratification, and high-risk patients should be considered candidates for aggressive pharmacological and lifestyle intervention.

While the use of office-based risk equations, such as the FRS, is the generally recommended approach to cardiovascular risk screening [2], it is not without shortcomings as a screening tool and seems to significantly underestimate risk in women and younger individuals. In a retrospective study, Akosah et al. showed that among adults aged <65 years with an acute MI with no previous history of CHD, only 25% of patients would have met the criteria for preventive treatment based on the FRS, had they presented 1 day before this event. The tendency of an FRS-based approach to underappreciate the risk of CHD was even more pronounced in women, with only 18% of women qualifying for pharmacotherapy for primary prevention: 58% of these patients had LDL-C < 130 mg/dl, and 40% had LDL-C < 100 mg/dl [4] (Fig. 1).

HOW CAN WE IMPROVE ON CURRENT PRACTICES OF CARDIOVASCULAR RISK ASSESSMENT?

Efforts have been made to develop noninvasive diagnostic tools to help determine the extent of underlying subclinical diseases atherosclerosis in asymptomatic patients. Improved precision in detecting these high-risk individuals may aid in more targeted preventive therapy.

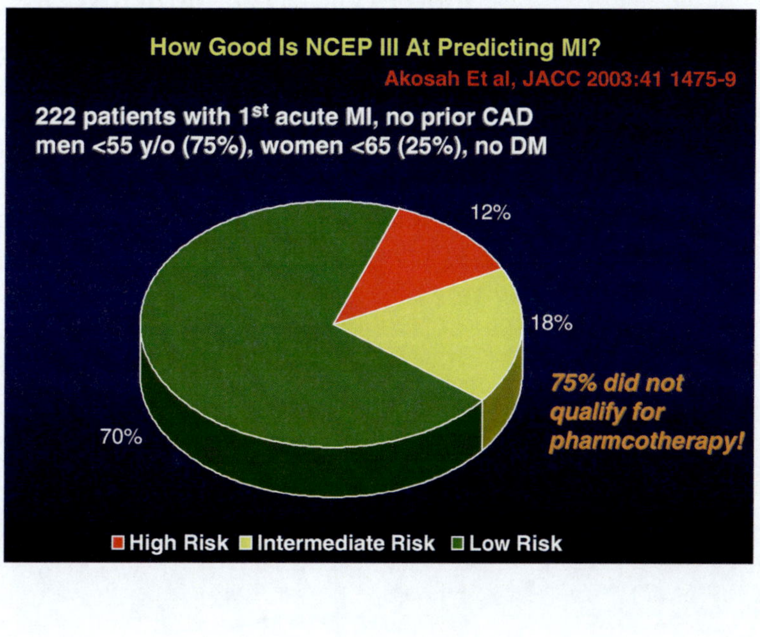

Fig. 1. Risk assessment based solely on risk factors misclassifies patients at immediate risk of coronary events.

ATHEROSCLEROTIC PLAQUE MEASUREMENT (IMAGING)

To go beyond risk factors in the assessment of the asymptomatic population, screening for subclinical atherosclerosis has been proposed. The assessment of an individual's vascular structure, which itself is representative of the accumulation of risk factors and their interaction with protective factors, is seen to be advantageous, i.e., looking at an individual's actual vasculature rather than an estimation of future cardiovascular risk based on epidemiological studies and risk calculators. A structural assessment of subclinical plaque is achieved with *imaging* modalities.

CORONARY ARTERY CALCIUM SCORE

One way to detect subclinical atherosclerosis is by measuring the coronary artery calcium (CAC) using either electron Beam Computed Tomography (EBCT) or multidetector CT (MDCT). A strong relationship ($r = 0.8–0.9$) between CAC measured by CT with histologic plaque areas at autopsy, both in whole arteries and whole hearts, has been established [5]. According to ACC/AHA guidelines, there is a graded increased in risk of CHD events in the range of 4–11 times if CAC score ranges from 100 to >1,000, compared to those without any CAC [6]. In addition, those with absent CAC have a very low rate of CHD death or MI (0.4%) over 3 to 5 years of observation [6].

CIMT

Carotid Intima Media Thickness, CIMT, refers to an imaging test of the carotid artery. A high-resolution b-mode ultrasound transducer is placed on the neck, and the carotid artery is imaged by a sonographer. From the resulting image, the thickness of the intim-a and media layers, those between the adventitia and lumen, of the artery, as well as the presence of any plaques are measured.

It has been shown that an increased carotid intima-medial thickness is associated with increased risk factors, and can be used as an indicator of generalized atherosclerosis [7, 14]. The advantages are its totally noninvasive nature and lack of radiation exposure.

LIMITATIONS OF IMAGING MODALITIES

The limitations of imaging modalities which are used in screening for subclinical atherosclerosis are many. CT scanning of coronary artery calcium poses hazardous radiation and the cost is high. In addition, the CT scanning of coronary calcium will not display any regression of plaques, only the slowing or halting of progression; thus, using it to monitor the effect of therapy is not ideal.

Carotid intima media thickness (CIMT) requires an expensive ultrasound device and, perhaps more importantly, a skilled ultrasonographer to perform the technique. Because of the dependence on a human operator as well as the low resolution of the ultrasound imaging, the procedure is prone to misclassifications.

BIOMARKERS

Recent advances in assay development have witnessed the introduction of cardiac risk in vitro diagnostics (blood tests) assessing risk factors such as hsCRP (high sensitivity C-reactive protein), fibrinogen, homocysteine, inflammation markers, blood coagulation markers, and genetic markers

HS-CRP

High sensitivity C-reactive Protein is an acute phase protein which has been most widely studied for risk of future CHD. In systemic inflammation, levels of hs-CRP are raised. Blood assays are available to measure the levels of hs-CRP and in turn be used as an aid in the prediction of cardiovascular disease. Some studies have found that the higher the hs-CRP levels, the higher the risk of having a heart attack [9]. However these findings have not been replicated in all studies. In fact, when all the established cardiovascular risk factors are controlled, there is no additional benefit for assessment of this inflammatory biomarker. Although it has been postulated that it will guide lipid-lowering therapy among those with normal cholesterol, the results of the trial are awaited to establish its potential role in primary CHD preventive strategies.

LP-PLA2

Lipoprotein-associated phospholipase A2 is an enzyme which has been identified as another novel risk factor. However, unlike hs-CRP, LP-PLA2 assays report consistent values that do not typically fluctuate during acute systemic inflammation. The enzyme is involved in the formation of vulnerable plaques and has been shown to be an independent predictor of stroke, even after adjusting for traditional risk factors [10]. Similarly, it has been found to identify future risk independent of all risk factors in an elderly population [10]. Whether this would identify a younger, at high-risk patient population in whom preemptive employment of preventive medication will reduce long-term CHD risk is yet to be determined.

VASCULAR FUNCTION MEASUREMENT CAN COMPLEMENT STRUCTURAL/ ANATOMICAL ASSESSMENT

It is logical that a structural assessment alone, such as those performed with imaging modalities, is not sufficient to predict the true risk of any patient. These structural assessments require a complementary component which can describe an individual's *vascular function.* Thus, the quest began for a vascular function assessment methodology, one which would interrogate the vessels themselves and observe their reaction in order to quantify their function (Fig. 2).

VASCULAR REACTIVITY AND ENDOTHELIAL FUNCTION

The endothelium, the monocellular inner layer of blood vessels, is a key player in vascular biology. The endothelium not only acts as a barrier, but regulates transport into smooth muscles surrounding blood vessels and controls vascular homeostasis.

However, in the presence of aforementioned cardiovascular risk factors, the endothelial layer facilitates inflammation, thrombosis, and vascular constriction. The endothelium can be considered as a barometer for cardiovascular disease [11] (Fig. 3).

Vascular reactivity is a vital component of vascular function that enables the circulatory system to respond to physiologic and pharmacologic stimuli that require adjustments of blood flow and alterations of vessel tone and diameter. Vascular reactivity occurs in two forms – vasoconstrictive and vasodilative – and can be exhibited at both the macrovascular and the microvascular levels.

"Macrovascular" pertains to large, conduit arteries with an internal diameter greater than 100 microns. "Microvascular" refers to small, resistance vessels (precapillary arterioles) with an internal diameter of less than 100 microns. It is estimated that the microvasculature accounts for over 95% of the total body vasculature.

Fig. 2. Methods of screening for atherosclerosis. From Naghavi et al., American Journal of Cardiology, 2006.

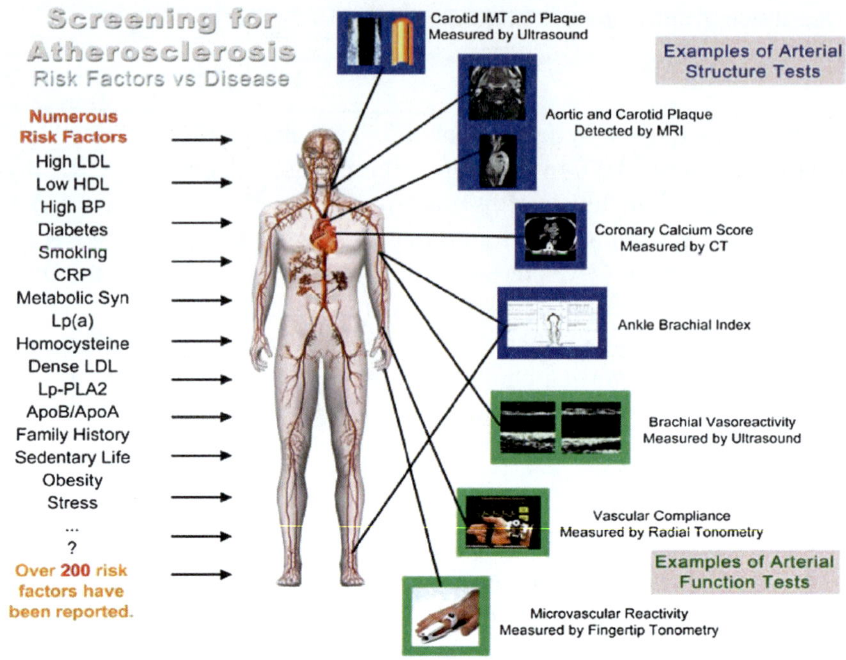

Fig. 3. Clinical conditions associated with vascular dysfunction.

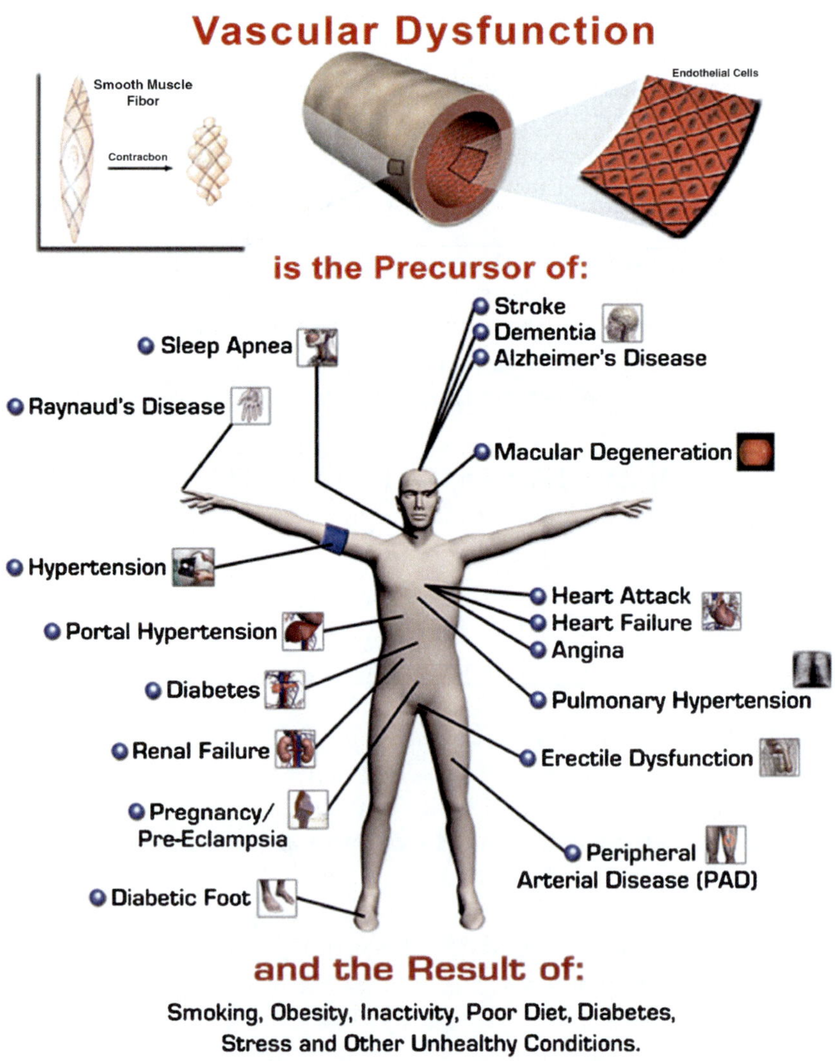

Microvascular reactivity (here, vasodilative reactivity) *causes* reactive hyperemia (increased blood flow in response to ischemia or similar pharmacologic stimuli), whereas macrovascular reactivity (flow mediated dilatation, or FMD) results *from* reactive hyperemia. Both macro- and microvascular reactivity are governed by multiple physiologic (endothelium-dependent and -independent) regulatory mechanisms and are mediated by a number of biochemical agents, such as nitric oxide (NO), endothelium-derived hyperpolarizing factor (EDHF), prostaglandins, adenosine, bradykinin, histamine, and other vasoactive substances. It is believed that macrovascular reactivity is predominantly mediated by endothelium-derived NO, whereas microvascular reactivity is only partially mediated by NO. Traditionally, assessment of macrovascular reactivity (FMD) at the brachial artery level by high-resolution ultrasound imaging has been described as an endothelial function test. However, some key opinion leaders believe that "endothelial function" is a misnomer because endothelial cells have numerous functions. Moreover, endothelial cells exist in all vascular beds and play critical roles at both macro- and microvascular levels.

DIGITAL THERMAL MONITORING (DTM)

Digital thermal monitoring (DTM) is a novel, noninvasive, nonimaging test of vascular reactivity. This simple yet promising technique of measuring vascular function is anticipated to yield information relevant to improving risk stratification and monitoring response to therapies. Therapies are currently being targeted at improving vascular function, and physicians are seeking biomarkers which will aid in the assessment of this vascular response. However, the aforementioned techniques are limited either by their operator dependence or their cost and are confined to the research setting. DTM brings vascular function assessment to clinical practice and enables the move from "bench to bedside."

DTM monitors, records, and analyzes fingertip temperature, which serves as a surrogate marker of blood flow changes that result from vascular reactivity. DTM operates on the premise that temperature can be used as a surrogate marker of blood flow, as blood itself is the source of heat. The skin surface is a window to the function of the cutaneous microvessels. The finger was chosen as the site of measurement for several reasons: (1) it is distal to cuff occlusion at the elbow or even at the wrist, (2) the fingers are highly vascularized, and thus representative of this vast, cutaneous vascular bed, and (3) the high surface area to mass ratio means that changes in temperature are amplified and well pronounced.

The DTM test begins with an automated blood pressure measurement in the left arm, followed by a period of suprasystolic cuff occlusion of the right arm (usually 5 min). During the cuff occlusion, fingertip temperature in the right hand falls because of the absence of warm circulating blood. The occlusion of blood flow elicits a vasodilatory response in the ischemic area. Once the cuff is released, blood flow rushes into the forearm and hand, causing a temperature rebound (TR) in the fingertip which is directly proportional to the reactive hyperemia response. The higher the temperature rebound, the better the vascular reactivity (Figs. 4 and 5).

BRACHIAL ARTERY ULTRASOUND (BAUS/BART)

In 1992, Celermajer and colleagues developed the technique of Brachial Artery Ultrasound (BAUS or BART) to measure flow-mediated dilation (FMD) of the brachial artery by ultrasound imaging, which they described to be a measure of endothelial function [12]. Brachial artery imaging with high-resolution ultrasound during reactive hyperemia has been widely studied in experimental settings to determine peripheral vascular function in various studies. In the procedure of cuff reactive hyperemia, an upper arm cuff is inflated above systolic blood pressure to occlude arterial inflow and briefly render the forearm and hand ischemic (blood- and oxygen-deprived). After the cuff is released, blood

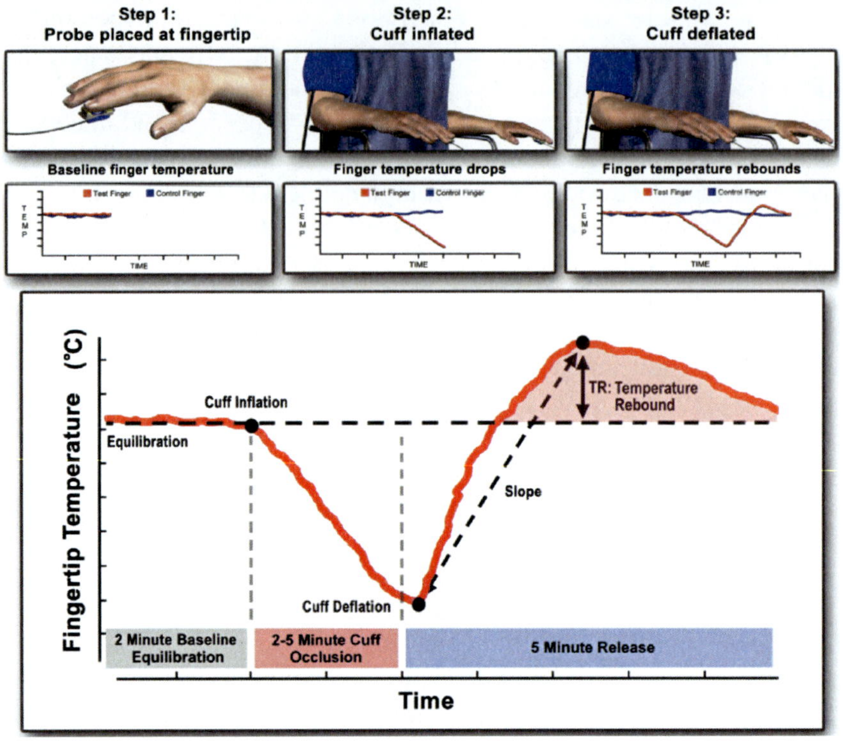

Fig. 4. An illustration of Digital Thermal Monitoring (DTM) of Vascular Reactivity.

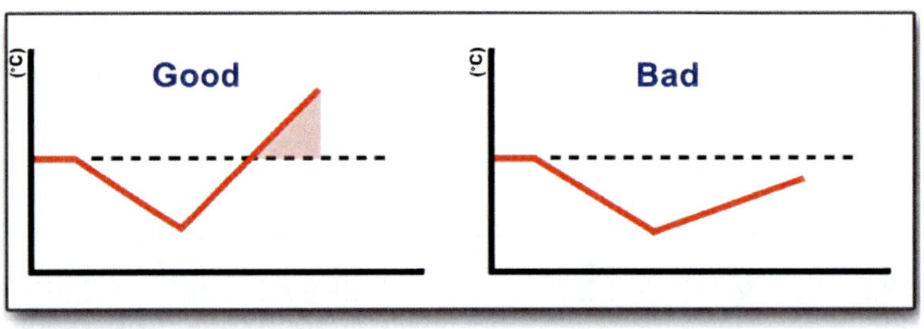

Fig. 5. Schematic graphs of Digital Thermal Monitoring (DTM) of vascular reactivity shows the higher the fingertip temperature rebound the better the vascular function.

enters the distal part of the arm at a rate determined by the relaxant capacity of the microvessels. In turn, the resultant bolus of blood causes shear stress to be applied to the endothelium of the macroconduit arteries, resulting in the release of nitric oxide and arterial dilatation. However, because of the difficulty of the technique, the price of the device (approx. \$150,000 for an imaging ultrasound device) and the dependence on a skilled operator, the brachial artery ultrasound technique has been confined to the research laboratory. In addition, this technique has poor reproducibility, limiting its clinical utility.

LASER DOPPLER FLOWMETRY

Rather than focusing on the response of large blood vessels to cuff occlusion, other methods have been developed that use micro (small)-vessel function as the indicator of overall blood vessel function; one such method is laser Doppler flowmetry (LDF). The skin surface is a window to measure microvessels and their function. However, similar to the previously mentioned BAUS technique, LDF has mostly been confined to research labs because it is quite costly and the measurement process is very slow and very dependent on precise probe location.

Several studies have shown that skin temperature (measured by DTM) correlates strongly with skin blood flow (measured by LDF). However, unlike LDF, which is sensitive to red blood cell motion only at the skin level (1–2 mm depth), DTM temperature signals can reflect blood flow changes in both skin and subcutaneous tissues simply because the heat from the inrush of warm blood travels from deep tissues to the skin surface. Also, LDF is markedly sensitive to any movement at the measurement site, whereas DTM is not affected by finger motion.

PERIPHERAL ARTERIAL TONOMETRY

The PAT device measures a pulse amplitude signal, termed peripheral arterial tonometry PAT. One study reported a significant correlation between PAT signals and coronary endothelial function [13]. Although both PAT and DTM measure vascular reactivity at the fingertip and employ a similar cuff-induced reactive hyperemia procedure, the PAT probe includes a fingertip cuff that obstructs microvasculature at the point of measurement; therefore, PAT may not be able to accurately evaluate microvascular reactivity at the fingertip. Studies have shown a modest correlation ($r=0.29$, $p=0.01$) between PAT reactive hyperemia index (RHI) and DTM temperature rebound (TR).

ADVANTAGES OF DTM OVER RESEARCH MODALITIES

Using simple skin temperature measurements as a surrogate for blood flow instead of costly imaging methods enables the science to move "from bench to bedside." Furthermore, the operator-independent procedure allows for the potential of using DTM as a screening device [14]. By removing the imaging component, reducing the cost, and omitting the dependence on a skilled operator, the development of the DTM device will allow the measurement of vascular function to be moved out of the research laboratory and into mainstream clinical practice. In addition, when measuring physical parameters, temperature measurements are the easiest, least expensive, and least prone to error.

CLINICAL UTILITY OF DTM

Research studies [16–27] have found DTM indices of vascular reactivity to correlate strongly with:

- Burden of cardiovascular risk factors, measured by Framingham Risk Score (Fig. 6)
- Burden of subclinical coronary atherosclerosis, measured by coronary calcium score (Fig. 7 and Fig. 8)
- Degree of coronary stenosis, measured by coronary CT angiography (Fig. 9)

Moreover, DTM has been shown to provide incremental predictive value over risk assessment (measured by Framingham Risk Score) for identification of high-risk asymptomatic patients (Fig. 10), and to predict response to therapy at 12-month follow up (Fig. 11)

Finally, DTM indices displayed

- Intraindividual reproducibility comparable to blood pressure measurements (Fig. 12)
- How Reproducible Are DTM DTM Results? (Intraindividual and Interobserver Variability)

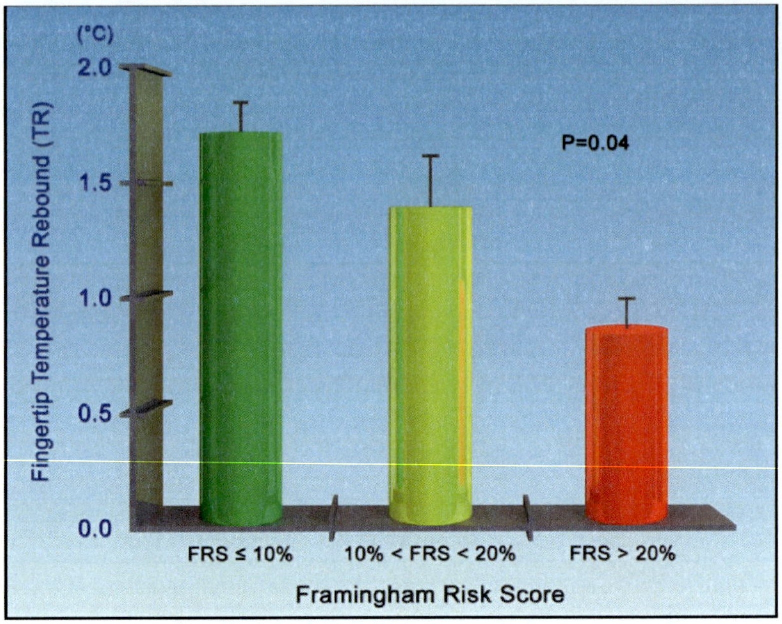

Fig. 6. Lower fingertip temperature rebound (TR) is associated with higher burden of cardiovascular risk factors measured by Framingham risk score (FRS).

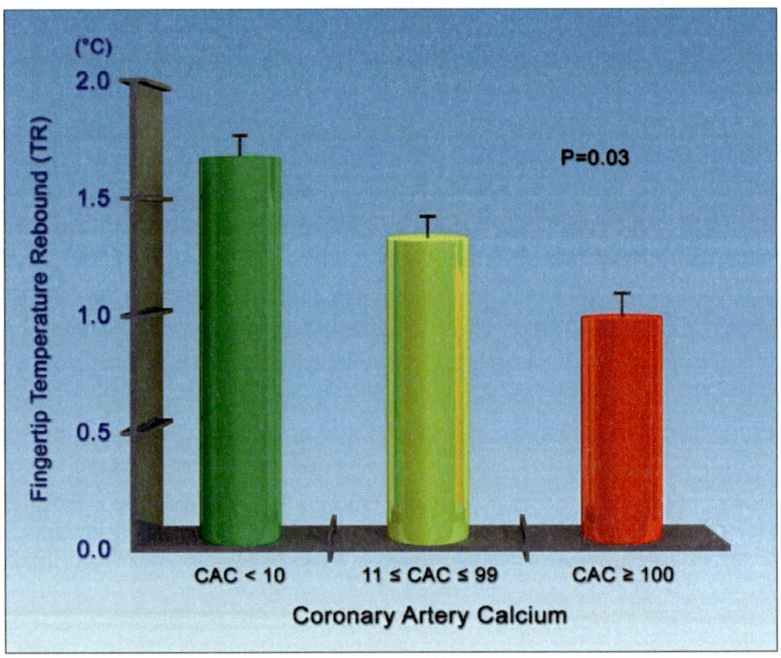

Fig. 7. Lower fingertip temperature rebound (TR) is associated with higher burden of atherosclerotic plaques measured by coronary artery calcium (CAC) score.

Our intraindividual repeatability studies (24-h interval) in apparently healthy individuals have shown that DTM parameters, TR (temperature rebound) and AUC (Area Under Curve), are reproducible when performed under the recommended standard test conditions [25–27]. The coefficient of variation (CV) was 5.7% for temperature rebound (TR), 8.7% for mean arterial pressure (MAP), and 11.4% for heart rate (HR). These data indicate that TR reproducibility fits within the accepted reproducibility range for methods that have been widely adopted in clinical practice, namely blood pressure and heart rate.

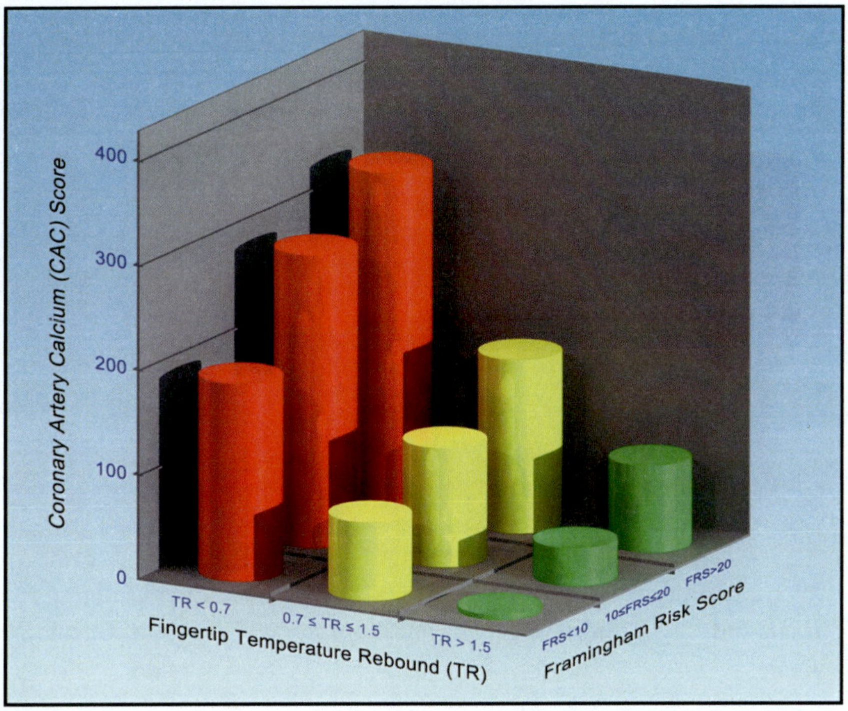

Fig. 8. The combination of lower fingertip temperature rebound and high Framingham Risk Score is associated with high risk coronary artery calcium score.

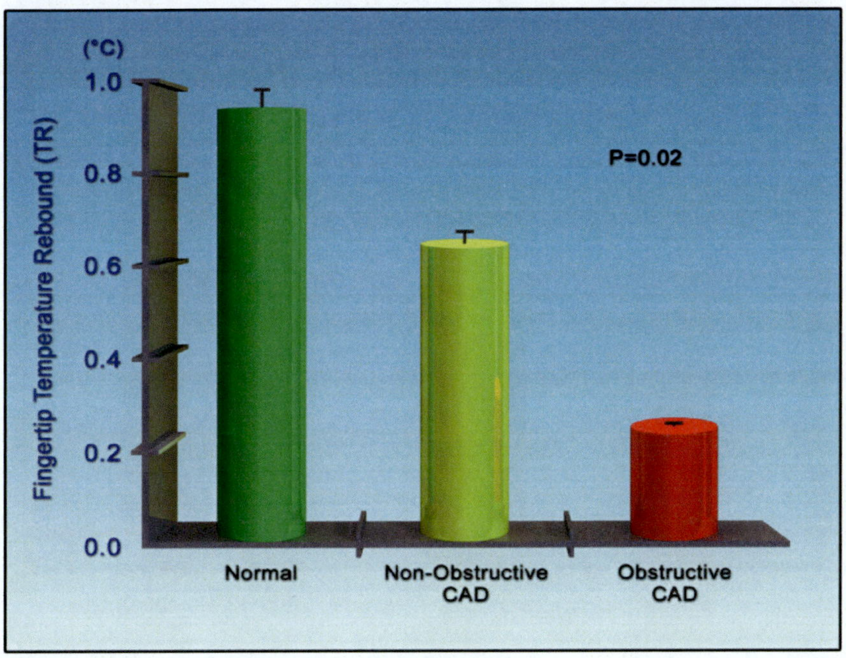

Fig. 9. In patients with chest discomfort, low fingertip temperature rebound (TR) is associated with coronary artery disease diagnosed by CT angiography.

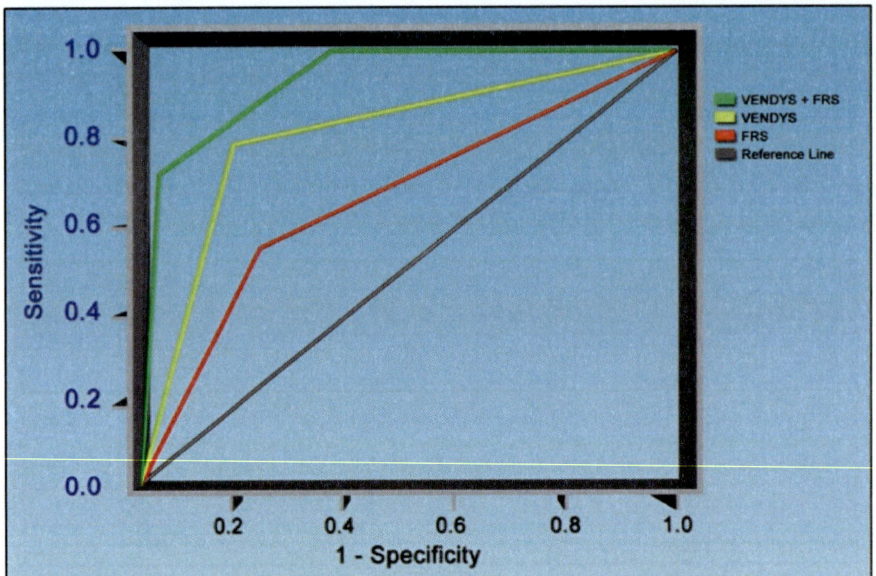

Variable	AUC ± S.D.	95% CI	P (compared to FRS)
VENDYS + FRS	0.89 (0.02)	0.84 - 0.93	0.001
VENDYS	0.79 (0.03)	0.72 - 0.84	0.001
FRS	0.66 (0.04)	0.57 - 0.77	---

Fig. 10. The combination of low fingertip temperature rebound (TR) and high Framingham risk score (FRS) provides larger area under the ROC curve compared to either TR or FRS alone.

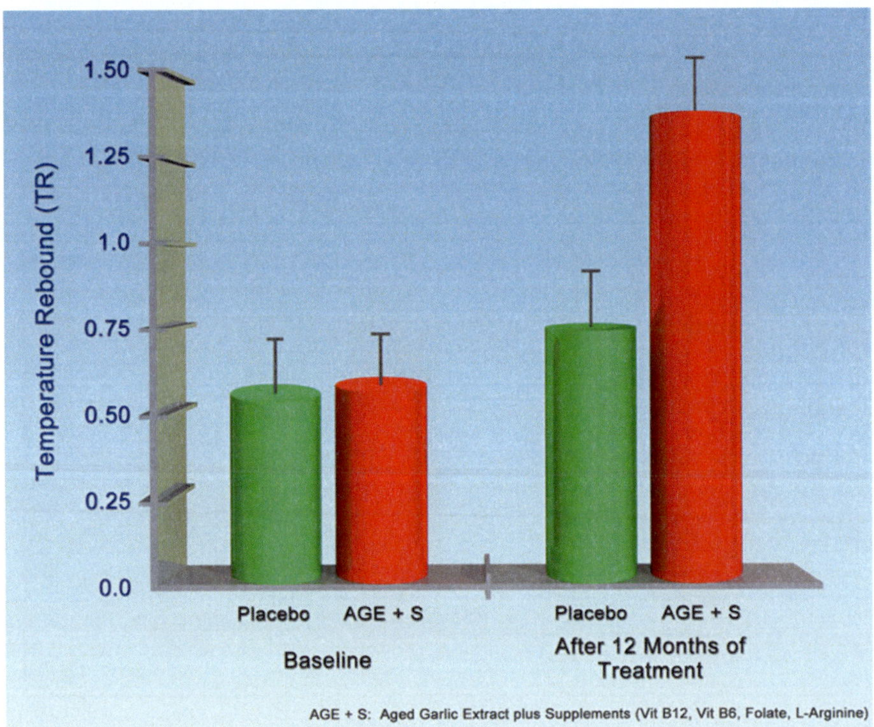

Fig. 11. One year treatment with Aged Garlic Extract was associated with lower coronary calcium progression and higher fingertip temperature rebound.

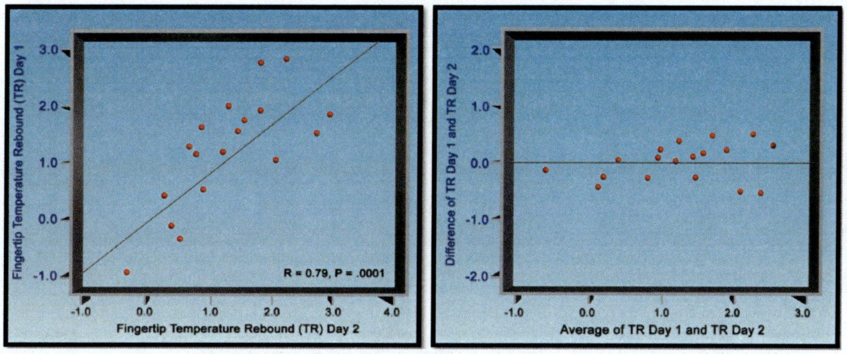

Fig. 12. Correlation plot (*left*) and Bland Altman graph (*right*) of TR values obtained 24 h apart.

Table 1
Digital thermal monitoring (DTM) indices of vascular function are reproducible and comparable to those of blood pressure measurements

Variable	*D*	SD_D	*CV (%)*	*CR (%)*	*ICC*	*P value*
Heart rate	0.47	0.054	11.4	10.6	0.7	0.01
Mean arterial pressure	0.44	0.038	8.7	7.5	0.79	0.0005
Start temperature	0.51	0.036	7.1	7.1	0.81	0.0001
DTM indices of vascular function						
TR (°C)	0.209	0.012	5.7	2.4	0.82	0.0001
AUC	0.292	0.014	4.8	2.8	0.83	0.0001

D mean absolute difference; SD_D SD of mean differences; *CV* coefficient of variability $[(SD_D/D)\times 100]$; *CR* coefficient of repeatability $[(SD_D\times 1.96)\times 100)]$; *ICC* Intraclass correlation coefficient

It is important to realize that DTM indices, like other cardiovascular physiologic markers (e.g., blood pressure and heart rate), are sensitive to factors such as autonomic nervous system activity and postprandial metabolic changes. Therefore, for maximum reproducibility, DTM tests should be performed under optimum conditions with minimum disturbing factors that would influence the cardiovascular system. Recommended subject and testing conditions are listed in the International Brachial Artery Reactivity Task Force guidelines (J Am Coll Cardiol 2002 Jan;39(2):257–65) (Table 1).

DTM AND NEUROVASCULAR REACTIVITY

Findings in Contralateral Fingers (Nonoccluded Arm)

Infrared cameras have been utilized to display thermal energy emitted by the entire hand before, during and after a standard cuff occlusion procedure. The infrared camera is able to display a temperature map of both hands. This noncontact probe was used to vividly display the changes in skin blood flow in the contralateral (nonoccluded) hand during cuff occlusion. Screen shots shown below from the video of the experiment display the aforementioned neurovascular response in the left hand, with significant warming (white portions) occurring in the left hand, as well as the expected hyperemia after cuff deflation in the study (right) arm (Fig. 13).

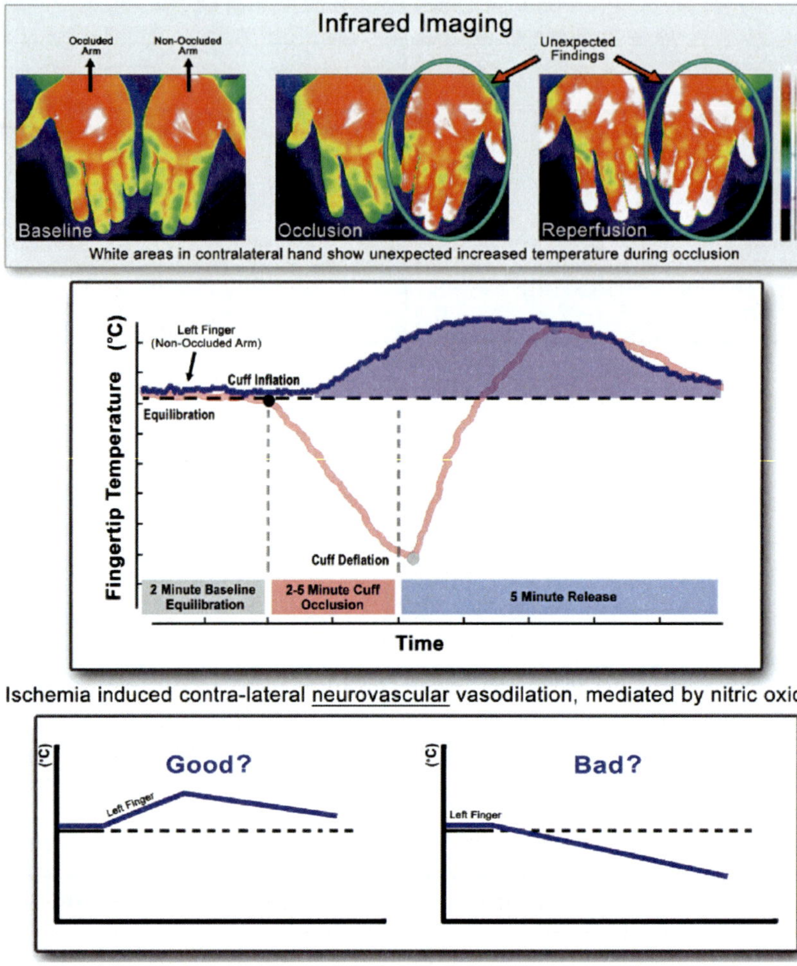

Fig. 13. DTM and neurovascular reactivity.

The second probe monitors fingertip temperature changes on the contralateral, nonoccluded hand. Temperature data from the second probe were originally intended to serve as a relatively stable, reference curve. However, recent studies have revealed that temperature changes in the nonoccluded hand may provide additional insight into the subject's vascular function. It is hypothesized that increased fingertip temperature in the contralateral hand is a physiologic, neurally mediated, systemic response to the ischemic stimulus. It is further hypothesized that this response would be vasodilatory in healthy individuals and hampered in individuals with cardiovascular risk factors and sympathetic overactivity.

The response that is seen in the left finger during inflation cannot be the result of circulating vasodilators from the distal part of the cuffed arm, since they could not pass the brachial cuff. Therefore, it follows that what is seen in the left arm during cuff inflation is a neurovascular response to the cuff-induced pain and the ischemic portion. The contralateral arm temperature increases during inflation in healthy people, which seems to be a systemic response to vasodilate the resistance vessels in an attempt to bring more blood into the ischemic portion. It is hypothesized that the body attempts to dilate the vessels distal to the cuff, but since it is a systemic response, the resistance vessels elsewhere dilate, i.e., in the contralateral arm, as well as the toes and indeed, the face. The dilation is hidden during inflation in the study (cuffed arm) as no blood flow can occur during inflation, but the systemic response adds to the local vasodilatory response of adenosine, prostaglandins, etc. to provide an augmented response in study arm postcuff deflation.

It seems that the ability to dilate the contralateral (as well as the study arm and remote sites) during inflation is indicative of a healthy neurovascular response to ischemia and can become attenuated with risk factors/disease. Certainly, more research is required to elucidate these findings.

CONCLUSIONS

Measuring risk factors alone is insufficient for assessment of the status of vascular health in an individual. A comprehensive, stepwise evaluation of cardiovascular risk requires measurement of risk factors along with functional and structural assessment of the cardiovascular system, as illustrated in the "Cardiovascular Screening Pyramid" (Fig. 14).

The findings described in this document, although promising, are preliminary and subject to corroboration by other cardiovascular researchers, particularly in long-term, prospective studies and clinical trials. It is important to emphasize that DTM is not intended to replace imaging and advanced diagnostic modalities or to disregard traditional risk factor assessment; rather, it is an inexpensive, noninvasive, and easy-to-use solution that can complement both risk factors and imaging modalities.

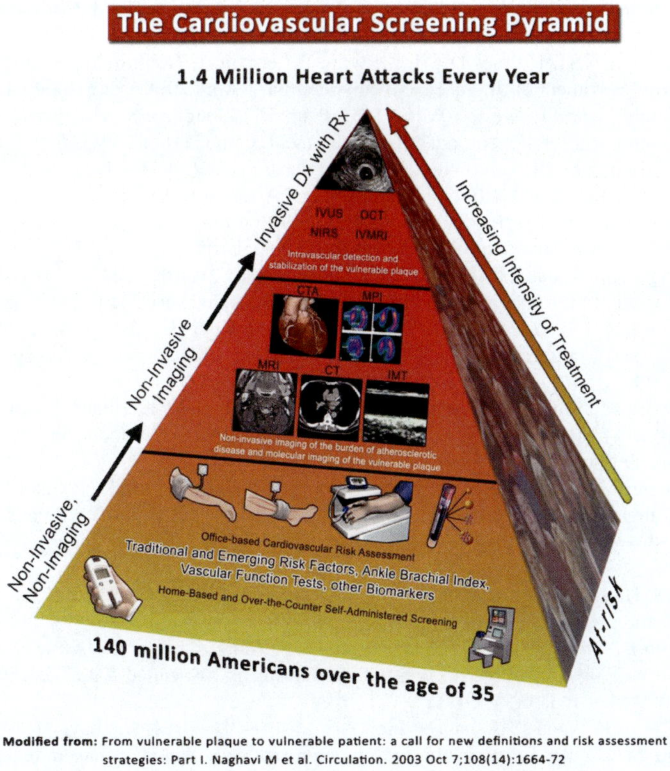

Fig. 14. The cardiovascular screening pyramid illustrates a new strategy for early detection and prevention of sudden cardiovascular events.

REFERENCES

1. Zipes DP, Wellens HJ. Sudden cardiac death. Circulation 1998;98(21):2334–51.
2. Grundy SM, Pasternak R, Greenland P, Smith S, Jr., Fuster V. AHA/ACC scientific statement: assessment of cardiovascular risk by use of multiple-risk-factor assessment equations: a statement for healthcare professionals from the American Heart Association and the American College of Cardiology. J Am Coll Cardiol 1999;34(4):1348–59.
3. Third Report of the National Cholesterol Education Program (NCEP) Expert Panel on Detection, Evaluation, and Treatment of High Blood Cholesterol in Adults (Adult Treatment Panel III) final report. Circulation 2002;106(25):3143–421.
4. Akosah KO, Schaper A, Cogbill C, Schoenfeld P. Preventing myocardial infarction in the young adult in the first place: how do the National Cholesterol Education Panel III guidelines perform? J Am Coll Cardiol 2003;41(9):1475–9.
5. Rumberger JA, Simons DB, Fitzpatrick LA, Sheedy PF, Schwartz RS. Coronary artery calcium area by electron-beam computed tomography and coronary atherosclerotic plaque area. A histopathologic correlative study. Circulation 1995;92(8):2157–62.
6. Greenland P, Bonow RO, Brundage BH, Budoff MJ, Eisenberg MJ, Grundy SM, et al. ACCF/AHA 2007 clinical expert consensus document on coronary artery calcium scoring by computed tomography in global cardiovascular risk assessment and in evaluation of patients with chest pain: a report of the American College of Cardiology Foundation Clinical Expert Consensus Task Force (ACCF/AHA Writing Committee to Update the 2000 Expert Consensus Document on Electron Beam Computed Tomography) developed in collaboration with the Society of Atherosclerosis Imaging and Prevention and the Society of Cardiovascular Computed Tomography. J Am Coll Cardiol 2007;49(3):378–402.
7. Bots ML, Hoes AW, Koudstaal PJ, Hofman A, Grobbee DE. Common carotid intima-media thickness and risk of stroke and myocardial infarction: the Rotterdam Study. Circulation 1997;96(5):1432–7.
8. Adams MR, Nakagomi A, Keech A, Robinson J, McCredie R, Bailey BP, et al. Carotid intima-media thickness is only weakly correlated with the extent and severity of coronary artery disease. Circulation 1995;92(8):2127–34.
9. Ridker PM, Buring JE, Rifai N, Cook NR. Development and validation of improved algorithms for the assessment of global cardiovascular risk in women: the Reynolds Risk Score. JAMA 2007;297(6):611–9.
10. Ballantyne C, Cushman M, Psaty B, Furberg C, Khaw KT, Sandhu M, et al. Collaborative meta-analysis of individual participant data from observational studies of Lp-PLA2 and cardiovascular diseases. Eur J Cardiovasc Prev Rehabil 2007;14(1):3–11.
11. Vita JA, Keaney JF, Jr., Larson MG, Keyes MJ, Massaro JM, Lipinska I, et al. Brachial artery vasodilator function and systemic inflammation in the Framingham Offspring Study. Circulation 2004;110(23):3604–9.
12. Celermajer DS, Sorensen KE, Gooch VM, Spiegelhalter DJ, Miller OI, Sullivan ID, et al. Non-invasive detection of endothelial dysfunction in children and adults at risk of atherosclerosis. Lancet 1992;340(8828):1111–5.
13. Bonetti PO, Pumper GM, Higano ST, Holmes DR, Jr., Kuvin JT, Lerman A. Noninvasive identification of patients with early coronary atherosclerosis by assessment of digital reactive hyperemia. J Am Coll Cardiol 2004;44(11):2137–41.
14. Stein JH, Fraizer MC, Aeschlimann SE, Nelson-Worel J, McBride PE, Douglas PS. Vascular age: integrating carotid intima-media thickness measurements with global coronary risk assessment. Clin Cardiol 2004;27(7):388–92.
15. Corretti MC, Anderson TJ, Benjamin EJ, Celermajer D, Charbonneau F, Creager MA, Deanfield J, Drexler H, Gerhard-Herman M, Herrington D, Vallance P, Vita J, Vogel R;International Brachial Artery Reactivity Task Force. Guidelines for the ultrasound assessment of endothelial-dependent flow-mediated vasodilation of the brachial artery: a report of the International Brachial Artery Reactivity Task Force. J Am Coll Cardiol. 2002 Jan 16;39(2):257–65.
16. Gul KM, Ahmadi N, Wang Z, Jamieson C, Nasir K, Metcalfe R, Hecht HS, Hartley CJ, Naghavi M. Digital thermal monitoring of vascular function: a novel tool to improve cardiovascular risk assessment. Vasc Med. 2009 May;14(2):143–8.
17. Budoff MJ, Ahmadi N, Gul KM, Liu ST, Flores FR, Tiano J, Takasu J, Miller E, Tsimikas S. Aged garlic extract supplemented with B vitamins, folic acid and L-arginine retards the progression of subclinical atherosclerosis: A randomized clinical trial. Prev Med. 2009 Aug-Sep;49(2-3):101–7
18. Ahmadi N, Hajsadeghi F, Gul K, Leibfried M, DeMoss D, Lee R, Flores F, Nasir K, Hecht H, Naghavi M, Budoff MJ. Vascular function measured by fingertip thermal reactivity is impaired in patients with metabolic syndrome and diabetes mellitus. J Clin Hypertens (Greenwich). 2009 Nov;11(11):678–84.
19. Ahmadi N, Nabavi V, Nuguri V, Hajsadeghi F, Flores F, Akhtar M, Kleis S, Hecht H, Naghavi M, Budoff MJ. Low fingertip temperature rebound measured by digital thermal monitoring strongly correlates with the presence and extent of coronary artery disease diagnosed by 64-slice multi-detector computed tomography. Int J Cardiovasc Imaging. 2009 Oct;25(7):725–38. Epub 2009 Jul 26.
20. Ahmadi N, Tirunagaram S, Hajsadeghi F, Flores F, Saeed A, Hecht H, Naghavi M, Budoff MJ. Concomitant insulin resistance and impaired vascular function is associated with increased coronary artery calcification. Int J Cardiol. 2009 Feb 2.
21. Ahmadi N, Usman N, Shim J, Nuguri V, Vasinrapee P, Hajsadeghi F, Wang Z, Foster GP, Nasir K, Hecht H, Naghavi M, Budoff MJ. Vascular dysfunction measured by fingertip thermal monitoring is associated with the extent of myocardial perfusion defect. J Nucl Cardiol. 2009 May-Jun;16(3):431–9.
22. Ahmadi N, Hajsadeghi F, Gul K, Vane J, Usman N, Flores F, Nasir K, Hecht H, Naghavi M, Budoff MJ. Relations between digital thermal monitoring of vascular function, the Framingham risk score, and coronary artery calcium score. J Cardiovasc Comput Tomogr. 2008 Nov;2(6):382–8.
23. Kuvin JT. Anatomy, physiology, or epidemiology: which is the best target for assessing vascular health? J Cardiovasc Comput Tomogr. 2008 Nov;2(6):389–91.

24. Dhindsa M, Sommerlad SM, DeVan AE, Barnes JN, Sugawara J, Ley O, Tanaka H. Interrelationships among noninvasive measures of postischemic macro- and microvascular reactivity. J Appl Physiol. 2008 Aug;105(2):427–32.
25. McQuilkin GL, Panthagani D, Metcalfe RW, Hassan H, Yen AA, Naghavi M, Hartley CJ. Digital Thermal Monitoring (DTM) of Vascular Reactivity Closely Correlates with Doppler Flow Velocity. IEEE: Engineering in Medicine and Biology. 31st Annual International Conference of the IEEE EMBS, Minneapolis, Minnesota, USA, September 2–6, 2009
26. Akhtar MW, Kleis SJ, Metcalfe R. Sensitivity of Digital Thermal Monitoring Parameters to Reactive Hyperemia, ASME Journal of Biomechanical Engineering. In Press
27. Ahmadi N, Mcquilkin G, Kleis S, Akhtar MW, Metcalfe RW, Hartley CJ. Naghavi M, Budoff MJ. Reproducibility and Variability of Digital Thermal Monitoring of Vascular Reactivity. Therapy - In Press

19 Assessment of Macro- and Microvascular Function and Reactivity

Craig J. Hartley and Hirofumi Tanaka

CONTENTS

ABSTRACT

The arterial system consists of large conduit vessels that branch continuously into smaller and smaller vessels ending in arterioles and capillaries. The role of the larger (macro) arteries is to distribute flow to various organs and to provide compliance to minimize the load on the heart and to maximize pressure during diastole. The role of the smaller (micro) vessels is to control regional blood flow by varying their resistance in response to local demand. When all the cardiovascular sensors, control mechanisms, and actuators are working properly, the input impedance of the vascular system remains matched to the output impedance of the heart to maximize efficiency and energy transfer both at rest and during exercise or stress. When disease or aging alters part of the system, overall function is compromised and other parts adapt to maintain basic function but at reduced efficiency and reserve. Thus, when evaluating macrovascular versus microvascular function, reserve, and reactivity to isolate the primary culprit, one must recognize that the entire arterial system may be altered. There are a number of methods and techniques available for assessing vascular function and reactivity, the most accepted being flow-mediated dilation. In this method, microvessels in a limb are stimulated via ischemia during inflation of a blood pressure cuff and assessed by measuring flow or velocity during reactive hyperemia after cuff deflation. Macrovessels are stimulated during the reactive hyperemia and assessed by measuring the change in diameter induced by the increased flow. Other methodologies evaluate different aspects of macrovascular and microvascular function and reactivity, and macrovascular may not be separated from microvascular function unambiguously. Thus, a multifaceted approach may be necessary for a comprehensive assessment of peripheral vascular function.

From: *Asymptomatic Atherosclerosis: Pathophysiology, Detection and Treatment*
Edited by: M. Naghavi (ed.), DOI 10.1007/978-1-60327-179-0_19

Key words: Arterial stiffness; Endothelial function; Flow-mediated dilation; Hyperemia

KEY POINTS

- Large macrovessels control regional vascular compliance, are named, and distribute flow from the heart.
- Small microvessels control local vascular resistance and regulate flow to organs and tissues.
- Macrovascular and microvascular functions are tightly coupled through compensatory mechanisms that attempt to maintain global pressure and regional flow at rest, during exercise, and in the face of disease.
- Vascular reactivity, function, and reserve are related concepts, but have different meanings and may not always correlate with one another.
- Static tests can measure the state of a parameter, but not necessarily vascular function or the ability to change the parameter.
- Provocative tests can measure vascular reserve or the ability to change a parameter, but not necessarily vascular function.
- An abnormal result from a vascular test indicates a problem but may not isolate the cause or determine if the problem is of vascular origin.

INTRODUCTION

Cardiovascular disease (CVD) remains the leading cause of morbidity and premature mortality in the United States, most of the industrialized world, and many developing countries [1]. While the traditional risk factors for CVD are widely recognized as the primary causes of CVD, a number of studies have documented that clinically abnormal risk factors are often absent in individuals who develop CVD [2,3]. Among relatively young adults hospitalized for acute myocardial infarction, mean lipid levels were all within the normal range, and 70% of patients fell into the lowest two risk categories based on the National Cholesterol Education Program guidelines [2]. These research findings that clinical CVD often occurs in the absence of prior exposure to major/traditional CVD risk factors would justify and prompt the search for new and currently unrecognized factors accounting for CVD risks.

Vascular abnormalities play an important role in the pathophysiology of CVD [4–7]. For this reason, a quest for a novel marker to identify and detect subclinical or presymptomatic CVD has focused on the vasculature, in particular easily accessible peripheral arteries. Because abnormality and dysfunction appear to manifest themselves more easily when the system is stressed, peripheral vascular reactivity has emerged as an early marker of atherosclerosis. To assess vascular reactivity, some form of stimulus, intervention, or stress is needed. Some of the maneuvers that have been used include: ischemia [8], Valsalva maneuver [9], heating or cooling, exercise or physical stress [10], mental stress, and administration of vasoactive agents [11]. One of the most commonly used tests is to occlude blood flow to the arm with a blood pressure cuff for several minutes and then release the cuff while measuring vascular parameters of interest [7,8]. Microvessels are stimulated via ischemia during occlusion and assessed by measuring flow during reactive hyperemia after release [12], and macrovessels are stimulated during the hyperemia and assessed by measuring flow-mediated dilation (FMD) [8]. A number of established and emerging techniques have been employed to measure peripheral vascular reactivity [4,7,8,13–16]. Vascular reactivity assessed by these various methodologies is assumed to provide similar information regarding the arterial health, more specifically endothelial function [17]. However, this may not be the case considering that the heterogeneity of the arterial tree spans from macro- to microvasculature, and different physiological factors modulate the responses.

This chapter reviews currently available measures of macro- and microvascular function and reactivity. As the focus of this chapter is to describe macro- and microvascular “function,” imaging of macrovascular structure (e.g., arterial wall thickness) is excluded. Although we classified each technique into either macro- or microvascular function test, the distinction is often vague and probably the measured values would reflect a combination of both macro- and microvascular function.

MACRO- AND MICROVASCULAR CLASSIFICATION

The systemic vascular system consists of large conduit arteries that branch continuously into smaller and smaller vessels and finally into arterioles and capillaries. The role of the larger (macro or conduit) arteries is to distribute flow from the heart to the various organs and to provide compliance to absorb each stroke volume delivered by the heart to minimize the load on the heart and to maximize pressure during diastole. The role of the smaller (micro or resistance) vessels is to control regional blood flow by varying their resistance in response to local demand. When all the cardiovascular sensors, control mechanisms, and actuators are working properly, the input impedance of the vascular system remains matched to the output impedance of the heart to maximize efficiency and energy transfer both at rest and during exercise or stress. Table 1 describes some general distinctions between macro- and microvascular characteristics (Table 1).

It is often assumed that resistance vessels which control the flow to the various beds operate normally even with vascular diseases such as hypertension, and that most of the vascular problems associated with aging and disease are with compliance vessels. Hypertension is usually related to high total peripheral resistance, but the cause and effect relation is unclear. Mean pressure is the product of cardiac output and total peripheral resistance, while pulse pressure is a function of both total arterial compliance and resistance. In general, high mean pressure indicates high resistance, and high pulse pressure indicates low compliance. To keep pressure and regional flow adequate and within normal ranges, both resistance and compliance must be adjustable on a regional level and responsive to changing conditions and stress. Blood pressure, regional flows, and cardiac output can vary considerably during daily activity, making it difficult to establish "normal" values for pressure and other parameters and indices of vascular status.

Measurements made at rest can only assess baseline characteristic values and cannot assess controllability. To do that requires an intervention designed to alter resistance, compliance, or both via known pathways so that the results can be interpreted. This is a challenging task. As an example, consider reactive hyperemia induced by inflation and deflation of a blood pressure cuff on the upper arm. The occlusion causes hypoxia, which stimulates dilation of resistance vessels but with little change in compliance. Upon cuff deflation, the high flow, velocity, and perfusion during reactive hyperemia are measures of microvascular function. The higher flow and higher shear stress in the macrovessels supplying the arm during hyperemia induces FMD, and the changes in vessel diameter, diameter pulsations, or pulse wave velocity (PWV) are measures of macrovascular function.

Table 1
Distinction between macro- and microvascular characteristics

	Microvasculature	*Macrovasculature*
Alternative name	Resistance	Conduit
Role in blood supply	Control	Distribution
Vessel size and volume	Small	Large
Vascular impedance	Resistance	Compliance
Effect on pressure and flow	Mean or average	Pulsatility or wave shape
Assessment method	Velocity or flow	Diameter

The assessment of macrovascular function via FMD requires an increase in flow or shear stress (microvascular function), and one has to assume that mean and pulsatile blood pressure are unchanged during the test.

MACROVASCULAR FUNCTION

It is apparent that there are many potential but complex ways to use the relations between pressure, flow, velocity, and diameter to characterize the vascular system in whole or in part, but all these require precision and high-fidelity waveforms of pressure or diameter and flow or velocity. In an attempt to simplify the measurements and analyses, investigators have developed several useful measures and indices of macrovascular function, including the pressure augmentation index (AI), the velocity pulsatility (PI) and resistance (RI) indices, and PWV which can be applied to suboptimal signals measured at one or more sites.

Arterial Stiffness/Pulse Wave Velocity

Pressure pulses generated by the heart propagate along the arteries at a finite speed called the PWV [18]. Because the transmission of the arterial pressure wave occurs along the arterial wall and is influenced primarily by the biomechanical property of the arterial wall, PWV has been used as an index of arterial stiffness [19,20]. PWV can be measured directly by timing the arrival of pressure or velocity pulses at two sites separated by a known distance. PWV is different from, and is faster than, the velocity of blood flow and is typically 4–10 m/s. PWV is related to the mechanical properties of the vessel segment by the Moens-Korteweg equation [4]:

$$\mathrm{PWV}^2 = Eh/d\rho,$$

where E is Young's modulus of elasticity, h is vessel wall thickness, d is vessel diameter, and ρ is the density of blood.

If there were no reflections, the time-varying pulsatile (or AC) part of pressure and flow (or velocity) waves would be identical and be related to the characteristic impedance (Z_0) of the vessel [21]. Interestingly, when Z_0 is expressed as the ratio of pressure to velocity rather than flow [4]:

$$Z_0 = \rho\mathrm{PWV}.$$

Thus, Z_0 can be estimated by measuring PWV since the density of blood is relatively constant at 1.06.

A number of epidemiological studies have demonstrated an independent association between aortic PWV and cardiovascular events in a variety of populations, including end-stage renal disease [6], hypertension [5], and the well-functioning older adults [22]. In marked contrast to the prevailing thought that arterial stiffness is a relatively static property, arterial stiffness has a large reserve and can be altered over a relatively short period of time [23,24]. Interventional studies have shown that arterial stiffness can be improved or reversed with a variety of interventions, including regular aerobic exercise [25], salt restriction [26], and a variety of drug therapies [27].

Vascular Impedance

The load that the vascular system provides to the heart can be described and quantified in terms of its mechanical impedance (Z) consisting of resistance (R) and compliance (C) terms [28]. Thus flow (Q) is pressure (P) divided by impedance ($Q = P/Z$), where Z is a complex term and is a function of frequency. When pressure and flow are measured at the aortic valve, R is total peripheral resistance, C is total arterial compliance, and Z_i is the input impedance. When P and Q are measured at more peripheral sites, *R* and *C* represent the resistance and compliance distal to the measurement site. Compliance is a measure of volume (or area since the length is relatively fixed) versus pressure of an arterial segment, and *R* is a measure of mean pressure divided by mean flow. In general, compliance dominates in large (macro) vessels and resistance dominates in small (micro) vessels. Vascular impedance is typically expressed either as modulus (amplitude of *P* divided by amplitude of *Q*) or phase (delay of *Q after P*) [4]. Vascular impedance has been used to characterize the hydraulic load provided by the arterial system to the left ventricle throughout the ventricular ejection [4,28].

Arterial Wave Reflection and Characteristic Impedance

Pressure pulses propagating into a vessel are reflected at sites of branching and by the terminal microvessels [28,29]. The sum of the waves reflected at each site and returning to the measurement site (backward wave) adds to the forward or incident wave, and the pressure measured at any site is actually the sum of forward and backward traveling waves at that site [29]. Indeed, many of the inflections seen in pressure waves are caused by reflections [30]. Flow or velocity waves are also reflected, but the reflected velocity waves subtract from the forward wave such that the flow or velocity measured at any site is the difference between the forward and backward traveling waves at that site [21]. The reason that flow and velocity waves peak before pressure waves and decelerate while pressure is still rising is because of wave reflections.

The equations for the measured pressure (P) and velocity (V) in terms of the forward (P_f) and backward (P_b) pressure waves and the characteristic impedance (Z_o) are [21]:

$$Z_o = P_f / V_f = P_b / V_b$$

$$P = P_f + P_b$$

$$V = V_f - V_b = (P_f - P_b) / Z_o$$

By rearranging the equations, it is possible to solve for P_f and P_b in terms of the measured pressure, velocity, and Z_o at a given site:

$$P_f = (P + Z_o V)/2$$

$$P_b = (P - Z_o V)/2$$

Another method to estimate Z_o is by the ratio of the derivatives of pressure (dP/dt) and velocity (dV/dt) in early systole before the return of any reflections [21,31]. Thus:

$$Z_o = d\,P_s/d\,V_s$$

The reflection coefficient (Γ) can be defined as the ratio of the backward to the forward waves or:

$$\Gamma(f) = P_b/P_f = |\Gamma|e^{j\phi}\,Z$$

where j is the square root of -1, φ is the phase angle, and Γ is a function of frequency since the forward and backward waves have different shapes. The input impedance (Z_i) is also a function of frequency since pressure and velocity waves have different shapes [4].

$$Z_i\,(f) = |P/V|\,e^{j\phi}$$

It must be noted that the analysis is only valid for the pulsatile or *AC* part of pressure and velocity (the waveforms) and not for the mean or *DC* part. Because of the similarities in waveforms between velocity and flow and between pressure and diameter, it is possible to substitute diameter for pressure signals and velocity for flow signals in analyzing vascular mechanics, impedance, PWV, wave reflections, and forward and backward waves [32–35]. This is especially true for dimensionless indices that are sensitive to the shape and timing of the waveforms rather than the magnitude.

The arterial system of mammals is designed so that reflected waves return to the heart after closure of the aortic valve to augment diastolic pressure and coronary blood flow while minimizing the load seen by the heart during systole [36]. As the arterial system ages and becomes stiffer and often diseased, PWV increases, and reflected waves arrive at the heart earlier in the cardiac cycle increasing cardiac work [4]. The augmentation index is based on the timing and magnitude of inflections during the upstroke of arterial pressure and is used to quantify the early return of reflected waves [13,37]. In large-scale clinical studies, augmentation index is typically measured by applying an arterial applanation tonometer perpendicular to the arterial surface to indent the vessel wall. When the artery is flattened into ellipsoidal geometry, pressure waveforms can be assessed accurately by the sensor [13]. Carotid and radial arteries are the most commonly assessed with this method. Higher augmentation index is associated with left ventricular hypertrophy [38], a lower peak aerobic capacity [20], and a more rapid onset of exercise-induced ischemia [39].

Pulsatility and Resistance Indices

PI and RI calculated from Doppler blood velocity (BV) signals are used to characterize the impedance of certain vascular beds distal to measurement sites [40,41].

$$\text{PI} = (\text{maximum BV} - \text{minimum BV})/\text{mean BV}$$

$$\text{RI} = (\text{maximum BV} - \text{end - diastolic BV})/\text{maximum BV}$$

RI is often used to assess perfusion in the umbilical or placental arteries during pregnancy where low resistance is favorable and high resistance is unfavorable [40]. PI is often used to assess flow in femoral arteries where a high pulsatility indicates high compliance (and resistance), and low pulsatility indicates low compliance and is suggestive of a flow-limiting stenosis in the femoral artery [41,42]. This index combines both macro- and microvascular values. Although these Doppler indices are sensitive to peripheral resistance and compliance, they are not commonly used in evaluating endothelial function.

Flow-Mediated Dilation

FMD reflects the endothelium-dependent change in arterial diameter in response to reactive hyperemia and is measured by comparing the lumen diameter of the brachial artery before and after a period of ischemia induced in the forearm. Since Celermajer and colleagues developed this technique in 1992 [8], FMD has been widely used as a noninvasive measure of endothelial function in various studies, and the guidelines for the FMD procedure have been published [7]. However, because of technical difficulty, reliance on expensive equipment, and a large interindividual variability, the technique has not been incorporated in a routine clinical setting [7].

Physiological mechanisms underlying FMD have not been well characterized. Several studies have demonstrated a role of nitric oxide (NO) in evoking FMD, as the infusion of NO synthase blocker abolishes the increase in arterial diameter following reactive hyperemia [17]. However, blood vessels of eNOS knockout mice still experience FMD by responding to shear stress, most likely mediated by prostaglandins [43]. Nervous system regulation of vascular tone has also been implicated in FMD [44,45].

Aside from the FMD, another popular methodology to examine endothelial-dependent vasodilation is the increase in forearm blood flow caused by intrabrachial artery infusions of endothelial dilators like acetylcholine [46]. If the acetylcholine infusion and FMD are measuring similar or common properties of peripheral vascular endothelial vasodilatory capacity, they will be expected to correlate with each other. However, these two methodologies do not significantly relate to each other [11,47]. Although there are a number of possible explanations for the divergent results produced by the use of these two techniques, one possibility is different levels of major contributions from macro- versus microvascular properties affecting each technique. The acetylcholine infusion examines resistance (micro) vessel endothelial-dependent vasodilation in response to a pharmacological stimulus, whereas the FMD assesses large conduit (macro) artery endothelial function in response to the physiological stimulus of increased shear stress.

An interesting question is why FMD occurs in the brachial (conduit) artery. Dilation of macrovessels has little effect on the pressure drop or on vascular resistance, so there must be another reason for this well-observed and well-documented effect. Vasodilation does increase compliance and may improve matching between the peripheral resistance and the characteristic impedance of the vessel thus minimizing wave reflections and easing the load on the heart during periods of increased flow and cardiac output [48].

MICROVASCULAR FUNCTION

Basal Peripheral Blood Flow

Basal limb blood flow can be measured by a variety of ways: dye dilution or thermodilution technique, Doppler flowmeters, venous occlusion plethysmography, etc. Basal limb perfusion is known to decrease with advancing age [49]. Reduction in limb perfusion in peripheral tissues is associated with a reduction in the clearance of atherogenic lipids and lipoproteins [50]. Chronic reductions in basal limb blood flow have been associated with reduced muscle glucose uptake and contribute to insulin resistance in aging adults [51]. Decreased blood flow has been implicated in the pathogenesis of metabolic syndrome, a major precursor to coronary, cerebral, and peripheral vascular occlusive disease [50].

Reactive Hyperemia

Reactive hyperemia is a complex hemodynamic response of the vasculature that aims to accelerate the delivery of oxygen to tissues as well as the removal of metabolic byproducts after a period of ischemia. Blood flow is typically measured with venous occlusion plethysmography or ultrasound Doppler flowmeters. Because nitric oxide does not appear to be involved in modulating peak reactive hyperemia as the infusion of L-NMMA does not affect the level of peak reactive hyperemia [12,52], much less attention has been given to peak reactive hyperemia as a clinical tool to detect subclinical atherosclerotic disease. However, there has been controversy surrounding the relative clinical utility of reactive hyperemia and FMD [53,54]. A recent report from the Framingham study suggested that hyperemic shear stress may be a better predictor because hyperemic shear stress was more strongly correlated with risk factors than FMD [54]. Additionally, adjusting for hyperemic shear stress in multivariate models greatly attenuated the association between FMD and risk factors [54]. Because reactive hyperemia and shear stress are the stimulus for FMD, impaired FMD previously observed in some patient populations may be attributed to a lesser stimulus to NO release. Therefore, it is essential that the magnitude of the stimulus imposed (blood flow and shear stress) is also considered when interpreting the FMD response [55].

The reactive hyperemic response depends on a number of physiological factors, including nitric oxide, adenosine, prostaglandin, endothelium-derived hyperpolarizing factors, potassium, pH, hydrogen peroxide, the myogenic response, and microvascular structure [12,56,57]. Nitric oxide appears to play a minor to modest role in peak vasodilation [12,52], and prostaglandins seem to be a more important determinant of peak blood flow [12]. In addition to the biochemical factors, reactive hyperemia may also reflect the structure of the microvasculature as peak limb vasodilatory capacity has been used as a bioassay of structural changes in the resistance arteries [10]. The idea behind this experimental approach is that, under conditions of peak vasodilation, vascular conductance becomes a direct function of the arterial structure in general and the arterial wall/lumen ratio in particular [58,59].

Skin Reactive Hyperemia

Skin and cutaneous circulation have been used as a model to investigate vascular reactivity in a variety of diseases, such as hypercholesterolemia, renal disease, diabetes, peripheral vascular disease, and systemic sclerosis [14,60]. The common technique to assess microvascular function during reactivity tests is through the use of laser Doppler flowmetry (LDF). LDF signals provide a relative measure of cutaneous perfusion using the Doppler shift of the scattered laser light; LDF provides a technique to assess hyperemic responses. Although LDF has been widely used in the research settings, it provides only relative perfusion measurements, the equipment has inherently high cost, the measurement is dependent on the optical properties of the tissue, which can vary greatly with anatomical location and amongst subjects. Moreover, initial skin temperature, level of ischemia produced by either occlusion time or occlusion pressure, and the presence of pain or discomfort are known to affect hyperemic response as well as the reproducibility of the response.

Peripheral Artery Tonometry

A peripheral artery tonometry device measures digital volume changes with each pulse wave with a probe that has a pneumatic cuff which encapsulates the fingertip [15]. In this technique, the probes are placed on the middle finger of both hands and the data are recorded continuously before, during, and after cuff deflation. Changes in pulse wave amplitude in response to reactive hyperemia are expressed as reactive hyperemia index. Reactive hyperemia index score has been shown to exhibit an excellent association with measures of coronary and peripheral endothelial dysfunction [15]. This technique is discussed in more detail in Dr. Lehman's chapter in this book.

Digital Thermal Monitoring

Digital Thermal Monitoring (DTM) is a noninvasive measurement of vascular responsiveness that assesses changes in fingertip temperature in response to blood flow changes in the fingertips [16]. Tissue temperature is a direct function of blood perfusion. Limb and digit temperatures are affected during brachial artery occlusion and subsequent hyperemia. The time required by the digits to return to normal temperature as well as the temperature change experienced depend on the capacity of the arteries to dilate and restore normal circulation. In this technique, fingertip skin temperature is measured by the probes placed on the index finger of both hands. During ischemia, the temperature drops toward room temperature, and upon cuff release, the temperature rapidly returns to and exceeds the baseline fingertip skin temperature. The increase in fingertip temperature after cuff deflation above the starting finger temperature (designated as the temperature rebound) is used as an index of vascular reactivity. This technique is very simple and is a promising tool for use in routine clinical settings, but clinical studies to validate the technique are currently lacking.

SUMMARY

There are a number of methods and techniques available for assessing vascular function and reactivity. Each methodology evaluates different aspects of macrovascular and microvascular function and reactivity, and macrovascular function may not be separated from microvascular function unambiguously. Thus, a multifaceted approach may be necessary for the comprehensive assessment of peripheral vascular function.

REFERENCES

1. Rosamond W, Flegal K, Friday G, Furie K, Go A, Greenlund K, Haase N, Ho M, Howard V, Kissela B, Kittner S, Lloyd-Jones D, McDermott M, Meigs J, Moy C, Nichol G, O'Donnell CJ, Roger V, Rumsfeld J, Sorlie P, Steinberger J, Thom T, Wasserthiel-Smoller S, Hong Y. Heart disease and stroke statistics – 2007 update: a report from the American Heart Association Statistics Committee and Stroke Statistics Subcommittee. Circulation 2007;115(5):e69–e71.
2. Akosah KO, Schaper A, Cogbill C, Schoenfeld P. Preventing myocardial infarction in the young adult in the first place: how do the National Cholesterol Education Panel III guidelines perform? J Am Coll Cardiol 2003;41(9):1475–1479.
3. Kullo IJ, Ballantyne CM. Conditional risk factors for atherosclerosis. Mayo Clin Proc 2005;80(2):219–230.
4. Nichols WW, O'Rourke MF. McDonald's Blood Flow in Arteries: Theoretical, Experimental and Clinical Principles, Fourth Edition. Third ed. London: Arnold; 1998.
5. Blacher J, Asmar R, Djane S, London GM, Safar ME. Aortic pulse wave velocity as a marker of cardiovascular risk in hypertensive patients. Hypertension 1999;33(5):1111–1117.
6. Blacher J, Guerin AP, Pannier B, Marchais SJ, Safar ME, London GM. Impact of aortic stiffness on survival in end-stage renal disease. Circulation 1999;99(18):2434–2439.
7. Corretti MC, Anderson TJ, Benjamin EJ, Celermajer D, Charbonneau F, Creager MA, Deanfield J, Drexler H, Gerhard-Herman M, Herrington D, Vallance P, Vita J, Vogel R. Guidelines for the ultrasound assessment of endothelial-dependent flow-mediated vasodilation of the brachial artery. A report of the International Brachial Artery Reactivity Task Force. J Am Coll Cardiol 2002;39(2):257–265.
8. Celermajer DS, Sorensen KE, Gooch VM, Spiegelhalter DJ, Miller OI, Sullivan ID, Lloyd JK, Deanfield JE. Non-invasive detection of endothelial dysfunction in children and adults at risk of atherosclerosis. Lancet 1992; 340:1111–1115.
9. Murgo JP, Westerhof N, Giolma JP, Altobelli SA. Manipulation of ascending aortic pressure and flow wave reflections with the Valsalva maneuver: relationship to input impedance. Circulation 1981;63(1):122–132.
10. Tanaka H, Reiling MJ, Seals DR. Regular walking increases peak limb vasodilatory capacity of older hypertensive humans: implications for arterial structure. J Hypertens 1998;16:423–428.
11. Eskurza I, Seals DR, DeSouza CA, Tanaka H. Pharmacological vs. flow-mediated assessments of peripheral vascular endothelial vasodilatory function in humans. Am J Cardiol 2001;88:47–49.
12. Engelke KA, Halliwill JR, Proctor DN, Dietz NM, Joyner MJ. Contribution of nitric oxide and prostaglandins to reactive hyperemia in the human forearm. J Appl Physiol 1996;81(4):1807–1814.
13. Kelly R, Hayword C, Ganis J, Daley J, Avolio A, O'Rourke M. Noninvasive registration of the arterial pressure pulse waveform using high-fidelity applanation tonometry. J Vascul Med Biol 1989;1(3):142–149.
14. Shamim-Uzzaman QA, Pfenninger D, Kehrer C, Chakrabarti A, Kacirotti N, Rubenfire M, Brook R, Rajagopalan S. Altered cutaneous microvascular responses to reactive hyperaemia in coronary artery disease: a comparative study with conduit vessel responses. Clin Sci (Lond) 2002;103(3):267–273.
15. Kuvin JT, Patel AR, Sliney KA, Pandian NG, Sheffy J, Schnall RP, Karas RH, Udelson JE. Assessment of peripheral vascular endothelial function with finger arterial pulse wave amplitude. Am Heart J 2003;146(1):168–174.
16. Kozlemeny E. Examination of flow mediated dilation with thermometry in case of patients with high cardiovascular risk. Cardiologia Hungarica 2005;35:11–16.
17. Joannides R, Haefeli WE, Linder L, Richard V, Bakkali EH, Thuillez C, Luscher TF. Nitric oxide is responsible for flow-dependent dilatation of human peripheral conduit arteries in vivo. Circulation 1995;91:1314–1319.

18. Bramwell JC, Hill AV. The velocity of the pulse wave in man. Proc R Soc Lond 1922;93:298–306.
19. Avolio AP, Fa-Quan D, Wei-Qiang L, Yao-Fei L, Zhen-Dong H, Lian-Fen X, O'Rourke MF. Effects of aging on arterial distensibility in populations with high and low prevalence of hypertension: comparison between urban and rural communities in China. Circulation 1985;71(2):202–210.
20. Tanaka H, DeSouza CA, Seals DR. Absence of age-related increase in central arterial stiffness in physically active women. Arterioscler Thromb Vasc Biol 1998;18(1):127–132.
21. Westerhof N, Sipkema P, Bos GCvd, Elzinga G. Forward and backward waves in the arterial system. Cardiovasc Res 1972;6(6):648–656.
22. Sutton-Tyrrell K, Najjar SS, Boudreau RM, Venkitachalam L, Kupelian V, Simonsick EM, Havlik R, Lakatta EG, Spurgeon H, Kritchevsky S, Pahor M, Bauer D, Newman A. Elevated aortic pulse wave velocity, a marker of arterial stiffness, predicts cardiovascular events in well-functioning older adults. Circulation 2005;111(25):3384–3390.
23. Barenbrock M, Spieker C, Witta J, Evers S, Hoeks APG, Rahn KH, Zidek W. Reduced distensibility of the common carotid artery in patients treated with ergotamine. Hypertension 1996;28:115–119.
24. Boutouyrie P, Locolley P, Girerd X, Beck L, Safar M, Laurent S. Sympathetic activation decreases medium-sized arterial compliance in humans. Am J Physiol 1994;267(36):H1368–H1376.
25. Tanaka H, Dinenno FA, Monahan KD, Clevenger CM, DeSouza CA, Seals DR. Aging, habitual exercise, and dynamic arterial compliance. Circulation 2000;102:1270–1275.
26. Gates PE, Tanaka H, Hiatt WR, Seals DR. Dietary sodium restriction rapidly improves large elastic artery compliance in older adults with systolic hypertension. Hypertension 2004;44(1):35–41.
27. Franklin SS. Is there a preferred antihypertensive therapy for isolated systolic hypertension and reduced arterial compliance? Curr Hypertens Rep 2000;2(3):253–259.
28. O'Rourke MF, Taylor MG. Input impedance of the systemic circulation. Circ Res 1967;20(4):365–380.
29. O'Rourke MF, Yaginuma T. Wave reflections and the arterial pulse. Arch Intern Med 1984;144(2):366–371.
30. Latham RD, Westerhof N, Sipkema P, Rubal BJ, Reuderink P, Murgo JP. Regional wave travel and reflections along the human aorta: a study with six simultaneous micromanometric pressures. Circulation 1985;72(6):1257–1269.
31. Meinders JM, Kornet L, Brands PJ, Hoeks AP. Assessment of local pulse wave velocity in arteries using 2D distension waveforms. Ultrason Imaging 2001;23(4):199–215.
32. Brands PJ, Hoeks AP, Rutten MC, Reneman RS. A noninvasive method to estimate arterial impedance by means of assessment of local diameter change and the local center-line blood flow velocity using ultrasound. Ultrasound Med Biol 1996;22(7):895–905.
33. Hartley CJ, Reddy AK, Madala S, Entman ML, Michael LH, Taffet GE. Noninvasive ultrasonic measurement of arterial wall motion in mice. Am J Physiol Heart Circ Physiol 2004;287(3):H1426–H1432.
34. Meinders JM, Hoeks AP. Simultaneous assessment of diameter and pressure waveforms in the carotid artery. Ultrasound Med Biol 2004;30(2):147–154.
35. Van Bortel LM, Balkestein EJ, van der Heijden-Spek JJ, Vanmolkot FH, Staessen JA, Kragten JA, Vredeveld JW, Safar ME, Struijker Boudier HA, Hoeks AP. Non-invasive assessment of local arterial pulse pressure: comparison of applanation tonometry and echo-tracking. J Hypertens 2001;19(6):1037–1044.
36. Westerhof N, Elzinga G. Normalized input impedance and arterial decay time over heart period are independent of animal size. Am J Physiol 1991;261(1 Pt 2):R126–133.
37. Murgo JP, Westerhof N, Giolma JP, Altobelli SA. Aortic input impedance in normal man: relationship to pressure wave forms. Circulation 1980;62(1):105–116.
38. Marchais SJ, Guerin AP, Pannier BM, Levy BI, Safar ME, London GM. Wave reflections and cardiac hypertrophy in chronic uremia: influence of body size. Hypertension 1993;22(6):876–883.
39. Kingwell BA, Waddell TK, Medley TL, Cameron JD, Dart AM. Large artery stiffness predicts ischemic threshold in patients with coronary artery disease. J Am Coll Cardiol 2002;40(4):773–779.
40. Evans DH, McDicken WN, Skidmore R, Woodcock JP. Doppler Ultrasound: Physics, Instrumentation, and Clinical Applications. New York, NY: Wiley; 1989.
41. Skidmore R, Woodcock JP, Wells PN. Physiological interpretation of Doppler-shift waveforms – III. Clinical results. Ultrasound Med Biol 1980;6(3):227–231.
42. Riehl J, Schmitt H, Bongartz D, Bergmann D, Sieberth HG. Renal artery stenosis: evaluation with colour duplex ultrasonography. Nephrol Dial Transplant 1997;12(8):1608–1614.
43. Sun D, Huang A, Smith CJ, Stackpole CJ, Connetta JA, Shesely EG, Koller A, Kaley G. Enhanced release of prostaglandins contributes to flow-induced arteriolar dilation in eNOS knockout mice. Circ Res 1999;85(3):288–293.
44. Thijssen DH, de Groot P, Kooijman M, Smits P, Hopman MT. Sympathetic nervous system contributes to the age-related impairment of flow-mediated dilation of the superficial femoral artery. Am J Physiol Heart Circ Physiol 2006;291(6):H3122–H3129.

45. Hijmering ML, Stroes ES, Olijhoek J, Hutten BA, Blankestijn PJ, Rabelink TJ. Sympathetic activation markedly reduces endothelium-dependent, flow-mediated vasodilation. J Am Coll Cardiol 2002;39(4):683–688.
46. DeSouza CA, Shapiro LF, Clevenger CM, Dinenno FA, Monahan KD, Tanaka H, Seals DR. Regular aerobic exercise prevents and restores age-related declines in endothelium-dependent vasodilation in healthy men. Circulation 2000;102:1351–1357.
47. Gori T, Di Stolfo G, Sicuro S, Dragoni S, Lisi M, Parker JD, Forconi S. Correlation analysis between different parameters of conduit artery and microvascular vasodilation. Clin Hemorheol Microcirc 2006;35(4):509–515.
48. Segers P, Stergiopulos N, Westerhof N. Relation of effective arterial elastance to arterial system properties. Am J Physiol Heart Circ Physiol 2002;282(3):H1041–1046.
49. Dinenno FA, Jones PP, Seals DR, Tanaka H. Limb blood flow and vascular conductance are reduced with age in healthy humans: relation to elevations in sympathetic nerve activity and declines in oxygen demand. Circulation 1999;100:164–170.
50. Lind L, Lithell H. Decreased peripheral blood flow in the pathogenesis of the metabolic syndrome comprising hypertension, hyperlipidemia, and hyperinsulinemia. Am Heart J 1993;125:1494–1497.
51. Baron AD, Laakso M, Brechtel G, Hoit B, Watt C, Edelman SV. Reduced postprandial skeletal muscle blood flow contributes to glucose intolerance in human obesity. J Clin Endocrinol Metab 1990;70:1525–1533.
52. Tagawa T, Imaizumi T, Endo T, Shiramoto M, Harasawa Y, Takeshita A. Role of nitric oxide in reactive hyperemia in human forearm vessels. Circulation 1994;90:2285–2290.
53. Huang AL, Silver AE, Shvenke E, Schopfer DW, Jahangir E, Titas MA, Shpilman A, Menzoian JO, Watkins MT, Raffetto JD, Gibbons G, Woodson J, Shaw PM, Dhadly M, Eberhardt RT, Keaney JF, Jr., Gokce N, Vita JA. Predictive value of reactive hyperemia for cardiovascular events in patients with peripheral arterial disease undergoing vascular surgery. Arterioscler Thromb Vasc Biol 2007;27(10):2113–2119.
54. Mitchell GF, Parise H, Vita JA, Larson MG, Warner E, Keaney JF, Jr., Keyes MJ, Levy D, Vasan RS, Benjamin EJ. Local shear stress and brachial artery flow-mediated dilation: the Framingham Heart Study. Hypertension 2004;44(2): 134–139.
55. Pyke KE, Tschakovsky ME. The relationship between shear stress and flow-mediated dilatation: implications for the assessment of endothelial function. J Physiol 2005;568:357–369.
56. Miura H, Wachtel RE, Liu Y, Loberiza FR, Jr., Saito T, Miura M, Gutterman DD. Flow-induced dilation of human coronary arterioles: important role of Ca(2+)-activated K(+) channels. Circulation 2001;103(15):1992–1998.
57. Carlsson I, Sollevi A, Wennmalm A. The role of myogenic relaxation, adenosine and prostaglandins in human forearm reactive hyperaemia. J Physiol 1987;389:147–161.
58. Agabiti-Rosei E, Rizzoni D, Castellano M, Porteri E, Zulli R, Muiesan ML, Bettoni G, Salvetti M, Muiesan P, Giulini SM. Media:lumen ratio in human small resistance arteries is related to forearm minimal vascular resistance. J Hypertens 1995;13:341–347.
59. Folkow B. Hypertensive structural changes in systemic precapillary resistance vessels: how important are they for in vivo haemodynamics? J Hypertens 1995;13:1546–1559.
60. Vuilleumier P, Decosterd D, Maillard M, Burnier M, Hayoz D. Postischemic forearm skin reactive hyperemia is related to cardiovascular risk factors in a healthy female population. J Hypertens 2002;20(9):1753–1757.

III

Non Invasive Structural Imaging of Asymptomatic Atherosclerotic Cardiovascular Disease

20 Coronary Artery Calcium Imaging

Harvey S. Hecht

Contents

Abstract

Coronary artery calcium imaging (CAC) in the asymptomatic population has been investigated in tens of thousands of primary prevention patients. The consistent results in both retrospective and prospective studies have confirmed the vast superiority of CAC to all risk-factor based predictive paradigms, e.g., Framingham Risk Score. Nonetheless, CAC screening has not yet been implemented. Future directions will include a lower radiation dose, and a concerted effort to incorporate CAC screening into routine preventive care.

Key words: Coronary artery calcium; Coronary artery disease; Screening

TOPIC PEARLS

- CAC is the most powerful predictor of coronary risk in the primary prevention population.
- Conventional risk factor based predictive paradigms are completely inadequate.
- Widespread screening by CAC offers the best hope for decreasing cardiac risk.

Coronary artery calcium (CAC) can be measured by two technologies. Electron beam computed tomography (EBCT) utilizes a rotating electron beam to acquire triggered, tomographic 100 ms X-ray images at 3 mm intervals in the space of a 30–40-s breath-hold, and precisely quantifies the calcified plaque in the epicardial coronary arteries. Multidetector computed tomography (MDCT) employs a rotating gantry with a special X-ray tube and variable number of detectors (from 4 to 64), with 165–500 ms

From: *Asymptomatic Atherosclerosis: Pathophysiology, Detection and Treatment*
Edited by: M. Naghavi (ed.), DOI 10.1007/978-1-60327-179-0_20

images at 0.5,1.5, 2.0, or 3.0 mm intervals, depending on the protocol and manufacturer. CAC is always associated with mural atheromatous plaque [1, 2]. A direct relationship has been established between CAC as measured by EBCT, and both histologic [3] and in-vivo intravascular ultrasound measures of atherosclerotic plaque [4, 5]. CAC provides an accurate estimate of total plaque burden, the most powerful predictor of cardiac events [6].

CORONARY CALCIUM SCORE

The original calcium score developed by Agatston et al. [7] is an index of plaque quantity, determined by plaque area and calcium lesion density. Scores of 1–100 are considered mild; 101–400, moderate; and greater than >400, severe. The calcium volume score [8] is a more reproducible parameter (SEM = 8%) that is independent of calcium density, and is considered to be the parameter of choice for serial studies to track progression or regression of atherosclerosis. By comparing a subject's calcium score to that of others of the same age and gender through the use of large databases of asymptomatic subjects (Table 1), a calcium percentile rank for any given individual patient can be determined [9, 10]. This is an index of the prematurity or, alternatively, the latency of atherosclerosis.

PREDICTIVE VALUE

Table 2 summarizes the relevant predictive studies.

The final report of the NCEP guidelines [26] made the following recommendation on the basis of existing data at the time of publication (2002): "Therefore, measurement of coronary calcium is an option for advanced risk assessment in appropriately selected persons. In persons with multiple risk factors, high coronary calcium scores (e.g., >75th percentile for age and sex) denotes advanced coronary atherosclerosis and provides a rationale for intensified LDL-lowering therapy."

Subsequent to the NCEP guidelines, several major reports have highlighted the incremental value of CAC to conventional risk factor assessment. In a retrospective analysis, Kondos et al. [16], in 5,635

Table 1
Database coronary artery calcium scores of asymptomatic subjects as a function of age and gender

		EBCT coronary calcium scores in asymptomatic patients as a function of patient age at the time of the examination					
		46–50	*51–55*	*56–60*	*61–65*	*66–70*	*70+*
Men (n = 28,250)							
10	0	0	0	1	1	3	3
25	0	1	2	5	12	30	69
50	2	3	15	54	117	166	350
75	11	36	110	229	386	538	844
90	69	151	346	588	933	1151	1650
Women (n = 14,540)							
10	0	0	0	0	0	0	0
25	0	0	0	0	0	1	4
50	0	0	1	1	3	25	51
75	1	2	6	22	68	148	231
90	4	21	61	127	208	327	698

Table 2
Characteristics and risk ratio for follow-up studies using electron beam computed tomography in asymptomatic persons

Author	*N*	*Mean age (years)*	*Follow-up duration (years)*	*Calcium score cutoff*	*Comparator group for RR calculation*	*Relative risk ratio*
Arad [11]	1,173	53	3.6	CAC>160	CAC<160	20.2
Detrano [12]	1,196	66	3.4	CAC>44	CAC<44	2.3
Park [13]	967	67	6.4	CAC>142.1	CAC<3.7	4.9
Raggi [14]	632	52	2.7	Top quartile	Lowest quartile	13
Wong [15]	926	54	3.3	Top quartile (>270)	First score quartile	8.8
Kondos [16]	5,635	51	3.1	CAC	No CAC	10.5
Greenland[17]	1,312	66	7.0	CAC>300	No CAC	3.9
Shaw [18]	10,377	53	5	CAC³400	CAC£10	8.4
Arad [19]	5,585	59	4.3	CAC³100	CAC<100	10.7
Taylor [20]	2,000	40–50	3.0	CAC>44	CAC=0	11.8
Vliegenthart [21]	1,795	71	3.3	CAC>1,000	CAC<100	8.3
				CAC 400–1,000	CAC<100	4.6
Budoff [22]	25,503	56	6.8	CAC>400	CAC 0	9.2
Lagoski [23]	3,601	45–84	3.75	CAC>0	CAC 0	6.5
Becker [24]	1,726	57.7	3.4	CAC>400	CAC 0	6.8 men7.9 women
Detrano [25]	6,814	62.2	3.8	CAC>300	CAC 0	14.1

CAC Coronary artery calcium score

asymptomatic, predominantly low to moderate risk, largely middle-aged patients followed for 37 ± 12 months, found that the presence of any CAC by EBCT was associated with a relative risk for events of 10.5, compared to 1.98 and 1.4 for diabetes and smoking, respectively. In women, only CAC was linked to events, with a relative risk of 2.6; traditional risk factors were not related. The presence of CAC provided prognostic information, incremental with age and other risk factors.

Shaw et al. [18] retrospectively analyzed 10,377 asymptomatic patients with a 5-year follow up after an initial EBCT evaluation. All-cause mortality increased proportionally to increasing CAC, which was an independent predictor of risk after adjusting for all of the Framingham risk factors ($p<0.001$). Superiority of CAC to conventional Framingham risk factor assessment was demonstrated by a significantly greater area under the ROC curves (0.73 vs. 0.67, $p<0.001$). Incremental value of CAC to Framingham risk was also established by a significant increase of the area under the ROC curves, from 0.72 for Framingham risk to 0.78 with the addition of CAC ($p<0.001$). In addition, Greenland et al. [17] prospectively followed 1,461 asymptomatic, predominantly moderate to high risk population based patients and found that CAC scores of >300 significantly added prognostic information to Framingham risk analysis in the 10–20% Framingham risk category.

The results of the St Francis Heart Study by Arad et al. [19] in a prospective, population based study of 5,585 asymptomatic, predominantly moderate to moderately high risk men and women, mirrored previous retrospective studies [11–15], and confirmed the higher event rates associated with increasing CAC scores. CAC scores of >100 were associated with relative risk ranging from 12 to 32, and secondary prevention equivalent to event rates of >2%/year. The areas under the ROC curves were 0.81 for CAC and 0.71 for Framingham ($p<0.01$). Moreover, classification by CAC tertiles changed approximately 67% of patients classified in the Framingham 10–20%, 10-year event rate group to either lower or higher risk as determined by actual outcome. In the Framingham high risk category (>20%, 10-year event rate), 45% were moved to lower risk categories by CAC tertile reclassification. Finally, in the Framingham <10%, 10-year risk group, 29% had scores of >100 with an associated 1.7%/year event rate.

Taylor et al. [20] demonstrated the powerful predictive value of CAC in a younger cohort of 2,000 asymptomatic Army personnel. There was a relative risk of 11.8 in patients with CAC of >44 compared to those with 0 CAC, after correcting for the Framingham Risk Score. In a much more elderly population (71 years), Vliegenthart et al. found a hazard ratio of 4.6 for CAC of 400–1,000 compared to <100, after 3.3 years of follow up [21].

Based upon the accumulated evidence, the ACCF/AHA 2007 Clinical Expert Consensus Document [27] judged that in the intermediate risk population "it may be reasonable to consider use of CAC measurement in such patients, based on available evidence that demonstrates incremental risk prediction information in this selected (intermediate risk) patient group."

Subsequently, even more powerful data have emerged, which have not yet been incorporated into a new societal recommendation. Budoff et al. [22], in another all cause mortality study, with retrospective analysis of 25,203 asymptomatic patients after 6.8 years, found that CAC>400 was associated with a hazard ratio of 9.2. In the female component of the prospective Multiethnic Study of Atherosclerosis (MESA), Lagoski et al. reported a 6.5 hazard ratio for a CAC of >0 vs. 0. In the full MESA cohort of 6,814 patients followed for 3.8 years [23], Detrano et al. noted a hazard ratio of 14.1 for CAC>300 [24]. In the largest study using coronary calcium percentile rather than absolute scores, Becker et al., in 1,724 patients followed prospectively for 3.4 years, reported hazard ratios for CAC percentile of >75% vs. 0% of 6.8 for men and 7.9 for women. CAC percentile was significantly superior to the Framingham, European Society of Cardiology and PROCAM risk scores [25].

In all of these studies, receiver operator characteristic curves for CAC were superior to the Framingham Risk Score and the annual event rate for CAC>100–400 exceeded the coronary artery disease equivalent of >2%/year. Table 20.1 summarizes the relative risk results of the largest published outcome studies.

0 CAC

Individuals with 0 CAC scores have not yet developed detectable, calcified coronary plaque. It must be understood that a zero score does not mean that there is no plaque; there is not an invariably benign outcome. Fatty streaking and early stages of plaque are present in many young adults [28], and events occur in patients with 0 CAC scores [14, 17–19, 24]. However, Raggi et al. [14] have demonstrated a very low annual event rate of 0.11% in asymptomatic subjects with 0 scores, and in the St. Francis Heart Study [19], scores of 0 were associated with a 0.12% annual event rate over the ensuing 4.3 years. Greenland et al. [17], in a higher risk asymptomatic cohort, noted a higher annual event rate (0.62%) with 0 CAC scores; a less sensitive CAC detection technique may have contributed to their findings [29]. Subsequent reports have confirmed the benign prognosis of 0 CAC, with a 0% event rate reported by Becker et al. [25], and a.0.4% annual event rate in the MESA study [24].

PARADIGM SHIFT

The consistently demonstrated superiority of CAC scoring to the conventional risk-factor based prediction of outcomes in the primary prevention population, establishes the rationale for its wide application in males 45 years and older, and females 55 years and older. Paradigms for modification by CAC scores of the NCEP ATP-III guidelines for initiation of lipid lowering therapy have been developed, particularly in the intermediate risk population. Selective utilization in lower risk younger patients with a premature family history of coronary disease is appropriate, as well as in higher risk patients in whom determination of the calcified plaque burden is critical to decision making.

LIMITATIONS

EBCT scanners are relatively few in number (~100) and will likely decrease further. MDCT scanners number in the thousands and are rapidly increasing. Current charges for coronary scanning range from $300 to $500, and will likely decrease to ~$100, especially when widespread partial or full insurance coverage is implemented. Radiation is implicit in the test and ranges from 0.9 mSv for EBCT to ~1.2 mSv for MDCT. Comparability of measurements between EBCT and MDCT, and between different MDCT scanners may vary; the development of a mass score may ensure widespread comparability. CAC measurement is easily, accurately, and reproducibly accomplished within several minutes [30].

FUTURE

CAC scanning is a mature technology, and CT will become the modality of choice for risk stratification, particularly in intermediate risk patients, with selective application in the lower and higher risk groups. The persistent obstacle to stronger societal screening recommendations has been the demand for studies demonstrating the effect of CAC on outcomes, a prerequisite not satisfied by any risk factor based predictive model, or by any other technology.

Further developments will include decreasing radiation, shorter acquisition times, a universal scoring system, and plaque characterization beyond calcification. A priori, CAC scores will not detect non-calcified plaques. CT angiography is better suited for the non-invasive detection of the non-calcified component of coronary atherosclerotic plaques, and will hopefully be intrumental in the classification of plaques along the spectrum of stable to vulnerable.

REFERENCES

1. Rifkin RD, Parisi AF, Folland E. Coronary calcification in the diagnosis of coronary artery disease. *Am J Cardiol* 1979;44:141–147.
2. McCarthy JH, Palmer FJ. Incidence and significance of coronary artery calcification. *Br Heart J* 1974;36:499–506.
3. Rumberger JA, Simons DB, Fitzpatrick LA, et al. Coronary artery calcium areas by electron beam computed tomography and coronary atherosclerotic plaque area: A histopathologic correlative study. *Circulation* 1995;92:2157–2162.
4. Baumgart D, Schmermund A, Goerge G, et al. Comparison of electron beam computed tomography with intracoronary ultrasound and coronary angiography for detection of coronary atherosclerosis. *J Am Coll Cardiol* 1997;30:57–64.
5. Schmermund A, Baumgart D, Gorge G, et al. Coronary artery calcium in abute coronary syndromes: A comparative study of electron beam CT, coronary angiography, and intracoronary ultrasound in survivors of acute myocardial infarction and unstable angina. *Circulation* 1997;96:1461–1469.
6. Roberts WC, Jones AA: Quantization of coronary arterial narrowing at necropsy in sudden coronary death: Analysis of 31 patients and comparison with 25 control subjects. *Am J Cardiol* 1979;44:39–45.
7. Agatston AS, Janowitz WR, Hildner FJ, et al. Quantification of coronary artery calcium using ultrafast computed tomography. *J Am Coll Cardiol* 1990;15:827–832.
8. Callister TQ, Cooil B, Raya SP, et al. Coronary artery disease: Improved reproducibility of calcium scoring with an electron-beam CT volumetric method. *Radiology* 1998;208:807–814.
9. Hoff JA, Chomka EV, Krainik AJ, et al. Age and gender distributions of coronary artery calcium detected by electron beam tomography in 35,246 adults. *Am J Cardiol* 2001;87:1335.

10. Schmermund A, Erbel R, Silber S. Age and gender distribution of coronary artery calcium measured by four-slice computed tomography in 2,030 persons with no symptoms of coronary artery disease. *Am J Cardiol* 2002;90:169–173.
11. Arad Y, Spadaro L, Goodman K, et al. Prediction of coronary events with electron beam computed tomography. *J Am Coll Cardiol* 2000;36:1253–1260.
12. Detrano RC, Wong ND, Doherty TM, et al. Coronary calcium does not accurately predict term coronary events in high-risk adults. *Circulation* 1999;99:2633–2638.
13. Park, R, Detrano R, Xiang M, et al. Combined use of computed tomography coronary calcium scores and C-reactive protein levels in predicting cardiovascular events in non-diabetic individuals. *Circulation* 2002;106:2073–2077.
14. Raggi P, Callister TQ, Cooil B, et al. Identification of patients at increased risk of first unheralded acute myocardial infarction by electron beam computed tomography. *Circulation* 2000;101:850–885.
15. Wong ND, Hsu JC, Detrano RC, et al. Coronary artery calcium evaluation by electron beam computed tomography and its relation to new cardiovascular events. *Am J Cardiol* 2000;86:495–498.
16. Kondos GT, Hoff JA, Sevrukov A, et al. Coronary artery calcium and cardiac events electron-beam tomography coronary artery calcium and cardiac events: A 37-month follow-up of 5,635 initially asymptomatic low to intermediate risk adults. *Circulation* 2003;107:2571–2576.
17. Greenland P, LaBree L, Azen SP, et al. Coronary artery calcium score combined with Framingham score for risk prediction in asymptomatic individuals. *JAMA* 2004;291:210–215.
18. Shaw LJ, Raggi P, Schisterman E, et al. Prognostic value of cardiac risk factors and coronary artery calcium screening for all-cause mortality. *Radiology* 2003;28:826–833.
19. Arad Y, Goodman K, Roth M, Newstein D, Guerci AD. Coronary calcification, coronary disease risk factors, C-reactive protein, and atherosclerotic cardiovascular disease events: The St. Francis Heart Study. *J Am Coll Cardiol* 2005;46:158–165.
20. Taylor AJ, Bindeman J, Feuerstein I, et al. Coronary calcium independently predicts incident premature coronary heart disease over measured cardiovascular risk factors: Mean three-year outcomes in the Prospective Army Coronary Calcium (PACC) project. *J Am Coll Cardiol* 2005;46:807–814.
21. Vliegenthart R, Oudkerk M, Hofman A, et al. Coronary calcification improves cardiovascular risk prediction in the elderly. *Circulation* 2005;112:572–577.
22. Budoff MJ, Shaw LJ, Liu ST, et al. Long-term prognosis associated with coronary calcification: Observations trom a registry of 25,253 patients. *J Am Coll Cardiol* 2007;49:1860–1870.
23. Lakoski SG, Greenland P, Wong ND, et al. Coronary artery calcium scores and risk for cardiovascular events in women classified as "Low Risk" based on Framingham risk score. The Multi-Ethnic Study of Atherosclerosis (MESA). *Arch Intern Med* 2007;167(22):2437–2442.
24. Detrano R,Guerci AD, Carr JJ. et al. Coronary calcium as a predictor of coronary events in four racial or ethnic groups. *N Engl J Med* 2008;358:1336–1345.
25. Becker A ,Leber A, Becker C, Knez A. Predictive value of coronary calcifications for future cardiac events in asymptomatic individuals. *Am Heart J* 2008;155:154–160.
26. Third Report of the National Cholesterol Education Program (NCEP) Expert Panel on Detection, Evaluation, and Treatment of High Blood Cholesterol in Adults (Adult Treatment Panel III). Final Report. *NIH Publication* No. 02-5215. September 2002.
27. Greenland P, Bonow RO, Brundage BH, et al. Clinical expert consensus document on coronary artery calcium scoring by computed tomography in global cardiovascular risk assessment and in evaluation of patients with chest pain. *J Am Coll Cardiol* 2007;49(3):378–402.
28. Tuzcu EM, Kapadia SR, Tutar E, et al. High prevalence of coronary atherosclerosis in asymptomatic teenagers and young adults: Evidence from intravascular ultrasound. *Circulation* 2001;103:2705–2710.
29. Budoff MJ, Ehrlich J, Hecht HS, Rumberger JR. Letter to the editor. *JAMA* 2004;291:1822.
30. Nasir K, Budoff MJ, Post WS et al. Electron beam CT versus helical CT scans for assessing coronary calcification: Current utility and future directions. *Am Heart J* 2003;146:969–977.

21 Noninvasive Ultrasound Imaging of Carotid Intima Thickness

Tasneem Z. Naqvi

CONTENTS

From: *Asymptomatic Atherosclerosis: Pathophysiology, Detection and Treatment*
Edited by: M. Naghavi (ed.), DOI 10.1007/978-1-60327-179-0_21

Abstract

Atherosclerotic cardiovascular disease is the leading cause of mortality in the West and is a rapidly growing problem worldwide. Long subclinical incubation period of atherosclerosis and earliest involvement of the vessel wall provide an opportunity to evaluate the presence of atherosclerosis by imaging arterial wall and initiate treatment measures. Assessment of thickness of intima-media layer of the vessel wall as well as early plaques by ultrasound is the most sensitive, reliable, noninvasive, and safe method to detect those at risk. Carotid artery vessel wall assessment in the form of intima-media thickness (IMT) has been identified since the late 1970s as a sensitive tool to detect atherosclerosis, predict its sequelae, and detect its progression and regression. Recent studies have shown that the presence of carotid plaques is also a strong predictor of disease, independent of carotid IMT. The technique has been recommended by writing groups such as American Heart Association as a useful tool for risk stratification in those with unclear or intermediate risk of cardiovascular disease. Validated reference databases exist for reporting purposes. Several automated robust softwares are now available that allow automated measurement of IMT by edge detection algorithms.

Key words: Carotid Artery; Intima-media thickness; Plaque; Ultrasound; Vessel

TOPIC PEARLS

- Anatomic measures of intima-media thickness (IMT) of the carotid artery wall represent the cumulative effects of an individual's exposure over years to identified and unidentified risk factors, and provide a snapshot of atherosclerotic disease in evolution.
- Elevated carotid IMT or the presence of carotid plaques, in addition to clinical risk factor assessment is the most sensitive method to assess future cardiovascular risk.
- The AHA suggested consideration of IMT determinations for patients older than 45 years who are at intermediate risk.
- Availability of population norms based on several NIH-sponsored multicenter studies, recent AHA clinical guidelines on the use of IMT, portable, safe and economic nature of this ultrasound test, improved image resolution and availability of computerized, automated edge detection algorithms now have made this technique ripe for clinical use.

WHAT IS IMT AND HOW IS IT MEASURED?

Carotid IMT (CIMT) uses conventional B-mode ultrasound to measure the thickness of the arterial wall. M-mode assessment provides better temporal resolution and provides comparable assessment of IMT [1]. IMT is defined as the distance between the lumen–intima interface and the media–adventitia interface (Fig. 1). Since the current ultrasound technology does not allow measurement of the intima alone, both intima and surrounding media are measured. Combined use of intima and media as IMT therefore represents a combination of the manifestations of early atherosclerosis. IMT may also represent

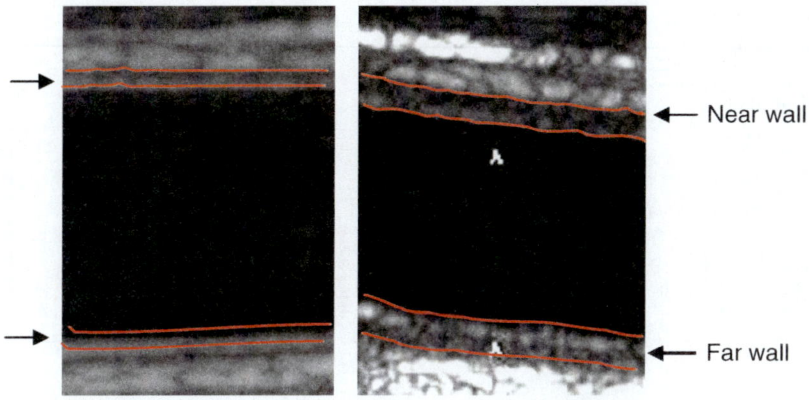

Fig. 1. Example of a normal and abnormal carotid artery intima-media thickness.

smooth muscle hypertrophy and/or hyperplasia, which may be induced by pressure overload [2] and/or age-related sclerosis.

Current equations to predict cardiovascular events include Framingham [3, 4], PROCAM [5], Sheffield table system [6], and BRHS scoring systems [7]. All these have very low specificity because of several emerging, genetic and unknown risk factors that these equations do not consider. Thus, although these scoring systems identify high-risk group (greater than 20% events over 10 years), they fail to identify the majority of patients who develop CV events despite being classified as "low risk." Controlling risk factors has been shown to reduce CV events in symptomatic [8] as well as asymptomatic subjects [9]. Similar effect may be found in individuals with diseased vessels and therefore "subclinical atherosclerosis" who have not yet developed evidence of symptomatic atherosclerosis. Ultrasound of major vessels (carotid and femoral arteries) can measure the thickness of artery wall as well as can detect the presence, size and nature of plaques each of which incrementally increases the risk of cardiovascular events. Unlike risk factors, anatomic measures of intima-media thickness (IMT) of the carotid artery wall in adulthood represent the cumulative effects of an individual's exposure over years to identified and unidentified risk factors, and measure that person's own response to such an exposure. In essence, imaging of the vessel wall itself allows a snapshot of disease in evolution, or preclinical disease that is of greater value than conventional risk factors such as low-density lipoprotein (LDL) cholesterol (LDL-C), high-density lipoprotein (HDL) cholesterol (HDL-C), total cholesterol, systolic and diastolic pressure [10, 11] diabetes, fasting glucose and insulin, reduced insulin sensitivity [12], and active and passive smoking in both genders [13–16], and body mass index, and triglycerides in women [14, 15, 17]. In addition, IMT is not only associated with coronary artery disease (CAD), it is predictive of cerebrovascular disease [18], left ventricular hypertrophy [19], albuminuria [20], ankle brachial index [21], CAD [11–16], endothelial function [22] and coronary artery calcium (CAC) score [23, 24]. Several studies have shown the association of IMT with conventional [25] as well as emerging [6] CV risk factors. Excellent reviews detail the predictive value of IMT for prevalent and incident cardiovascular disease (CVD) [26–31].

CIMT can be measured reliably by ultrasound and correlates with autopsy measurements [32]. In healthy adults, mean CIMT ranges from 0.25 to 1.5 mm [33], and values of 1.0 mm are often regarded as abnormal. Normal values based on age and gender for black and white races have been derived [34, 35] (Figs. 2–4).

Fig. 2. Carotid plaque and intima-media thickness assessed by B-mode ultrasonography in subjects ranging from young adults to centenarians. (Reproduced from Homma S, et al. Stroke 2001 32: 830–835).

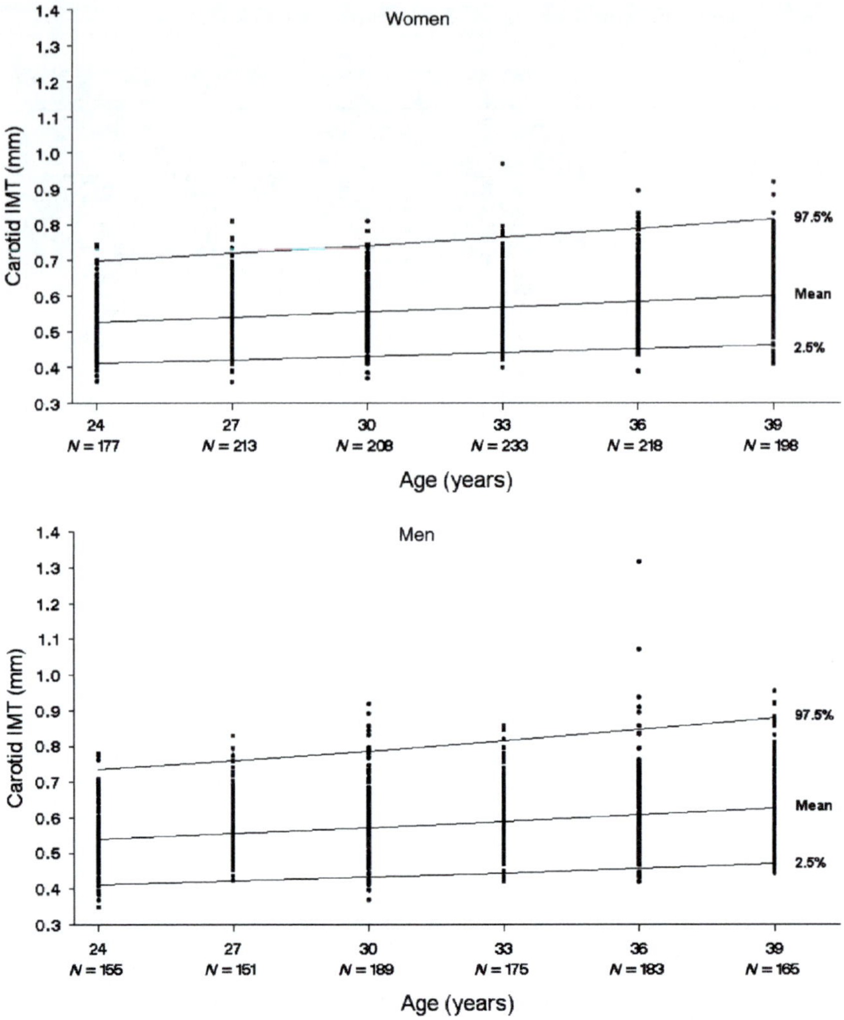

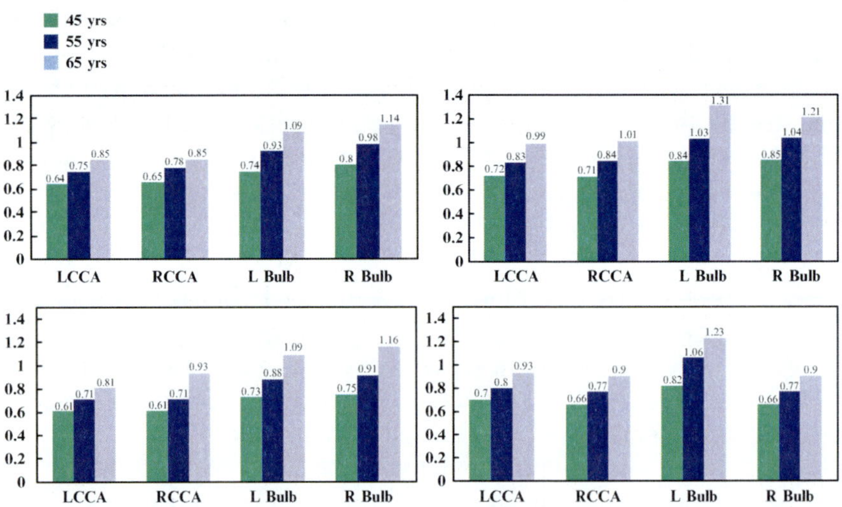

Fig. 3. Bar graph of 75th percentiles of common carotid artery (CCA) and carotid artery bifurcation IMT in men and women stratified according to decade of age (45 years green, 55 years dark blue, 65 years light blue and race). (Adapted from Howard G, et al. Stroke 1993; 24:1297–304.)

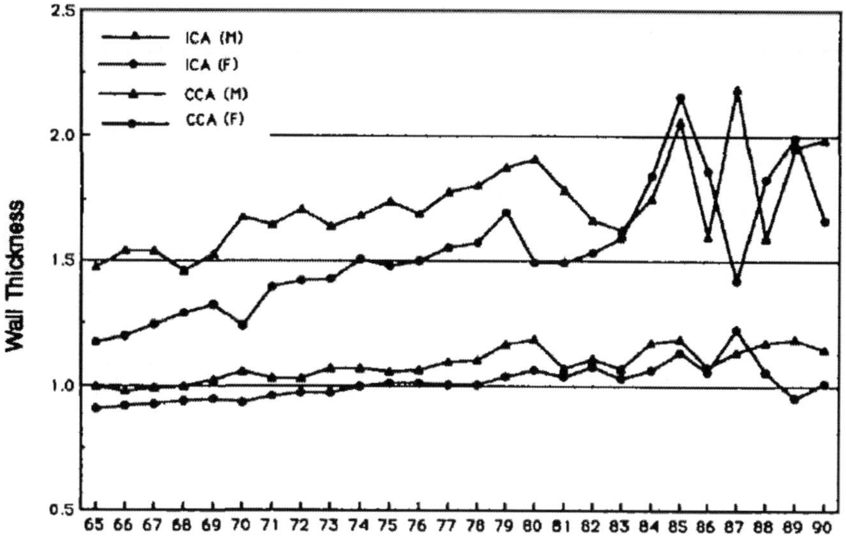

Fig. 4. Line graph of maximum internal carotid artery (ICA) and CCA wall thickness by age for women (F) and men (M). (Reproduced from O'Leary DH, et al. Stroke 1992; 23:1752–1760.)

DISTRIBUTION OF IMT IN NORMAL POPULATION

Cross-sectional analysis suggests that age-related increases in wall thickness average approximately 0.015 mm/year in women and 0.018 mm/year in men in the carotid bifurcation, 0.010 mm/y for women and 0.014 mm/year for men in the internal carotid artery (ICA), and 0.010 mm/year in both sexes in the common carotid artery (CCA; ARIC) [34]. Very close results are observed in older populations with estimates around 0.008–/0.010 mm/year in both sexes [36]. Men have uniformly larger wall thickness than women and IMT increases progressively with age. Individuals tend to have a larger wall thickness in the carotid bifurcation than in CCA. ICA values are more variable. African-Americans have modestly higher CCA IMT values than Caucasians [34]. On average, a healthy person reaches an IMT of 0.78 mm at the age of 76 years. In the Community Health Study (CHS) population aged >65 years, 80th percentile of CCA IMT was 1.18 mm [37]. Thickening of the intima-media is accelerated and enhanced in the presence of risk factors of atherosclerosis. In familial hypercholesterolemia patients, this IMT is already reached at the age of 40 years [38]. Thus, IMT is used as a tool to investigate normal aging and preclinical atherosclerosis. One study found that mean IMT in plaque-free sites correlates linearly with age from young adults to centenarians [39] (Fig. 5).

IMT in the Young: Appendix 1 and Fig. 2 detail the distribution of IMT in young adults on the basis of Bogolusa Study [40]. In a study of healthy 10–20 year olds, femoral and CCA IMT was measured [41].

Appendix 2 and Fig. 3 represent the distribution of IMT in middle-aged adults on the basis of ARIC study [34] and Fig. 4 represents the distribution of IMT in older adults greater than 65 years on the basis of CHS study [36]. In the CHS study, IMT of the CCA increased by 0.01 mm for each year beyond 65 in both sexes and that of ICA by 0.02 mm.

PREDICTIVE VALUE OF IMT IN PRIMARY RISK STRATIFICATION

Seven important studies measured CIMT in adults [10, 34, 42–49] and four studies measured CIMT in children and young adults [50–53]. Although the studies measured IMT in different segments – CCA, bulb or bifurcation, and ICA, near or far wall – all of them measured the CCA far-wall IMT. Two different measurements were used – mean and maximum IMT. Most of these studies reported the mean

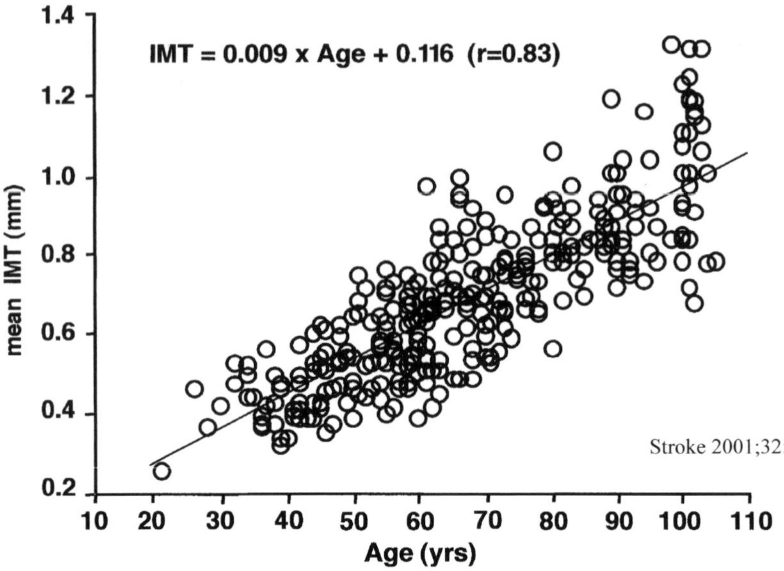

Fig. 5. Scatter plot of mean carotid artery thickness in young healthy adults. (Reproduced from Juonala M, et al. Eur Heart J 2008; 29:1198–1206)

IMT based on the right and left CCA. These studies include the EVA (Etude sur Ie vieillissement arreriel, Vascular Aging Study), ARIC (Atherosclerosis Risk in Communities), "Rotterdam," and AXA (name of a French insurance company) studies. The EAS (Edinburgh Artery Study) reported the greatest maximum measure on either the right or left CCA. KIHD (Kuopio Ischemic Heart Disease) and CHS (Cardiovascular Health Study) studies measured mean maximum IMT.

Increased IMT might occur in an earlier phase of the atherosclerotic process [54]. This is suggested by findings of EVA study where propensity for plaques development increased incrementally based on baseline abnormality in IMT over 4-year follow up in subjects 59–71 years old. However majority of plaques formed at the bulb and ICA during follow up and not at CCA where baseline IMT was measured; hence, CIMT and plaque are likely different phenotypes of atherosclerosis. In the Rotterdam nested case control study (374 subjects, 1,496 controls) [48], CIMT (CCA, bulb or ICA max, sensitivity 14%, specificity 96%) did not improve prediction of future stroke or Myocardial Infarction (MI) over and above conventional risk factors (sensitivity 17%, specificity 95%), however in this study, subjects with previous MI or stroke were also included. This history of previous CV disease was used as a variable in multivariate analysis. This may explain why the Rotterdam investigators were unable to show a strong association between CCA IMT and the risk of MI [55]. In a separate analysis in the same study that excluded patients with symptomatic atherosclerosis both CIMT and carotid plaques predicted incident MI independent of risk factors [56]. A separate report from the same study in 7,983 subjects in whom subjects with a previous MI or stroke were excluded, odds ratio of CIMT was 1.57 for stroke and 1.51 for MI [57]. In the CHS study [58] in previously asymptomatic elderly subjects >65 years old, each quintile of increased CIMT was associated with incremental risk of future stroke or MI, relative risk of 1.54, 1.84, 2.01, and 3.15 for second, third, fourth, and fifth quintiles, respectively, after adjusting for traditional CV risk factors.

IMT PROGRESSION RATES

Smoking was a statistically significant predictor of common and composite CIMT progression in both sexes in the Bogolusa Heart Study (Table 1). In men, systolic blood pressure (SBP) was an independent predictor of internal carotid and composite CIMT progression, fasting glucose predicted com-

Table 1
Predictors of CIMT Progression in healthy young adults (Bogolusa Study)

	Men				*Women*			
Variable	*β*	*95%*	*CI*	P_{adj}	*β*	*95%*	*CI*	P_{adj}
Intercept	−0.0242	−0.0833	0.0348	0.417	−0.0424	−0.0825	−0.0023	0.038
Age	0.0001	−0.0013	0.0015	0.874	0.0009	− 0.0001	0.0018	0.065
BMI	0.0006	−0.0004	0.0017	0.221	0.0001	−0.0004	0.0007	0.640
Current drinker	−0.0089	−0.0181	0.0004	0.059	−0.0009	−0.0070	0.0053	0.777
Current smoker	0.0092	0.0007	0.0177	0.035	0.0064	0.0003	0.0125	0.039
Family history	0.0016	−0.0062	0.0094	0.687	0.0013	−0.0048	0.0073	0.682
Glucose	0.0005	0.0001	0.0010	0.025	0.0000	−0.0003	0.0003	0.979
Log insulin	−0.0021	−0.0247	0.0205	0.854	0.0034	−0.0140	0.0208	0.701
SBP	−0.0002	−0.0005	0.0002	0.351	0.0001	−0.0001	0.0004	0.301
Total/HDL cholesterol ratio	0.0005	−0.0018	0.0028	0.652	0.0014	−0.0009	0.0037	0.234
(b) Carotid bulb								
Intercept	−0.0248	−0.1849	0.1353	0.758	0.0350	−0.0714	0.1414	0.517
Age	0.0005	−0.0032	0.0042	0.789	0.0013	−0.0011	0.0038	0.281
BMI	−0.0007	−0.0035	0.0021	0.621	−0.0003	−0.0019	0.0013	0.748
Current drinker	0.0050	−0.0188	0.0289	0.675	−0.0125	−0.0290	0.0041	0.138
Current smoker	0.0171	−0.0053	0.0395	0.133	0.0157	−0,0007	0.0320	0.060
Family history	0.0184	−0.0022	0.0389	0.079	0.0008	−0.0155	0.0172	0.920
Glucose	−0.0004	−0.0016	0.0009	0.534	−0.0001	−0.0008	0.0006	0.771
Log insulin	0.0361	−0.0225	0.0948	0.223	0.0275	−0.0200	0.0749	0.254
SBP	0.0002	−0.0006	0.0011	0.564	−0.0007	−0.0013	0.0000	0.052
TotaL/HOL cholesterol ratio	−0.0005	−0.0064	0.0055	0.872	0.0019	−0.0042	0.0080	0.532
(c) Internal carotid artery								
Intercept	−0.1409	−0.2931	0.0113	0.069	−0.0712	−0.1556	0.0131	0.097
Age	−0.0003	−0.0038	0.0031	0.842	0.0012	−0.0007	0.0031	0.208
BMI	−0.0022	−0.0049	0.0004	0.095	−0.0002	−0.0014	0.0011	0.809
Current drinker	0.0028	−0.0209	0.0264	0.815	0.0051	−0.0079	0.0181	0.436
Current smoker	0.0131	−0.0088	0.0350	0.237	0.0095	−0.0038	0.0229	0.160
Family history	0.0183	−0.0015	0.0382	0.069	0.0045	−0.0086	0.0175	0.502
Glucose	0.0009	−0.0003	0.0022	0.133	0.0003	−0.0002	0.0009	0.233
Log insulin	−0.0025	−0.0599	0.0549	0.931	0.0001	−0.0368	0.0370	0.996
SBP	0.0011	0.0003	0.0020	0.008	−0.0001	−0.0006	0.0005	0.831
Total/HDL cholesterol ratio	0.0014	−0.0043	0.0072	0.620	0.0034	−0.0024	0.0093	0.245
(d) Composite								
Intercept	−0.0765	−0.1560	0.0031	0.059	−0.0248	−0.0785	0.0290	0.363
Age	−0.0001	−0.0019	0.0017	0.931	0.0011	−0.0001	0.0023	0.082
BMI	−0.0006	−0.0020	0.0008	0.380	0.0001	−0.0007	0.0009	0.867
Current drinker	−0.0013	−0.0134	0.0108	0.832	−0.0030	−0.0113	0.0053	0.474
Current smoker	0.0173	0.0059	0.0286	0.003	0.0110	0.0027	0.0194	0.010
Family history	0.0138	0.0036	0.0241	0.008	0.0020	−0.0064	0.0104	0.631
Glucose	0.0003	−0.0003	0.0009	0.342	0.0001	−0.0003	0.0004	0.726
Log insulin	0.0093	−0.0200	0.0387	0.527	0.0053	−0.0187	0.0294	0.662
SBP	0.0006	0.0001	0.0010	0.009	−0.0002	−0.0005	0.0002	0.303
Total/HDL cholesterol ratio	0.0007	−0.0023	0.0036	0.652	0.0023	−0.0007	0.0054	0.134

mon CIMT progression, and family history predicted composite CIMT progression [59]. In middle-aged and older women, serum triglycerides, presence of the metabolic syndrome, and pulse pressure predicted CIMT progression compared with men, whereas physical activity and fibrinogen levels independently predicted CIMT in middle-aged and older men but not in women [60–62]. Age, SBP, fasting glucose, and smoking predicted CIMT progression in both middle-aged and older men and women [63]. In middle-aged adults in the Atherosclerosis Risk in Communities study, there was a linear relation between total pack-years of smoking and increased CIMT that persisted with adjustment for age and sex [64]. Statistically significant associations were found between change in IMT and change in LDL cholesterol (LDL-C) and triglycerides and with onset of diabetes and hypertension.

PREDICTIVE VALUE OF PLAQUE IN PRIMARY RISK STRATIFICATION

Plaque is defined as a focal structure of at least 0.5 mm or 50% of the surrounding IMT value that encroaches into the arterial lumen or demonstrates a thickness of ≥1.5 mm as measured from the media–adventitia interface to the intima–lumen interface [65]. Roughness of the boundary and inconsistency in the visualization of the boundary and bright echoes, and/or shadowing in wall texture are other criteria to define plaque. The size of a single plaque or overall plaque burden is difficult to quantify, although number of carotid plaques appears to quantify CV risk [66]. The prediction of cardiac and cerebral events is different for IMT and plaque. CCA IMT appears to be primarily determined by age and blood pressure, and reflects not only early atherosclerosis, but also nonatherosclerotic intimal reactions such as intimal hyperplasia and intimal fibrocellular hypertrophy [67]. Plaque on the other hand is an early manifestation of atherosclerosis and generally forms in the near as well far wall of bulb and the ICA [68]. Only 15–20% of plaques form at CCA; hence, CCA is less likely to be optimal segment to study compared to bifurcation and internal segments in predicting prevalent and incident atherosclerosis in individual patients. This explains part of the reason for discrepancy among different studies, majority of which used CCA far wall IMT for evaluation of atherosclerosis [42]. Other studies reported composite IMT of CCA, bulb, and ICA inclusive of plaque [34], while others evaluated CCA and ICA IMT [36] or reported plaques separately [69]. Data suggest differential impact of risk factor on IMT vs plaque [85]; however, IMT appears to be the most important determinant of development of future plaques [86]. The plaque score, which is computed by summing the maximum thickness of all the CIMT complexes in the carotid artery [87] or as a sum of all plaques in all segments of the carotid artery, may be a more sensitive measure of the extent and severity of atherosclerosis than summation of CIMT. However, few data are available on the use of plaque score as a marker of atherosclerosis progression. Large prospective studies such as ARIC, CHS, and Rotterdam studies do not report the incremental predictive nature of focal plaque separate from IMT. A number of studies have reported on the high predictive value of plaque as an independent predictor of CV events [70], whereas association of CIMT with future events is not very strong. IMT is strongly influenced by genetic determinants whereas plaque appears to be determined by common CAD risk factors such as age, sex, hypertension, diabetes mellitus, hypercholesterolemia, amount of nicotine consumed, factor VIII, and vWF and not by genetic inheritance [71].

CCA IMT, bifurcation IMT, and plaque are correlated with each other but show differing patterns of association with risk factors and prevalent disease. CCA IMT is strongly associated with risk factors for stroke and with prevalent stroke, whereas IMT of carotid bifurcation and plaque are more directly associated with ischemic heart disease risk factors and prevalent ischemic heart disease [25]. In subjects aged 59–71 years with family history of premature CAD, the odds ratio of atheromatous plaques (defined as >1.0 mm) associated with parental history of premature death from CAD after adjusting for age, gender, and CV risk factors was 2.70. In contrast, CCA IMT was not associated with parental history of premature death from CAD [72]. A recent cross-sectional study found independent prognostic value of risk factors, IMT, and plaques to predict stroke risk [73]. Inclusion of plaque thickness in IMT measurement may be confounding two qualitatively different pathological processes: smooth muscle hypertrophy and plaque formation. Studies such as ARIC reported mean IMT value inclusive of plaque. The studies by Balcero et al. graded severity of atherosclerosis from grade I to grade IV based on normal IMT to intima-media granulation (or increased IMT >1 mm) to nonstenotic and stenotic plaque. In the first study [74], asymptomatic nondiabetic and nonhypercholesterolemic subjects underwent evaluation of carotid and femoral arteries and followed for 6 years. Less than 1% of patients (0.6%) with no plaque, or increased IMT had CV events compared to 27% in those with at least one plaque in the CCA and femoral arteries. Among those with plaques event rate was 18% with small plaque and 42% with large >50% stenotic plaques. Another study [75] involving both carotid and femoral IMT and plaque found that in 13,221 low-risk asymptomatic subjects 99% of events occurred in patients with class II–IV artery (irregularity of IMT, focal plaque >2 mm, nonstenotic plaque, stenotic plaque) morphology. Event rate was 0.12% in subjects in class I category, 9% with class II anatomy, 39% with class III, and 81% with class IV anatomy. In addition the study found that a normal CCA IMT was observed in 74% of subjects in class II, in 54% of subjects in class III and in 44% of subjects in class IV, implying that presence of plaque in the bifurcation in the presence of normal CCA IMT still carries a high risk. Furthermore, 30% of patients with normal carotid arteries had femoral arteriosclerotic lesions. Hence, the assessment of carotid as well as femoral bifurcations offers a more global view of the arteriosclerotic status of the subject, and it is possibly a better and earlier indication of subclinical arteriosclerosis than CCA IMT measurements. A recent meta-analysis of 37,197 subjects who were followed up for a mean 5.5 years found that CIMT can be used to predict MI and stroke in the general population [76]. For an absolute CIMT difference of 0.1 mm, the future risk of MI increased by 10–15%, and that of stroke increased by 13–18% [76].

PLAQUES IN SYMPTOMATIC PATIENTS

While a number of studies have assessed predictive role of IMT and plaques in those with no clinical CV disease, few studies have evaluated the utility of this approach in those with established CV disease. In 558 patients with stable angina who participated in the Angina Prognosis Study in Stockholm (APSIS), CIMT after adjustment for age, sex, smoking, previous CV disease and lipid status failed to predict any CV event, whereas carotid plaques tended ($P=0.056$) to predict the risk of CV death or MI and femoral IMT ($P<0.01$) and plaques ($P<0.05$) were also related to the risk of revascularization after adjustment for risk factors. There was a weak correlation between carotid and femoral plaques and among 508 subjects, 68 patients had plaque only in the carotid artery and 127 patients had plaques only in the femoral artery. These data highlight the need to evaluate both carotid artery and femoral artery vascular beds to perform a more accurate assessment of subclinical atherosclerosis. In symptomatic patients without known CAD CIMT in the >75th percentile was associated with increased likelihood of presence of significant single vessel CAD (≥50%) 74% vs 44%, $P=0.047$) and with presence of carotid plaque (96% vs 59%, $P=0.003$ [77].

EVALUATION OF PLAQUE COMPOSITION

Echolucency of carotid plaques on ultrasound B-mode imaging was associated with increased risk for stroke. Echolucent plaques are associated with increased lipid content and macrophage density and are prone to rupture [78]. Surface irregularity is another feature associated with higher risk for future ischemic stroke [79]. Echolucent carotid artery plaques are associated with lipid-rich core with thin fibrous cap [80], low HDL-C [81] and predict future strokes [82]. Plaque lucency is more reproducible than plaque thickness measurement [83]. The size of a single plaque or overall plaque burden is difficult to quantify, although the number of carotid plaques appears to quantify CV risk [66]. Presence of calcified carotid plaque increases risk of vascular events [84]. However the clinical association is not strong enough to be useful in reliable clinical prediction for the individual patient. Clinical utility of ultrasound will increase exponentially if it can accurately detect echolucent rupture-prone plaques in the individual patient.

Plaques not only offer the opportunity to evaluate changes in plaque size but more importantly in composition in response to lipid-lowering treatment. Changes in plaque volume by three-dimensional ultrasound appear to be more sensitive than changes in CIMT over time and its use may reduce sample size for future interventional studies [88]. Techniques used to evaluate plaque composition have included spectral analysis of backscattered radio-frequency signals [89, 90]. Early data suggest that despite no significant decrease in plaque size, changes in plaque characteristics occur on lipid-lowering treatment thus making these more echodense [91]. Gray-scale median of plaque images is another technique such that plaques with a high lipid and hemorrhage content as established histologically had a low gray-scale median and those with a high fibrous content had a high gray-scale median [92]. Another promising area in determining plaque activity is use of ultrasound contrast agents. Limited reports suggest detection of increased *vasa vasorum* flow in active plaques which may be decreased by lipid lowering [93]. Use of tagged ultrasound contrast agents may assist in identifying inflammation within the plaque in future [94]. Evaluation of plaque volume by three-dimensional ultrasound may be even stronger predictor of risk of CVD and effect of lipid-lowering treatment [95]. In vitro studies using excised human carotid artery plaque using ultrasound texture classification showed a good match with histology in the location of fibrin, elastin, calcium, lipid, or hemorrhage [96, 97].

Further development of imaging techniques to determine plaque volume and composition will assist in studying effect of novel lipid altering drugs in future trials.

IMT IN THE YOUNG

It is widely accepted that CVD begins in childhood, but the best way to target children at risk remains incompletely defined [98]. CIMT is increased in obese children [99–101]. Increased vascular mass was found in children with metabolic syndrome [102] and that blood pressure and body mass index and NOT total and LDL-C were associated with vascular remodeling. Others have found that impaired glucose tolerance demonstrates higher association with increased IMT in children than metabolic syndrome [103]. A number of studies have shown that exposure to the level of risk factors such as LDL-C and HDL-C during childhood years increases IMT [104]. IMT is increased in children with familial hypercholesterolemia [105]. Children with hypercholesterolemia and diabetes show increased IMTs compared with healthy controls, with a relatively greater increase in the aortic IMT than in the CIMT [106]. Triglycerides are associated with increased IMT in young females [15]. Based on epidemiological data, demonstrating the continuing and significant increase in incidence of overweight and obesity in childhood and adolescence, comprehensive strategies for the long-term prevention and the treatment of risk factors should be emphasized from childhood.

REPRODUCIBILITY OF IMT

Edge detection systems that are properly calibrated provide accurate measurements of IMT and can provide the mean maximal value of 150 measurements performed on 10 mm of CCA in a very short time. IMT image is frozen in late diastole by EKG triggering to ensure uniform data acquisition at baseline and follow up. These in general use determination of gray-level density recognition tissue algorithms thereby allowing an automated measurement of IMT to be performed without reader dependence. Some softwares are semiautomated allowing manual trace of IMT. In a small sample of 44 subjects aged 18–83 years, the change in IMT of CCA during the heart cycle averaged 25 μm [107]; hence, some believe that timing of cardiac cycle is not important and the frame that shows best IMT during cardiac cycle can be used without sacrificing accuracy.

These computerized procedures improve the precision and reproducibility rate of the IMT measurement, providing approximately 3% of relative difference between two successive measures [108]. Compared with an optical method of measurement of interface distance, the computerized ultrasound method had a high reliability coefficient (*R*) of 0.99 [109]. In one study, the absolute difference between optical and ultrasound measurements varied from 0.03±0.05 mm without any systematic error [108, 110]. If one adjusts for the baseline difference in IMT between CCA, bulb, and ICA, the percentage variability between two repeated measurements is similar (approximately 7%) for the CCA and for the 12 multiple sites measurement [111]. For the CCA absolute difference between repeated measures is as low as 0.02 mm [112], i.e., a percentage variability of less than 4%. However, these softwares require excellent image quality to work effectively and are appropriate for the CCA segment only since totally automatic methods have not been developed for bifurcation and for ICA segments. Although the computerized ultrasound method allows the assessment of changes in distance between echogenic interfaces that are ten times smaller than the axial resolution of the ultrasound transducers thereby reduced reader variability, the axial resolution of current generation ultrasound systems of 0.2±0.4 mm [110], is a limiting factor in detecting progression rates in individual patients.

Precision of measurement depends on the underlying population being studied. For example in age ranges 55 and above, rounding off the mean value of 12 segments far wall to nearest 0.1 mm does not affect centile of risk based on ARIC data. On the other hand in young subjects less than 30 years old rounding off to nearest 0 is not acceptable since change of IMT of 0.05 mm from far wall of R CCA may place women from 25 to 75th centile (AXA study) [35].

USE OF IMT FOR SCREENING ASYMPTOMATIC SUBJECTS

A European consensus panel concluded that although IMT is an important risk marker, it cannot be classified as a risk factor because positive and negative predictive value for a given population has not been established [65]. Other studies have reported its positive predictive value (max IMT ≥ 0.9 mm) somewhere around 21% and negative predictive value around 87% similar to that of ankle brachial index; however, this represents prediction based on CCA IMT and not bulb or ICA IMT. Combining risk factors with atherosclerosis burden may be a useful clinical risk stratification method. Replacing biologic age in clinical risk stratification algorithms such as Framingham index with vascular age derived from CIMT has been proposed to provide a more robust clinical risk stratification tool [113]. Preliminary data are emerging on the utility of this approach in patients with intermediate risk on clinical screening [114]. Figure 6a shows example of a patient whose cardiovascular risk was downgraded and Fig. 6b that of another patient whose cardiovascular risk was upgraded after assessment of IMT.

IMT has thus far been largely used as a research method in large multicenter studies. No consensus has been developed regarding methodology, analysis, and interpretation and no agreed upon clinical protocol exists. This is because of varying sites of assessment and reporting methods used in earlier research studies. In addition, despite this wealth of information on the predictive value of atherosclerosis imaging, it remains to be established whether such screening tests lead to improved clinical outcomes and hence, major health insurance bodies consider this test for use in clinically asymptomatic individuals investigational as specifically stated in the insurance carrier policy

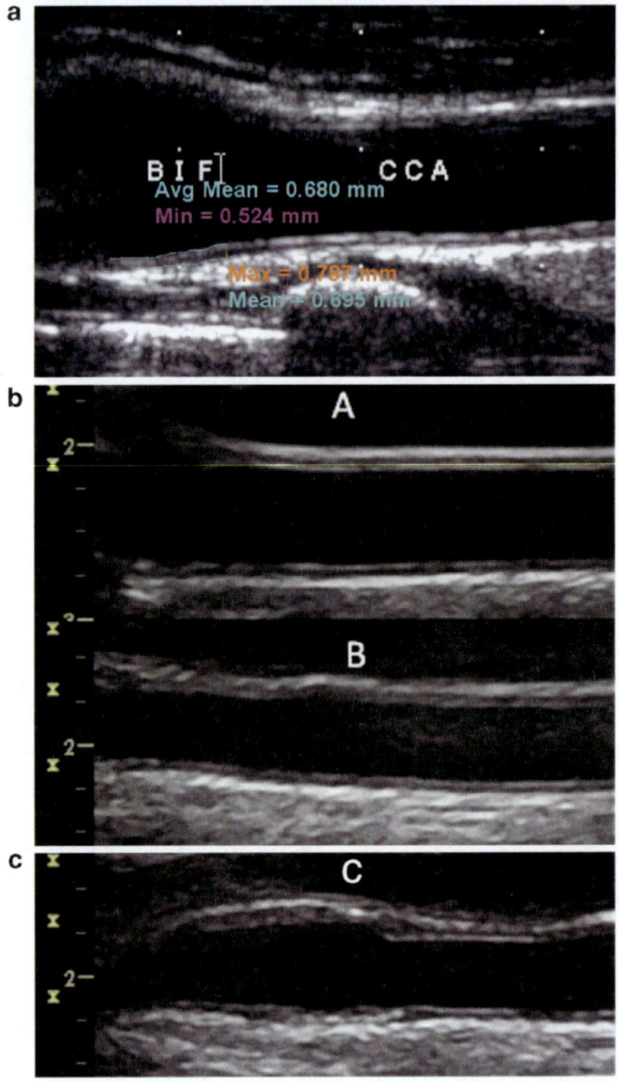

Fig. 6. (**a**) Common carotid IMT in a 53-year-old male with a total cholesterol of 251, HDL 53, LDL 167 and triglycerides 70 mg/dL, and Framingham risk score of 11%. CCA IMT was 45th centile for age, race, and gender. (**b**) Right CCA IMT (A), right bulb and ICA IMT (B) and left CCA, bulb and ICA (**c**) IMT in a 53-year-old female with a Framingham risk score of 5%. CCA IMT was 80th centile for age, race, and gender.

"However, at the present time there appears to be no scientific literature that directly and experimentally test the hypothesis that measurement of CIMT results in improved patient outcomes, and no specific guidance on how measurements of CIMT should be incorporated into risk assessment and risk management [115]." On the other hand, the AHA Prevention Conference V recommended that "In asymptomatic persons >45 years old, carefully performed carotid ultrasound examination with IMT measurement can add incremental information to traditional risk factor assessment and that in experienced laboratories, this test can now be considered for further clarification of coronary heart disease (CHD) risk assessment at the request of a physician [116]." It is also widely accepted that at this time IMT is the only surrogate end point for CAD that is endorsed for clinical studies. US Food and Drug Administration considers IMT as valid end point in the evaluation of new medications [117]. The 2003 European Society of Hypertension–European Society of Cardiology guidelines recommend IMT assessment particularly in those patients in whom target organ damage is not discovered by routine investigations, including an electrocardiogram [118]. Screening for Heart Attack Prevention and Education Task Force published guidelines in which screening for subclinical atherosclerosis of all asymptomatic middle-aged persons, "except those defined as very low risk," was called for [119]. Medicare Current Procedural Terminology code has been created for CIMT. Insurance reimbursement has been requested for CIMT and coronary artery calcium tests by a state bill introduced in the Texas Legislature. This bill was called "a first legislative effort in the US" to encourage the identification of "apparently healthy individuals who are at risk of a near-future heart attack [125].

EFFECT OF CAROTID IMT ON PHYSICIAN PRESCRIBING PATTERNS AND PATIENT CORONARY RISK BEHAVIOR

Evidence on the effect of IMT on patient management is beginning to emerge. Ultrasound screening for carotid plaque in an office setting in 50 middle-aged patients (mean age: 54 years) with a Framingham risk score (FRS) of 8 was shown to alter physician treatment plans with increased prescriptions for aspirin and lipid-lowering therapy in subjects with plaque (found in 58% of the study subjects). The study found that although the presence of plaque increased patient perception of cardiovascular risk, it did not motivate patients to make lifestyle changes [120]. Another study found improved success at smoking cessation when patients were given an image of their carotid plaque [121]. Studies have demonstrated that a personalized picture of the artery is an effective method of ensuring patient compliance with diet, exercise, and smoking cessation. Improvement in compliance rates from 40 to 76% has been shown. Thus among 210 participants after 12 months blood pressure normalized in 26 out of 40 subjects, hypercholesterolemia resolved in 45 out of 55 subjects, and the number of subjects who smoked decreased in 9 out of 22. This was associated with a significant decrease in IMT among those given the image of the artery [122]. Data collected in high school students found that CIMT was related to diet and traditional risk factors for heart diseases [123]. Overall cumulative data suggest against a large attributable effect of atherosclerosis imaging on patient motivation, on a long-term basis. Incorporating these data into a recurring clinical patient/physician relationship could lead to behavioral modification [124].

IMAGING PROTOCOL FOR IMT

When adopting this new technology, training and certification of sonographers and physicians on IMT acquisition and measurement are required. Each lab should perform its own inter- and intraobserver and subject variability. Phantom scanning should be performed at least monthly to ensure appropriate system calibration. Assignment of labor is required to ensure adequate time for scanning, measuring, and reporting of high-quality data.

Studies that have used IMT show variations both in scanning and reading methods. The difference concerns the arterial segment evaluated, the site-specific measurement, and the variables used which can be single or aggregates including values from very different sites. Near and far walls can be visualized on B-mode scanning, but B-mode evaluation of the near wall is less reliable than the far wall. A number of epidemiologic studies have used IMT of far wall of distal CCA as the surrogate end point for atherosclerosis largely due to a measurement yield of >90% at CCA. While this approach provides accurate and reproducible data, the approach has limitations since far wall of CCA may miss atherosclerosis. ICA IMT appears to have the strongest independent correlate of prevalent CHD; however, measurement yield is lowest at 30–50%, compared to 65–80% for the bulb. In the CHS study predictive value of events increased after CCA near wall IMT was included. Thus, IMT has a higher predictive value when it is measured at multiple extracranial carotid sites as in the ARIC study protocol [13] than solely in the distal CCA. For clinical purposes, at least two angles (anterior and posterior) should

Table 2
Equipment and supplies for IMT

1. Ultrasound system with high frequency 7–15 MHz vascular transducer and two dimensional, Doppler imaging as well as online measurement capability.
2. Bed which allows subject's head to be at zero degree angle and have adjustable height for sonographer comfort.
3. Chair with back rest and adjustable height placed at the head end of the bed.
4. Space that is able to house ultrasound system to the subjects left and right sides. When the ultrasound is positioned only on the left side of the subject, scanning is done with the right hand on the right side, and with the left hand on the left side. Machine controls are handled with left hand for the right sided scan and with the right hand for the left sided scan. Ultrasound platform can be placed on the subject's right side for scanning left side of the neck. In that case scanning is performed with left hand and right hand is used to operate machine controls.
5. Other routine accessories for ultrasound including multiple small towels to be placed around the neck. A foam wedge placed under the subject's neck and a pillow under the subject's knee increases subject's comfort.
6. Digital acquisition capability. Image downloading to a computer station directly or remotely via Ethernet or by optical disc, CD-ROM, or DVD.
7. Neck Arc with angles placed around patient's neck if multiple angles desired.
8. Edge detection software on a computer station.

be used and both near and far walls should be evaluated since disease may be confined to the near wall, irrespective of whether bulb and ICA are incorporated.

Because IMT varies by age, gender, race, and blood pressure, use of a cut off value for abnormality, e.g., 1 mm, may result in systematic underdetection of abnormality in younger individuals and over-detection in older individuals. Age, gender, and race-adjusted values need to be used. Such values are available through large databases of asymptomatic subjects (Appendixes 1 and 2 and Figs. 2–4). Vascular age along with alteration in CV risk category for any given individual patient can be determined based on these values [126].

Table 2 details equipment needed for IMT assessment. Table 3 describes full IMT protocol.

Carotid ultrasound is performed using standard ultrasound machines equipped with high-frequency transducers (usually 5–12 MHz linear array) and appropriate software. In brief, the patient should be supine with slight hyperextension and rotation of the neck in the direction opposite the probe. Scanning is performed in the transverse and longitudinal planes and from multiple angles to evaluate the near and far walls of CCA, bulb, and ICA. The time needed for a thorough and complete examination is dependent on the protocol and sonographer experience, but typically is 30–60 min for a comprehensive IMT evaluation.

IMT is usually measured in the CCA (usually the distal 1 cm), the bifurcation (bulb) (usually 1 cm in length) and the ICA (proximal 1 cm), and then averaged so that a mean of 2–12 segments (near and far wall of CCA, bulb, ICA) or mean of distal common IMT are obtained (Fig. 7). Cyclic variations in IMT and lumen diameter should be taken into account by ECG-gating and/or determination of minimal (end-diastolic) and maximal (peak-systolic) diameters. If a significant plaque is identified, Pulsed Wave (PW) Doppler of ICA is obtained within and beyond the narrowest segment as directed by aliasing on color flow Doppler, followed by PW Doppler of CCA. Systolic and diastolic velocity criteria are used to report % stenosis severity [127].

Table 4 describes abbreviated IMT protocol. This IMT protocol is designed to be performed and completed within 15 min. Substantially lesser times (less than 5 min) may be required if overt plaque

Table 3
IMT protocol – comprehensive

1. Sonographer is seated behind patient's head. An arc with angles placed around patient's neck.
2. Patients are asked to assume a supine position, lying recumbent on the flat exam table with the neck in a comfortable position. The subject's face is turned about 50° to the side opposite to the side being imaged. EKG leads are placed and displayed on the ultrasound monitor.
3. A high-resolution B-mode system is used, with a linear ultrasound transducer operating at frequencies 8/13 MHz or greater, appropriate depth of focus (e.g., 30–40 mm), frame rate (>15 Hz), and gain settings (minimal intraluminal artifacts) are used. The depth is kept constant throughout the study.
4. Interrogate common/bulb/internal carotid sequentially assess for the presence of plaque and then for increased carotid IMT.
5. Short-axis imaging is performed from the base of the neck to the carotid bifurcation to the internal carotid artery (ICA) as far in the neck as possible. Look for plaque and get a circumferential map.
6. Long-axis imaging is then performed at anterior (R 180–150°, L 180–210°), middle, (R 150–120°, L 210–240°), and posterior (R 120–90°, L 240–270° angles).
7. In each angle near and far walls of common carotid artery (CCA) are imaged followed by near wall of bulb, near wall of ICA, far wall of ICA, and far wall of bulb. An electronic caliper may be placed over the segment and its side being imaged. Near wall of bulb is shown in continuation with the near wall of the distal vessel, i.e., ICA or ECA and similarly far wall of bulb is imaged in continuation with the far wall of the distal vessel – ICA or ECA. Pulsed wave Doppler is performed in the ICA and ECA to differentiate ICA from ECA.

Adapted from protocols used in multicenter studies. A perpendicular angle to the target structure is recommended for all IMT data acquisition measurements. Setting the focal position on the far CCA wall and using overall gain, time gain compensation, and postprocessing functions (e.g., dynamic range, edge, space/time) can further enhance the quality of the images. The morphology of plaque is noted as well as its shape, focal or circumferential nature, location and extension. An M-mode measurement may be performed across short axis at the site of maximum IMT or plaque if feasible. Perpendicular ultrasound beam to the artery wall should be the goal. For CCA both walls should be clearly visualized to ensure perpendicular beam alignment. Since IMT success rate at CCA is high and plaque usually does not form at CCA and since IMT success rate at bulb is intermediate and ICA IMT success rate is low, mean IMT measurement is more feasible at CCA and max IMT and plaque measurement are more feasible at the bulb and ICA. Alternatively once abnormal IMT and nonobstructive plaque are found on one side on detailed scanning, screening short-axis scan and one long axis for CCA, bulb, and ICA may be performed for contralateral side so as not to miss significant stenotic disease. Since 20–30% of atherosclerotic disease may be missed if femoral arteries are not examined, it is recommended to perform femoral IMT and plaque assessment if the carotid IMT (CIMT) is normal in a subject with CV risk factors. The incremental role of IMT in risk prediction in the presence of plaque is unclear. There should be no harmonic or compound imaging as this will "bloom" the returning signals and can create a falsely thickened CIMT.

is present on initial scans of either carotid artery. (Prognostic value for predicting CVD is at least twofold higher than that of thickened IMT.) In those in whom plaque is not identified: Measure highest IMT in the bulb in any of the two angles (irrespective of whether or not there is a bulb plaque). Short- or long-axis view with suspected plaque should be stored as an image file. Near wall of CCA is not measured since near wall IMT does not have same image resolution as far wall; however, it should be measured if it appears thicker than far wall. Plaque and maximum IMT assessment can be done online using electronic calipers on the ultrasound system.

In contrast to research-based IMT procedures, the abbreviated IMT protocol is easy to use, and therefore can be more readily adopted as a risk assessment tool for detection of early atherosclerosis in office settings and in community screening programs. This method can still provide improved sensitivity to detect CV risk, as compared with classic FRS, as well as be a cost-effective and practical method for use in office-based practice or mobile screening programs on the other hand. The rapid data acquisition may provide an incomplete assessment of all carotid segments as compared to research-based protocols. Thus, the results may not be directly comparable with the published IMT

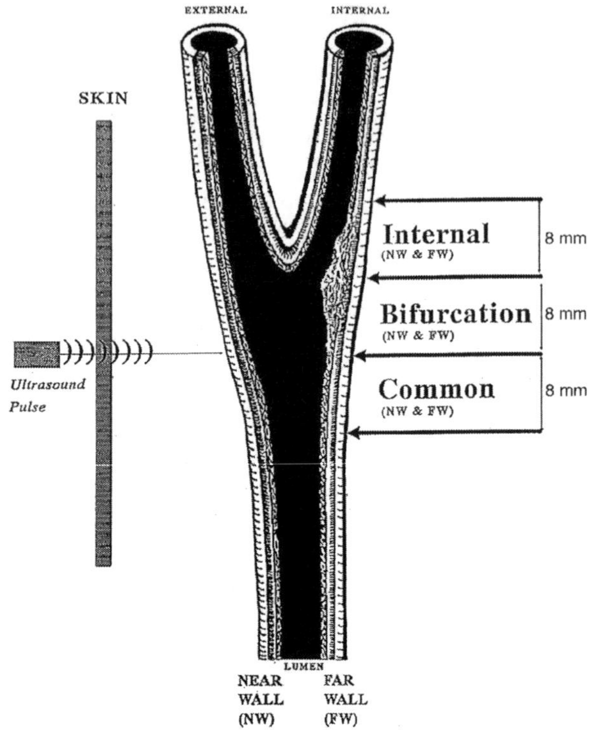

Fig. 7. Diagram showing common sites of atherosclerosis development in the carotid arteries at the bulb and approximately 1-cm segments above and below it that are the target of ultrasound evaluation of intima-media thickness and plaque.

Table 4
IMT protocol abbreviated

Interrogate the common/bulb/internal carotid sequentially. Assess for the presence of plaque and then for increased carotid IMT, as noted below.
1. *Bilateral carotid plaque assessment*
Obtain transverse images to identify plaque.
An initial short-axis view of the CCA, carotid bifurcation, and ICA is followed by use of a longitudinal view to evaluate for the presence of any obvious plaque bilaterally.
Obtain long-axis views in the anterior (180–90°) and posterior angles (≤90°).
Select one optimal image in each of these angles.
Measure IMT from each of these views bilaterally.
If plaque is present, both short-axis still image and long-axis views should be recorded (four or more per patient). Any suspected plaque should be included in the stored image file.
2. *Bilateral IMT assessment*
For rapid data acquisition, only the CCA far wall IMT is assessed. Using images obtained perpendicular to the ultrasound beam, obtain the CCA images for a minimum of 10 mm in length and proximal to the bifarcation.
For IMT, optimizing the best visual imaging of the far wall double-pattern, long-axis view is obtained from the anterior (180–90°) and posterior angles (≤90°). Obtain one measurement from each of these views bilaterally.

An image is considered "diagnostic" if the visual IMT double-pattern of the CCA far wall is obtained in *any* of the two views. Acquire image loops or still frames at end diastole (onset of R wave). For loops, using EKG as the trigger freeze the image in end-diastolic frame for making measurements

data, as provided by the ARIC study. A limited sampling of carotid segments may potentially be associated with a lesser sensitivity of the technique to measure progression or regression of IMT in future prospective interventional studies.

MEASUREMENT METHOD

Accurate data collection methodology and measurement precision are essential, as such a method that is sensitive yet not cumbersome is required for clinical utility. While electronic caliper measurement is adequate for plaque or maximum IMT, automated measurements should be used for assessment of mean IMT. Average mean or mean max of measurement at anterior and posterior angles of appropriate images each for CCA, bulb, and ICA should be used.

EKG triggering: Studies have shown that the variation in IMT measurement in different phases of cardiac cycle is less than 4%. Although measurement of IMT at a fixed time point during the cardiac cycle will decrease variability between data, for an average IMT of 660 μm, the maximal error due to IMT changes during the cardiac cycle is 3.8% and the difference between diastolic and mean IMT is 1.3%.

Other issues: Adjustment for vessel lumen may be important in hypertensives on treatment, since lowering of blood pressure affects lumen expansion and stretch.

REPORTING METHOD

No standardized reporting system for IMT exists. Given different methods used in clinical trials, it is difficult to compare a given patient results against published norms. Mean IMT (of near and far wall) of R and L CCA, bulb, and ICA may be reported as absolute as well as percentiles and plotted on graphs. Plaques may also reported separately along with plaque characteristics, i.e., echolucent, calcified, homogeneous, heterogeneous, smooth, irregular.

The reporting method has to be able to communicate information to the physician effectively. Percentiles value of patients' IMT compared to established norm is effective along with separate description of plaques. Risk ratios incurred by increased IMT and presence and characteristics of plaque based on published studies should be reported. Plaque may be report as a categorical variable (yes or no) or maximum plaque thickness may be measured. The report not only needs to educate physicians but also patients.

Reporting based on age: ARIC data report mean IMT values of subjects between 45 and 65 years age. Rotterdam study included patients >60 years but reported maximum IMT. Bogalusa study included patients up to 25–45 years but reported maximum IMT. Mean or maximum values of patients IMTs may be compared against nomograms based on these studies provided the method followed in each study is adopted.

Since IMT increases with age a single threshold value of IMT when IMT becomes abnormal is inaccurate. For simplification of reporting and based on published studies mean IMT of 1 mm may be used as threshold abnormal value for men and women greater than 45 years (Fig. 8). In general subjects with IMT > 75th percentile of the age and gender IMT distribution are classified as abnormal. AEHA proposed risk of CV disease based on IMT and coronary calcium score. IMT of <50th centile classified subjects as low risk in the absence of known cardiovascular risk factors and moderate risk in the presence of these risk factors. CCA IMT of <1 mm and <75th centile in the absence of plaque classified subjects as moderately high risk, CCA IMT of ≥1 mm or >75th centile classified subjects as high risk, whereas 75% stenotic plaque classified subjects as very high risk [119].

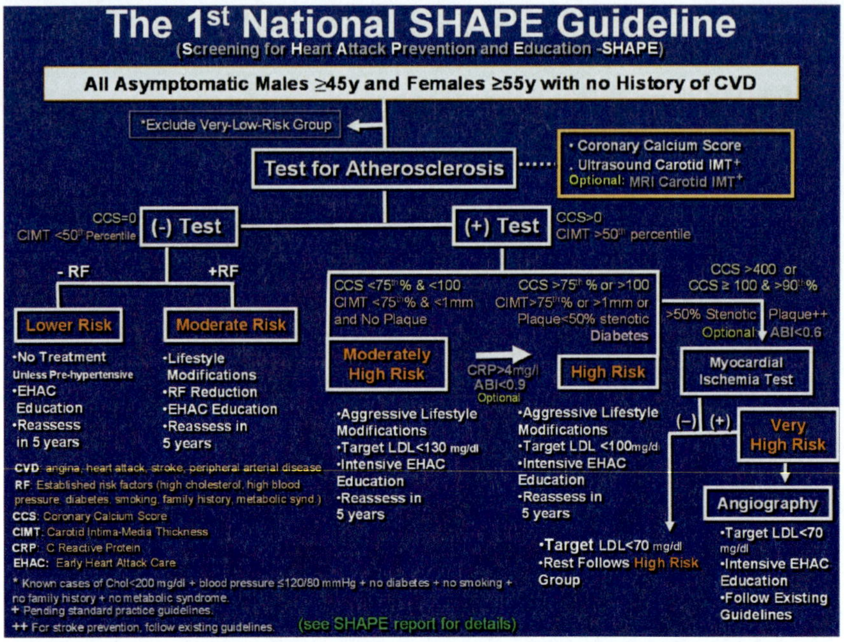

Fig. 8. Flow chart of the First Screening for Heart Attack Prevention and Education (SHAPE) Guideline. *ABI* ankle brachial index, *CACS* coronary artery calcium score, *CIMT* carotid intima-media thickness, *CRP* C-reactive protein, *LDL* low-density lipoprotein.*No history of angina, heart attack, stroke, or peripheral arterial disease. †Population aged >75 years is considered high risk and must receive therapy without testing for atherosclerosis. ‡Must not have any of the following: total cholesterol level 200 mg/dL (5.18 mmol/L), blood pressure >120/80 mmHg, diabetes mellitus, smoking, family history of coronary heart disease (CHD), or the metabolic syndrome. §Pending the development of standard practice guidelines. ¶High cholesterol, high blood pressure, diabetes, smoking, family history of CHD, or the metabolic syndrome. For stroke prevention, follow existing guidelines.

Table 5
Associations between BI and FCRS, CCA IMT, and carotid plaques

	OR (95% CI)	*P*	*OR (95% CI)*[a]
Univariate analysis			
FCRS	2.46 (1.83–3.29)	<0.0001	2.31 (1.58–3.37)
CCA IMT	2.05 (1.57–2.66)	<0.0001	2.10 (1.49–2.94)
Carotid plaques	3.49 (2.25–5.43)	<0.0001	3.37 (1.95–5.83)
Multivariate analysis			
FCRS	2.16 (1.57–2.98)	<0.0001	1.98 (1.31–2.98)
CCA IMT	1.68 (1.25–2.26)	0.0006	1.76 (1.20–2.58)
Carotid plaques	2.73 (1.68–4.44)	<0.0001	2.67 (1.47–4.86)

ORs were computed using conditional logistic regression for matched sets
[a]In cases and matched controls free of cardiovascular and cerebrovascular history ($n = 155$)
[b]OR per 1 SD increase of FCRS (12.1%)
[c]OR per 1 SD increase of CCA IMT (0.153 mm)

Maximal IMT of CCA IMT value may also be used as was done in the cardiovascular health study (>65 years) and Bogolusa Study (25–40 years).

Plaque has a higher predictive role for stroke compared to IMT as in study by Touboul et al. [73] (Table 5).

ULTRASOUND CAROTID ARTERY INTIMA-MEDIA THICKNESS ASSESSMENT FOR PROGRESSION OF ATHEROSCLEROSIS IN LIPID INTERVENTION STUDIES

Data support limitation of clinical CV risk assessment in identification of individuals who are at high risk of developing CVD [128]. Assessment of subclinical atherosclerosis by imaging methods which identify effect of various known and unknown risk factors has gained wider attention in more recent recommendations and consensus opinions on CVD prevention. Ultrasound assessment of IMT and presence of early nonobstructive plaques has been shown to detect prevalent as well as incident CVD [76]. IMT predicts both incident MI and stroke [129, 130]. In fact recent data support discordance between IMT assessed subclinical atherosclerosis and FRS in about 60% of patients [131]. IMT and plaque assessment adjust the risk strata of over 60% of patients deemed as having intermediate risk by FRS [132]. In particular a high prevalence of subclinical atherosclerosis in the low Framingham risk category has been noted. Sensitive ultrasonographic measurement over time at fixed points can allow the increase in IMT to be followed. IMT is now accepted as a validated marker of progression for the purposes of drug development [133]. Most studies have used carotid artery IMT, however femoral artery IMT has been used in some studies, although measurements of femoral artery IMT are less reproducible than those of CIMT [134]. Recent studies have shown a high reproducibility of measurement with intraclass correlation coefficient of 0.8–0.95 [135]. Thus far ultrasound assessment of subclinical atherosclerosis has been largely limited to research studies; however, it has the potential for broad clinical application due to its low cost and risk, portability, and ready availability. The caveat is, however, that data acquisition, measurement, and analysis need to be performed by dedicated staff with adequate training, equipment, and expertise as well as regular quality control [136].

Increased reproducibility of IMT in large prospective randomized studies led to its use for evaluation of effect of pharmacologic agents on atherosclerosis progression [137]. Measurement of the change in atherosclerosis burden by IMT allows the clinical benefits of a therapy to be established in a relatively short time and with fewer subjects compared with clinical outcome trials. IMT has been used as an intermediate endpoint to evaluate the effect of lipid-lowering agents, antioxidants, diet treatment, antihypertensive agents, and glucose-lowering agents on subclinical atherosclerosis.

Most studies on IMT have been single or multicenter clinical studies that have evaluated CIMT. Few studies evaluated both carotid and femoral IMT. There has been variation in the methodology used for IMT evaluation in previous studies. This includes evaluation of segment used, i.e., CCA, carotid bulb or ICA, measurement of far wall, near wall or both, inclusion or exclusion of plaque within IMT measurement, measurement of maximum or mean thickness, and finally in the expression of results as: IMT ≥ 1 mm, risk per 0.1 mm, quintiles, or standard deviation increase. This has led to difficulty in comparing data from different studies. Despite this limitation, strength of data suggests that aggressive lipid lowering prevents progression of atherosclerosis and that lowering of LDL levels below 70 mg/dL or by 50% or so from baseline may lead to regression. Improvement in imaging methods and measurement and consensus on reported methods would allow the results of these studies to be applied to individuals [138]. LDL Cholesterol reduction with statins reduces coronary events and improves rates of transient ischemic attacks and strokes by 25–30% [139–143]. Earlier studies compared effect of lipid-lowering agents vs placebo. Once the effect of statins in subjects at risk for CV events was established, studies compared high dose vs moderate dose lipid lowering, or combination vs monotherapy or evaluated subjects with low risk of CV events. Aggressive LDL lowering and/or raising HDL Cholesterol has been the subject of the most recent studies.

EFFECT OF NONPHARMACOLOGICAL INTERVENTIONS ON IMT PROGRESSION

The Monitored Atherosclerosis Regression Study found that reducing body mass index by 5 kg/m^2, quitting a 10-cigarette/day smoking habit, and reducing dietary cholesterol intake by 100 mg/day on average reduced the annual rate of CIMT progression by 0.13 mm year [144]. In the Women's Healthy Lifestyle Project, CIMT progression was accelerated during the menopause transition and a diet/exercise intervention slowed this progression [145]. The Los Angeles Atherosclerosis Study found that increased activity level [146] and increased fiber intake [147] was associated with a decreased progression rate of CIMT. Good cardiorespiratory fitness assessed by maximal oxygen uptake (mL/kg/min) was associated with slower progression of early atherosclerosis in middle-aged men [148]. Weight loss after gastric bypass has also been shown to decrease the rate of progression of CIMT [149], and improved glycemic control has been shown to slow CIMT progression in diabetic patients [150].

LIPID INTERVENTION TRIALS THAT HAVE EVALUATED CIMT

A number of studies have evaluated the effect of moderate to aggressive LDL Cholesterol lowering on IMT progression. Statins are the primary therapy used to reduce atherosclerosis and CV events including MI, strokes, and transient ischemic attacks. In contrast, data for other agents including fibrates and nicotinic acid in reducing the progression of atherosclerosis are less extensive. Few have specifically examined the effect of HDL Cholesterol raising on IMT progression. These studies are summarized in Table 6 [154].

A meta-analysis including nine trials (2,792 subjects in total) investigating the effect of statin therapy on CIMT progression showed a strong correlation between LDL Cholesterol lowering and CIMT reduction ($r=0.65$, $P=0.004$) [140]. Each 10% reduction in LDL Cholesterol was estimated to reduce the CIMT by 0.73% per year (95% CI: 0.27–1.19). Another meta-analysis including ten trials and a total of 3,443 individuals also showed that statin therapy significantly reduces the rate of carotid atherosclerosis progression [155]. The total weighted mean difference of CIMT progression between patients receiving statins vs placebo was −22.35% (95% CI: −18.14 to 26.56%, $P<0.00001$). The results of these meta-analyses strongly suggest that statin therapy offers significant advantages to patients with carotid artery disease.

A long-term follow-up at 8.8 years of 146 men who completed the CLAS study [156] found that for each 0.03-mm increase per year in CIMT, there was over twofold increase in risk for nonfatal MI or coronary death and a threefold increase in relative risk for any coronary event. Absolute thickness and progression in thickness predicted risk for coronary events beyond that predicted by angiographic coronary arterial measures of atherosclerosis and lipid measurements. This is the only study that explored the relationship between change in CIMT and CV event rates following therapeutic intervention.

Table 6
Clinical trials that evaluated the effect of LDL-C lowering and HDL cholesterol raising on subclinical atherosclerosis by carotid IMT

Trial	*Year*	*Ref.*	*Method*	*N*	*Treatment*	*FU (months)*	*% LDL*	*Change in IMT*	*Treatment Placebo*	*P*
LDL lowering										
ACAPS [174]	1994	22	MnMx 12	919	Lovastatin 20–40	36	−28	−0.009	+0.006	0.001
REGRESS [175]	1995	15	MnCCA/F	255	Pravastatin 40	24	−29	−0.05	+0.0456	0.0085
PLAC II[a] [176]	1995	16	MnMx12	151	Pravastatin 10–40	36	−28	+0.059	+0.068	NS
KAPS [177]	1995	17	MnMxCCA/b/F	447	Pravastatin 40	36	−27	+0.017	+0.031	0.005
MARS [178]	1996	18	MnCCA	188	Lovastatin 80	48	−45	−0.038	+0.009	0.001
CAIUS [179]	1996	19	MnMx12	305	Pravastatin 40	36	−22	−0.0043	+0.031	0.005
LIPID[a] [180]	1998	20	MaxCCA	522	Pravastatin 40	48	−27	−0.014	+0.019	<0.001
BCAPS [181]	2001	161	MnCCAMxbulb	793	Fluvastatin 40	36	−23	−0.009	0.013	0.002
FH	2003	21	MnCA/F	153	Simvastatin 80	24	−44	−0.043	–	
ARBITER1 [182]	2002	23	MnCCA	161	AT80/Pravastatin 40	12	−49/−27	−0.160	+0.0021	0.08
FAST [183]	2002	165	MnCCA6	246	Pravastatin 10/diet	24	−36 to 12	−13.9%	23.9	<0.05
ASAP (FH) [184, 185]	2005	25	MnC/B/I	325	Simvastatin 40/A80	24	−51/−41	−0.02	+0.02	0.001
METEOR [186]	2007	26	MnMx12	984	Rosuvastatin 80	24	−48.8	−0.0014	+0.131	<0.0001
HDL raising										
CLAS[a] [187, 188]	1993	14	MnCCA	188	Cholestipol/Niacin	12	−47/+41	−0.02	+0.01	0.01
ARBITER II[a] [189]	2004	27	MnCCA12	167	Niacin 1000 /Statin>20	12	+17	+0.014	+0.044	0.08
RADIANCE1 (FHH) [190]	2007	29	MnMx 12	850	Torcetr. 60/AT 20–80	24	+54	+0.0038	−0.0014	0.0052
RADIANCE II (MH) [191]	2007	30	MnMx 12	758	Torcetr. 60/AT 10–80	24	+62	+0.0126	+0.0076	0.0050

ACAPS Asymptomatic Carotid Artery Progression Study, *IMT* intima media thickness, *PLAC-II*, Pravastatin Lipids and Atherosclerosis in the Carotid Arteries-II Study, *CCA* common carotid artery, *KAPS* Kuopio Atherosclerosis Prevention Study, *CI* confidence interval, *CAIUS* Carotid Atherosclerosis Italian Ultrasound Study, *MARS* Monitored Atherosclerosis Regression Study, *LIPID* Long-term Intervention with Pravastatin in Ischemic Disease Study, *SE* standard error, *REGRESS* Regression Growth Evaluation Statin Study, *BCAPS* Beta-Blocker Cholesterol-Lowering Asymptomatic Plaque Study, *ASAP* Atorvastatin vs Simvastatin on Atherosclerosis Progression, *ARBITER* Arterial Biology for the Investigation of the Treatment Effects of Reducing Cholesterol, *FAST* Fukuoka Atherosclerosis Trial, *MnCCA* mean of mean IMT measurements at multiple sites, *F* femoral IMT, *AT* atorvastatin, *Torcetr.* torcetrapid, *FH* familial hypercholesterolemia, *FHH* familial heterozygous hypercholesterolemia, *MH* mixed hypertipidemia, METEOR Measuring effects on intima-media thickness: An Evaluation Rosuvastatin

[a]Studies in subjects with established coronary artery disease

Another single center nonplacebo controlled study showed decrease in CIMT in 153 subjects with familial hypercholesterolemia by aggressive lipid lowering using simvastatin 80 mg [157].

In ARBITER 3 study Niacin SR was extended to 2 years. Further regression of CIMT occurred during 12–24 months of treatment with niacin. Regression was 25.4% with placebo and 52.8% with niacin at 12 months and 59.6% at 24 months [158].

Ezetimibe and simvastatin in hypercholesterolemia enhances atherosclerosis regression (ENHANCE) trial evaluated the effect of simvastatin 80 mg and placebo vs simvastatin and 10 mg ezetimibe on mean change in CIMT at 2 years and found no significant difference in the 2gps [159]. The Carotid Atorvastatin Study in Hyperlipidemic post-Menopausal women (CASHMERE) trial is another ongoing double-blind, randomized trial, which aims to investigate the effect of statin and hormone replacement therapy in reducing the early progression of atherosclerosis in postmenopausal women [160]. It aims to compare the effects of 12-month atorvastatin (80 mg/day) therapy alone, oral 17 beta-estradiol (1 or 2 mg/day) plus cyclic dydrogesterone (10 mg) alone, and their combination vs placebo on the progression of CIMT by using a high-definition echotracking device.

Generally a 1% reduction in LDL-C reduces coronary events by 1% [30]. Meta-analysis of the statin studies suggests that a 1 mmol/L reduction in LDL-C reduces atherosclerotic events by 20–25% [161]. Studies suggest that an equivalent proportional rise in HDL-C translates into a 2–3% benefit [162, 163]. In general, statin-induced lipid changes correlated relatively poorly with statin-induced changes in vascular structure and function, supporting the hypothesis that statins act on factors not directly related to lipids. Statin-mediated improvements in vascular structure and function correlate poorly with effects on circulating lipids, suggesting that the mechanisms that underlie the vascular changes are likely complex and due to more than lipid-lowering effects [164].

While there are considerable data from aforementioned clinical trials of cardiovascular therapies to show that active treatment retards the progression of CIMT, these trials did not relate changes in CIMT with cardiovascular event rates. No study showed a correlation between vascular effect and clinical outcome. A recent meta-analysis of seven statin studies in which both CIMT was measured and the frequency of cardiovascular events was reported found that a mean change in CIMT progression of –0.012 mm/year (95% CI: –0.016 to –0.007) was associated with an odds ratio of 0.48 (95% CI: 0.30–0.78) for the reduction in cardiovascular events [165].

Statin therapy (pravastatin) in children with familial hypercholesterolemia was associated with a smaller IMT at 2-year follow up [166]. Further extension of the study to 4.5-year follow up found that earlier initiation of statin was associated with a lower IMT [167]. Studies with FDA approved statins in children including lovastatin, simvastatin, pravastatin, and atorvastatin have been conducted in over 1,000 children with familial hypercholesterolemia thus far [168–171]. Between these four statins, randomized placebo-controlled trials of at least 24 weeks have been reported in >750 male and female children. The scientific statement on drug therapy of high-risk lipid abnormalities in children and adolescents from the American Heart Association Atherosclerosis, Hypertension, and Obesity in Youth Committee, Council of Cardiovascular Disease in the Young [172] states: "In general, do not start (drug therapy) before 10 years of age in boys and preferably after the onset of menses in girls. Patients should ideally be at Tanner stage II or higher."

Lipid lowering studies vary in the number of carotid artery segments that were evaluated. While all studies evaluated far wall of CCA, some evaluated near wall of CCA and bulb with or without far and near wall of ICA as well. There is in addition variation in studies on whether mean CIMT was measured or mean maximum of 1–12 segments. Image analysis also varied including caliper measurement vs automated edge detection methods. Finally statistical analysis method of <1 vs >1 mm IMT, every 0.1 mm increase in IMT, standard deviation increase in IMT or quintiles and tertiles of

IMT make it difficult to compare IMT data from different statin intervention studies. These studies however confirm the utility of CIMT as a surrogate endpoint for lipid-lowering drug trials. The weight of evidence indicates that a greater magnitude of plasma LDL Cholesterol lowering is associated with a greater beneficial impact in terms of atherosclerotic regression. Findings from these studies confirm that CIMT is an effective intermediate endpoint in lipid altering studies and that evaluation of vessel wall for atherosclerosis predicts clinical events. In general moderate LDL Cholesterol reduction appears to reduce progression and aggressive LDL Cholesterol lowering leads to regression of subclinical atherosclerosis. The effect on CIMT became evident at 6 months and greater baseline LDL Cholesterol leads to greater effect on CIMT. Findings of METEOR study [186] suggest that CIMT may be used for evaluation of subclinical atherosclerosis in patients with low FRS who nevertheless have 1 or 2 CV factors in a clinical setting since aggressive LDL Cholesterol lowering prevents atherosclerotic progression in this low-risk group.

CONCLUSIONS

Ultrasound assessment of vessel wall structure as IMT is a powerful tool for CV risk stratification. Its predictive value in particular in the presence of plaque is greater than FRS and the test has been recommended by AHA for further risk stratification in individual patients. Unification of protocols to be adopted for quick screening as well as for detailed evaluation of CV risk, publication of standard nomograms of IMT values from young adulthood to old age, and finally agreement on reporting method will make this a useful screening test for clinical practice. Primary prevention represents the only hope of reducing the burden of atherosclerotic disease in society. Evaluation of carotid artery wall for early stages of atherosclerosis by measurement of IMT, and presence and size of plaques offers a reliable noninvasive method for evaluation of atherosclerosis and of the effect of lipid-altering medications on atherosclerosis. With sonographer training, quality control and evaluation of studies in a core lab, the technology is robust enough at present to evaluate subclinical disease presence in individuals. Utility of assessment of carotid vessel wall for detecting progression and regression of atherosclerosis has been shown by several large multicenter studies. Consensus on imaging methodology, measurement and reporting will improve evaluation of data across different studies. The multiple measurements used in studies of CIMT highlight the difficulty of comparing dissimilar studies. Alteration of composition of atherosclerotic plaques leading to plaque stabilization and decreased vulnerability to rupture may be one of the mechanisms of differences observed on CV vs IMT by statins. Further development in tissue characterization of plaques and contrast imaging has a promise to decrease sample size in drug intervention studies and obtain endpoints at a shorter-term follow up. Improvement in imaging technology as well as in measurement precision would allow results of population studies on regnertion of atherosclerosis to be extrapolated to individual patients at risk. Development of pharmacogenomics would further facilitate this individualized treatment approach. Framingham risk is not applicable to individuals not on lipid-lowering therapy. Advent of three-dimensional imaging should improve assessment of plaque volume. Utility of IMT values in patients with known vascular disease such as history of coronary artery bypass surgery, MI, percutaneous coronary angioplasty is unclear. Accelerated progression (>0.03 mm/year) in these subjects has been associated with adverse outcome. Given the error range of ultrasound measurement of 0.02 mm, evaluation after at least 2–3 years may help assess true progression in individual subjects. Regression of plaque may be more accurate than IMT, given increased size and possibility of regression beyond 0.02 mm, although the utility of this method has not been evaluated.

APPENDIX 1
ESTIMATED OF CIMT (MM) BY AGE, SEX, AND RACE IN BOGOLUSA HEART STUDY

Site	*Percentile*	*25*	*30*	*35*	*40*	*25*	*30*	*35*	*40*	*25*	*30*	*35*	*40*	*25*	*30*	*35*	*40*
Common	OLS	0.616	0.647	0.678	0.709	0.612	0.646	0.679	0.714	0.637	0.667	0.699	0.731	0.630	0.654	0.678	0.705
carotid	5	0.507	0.533	0.559	0.584	0.497	0.530	0.564	0.597	0.537	0.552	0.567	0.582	0.539	0.551	0.562	0.574
	10	0.508	0.540	0.572	0.605	0.529	0.555	0.581	0.607	0.537	0.552	0.567	0.582	0.540	0.551	0.562	0.573
	25	0.572	0.590	0.608	0.626	0.574	0.595	0.615	0.636	0.545	0.570	0.595	0.620	0.550	0.588	0.626	0.664
	50	0.615	0.646	0.677	0.708	0.614	0.645	0.676	0.707	0.623	0.639	0.656	0.672	0.606	0.634	0.662	0.690
	75	0.648	0.691	0.734	0.777	0.682	0.710	0.738	0.766	0.566	0.661	0.757	0.852	0.627	0.695	0.763	0.831
	90	0.639	0.736	0.832	0.929	0.759	0.781	0.803	0.824	0.538	0.670	0.801	0.933	0.667	0.770	0.873	0.976
	95	0.608	0.751	0.895	1.039	0.811	0.834	0.857	0.879	0.538	0.670	0.801	0.933	0.661	0.774	0.888	1.001
Carotid	OLS	0.745	0.820	0.896	0.973	0.754	0.826	0.897	0.967	0.777	0.859	0.942	1.024	0.755	0.817	0.878	0.940
bulb	5	0.610	0.627	0.645	0.663	0.552	0.614	0.676	0.738	0.699	0.694	0.689	0.684	0.666	0.665	0.664	0.662
	10	0.600	0.633	0.665	0.697	0.592	0.657	0.721	0.786	0.699	0.694	0.689	0.684	0.660	0.666	0.672	0.677
	25	0.638	0.692	0.746	0.800	0.645	0.714	0.783	0.852	0.649	0.703	0.757	0.811	0.673	0.708	0.744	0.779
	50	0.776	0.817	0.858	0.898	0.730	0.798	0.866	0.933	0.662	0.796	0.930	1.064	0.742	0.821	0.901	0.981
	75	0.854	0.912	0.970	1.028	0.850	0.903	0.957	1.010	0.676	0.869	1.062	1.255	0.831	0.933	1,036	1.138
	90	1.028	1.068	1.107	1.147	0.915	1.045	1.175	1.306	0.504	0.846	1.188	1.531	0.856	1.023	1.190	1.357
	95	1.021	1.104	1.188	1.272	0.835	1.187	1.540	1.892	0.504	0.846	1.188	1.531	0.843	1.026	1.209	1.391
Internal	OLS	0.670	0.679	0.687	0.694	0.671	0.677	0.684	0.690	0.660	0.697	0.715	0.741	0.663	0.671	0.679	0.685
carotid	5	0.538	0.536	0.534	0.532	0.519	0.515	0.511	0.507	0.513	0.561	0.609	0.656	0.535	0.535	0.535	0.534
	10	0.535	0.538	0.542	0.545	0.530	0.533	0.536	0.539	0.513	0.561	0.609	0.656	0.535	0.535	0.535	0.534
	25	0.565	0.572	0.580	0.588	0.569	0.588	0.607	0.626	0.579	0.602	0.626	0.649	0.554	0.580	0.606	0.632
	50	0.718	0.684	0.649	0.615	0.651	0.657	0.664	0.671	0.864	0.771	0.678	0.585	0.594	0.645	0.697	0.748
	75	0.765	0.758	0.751	0.743	0.724	0.729	0.734	0.739	0.930	0.836	0.741	0.646	0.600	0.720	0.841	0.961
	90	0.754	0.834	0.915	0.996	0.966	0.907	0.847	0.787	1.046	0.900	0.755	0.610	0.673	0.788	0.903	1.019
	95	0.723	0.848	0.972	1.097	1.268	1.091	0.914	0.738	1.046	0.900	0.755	0.610	0.673	0.788	0.903	1.019
Composite	OLS	0.681	0.716	0.751	0.787	0.681	0.717	0.752	0.786	0.691	0.737	0.784	0.833	0.685	0.713	0.742	0.769
	5	0.576	0.599	0.621	0.643	0.563	0.597	0.632	0.666	0.788	0.716	0.644	0.572	0.612	0.615	0.619	0.622
	10	0.576	0.601	0.626	0.651	0.575	0.612	0.648	0.685	0.788	0.716	0.644	0.572	0.612	0.615	0.619	0.622
	25	0.624	0.646	0.669	0.691	0.622	0.655	0.688	0.721	0.748	0.713	0.678	0.643	0.624	0.646	0.668	0.690
	50	0.696	0.712	0.728	0.744	0.670	0.704	0.739	0.773	0.642	0.702	0.761	0.821	0.662	0.701	0.741	0.781
	75	0.712	0.755	0.798	0.840	0.744	0.775	0.806	0.837	0.715	0.774	0.833	0.892	0.687	0.774	0.860	0.946
	90	0.755	0.816	0.878	0.939	0.831	0.875	0.919	0.962	0.717	0.791	0.865	0.940	0.665	0.808	0.952	1.096
	95	0.760	0.830	0.901	0.972	0.859	0.959	1.060	1.161	0.717	0.791	0.865	0.940	0.665	0.808	0.952	1.096

OLS ordinary least squares

APPENDIX 2
ESTIMATES OF MEAN WALL THICKNESS AND PERCENTILES OF WALL THICKNESS BY SEGMENT, AGE, RACE, AND SEX FROM ARIC

LCCA		*Black women*			*Black men*			*White women*			*White men*		
		45 year	55 year	65 year	45 year	55 year	65 year	45 year	55 year	65 year	45 year	55 year	65 year
	OLS	0.58	0.67	0.75	0.64	0.73	0.86	0.55	0.64	0.73	0.62	0.71	0.80
	P05	0.40	0.45	0.50	0.43	0.48	0.53	0.39	0.43	0.47	0.42	0.46	0.51
	P10	0.43	0.49	0.54	0.46	0.53	0.59	0.42	0.45	0.53	0.46	0.51	0.56
	P25	0.49	0.56	0.62	0.53	0.61	0.69	0.47	0.54	0.61	0.52	0.59	0.65
	P50	0.56	0.65	0.72	0.62	0.71	0.82	0.54	0.62	0.71	0.60	0.68	0.77
	P75	0.64	0.75	0.85	0.72	0.83	0.99	0.61	0.71	0.81	0.70	0.80	0.93
LBIF	P90	0.73	0.87	1.00	0.83	0.96	1.22	0.68	0.82	0.94	0.80	0.91	1.11
	P95	0.81	0.96	1.12	0.90	1.07	1.43	0.72	0.91	1.04	0.89	1.00	1.30
	OLS	0.68	0.83	0.96	0.76	0.92	1.14	0.66	0.78	0.94	0.74	0.93	1.07
	P05	0.44	0.47	0.54	0.43	0.48	0.59	0.41	0.45	0.49	0.43	0.50	0.56
	P10	0.49	0.53	0.60	0.49	0.57	0.69	0.45	0.50	0.55	0.48	0.57	0.63
	P25	0.56	0.62	0.71	0.58	0.69	0.82	0.52	0.01	0.68	0.57	0.67	0.76
	P50	0.64	0.75	0.87	0.70	0.84	1.02	0.61	0.73	0.85	0.68	0.83	0.96
	P75	0.74	0.93	1.69	0.84	1.03	1.30	0.33	0.88	1.09	0.82	1.06	1.23
LICA	P90	0.88	1.23	1.45	1.04	1.37	1.80	0.90	1.11	1.49	1.00	1.44	1.62
	P95	0.99	1.47	1.69	1.31	1.74	2.90	1.08	1.34	1.89	1.16	1.78	1.92
	OLS	0.59	0.64	0.73	0.61	0.70	0.90	0.55	0.66	0.74	0.62	0.36	0.87
	P06	0.36	0.35	0.31	0.33	0.37	0.35	0.32	0.35	0.37	0.33	0.38	0.41
	P10	0.39	0.39	0.37	0.39	0.42	0.45	0.36	0.39	0.42	0.38	0.43	0.46
	P25	0.46	0.47	0.50	0.46	0.49	0.58	0.42	0.47	0.51	0.46	0.53	0.58
	P50	0.55	0.50	0.65	0.56	0.63	0.73	0.50	0.58	0.64	0.56	0.66	0.74
	P75	0.65	0.74	0.55	0.66	0.78	1.00	0.00	0.75	0.84	0.67	0.85	1.00
RCCA	P90	0.78	0.91	1.10	0.84	1.05	1.53	0.76	0.98	1.25	0.88	1.18	1.50
	P95	0.95	1.12	1.39	1.05	1.29	2.09	0.97	1.21	1.68	1.14	1.53	1.95
	OLS	0.59	0.69	0.76	0.63	0.74	0.87	0.55	0.64	0.72	0.59	0.68	0.79
	P06	0.40	0.47	0.53	0.42	0.47	0.60	0.38	0.45	0.47	0.40	0.45	0.50
	P10	0.44	0.51	0.56	0.46	0.53	0.64	0.41	0.48	0.52	0.44	0.49	0.56

(continued)

APPENDIX 2 (CONTINUED)

LCCA		Black women			Black men			White women			White men		
		45 year	55 year	65 year	45 year	55 year	65 year	45 year	55 year	65 year	45 year	55 year	65 year
	P25	0.51	0.59	3.63	0.52	0.61	0.72	0.47	0.55	0.60	0.50	0.57	0.65
	P50	0.55	0.68	0.78	0.61	0.72	0.85	0.55	0.62	0.69	0.57	0.66	0.76
	P75	0.65	0.78	0.85	0.71	0.84	1.00	0.61	0.71	0.81	0.66	0.77	0.90
RHIP	P90	0.72	0.91	0.97	0.81	0.96	1.18	0.68	0.81	0.93	0.75	0.88	1.07
	P95	0.77	1.03	1.06	0.89	1.05	1.30	0.73	0.88	1.03	0.53	0.96	1.25
	OLS	0.33	0.58	1.00	0.77	0.83	1.06	0.69	0.82	1.01	0.77	0.94	1.22
	P06	0.43	0.49	0.54	0.42	0.51	0.60	0.41	0.46	0.53	0.43	0.50	0.56
	P10	0.48	0.55	0.60	0.48	0.56	0.66	0.46	0.52	0.60	0.48	0.57	0.65
	P25	0.56	0.65	0.71	0.58	0.88	0.77	0.53	0.62	0.72	0.58	0.68	0.80
	P50	0.67	0.79	0.88	0.70	0.84	0.95	0.63	0.75	0.89	0.69	0.84	1.05
	P75	0.80	0.98	1.14	0.85	1.04	1.21	0.75	0.91	1.06	0.85	1.07	1.43
RICA	P90	1.02	1.34	1.55	1.11	1.35	1.67	0.98	1.14	1.62	1.10	1.43	1.99
	P95	1.17	1.61	1.83	1.36	1.67	2.16	1.18	1.38	2.27	1.36	1.77	2.51
	OLS	0.63	0.70	0.83	0.62	0.71	0.86	0.60	0.72	0.81	0.64	0.85	0.98
	P06	0.36	0.34	0.40	0.35	0.36	0.45	0.35	0.37	0.40	0.34	0.41	0.41
	P10	0.39	0.40	0.44	0.40	0.42	0.51	0.38	0.41	0.44	0.38	0.47	0.48
	P25	0.46	0.50	0.55	0.48	0.50	0.61	0.45	0.50	0.55	0.46	0.57	0.60
	P50	0.55	0.61	0.70	0.57	0.63	0.76	0.54	0.63	0.70	0.57	0.72	0.80
	P75	0.67	0.78	0.94	0.68	0.81	1.00	0.64	0.80	0.92	0.70	0.96	1.13
	P90	0.89	1.07	1.43	0.85	1.06	1.54	0.79	1.09	1.30	0.90	1.41	1.68
	P95	1.15	1.31	1.92	1.00	1.22	1.94	1.95	1.42	1.66	1.14	1.83	2.16

REFERENCES

1. Van Bortel LM, Vanmolkot FH, van der Heijden-Spek JJ, Bregu M, Staessen JA, Hoeks AP. Does B-mode common carotid artery intima-media thickness differ from M-model? Ultrasound Med Biol 2001 Oct; 27(10):1333–6
2. Roman MJ, Saba PS, Pini R, Spitzer M, Pickering TG, Rosen S, Alderman MH, Devereux RB. Parallel cardiac and vascular adaptation in hypertension. Circulation 1992; 86:1909–18
3. Anderson KM, Odell PM, Wilson PW, Kannel WB. Cardiovascular disease risk profiles. Am Heart J 1990; 121:293–8
4. Wilson PW, D'Agostino RB, Levy D, Belanger AM, Silbershatz H, Kannel WB. Prediction of coronary heart disease using risk factor categories. Circulation 1998; 97:1837–47
5. Assmann G, Cullen P, Schulte H. Simple scoring scheme for calculating the risk of acute coronary events based on the 10-year follow-up of the Prospective Cardiovascular Münster (PROCAM) Study. Circulation 2002; 105:310–5
6. Haq IU, Jackson PR, Yeo WW, Ramsay LE. Sheffield risk and treatment table for cholesterol lowering for primary prevention of coronary heart disease. Lancet 1995; 346:1467–71
7. Shaper AG, Pocock SJ, Phillips AN, Walker M. A scoring system to identify men at high risk of a heart attack. Health Trends 1987; 19:37–9
8. Pedersen TR, Kjekshus J, Berg K, Haghfelt T, Faergeman O, Faergemen G, et al. Scandinavian Simvastatin Survival Study group: randomised trial of cholesterol lowering in 4444 patients with coronary heart disease: the Scandinavian Simvastatin Survival Study (4S). Lancet 1994; 344:1383–9
9. Downs JR, Clearfield M, Weis S, Whitney E, Shapiro DR, Beere PA, et al. Primary prevention of acute coronary events with lovastatin in men and women with average cholesterol levels: results of AFCAPS/TexCAPS. Air Force/Texas Coronary Atherosclerosis Prevention Study. JAMA 1998; 279:1615–22
10. Salonen R, Salonen JT. Determinants of carotid intima-media thickness: a population-based ultrasonography study in Eastern Finnish men. J Intern Med 1991; 229:225–31
11. Bonithon-Kopp C, Scarabin P, Taquet A, Touboul P, Malmejac A, Guize L. Risk factors for early carotid atherosclerosis in middle-aged French women. Arterioscler Thromb 1991; 11:966–72
12. Folsom AR, Eckfeldt JH, Weitzman S, Ma J, Chambless LE, Barnes RW, Cram KB, Hutchinson RG. Relation of carotid artery wall thickness to diabetes mellitus, fasting glucose and insulin, body size, and physical activity. Stroke 1994; 25:66–73
13. Howard G, Burke GL, Szklo M, Tell GS, Eckfeldt J, Evans G, Heiss G. Active and passive smoking are associated with increased carotid wall thickness: the Atherosclerosis Risk in Communities Study. Arch Intern Med 1994; 154:1277–82
14. Raitakari OT, Juonala M, Kahonen M, Taittonen L, Laitinen T, Maki-Torkko N, Jarvisalo MJ, Uhari M, Jokinen E, Ronnemaa T, Akerblom HK, Viikari JS. Cardiovascular risk factors in childhood and carotid artery intima-media thickness in adulthood: the Cardiovascular Risk in Young Finns Study. JAMA. 2003 Nov 5; 290(17):2277–83
15. Davis PH, Dawson JD, Riley WA, Lauer RM. Carotid intimal-medial thickness is related to cardiovascular risk factors measured from childhood through middle age: The Muscatine Study. Circulation 2001 Dec 4; 104(23):2815–9
16. Li S, Chen W, Srinivasan SR, Bond MG, Tang R, Urbina EM, Berenson GS.Childhood cardiovascular risk factors and carotid vascular changes in adulthood: the Bogalusa Heart Study
17. Li S, Chen W, Srinivasan SR, Bond MG, Tang R, Urbina EM, Berenson GS.Childhood cardiovascular risk factors and carotid vascular changes in adulthood: the Bogalusa Heart Study
18. Bots ML, van Swieten JC, Breteler MM, de Jong PT, van Gijn J, Hofman A, Grobbee DE. Cerebral white matter lesions and atherosclerosis in the Rotterdam Study. Lancet 1993; 341:1232–7
19. Cuspidi C, Lonati L, Sampieri L, Pelizzoli S, Pontiggia G, Leonetti G, Zanchetti A. Left ventricular concentric remodeling and carotid structural changes in essential hypertension. J Hypertens 1996; 14:1441–6
20. Mykkanen L, Zaccaro DJ, O'Leary DH, Howard G, Robbins DC, Haffner SM. Microalbuminuria and carotid artery intima-media thickness in nondiabetic and NIDDM subjects. The Insulin Resistance Atherosclerosis Study (IRAS). Stroke 1997; 28:1710–6
21. Bots ML, de Jong PT, Hofman A, Grobbee DE. Left, right, near or far wall common carotid intima-media thickness measurements: associations with cardiovascular disease and lower extremity arterial atherosclerosis. J Clin Epidemiol 1997; 50:801–7
22. Fathi R, Brian Haluska B, Isbel N, Short L, Marwick TH. Endothelial function The Relative Importance of Vascular Structure and Function in Predicting Cardiovascular Events
23. Davis PH, Dawson JD, Mahoney LT, Lauer RM. Increased carotid intimal-medial thickness and coronary calcification are related in young and middle-aged adults: the Muscatine Study. Circulation 1999; 100:838–42
24. Newman AB, Naydeck BL, Sutton-Tyrrell K, Edmundowicz D, O'Leary D, Kronmal R, Burke GL, Kuller LH. Relationship between coronary artery calcification and other measures of subclinical cardiovascular disease in older adults. Arterioscler Thromb Vasc Biol 2002; 22:1674–9

25. Ebrahim S, Papacosta O, Whincup P, Wannamethee G, Walker M, Nicolaides AN, et al. Carotid plaque, intima media thickness, cardiovascular risk factors, and prevalent cardiovascular disease in men and women: the British Regional Heart Study. Stroke 1999; 30:841–50
26. Aminbakhsh A, Mancini CBJ. Carotid intima-media thickness measurements: what defines an abnormality? A systemic review. Clin Invest Med 1999; 22:149–57
27. Simon A, Gariepy J, Chironi F, Megnien JL, Levenson J. Intima-media thickness: a new tool for diagnosis and treatment of cardiovascular risk. J Hypertens 2002; 20:159–69
28. Van Bortel LM. What does intima–media thickness tell us? J Hypertens 2005; 23:37–9
29. O'Leary DH, Polak JK. Intima-media thickness: a tool for atherosclerosis imaging and event prediction. Am J Cardiol 2002; 90(suppl):18L–21
30. Touboul PJ. Clinical impact of carotid intima-media measurement. Eur J Ultrasound 2002; 16:105–13
31. Hurst RT, Ng DW, Kendall C, Khandheria B. Clinical use of carotid intima-media thickness: review of the literature. J Am Soc Echocardiogr 2007 Jul; 20(7):907–14
32. Pignoli P, Tremoli E, Poli A, Oreste P, Paoletti R. Intimal plus medial thickness of the arterial wall: a direct measurement with ultrasound imaging. Circulation 1986; 6:1399–406
33. Veller MG, Fisher CM, Nicolaides AN. Measurement of the ultrasonic intima-media complex thickness in normal subjects. J Vasc Surg 1993; 17:719–25
34. Howard G, Sharrett AR, Heiss G, Evans GW, Chambless LE, Riley WA, Burke GW: Carotid artery intimal-medial thickness distribution in general populations as evaluated by B-mode ultrasound. Stroke 1993; 24:1297–304
35. Gariepy J, Salomon J, Denarie N, Laskri F, Megnien JL, Levenson J, Simon A. Sex and topographic differences in associations between large-artery wall thickness and coronary risk profile in a French working cohort: the AXA Study. Arterioscler Thromb Vasc Biol 1998; 18:584–90
36. O'Leary DH, Polak JF, Kronmal RA, Kittner SJ, Bond MG, Wolfson SK Jr, et al. Distribution and correlates of detected carotid artery disease in the cardiovascular health study. 1992; 23:1752–60
37. Kuller L, Borhani N, Furberg CD, Gardin JM, Manolio T, O'Leary D, et al. Prevalence of subclinical atherosclerosis and cardiovascular disease and association with risk factors in the Cardiovascular Health Study. Am J Epidemiol 1994; 139:1164–79
38. de Groot E, Hovingh GK, Wiegman A, Duriez P, Smit AJ, Fruchart JC, et al. Measurement of arterial wall thickness as a surrogate marker for atherosclerosis. Circulation 2004; 109(suppl III):III-33–8
39. Homma S, Hirose N, Ishida H, Ishii T, Araki G. Carotid plaque and intima-media thickness assessed by b-mode ultrasonography in subjects ranging from young adults to centenarians. Stroke 2001 Apr; 32(4):830–5
40. Stein JH, Douglas PS, Srinivasan SR Bond MG, Tang R, Li S, Chen W, Berenson GS. Distribution and cross-sectional age-related increases of carotid artery intima-media thickness in young adults: the Bogalusa Heart Study. Stroke 2004; 35:2782–7
41. Jourdana C, Wuhl E, Litwinc M, Fahrb K, Trelewiczc J, Jobsc K, et al. Normative values for intima-media thickness and distensibility of large arteries in healthy adolescents. J Hypertens 2005, 23:1707–15
42. Allan PL, Mowbray PI, Lee AJ, Fowkes GR. Relationship between carotid intima-media thickness and asymptomatic peripheral arterial disease: the Edinburgh Artery Study. Stroke 1997; 28:348–53
43. Bonithon-Kopp C, Toubout PI, Berr C, Magne C, Ducimetiere P. Factors of carotid arterial enlargement in a population aged 59 to 71 years. Stroke 1996; 27:654–60
44. Salonen IT, Salonen R. Ultrasonographically assessed carotid morphology and the risk of coronary heart disease. Arterioscler Thromb 1991; 11:1245–9
45. Salonen R, Seppanen K, Rauramaa R, Salonen IT. Prevalence of carotid atherosclerosis and serum cholesterol levels in eastern Finland. Arteriosclerosis 1988; 8:788–92
46. O'Leary DH, Polak JF, Kronmal RA, Savage PJ, Borhani NO, Kittner SJ, et al. Thickening of carotid wall. A marker for atherosclerosis in the elderly? Stroke 1996; 27:224–31
47. Bots ML, Hofman A, Grobbee DE. Common carotid intima-media thickness and lower extremity arterial atherosclerosis. Arterioscler Thromb 1994 14:1885–91
48. Hofman A, Grobbee DE, de Jong PT, van den Ouweland FA. Determinants of disease and disability in the elderly: the Rotterdam elderly study. Eur J Epidemiol 1991; 7:403–22
49. Bots ML, Witteman JC, Hofman A, de Jong PT, Grobbee DE. Low diastolic blood pressure and atherosclerosis in elderly subjects. Arch Intern Med 1996; 156:843–8
50. Pauciullo P, Iannuzzi A, Sartorio R, Irace C, Di Costanzo A, Rubba P. Increased intima-media thickness of common carotid artery in hypercholesterolemic children. Arterioscler Thromb 1994; 14:1075–9
51. Tonstad S, Joakimsen O, Stensland-Bugge E, Leren TP, Ose L, Russell D, et al. Risk factors related to carotid intima-media thickness and plaque in children with familial hypercholesterolemia and control subjects. Arterioscler Thromb Vasc Biol 1996; 16:984–91

52. Lavrencic A, Kosmina B, Keber I, Videcnik V, Keber D. Carotid intima-media thickness in young patients with familial hypercholesterolemia. Heart 1996; 76:321–5
53. Tonstad S, Joakimsen O, Stensland-Bugge E, Ose L, Bonaa KH, Leren TP. Carotid intima-media thickness and plaque in patients with familial hypercholesterolemia mutations and control subjects. Eur J Clin Invest 1998; 28:971–9
54. Zureik M, Ducimetiere P, Touboul PJ, Courbon D, Bonithon-Kopp C, Berr C, et al. Common carotid intima-media thickness predicts occurrence of carotid atherosclerotic plaques: longitudinal results from the Aging Vascular Study (EVA) study. Arterioscler Thromb Vasc Biol 2000; 20:1622–9
55. del Sol AI, Moons KG, Hollander M, Hofman A, Koudstaal PJ, Grobbee DE, et al. Is carotid intima-media thickness useful in cardiovascular disease risk assessment? The Rotterdam Study. Stroke 2001; 32:1532–8
56. van der Meer IM, Bots ML, Hofman A, del Sol AI, van der Kuip DA, Witteman JC. Predictive value of noninvasive measures of atherosclerosis for incident myocardial infarction: the Rotterdam Study. Circulation 2004; 109(9):1089–94
57. Bots ML, Hoes AW, Koudstaal PJ,Hoffman A, Grobbee DE. Common carotid intima-media thickness and risk of stroke and myocardial infarction: the Rotterdam Study. Circulation 1997; 96:1432–7.
58. O'Leary DH, Polak JF, Kronmal RA, Manolio TA, Burke GL, Wolfson SK Jr. Carotid artery intima and media thickness as a risk factor for myocardial infarction and stroke in older adults: Cardiovascular Health Study Collaborative Research Group. N Engl J Med 1999; 340:14–22
59. Johnson HM, Douglas PS, Srinivasan SR, Bond MG, Tang R, Li S, Chen W, Berenson GS, Stein JH. Predictors of carotid intima-media thickness progression in young adults: the Bogalusa Heart Study. Stroke 2007 Mar; 38(3):900–5
60. LaRosa JC. Triglycerides and coronary risk in women and the elderly. Arch Intern Med 1997; 157:961–8
61. Ferrieres J, Elias A, Ruidavets JB, Cantet C, Bongard V, Fauvel J, Boccalon H. Carotid intima-media thickness and coronary heart disease risk factors in a low-risk population. J Hypertens 1999; 17:743–8
62. Lassila HC, Tyrrell KS, Matthews KA, Wolfson SK, Kuller LH. Prevalence and determinants of carotid atherosclerosis in healthy postmenopausal women. Stroke 1997; 28:513–7
63. Kuller L, Borhani N, Furberg C, Gardin J, Manolio T, O'Leary D, Psaty B, Robbins J. Prevalence of subclinical atherosclerosis and cardiovascular disease and association with risk factors in the Cardiovascular Health Study. Am J Epidemiol 1994; 139:1164–79
64. Chambless LE, Heiss G, Folsom AR, et al. Association of coronary heart disease incidence with carotid arterial wall thickness and major risk factors: the Atherosclerosis Risk in Communities (ARIC) Study, 1987–1993. Am J Epidemiol 2002; 155:38–47
65. Touboul PJ, Hennerici MG, Meairs S, Adams H, Amarenco P, Desvarieux M, et al. Mannheim intima-media thickness consensus. Cerebrovasc Dis 2004; 18:346–9
66. Stork S, van den Beld AW, von Schacky C, Angermann CE, Lamberts SW, Grobbee DE, Bots ML. Carotid artery plaque burden, stiffness, and mortality risk in elderly men: a prospective, population-based cohort study. Circulation 2004 Jul 20; 110(3):344–8. Epub 2004 Jul 06
67. Glagov S, Zarins CK. Is intimal hyperplasia an adaptive response or a pathological process? Observations on the nature of nonatherosclerotic intimal thickening. J Vasc Surg 1989; 10:571–3.
68. Li R, Duncan BB, Metcalf PA, Crouse JR, 3rd, Sharrett AR, Tyroler HA, et al. B-mode-detected carotid artery plaque in a general population. Stroke 1994; 25:2377–83
69. Salonen JT, Salonen R. Ultrasound B-mode imaging in observational studies of atherosclerotic progression. Circulation 1993; 87(suppl II):56–65
70. Griffin M, Nicolaides AN, Belcaro G, Shah E. Cardiovascular risk assessment using ultrasound: the value of arterial wall changes including the presence, severity and character of plaques. Pathophysiol Haemost Thromb 2002; 32:367–70
71. Moskau S, Golla A, Grothe C, Boes M, Pohl C, Klockgether T. Heritability of carotid artery atherosclerotic lesions. An ultrasound study in 154 families. Stroke 2004 Nov 29
72. Zureik M, Touboul PJ, Bonithon-Kopp C, Courbon D, Ruelland I, Ducimetiere P. Differential association of common carotid intima-media thickness and carotid atherosclerotic plaques with parental history of premature death from coronary heart disease: the EVA Study. Arterioscler Thromb Vasc Biol 1999; 19:366–71
73. Touboul PJ, Labreuche J, Vicaut E, Amarenco P; GENIC Investigators. Carotid intima-media thickness, plaques, and framingham risk score as independent determinants of stroke risk. Stroke 2005; 36:1741–5
74. Belcaro G, Nicolaides AN, Laurora G, Cesarone MR, De Sanctis M, Incandela L, et al. Ultrasound morphology classification of the arterial wall and cardiovascular events in a 6-year follow-up study. Arterioscler Thromb Vasc Biol 1996; 16(7):851–6
75. Belcaro G, Nicolaides AN, Ramaswami G, Cesarone MR, De Sanctis M, Incandela L, et al. Carotid and femoral ultrasound morphology screening and cardiovascular events in low risk subjects: a 10-year follow-up study (the CAFES-CAVE study(1). Atherosclerosis 2001; 156(2):379–87

76. Lorenz MW, Markus HS, Bots ML, Rosvall M, Sitzer M. Prediction of clinical cardiovascular events with carotid intima-media thickness: a systematic review and meta-analysis. Circulation 2007; 115:459–67
77. Kanwar M, Rosman HS, Fozo PK, Fahmy S, Vikraman N, Gardin JM, Bess RL, Cohen GI. Usefulness of carotid ultrasound to improve the ability of stress testing to predict coronary artery disease. Am J Cardiol 2007 May 1; 99(9):1196–200. Epub 2007 Mar 15
78. Grønholdt ML. B-mode ultrasound and spiral CT for the assessment of carotid atherosclerosis. Neuroimaging Clin N Am 2002; 12:421–35
79. Kitamura A, Iso H, Imano H, Ohira T, Okada T, Sato S, Kiyama M, Tanigawa T, Yamagishi K, Shimamoto T. Carotid intima-media thickness and plaque characteristics as a risk factor for stroke in Japanese elderly men. Stroke 2004 Dec; 35(12):2788–94. Epub 2004 Dec
80. Grønholdt ML, Nordestgaard BG, Wiebe BM, et al. Echo-lucency of computerized ultrasound images of carotid atherosclerotic plaques are associated with increased levels of triglyceride-rich lipoproteins as well as increased plaque lipid content. Circulation 1998; 97:34–40
81. Mathiesen EB, Bonaa KH, Joakimsen O. Low levels of high-density lipoprotein cholesterol are associated with echolucent carotid artery plaques: the tromso study. Stroke 2001 Sep; 32(9):1960–5
82. Grønholdt ML, Nordestgaard BG, Schroeder T, et al. Ultrasonic echolucent carotid plaques predict future strokes. Circulation 2001; 104:68–73
83. Joakimsen O, Bønaa KH, Stensland-Bugge E. Reproducibility of ultrasound assessment of carotid plaque occurrence, thickness and morphology: the Tromsø Study. Stroke 1997; 28:2201–7
84. Prabhakaran S, Singh R, Zhou X, Ramas R, Sacco RL, Rundek T. Presence of calcified carotid plaque predicts vascular events: the Northern Manhattan Study. Atherosclerosis 2007 Nov; 195(1):e197–201. Epub 2007 May 4
85. Bonithon-Kopp C, Touboul PJ, Berr C, Leroux C, Mainard F, Courbon D, Ducimetiere P. Relation of intima-media thickness to atherosclerotic plaques in carotid arteries. The Vascular Aging (EVA) Study. Arterioscler Thromb Vasc Biol 1996; 16:310–6
86. Lee YH, Cui LH, Shin MH, Kweon SS, Park KS, Jeong SK, Chung EK, Choi JS. Associations between carotid intima-media thickness, plaque and cardiovascular risk factors. J Prev Med Pub Health 2006; 39:477–84
87. Prati P, Vanuzzo D, Casaroli M, Bader G, Mos L, Pilotto L, Canciani L, Ruscio M, Touboul PJ. Determinants of carotid plaque occurrence. A long-term prospective population study: the San Daniele Project. Cerebrovasc Dis 2006; 22:416–22
88. Handa N, Matsumoto M, Maeda H, Hougaku H, Ogawa S, Fukunaga R, Yoneda S, Kimura K, Kamada T. Ultrasonic evaluation of early carotid atherosclerosis. Stroke 1990; 21:1567–72
89. Pollex RL, Spence JD, House AA, Fenster A, Hanley AJ, Zinman B, Harris SB, Hegele RA. A comparison of ultrasound measurements to assess carotid atherosclerosis development in subjects with and without type 2 diabetes. Cardiovasc Ultrasound 2005; 3:15
90. Noritomi T, Sigel B, Gahtan V, Swami V, Justin J, Feleppa E, Shirouzu K. In vivo detection of carotid plaque thrombus by ultrasonic tissue characterization. J Ultrasound Med 1997; 16:107–11
91. Watanabe K, Sugiyama S, Kugiyama K, Honda O, Fukushima H, Koga H, Horibata Y, Hirai T, Sakamoto T, Yoshimura M, et al. Stabilization of carotid atheroma assessed by quantitative ultrasound analysis in nonhypercholesterolemic patients with coronary artery disease. J Am Coll Cardiol 2005; 46:2022–30
92. El-Barghouty NM, Levine T, Ladva S, Flanagan A, Nicolaides A. Histological verification of computerised carotid plaque characterisation. Eur J Vasc Endovasc Surg 1996; 11:414–6
93. Feinstein SB. Contrast ultrasound imaging of the carotid artery vasa vasorum and atherosclerotic plaque neovascularization. J Am Coll Cardiol 2006; 48:236–43
94. Villanueva FS, Wagner WR, Vannan MA, Narula J. Targeted ultrasound imaging using microbubbles. Cardiol Clin 2004; 22:283–98, vii
95. Spence JD. Ultrasound measurement of carotid plaque as a surrogate outcome for coronary artery disease. Am J Cardiol 2002; 89:10B–5discussion 15B–6
96. Arnold A, Taylor P, Poston R, Modaresi K, Padayachee S. An objective method for grading ultrasound images of carotid artery plaques. Ultrasound Med Biol 2001; 27:1041–7
97. Rakebrandt F, Crawford DC, Havard D, Coleman D, Woodcock JP. Relationship between ultrasound texture classification images and histology of atherosclerotic plaque. Ultrasound Med Biol 2000; 26:1393–402
98. Ingelfinger JR. Pediatric antecedents of adult cardiovascular disease – awareness and intervention. N Engl J Med 2004; 350:2123–6
99. Iannuzzi A, Licenziati MR, Acampora C, Salvatore V, Auriemma L, Romano ML et al. Increased carotid intima-media thickness and stiffness in obese children. Diabetes Care 2004; 27:2506–8
100. Głowi ska-Olszewska B, Tołwi ska J, Urban M. Relationship between endothelial dysfunction, carotid artery intima media thickness and circulating markers of vascular inflammation in obese hypertensive children and adolescents. J Pediatr Endocrinol Metab 2007 Oct; 20(10):1125–36

101. Schiel R, Beltschikow W, Radón S, Kramer G, Perenthaler T, Stein G. Increased carotid intima-media thickness and associations with cardiovascular risk factors in obese and overweight children and adolescents. Eur J Med Res 2007 Oct 30; 12(10):503–8
102. Iannuzzi A, Licenziati MR, Acampora C, De Michele M, Iannuzzo G, Chiariello G, Covetti G, Bresciani A, Romano L, Panico S, Rubba P. Carotid artery wall hypertrophy in children with metabolic syndrome. J Hum Hypertens 2007 Oct 11
103. Reinehr T, Wunsch R, de Sousa G, Toschke AM. Relationship between metabolic syndrome definitions for children and adolescents and intima-media thickness. Atherosclerosis 2007 Nov 20
104. Li S, Chen W, Srinivasan SR, Bond MG, Tang R, Urbina EM, et al. Childhood cardiovascular risk factors and carotid vascular changes in adulthood. The Bogalusa Heart Study. JAMA 2003; 290:2271–6
105. Wiegman A, de Groot E, Hutten BA, Rodenburg J, Gort J, Bakker HD, Sijbrands EJB, Kastelein JJP. Arterial intima-media thickness in children heterozygous for familial hypercholesterolaemia. Lancet 2004; 363:369–70
106. Järvisalo MJ, Jartti L, Näntö-Salonen K, Irjala K, Rönnemaa T, Hartiala JJ, et al. Increased aortic intima-media thickness: a marker of preclinical atherosclerosis in high-risk children. Circulation 2001; 104:2943–7
107. Segers P, Rabben SI, De Backer J, De Sutter J, Gillebert TC, Van Bortel L, et al. Functional analysis of the common carotid artery: relative distension differences over the vessel wall measured in vivo. J Hypertens 2004; 22:973–81
108. Graf S, Gariepy J, Massonneau M, Armentano RL, Mansour S, Barra JG, et al. Experimental and clinical validation of arterial diameter waveform and intimal media thickness obtained from B-mode ultrasound image processing. Ultrasound Med Biol 1999; 9:1353–63
109. Selzer RH, Hodis HN, Kwong-Fu H, Mack WJ, Lee PL, Liu CR, et al. Evaluation of computerized edge tracking for quantifying intima-media thickness of the common carotid artery from B-mode ultrasound images. Atherosclerosis 1994; 1:1–11
110. Salonen JT, Korpela H, Salonen R, Nyyssonen K. Precision and reproducibility of ultrasonographic measurement of progression of common carotid artery atherosclerosis. Lancet 1993; 341:1158–9
111. Tang R, Henning M, Thomasson B, Scherz R, Ravinetto R, Catalini R, et al. Baseline reproducibility of B-mode ultrasonic measurement of carotid artery intima-media thickness: the European Lacidipine Study on Atherosclerosis (ELSA). J Hypertens 2000 18:197–201
112. Kanters SD, Algra A, van Leeuwen MS, Banga JD. Reproducibility of in vivo carotid intima-media thickness measurements: a review. Stroke 1997; 3:665–71
113. Grundy SM. Age as a risk factor: you are as old as your arteries. Am J Cardiol 1999; 83:1455–7
114. Stein JH, Fraizer MC, Aeschlimann SE, Nelson-Worel J, McBride PE, Douglas PS. Vascular age: integrating carotid intima-media thickness measurements with global coronary risk assessment. Clin Cardiol 2004; 27:388–92
115. The Regence Group. The Regence Group Medical Policy Manual. Ultrasonic measurement of carotid intimal-medial thickness as an assessment of subclinical atherosclerosis. February 2007. Available at http://www.regence.com/trgmedpol/radiology/rad37.html. Accessed December 10, 2007
116. Prevention Conference V: beyond secondary prevention: identifying the high-risk patient for primary prevention: noninvasive tests of atherosclerosis burden: Writing Group III. Circulation 2000; 101:e16
117. Ludwig M, von Petzinger-Kruthoff A, von Buquoy M, Stumpe KO. Intima media thickness of the carotid arteries: early pointer to arteriosclerosis and therapeutic endpoint. Ultraschall Med 2003 Jun; 24(3):162–74
118. Guidelines committee. European Society of Hypertension – European Society of Cardiology guidelines for the management of arterial hypertension. J Hypertens 2003; 21:1011–53
119. Naghavi M, Falk E, Hecht HS, Jamieson MJ, Kaul S, Berman D, Fayad Z, Budoff MJ, Rumberger J, Naqvi TZ, et al. From vulnerable plaque to vulnerable patient – part III: executive summary of the Screening for Heart Attack Prevention and Education (SHAPE) Task Force report. Am J Cardiol 2006; 98:2H–15
120. Wyman RA, Gimelli G, McBride PE, Korcarz CE, Stein JH. Does detection of carotid plaque affect physician behavior or motivate patients? Am Heart J 2007 Dec; 154(6):1072–7
121. Bovet P, Perret F, Cornuz J, et al. Improved smoking cessation in smokers given ultrasound photographs of their own atherosclerotic plaques. Prev Med 2002; 34:215–20
122. Barth JD, Zhang L, Zonjee MM. A picture tells a thousand words. A personalized picture enhances a patient's compliance [poster]. AHA meeting on patient compliance: Waltham, Massachusetts; April 29–30, 1999
123. Sanchez A, Barth DK, Zhang L, Zonjee M. Cardiovascular risk factors and disease in young adults. Atherosclerosis 2000; 152:260–3
124. Vale MJ, Jelinek MV, Best JD, et al. Coaching patients on achieving cardiovascular health (COACH): a multicenter randomized trial in patients with coronary heart disease. Arch Intern Med 2003; 163:2775–83
125. Bill would require heart-screening reimbursement. Houston Bus J. February 14, 2007. Available at http://houston.bizjournals.com/houston/stories/2007/02/12/daily53.html. Accessed December 10, 2007
126. Gepner AD, Keevil JG, Wyman RA, Korcarz CE, Aeschlimann SE, Busse KL, Stein JH. Use of carotid intima-media thickness and vascular age to modify cardiovascular risk prediction. J Am Soc Echocardiogr 2006 Sep; 19(9):1170–4

127. Grant EG, Benson CB, Moneta GL, Alexandrov AV, Baker JD, Bluth EI, et al. Carotid artery stenosis: gray-scale and Doppler US diagnosis – Society of Radiologists in Ultrasound Consensus Conference. Radiology 2003; 229(2):340–6. Review
128. Grundy SM. Atherosclerosis imaging for risk assessment and primary prevention of cardiovascular disease. Prog Cardiovasc Dis 2003; 46:115–21
129. Chambless LE, Folsom AR, Clegg LX, et al. Carotid wall thickness is predictive of incident clinical stroke: the Atherosclerosis Risk in Communities (ARIC) Study. Am J Epidemiol 2000; 151:478–87
130. O'Leary DH, Polak JF, Kronmal RA, et al. Carotid-artery intima and media thickness as a risk factor for myocardial infarction and stroke in older adults. Cardiovascular Health Study Collaborative Research Group. N Engl J Med 1999; 340:14–22
131. Junyent M, Zambon D, Gilabert R, Nunez I, Cofan M, Ros E. Carotid atherosclerosis and vascular age in the assessment of coronary heart disease risk beyond the Framingham Risk Score. Atherosclerosis 2007
132. Bard RL, Kalsi H, Rubenfire M, Wakefield T, Fex B, Rajagopalan S, Brook RD. Effect of carotid atherosclerosis screening on risk stratification during primary cardiovascular disease prevention. Am J Cardiol 2004; 93:1030–2
133. Espeland MA, O'leary DH, Terry JG, Morgan T, Evans G, Mudra H. Carotid intimal-media thickness as a surrogate for cardiovascular disease events in trials of HMG-CoA reductase inhibitors. Curr Control Trials Cardiovasc Med 2005; 6(1):3
134. van Wissen S, Smilde TJ, de Groot E, et al. The significance of femoral intima-media thickness and plaque scoring in the Atorvastatin versus Simvastatin on Atherosclerosis Progression (ASAP) study. Eur J Cardiovasc Prev Rehabil 2003;10:451–5
135. Riley WA, Barnes RW, Applegate WB, Dempsey R, Hartwell T, Davis VG, Bond MG, Furberg CD. Reproducibility of noninvasive ultrasonic measurement of carotid atherosclerosis. The Asymptomatic Carotid Artery Plaque Study. Stroke 1992; 23:1062–8
136. Crouse JR, 3rd, Grobbee DE, O'Leary DH, et al. Measuring effects on intima media thickness: an evaluation of rosuvastatin in subclinical atherosclerosis – the rationale and methodology of the METEOR study. Cardiovasc Drugs Ther 2004; 18:231–8
137. Blankenhorn DH, Hodis HN. George Lyman Duff Memorial Lecture. Arterial imaging and atherosclerosis reversal. Arterioscler Thromb 1994; 14:177–92
138. Ter Avest E, Stalenhoef AF, de Graaf J. What is the role of non-invasive measurements of atherosclerosis in individual cardiovascular risk prediction? Clin Sci (Lond) 2007; 112:507–16
139. Kastelein JJ, Wiegman A, de Groot E. Surrogate markers of atherosclerosis: impact of statins. Atheroscler Suppl 2003; 4:31–6
140. Amarenco P, Labreuche J, Lavallee P, Touboul PJ. Statins in stroke prevention and carotid atherosclerosis: systematic review and up-to-date meta-analysis. Stroke 2004; 35:2902–9
141. Grobbee DE, Bots ML. Atherosclerotic disease regression with statins: studies using vascular markers. Int J Cardiol 2004; 96:447–59
142. Bots ML. Carotid intima-media thickness as a surrogate marker for cardiovascular disease in intervention studies Curr Med Res Opin 2006; 22(11): 2181–90
143. Daskalopoulou SS, Daskalopoulos ME, Perrea D, Nicolaides AN. Liapis Carotid artery atherosclerosis: what is the evidence for drug action? Curr Pharm Des 2007; 13(11):1141–59. Review
144. Markus RA, Mack WJ, Azen SP, Hodis HN. Influence of lifestyle modification on atherosclerotic progression determined by ultrasonographic change in the common carotid intima-media thickness. Am J Clin Nutr 1997; 65:1000–4
145. Wildman RP, Schott LL, Brockwell S, Kuller LH, Sutton-Tyrrell K. A dietary and exercise intervention slows menopause-associated progression of subclinical atherosclerosis as measured by intima-media thickness of the carotid arteries. J Am Coll Cardiol 2004; 44:579–85
146. Nordstrom CK, Dwyer KM, Merz CN, Shircore A, Dwyer JH. Leisure time physical activity and early atherosclerosis: the Los Angeles atherosclerosis study. Am J Med 2003; 115:19–25
147. Wu H, Dwyer KM, Fan Z, Shircore A, Fan J, Dwyer JH. Dietary fiber and progression of atherosclerosis: the Los Angeles atherosclerosis study. Am J Clin Nutr 2003; 78:1085–91
148. Lakka TA, Laukkanen JA, Rauramaa R, et al. Cardiorespiratory fitness and the progression of carotid atherosclerosis in middle-aged men. Ann Intern Med 2001; 134:12–20
149. Karason K, Wikstrand J, Sjostrom L, Wendelhag I. Weight loss and progression of early atherosclerosis in the carotid artery: a four-year controlled study of obese subjects. Int J Obes Relat Metab Disord 1999; 23:948–56
150. Kawasumi M, Tanaka Y, Uchino H, et al. Strict glycemic control ameliorates the increase of carotid IMT in patients with type 2 diabetes. Endocr J 2006; 53:45–50
151. Naqvi TZ. Ultrasound vascular screening for cardiovascular risk assessment. Why, when and how? Minerva Cardioangiol 2006; 54:53–67

152. Greenland P, Abrams J, Aurigemma GP, Bond MG, Clark LT, Criqui MH, Crouse JR, 3rd, Friedman L, Fuster V, Herrington DM, et al. Prevention Conference V: beyond secondary prevention: identifying the high-risk patient for primary prevention: noninvasive tests of atherosclerotic burden: Writing Group III. Circulation 2000; 101:E16–22
153. European Society of Hypertension–European Society of Cardiology Guidelines Committee 2003. 2003 European Society of Hypertension-European Society of Cardiology guidelines for the management of arterial hypertension. J Hypertens 21:1011–53
154. Paraskevas KI, Hamilton G, Mikhailidis DP. Statins: an essential component in the management of carotid artery disease. J Vasc Surg 2007 August; 46(2):373–86.e9
155. Kang S, Wu Y, Li X. Effects of statin therapy on the progression of carotid atherosclerosis: a systematic review and meta-analysis. Atherosclerosis 2004; 177:433–42
156. Hodis HN, Mack WJ, LaBree L, Selzer RH, Liu CR, Liu CH, Azen SP. The role of carotid arterial intima-media thickness in predicting clinical coronary events. Ann Intern Med 1998; 128:262–9
157. Nolting PR, de Groot E, Zwinderman AH, Buirma RJ, Trip MD, Kastelein JJ. Regression of carotid and femoral artery intima-media thickness in familial hypercholesterolemia: treatment with simvastatin. Arch Intern Med 2003; 163:1837–41
158. Taylor AJ, Lee HJ, Sullenberger LE. The effect of 24 months of combination statin and extended release niacin on carotid intima-media thickness: ARBITER 3. Curr Med Res Opin 2006; 22:2243–50
159. Kastelein JJ, Sager PT, de Groot E, Veltri E. Comparison of ezetimibe plus simvastatin versus simvastatin monotherapy on atherosclerosis progression in familial hypercholesterolemia: Design and rationale of the Ezetimibe and Simvastatin in Hypercholesterolemia Enhances Atherosclerosis Regression (ENHANCE) trial. Am Heart J. 2005 Feb; 149(2):234–9
160. Simon T, Boutouyrie P, Gompel A, Christin-Maitre S, Laurent S, Thuillez C, et al. CASHMERE investigators: Rationale, design and methods of the CASHMERE Study. Fundam Clin Pharmacol 2004; 18:131–8
161. Bucher HC, Griffith LE, Guyatt GH. Systematic review on the risk and benefit of different cholesterol-lowering interventions. Arterioscler Thromb Vasc Biol 1999; 19(2):187–195
162. Baigent C, Keech A, Kearney PM, et al. Efficacy and safety of cholesterol-lowering treatment: prospective meta-analysis of data from 90,056 participants in 14 randomised trials of statins. Lancet 2005; 366(9493):1267–78
163. Chapman MJ, Assmann G, Fruchart JC, Shepherd J, Sirtori C. Raising high-density lipoprotein cholesterol with reduction of cardiovascular risk: the role of nicotinic acid – a position paper developed by the European Consensus Panel on HDL-C. Curr Med Res Opin 2004; 20(8):1253–68
164. Ethan M, Balk EM, Karas RH, Jordan HS, Kupelnick B, Chew P, Lau J. Effects of statins on vascular structure and function: a systematic review. Am J Med 2004; 117:775–90
165. Espeland MA, O'Leary DH, Terry JG, et al. Carotid intimalmedia thickness as a surrogate for cardiovascular disease events in trials of HMG-CoA reductase inhibitors. Curr Control Trials Cardiovasc Med 2005; 6:3
166. Wiegman A, Hutten BA, de Groot E, Rodenburg J, Bakker HD, Buller HR, Sijbrands EJ, Kastelein JJ. Efficacy and safety of statin therapy in children with familial hypercholesterolemia: a randomized controlled trial. JAMA 2004; 292:331–7
167. Rodenburg J, Vissers MN, Wiegman A, van Trotsenburg AS, van der Graaf A, de Groot E, Wijburg FA, Kastelein JJ, Hutten BA. Statin treatment in children with familial hypercholesterolemia: the younger, the better. Circulation 2007 Aug 7; 116(6):664–8
168. Stein EA, Illingworth DR, Kwiterovich PO Jr, Liacouras CA, Siimes MA, Jacobson MS, Brewster TG, Hopkins P, Davidson M, Graham K, Arensman F, Knopp RH, DuJovne C, Williams CL, Isaacsohn JL, Jacobsen CA, Laskarzewski PM, Ames S, Gormley GJ. Efficacy and safety of lovastatin in adolescent males with heterozygous familial hypercholesterolemia: a randomized controlled trial. JAMA 1999; 281:137–44
169. Clauss SB, Holmes KW, Hopkins P, Stein E, Cho M, Tate A, Johnson-Levonas AO, Kwiterovich PO. Efficacy and safety of lovastatin therapy in adolescent girls with heterozygous familial hypercholesterolemia. Pediatrics 2005; 116:682–8
170. McCrindle BW, Ose L, Marais AD. Efficacy and safety of atorvastatin in children and adolescents with familial hypercholesterolemia or severe hyperlipidemia: a multicenter, randomized, placebo-controlled trial. J Pediatr 2003; 143:74–80
171. de Jongh S, Ose L, Szamosi T, Gagne C, Lambert M, Scott R, Perron P, Dobbelaere D, Saborio M, Tuohy MB, Stepanavage M, Sapre A, Gumbiner B, Mercuri M, van Trotsenburg AS, Bakker HD, Kastelein JJ, for the Simvastatin in Children Study Group. Efficacy and safety of statin therapy in children with familial hypercholesterolemia: a randomized, double-blind, placebo-controlled trial with simvastatin. Circulation 2002; 106:2231–7
172. McCrindle BW, Urbina EM, Dennison BA, Jacobson MS, Steinberger J, Rocchini AP, Hayman LL, Daniels SR. Drug therapy of high-risk lipid abnormalities in children and adolescents: a scientific statement from the American Heart Association Atherosclerosis, Hypertension, and Obesity in Youth Committee, Council of Cardiovascular Disease in the Young, with the Council on Cardiovascular Nursing. Circulation 2007; 115:1948–67

173. Byington RP, Evans GW, Espeland MA, Applegate WB, Hunninghake DB, Probstfield J, et al. Effects of lovastatin and warfarin on early carotid atherosclerosis: sex-specific analysis: Asymptomatic Carotid Atherosclerosis Progression Study (ACAPS) Research Group. Circulation 1999; 100:e14–7
174. de Groot E, Jukema JW, van Boven AJ, Reiber JH, Zwinderman AH, Lie KI, Ackerstaff RA, Bruschke AV. Effect of pravastatin on progression and regression of coronary atherosclerosis and vessel wall changes in carotid and femoral arteries: a report from the Regression Growth Evaluation Statin Study. Am J Cardiol 1995; 76:40C–6
175. Crouse JR, 3rd. Pravastatin, lipids and atherosclerosis in the carotid arteries (PLAC II). Am J Cardiol 1995; 75:455–9
176. Salonen R, Nyyssonen K, Porkkala E, Rummukainen J, Belder R, Park JS, Salonen JT. Kuopio Atherosclerosis Prevention Study (KAPS). A population-based primary preventive trial of the effect of LDL lowering on atherosclerotic progression in carotid and femoral arteries. Circulation 1995; 92:1758–64
177. Hodis HN, Mack WJ, LaBree L, Selzer RH, Liu C, Liu C, Alaupovic P, Kwong-Fu H, Azen SP. Reduction in carotid arterial wall thickness using lovastatin and dietary therapy: a randomized controlled clinical trial. Ann Intern Med 1996; 124:548–56
178. Mercuri M, Bond MG, Sirtori CR, Veglia F, Crepaldi G, Feruglio FS, Descovich G, Ricci G, Rubba P, Mancini M, et al. Pravastatin reduces carotid intima-media thickness progression in an asymptomatic hypercholeste rolemic mediterranean population: the Carotid Atherosclerosis Italian Ultrasound Study. Am J Med 1996; 101:627–34
179. MacMahon S, Sharpe N, Gamble G, Hart H, Scott J, Simes J, White H. Effects of lowering average of below-average cholesterol levels on the progression of carotid atherosclerosis: results of the LIPID Atherosclerosis Substudy. LIPID Trial Research Group. Circulation 1998; 97:1784–90
180. Hedblad B, Wikstrand J, Janzon L, Wedel H, Berglund G. Low-dose metoprolol CR/XL and fluvastatin slow progression of carotid intimamedia thickness: main results from the Beta-Blocker Cholesterol-Lowering Asymptomatic Plaque Study (BCAPS). Circulation 2001; 103:1721–6
181. Taylor AJ, Kent SM, Flaherty PJ, Coyle LC, Markwood TT, Vernalis MN. ARBITER: Arterial Biology for the Investigation of the Treatment Effects of Reducing Cholesterol: a randomized trial comparing the effects of atorvastatin and pravastatin on carotid intima medial thickness. Circulation 2002; 106:2055–60
182. Sawayama Y, Shimizu C, Maeda N, Tatsukawa M, Kinukawa N, Koyanagi S, Kashiwagi S, Hayashi J. Effects of probucol and pravastatin on common carotid atherosclerosis in patients with asymptomatic hypercholesterolemia. Fukuoka Atherosclerosis Trial (FAST). J Am Coll Cardiol 2002 Feb 20; 39(4):610–6
183. Smilde TJ, van Wissen S, Wollersheim H, Trip MD, Kastelein JJ, Stalenhoef AF. Effect of aggressive versus conventional lipid lowering on atherosclerosis progression in familial hypercholesterolaemia (ASAP): a prospective, randomised, double-blind trial. Lancet 2001; 357:577–81
184. van Wissen S, Smilde TJ, Trip MD, Stalenhoef AF, Kastelein JJ. Long-term safety and efficacy of high-dose atorvastatin treatment in patients with familial hypercholesterolemia. Am J Cardiol 2005; 95:264–6
185. Crouse JR, 3rd, Raichlen JS, Riley WA, Evans GW, Palmer MK, O'Leary DH, Grobbee DE, Bots ML. Effect of rosuvastatin on progression of carotid intima-media thickness in low-risk individuals with subclinical atherosclerosis: the METEOR Trial. JAMA 297:1344–53
186. Mack WJ, Selzer RH, Hodis HN, Erickson JK, Liu CR, Liu CH, Crawford DW, Blankenhorn DH. One-year reduction and longitudinal analysis of carotid intima-media thickness associated with colestipol/niacin therapy. Stroke 1993; 24:1779–83
187. Blankenhorn DH, Selzer RH, Crawford DW, Barth JD, Liu CR, Liu CH, Mack WJ, Alaupovic P. Beneficial effects of colestipol-niacin therapy on the common carotid artery. Two- and four-year reduction of intima-media thickness measured by ultrasound. Circulation 1993; 88:20–8
188. Taylor AJ, Sullenberger LE, Lee HJ, Lee JK, Grace KA. Arterial Biology for the Investigation of the Treatment Effects of Reducing Cholesterol (ARBITER) 2: a double-blind, placebo-controlled study of extended-release niacin on atherosclerosis progression in secondary prevention patients treated with statins. Circulation 2004; 110:3512–7
189. Lewis GF, Rader DJ. New insights into the regulation of HDL metabolism and reverse cholesterol transport. Circ Res 2005; 96:1221–32
190. Bots ML, Visseren FL, Evans GW, Riley WA, Revkin JH, Tegeler CH, Shear CL, Duggan WT, Vicari RM, Grobbee DE, Kastelein JJ; RADIANCE 2 Investigators. Torcetrapib and carotid intima-media thickness in mixed dyslipidaemia (RADIANCE 2 study): a randomised, double-blind trial. Lancet 2007 Jul 14; 370(9582):153–60

22 Carotid Intima-Media Thickness: Clinical Implementation in Individual Cardiovascular Risk Assessment

Ward A. Riley

CONTENTS

ABSTRACT

The approach briefly outlined in this chapter for obtaining accurate measurements of carotid intima-media thickness (CIMT) measurements is proposed for consideration in the practice of the SHAPE atherosclerosis-screening program. While this protocol is more detailed than some would prefer from a time and cost perspective, it provides a more valid and reliable estimate of risk in an individual subject than other protocols that focus on fewer anatomical segments, fewer ultrasonic interrogation angles, and on only the far (deeper) walls. Cost-effective analyses should be performed to determine if this protocol can be further condensed while maintaining the accuracy of the risk estimate for an individual patient. In summary, images of both near and far wall segments are optimized in sequence for measurement at each interrogation angle and anatomical site. A minimum of five complete cardiac cycles of images are stored for later offline measurement for each wall-angle-site combination. An examination with complete data will include a total of 36 carotid wall image sequences for measurement. As the sonographer reaches a high skill level, total scan time should not exceed 30 min. Before proceeding with the detailed examination of the carotid arteries, an initial rapid scan of the defined carotid segments is performed including a transverse scan of the

From: *Asymptomatic Atherosclerosis: Pathophysiology, Detection and Treatment*
Edited by: M. Naghavi (ed.), DOI 10.1007/978-1-60327-179-0_22

entire 30 mm length. If one or more focal plaques greater than about 1.3–1.5 mm in thickness are observed, or consistent CIMT thickening greater than 1.2 mm is observed, the individual will have a mean CIMT exceeding the 95th percentile, corresponding to the very high-risk category of the SHAPE guideline. In such an individual, a detailed CIMT assessment may not required. A simple algorithm derived from results of the Atherosclerosis Risk in Communities study is used to compute an estimate of absolute cardiovascular risk (percent chance of experiencing a heart attack or stroke within 10 years) from the composite mean CIMT calculation.

Key words: Carotid Intima-Media Thickness – CIMT; Carotid Atherosclerosis; Carotid Plaque; Carotid Ultrasound

KEY POINTS

- A thorough analysis of carotid near and far wall images are needed to obtain an accurate CIMT measurement.
- An experienced sonographer is needed to conduct the detailed measurements within 30 min.
- A cost-effective analysis of the protocol proposed in this chapter versus other protocols is needed to define the most optimized method for clinical practice of CIMT screening as outlined in the SHAPE guideline.

INTRODUCTION

This chapter outlines the key elements of a standard approach for obtaining estimates of absolute cardiovascular risk (percent chance of experiencing a heart attack or stroke within 10 years) in adult individuals from measurements of carotid intima-media thickness (CIMT). The method is proposed for consideration as an important element in the overall SHAPE atherosclerosis-screening program. More detailed publications provide additional insight into the rationale and methodology of this approach and contain important references on the topic [1, 2].

ULTRASONIC IMAGING EQUIPMENT

A routinely serviced, late-model, high-frequency (7.0–10 MHz) digital ultrasound imaging system is required with axial resolution of the order of 0.20–0.30 mm, lateral resolution at the measurement depth of approximately 1.0 mm, and a comparable azimuthal (slice thickness) resolution of the order of 1.0 mm. The routine performance of scans of widely available tissue equivalent ultrasound phantoms provides a quantitative basis for demonstrating these resolution requirements. The use of ultrasound systems with poorer resolution characteristics can result in less accurate measurements of CIMT and consequently less accurate estimates of absolute cardiovascular risk.

CAROTID SCANNING PROTOCOL

The right and left carotid systems including 10 mm segments of the common carotid artery, the carotid bulb (or bifurcation region), and the internal carotid artery are scanned longitudinally from three angles of interrogation using the Meijer Arc as a guide for transducer placement [2]. The three interrogation angles on each side are separated by an interval of approximately 50° to sample the circumferential variation of CIMT within each arterial segment. These segments are referenced to the tip of the flow divider separating the external and internal carotid arteries [1, 2]. The maximum imaging depth is set at approximately 40 mm and consistently maintained when imaging all segments to ensure a constant image calibration factor for all measurements.

Images of both near and far wall segments are optimized in sequence for measurement at each interrogation angle and anatomical site. A minimum of five complete cardiac cycles of images is stored for later offline measurement for each wall-angle-site combination. An EKG signal is displayed on the stored images for reference during the CIMT measurement process.

An examination with complete data will include a total of 36 carotid wall image sequences for measurement. In general, data will be missing from some segments due to anatomical constraints or other patient-specific factors. An adequate study should include data from at least 25 of the 36 segments.

INITIAL OVERVIEW SCAN

Before proceeding with the detailed examination of the carotid arteries described, "Carotid Scanning Protocol," an initial rapid scan of the defined carotid segments is performed including a transverse scan of the entire 30 mm length. If one or more focal plaques greater than about 1.3–1.5 mm in thickness are observed, or consistent CIMT thickening greater than 1.2 mm is observed, the individual will have a mean CIMT exceeding the 95th percentile in the general population and a high corresponding cardiovascular risk exceeding 20% per 10 years. Since a high-risk classification has already been determined, a detailed CIMT assessment is not required in this individual. In all other subjects, the detailed scan defined above should be performed.

MEASUREMENT OF CIMT

The best quality image frame in each of the up to 36 stored image sequences of the carotid segments are measured at minimum diastole using a suitable software program. After the mean CIMT within each segment is measured, the composite mean of all of the segments measured is computed. This composite or global mean CIMT is used to obtain an estimate of absolute cardiovascular risk and contains information on the circumferential variation of CIMT as well as its variation with anatomical site.

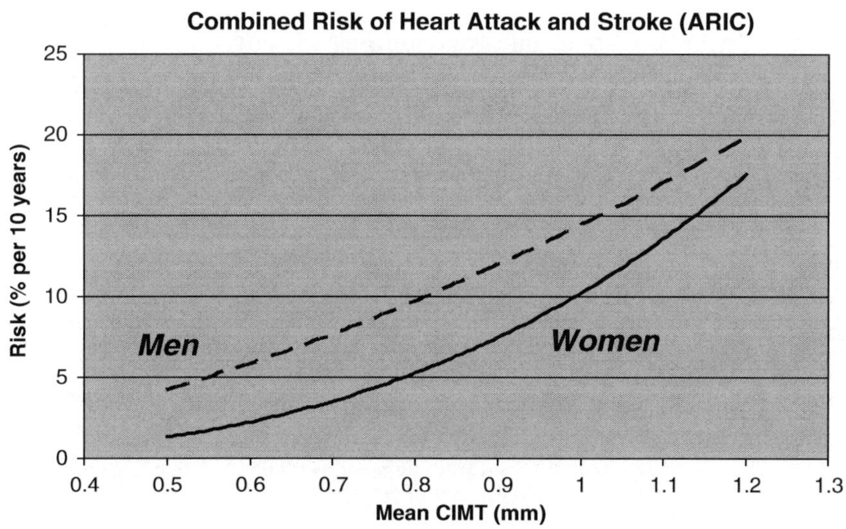

CALCULATION OF ABSOLUTE CARDIOVASCULAR RISK

A simple algorithm derived from results of the Atherosclerosis Risk in Communities (ARIC) Study is used to compute an estimate of absolute cardiovascular risk (percent chance of experiencing a heart attack or stroke within 10 years) from the composite mean CIMT calculation. These data are derived from the long-term follow-up of an initial population sample of 16,000 men and women between 45 and 65 years of age [3, 4]. This risk estimate should be accurate to within approximately ±2.5% per 10 years if the accuracy and reliability of the CIMT measurement is of the order of 0.10 mm. A specific CIMT-based risk cutpoint can be selected to optimize the cost effectiveness of the atherosclerosis-screening program.

CERTIFICATION OF SONOGRAPHERS AND READERS

Completion of a standardized CIMT scanning and reading certification program is required to demonstrate the ability of a clinical laboratory to meet this high level of measurement quality and consistency. Experienced CIMT investigators from core medical research laboratories in the United States and Europe can be contacted for information on current training and certification programs [1, 2]. Investigators at these sites have played major roles in the conduct of many major CIMT research studies over the last two decades including ARIC, Rotterdam, ACAPS, PREVENT, OPAL, METEOR, APPLE, RADIANCE 1, and RADIANCE 2.

DURATION OF EXAMINATION AND MEASUREMENT PROCESS

As the sonographer reaches a high skill level, total scan time should not exceed 30 min. While total reading time may approach 60 min in difficult subjects, average reading time should approach 30–45 min as a high level of skill is reached.

CONCLUSION

The approach outlined here for obtaining absolute estimates of cardiovascular risk from CIMT measurements is proposed for consideration in the SHAPE atherosclerosis-screening program. While this protocol is more detailed than some would prefer from a time and cost perspective, it provides a more valid and reliable estimate of risk in an individual subject than protocols that focus on fewer anatomical segments, fewer ultrasonic interrogation angles, and on only the far (deeper) walls. Cost-effective analyses should be performed to determine if this protocol can be further condensed while maintaining the accuracy of the risk estimate for an individual patient.

REFERENCES

1. Riley WA. Cardiovascular risk assessment in individual patients from carotid intimal-medial thickness measurements. Curr Atheroscler Reports 2004;6:225–231.
2. Bots ML, Evans GW, Riley WA, Grobbee DE. Carotid intimal-medial thickness measurements in intervention studies: design options, progression rates, and sample size considerations: a point of view. Stroke 2003;34:2985–2994.
3. Chambless LE, Heiss G, Folsom AR, et al. Association of coronary heart disease incidence with carotid arterial wall thickness and major risk factors: the atherosclerosis risk in communities (ARIC) study, 1987–1993. Am J Epidemiol 1997;146:483–494.
4. Chambless LE, Folsom AR, Clegg LX, et al. Carotid wall thickness is predictive of incident clinical stroke: the atherosclerosis risk in communities (ARIC) study. Am J Epidemiol 2000;151:478–487.

23 Computed Tomographic Angiography

Detection, Treatment, and Monitoring of Asymptomatic Individuals Susceptible to Atherosclerosis and Vulnerable to Cardiovascular Events

Harvey S. Hecht

CONTENTS

ABSTRACT

Sixty four slice coronary computed tomographic angiography (CTA), while traditionally employed as a substitute for stress testing in symptomatic patients, has increasing application in the "asymptomatic" population, and is additive to coronary artery calcium scanning.

1. Patients with atypical symptoms are often misclassified as "symptomatic"; CTA provides accurate information regarding obstruction, as well as risk stratification based on calcified and non-calcified plaque.
2. Using tomographic intravascular analysis (TIVA), CTA provides non-calcified and calcified plaque characterization, similar to intravascular ultrasound. High risk plaques, including thin cap fibroatheromas and plaque rupture, may be identified, as well as totally non-calcified plaque that may or may not result in measurable narrowing.
3. In the truly asymptomatic population, CTA is appropriate in younger patients with a family history of premature coronary disease, in whom coronary calcium screening is not even recommended and whose risk may be established by demonstration of non-calcified plaque. Stress testing is often used for risk stratification in patients with multiple risk factors; CTA is a more appropriate tool and should replace stress testing in this capacity.
4. Totally non-calcified plaque resulting in any measurable narrowing justifies aggressive medical treatment.
5. Non-calcified plaque quantitation and reduction in radiation and contrast will be required for CTA to replace coronary calcium screening.

From: *Asymptomatic Atherosclerosis: Pathophysiology, Detection and Treatment*
Edited by: M. Naghavi (ed.), DOI 10.1007/978-1-60327-179-0_23

Key words: Asymptomatic and symptomatic population; Calcified and non-calcified plaque; Computed tomographic angiography; Coronary artery disease; Plaque characterization, SHAPE guidelines

TOPIC PEARLS

- Coronary CTA has IVUS plaque characterization capability and may identify vulnerable plaques.
- Screening with lower dose coronary CTA is appropriate for younger patients with a family history of premature coronary disease.
- Coronary CTA is always preferable to stress testing for risk stratification in the asymptomatic population.

Coronary computed tomographic angiography (CTA) offers the practicing physician a unique combination of data heretofore available only through invasive coronary angiography and intravascular ultrasound [1, 2]. Although it has been used primarily as an alternative to stress testing for the evaluation of symptomatic patients, there is an increasing appreciation of its value in areas related to plaque characterization and risk assessment, irrespective of symptoms.

CLINICAL CONCEPTS

Unlike coronary artery calcium scanning, which is well suited for screening large segments of the asymptomatic population [3, 4], CTA, by virtue of its higher radiation exposure, intravenous contrast, and cost, must be used more selectively.

"Symptomatic" and "Asymptomatic" Patients: Clinical Scenario

A 44 year old male presented himself to his internist with complaints of mild left sided chest discomfort of 3 months duration. The symptom was mild in intensity and present almost continually; it was occasionally worsened by effort. There was no history of hypertension, diabetes or tobacco use, and he exercised regularly and followed a balanced diet. The patient's father died 2 days after an acute myocardial infarction at age 56, and any chest discomfort, even non-exercise related, provoked extreme anxiety. Physical examination was entirely benign. Laboratory values were pertinent for a fasting blood sugar of 86 mg/dl, total cholesterol 176 mg/dl, LDL 105 mg/dl, HDL 62 mg/dl and triglycerides 45 mg/dl.

Risk assessment was performed by Framingham Risk Score recommendations [5]; the absence of risk factors did not even qualify him for calculation of a Framingham Risk Score. His physician ordered a treadmill stress test for evaluation of his atypical symptoms; it was entirely normal. For more extensive risk assessment, he underwent a coronary artery calcium scan; once again, the results were normal, without evidence for coronary or aortic calcified plaque, and the patient was reassured of his benign cardiovascular prognosis. However, the atypical symptoms persisted, and the patient was referred to a cardiologist, who ordered a coronary CTA. The results are shown in Fig. 1. There was a 25–50% stenosis in the proximal left anterior descending coronary artery and a large amount of non-calcified plaque responsible for the narrowing. Further analysis of the CTA through tomographic intravascular analysis (TIVA) revealed a very low density lipid component with negative Hounsfield units (HU), consistent with a thin cap fibroatheroma (TCFA).

The cardiologist concluded that while the narrowing was not significant enough to produce ischemic symptoms, the presence of sufficient non-calcified plaque to produce measurable stenosis, as well as a TCFA, placed the patient in a high risk coronary disease equivalent category. Accordingly, the patient was started on a statin for LDL reduction to <70 mg/dl [6], and aspirin.

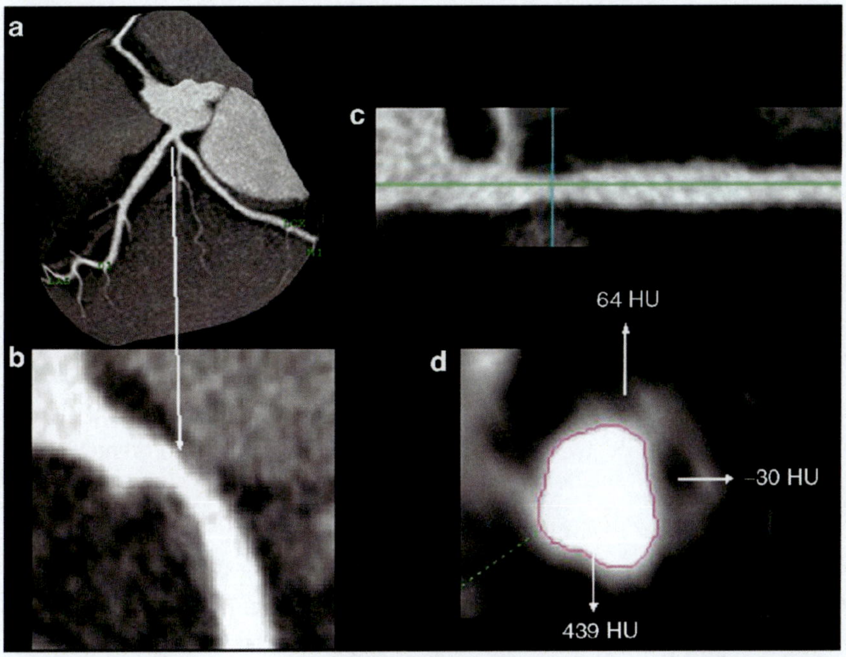

Fig. 1. A 44 year old male underwent CTA for reasons described in the text. CTA global coronary representation (**a**) revealed ostial LAD narrowing of 25–50% (arrow) on the curved MPR (**b**). TIVA of the straightened MPR (**c**) demonstrated contrast (439 HU), non-calcified plaque (84 HU) and a lipid core (−30 HU) consistent with a TCFA. Abbreviations: *CTA* Computed tomographic angiography, *HU* Hounsfield units, *LAD* Left anterior descending, *MPR* Multiplanar reconstruction, *TCFA* Thin cap fibroatheroma, *TIVA* Tomographic intravascular analysis.

Discussion: While the focus of this textbook is on subclinical atherosclerosis in the asymptomatic population, an undetermined, but undoubtedly substantial proportion of "symptomatic" patients could more correctly be classified as "asymptomatic" if more stringent criteria were applied. The clinical scenario described above was so atypical of ischemic heart disease that, even though the patient was "symptomatic", the term is more a misnomer than a truly accurate description. Patients with any kind of chest discomfort or dyspnea or fatigue are labeled "symptomatic" and undergo stress testing or invasive angiography to rule out a cardiac etiology, despite a low pretest likelihood of obstructive coronary disease. Evaluation of these patients must, by medical, psychological or legal necessity, answer the question raised by these "symptoms". However, the more important question is the evaluation of risk determined by subclinical rather than obstructive disease. CTA is uniquely suited to answer all of these issues. Thus, the patient warranted aggressive medical treatment by secondary prevention criteria on the basis of extensive non-obstructive non-calcified plaque with a high risk TCFA.

Obstructive Disease: Clinical Scenario

A 66 year old asymptomatic female with multiple risk factors was evaluated by her cardiologist. She had a history of well controlled hypertension, obesity, ongoing cigarette use, and abnormal lipids treated with a statin. She underwent treadmill stress testing as part of her risk evaluation; 1 mm ST segment depression was noted and was deemed to be an equivocal finding. CTA was then performed

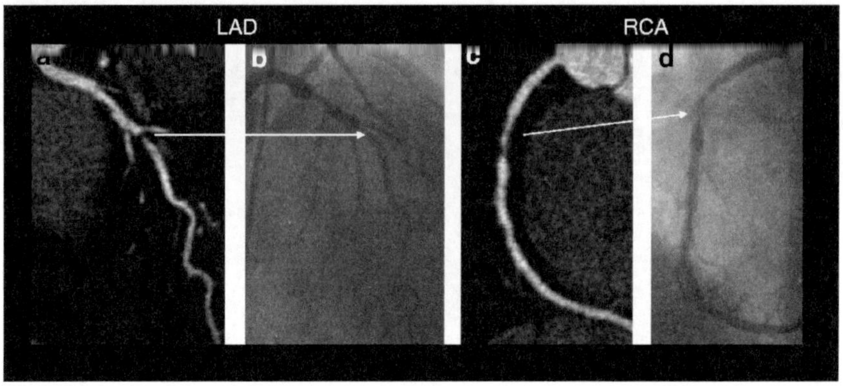

Fig. 2. A 66 year old female underwent CTA after equivocal stress testing. Curved MPR of the LAD and RCA (**a**, **c**) revealed subtotal occlusions, confirmed by invasive coronary angiography (**b**, **d**) Abbreviations: *CTA* Computed tomographic angiography, *LAD* Left anterior descending, *MPR* Multiplanar reconstruction, *RCA* Right coronary artery.

(Fig. 2) and demonstrated subtotal occlusions of both the left anterior descending and right coronary arteries, secondary to totally non-calcified plaque. Invasive angiography confirmed the findings and she underwent percutaneous intervention on both vessels.

Discussion: The definition of the coronary anatomy by CTA, is sufficient to function as a substitute for stress testing and invasive coronary angiography, as the first test in almost all clinical scenarios. The sensitivity, specificity and negative predictive accuracy compared to invasive coronary angiography are 90, 95 and 98% respectively [1]. However, stress testing yields no information regarding subclinical atherosclerosis; 56% of patients with normal myocardial perfusion tests had coronary calcium scores exceeding 100, placing them in a high risk category despite the normal nuclear test [7]. In the clinical scenario, the patient was asymptomatic and underwent CTA after a stress test performed for risk assessment yielded equivocal findings. The presence of two subtotally obstructed vessels by totally non-calcified plaque was quite surprising and was appropriately followed by percutaneous intervention. Coronary calcium scoring alone would have missed the diagnosis, but this still does not justify CTA screening in the population covered by the SHAPE guidelines [3], as discussed below.

The discovery of significant obstructive disease in truly asymptomatic or clearly atypically symptomatic patients identifies them as high risk and deserving of the most aggressive medical therapy. Percutaneous or surgical intervention in this group has no evidence base, but is frequently implemented if the disease is felt to be life threatening, as demonstrated in the clinical scenario.

Calcified and Non-calcified Plaque

Coronary artery calcium, as discussed in an earlier chapter, is the most powerful prognosticator of cardiovascular events [3], and there are extensive data documenting the very benign prognosis of patients with 0 coronary calcium scores [8–10]. While there are no data regarding the prognostic importance of exclusively non-calcified plaque, the following pertinent observations have been made:

1. Significant obstructive disease has been found in 1% of asymptomatic patients (11] and in 7% of symptomatic patients [12) with 0 coronary calcium scores.

2. Exclusively non-calcified significant obstructive disease was noted in 5% of patients with myocardial infarction or unstable angina, in both older (57 ± 11 years) [13] and younger (41 ± 11 years) populations [14].
3. With 500,000 patients presenting annually with a myocardial infarction as the first symptom of coronary disease [15], 25,000 would presumably escape identification by coronary artery calcium screening.

Clinical Applications

These observations lead to the following clinical questions:

1. Can those at-risk patients who would escape detection by coronary artery calcium screening, i.e., those with totally non-calcified plaque who will develop totally non-calcified symptomatic obstructive disease, be identified?

Plaque Characterization: CTA is well suited for characterization of both non-calcified and calcified plaque. CTA plaque evaluation is dependent on density measurements, using X-ray attenuation defined by HU. Lipid is defined as tissue with an HU range of 0 to –150, non-calcified plaque from 0 to 130 with values increasing as the content increases from fat to fibrous tissue, and calcified plaque as >130 HU. Contrast ranges in density, depending on the degree of dilution and the size of the patient; typically, it ranges from 250 to 500 HU in proximal vessels. The CTA in Fig. 3, in a symptomatic patient with significant obstructive disease in the left main and circumflex coronary arteries, demonstrates complex obstructive plaque with calcified and non-calcified components. Intravascular ultrasound of the same areas confirms the TIVA findings, and virtual histology using radiofrequency backscatter analysis of the IVUS further supports the CTA plaque characterization. The minimum luminal area measurements which are readily available from TIVA, were also confirmed by the intravascular ultrasound. The plaque characterization [16–23] and area measurements [24, 25] confer on CT the intravascular ultrasound properties that greatly enhance its diagnostic value.

The absolute HU criteria are truly accurate only in vitro; in the real world of in vivo imaging, apparent tissue density is profoundly affected by the "company it keeps" by two mechanisms.

Volume Averaging: Volume averaging, or the partial volume effect, will increase the HU of low density tissue that is adjacent to denser material (e.g., contrast, calcified plaque) by sharing voxels with the higher density tissue, with a resultant increase in the average HU of the sample. Thus, lipid measuring –50 HU in vitro, may measure 100 HU next to a 500 HU calcified plaque, and will no longer be classified as lipid. In addition, volume averaging produces a symmetrical "halo" surrounding the luminal contrast. It varies in thickness from patient to patient depending on technical factors, and is a normal finding. When the halo is asymmetrical, the asymmetrical component represents non-calcified plaque.

Shadowing: At the other extreme, "shadowing", manifested by extremely dense material blocking photons from reaching adjacent tissue, may transform contrast with an in vitro HU of 350 to the negative density of lipid (0 to –150), if it is adjacent to a densely calcified plaque (HU>1000), and would lead to an erroneous classification. There is currently no acceptable solution; absolute HU cannot be used for plaque characterization across the wide variety of complex plaque typically encountered in the average diseased vessel. Algorithms employing HU gradients between adjacent structures are under evaluation and may provide solutions, as dual source imaging advances.

Despite these limitations, CTA offers the best noninvasive hope for coronary plaque analysis; magnetic resonance angiography, while excellent for carotid and aortic plaque evaluation, is inadequate for the rapidly moving coronary circulation. Substantial IVUS correlated data supports the ability of CTA to reasonably assess plaque eccentricity, remodeling, volume, calcified and non-calcified plaque in both stable and unstable patients [16–23, 26].

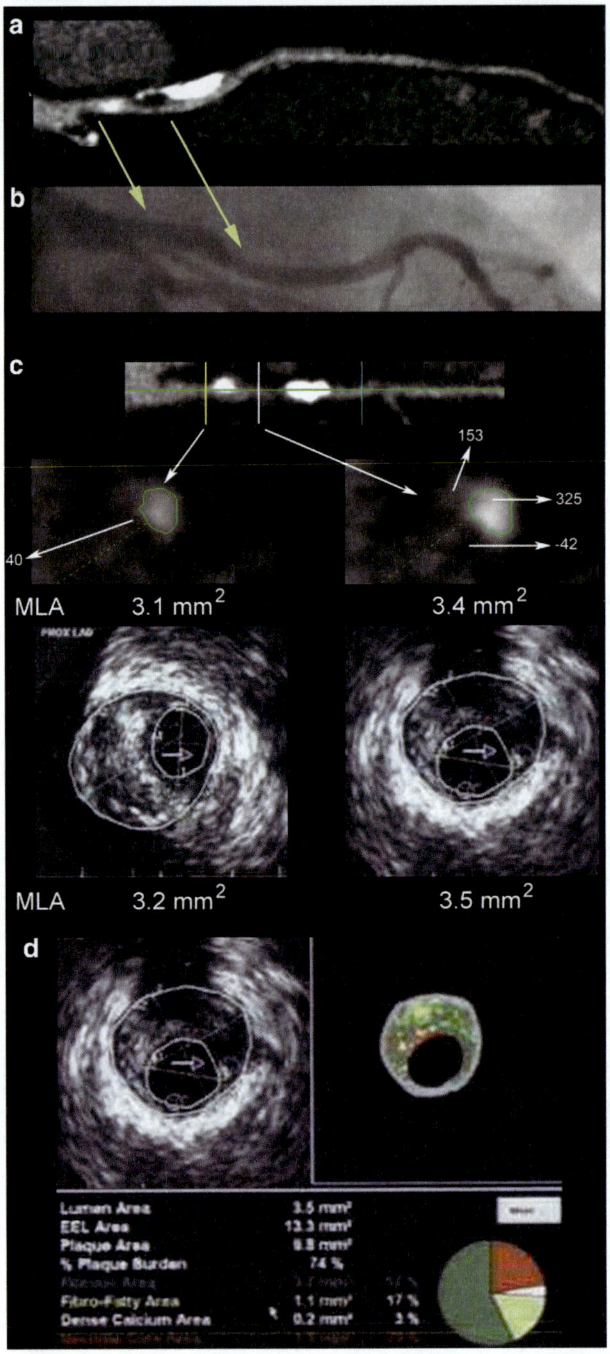

Fig. 3. An asymptomatic 71 year old male with peripheral vascular disease underwent CTA which revealed significant ostial and proximal LAD disease (arrows). The ostial lesion was less impressive on CA (**b**). TIVA of the straightened MPR (**c**) revealed significant equally reduced MLA at both sites (upper left and right), confirmed by IVUS (lower left and right). PCI of both lesions was performed in the proximal LAD (upper left), a moderate sized low density (−42 HU) lipid laden plaque was noted, consistent with a TCFA. Virtual histology of the proximal LAD lesion (**d**) revealed a large necrotic core (23% of total plaque volume), confirming the presence of a TCFA. Reproduced from Hecht, 2008 with permission from Wiley InterScience [2].Abbreviations: *CA* Conventional angiography, *CTA* Computed tomographic angiography, *HU* Hounsfield units, *LAD* Left anterior descending, *MLA* Minimum luminal area, *MPR* Multiplanar reconstruction, *TCFA* Thin cap fibroatheroma, *TIVA* Tomographic intravascular analysis.

HIGH RISK PLAQUES

a. Thin cap fibroatheroma: The noninvasive identification of high risk TCFA [27, 28] would provide a powerful tool for risk reduction, particularly if ongoing studies confirm a convincing association of future clinical events with TCFA's identified by IVUS virtual histology analysis at the time of the initial presentation with an acute coronary syndrome. TCFA may be diagnosed by CTA with a reasonable degree of certainty when a lipid core can be identified despite the above limitations. While there have been no studies correlating CTA defined TCFA with histology, the classic TCFA characteristics may be observed on TIVA cross sectional evaluation (Fig. 1): (1) focal (adjacent to non-TCFA); (2) lipid core ≥10%: (3) direct contact with the lumen; (4) percent area obstruction ≥40%. In a more complex case (Fig. 4), in a patient with significant obstructive disease, tandem stenoses were noted in the left anterior descending coronary artery. TIVA revealed complex plaque with a low density lipid core in the second plaque consistent with a TCFA. Intravascular ultrasound with virtual histology confirmed the findings. The minimum luminal area measurements were also confirmed by the intravascular ultrasound.

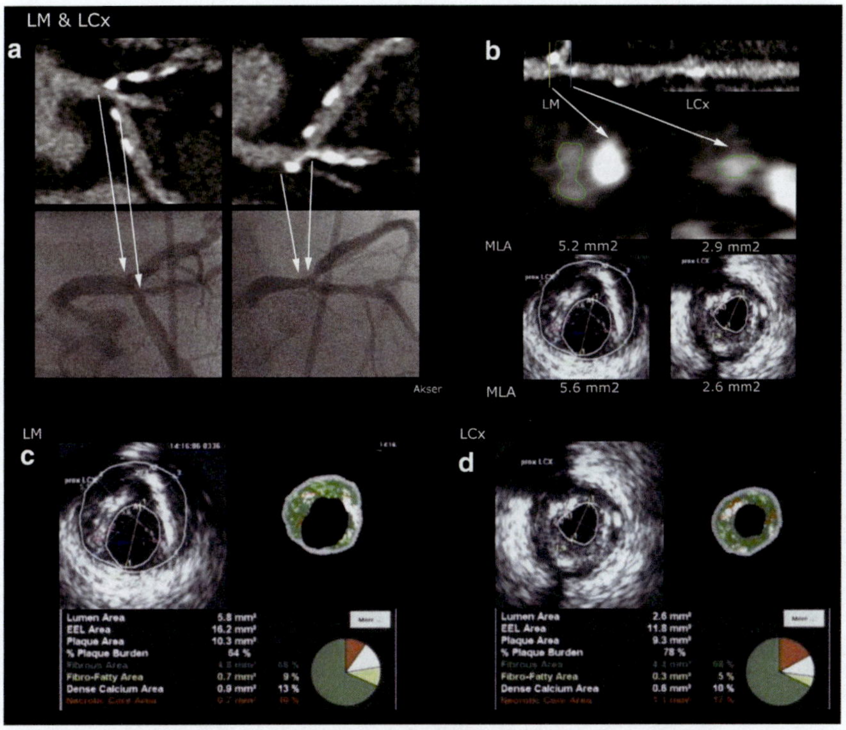

Fig. 4. An asymptomatic 71 year old male with peripheral vascular disease underwent CTA which revealed significant ostial and proximal LAD disease (arrows). The ostial lesion was less impressive on CA (**b**). TIVA of the straightened MPR (**c**) revealed significant equally reduced MLA at both sites (upper left and right), confirmed by IVUS (lower left and right). PCI of both lesions was performed in the proximal LAD (upper left), a moderate sized low density (−42 HU) lipid laden plaque was noted, consistent with a TCFA. Virtual histology of the proximal LAD lesion (**d**) revealed a large necrotic core (23% of total plaque volume), confirming the presence of a TCFA. Reproduced from Hecht, 2008 with permission from Wiley InterScience [2]. Abbreviations: *CA* Conventional angiography, *CTA* Computed tomographic angiography, *HU* Hounsfield units, *LAD* Left anterior descending, *MLA*, Minimum luminal area, *MPR* Multiplanar reconstruction, *TCFA* Thin cap fibroatheroma, *TIVA* Tomographic intravascular analysis.

The impact on PCI is hypothetical at this point. If early PCI for non-obstructive TCFA containing lesions proves beneficial, CTA may provide an ideal noninvasive identification of the high risk patient; i.e., the patient with either single or multiple proximal TCFA's.

b. Plaque rupture: A more readily identifiable high risk characteristic is plaque rupture (Fig. 5) which is associated with an increased risk of acute coronary events [29]. Data justifying PCI for non-obstructive lesions with these characteristics in the asymptomatic patient is still lacking, but the ability to identify them noninvasively provides a promising research avenue. Aggressive medical intervention is clearly appropriate for patients demonstrating high risk plaque characteristics.

2. Are there data to support treatment of patients with totally non-calcified plaque, and if so, at what volume of non-calcified plaque?

There are no data that justify the treatment of asymptomatic patients with totally non-calcified plaque, since their risk has not been clearly defined, and they have never been evaluated. Nonetheless, they are clearly associated with events [11–14], and treatment must be considered despite the absence of data. Presumably, high risk plaques, e.g., TCFA and ruptured plaque (Figs. 1, 4, and 5), are logical candidates for aggressive medical therapy as CAD equivalents. These are infrequently noted; the more common scenario is non-calcified plaque without particularly malignant characteristics which is present in varying amounts. Aggressive medical therapy for non-calcified plaque should be implemented if there is measurable obstructive disease, i.e., greater than luminal irregularities, since similar measures would be implemented if calcified plaque were responsible for the narrowing.

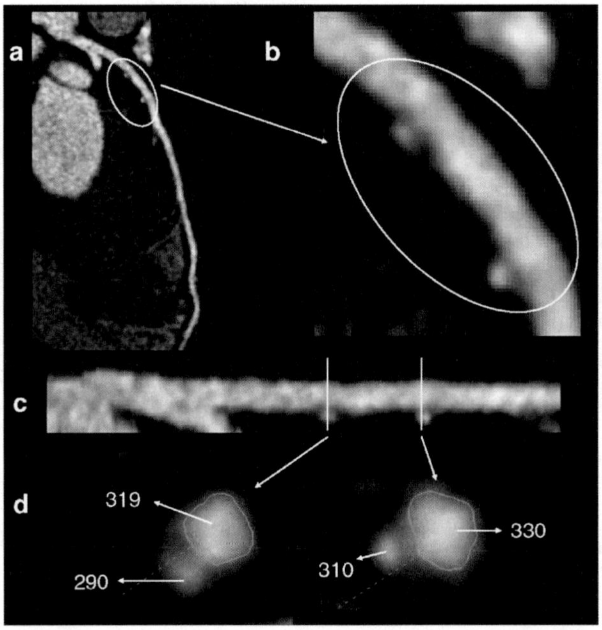

Fig. 5. An asymptomatic 33 year old male with a striking family history of premature coronary disease underwent CTA for risk evaluation. Curved MPR of the LAD revealed the absence of calcified plaque, and two extraluminal densities (**b**). TIVA of the straightened MPR (**c**) demonstrated HU of the densities to be similar to contrast (**d**), consistent with extravasation of contrast from ruptured noncalcified plaques. Abbreviations: *CTA* Computed tomographic angiography, *HU* Hounsfield units, *LAD* Left anterior descending, *MPR* Multiplanar reconstruction numbers = Hounsfield units, *TIVA* Tomographic intravascular analysis.

In the absence of measureable narrowing, reliance must be placed on extrapolation from coronary calcium evaluation. Even though non-calcified plaque presumably represents an earlier stage of atherosclerosis, there is no reason to assume it represents less of a threat than calcified plaque. There are currently no standardized quantitative analyses of non-calcified plaque similar to the Agataston score for calcified plaque, but attempts should be made to provide non-calcified volume data that can be equated to calcified plaque volume data, with therapeutic recommendations based on those measures.

3. Which patient subsets should be evaluated?

Coronary artery calcium screening by the SHAPE guidelines applies to men older than 45 and women older than 55, who are not in the very lowest risk category [3], and is supported by an ever increasing body of data. Until such time as CTA can be performed with a radiation exposure similar to calcium screening, the use of CTA for screening the SHAPE population cannot be justified. Nonetheless, there are two major categories of asymptomatic patients for whom CTA should be regularly employed.

CLINICAL SCENARIO

A 33 year old male sought evaluation because of his family history. His father died suddenly at age 39, presumably from a myocardial infarction, his 38 year old sister underwent stent placement and his 40 year old brother had coronary bypass surgery. The patient was entirely asymptomatic, exercised vigorously and followed a well balanced diet. There was no history of diabetes, hypertension or smoking. His lipid profile was as follows: total cholesterol 181 mg/dl, LDL 121 mg/dl, HDL 39 mg/dl, triglycerides 105 mg/dl. He was referred for a CTA (Fig. 5) which revealed total absence of calcified plaque; TIVA demonstrated two ruptured non-calcified plaques in the left anterior descending coronary artery, characterized by extraluminal densities with HU similar to contrast. There was no luminal narrowing. Aggressive medical therapy by secondary prevention standards was implemented, and the patient was started on a statin, niacin and aspirin.

1. Younger patients with a family history of premature coronary disease: Men younger than 45 and women younger than 55 are not included in the SHAPE screening guidelines. However, a family history of premature CAD, defined as a first degree relative with CAD prior to age 55 for men and 65 for women, is associated with markedly increased risk [30, 31]. The coronary calcium score in these patients may be 0 or trivial, and may be inadequate to truly define their risk. The use of CTA to supplement the coronary calcium score by evaluating the non-calcified plaque as described above offers an increased opportunity to implement appropriate aggressive treatment at an earlier stage. The patient in the clinical scenario would not have been screened by the SHAPE guidelines, and would have escaped detection by calcium screening even if he had been evaluated. CTA is an appropriate screening tool in this unique subset [32].

2. Patients undergoing stress testing: Stress testing for evaluation of atypical symptoms in otherwise asymptomatic patients is routinely performed, and stress testing for risk assessment of asymptomatic patients with multiple risk factors is a IIB indication by ACC/AHA Guidelines [33]. Since CTA is more accurate for the detection of obstructive disease, and provides the prognostic data from the coronary calcium component as well as the non-calcified plaque information, it should be substituted for stress testing for these clinical indications if coronary calcium screening has not already been performed. The patient described in Fig. 1 would have been better served by undergoing CTA as the first test.

Future Directions

Efforts are underway to dramatically reduce the radiation exposure from CTA by employing prospective gating techniques, in which radiation is only applied during a selected phase of the cardiac cycle rather than throughout the cycle with retrospective gating [34]. At the same time, the use of increasing numbers of detectors will decrease the amount of contrast. With these developments, and the ongoing work in the area of plaque characterization and quantitation of non-calcified plaque, CTA may supplant coronary artery calcium as a screening tool in larger segments of the population. Detection of high risk plaques may lead to percutaneous intervention in the asymptomatic patient, if further studies document the efficacy of such treatment.

REFERENCES

1. Hecht HS, Roubin G. Usefulness of computed tomographic angiography guided percutaneous coronary intervention. Am J Cardiol 2007;99:871–5.
2. Hecht HS. Applications of multislice coronary computed tomography to percutaneous coronary intervention: how did we ever do without it? Catheter Cardiovasc Interv 2008;71:490–503.
3. Naghavi M, Falk E, Hecht HS, et al. From vulnerable plaque to vulnerable patient – part III: executive Summary of the Screening for Heart Attack Prevention and Education (SHAPE) Task Force. Am J Cardiol 2006; 98:2H–15H.
4. Greenland P, Bonow RO, Brundage BH, et al. ACCF/AHA 2007 clinical expert consensus document on coronary artery calcium scoring by computed tomography in global cardiovascular risk assessment and in evaluation of patients with chest pain. J Am Coll Cardiol 2007; 49:378–402.
5. Executive summary of the third report of the National Cholesterol Education Program (NCEP) Expert panel on detection, evaluation, and treatment of high blood cholesterol in adults (Adult Treatment Panel III). JAMA 2001;285:2486–97.
6. Grundy SM, Cleeman JI, Merz CN, et al. Implications of recent clinical trials for the National Cholesterol Education Program Adult Treatment Panel III guidelines. Circulation 2004;110:227–39.
7. Berman DS, Wong, ND, Gransar H, et al. Relationship between stress-induced myocardial ischemia and atherosclerosis measured by coronary calcium tomography. J Am Coll Cardiol 2004;44:923–30.
8. Raggi P, Callister TQ, Cooil B, et al. Identification of patients at increased risk of first unheralded acute myocardial infarction by electron-beam computed tomography. Circulation 2000;101:850–5.
9. Arad Y, Goodman KJ, Roth M, et al. Coronary calcification, coronary risk factors, C-reactive protein and atherosclerotic cardiovascular disease events: the St. Francis Heart Study. J Am Coll Cardiol 2005;46:158–64.
10. Shaw LJ, Raggi P, Schisterman E, Berman DS, Callister TQ. Prognostic value of cardiac risk factors and coronary artery calcium screening for all-cause mortality. Radiology 2003;228:826–33.
11. Haberl R, Becker A, Leber A, et al. Correlation of coronary calcification and angiographically documented stenoses in patients with suspected coronary artery disease: results of 1,764 patients. J Am Coll Cardiol 2001;37:451–7.
12. Rubinshtein R, Tamar Gaspar T, Halon DA, et al. Prevalence and extent of obstructive coronary artery disease in patients with zero or low calcium score undergoing 64-Slice cardiac multidetector computed tomography for evaluation of a chest pain syndrome. Am J Cardiol 2007;99:472–5.
13. Schmeermund A, Baumgart D, Gorge G, et al. Coronary artery calcium in acute coronary syndromes. A comparative study of electron-beam computed tomography, coronary angiography, and intracoronary ultrasound in survivors of acute myocardial infarction and unstable angina. Circulation 1997;96:1461–9.
14. Pohle K, Ropers D, Maffert R, Geitner P, Moshage W, Regenfus M, Kusus M, Daniel WG, Achenbach S. Coronary calcifications in young patients with first, unheralded myocardial infarction: a risk factor matched analysis by electron beam tomography. Heart 2003;89:625–8.
15. Morbidity and mortality: 2002. Chart book on cardiovascular, lung, and blood diseases. National Institutes of Health, National Heart, Lung, and Blood Institute. Bethesda, MD.
16. Schroeder S, Kopp AF, Baumbach A, et al. Noninvasive detection and evaluation of atherosclerotic coronary plaques with multislice computed tomography. J Am Coll Cardiol 2001;37:1430–5.
17. Caussin C, Ohanessian A, Lancelin B, et al. Coronary plaque burden detected by multislice computed tomography after acute myocardial infarction with near-normal coronary arteries by angiography. Am J Cardiol 2003;92:849–52.
18. Caussin C, Ohanessian A, Ghostine S, et al. Characterization of vulnerable nonstenotic plaque with 16-slice computed tomography compared with intravascular ultrasound. Am J Cardiol 2004;94:99–104.
19. Leber AW, Knez A, Becker A, et al. Accuracy of multidetector spiral computed tomography in identifying and differentiating the composition of coronary atherosclerotic plaques: a comparative study with intracoronary ultrasound. J Am Coll Cardiol 2004;43:1241–7.

20. Achenbach S, Moselewski F, Ropers D, et al. Detection of calcified and noncalcified coronary atherosclerotic plaque by contrast enhanced, submillimeter multidetector spiral computed tomography: a segment-based comparison with intravascular ultrasound. Circulation 2004;109:14–7.
21. Hausleiter J, Meyer T, Hadamitzky M, et al. Prevalence of noncalcified coronary plaques by 64-slice computed tomography in patients with an intermediate risk for significant coronary artery disease. J Am Coll Cardiol 2006;48:312–8.
22. Hoffmann U, Moselewski F, Nieman K, et al. Noninvasive assessment of plaque morphology and composition in culprit and stable lesions in acute coronary syndrome and stable lesions in stable angina by multidetector computed tomography. J Am Coll Cardiol 2006;47:1655–62.
23. Leber AW, Becker A, Knez A, et al. Accuracy of 64-slice computed tomography to classify and quantify plaque volumes in the proximal coronary system. A comparative study using intravascular ultrasound. J Am Coll Cardiol 2006;47:672–7.
24. Moselewski F, Ropers D, Pohle K, et al. Measurement of cross-sectional coronary atherosclerotic plaque and vessel areas by 16-slice multi-detector CT: comparison to IVUS. Am J Cardiol 2004;94:1294–7.
25. Caussin C, Larchez C, Ghostine S, et al. Comparison of coronary minimal lumen area quantification by sixty-four-slice computed tomography versus intravascular ultrasound for intermediate stenosis. Am J Cardiol 2006;98:871–6.
26. Varnava AM, Mills PG, Davies MJ. Relationship between coronary artery remodeling and plaque vulnerability. Circulation 2002;105:939–43.
27. Kolodgie FD, Burke AP, Farb A, et al. The thin-fibrous cap fibroatheroma: a type of vulnerable plaque: the major precursor lesion to acute coronary syndromes. Curr Opin Cardiol 2001;16:285–92.
28. Virmani R, Kolodgie FD, Burke AP, Farb A, Schwartz SM. Lessons from sudden coronary death: a comprehensive morphological classification scheme for atherosclerotic lesions. Arterioscler Thromb Vasc Biol 2000;20:1262–75.
29. von Birgelen C, Klinkhart W, Mintz GS, et al. Plaque distribution and vascular remodeling of ruptured and nonruptured coronary plaques in the same vessel: an intravascular ultrasound study in vivo. J Am Coll Cardiol 2001;37:1864–70.
30. Sesso HD, Lee IM, Gaziano JM, et al. Maternal and paternal history of myocardial infarction and risk of cardiovascular disease in men and women. Circulation 2001;104:393–8.
31. Nasir K, Michos ED, Rumberger JAR, et al. Coronary artery calcification and family history of premature coronary heart disease: sibling history is more strongly associated than parental history. Circulation 2004;110:2150–6.
32. Poon M, Rubin GD, Achenbach SA, et al. Consensus update on the appropriate usage of cardiac computed tomographic angiography. J Inv Cardiol 2007:19:484–90.
33. Gibbons RJ, Balady GJ, Bricker JT, et al. ACC/AHA 2002 guideline update for exercise testing: summary article: a report of the American College of Cardiology/American Heart Association Task Force on Practice Guidelines (Committee to update the 1997 exercise testing guidelines). Circulation 2002;106:1883–92.
34. Paul JF, Abada HT. Strategies for reduction of radiation dose in cardiac multislice CT. Eur Radiol 2007;17:2028–37.

24 Role of Noninvasive Imaging using CT for Detection and Quantitation of Coronary Atherosclerosis

John A. Rumberger

Contents

Abstract

Cardiac CT began with electron beam CT in the early 1980s and continues now with multidetector CT in the twenty-first century. The major applications of noncontrast cardiac CT are currently for the quantification of coronary artery calcium – a reliable and repeatable means to estimate atherosclerotic plaque burden. The major applications of contrast-enhanced CT (CT angiography) is for more detailed estimation of total plaque burden by qualitatively defining "noncalcified" and complex plaque as well as ruling out obstructive coronary artery disease. Both of these applications are discussed, along with historical perspectives, in this review.

Key words: Atherosclerotic Plaque; Coronary Angiography; Coronary Artery; Coronary Calcification; Electron beam CT (EBT); Multidetector CT (MDCT)

From: *Asymptomatic Atherosclerosis: Pathophysiology, Detection and Treatment*
Edited by: M. Naghavi (ed.), DOI 10.1007/978-1-60327-179-0_24

KEY POINTS

- Coronary artery calcium (CAC) scanning using CT began in the 1990s
- CAC score or calcified area provides a direct, but underestimated measure of the coronary atherosclerotic burden in a given individual.
- A zero CAC score is consistent with a very low cardiac risk in the next decade regardless of age, gender, or race.
- A high CAC score (>400 or above the 90th percentile for age) is associated with a very high cardiac risk in the next decade of myocardial infarction or sudden cardiac death.
- CT noninvasive coronary angiography (CCTA) provides an ability to also assess the coronary lumen.
- Noncalcified or complex plaque found by CCTA provides a further measure of the true coronary atherosclerotic plaque burden.
- The clinical value of CCTA lies in the ability to rule out the presence of atherosclerosis or to rule out the presence of obstructive coronary disease in symptomatic patients.

HISTORICAL ASPECTS OF CT DEVELOPMENT AND CARDIAC CT

Sir Godfrey Hounsfield and colleagues, under the auspices of EMI (Electronic and Musical Industries, Ltd.), produced the first commercially viable X-ray computed tomography (CT) scanner in 1971, installed at the Atkinson-Morley Hospital, London. A number of clinical scans, mostly of the brain, were performed, and by 1973 [1, 2], the first EMI scanner was ready for delivery to the Mayo Clinic, Rochester, Mn., USA. A young electrical engineer, David King, a recent graduate of Sheffield College, was selected to perform the installation and lead the clinical development for EMI.

Working independent of Hounsfield, D. Boyd and M. Goiten introduced in 1971 the concept of the pure rotary scanner using a position sensitive Xenon detector, which was the subsequent standard of CT scanner design for the next 20 years (until Xenon was replaced by a scintillator-photodiode array, as is the case for all current CT scanners).

Imaging of stationary objects (e.g., the brain or during a breath-hold for the chest) using commercial CT scanners quickly became the clinical norm in the later 1970s and early 1980s – as image reconstruction times reduced from the original 5 days (1969) to less than a minute (1980).

During the late 1970s, it seemed clear that rotary mechanical gantry CT systems (at least as imagined at the time) would never become fast enough to allow diagnostic imaging of objects in constant motion – i.e., the heart. In 1979, an alternative approach to CT using a scanning electron beam (cine CT) was proposed [3] and later commercially introduced by D. Boyd and the Imatron Corporation in 1987 [4].

EBT (electron beam CT) was capable of very rapid cardiac imaging (50–100 ms per image), at up to eight levels nearly simultaneously, at frame rates of 17/s and ushered in the era of CT imaging for cardiac anatomy, cardiac perfusion, and cardiac function [5, 6]. Between 1985 and the latter 1990s, literally, hundreds of papers from researchers around the world were published validating the cardiac application of EBT. Cine-CT/Ultrafast CT (EBT) was used to define left and right ventricular volumes/function [6] to evaluate valvular pathology [6], to quantify myocardial perfusion [7], and to define the consequences of postinfarction cardiac remodeling [8].

Coronary artery calcification had long been recognized as a marker for coronary atherosclerosis, but defined for years only in pathologic specimens or qualitatively for clinical evaluation using fluoroscopy. David King, now Science Director for Imatron, was the first to develop the application of EBT to coronary imaging, developing "scoring" methods later published by Agatston and Janowitz [9] in 1990. Coronary imaging in contrast-enhanced EBT scans was later introduced by S. Achenbach [10] from Germany in 1995, performing the first noninvasive CT angiogram (CTA) of the coronary arteries which was extended to details of coronary segmental disease by Rumberger et al. [11] in 1998 at the Mayo Clinic, USA.

Despite the maturity of the EBT technology, the number of scanners worldwide, due to a number of issues including very expensive manufacturing requirements, remained at most at 100–125. At the same time traditional translate-rotate, mechanical, commercial CT scanners, even after the introduction of the "slip-ring" technology in the 1990s, were not able to provide anything more than blurred images of the heart, but their broad based worldwide availability, now in the tens of thousands, spurred more research dollars to develop a true cardiac scanner. The concept of "multiple" slices per rotation of the X-ray source sped up traditional imaging by acquiring variable numbers of thin tomographic segments and several manufacturers introduced 2-, 4-, and 8-slice CT scanners in the late 1990s and up to 2001. Despite these efforts, imaging of the entire heart took too long (up to a minute), rotational speeds were too slow (0.75–1.0 s), and spatial resolution was too coarse for coronary evaluation (1.0–2.0 mm). However, beginning in 2002 and up to the present day, a number of developmental events occurred in CT imaging physics. In particular the development of 16-, 32-, and 64+-MDCT (multidetector CT) shortened imaging of the heart to as little as 5 s – but importantly other improvements in image reconstruction time (essentially "real time"), faster rotational speeds (1/3 s or less), improved spatial resolution (0.4–0.6 mm), and the utilization of beta-blocker medications in patients fostered a rapid realization of cardiac and, in particular, coronary artery imaging by commercial, broadly available, CT scanners.

At the present time, EBT is no longer manufactured (although manuscripts using the installed base continue to appear in the literature) and MDCT has emerged as the broad-based method of choice for clinical CT cardiac imaging throughout the world. At the present time, further developments beyond 64-slice MDCT are continuing with dual-source (128-slice), 256-slice, and even 320-slice scanners, capable of imaging the entire heart volume in real time during a single cardiac cycle.

CORONARY ARTERY CALCIFICATION

EBT utilizes a rotating electron beam to acquire triggered, tomographic 50–100 ms X-ray images at 3 mm intervals in the space of a 30–40 s breath-hold. Current state of the art MDCT employs a rotating gantry with a special X-ray tube and 64 (or more) rows of detectors, with 165 ms images at 3 mm intervals. Cardiac scans using <64 slice MDCT remain suspect as to their accuracy to quantify coronary calcium (CAC), due to motion and scan timing issues.

CAC is virtually always associated with mural atheromatous plaque [12, 13]. A strong direct relationship has been established between CAC as measured by EBT, and both histologic [14] and in vivo intravascular ultrasound (IVUS) [15, 16] measures of combined calcified and noncalcified plaque. Thus, CAC provides a viable estimate of total coronary plaque burden [14–16].

The original coronary calcium score developed by David King (then an employee of the developer of EBT, Imatron, Inc) was published (as noted above) by Agatston and Janowitz [9] and is determined by calcified plaque area and calcium lesion density; it is generally referred to as the "Agatston calcium score". It requires a 3 mm CT slice thickness and a threshold for CAC of >130 Hounsfield units (CT density) involving ≥1 mm^2. It is important to note that the original application was defined using EBT and it is essential that current MDCT scanners be standardized to these parameters for any confident comparison to established scoring guidelines and for application of scoring based upon prior published works. MDCT scanners set to <3 mm slice thickness result in "over-sampling" and calculated scores higher than that from EBT, and scanners set to >3 mm slice thickness result in "under-sampling" and calculated scores less than that of the EBT published standards. Conventional categories for CAC scoring was originally put forward by Rumberger et al.

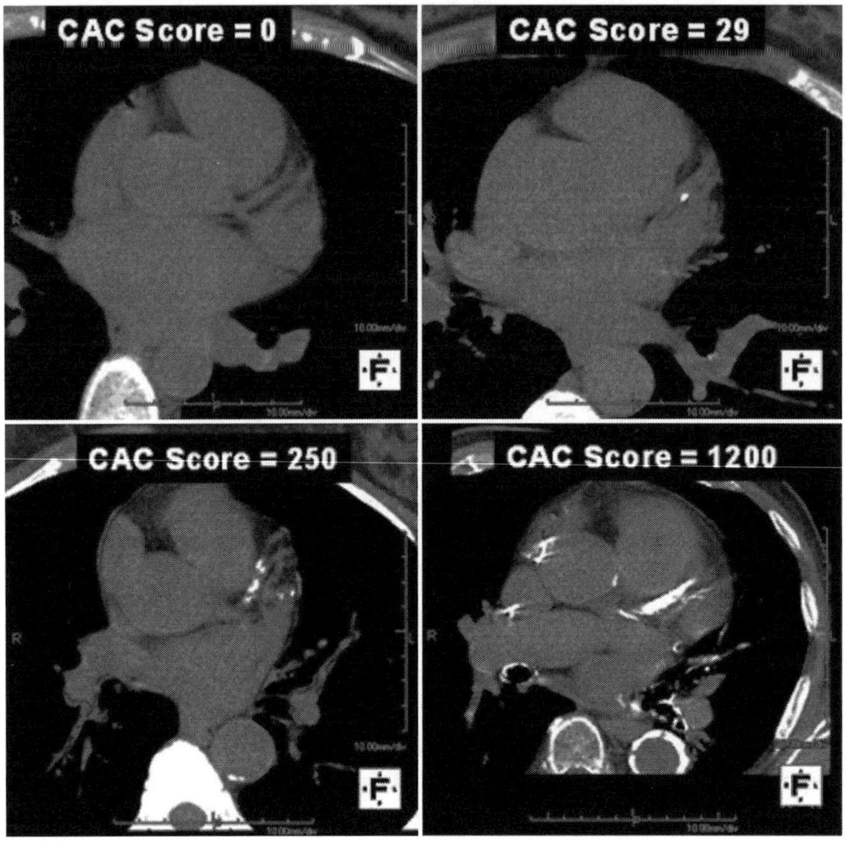

Fig. 1. Example noncontrast CT scans of the heart demonstrating calcified coronary plaque of increasing severity. CAC Score refers to the standardized Agatston calcium score. See text for details.

[17] and the plaque burden quantitatively characterized as follows: scores of 1–10 as minimal, 11–100 as mild, 101–400 as moderate and >400 as extensive. Example CT images representing increasing severity of the Agatston CAC score are shown in Fig. 1. The calcium volume score [18] is a more reproducible parameter that is independent of calcium density and considered to be better suited for serial studies to track progression or regression of atherosclerosis. By comparing a subject's calcium score to others of the same age and gender through the use of large databases of asymptomatic subjects, a calcium score percentile rank for any given individual patient can be determined [19, 20]. This is an index of the severity but also prematurity or, alternatively, the latency of atherosclerosis development at a given chronological age. Although these widely utilized nomograms are useful, it should be understood that variations according to ethnicity have been described [21–24] and data regarding these variations are still being collected and separated. However, recent data have confirmed the predictive power of CAC scoring across large populations [25], but another recent study has also indicated further risk awareness in African Americans with a positive CAC score [26].

The report of the NCEP ATP III guidelines [27] made the following recommendation on the basis of existing data at the time of its publication (2002): *"Therefore, measurement of coronary calcium is an option for advanced risk assessment in appropriately selected persons. In persons with multiple* *risk factors, high coronary calcium scores (e.g., >75th percentile for age and sex) denotes advanced coronary atherosclerosis and provides a rationale for intensified LDL-lowering therapy.*"

Subsequent to the NCEP guidelines, several major reports have highlighted the incremental value of CAC to conventional risk factor assessment. In a retrospective analysis, Kondos et al. [28], in 5,635 asymptomatic, predominantly low to moderate conventional (Framingham) risk, largely middle-aged patients followed for 37 ± 12 months, found that the presence of any CAC by EBT was associated with a relative risk for future cardiac events of 10.5, compared to 1.98 and 1.4 for diabetes and smoking, respectively. In women, only CAC was linked to future events, with a relative risk of 2.6; conventional risk factors were not related. The presence of CAC also provided prognostic information incremental to age and other more conventional risk factors.

Shaw et al. [29] retrospectively analyzed 10,377 asymptomatic patients with a 5 year follow up after an initial EBT evaluation. All-cause mortality (National Death Index listing at follow up) increased proportionally to baseline CAC score, which was an independent predictor of risk after adjusting for all Framingham risk factors ($p<0.001$). Superiority of CAC to conventional Framingham risk factor assessment was also demonstrated by a significantly greater area under the ROC curves (0.73 vs. 0.67, $p<0.001$). Incremental value of CAC to Framingham risk was also established by a significant increase of the area under the ROC curves, from 0.72 for Framingham risk to 0.78 with the addition of CAC ($p<0.001$). Stratification of mortality risk by CAC score was as effective in women as in men. A recent study published by Budoff and colleagues used the same approach to examine the National Death Index and define all cause mortality in >25,000 initially asymptomatic subjects and found similar data for prognostication using the baseline or initial CAC score defined in EBT examination [25].

Greenland et al. [30] analyzed a population based study of 1,461 prospectively followed, older asymptomatic subjects, who were predominantly moderate to high risk, and found that CAC scores >300 significantly added prognostic information to Framingham risk analysis in the 10–20% Framingham risk category.

In the St Francis Heart Study [31], a prospective, population based study of 5,585 asymptomatic patients, CAC scores >100 were associated with relative risks from 10.4 to 32, and transformed conversion of Framingham intermediate risk individuals to high or very high risk status. In a subset of 1,817 patients with risk factor data, incremental information over Framingham scores was documented, with areas under the ROC curves of 0.79 for CAC and 0.69 for Framingham ($p=0.0006$). The greatest separation of patients who developed nonfatal MI or cardiac death in follow-up, from those who did not, was at the CAC score of 100; which has for nearly the past decade been considered the dividing point between mild and moderate coronary atherosclerosis [17]. Importantly, the 15% of patients in the Saint Francis study with initial CAC scores in the 100–400 range had a 10-fold increase in relative risk for any cardiovascular event compared to the 33% of individuals entered into the study protocol with a zero CAC score.

The previously noted and most recent study by Budoff and colleagues performed a retrospective analysis of >25,000 initially asymptomatic individuals, using the National Death Index, to define all cause mortality [25]. Again, these data have essentially reconfirmed information published within the prior decade on the predictive power of CAC scoring, across broad categories of Americans.

Individuals with 0 CAC scores have not yet developed detectable, calcified coronary plaque, but they may have fatty streaking and early stages of plaque in <1% obstructive disease. Atherosclerotic plaques are present in many young adults [32], but the event rate in patients with CAC score 0 is very low [28, 30, 31, 33]. Raggi et al. [33] have demonstrated an annual event rate of 0.11% in asymptomatic subjects with 0 scores, and in the St. Francis Heart Study [31], scores of 0 were associated with a 0.12% annual event rate over the ensuing 4.3 years. Greenland et al. [30], in a higher risk asymptomatic cohort, noted a higher annual event rate (0.62%) with 0 CAC scores; however a less sensitive CAC detection technique (significant "under sampling" by using higher thresholds for positive scans – i.e. nonstandard Agatston scoring) and marked ethnic heterogeneity may have contributed to their different findings [34]. However, regardless of the sampling method, multiple published studies demonstrate that a CAC score of zero confers a low to very low, medium to long term cardiovascular event risk.

CORONARY CT ANGIOGRAPHY

CTA (CT contrast-enhanced coronary angiography) has advanced significantly from the original studies by Achenbach and Rumberger using EBT. The ability to have "isotropic" voxels (volume element which are the same dimension in all 3-dimensions) using 64+-slice MDCT images greatly facilitates the ability to provide high fidelity noninvasive imaging of the coronary arteries and plaque.

The goal of CT angiography is to have the "look and feel" of standard invasive angiography but provide the advantage of not only viewing the lumen, but also the mural surfaces to allow a more complete quantitation of plaque location, plaque composition, and plaque severity.

Both EBT and 16 slice or greater MDCT have been validated against the reference standard of invasive coronary angiography for native coronary arteries and for bypass grafts. Using a 50% or greater stenosis as the definition of obstructive coronary/bypass disease, the overall accuracy for EBT is now in the order of 92–93%; for MDCT the accuracy is in the order of 94–95%. The negative predictive value for both approaches is 100% in multiple studies. Table 1 lists summary statistics for published studies. Please note that the numbers of "nonevaluable" segments was greater in the earlier studies compared to the more recent. This is due to improvements in scanner technology, thinner CT slice thicknesses, improvements in CT angiography contrast and acquisition protocols, and most importantly to newer workstations. The changes to thinner CT scanning for all current systems have allowed visualization in nearly all studies to include the proximal and distal portions of the LCX and distal branches of the RCA. Views of the LCX and to some extent the posterior descending artery (PDA) were hindered for some time in the original studies by 3-D rendering tools that did not allow sufficient navigation to facilitate "unveiling" of the anterior cardiac vein/coronary sinus, or the middle cardiac veins which course across and often parallel to these vessels, respectively. As with all things in digital imaging, CT angiography methods have improved and the 3-D rendering and workstation tools have advanced considerably.

Currently, definition of coronary in-stent stenosis remains problematic, although stent patency is straightforward in nearly all cases. Although there have been individual case reports of performing very thin CT sectioning through coronary stents, demonstrating in-stent narrowing, these methods remain currently clinically impractical. In addition, extensive coronary mural calcification can also confound focal stenosis definition. Although there are no set rules for when there is too much coronary calcification to provide global native coronary accuracy with CT angiography, a good rule of thumb is that the value of the test reduces as the coronary scores (Agatston scale) becomes >400. Additionally, in a symptomatic patient, data have shown that high coronary calcium scores have specificity for significant coronary obstructive disease above 90%, even in the absence of performing a companion CT angiography study.

Contrast enhanced CT using both EBT and MDCT has been shown to potentially define noncalcified (falsely called *"soft"*) plaque on a segmental basis (Fig. 2). There have been three studies published to date in this regard. Achenbach and colleagues [35] compared IVUS obtained during cardiac catheterization with noninvasive contrast enhanced coronary studies using MDCT. They found that

Table 1
Correlations of CT angiography with conventional Angiography for detection of luminal coronary stenoses >50% (EBT and MDCT)

Reference	*Year published*	*No. of Subjects*	*Se (%)*	*Sp (%)*	*NE (%)*
EBT					
Nakanishi [56]	1997	37	74	91	–
Schmermund [11]	1998	28	82	88	12
Reddy [57]	1998	23	88	79	8
Rensing [58]	1998	37	77	94	19
Achenbach [59]	1998	125	92	94	25
Budoff [60]	1999	52	78	71	11
Achenbach [61]	2000	36	92	93	20
Leber [62]	2001	87	78	93	24
Ropers [63]	2002	118	90	82	24
Nikolau [64]	2002	20	85	77	11
Rasouli [65]	2003	10	94	88	8
MDCT					
Nieman [66]	2003	59	95	86	–
Ropers [67]	2003	77	92	93	12
Mollet [68]	2004	128	94	91	0
Bypass grafts – EBT					
Achenbach [69]	1999 (occlusion)	56	100	100	0
	1999 (stenosis)		100	97	16
Bypass Grafts – MDCT					
Ropers [70]	2002 (occlusion)	65	97	98	0
	2002 (stenosis)		75	92	–
Schlosser [71]	2004(occlusion and stenosis)	51	96	95	6
Martuscelli [72]	2004(occlusion and stenosis)	84	97	100	9

Se Sensitivity, *Sp* Specificity, *NE* Nonevaluable coronary segments

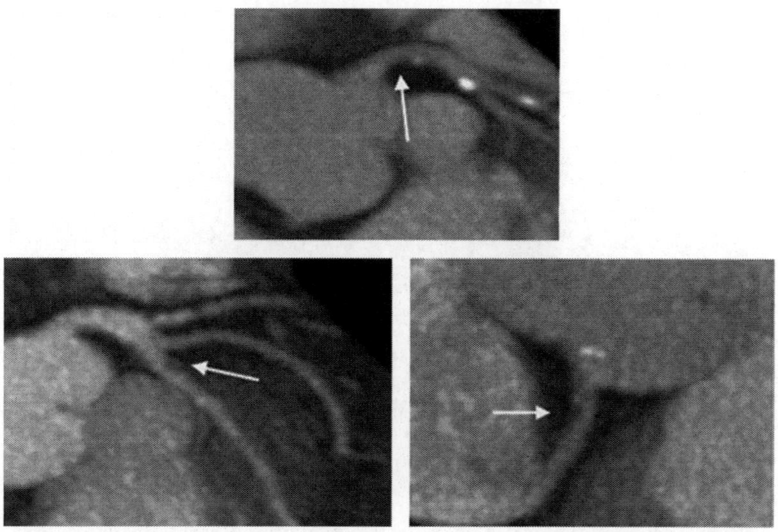

Fig. 2. Representative examples of noncalcified plaque from coronary CTA studies using EBT.

CT had a sensitivity of about 82% to detect coronary segments with atherosclerotic plaque, but had only a 53% sensitivity of defining segments with noncalcified atherosclerotic plaque. Thus combining CAC and contrast enhanced segmental definition of "soft" plaque still resulted in significant underestimation of true total atherosclerotic plaque burden.

Leber et al. [36] also performed a comparison between IVUS and contrast enhanced CT. They reported a sensitivity for "soft" plaque at about 78%, a sensitivity for fibrous plaque at about 78%, while maintaining a sensitivity for "calcified" plaque (as had been shown in prior EBT noncontrast enhanced studies) of about 95%. Thus in about 80% of the cases, contrast enhanced CT can be used to provide additional information about noncalcified plaque, but the total "atherosclerotic plaque burden" remains under defined. Leber and colleagues [37] extended this work to 64-slice CT, demonstrating an even greater accuracy in determining "global" coronary plaque burden.

Studies attempting to define global atherosclerotic plaque burden studies are possible using both EBT and MDCT, but both have specific deficiencies. EBT is limited currently by spatial resolution on the order of 1–1.5 mm, as compared with sub millimeter definition by MDCT; conversely, EBT can be used across heart rates from 50 to 120 beats/min without the need for beta-blockade to lower resting heart rate, due to temporal resolution 2–3 times superior to MDCT. All published studies to date using MDCT have required resting heart rates <65 beats/min for adequate image resolution.

Contrast enhanced CT, although possessing great potential as a diagnostic catheterization for defining the absence or presence of "significant" coronary stenotic lesions, is still somewhat limited in defining "noncalcified" plaque and has not been shown currently to provide incremental value in predicting the potential for preventing heart attack. An example of the power of 64-slice MDCT in defining regional plaque burden is shown in Fig. 3 in which there is nonobstructive lumen narrowing, but in the presence of laminated noncalcified plaque, calcified plaque, and possible ulcerated plaque. Standard "lumenography" by traditional coronary angiography would likely have missed such a potential unstable plaque which is quickly realized using contrast-enhanced cardiac CT.

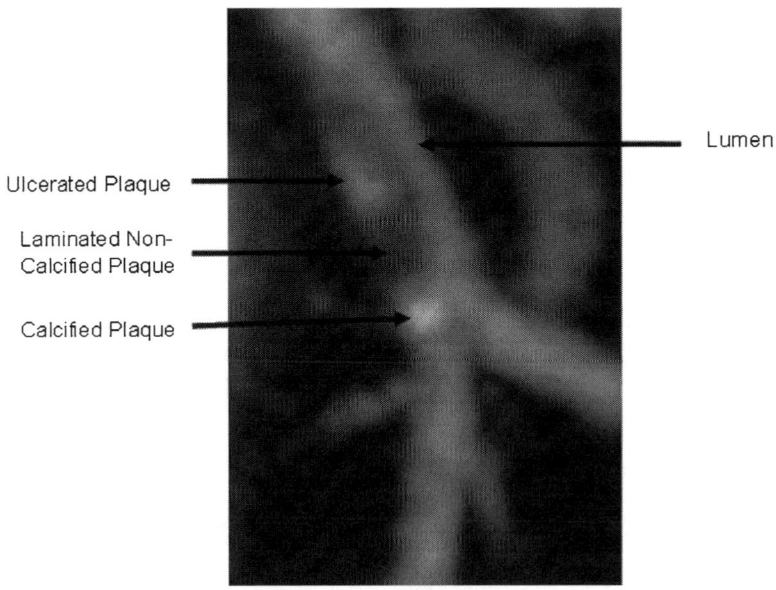

Fig. 3. Example of eccentric, very complex atherosclerotic plaque with possible ulceration from coronary CTA done using 64-slice CT. This type of plaque is potentially very unstable.

CLINICAL APPLICATIONS OF CARDIAC CT

Noncontrast-enhanced CT of the heart and contrast-enhanced CT of the heart provide incremental information regarding atherosclerotic plaque burden. The quantification of CAC volume (noncontrast CT) provides a reliable, repeatable, simple, low radiation approach to estimating plaque burden, but defines at best about 20%. A contrast-enhanced CTA provides additional information about noncalcified plaque and can account for up to 80% of the total atherosclerotic burden, but at the risk of higher radiation doses and the use of intravenous contrast media. Both have distinct roles in risk stratification in patients and the CAC scan can stand alone, but, in my opinion, the contrast study (CTA) is totally incomplete unless accompanied by a noncontrast (CAC) scan.

CAC SCANS

Recommendations for CAC scanning are not based on age and gender alone. Rather, the Framingham Risk Score, which incorporates both age and gender, is recommended as the initial step in selecting the appropriate test populations. Asymptomatic patients in the 10–20% Framingham 10 year risk category (intermediate risk) comprise the group that presents the greatest challenge to the treating physician, and are those in whom the application of CAC scoring is considered most appropriate. This group represents up to 40% of the population that might be seen sitting in the waiting room of the average Internist [38]. While this application was proposed as being reasonable in the early ACC/AHA consensus statement [39], the recent additional evidence of risk-stratification by CAC in this group has resulted in a greater acceptance of its benefits, and was included in the 2005 AHA Scientific Statement on noninvasive testing in women for use in the intermediate risk population [40].

Selected patients with less than intermediate Framingham risk may also benefit. For instance, most young patients with a family history of premature CAD (first degree relatives with documented heart disease below the age of 55) will not have sufficient risk factors to even warrant Framingham scoring (lower NCEP risk), or will be in the low (1–10%) 10 year Framingham risk group [41, 42]. Data from Schmermund et al. [16] and Pohle et al. [43] indicate that 95% of acute MI patients would have been identified by EBT plaque imaging, even in those with a mean age of 41 years. On the basis of these observations, the use of CAC scoring should be considered in patients with a family history of premature CAD, especially if their Framingham risk is intermediate (although many would advocate this use even if the initial Framingham risk was calculated as low; since family history remains one of the most positive risk factors and is NOT included in conventional Framingham scoring).

Selective application of CAC scanning to patients with Framingham high risk may also be warranted. For instance, some Framingham high risk patients may be intolerant of statins or may strongly prefer alternative-medicine approaches. In these patients, CAC evidence of high risk may be used to reinforce the necessity for finding a statin that can be tolerated and for persuading the refractory patient of the need for aggressive treatment. Conversely, the absence of significant CAC may permit relaxation of the treatment goals, an approach that appears justified by the low event rate in the 0 score CAC group [28–31, 33].

The presence or absence and the amount of CAC can be useful for clinical decision making, as previously recommended in the AHA Prevention V Update [44]. As an extension of this report, based on recent data, Table 2 provides simple, easily implemented treatment paradigms for combining risks of varying CAC scores with the most recent NCEP recommendations. Patients in the 10–20% 10 year risk category who are identified to be at higher risk by CAC become candidates for secondary prevention lipid goals regardless of their baseline lipid level. This would apply even for patients with LDL

Table 2
Guidelines for treatment in asymptomatic individuals classified as intermediate risk patients by NCEP (Framingham 10–20% 10 year risk)

CAC score and percentile ranking	*Framingham risk group equivalent*	*Target LDL goal (mg/dl)*	*Pharmacologic therapy indicated (mg/dl)*
Zero	Lowest risk (10 year risk <5%)	<160	≥190
>0, <10 AND <75th percentile	Low risk (10 year risk <10%)	<130	≥160
11–100 AND <75th percentile	Intermediate risk (10 year risk >10% but <20%)	<130	≥130
101–400 OR ≥75th but <90th percentile	High risk (coronary disease risk equivalent; 10 year risk ≥20%)	<100	≥100
>400 OR ≥90th percentile	Very high risk (10 year risk >30%)	<50–70	Any LDL level

cholesterol <100 mg/dl, as implied by the Heart Protection Study [45] and stated in the prior NCEP report.

Based on prognostic data, CAC >100 or >75th percentile serves to define a CAD risk equivalent (i.e. >20% over the next decade). In the St. Francis Heart Study [31], the CAC dividing point for secondary prevention risk equivalency in the Framingham 10–20% 10 year risk group was a score >100; or, additionally at a score >75th percentile for age as suggested by the NCEP guidelines. In this regard, CAC scores >400 or >90th percentile are associated with a very high annual risk (4.8 and 6.5% respectively) [33, 46], and these individual are candidates for an even more aggressive approach (i.e. LDL <70 mg/dl as suggested by the latest update to the NCEP [47]) and possibly further stratification with stress testing (see discussion below).

In the Framingham 10–20% 10 year risk population, patients with CAC scores ≤100 and ≤75th percentile remain in the same risk group or are transformed to lower risk categories depending on the score. A reasonable approach is to leave the patients with CAC scores from 10 to 100 and <75th percentile in the intermediate risk (10–20% 10 year risk), and reclassify patients with CAC scores from 1 to 10 and <75th percentile as low risk (<10% 10 year risk) and treat accordingly. CAC scores of 0 would reclassify the patient to the very low risk category.

As noted above, some patients in the lower risk groups based on Framingham scores, such as younger patients (35–45 years of age) with a strong family history of premature coronary heart disease, may be appropriately tested with CAC scanning. In such patients, the recommendations in Table 2 would also apply. While it is widely accepted that high CAC scores increase the intensity of medical therapy, how low CAC scores should affect therapy is not yet clear. It would appear reasonable that in high risk asymptomatic patients who have undergone imaging, CAC scores ≤100, and, in particular, ≤10, imply a lower than expected risk and maybe a reduction in the intensity of therapy. The rationale for this lowest category is as follows. If the use of cholesterol lowering medications (such as statins) can across the board, lower the risk of an MI by 1/3 – this is significantly of value when the risk is found to be high, but is less practical when the risk is very low. For instance, if the "risk" of a cardiovascular event is 0.1% for a zero CAC score (as supported by the published literature), then using a cholesterol medication may be of limited incremental value if the risk reduces to 0.07%.

It is important to note, however, that a CAC score of 0 does not imply that no treatment is necessary. Rather, it is used to shift the patient to a lowest risk group. For example, early information has shown that the event rate in diabetics with 0 CAC scores is as low as in nondiabetics with 0 scores [48], potentially creating a group of diabetics who would not have to be considered to have "coronary heart disease" equivalence. More data are needed in these groups for determining the therapeutic implications of the absence of CAC.

The use of changes in CAC score rather than changes in lipid values to track treatment effects has been under investigation. Serial EBT scanning has shown that aggressive lipid lowering therapy may slow progression of calcified plaque [49–54], although it is far from infallible [55]. Clearly, a noninvasive tool with which sequential testing could be performed safely and reliably would be highly desirable provided the results are associated with significant prognostic value. Raggi et al. have demonstrated that CAC progression is greater in patients with future MI [54], whereas LDL levels on treatment were similar in patients with and without events. Progression was associated with a worse prognosis compared to stabilization, irrespective of baseline CAC score. However, more studies are required to justify the broad based use of serial CAC scanning to monitor treatment efficacy.

CORONARY CTA

As has been shown, CTA provides a reasonable accurate means to define the anatomic severity of epicardial coronary artery disease. Its positive predictive value (PPV) for significant coronary disease (defined as >50% narrowing on direct coronary angiography) is good, but currently at about 65%. One has to ask oneself if the promise of CTA is in finding a better "angiogram" or in another more clinically important situation, of defining the extent of atherosclerotic heart disease, and thus refining risk stratification beyond that provided by measures of conventional risk factors.

CAC defines, as stated, only about 20% of the total coronary atherosclerotic plaque burden, and better stratification can be found by having better estimates of total plaque severity. The additional ability to at least semiquantitatively define the noncalcified plaque burden is a great advantage to CTA. Although the PPV is moderate, the negative predictive valve (NPV) is approaching 100% and the PPV for "atherosclerotic plaque" is also nearly at 100%. If the true estimate of "risk" is best defined by quantification of the "plaque burden" (as suggested by the CAC studies) then the incremental value of defining plaque burden by CTA is likely to be substantial when applied to the correct patient population.

CAC is a wonderful method, especially in the asymptomatic, intermediate risk patient – but CTA is also a wonderful method in the symptomatic, but also intermediate risk patient. In fact the best predictive power for a test with nearly a 100% NPV is to apply this in patients with low to intermediate likelihood – that is the power of CTA.

FUTURE DEVELOPMENTS

Cardiac CT has been in constant progressive mode for greater than 24 years and has been validated for numerous cardiovascular applications. At present, it rivals or exceeds the ability of magnetic resonance imaging in assessing cardiac anatomy and function. Furthermore, cardiac CT, after a short apprentice period, can be performed using current CT scanners on a worldwide basis eclipsing many of the currently available and more traditional cardiac imaging methods, including invasive coronary angiography.

However, there remain several issues that require resolution. In particular, the radiation dose from cardiac CT can be significantly higher than that of a standard CT chest exam, with doses likely exceeding those of diagnostic cardiac catheterization, but less than what would be required for a standard nuclear stress test. Further reducing radiation doses however, would be of major importance. Already some of the CT manufacturers have developed methods to allow maintenance of diagnostic accuracy while reducing radiation doses to 1/3 or less – continued efforts in this regard are necessary for broad based utilization of CT in common coronary diagnostics.

An additional matter is spatial resolution. There have been considerable improvements in CT slice thickness from the 1.5 to 3.0 mm EBT scanners to the current 0.4–0.5 mm MDCT scanners. However, conventional coronary angiography has a spatial resolution in the order of 0.1 mm. In order for CT to even approach this equivalency (and to then assess total atherosclerotic burden), more research is needed. Adding on more slices, as some manufacturers have done, does not actually improve spatial resolution, but only improved the coverage of each scan (and thus shortens the imaging time and thus reduces radiation dose). All current CT scanners use detectors that are made of ceramics and further improvements in these fundamental detector material is needed prior to any further significant improvements in CT spatial resolution.

EXECUTIVE SUMMARY

1. Historical aspects of cardiac CT development
   (a) Cardiac CT began with the use of EBT in 1984 and remained the dominant method for nearly 20 years – setting the stage for applications in cardiac anatomy, function, and perfusion.
   (b) CAC studies emerged in the 1990s and CT coronary angiography by 1995.
   (c) Today, due to considerable improvements in CT physics, 64+-slice MDCT has emerged as the leader in cardiac and coronary applications.
2. Coronary artery calcification
   (a) CAC by CT was validated as a means to estimate total coronary atherosclerotic burden.
   (b) Additional research has demonstrated coronary calcium score and percentile rank to be a powerful predictor of cardiovascular risk in asymptomatic individuals, significantly improving risk predictions compared to conventional Framingham risk models.
3. CT coronary angiography
   (a) Studies using EBT first demonstrated the ability to define segmental coronary stenoses.
   (b) Numerous validation studies, in particular using the MDCT systems have validated the value of CT angiography in predicting coronary stenoses but also in defining coronary atherosclerotic burden incremental to that defined by coronary calcium.
4. Clinical applications of cardiac CT
   (a) CAC Scans
      - The application of coronary calcium in asymptomatic individuals is best utilized in low to intermediate risk patients to refine risk calculations and determine the need for or aggressiveness of medical therapy.
   (b) Coronary CTA
      - The major applications for coronary CTA is in the nearly 100% negative predictive value for ruling out obstructive coronary disease and in the high PPV for atherosclerotic plaque.
      - CT angiography aids in particular in defining atherosclerotic burden in intermediate risk patients and aids in defining complex coronary disease that would otherwise be missed by traditional cardiac imaging methods.
5. Future developments
   (a) The future for cardiac CT is very bright as the method is straightforward and widely available.
   (b) Additional improvements however are needed in two important areas: reducing the radiation dose and further improvements in spatial resolution.

REFERENCES

1. Hounsfield GN. Computerized transverse axial scanning (tomography). Par 1. Description of system. Br J Radiol 1973;46: 1016–22
2. Ambrose J. Computerized transverse axial scanning (tomography). Part II. Clinical applications. Br J Radiol 1973;46: 1023–27
3. Boyd D. A proposed dynamic cardiac 3-D densitometer for early detection and evaluation of heart disease. IEEE Trans Nuc/ Sci 1979;N26:2724
4. Boyd DP, Couch JL, Napel SA, Peschmann KR, Rand RE. Ultrafast cine CT: where have we been? What lies ahead? Am J Cardiac Imaging 1987;1:175–85
5. Rumberger JA, Lipton MJ. Ultrafast cardiac CT scanning. Cardiol Clin 1989;7:713–34
6. Rumberger JA, Sheedy PF, Breen JF (1996) Use of ultrafast (cine) X-ray computed tomography in cardiac and cardiovascular imaging. In: Giuliani ER, Gersh BJ, McGoon MD, Hayes DL, Schaff HF (eds), Mayo clinic practice of cardiology, 3rd edn. Mosby, St. Louis, Chapter 8, pp 303–324.
7. Rumberger JA, Feiring AJ, Lipton MJ, Higgins CB, Marcus ML. Measurement of myocardial perfusion by ultrafast CT. J Am Coll Cardiol 1985;5(2):500
8. Rumberger JA, Gersh BJ. Non-parallel changes in global chamber volume and muscle mass during the first year following transmural myocardial infarction in man: letter to the editor. J Am Coll Cardiol 1993;22:2060-1
9. Agatston AS, Janowitz WR, Hildner FJ, Zusmer NR, Viamonte M, Detrano R. Quantification of coronary artery calcium using ultrafast computed tomography. J Am Coll Cardiol 1990;15:827–32
10. Moshage WE, Achenbach S, Seese B, Bachmann K, Kirchgeorg M. Coronary artery stenoses: three-dimensional imaging with electrocardiographically triggered, contrast-enhanced, electron beam CT. Radiology 1995;196:707–14
11. Schmermund A, Rensing BJ, Sheedy PF, Bell MR, Rumberger JA. Intravenous electron-beam CT coronary angiography for segmental analysis of coronary artery stenoses. J Am Coll Cardiol 1998;31:1547–54
12. Rifkin RD, Parisi AF, Folland E. Coronary calcification in the diagnosis of coronary artery disease. Am J Cardiol 1979;44:141–7
13. McCarthy JH, Palmer FJ. Incidence and significance of coronary artery calcification. Br Heart J 1974;36:499–506
14. Rumberger JA, Simons DB, Fitzpatrick LA, et al. Coronary artery calcium areas by electron beam computed tomography and coronary atherosclerotic plaque area: a histopathologic correlative study. Circulation 1995;92:2157–62
15. Baumgart D, Schmermund A, Goerge G, et al. Comparison of electron beam computed tomography with intracoronary ultrasound and coronary angiography for detection of coronary atherosclerosis. J Am Coll Cardiol 1997;30:57–64
16. Schmermund A, Baumgart D, Gorge G, et al. Coronary artery calcium in acute coronary syndromes: a comparative study of electron beam CT, coronary angiography, and intracoronary ultrasound in survivors of acute myocardial infarction and unstable angina. Circulation 1997;96:1461–9
17. Rumberger JA, Brundage BH, Rader DJ, Kondos G. Electron beam CT coronary calcium scanning: a review and guidelines for use in asymptomatic individuals. Mayo Clin Proc 1999;74:243–52
18. Callister TQ, Cooil B, Raya SP, et al. Coronary artery disease: improved reproducibility of calcium scoring with an electron-beam CT volumetric method. Radiology 1998;208:807–14
19. Hoff JA, Chomka EV, Krainik AJ, et al. Age and gender distributions of coronary artery calcium detected by electron beam tomography in 35,246 Adults. Am J Cardiol 2001;87:1335–9
20. Schmermund A, Erbel R, Silber S. Age and gender distribution of coronary artery calcium measured by four-slice computed tomography in 2,030 persons with no symptoms of coronary artery disease. Am J Cardiol 2002;90:169–73
21. Budoff MJ, Yang TP, Shavelle RM. Ethnic differences in coronary atherosclerosis. J Am Coll Cardiol 2002;39:408–12
22. Newman AB, Naydeck BL, Whittle J, et al. Racial differences in coronary artery calcification in adults. Arterioscler Thromb Vasc Biol 2002;22:424–30
23. Khuran C, Rosenbaum CG, Howard BV, et al. Coronary artery calcification in black women and white women. Am Heart J 2003;145:724–9
24. Jain T, Peshock R, Darren K. McGuire DK, et al. African Americans and Caucasians have a similar prevalence of coronary calcium in the Dallas Heart Study. J Am Coll Cardiol 2004;44:1011–7
25. Budoff MJ, Shaw LJ, Liu ST, Weinstein SR, Mosler TP, Tseng PH, Flores FR, Callister TR, Raggi P, Berman DS. Long term prognosis associated with coronary calcium: observations from a registry of 25,253 patients. JACC 2007;49:1860–70
26. Nasir K, Shaw LJ, Liu ST, Weinstein SR, Mosler TR, Flores PR, Flores FR, Raggi P, Berman DS, Blumenthal RS, Budoff MJ. Ethnic differences in the prognostic value of coronary artery calcification for all-cause mortality. JACC 2007;50:953–60
27. Third report of the National Cholesterol Education Program (NCEP) Expert panel on detection, evaluation, and treatment of high blood cholesterol in adults (Adult Treatment Panel III) Final Report. NIH Publication No. 02-5215. September 2002.
28. Kondos GT, Hoff JA, Sevrukov A, et al. Coronary artery calcium and cardiac events electron-beam tomography coronary artery calcium and cardiac events: a 37-month follow-up of 5,635 initially asymptomatic low to intermediate risk adults. Circulation 2003;107:2571–6
29. Shaw LJ, Raggi P, Schisterman E, et al. Prognostic value of cardiac risk factors and coronary artery calcium screening for all-cause mortality. Radiology 2003;28:826–33

30. Greenland P, LaBree L, Azen SP, et al. Coronary artery calcium score combined with Framingham score for risk prediction in asymptomatic individuals. JAMA 2004;291:210–5
31. Arad Y, Goodman KJ, Roth M, et al. Coronary calcification, coronary risk factors, C-reactive protein and atherosclerotic cardiovascular disease events: the St. Francis Heart Study. J Am Coll Cardiol 2005;46:158–65
32. Tuzcu EM, Kapadia SR, Tutar E, et al. High prevalence of coronary atherosclerosis in asymptomatic teenagers and young adults: evidence from intravascular ultrasound. Circulation 2001;103:2705–10
33. Raggi P, Callister TQ, Cooil B, et al. Identification of patients at increased risk of first unheralded acute myocardial infarction by electron beam computed tomography. Circulation 2000;101:850–5
34. Budoff MJ, Ehrlich J, Hecht HS, Rumberger JR. Letter to the editor. JAMA 2004;291:1822
35. Achenbach S, Moselewski F, Ropers D, Ferencik M, Hoffman U, MacNeill B, Phole K, Baum U, Anders K, Jang IK, Daniel WG, Brady TJ. Detection of calcified and noncalcified coronary atherosclerotic plaque by contrast-enhanced submillimeter multidetector spiral computed tomography. Circulation 2004;109:14–7
36. Leber AW, Knez A, Becker A, Becker C, Ziegler F, Nikolaou K, Rist C, Reiser M, White C, Steinbeck G, Boekstegers P. Accuracy of multidetector spiral computed tomography in identifying and differentiating the composition of coronary atherosclerotic plaques. JACC 2004;43:1241–7
37. Leber AW, Becker A, Knez A, et al. Accuracy of 64-slice CT to classify and quantify plaque volume in the proximal coronary system: a comparison study with intravascular ultrasound. J Am Coll Cardiol 2006;47:672–7
38. Greenland P, Smith SC, Grundy SM. Improving coronary heart disease risk assessment in asymptomatic people: role of traditional risk factors and noninvasive cardiovascular tests. Circulation 2001;104:1863-7
39. O'Rourke RA, Brundage BH, Froelicher VF, et al. American College of Cardiology/American Heart Association expert consensus document on electron beam computed tomography for the diagnosis and prognosis of coronary artery disease. Circulation 2000;102:126–34
40. Mieres JH, Shaw LJ; Andrew Arai A, et al. AHA scientific statement: role of noninvasive testing in the clinical evaluation of women with suspected coronary artery disease. Consensus statement from the Cardiac Imaging Committee, Council on Clinical Cardiology, and the Cardiovascular Imaging and Intervention Committee, Council on Cardiovascular Radiology and Intervention, American Heart Association. Circulation 2005;111:682–96
41. Wilson PWF, D'Agostino B, Levy D, et al. Prediction of coronary heart disease using risk factor categories. Circulation 1998;97:1837–47
42. Expert panel on detection, evaluation, and treatment of high blood cholesterol in adults. Executive summary of the third report of the National Cholesterol Education Program (NCEP) (Adult Treatment Panel III). JAMA 2001;285:2486–97
43. Pohle K, Ropers D, Mäffert R, et al. Coronary calcifications in young patients with first, unheralded myocardial infarction: a risk factor matched analysis by electron beam tomography. Heart 2003;89:625–8
44. Smith SC, Greenland P, Grundy SM. Prevention conference V: beyond secondary prevention: identifying the high-risk patient for primary prevention. Executive summary. Circulation 2000;101:111–6
45. Heart Protection Study Collaborative Group. MRC/BHF Heart Protection Study of cholesterol lowering with simvastatin in 20 536 high-risk individuals: a randomized placebo-controlled trial. Lancet 2002;360:7–22
46. Raggi P, Cooil B, Callister TQ. Use of electron beam tomography data to develop models for prediction of hard coronary events. Am Heart J 2001;141:375–82
47. Grundy SM, Cleeman JI, Merz CN, et al. Implications of recent clinical trials for the National Cholesterol Education Program Adult Treatment Panel III Guidelines. Circulation 2004;110:227–39
48. Raggi P, Shaw LJ, Berman DS, Callister TQ. Prognostic value of coronary artery calcium screening in subjects with and without diabetes. J Am Coll Cardiol 2004;43:1663–9
49. Callister TQ, Raggi P, Cooil B, et al. Effect of HMG-CoA reductase inhibitors on coronary artery disease as assessed by electron beam computed tomography. N Engl J Med 1998;339:1972–8
50. Budoff MJ, Lane KL, Bakhsheshi H, et al. Rates of progression of coronary calcium by electron beam tomography. Am J Cardiol 2000;86:8–11
51. Achenbach S, Ropers D, Pohle K, et al. Influence of lipid-lowering therapy on the progression of coronary artery calcification: a prospective evaluation. Circulation 2002;106:1077–82
52. Shavelle DM, Takasu J, Budoff MJ, et al. HMG CoA reductase inhibitor (statin) and aortic valve calcium. Lancet 2002;359(9312):1125–6
53. Raggi P, Cooil B, Shaw L, et al. Progression of coronary calcification on serial electron beam tomography scanning is greater in patients with future myocardial infarction. Am J Cardiol 2003;92:827–9
54. Raggi P, Callister TQ, Shaw LJ. Progression of coronary artery calcium and risk of first myocardial infarction in patients receiving cholesterol-lowering therapy. Arterioscler Thromb Vasc Biol 2004;24:1–7
55. Hecht HS Harman SM. Changes in calcified plaque and serum lipoprotein values: evaluation by electron beam tomography in treated and untreated asymptomatic patients. Am J Cardiol 2003;91:1131–4
56. Nakinishi T, Ito K, Imazu M, Yamakido, M. Evaluation of coronary artery stenoses using electron-beam CT and mutiplanar reformation. J Comp Assist 1997;21:121–7
57. Reddy GP, Chernoff DM, Adams JR, Higgins CB. Coronary artery stenoses: 59 assessment with contrast-enhanced electron-beam CT and axial reconstructions. Radiology 1998;208:167–72

58. Rensing BJ, Bongaerts A, van Geuns RJ, van Ooijen P, Oudkerk M de Feyter PJ. Intravenous coronary angiography by electron beam computed tomography: a clinical evaluation. Circulation 1998;98:2509–12
59. Achenbach S, Moshage W. Ropers D, Nossen J, Daniel WG. Value of electron beam computed tomography for the noninvasive detection of high-grade coronary artery stenoses and occlusions. N Engl J Med 1998;339:1964–71
60. Budoff MJ, Oudiz RJ, Zalace CP, Bakhsdeshi H, Goldberg SL, French WJ, Rami TG, Brundage BH. Intravenous three-dimensional coronary angiography using contrast enhanced electron beam computed tomography. Am J Cardiol 1999;83:840–5
61. Achenbach S, Ropers D, Regenfus M, Uizheimer S, Derlien H, Schulte C, Wenkel E, Moshage W, Bautz W, Daniel WG. Contrast enhanced electron beam computed tomography to analyze the coronary arteries in patients after acute myocardial infarction. Heart 2000;84:489–93
62. Leber AW, Knez A, Mukherjee R, White C, Huber A, Becker A, Becker CR, Reiser M, Haberl R, Steinbeck G. Usefulness of calcium scoring using electron beam computed tomography and noninvasive coronary angiography in patients with suspected coronary artery disease. Am J Cardiol 2001;88:219–23
63. Ropers D, Regenfus M, Stilanakis N, Birke S, Kessler W, Moshage W, Laub G, Daniel WG, Achenbach S. A direct comparison of noninvasive coronary angiography by electron beam tomography and navigator-echobased magnetic resonance imaging for detection of restenosis following coronary angioplasty. Invest Radiol 2002;37:386–92
64. Nikolaou K, Huber A, Knez A, Breuning R, Reiser M. Intraindividual comparison of contrast-enhanced electron-beam computed tomography and navigator echo-based magnetic resonance imaging for noninvasive coronary artery angiography. Eur Radiol 2002;12:1663–71
65. Rasouli ML, Budoff M, Mao S, et al. Detection of coronary stenosis using e-Speed electron beam tomography. Circulation 2003;108:IV–527 (abstract)
66. Nieman K, Cademartiri F, Lemos P, Raaijmakers R, Pattynama P, de Feyter P. Reliable non-invasive coronary angiography sung sub-millimetre multislice spiral CT. Circulation 2002;106:2051–4
67. Ropers D, Baum U, Pohle K, Katharina MD, Anders K, Ulzheimer S, Ohnesorge B, Schlundt C, Bautz W, Daniel WG, Achenbach S. Detection of coronary artery stenoses with thin-slice multi-detector row spiral computed tomography and multiplanar reconstruction. Circulation 2003;107:664–6
68. Mollet NR, Cademartiri F, Nieman K, Saia F, Lemos PA, McFadden EP, Pattynama PMT, Serruys PW, Krestin GP, de Feyter P. MSCT coronary angiography in stable angina. J Am Coll Cardiol 2004;43:2265–70
69. Achenbach S, Giesler A, Moshage W, Ropers D, Nossen J, Bachmann K. Noninvasive three-dimensional visualization of coronary artery bypass grafts by electron beam tomography. Am J Cardiol 1997;88:792–5
70. Ropers D, Ulzheimer S, Wenkel E, Anders K, Ohnesorge B, Schlundt C, Bautz W, Daniel WG, Achenbach S. Investigation of aortocoronary artery bypass grafts by multislice spiral computed tomography with electrocardiographic-gated image reconstruction. Am J Cardiol 2001;88:792–5
71. Schlosser T, Konorza T, Hunold P, Huhl H. Schmermund A, Barkhausen J. Noninvasive visualization of coronary artery bypass grafts using 16-detector row computed tomography. J Am Coll Cardiol 2004;44:1224–9
72. Martuscelli E, Romagnoli A, D'Eliseo A, Tomassini M, Razzini C, Sperandio CM, Simonetti G, Romeo F, Mehta JL. Evaluation of venous and arterial conduit patency by 16-slice spiral computed tomography. Circulation 2004;110:3234–28

25 Noninvasive Coronary Plaque Characterization: CT Versus MRI

John A. Rumberger

CONTENTS

ABSTRACT

Magnetic resonance imaging (MRI) or magnetic resonance angiography (MRA) can potentially define atherosclerotic plaque in the aorta and the heart – however, the majority of information on looking at coronary plaque noninvasively comes from doing Cardiac CT. In particular, noncontrast CT can define a linear estimate of coronary atherosclerotic plaque by defining the coronary calcium "score." Adding on contrast-enhanced CT coronary angiography also provides a means to define the present of noncalcified, "soft," and potentially vulnerable plaque over and above that of just the calcium score.

Key words: Computed tomography (CT); Coronary artery calcification; CT coronary angiography; Noncalcified atherosclerotic plaque

KEY POINTS

- MRI can potentially define noncalcified plaque, but has not been shown to quantify overall plaque burden
- Cardiac CT can define a reproducible measure of the coronary calcium score, an estimate of overall plaque burden
- Using contrast-enhanced cardiac CT angiography, additional information regarding noncalcified, "soft" or potentially vulnerable plaque can also be estimated

Imaging plays a major role in the detection of atherosclerotic plaque, as has been discussed and detailed elsewhere in this report. Ultrasound provides information on plaque type in selected regions in which images can be obtained. The same can be said for MRI. However, specific details of coronary

From: *Asymptomatic Atherosclerosis: Pathophysiology, Detection and Treatment*
Edited by: M. Naghavi (ed.), DOI 10.1007/978-1-60327-179-0_25

plaque, except in limited views, are beyond noninvasive ultrasound. Characterizations also by MRI have been limited, except in specific clinical examples or in controlled experimental studies. CT (EBT and MDCT) on the other hand can provide information on calcified plaque that specifically applies to prediction of coronary artery plaque burden/extent. Histologic [1, 2], ultrasonic [3] and angiographic [4] studies have confirmed that coronary calcium quantified by X-ray CT is related to the extent of atherosclerotic plaque disease in a direct fashion, regardless of age or gender; although it is not a substitute for actual angiographic stenosis severity [5]. Furthermore, these measures have been shown to provide cardiac prognostic information that is separate and incremental to conventional-based risk factor analysis [6–8].

HARD VS. "SOFT" (NONCALCIFIED) ATHEROSCLEROTIC PLAQUE

A common issue of discussion however with regard to coronary artery calcium (CAC) quantitation by CT has been the general misunderstanding of what it actually measures: i.e., it defines only "hard" plaque, but provides no information of "soft" (and potentially vulnerable, noncalcified) plaque. Rumberger [2] initially studied autopsy hearts defining the use of CAC as an estimate of coronary atherosclerotic plaque burden, when looking at the coronary arteries as a whole. In nondecalcified coronary artery segments, using contact microradiography, the relationship between CAC and total atherosclerotic plaque area on a segment by segment basis, however, is variable where at times the tracking is intimate and at other times somewhat dissociated [9] (Fig. 1).

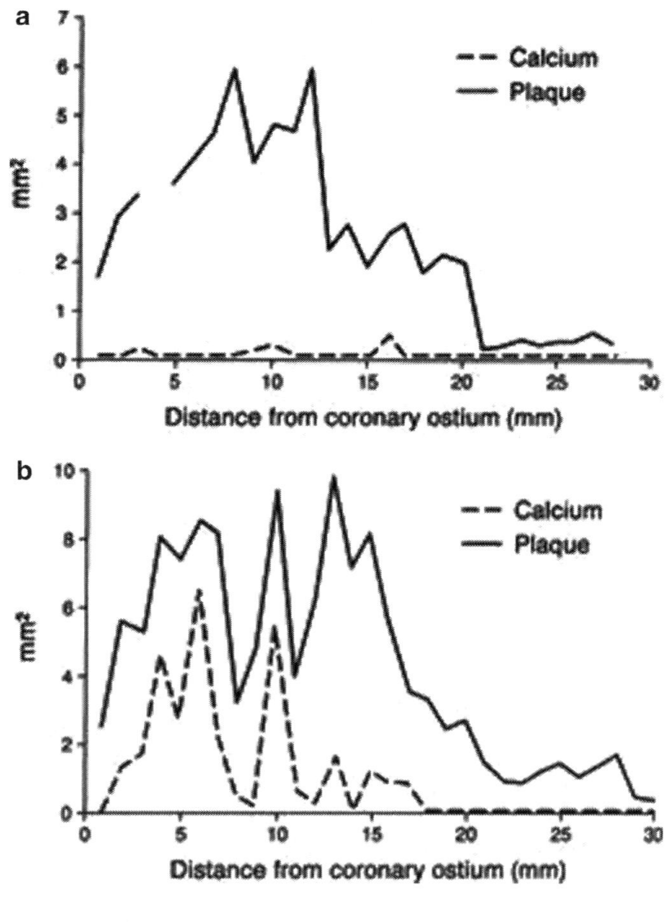

Fig. 1. Plaque area and coronary calcium area along the length of a coronary artery as determined by direct contact microradiography. (**a**) there is diffuse coronary artery plaque with little associated calcification. (**b**) there is diffuse segmental coronary plaque with an intimate association with coronary calcium in each segment.

Autopsy studies have shown that "scar" (sclerosis) is seen in about two-third of all coronary plaque and that the distribution of scar versus lipid-rich plaque in a 3:1 ratio is generally constant across all levels of coronary narrowing. Lipid-rich plaque, commonly referred to as "soft" plaque, is thus an intimate part of virtually all atherosclerotic plaque compositions.

Thus CAC, although a method to define or estimate global coronary atherosclerotic plaque burden, is not necessarily a method to define plaque burden on a segment by segment basis.

NONINVASIVE CORONARY ANGIOGRAPHY

Commencing with the work by Moshage in Germany [10] followed rapidly by the work of Schmermund and Rumberger at the Mayo Clinic [11] in the mid-1990s, the use of contrast-enhanced CT has been advocated as a noninvasive method to quantify coronary luminal stenoses. Improvements in MRI method in the 1990s also introduced another potential noninvasive method to potentially define coronary disease [12].

Budoff et al. reviewed the literature on the use of EBT/MDCT and MRI to noninvasively quantify epicardial coronary stenoses [13]. They concluded that EBT/MDCT can have sensitivities and specificities for defining obstructive coronary disease between 90 and 95%, while MRI fared somewhat less with sensitivity on the order of 77% and specificity of 71%. The general issues for coronary MRI are that spatial resolution is inversely related to temporal resolution and with the need for rapid imaging for coronary visualization, the overall accuracy falls below that of CT.

CONTRAST-ENHANCED CT AND "SOFT" PLAQUE

Contrast-enhanced CT using both EBT and MDCT has been shown to potentially define noncalcified (so called "soft") plaque on a segmental basis (Fig. 2).

The subject of this discussion is defining plaque and predicting heart attack. The question then is: can these methods be used to better define coronary artery plaque burden and/or the potential to define vulnerable pathology?

There have been two studies published to date in this regard. Achenbach and colleagues [14] compared intravascular ultrasound (IVUS) obtained during cardiac catheterization with noninvasive contrast-enhanced coronary studies using MDCT. They found that CT had a sensitivity of about 82% to detect coronary segments with atherosclerotic plaque, but had only a 53% sensitivity of defining segments with noncalcified atherosclerotic plaque. Thus combining CAC and contrast-enhanced segmental definition of "soft" plaque still resulted in significant underestimation of true total atherosclerotic plaque burden.

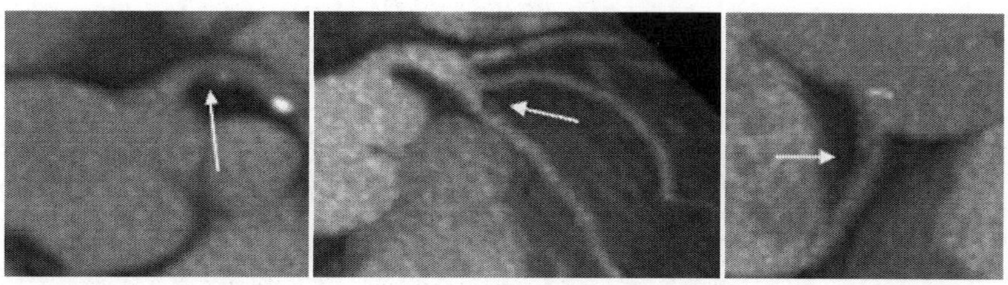

Fig. 2. EBT contrast-enhanced coronary artery scans demonstrating calcified as well as "soft" (noncalcified, low attenuation) plaque.

Leber et al. [15] also performed a comparison between IVUS and contrast-enhanced CT. They reported a sensitivity for "soft" plaque at about 78%, a sensitivity for fibrous plaque at about 78%, while maintaining a sensitivity for "calcified" plaque (as had been shown in prior EBT noncontrast-enhanced studies) of about 95%. Thus in about 80% of the cases, contrast-enhanced CT can be used to provide additional information about noncalcified plaque, but the total "atherosclerotic plaque burden" remains underdefined. Such studies are possible using both EBT and MDCT, but both have specific deficiencies. EBT is limited currently by spatial resolution on the order of 1–1.5 mm as compared with submillimeter definition by MDCT; conversely, EBT can be used across heart rates from 50 to 120 beats/min without the need for beta-blockade to lower resting heart rate due to temporal resolution 2–3 times superior to MDCT. All published studies to date using MDCT have required resting heart rates <65 beats/min for adequate image resolution.

CONCLUSIONS

Contrast-enhanced CT, although possessing great potential as a diagnostic catheterization for defining the absence or presence of "significant" coronary stenotic lesions, is still somewhat limited in defining "noncalcified" plaque and has not been shown currently to provide incremental value in predicting the potential for preventing heart attack. The same can be said for MRI – although there is much discussed on soft versus hard plaque – the characterization of any "soft" plaque as one that it is potentially "vulnerable" remains moot.

REFERENCES

1. Simons DB, Schwartz RS, Edwards WD, Sheedy PF, Breen JF, Rumberger JA: Non-Invasive Definition of Anatomic Coronary Artery Disease by Ultrafast CT: A Quantitative Pathologic Study. J Am Coll Cardiol 1992;20:1118-26
2. Rumberger JA, Simons DB, Fitzpatrick LA, Sheedy PF, Schwartz RS: Coronary Artery Calcium Areas by Electron Beam Computed Tomography and Coronary Atherosclerotic Plaque Area: A Histopathologic Correlative Study. Circulation 1995;92:2157–62
3. Baumgart D, Schmermund A, Goerge G, Haude M, Ge J, Adamzik M, Sehnert C, Altmaier K, Groenemeyer D, Seibel R, Erbel R: Comparison of Electron Beam Computed Tomography with Intracoronary Ultrasound and Coronary Angiography for Detection of Coronary Atherosclerosis. J Am Coll Cardiol 1997;30:57–64
4. Rumberger JA, Sheedy PF, Breen JR, Schwartz RS: Coronary Calcium as Determined by Electron Beam Computed Tomography, and Coronary Disease on Arteriogram: Effect of Patient's Sex on Diagnosis. Circulation 1995;91:1363–7
5. Rumberger JA, Sheedy PF, Breen JF, Schwartz RS: Electron Beam CT Coronary Calcium Score Cutpoints and Severity of Associated Angiography Luminal Stenosis. J Am Coll Cardiol 1997;29:1542–8
6. Wong ND, Hsu JC, Detrano RC, et al. Coronary Artery Calcium Evaluation by Electron Beam Computed Tomography and its Relation to New Cardiovascular Events. Am J Cardiol 2000, 86:495–8
7. Kondos GT, Hoff JA, Sevrukov A, et al. Coronary Artery Calcium and Cardiac Events Electron-Beam Tomography Coronary Artery Calcium and Cardiac Events: A 37-Month Follow- Up of 5,635 Initially Asymptomatic Low to Intermediate Risk Adults. Circulation 2003;107:2571–6
8. Arad Y, Roth M, Newstein D, et al. Coronary Calcification, Coronary Risk Factors, and Atherosclerotic Cardiovascular Disease Events. The St. Francis Heart Study. J Am Coll Cardiol 2003;41:6
9. Sangiorgi G, Rumberger JA, Severson A, Edwards WD, Gregoire J, Fitzpatrick LA, Schwartz RS: Arterial Calcification and Not Lumen Stenosis is Highly Correlated with Atherosclerotic Plaque Burden in Humans: A Histologic Study of 723 Coronary Artery Segments using Non-Decalcifying Methodology. J Am Coll Cardiol 1998;31:126–33
10. Moshage WE, Achenbach S, Seese B: Coronary Artery Stenosis: Three-dimensional Imaging with Electrocardiographically Triggered Contrast Agent Enhanced, Electron-beam CT. Radiology 1995;196:707–14
11. Schmermund A, Rensing BJ, Sheedy PF, Bell MR, Rumberger JA: Intravenous Electron-Beam CT Coronary Angiography for Segmental Analysis of Coronary Artery Stenoses. J Am Coll Cardiol 1998;31:1547–54
12. Manning WJ, Li W, Edelman RR: A Preliminary Report Comparing Magnetic Resonance Coronary Angiography with Conventional Angiography. N Engl J Med 1003;328:828–32
13. Budoff MJ, Achenbach S, Duerinckx A: Clinical Utility of Computed Tomography and Magnetic Resonance Techniques for Noninvasive Coronary Angiography. J Am Coll Cardiol 2003;42:167–78

14. Achenbach S, Moselewski F, Ropers D, Ferencik M, Hoffman U, MacNeill B, Phole K, Baum U, Anders K, Jang IK, Daniel WG, Brady TJ: Detection of Calcified and Noncalcified Coronary Atherosclerotic Plaque by Contrast-Enhanced Submillimeter Multidetector Spiral Computed Tomography. Circulation 2004;109:14–7
15. Leber AW, Knez A, Becker A, Becker C, Ziegler F, Nikolaou K, Rist C, Reiser M, White C, Steinbeck G, Boekstegers P: Accuracy of Multidetector Spiral Computed Tomography in Identifying and Differentiating the Composition of Coronary Atherosclerotic Plaques. JACC 2004;43:1241–7

26 Magnetic Resonance Imaging

Zahi A. Fayad

CONTENTS

Abstract

In the future, the use of imaging methods to quantify the progression and regression of atherothrombosis could play a very strong role in the management of patients. High-resolution, noninvasive cardiovascular magnetic resonance (CMR) imaging has the potential to provide three-dimensional anatomical information about the lumen and the vessel wall. Furthermore, CMR has the ability to characterize atherothrombotic plaque composition and micro-anatomy and therefore to identify lesions at risk to rupture or erosion. The high resolution of CMR and the development of sophisticated contrast agents offer the promise of in vivo molecular imaging of the plaque. This may aid early intervention in both primary and secondary treatment of vascular disease in all arterial beds.

Key words: Magnetic resonance imaging; Atherosclerosis; Noninvasive imaging

KEY POINTS

- Magnetic resonance imaging (MRI) can provide noninvasive assessment of atherosclerosis in the carotid arteries, aorta, and other peripheral vessels
- MRI can measure plaque morphology
- MRI can characterize the components of the plaque
- MRI can be used for the evaluation of regression after therapeutic management

From: *Asymptomatic Atherosclerosis: Pathophysiology, Detection and Treatment*
Edited by: M. Naghavi (ed.), DOI 10.1007/978-1-60327-179-0_26

Cardiovascular Magnetic Resonance (CMR) has emerged as one of the most promising noninvasive imaging modalities for atherosclerotic disease detection [1]. It directly images atherosclerotic lesions, measures atherosclerotic burden, and characterizes plaque components. Atherosclerotic lesion imaging requires the acquisition of high spatial (<1 mm) and contrast resolution, because of the small size of the vessels under consideration, the adjacent lumen, and the size of each plaque structure.

Noninvasive, in vivo high-resolution CMR is performed using dedicated external receiver coils and imaging sequences. Most CMR plaque imaging is currently being performed on a whole-body 1.5T MR system. In vivo CMR plaque imaging and characterization have been performed utilizing a multi-contrast approach with high-resolution black blood spin echo- and fast spin echo-based MR and bright blood sequences. In the black blood sequence, the signal from the flowing blood is rendered black through preparatory pulses. Another technique, bright blood imaging, can be employed in assessing fibrous cap thickness and morphological "integrity" of the carotid artery plaques [2].

PLAQUE BURDEN

Evidence from current studies shows that CMR provides excellent quantitative capabilities for the measurement of total plaque volume and disease burden. It was demonstrated that the error in vessel wall area measurement was 2.6% for aortic and 3.5% for carotid plaques [3]. Similar low measurement errors in plaque area and volume (4–6%) were reported by others, proving that plaque area and volume can be accurately assessed [4, 5]. Therefore, we estimate that changes in plaque size >5.2% or 9 mm^2 (for aortic lesions) and >7% or 3 mm^2 (for carotid lesions) are likely to be measured by MR.

In a longitudinal study of drug therapy, we estimate that to show a statistically significant change in vessel area by MR requires a rather small number of subjects. For example, a 12% true change in vessel wall area compared to baseline requires 15 patients with a power=0.8, and alpha=0.05. Similarly, a 6% true change will require 29 subjects, and a 3% true change will require 108 subjects.

CAROTID ARTERIES

Carotid arteries' superficial location and relative absence of motion present less of a technical challenge for imaging than that presented by the aorta or coronary arteries. Some of the MR studies of carotid arterial plaques include imaging and characterization of atherosclerotic plaques [6, 7], quantification of plaque size [8], and detection of fibrous cap "integrity" [2].

Yuan et al. showed that in vivo multi-contrast CMR of human carotid arteries had a sensitivity of 85% and specificity of 92% for the identification of lipid core and acute intraplaque hemorrhage [6]. Cai et al. demonstrated good agreement between the classification obtained by CMR and the American Heart Association classifications [7]. This study demonstrated that multi-contrast CMR is capable of in vivo classification of the human carotid atherosclerotic plaques.

A recent study demonstrated a strong association between fibrous cap thinning or rupture, as determined by CMR vessel wall imaging, and the history of recent transient ischemic attack (TIA) or stroke [9]. There was a strong and statistically significant trend showing a higher percentage of symptomatic patients for ruptured caps (70%) compared with that for thick caps (9%) (p=0.001 Mann-Whitney test for cap status vs. symptoms). Compared to patients with thick fibrous caps, patients with ruptured caps were 23 times more likely to have had a recent TIA or stroke (95% CI=3, 210). This study indicates that MR identification of a ruptured fibrous cap is highly associated with a recent history of TIA or stroke.

Blake et al. showed that in 46 carotid atherosclerotic patients, **an association existed between elevated plasma levels of soluble CD40 ligand and carotid plaques, as defined by T2W high-spatial resolution MR, and features of high risk without relation to the severity of stenosis [10].

AORTA

It has been shown by CMR that the wall thickness of the ascending aorta is increased in patients with homozygous familial hypercholesterolemia [11]. Thoracic aortic plaque composition and size were compared to match CMR and TEE cross-sectional aortic segments, and it was shown that a strong correlation was present for plaque composition and mean maximum plaque thickness.

A study of asymptomatic subjects from the Framingham Heart Study (FHS) by CMR showed that aortic atherosclerosis prevalence and burden (i.e., plaque volume/aortic volume) significantly increased with age and were higher in the abdominal aorta than in the thoracic aorta [12]. It was also found that long-term measures of risk factors and FHS coronary risk score are strongly associated with asymptomatic aortic atherosclerosis as detected by CMR [12].

In a subset study from the Multiethnic Study of Atherosclerosis (MESA), 196 participants (99 black, 97 white; 98 men, 98 women) who were 45–84 years old without clinical cardiovascular disease were recruited from six study centers in the United States. Average and maximal wall thickness as measured by CMR increased with age. Men had greater mean average wall thickness and mean maximal wall thickness than women. Blacks had greater mean maximal wall thickness than whites. This study shows that CMR is a feasible method to measure aortic wall thickness with high interobserver agreement. Aortic wall thickness increases with age and also varies by race and sex.

RISK FACTORS

Recently a study showing associations of risk factors and plasma inflammatory markers with plaques in both thoracic and abdominal aortas in 102 patients undergoing coronary angiography was performed [13]. Age and systolic blood pressure correlated with plaque extents in both the aortas. The LDL-cholesterol and smoking were characteristically associated with plaques in the thoracic and abdominal aortas, respectively. Regarding inflammatory markers, fibrinogen and C-reactive protein levels correlated with total plaque extent in the aortas. Although plaque extents in both the aortas correlated with the severity of CAD, only thoracic plaques were independently associated with CAD. The thoracic and abdominal aortas may have different susceptibilities to risk factors. However, plasma inflammatory markers appear to reflect total extent of aortic atherosclerosis. Although aortic plaques are common in patients with CAD, only thoracic plaques are an independent factor for CAD.

A study by Weiss et al. in 52 subjects (≥40 years old; average 40–79) showed that increased wall thicknesses on T2W signal and/or on gadolinium contrast enhanced MR in the carotid arteries and aorta were associated with elevated serum levels of the inflammatory markers interleukin 6, C-reactive protein, intercellular adhesion molecule-1, and vascular cell adhesion molecule-1 [14].

TREATMENT

In asymptomatic, untreated, hypercholesterolemic patients with carotid and aortic atherosclerosis, we have shown that MR can be used to measure the effects of lipid-lowering therapy (statins) on plaque regression [3]. Aortic and carotid artery plaques were evaluated in 51 patients at baseline. This work was the first to demonstrate that maintained lipid-lowering therapy with simvastatin is associated with significant regression of established atherosclerotic lesions in humans.

A case-controlled study demonstrated substantially reduced carotid plaque lipid content (with no substantial overall plaque area reduction) in patients treated for 10 years with an aggressive lipid-lowering regimen compared with untreated controls [15].

In an experimental rabbit study, Corti et al. demonstrated the beneficial effects of statins on atherosclerosis followed by MRI and additional anti-atherogenic benefits of combining a PPAR-gamma agonist with simvastatin [16].

FUTURE

Improvements in coronary plaque imaging by MR would be greatly welcomed and it would add to the evaluation of simultaneous multi-vessel (aorta, coronary arteries, carotid arteries, and other peripheral arteries) assessment of atherosclerosis [17]. Future, work may be carried out at 3.0T whole-body MR systems. New black blood techniques have been introduced for the simultaneous acquisition of multiple slices and shown to greatly reduce total examination time [18, 19]. Prospective studies are needed to determine the predictive value of fibrous cap characteristics, as visualized by MR, for risk of subsequent ischemic events [9].

Although early in the development of this noninvasive imaging tool, CMR use for serial monitoring of atherosclerotic plaque progression and regression in the carotid arteries and aorta is clearly progressing rapidly, and may be the noninvasive imaging technology of choice for this purpose in the future, given the high image quality and the sensitivity to small changes in plaque size and possible characterization. For other review papers see [20–22]. Further studies are needed for the correlation of the CMR based plaque imaging findings and prediction of future events.

REFERENCES

1. Fayad ZA, Fuster V, Nikolaou K, Becker C. Computed tomography and magnetic resonance imaging for noninvasive coronary angiography and plaque imaging: current and potential future concepts. Circulation 2002;106:2026–34.
2. Hatsukami TS, Ross R, Polissar NL, Yuan C. Visualization of fibrous cap thickness and rupture in human atherosclerotic carotid plaque in vivo with high-resolution magnetic resonance imaging. Circulation 2000;102:959–64.
3. Corti R, Fayad ZA, Fuster V, Worthley SG, Helft G, Chesebro J, Mercuri M, Badimon JJ. Effects of lipid-lowering by simvastatin on human atherosclerotic lesions: a longitudinal study by high-resolution, noninvasive magnetic resonance imaging. Circulation 2001;104:249–52.
4. Kang X, Polissar NL, Han C, Lin E, Yuan C. Analysis of the measurement precision of arterial lumen and wall areas using high-resolution MRI. Magn Reson Med 2000;44:968–72.
5. Chan SK, Jaffer FA, Botnar RM, Kissinger KV, Goepfert L, Chuang ML, O'Donnell CJ, Levy D, Manning WJ. Scan reproducibility of magnetic resonance imaging assessment of aortic atherosclerosis burden. J Cardiovasc Magn Reson 2001;3:331–338.
6. Yuan C, Mitsumori LM, Ferguson MS, Polissar NL, Echelard D, Ortiz G, Small R, Davies JW, Kerwin WS, Hatsukami TS. In vivo accuracy of multispectral magnetic resonance imaging for identifying lipid-rich necrotic cores and intraplaque hemorrhage in advanced human carotid plaques. Circulation 2001;104:2051–6.
7. Cai JM, Hatsukami TS, Ferguson MS, Small R, Polissar NL, Yuan C. Classification of human carotid atherosclerotic lesions with in vivo multicontrast magnetic resonance imaging. Circulation 2002;106:1368–1373.
8. Yuan C, Beach KW, Smith LH, Jr., Hatsukami TS. Measurement of atherosclerotic carotid plaque size in vivo using high resolution magnetic resonance imaging. Circulation 1998;98:2666–71.
9. Yuan C, Zhang SH, Polissar NL, Echelard D, Ortiz G, Davis JW, Ellington E, Ferguson MS, Hatsukami TS. Identification of fibrous cap rupture with magnetic resonance imaging is highly associated with recent transient ischemic attack or stroke. Circulation 2002;105:181–185.
10. Blake GJ, Ostfeld RJ, Yucel EK, Varo N, Schonbeck U, Blake MA, Gerhard M, Ridker PM, Libby P, Lee RT. Soluble CD40 ligand levels indicate lipid accumulation in carotid atheroma: an in vivo study with high-resolution MRI. Arterioscler Thromb Vasc Biol 2003;23:e11–e14.
11. Summers RM, Andrasko-Bourgeois J, Feuerstein IM, Hill SC, Jones EC, Busse MK, Wise B, Bove KE, Rishforth BA, Tucker E, Spray TL, Hoeg JM. Evaluation of the aortic root by MRI: insights from patients with homozygous familial hypercholesterolemia. Circulation 1998;98:509–518.
12. Jaffer FA, O'Donnell CJ, Larson MG, Chan SK, Kissinger KV, Kupka MJ, Salton C, Botnar RM, Levy D, Manning WJ. Age and sex distribution of subclinical aortic atherosclerosis: a magnetic resonance imaging examination of the Framingham Heart Study. Arterioscler Thromb Vasc Biol 2002;22:849–854.

13. Taniguchi H, Momiyama Y, Fayad ZA, Ohmori R, Ashida K, Kihara T, Hara A, Arakawa K, Kameyama A, Noya K, Nagata M, Nakamura H, Ohsuzu F. In vivo magnetic resonance evaluation of the associations between aortic atherosclerosis and both risk factors and coronary artery disease in patients referred for coronary angiography. Am Heart J 2004;148(1):137–143.
14. Weiss CR, Arai AE, Bui MN, Agyeman KO, Waclawiw MA, Balaban RS, Cannon RO. Arterial wall MRI characteristics are associated with elevated serum markers of inflammation in humans. J Magn Reson Imaging 2001;14:698–704.
15. Zhao XQ, Yuan C, Hatsukami TS, Frechette EH, Kang XJ, Maravilla KR, Brown BG. Effects of prolonged intensive lipid-lowering therapy on the characteristics of carotid atherosclerotic plaques in vivo by MRI: a case-control study. Arterioscler Thromb Vasc Biol 2001;21:1623–1629.
16. Corti R, Osende JI, Fallon JT, Fuster V, Mizsei G, Jneid H, Wright SD, Chaplin WF, Badimon JJ. The selective peroxisomal proliferator-activated receptor-gamma agonist has an additive effect on plaque regression in combination with simvastatin in experimental atherosclerosis: in vivo study by high-resolution magnetic resonance imaging. Journal of the American College of Cardiology 2004;43:464–473.
17. Fayad ZA, Fuster V, Fallon JT, Jayasundera T, Worthley SG, Helft G, Aguinaldo JG, Badimon JJ, Sharma SK. Noninvasive in vivo human coronary artery lumen and wall imaging using black-blood magnetic resonance imaging. Circulation 2000;102:506–510.
18. Itskovich VV, Mani V, Mizsei G, Aguinaldo JG, Samber DD, Macaluso F, Wisdom P, Fayad ZA. Parallel and nonparallel simultaneous multislice black-blood double inversion recovery techniques for vessel wall imaging. J Magn Reson Imaging 2004;19:459–67.
19. Mani V, Itskovich VV, Szimtenings M, Aguinaldo JG, Samber DD, Mizsei G, Fayad ZA. Rapid extended coverage simultaneous multisection black-blood vessel wall MR imaging. Radiology 2004;232(1):281–288.
20. Rudd JH, Myers KS, Sanz J, Fayad ZA. Multimodality imaging of atherosclerosis (magnetic resonance imaging/computed tomography/positron emission tomography-computed tomography). Top Magn Reson Imaging 2007;18(5):379–388.
21. Momiyama Y, Fayad ZA. Aortic plaque imaging and monitoring atherosclerotic plaque interventions. Top Magn Reson Imaging 2007;18(5):349–355.
22. Sanz J, Fayad ZA. Imaging of atherosclerotic cardiovascular disease. Nature 2008;451(7181):953–957.

27 The Role of MRI in Examining Subclinical Carotid Plaque

Chun Yuan, Hideki Ota, Xihai Zhao, and Tom Hatsukami

Contents

Abstract

Stroke is the third leading cause of death in the United States. The degree of luminal narrowing evaluated by angiography is the standard for assessing the risk of stroke in patients with carotid atherosclerosis and for determining the need for surgical intervention. However, multiple studies have shown that clinical events arise not from the degree of stenosis but from the morphologic characteristics and plaque composition. This is borne out by the difference in absolute risk reduction between symptomatic and asymptomatic patients who receive surgical carotid endarterectomy (CEA). Future clinical practice may diagnose patients with high-risk atherosclerosis, based on plaque characteristics and morphology rather than the degree of stenosis alone. Carotid MRI is a noninvasive imaging method that can provide information on atherosclerotic plaque morphology, composition, and progression or regression. This chapter describes the current capabilities of MRI for visualizing carotid atherosclerosis, including MRI protocols to appropriately evaluate carotid plaque, the image features of carotid arteries, and the future direction of carotid MR imaging and how it can be better used for the management of patients with subclinical atherosclerosis, resulting in a higher quality of life.

Key words: Atherosclerosis; Atherosclerosis biomarkers; Carotid; Heart disease; Imaging biomarkers; MRI; Plaque Imaging; Stenosis; Stroke

From: *Asymptomatic Atherosclerosis: Pathophysiology, Detection and Treatment*
Edited by: M. Naghavi (ed.), DOI 10.1007/978-1-60327-179-0_27

KEY POINTS

- Techniques and protocols for imaging atherosclerosis with Carotid MRI (CMRI)
- Key Features of Vulnerable Carotid Lesions and Their MR Characteristics
- Plaque Burden Measurement
- Future Directions of Plaque Imaging and Carotid MRI

INTRODUCTION

Each year, about 700,000 people in the United States experience a new or recurrent stroke [1], and stroke ranks third among all causes of death, after cancer and heart disease [2]. Even for survivors, stroke is a leading cause of serious long-term disability: 15–30% of stroke survivors are permanently disabled. Methods to evaluate arterial plaque and predict stroke would have a significant effect on lowering the impact of this disease.

Carotid luminal narrowing evaluated by angiography is the standard for assessing the risk of stroke in patients with carotid atherosclerosis and for determining the need for surgical intervention [3]. Although the risk of stroke increases with higher grades of stenosis, the fact that low-grade stenosis may also result in stroke implies that predicting future cerebrovascular ischemic events in patients with carotid atherosclerosis is not possible on the basis of the degree of stenosis alone [4]. Recent studies have consistently shown that individuals with extensive plaque burden have a very high risk of stroke regardless of their risk factor profile [5]. It is also known from past studies of coronary arteries that plaque rupture may occur in areas with low degrees of narrowing and that the degree of narrowing is a poor predictor of events [6]. The catastrophic ischemic events associated with atherosclerosis are most often related to sudden rupture or to the erosion of a vulnerable plaque. These plaques must progress to a substantial size before demonstrating significant stenosis by angiography [6].

Therefore, factors other than the degree of stenosis – including plaque composition, remodeling, and inflammation – should be taken into account when evaluating carotid atherosclerosis. An imaging modality that can identify vulnerable plaques is needed to produce a treatment plan for patients with atherosclerosis.

Carotid MRI is noninvasive, can provide morphological and progression or regression information, and has the potential to monitor systemic atherosclerosis, as increases in the thickness of the carotid intima were directly associated with an increased risk of myocardial infarction and stroke in older adults with no history of cardiovascular disease [7]. MRI is uniquely suited for atherosclerosis imaging. It is a noninvasive procedure, and has the ability to depict not only the degree of stenosis but also the arterial wall itself, including plaque morphology and composition. MRI has high soft tissue contrast resolution and can provide 3D distribution of lesions. For MR imaging of the carotid atherosclerotic plaque, many past studies have demonstrated good correlations between histology and MRI for the delineation of plaque tissue composition, including the lipid/necrotic cores, fibrous cap, dense and loose fibrous matrix, intraplaque hemorrhage, and calcification [8–13].

One aim of carotid MR imaging for patients with subclinical atherosclerosis is to screen and detect vulnerable patients, based on the identifying features of vulnerable plaque, in order to prevent future cerebrovascular ischemic events. In this chapter, we will describe the current aspects of MRI for carotid atherosclerosis, including MRI protocols to appropriately evaluate carotid plaque, the image features of carotid arteries, and the future direction of carotid MR imaging and how it can be better utilized for the management of patients with subclinical atherosclerosis, resulting in a higher quality of life. Also presented are three subclinical cases that demonstrate the practical value of current MRI techniques: carotid fibrous cap disruption, intraplaque hemorrhage, and expandable plaque burden with mild stenosis.

CAROTID PLAQUE MR IMAGING TECHNIQUES

Carotid Plaque Imaging Pulse Sequences

In general terms, the pulse sequences designed for carotid artery imaging use multicontrast-weighted MR techniques including "black-blood" and "bright-blood" techniques. These techniques either suppress or enhance the signal from flowing blood. Each of these two types of sequences offers specific advantages for carotid imaging.

Black-blood techniques refer to MR techniques which suppress the signal from flowing blood [14]. These sequences are good for plaque imaging, because the conspicuity of the vessel wall is increased when adjacent to a hypointense lumen and the echo and repetition times can be easily controlled to optimize visualization of specific plaque components. Common flow-suppression techniques used with black-blood imaging are Double Inversion Recovery (DIR) and Quadruple Inversion Recovery (QIR) sequences [15, 16]. DIR sequences tend to provide excellent flow suppression, as shown on T1-weighted (T1W) images [17]. A number of time-efficient versions of DIR have also been introduced [18]. QIR is an effective technique for black-blood imaging when T1 contrast agent is applied [16, 19]. These images typically allow the most accurate quantitative measurements of disease burden and are used to identify lipid rich necrotic cores in vivo [20].

Bright-blood techniques refer to the Gradient Recalled Echo (GRE) based imaging sequences used to acquire MR angiograms. These sequences, such as GRE and spoiled GRE, enhance the signal intensity of flowing blood; thus, the lumen appears hyperintense relative to the adjacent vessel wall. Compared with SE sequences, bright-blood techniques can produce images with shorter repetition and echo times. The lack of spin echo in these sequences creates a T2*-sensitive tissue signal improves the visibility of calcifications and the fibrous cap, which is generally a densely structured layer of collagen [10, 21]. Faster imaging also allows the acquisition of high-spatial-resolution 3D data sets, which should improve plaque characterization [22]. We currently incorporate a 3D TOF sequence to obtain transverse GRE images in protocols for carotid plaque characterization. These images have been useful for evaluating the in vivo state of the fibrous cap and for detecting large intraplaque hemorrhages [20].

Carotid Plaque Imaging Protocol

Most current carotid imaging is done with a 1.5T whole-body MR scanner. The superficial configuration of the carotid arteries is well suited for the use of phased-array surface coils, and a dedicated phased-array coil assembly [23] with overall dimensions of 6.4×10.8 cm was constructed for imaging. With this coil assembly, an effective longitudinal coverage of up to 5 cm can be achieved. This coil, initially designed over 10 years ago, remains indispensable for carotid MR Imaging. A standardized multicontrast-weighted MR imaging protocol was developed to reproducibly evaluate the in vivo morphology of carotid plaques. The protocol (a) allows the acquisition of high-spatial-resolution transverse images of bilateral carotid arteries, with both black-blood and bright-blood techniques; (b) provides an oblique view of the carotid artery to better demonstrate the location of the carotid bifurcation and the plaque distribution; (c) uses the bifurcation as an internal landmark to enable reproducible selection of section locations for serial studies; and (d) restricts the total examination time to 40 min or less. Currently, four imaging sequences (3D TOF, T1W QIR, T2-weighted DIR, and intermediate-weighted DIR) are performed to generate four contrast weightings at each section location. Signal characteristics of carotid atherosclerotic plaques in multicontrast-weighted MR imaging are summarized in Table 1. Furthermore, postcontrast T1W MR imaging using gadolinium as a contrast agent is helpful for detecting the necrotic core and fibrous cap [24]. By applying a zero-filled

Table 1
Signal characteristics of carotid atherosclerotic plaque

	TOF	*T1W*	*PDW*	*T2W*	*CE-*
Lipid-rich/necrotic core with					
Little or no hemorrhage	o	o/+	o/+	–/o	–
With Type I hemorrhage	+	+	–/o	–/o	–
With Type II hemorrhage	+	+	+	+	–
Calcium	–	–	–	–	–
Loose fibrous matrix	o	–/o	+	+	+

Note: + hyperintense; o iso-intense; – hypointense (this represents a range of SI); Contrast enhancement in CE-T1W present (+) or absent (–)

Fourier transform [24] applied to all sequences, a voxel size of 0.30×0.30×2.0 mm was achieved for the black-blood and bright-blood sequences. Chemical-selective fat saturation is used for all sequences to reduce the signal from the subcutaneous tissues [25, 26].

KEY FEATURES OF VULNERABLE CAROTID LESIONS AND THEIR MR CHARACTERISTICS

Fibrous Cap Disruption and Surface Rupture

A large necrotic core covered by a thin fibrous cap infiltrated by macrophages and lymphocytes is considered the hallmark of a plaque prone to rupture. When the fibrous cap ruptures the underlying necrotic thrombogenic material is exposed to flowing blood and a thrombus forms [27]. Spagnoli et al. [28] found that thrombosis associated with plaque rupture is one of the major determinants of ischemic stroke in patients affected by carotid atherosclerotic disease. In addition, they showed the presence of a fresh thrombus several months after the first cerebrovascular event, suggesting that the continuous vulnerable state of the plaque may trigger continuous release of embolic material if the plaque is not removed, which in turn may be related to subsequent cerebrovascular events.

Carotid MRI can evaluate fibrous cap status both qualitatively and quantitatively. Hatsukami et al. [10] were the first to report the use of a 3D TOF bright-blood imaging technique to identify a ruptured fibrous cap in vivo in atherosclerotic human carotid arteries. The in vivo state of the fibrous cap was characterized, on the basis of its appearance on MR images, as being "intact and thick" (defined as a uniform dark band between the bright lumen and the gray plaque core contents), "intact and thin" (defined as the absence of the dark band between the bright lumen and the gray plaque core), or "ruptured" (defined as the absence of the dark band between the lumen and the plaque core and the presence of a bright gray region adjacent to the lumen, corresponding to recent plaque hemorrhage or mural thrombus). They found that the appearance of the fibrous cap on MRI closely agreed with gross and histological findings, with Cohen kappa=0.83 (95% confidence interval=0.67, 1.00) and weighted kappa=0.87. Mitsumori et al. [29] demonstrated that in vivo MR imaging using a multisequence protocol generating four contrast weightings (3D TOF, T1, proton density, and T2) has a high test sensitivity (0.81) and specificity (0.90) for identifying a thin or ruptured cap, as compared with carotid endarterectomy specimens.

Trivedi et al. [30] used a short T1 inversion-recovery image sequence to quantify the fibrous cap and lipid-rich necrotic core of 25 recently symptomatic patients and correlated the results with the carotid endarterectomy specimens. The authors showed good agreement between MR- and histology-derived quantification of both fibrous cap and lipid core content (the mean % difference for the fibrous cap was –0.75%, and for the lipid core was –0.86%), with good interobserver agreement (intraclass correlation coefficients of 0.94 and 0.88 for the quantification of the fibrous cap and lipid core, respectively) [30].

It has been reported that gadolinium-enhanced postcontrast T1W MR images have helped discriminate the fibrous cap from the necrotic core [9, 31]. In a study of nine subjects with carotid atherosclerosis, Wassermann et al. [31] found that gadolinium-enhanced T1W images, based on selective enhancement of the fibrous cap relative to the lipid core, helped discriminate these two plaque components with a contrast-to-noise ratio as good as or better than that of T2-weighted MR images but with approximately twice the signal-to-noise ratio (postcontrast images, 36.6±3.6; T2-weighted images, 17.5±2.1; $P<0.001$). Yuan et al. demonstrated, in the comparison of pre- and post gadolinium enhanced T1W images of carotid MRI, statistically significant differences in the mean intensity change between tissues, with the largest increase for the fibrous tissue (79.5%) and the smallest for the necrotic core (28.6%) [9]. Cai et al. [24] showed a moderate to good correlation between findings from carotid MR imaging and the excised histological specimen for the maximal thickness ($r=0.78$, $P<0.001$), length ($r=0.73$, $P<0.001$), and area ($r=0.90$, $P<0.001$) of the intact fibrous cap, using unenhanced T1W and contrast-enhanced T1W images.

With the current MRI protocol, it is preferable to use multisequence imaging to evaluate fibrous cap status [32]. If gadolinium injection is available, postcontrast T1W images are useful, in addition to T2-weighted images, in differentiating between the thin or thick fibrous cap. TOF images are indispensable in detecting recent plaque hemorrhage due to a ruptured fibrous cap, though the irregular surface shape seen on the other black-blood images is also helpful (Fig. 1).

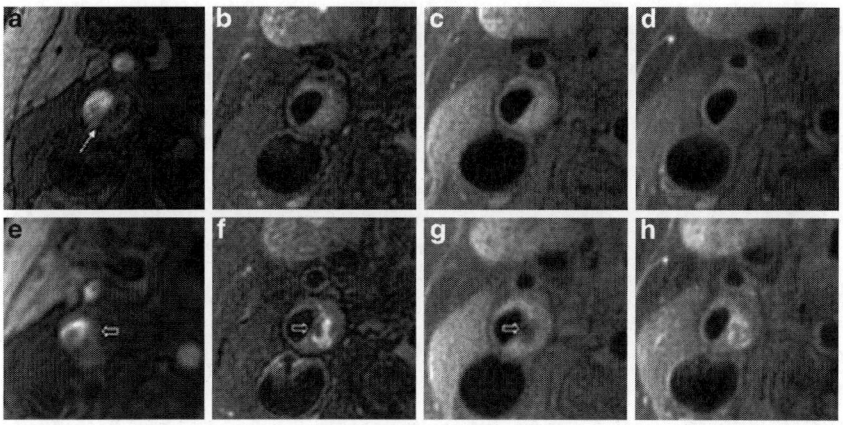

Fig. 1. (**a–d**), Matched baseline images ((**a**), 3-dimensional time of flight; (**b**), T_2-weighted; (**c**), precontrast-enhanced, T_1-weighted; and (**d**), postcontrast-enhanced, T_1-weighted, obtained by high-spatial-resolution MRI, demonstrate carotid atherosclerotic plaque and luminal stenosis in the right internal carotid artery. A dark band between the lumen and arterial wall (*arrow*, (**a**)) suggests intact fibrous cap (http://circ.ahajournals.org/cgi/content/full/113/12/e660#R1-173946). Hyperintense signal on images (**a**), (**b**), and (**c**) suggests presence of intraplaque hemorrhage (http://circ.ahajournals.org/cgi/content/full/113/12/e660#R2-173946). Follow-up MR images (**e**) through (**g**) (corresponding to images (**a**) through (**c**), respectively, in sequence and location) demonstrate surface disruption (*open arrows*) and a penetrating ulcer. The signal within the ulcer demonstrates hyperintense signal on (**e**), mixed hyperintense and hypointense signal on (**f**), hypointense signal on (**g**), and contrast enhancement on (**h**). This signal pattern suggests turbulent flow within the ulcer. Note slight location mismatch between postcontrast-enhanced T_1-weighted images at baseline (**d**) and follow-up (**h**). This mismatch resulted from the patient's minimum motion during image acquisition of image (**h**). Reprinted from [32].

Fibrous cap rupture detected by MRI is associated with multiple clinical symptoms. Yuan et al. [33] showed that the identification of a ruptured fibrous cap by MRI was highly associated with a recent history of TIA or stroke. In 28 symptomatic and 25 asymptomatic subjects, patients with a ruptured cap were 23 times more likely (95% confidence interval: 3,210) to have had a recent transient ischemic attack or stroke, compared to those with a thick fibrous cap. Takaya et al. [34] demonstrated in a prospective study that the presence of a thin or ruptured fibrous cap was associated with subsequent symptoms with a hazard ratio of 17.0 during a mean follow-up period of 38.2 months.

Intraplaque Hemorrhage

The precise mechanisms behind the development of intraplaque hemorrhage are not fully understood [35]. One likely explanation, based on the histological examination of coronary arteries from patients who had a sudden coronary death, is that plaque fissuring leads to the transfer of erythrocytes from the lumen into the plaque [27, 36]. Alternatively, intraplaque hemorrhage may arise from the disruption of thin-walled microvessels lacking smooth-muscle cells [37], as intraplaque hemorrhage is strongly associated with an increased density in microvessels [38].

Intraplaque hemorrhage can cause plaque progression and plaque rupture. Free cholesterol in the necrotic core can be derived from the apoptotic cell death of the foamy cells containing cholesterol in the plaque. On the other hand, in a histological study of coronary arteries, Kolodgie et al. [37] demonstrated that the accumulation of erythrocyte membranes within an atherosclerotic plaque may represent a potent atherogenic stimulus by contributing to the deposition of free cholesterol, macrophage infiltration, and enlargement of the necrotic core. Erythrocyte membranes are said to be a richer source of cholesterol than any other cell in the body [4]. These factors may increase the risk of plaque destabilization. In addition, the incidence of intraplaque hemorrhage detected histologically was higher in the plaques from symptomatic patients, and intraplaque hemorrhage correlated strongly with plaque rupture [39]. Therefore, detection of intraplaque hemorrhage may play an important role in discriminating unstable plaque.MRI is a reliable method for evaluating intraplaque hemorrhage in the carotid artery and has good accuracy when matched with the histology of carotid endarterectomy specimens [8, 40–42]. Intraplaque hemorrhage is typically detected as a high signal intensity area on a T1W sequence, presumably because of the formation of met-hemoglobin in red blood cells resulting in a shortening of T1 [42]. Moody et al. demonstrated that a T1W magnetization-prepared three-dimensional gradient echo sequence can detect met-hemoglobin within the intraplaque hemorrhage of carotid vessels, with a histology confirmation showing asensitivity and specificity of 84% [42]. Cappendijk et al. reported a sensitivity and specificity of 93% for the detection of carotid intraplaque hemorrhage using T1W turbo field echo imaging (95% confidence interval: 77%, 99%) and 96% [41].

On the other hand, intraplaque hemorrhage shows a variable signal pattern on proton density-weighted and T2-weighted sequences, based on hemorrhage types (Fig. 2). Type I hemorrhage, which is histologically discriminated by intact red blood cells with intracellular methemoblobin, appears iso- to hypointense on proton density weighted and T2-weighted images, whereas Type II hemorrhage, which is discriminated by histologically lytic red blood cells with extracellular methemoblobin, appears hyperintense on all weighted images [40, 43]. Chu et al. [40] demonstrated that MRI using multiple sequences of 3D TOF, T1W, proton density-weighted, and T2-weighted images visualized intraplaque hemorrhage of the carotid artery with a sensitivity of 90% and specificity of 74% as against histology, and also demonstrated moderate agreement between MRI and histology in classifying the stages of intraplaque hemorrhage.

The detection of intraplaque hemorrhage by MRI has the potential to become an important tool for characterizing carotid plaque and predicting future clinical conditions in patients. Saam et al. [43]

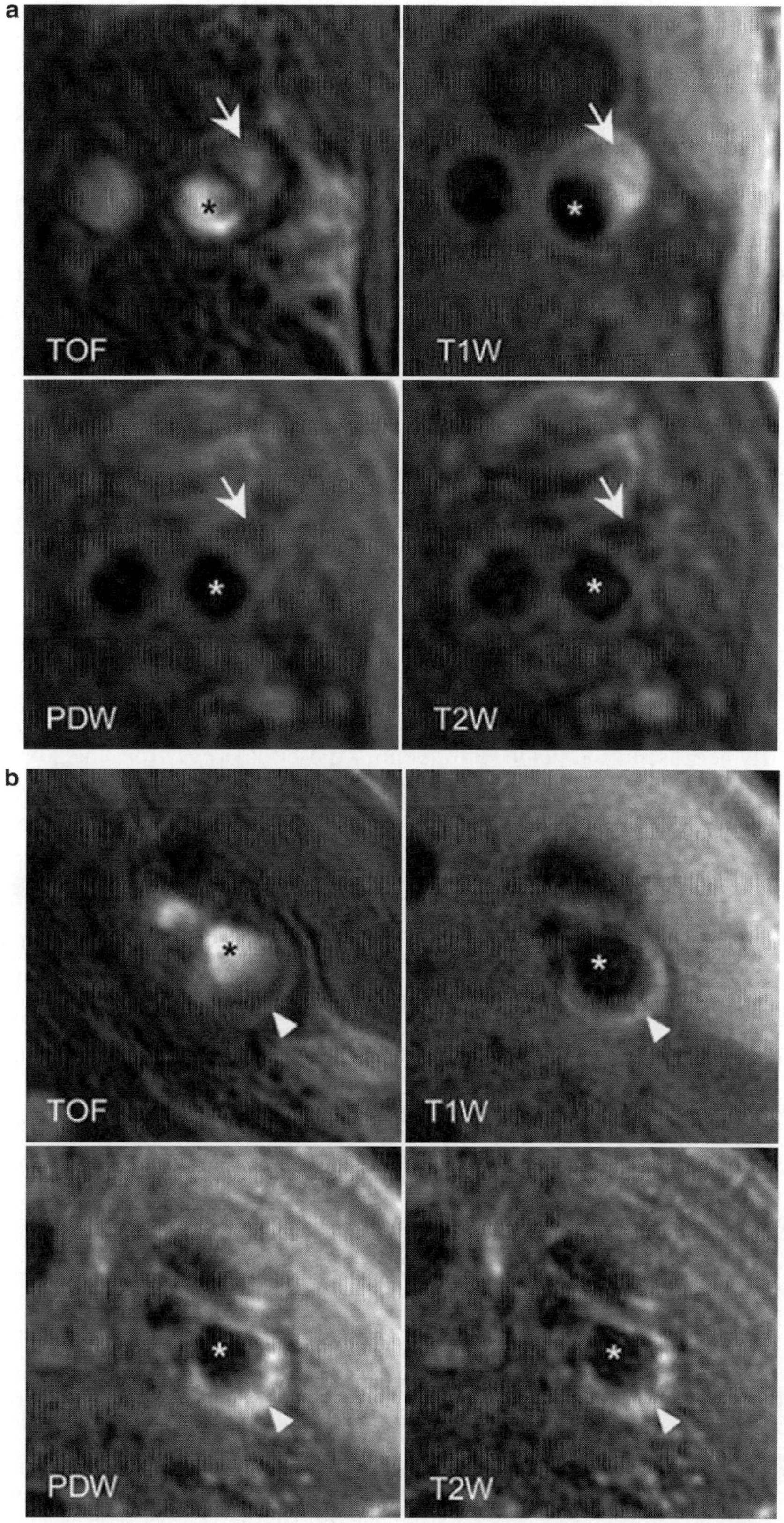

Fig. 2. Examples of lipid-rich necrotic core with intraplaque hemorrhage. (**a**) Type I hemorrhage. Signal intensity patterns are hyperintensity on TOF and T1W images and hypointensity on PD/T2 images (*arrows*). (**b**) Type II hemorrhage. Signal intensity patterns show hyperintensity on all four contrast weightings (*arrowheads*). Asterisks show location of lumen. Reprinted from [46].

demonstrated a significant correlation between Type I hemorrhage and recent transient ischemic attack or stroke. In a prospective longitudinal cohort study of 64 symptomatic patients with mild to moderate (30–69%) carotid stenosis, Altaf et al. [44] demonstrated that recurrent cerebrovascular events were more frequent in those with ipsilateral carotid intraplaque compared to those without during follow up, a period of a median of 28 months (hazard ratio=9.8, 95% confidence interval 1.3–75.1, $P=0.03$). These trends were also observed in a symptomatic patient cohort with high-grade carotid stenosis [45]. Intraplaque hemorrhage does not always occur in symptomatic patients and may be a significant factor in the plaque progression of asymptomatic patients.

Takaya et al. [46] demonstrated that the presence of intraplaque hemorrhage, detected by high-resolution MRI, stimulates the progression of carotid atherosclerotic plaques in asymptomatic patient groups. They revealed that the percent change in wall volume (6.8% vs. –0.15%; $P=0.009$) and lipid-rich necrotic core volume (28.4% vs. –5.2%; $P=0.001$) was significantly higher in the hemorrhage group than in the controls over an 18-month study period. Furthermore, those with intraplaque hemorrhage at baseline were much more likely to have new plaque hemorrhages at 18 months when compared with controls (43% vs. 0%; $P=0.006$). Therefore, the ability of MRI to detect intraplaque hemorrhage in carotid arteries may become a helpful tool for the management of patients with subclinical atherosclerosis (Fig. 3).

Plaque Burden and Low-Grade Carotid Stenosis

There have been no studies linking stroke to features of extracranial carotid atheroma causing low-grade stenosis, partly because of the inability to identify these features before the advent of MRI and because large plaques with little hemodynamic effect are overlooked. Not all culprit carotid plaques (plaques causing TIA or stroke) cause high-grade luminal stenosis. Nonetheless, low-grade carotid stenosis is very prevalent. The cardiovascular health study detected carotid stenosis of <50% in 68% of men and 57% of women over 64 years of age by ultrasound [47], and a study by Saam et al. [48]. showed that the prevalence of AHA lesion Type VI (complicated plaques) was 16.5% in the 97 arteries with <50% stenosis. The most common reason for a lesion to be classified as a Type VI lesion was hemorrhage (65.7%), followed by fibrous cap rupture (26.4%) and others (7.7%) [48]. Although the risk of stroke with <50% stenosis is low, the attributable risk for stroke resulting from <50% carotid

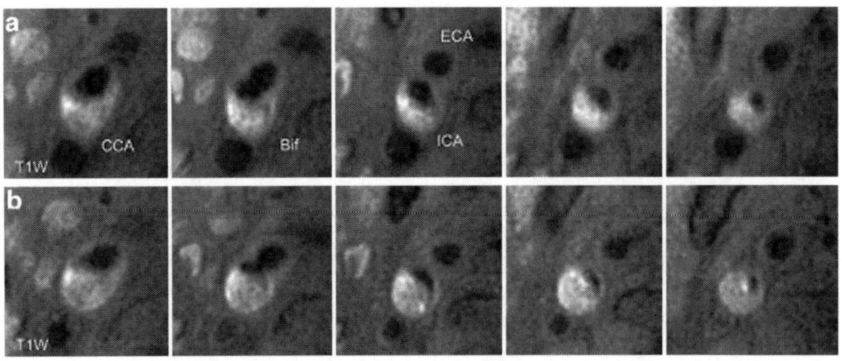

Fig. 3. T1-weighted images of progression of atherosclerosis with intraplaque hemorrhage (high signal intensity area) in right carotid artery. Each column presents matched cross-sectional locations in carotid artery of an asymptomatic patient from baseline MRI (**a**) and MRI obtained 18 months later (**b**). Lumen area decreased, and wall area increased in each section at the second examination. *CCA* indicates common carotid artery; *Bif* bifurcation; *ICA* internal carotid artery; and *ECA* external carotid artery. Reprinted from [34].

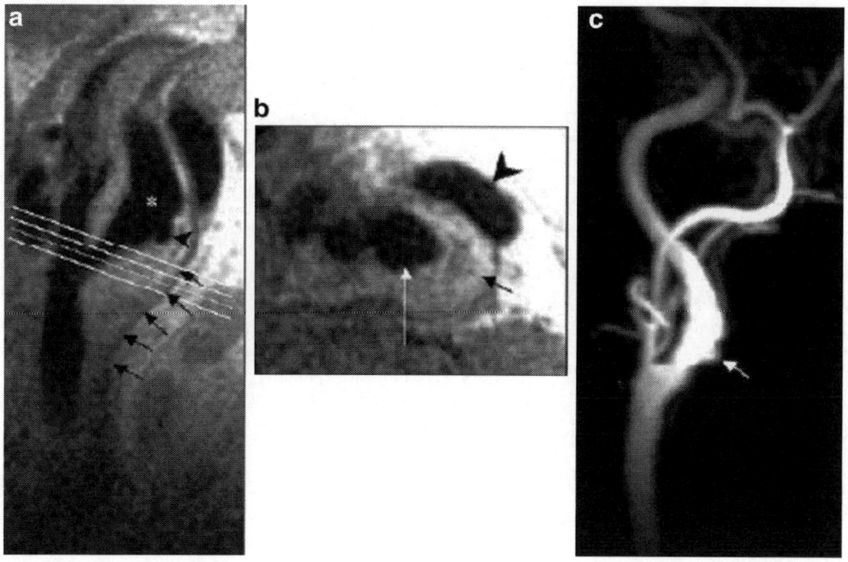

Fig. 4. High-resolution MRI examination from December 2001 of the left carotid artery of a 67-year-old man with hyperlipidemia and left cerebral ischemic events beginning in August 2001. (**a**) Long-axis Black-Blood MRI image through the carotid bifurcation reveals a large plaque along the outer wall of the bulb (*long arrows*) narrowing the internal carotid artery lumen (*) with a small ulceration along its distal margin (*arrowhead*). (**b**) Double oblique Black-Blood MRI image oriented through the plaque as shown in **a** (*dotted line*, **a**) demonstrates outward expansion of the plaque (*black arrow*) with compression of the adjacent jugular vein (*arrowhead*) and relative preservation of the internal carotid artery lumen (*white arrow*) corroborated by the insignificant narrowing seen on the CEMRA MIP (**c**). The small ulceration is again seen (*white arrow*). FD indicates flow divider. Reprinted from [6].

stenosis may be significant as result of the high prevalence of this finding. Wasserman et al. [6] established that for low-grade carotid stenosis, high-resolution MRI plays an important role in assessing plaque features in compensatory remodeling, in monitoring atherosclerotic plaque progression, and in identifying culprit lesions (Fig. 4). A challenge of evaluating low-grade carotid stenosis ipsilateral to a cerebrovascular ischemic event is in demonstrating whether the event is caused by the lesion. The aortic arch is another source of cerebrovascular ischemic events. Shimizu et al. [49] showed that an increase in carotid intima media thickness is associated with complex aortic atheromas which are more likely to lead to embolic events. Inzitari et al. [50] showed that stroke risk is substantially less in the territory of an asymptomatic carotid artery than in a symptomatic artery with a similar degree of stenosis.

FUTURE DIRECTIONS

Carotid artery high-resolution MRI can evaluate the vulnerability of atherosclerotic plaque and monitor the disease progression in patients with risk of heart attack and stroke. This technique may be able to provide valuable information about the progression of a lesion before it becomes a culprit lesion that causes clinical symptoms. With new techniques being developed and the advent of new MR scanner hardware and software, it is possible that the current scan protocols can be improved from 2D to 3D acquisition [51, 52] and converted to a more efficient screening tool that is economically feasible for a population-based study. Such screening may be used for finding patients who have significant lesion development, despite minimal lumen stenosis. We can study the risk factor associations with the features of carotid plaque of asymptomatic individuals using high-resolution MRI. A multiethnic study of atherosclerosis (MESA) established that plasma total cholesterol is strongly associated with lipid core presence by MRI [53]. This and other ongoing studies will help to establish MRI-based lesion features associated with increased risk of cardiovascular events among clinically silent plaques.

REFERENCES

1. Rosamond W, Flegal K, Furie K et al. Heart disease and stroke statistics – 2008 update: a report from the American Heart Association Statistics Committee and Stroke Statistics Subcommittee. Circulation. 2008, 117(4):e25–146
2. Prevalence of stroke–United States, 2005. Centers for Disease Control and Prevention (CDC). MMWR Morb Mortal Wkly Rep. 2007 May 18;56(19):469–74
3. Biller J, Feinberg WM, Castaldo JE et al. Guidelines for carotid endarterectomy: a statement for healthcare professionals from a Special Writing Group of the Stroke Council, American Heart Association. Circulation. 1998, 97(5):501–9
4. Virmani R, Ladich ER, Burke AP, Kolodgie FD. Histopathology of carotid atherosclerotic disease. Neurosurgery. 2006, 59:S219–27
5. Naghavi M. Preventive cardiology: the SHAPE of the future. A synopsis from the screening for heart attack prevention and education (SHAPE) task force report. Herz. 2007, 32:356–61
6. Wasserman BA, Wityk RJ, Trout HH 3rd et al. Low-grade carotid stenosis: looking beyond the lumen with MRI. Stroke. 2005, 36(11):2504–13
7. O'Leary DH, Polak JF, Kronmal RA et al. Carotid-artery intima and media thickness as a risk factor for myocardial infarction and stroke in older adults. Cardiovascular Health Study Collaborative Research Group. N Engl J Med. 1999, 340(1):14–22
8. Yuan C, Mitsumori LM, Ferguson MS et al. In vivo accuracy of multispectral magnetic resonance imaging for identifying lipid-rich necrotic cores and intraplaque hemorrhage in advanced human carotid plaques. Circulation. 2001, 104:2051–6
9. Yuan C, Kerwin WS, Ferguson MS et al. Contrast-enhanced high resolution MRI for atherosclerotic carotid artery tissue characterization. J Magn Reson Imaging. 2002, 15:62–67
10. Hatsukami TS, Ross R, Polissar NL et al. Visualization of fibrous cap thickness and rupture in human atherosclerotic carotid plaque in vivo with high-resolution magnetic resonance imaging. Circulation. 2000, 102:959–64
11. Cai JM, Hatsukami TS, Ferguson MS et al. Classification of human carotid atherosclerotic lesions with in vivo multicontrast magnetic resonance imaging. Circulation. 2002, 106:1368–73
12. Toussaint JF, LaMuraglia GM, Southern JF et al. Magnetic resonance images lipid, fibrous, calcified, hemorrhagic, and thrombotic components of human atherosclerosis in vivo. Circulation. 1996, 94:932–8
13. Clarke SE, Hammond RR, Mitchell JR et al. Quantitative assessment of carotid plaque composition using multicontrast MRI and registered histology. Magn Reson Med. 2003, 50:1199–208
14. Finn JP, Edelman RR. Black-blood and segmented k-space magnetic resonance angiography. Magn Reson Imaging Clin N Am. 1993, 1:349–57
15. Edelman RR, Chien D, Kim D, et al. Fast selective black blood MR imaging. Radiology. 1991, 181:655–60
16. Yarnykh VL, Yuan C. *T1*-insensitive flow suppression using quadruple inversion-recovery. Magn Reson Med. 2002, 48:899–905
17. Yuan C, Beach KW, Smith LH, Jr, Hatsukami TS. Measurement of atherosclerotic carotid plaque size in vivo using high resolution magnetic resonance imaging. Circulation. 1998, 98:2666–71
18. Yarnykh VL, Yuan C. Multi-slice double inversion-recovery black-blood imaging with simultaneous slice-re-inversion. J Magn Reson Imaging. 2003, 17:478–83.
19. Yarnykh VL, Yuan C. Simultaneous outer volume and blood suppression by quadruple inversion-recovery. Magn Reson Med. 2006, 55(5):1083–92
20. Mitsumori LM, Yuan C, Ferguson MS, Hatsukami TS. In vivo identification of lipid cores in advanced carotid atherosclerotic plaques by high resolution MR imaging (abstr). Circulation. 2000, 102(Suppl):II252
21. Aoki S, Aoki K, Ohsawa S et al. Dynamic MR imaging of the carotid wall. J Magn Reson Imaging. 1999, 9:420–7
22. Coombs BD, Ursell PC, Reilly LM et al. Carotid bifurcation plaque structure: high resolution MRI with histologic correlation (abstr) In: Proceedings of the sixth meeting of the international society for magnetic resonance in medicine. Berkeley, Calif: International Society for Magnetic Resonance in Medicine, 1998; 591
23. Hayes CE, Mathis CM, Yuan C. Surface coil phased arrays for high-resolution imaging of the carotid arteries. J Magn Reson Imaging 1996, 6:109–12
24. Cai J, Hatsukami TS, Ferguson MS et al. In vivo quantitative measurement of intact fibrous cap and lipid-rich necrotic core size in atherosclerotic carotid plaque: comparison of high-resolution, contrast-enhanced magnetic resonance imaging and histology. Circulation. 2005, 112(22):3437–44
25. Merickel MB, Carman CS, Brookeman JR et al. Identification and 3-D quantification of atherosclerosis using magnetic resonance imaging. Comput Biol Med. 1988, 18:89–102
26. Yuan C, Petty C, O'Brien KD et al. In vitro and in situ magnetic resonance imaging signal features of atherosclerotic plaque-associated lipids. Arterioscler Thromb Vasc Biol. 1997, 17:1496–503

27. Virmani R, Kolodgie FD, Burke AP, Farb A, Schwartz SM. Lessons from sudden coronary death: a comprehensive morphological classification scheme for atherosclerotic lesions. Arterioscler Thromb Vasc Biol. 2000, 20:1262–75
28. Spagnoli LG, Mauriello A, Sangiorgi G, Fratoni S, Bonanno E, Schwartz RS, Piepgras DG, Pistolese R, Ippoliti A, Holmes DR Jr. Extracranial thrombotically active carotid plaque as a risk factor for ischemic stroke. JAMA. 2004, 292:1845–52
29. Mitsumori LM, Hatsukami TS, Ferguson MS et al. In vivo accuracy of multisequence MR imaging for identifying unstable fibrous caps in advanced human carotid plaques. J Magn Reson Imaging. 2003, 17:410–20
30. Trivedi RA, U-King-Im J, Graves MJ et al. Multi-sequence in vivo MRI can quantify fibrous cap and lipid core components in human carotid atherosclerotic plaques. Eur J Vasc Endovasc Surg. 2004, 28:207–13
31. Wasserman BA, Smith WI, Trout HH 3rd et al. Carotid artery atherosclerosis: in vivo morphologic characterization with gadolinium-enhanced double-oblique MR imaging initial results. Radiology. 2002, 223:566–73
32. Chu B, Yuan C, Takaya N et al. Images in cardiovascular medicine. Serial high-spatial-resolution, multisequence magnetic resonance imaging studies identify fibrous cap rupture and penetrating ulcer into carotid atherosclerotic plaque. Circulation. 2006, 113: e660–1
33. Yuan C, Zhang SX, Polissar NL et al. Identification of fibrous cap rupture with magnetic resonance imaging is highly associated with recent transient ischemic attack or stroke. Circulation. 2002, 105:181–5
34. Takaya N, Yuan C, Chu B et al. Association between carotid plaque characteristics and subsequent ischemic cerebrovascular events: a prospective assessment with MRI--initial results. Stroke. 2006, 37(3):818–23
35. Saam T, Hatsukami TS, Takaya N, Chu B, Underhill H, Kerwin WS, Cai J, Ferguson MS, Yuan C. The vulnerable, or high-risk, atherosclerotic plaque: noninvasive MR imaging for characterization and assessment. Radiology. 2007, 244:64–77
36. Davies MJ, Thomas AC. Plaque fissuring–the cause of acute myocardial infarction, sudden ischaemic death, and crescendo angina. Br Heart J. 1985, 53:363–73
37. Kolodgie FD, Gold HK, Burke AP et al. Intraplaque hemorrhage and progression of coronary atheroma. N Engl J Med. 2003, 349:2316–25
38. Mofidi R, Crotty TB, McCarthy P et al. Association between plaque instability, angiogenesis and symptomatic carotid occlusive disease. Br J Surg. 2001, 88:945–50
39. Carr S, Farb A, Pearce WH, Virmani R, Yao JS. Atherosclerotic plaque rupture in symptomatic carotid artery stenosis. J Vasc Surg. 1996, 23:755–65
40. Chu B, Kampschulte A, Ferguson MS et al. Hemorrhage in the atherosclerotic carotid plaque: a high-resolution MRI study. Stroke. 2004, 35:1079–84
41. Cappendijk VC, Cleutjens KB, Kessels AG et al. Assessment of human atherosclerotic carotid plaque components with multisequence MR imaging: initial experience. Radiology. 2005, 234:487–92
42. Moody AR, Murphy RE, Morgan PS et al. Characterization of complicated carotid plaque with magnetic resonance direct thrombus imaging in patients with cerebral ischemia. Circulation. 2003, 107:3047–52
43. Saam T, Cai J, Ma L et al. Comparison of symptomatic and asymptomatic atherosclerotic carotid plaque features with in vivo MR imaging. Radiology. 2006, 240:464–72
44. Altaf N, Daniels L, Morgan PS et al. Detection of intraplaque hemorrhage by magnetic resonance imaging in symptomatic patients with mild to moderate carotid stenosis predicts recurrent neurological events. J Vasc Surg. 2008, 47(2):337–42
45. Altaf N, MacSweeney ST, Gladman J et al. Carotid intraplaque hemorrhage predicts recurrent symptoms in patients with high-grade carotid stenosis. Stroke. 2007, 38:1633–5
46. Takaya N, Yuan C, Chu B et al. Presence of intraplaque hemorrhage stimulates progression of carotid atherosclerotic plaques: a high-resolution magnetic resonance imaging study. Circulation. 2005, 111:2768–75
47. O'Leary DH, Polak JF, Kronmal RA et al. Distribution and correlates of sonographically detected carotid artery disease in the cardiovascular health study. The CHS Collaborative Research Group. Stroke. 1992, 23:1752–60
48. Saam T, Hatsukami TS, Underhill H et al. Prevalence of AHA type VI carotid lesions identified by MRI across different categories of stenosis measured by duplex ultrasound. Circulation. 2006, 114:II–776
49. Shimizu Y, Kitagawa K, Nagai Y et al. Carotid atherosclerosis as a risk factor for complex aortic lesions in patients with ischemic cerebrovascular disease. Circ J. 2003, 67:597–600
50. Inzitari D, Eliasziw M, Gates P et al. The causes and risk of stroke in patients with asymptomatic internal-carotid-artery stenosis. North American Symptomatic Carotid Endarterectomy Trial collaborators. N Engl J Med. 2000, 342:1693–700
51. Koktzoglou I, Chung YC, Carroll TJ et al. Three-dimensional black-blood MR imaging of carotid arteries with segmented steady-state free precession: initial experience. Radiology. 2007, 243(1):220–8
52. Koktzoglou I, Li D. Diffusion-prepared segmented steady-state free precession: Application to 3D black-blood cardiovascular magnetic resonance of the thoracic aorta and carotid artery walls. J Cardiovasc Magn Reson. 2007, 9(1):33–42
53. Wasserman BA, Sharrett AR, Lai S et al. Risk factor associations with the presence of a lipid core in carotid plaque of asymptomatic individuals using high-resolution MRI: the multi-ethnic study of atherosclerosis (MESA). Stroke. 2008, 39(2):329–35

28 Comprehensive Non-contrast CT Imaging of the Vulnerable Patient

Damini Dey, Ioannis A. Kakadiaris, Matthew J. Budoff, Morteza Naghavi, and Daniel S. Berman

CONTENTS

ABSTRACT

Atherosclerotic cardiovascular disease is the leading cause of death in developed countries. Every year, one million people in the US experience a heart attack or sudden cardiac death. A large percentage of these patients have no prior symptoms of any kind but suffer from silent heart disease, which may cause a heart attack at any time. Currently, there is no reliable screening method to identify the "vulnerable patient" who may have silent heart disease and therefore is at the risk of suffering a cardiovascular event such as a heart attack.

Non-contrast cardiac CT is used worldwide to assess coronary artery calcium, a subclinical marker of coronary atherosclerosis. It has been recommended for screening asymptomatic individuals with

From: *Asymptomatic Atherosclerosis: Pathophysiology, Detection and Treatment*
Edited by: M. Naghavi (ed.), DOI 10.1007/978-1-60327-179-0_28

intermediate-high Framingham risk, due to its high prognostic value, low radiation burden, and simplicity. In this chapter, we review technical aspects of imaging coronary calcium and techniques for "coronary calcium scoring" and review its value in prognostic studies.

The non-contrast cardiac CT scan provides three-dimensional images of the heart and contains important additional information regarding the patient's cardiovascular risk, beyond the coronary calcium score. These include pericardial and thoracic fat, aortic calcification, aortic and left ventricular size, spotty calcification pattern, and the number of calcified lesions. These markers are, however, not considered in routine clinical analysis. In this chapter, we summarize the methods to quantify these markers of cardiovascular risk and the growing evidence regarding their clinical and prognostic significance. Automated algorithms to identify and quantify these markers may help in identifying the vulnerable patient with silent heart disease.

Key words: Coronary calcium scoring; Non-contrast CT; Pericardial fat; Thoracic fat; Aortic calcium; Aortic size; Left ventricular size; Spotty calcification; Number of calcified lesions

TOPIC PEARLS

- Non-contrast cardiac CT
- Coronary Calcium Scoring
- Pericardial and thoracic fat
- Aortic calcification and size
- Left ventricular size
- Spotty calcification and number of calcified lesions

INTRODUCTION

Atherosclerotic cardiovascular disease is the leading cause of death in developed countries and is rapidly becoming the number-one killer in the world. From current estimates, more than 61 million Americans have one or more types of cardiovascular disease [1]. Every year, more than one million people in the United States and more than 19 million people worldwide experience a sudden acute coronary event (sudden cardiac death or myocardial infarction) [2]. A large percentage of this population (40–60%, approximately 500,000 people a year in the US) have no prior symptoms of cardiovascular disease [3, 4]. Since current therapy can reduce the frequency of heart attack by approximately 60–70%, there is a critical need to identify the patients who are asymptomatic but are at risk for coronary events. The culprit plaques that cause such coronary events are called "vulnerable plaques" [5]. A recent consensus statement from leading investigators in the field elaborated on different types of vulnerable plaques and called for the identification of the vulnerable patient,who is at risk of suffering a cardiovascular event [5, 6]. However, currently available screening, diagnostic, and risk assessment methods are still insufficient to identify a large proportion of vulnerable patients [5].

CARDIOVASCULAR RISK ASSESSMENT

Cardiovascular risk is typically defined as the probability of developing an adverse coronary event over a finite time period and can be qualified as high, intermediate, or low [7]. The first step in individual risk assessment is to identify the major causal risk factors for coronary artery disease. These include the smoking history and family history of CAD of the individual, systolic blood pressure, confirmation of the presence or absence of type 2 diabetes, and measuring the total, high-density lipoprotein (HDL), and low-density lipoprotein (LDL), blood cholesterol, and glucose in fasting blood plasma [7]. Individual cardiovascular risk can be quantified by the Framingham Risk Score [8, 9], which integrates age, gender, total and HDL cholesterol, systolic blood pressure, and the presence or absence of current smoking.

C-reactive Protein (CRP) is a blood marker of inflammation which has been shown to be an independent risk factor and a strong predictor of cardiovascular events in the asymptomatic population [10–12]. Although CRP is a non-specific marker of systematic inflammation, it has been suggested that it has an important role in plaque inflammation [13].

NON-CONTRAST CT

Non-contrast cardiac computed tomography (CT) has been increasingly used in the United States and other countries during the past 15 years, with the goal of identifying patients at risk of having obstructive coronary artery disease on the basis of the presence and severity of coronary artery calcium (CAC), a sub-clinical marker of coronary atherosclerosis. Non-contrast CT imaging uses the natural density of tissues within subjects, utilizing the different attenuation values of air, fat, tissue (muscle and blood), and calcium. It is a low-radiation exposure technique, and can determine the presence or absence of CAC within a single breath hold, without pre-medication or intravenous contrast. Figure 1 shows examples of non-contrast CT scans from 2 patients (both asymptomatic males, 59 years old, without prior CAD) with no and with substantial coronary calcium. To date, follow-up studies with thousands of patients have reported that the total CAC measured from non-contrast CT, usually quantified as the "Agatston score", predicts cardiovascular events beyond standard cardiovascular risk factors [14–28]. In large-scale observational studies, Shaw et al. [15] and Budoff et al. [29] have shown that CAC provides incremental information in addition to traditional risk factors in the prediction of all-cause mortality. Assessment of CAC or coronary calcium scoring (CCS) by non-contrast CT has been recommended as a screening test for asymptomatic individuals within specific age limits (males > 40 years of age and women > 50 years of age [30]) because of its high prognostic value, low radiation burden, and simplicity [31]. It has also been recommended for the assessment of symptomatic individuals, especially in the setting of equivocal treadmill or functional testing [31].

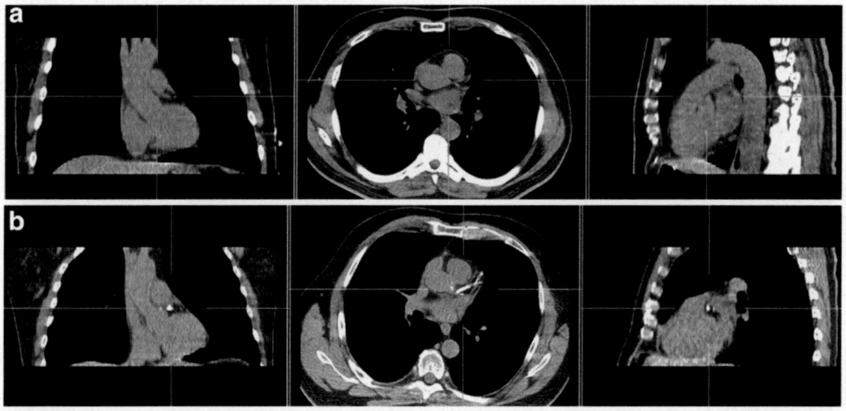

Fig. 1. Examples of non-contrast CT scans from two patients enrolled in the ongoing EISNER study at our institution. Both patients were asymptomatic, male, 59 years old, without prior cardiovascular disease. (**a**) Coronal, shows coronal, transverse, and sagittal views from the non-contrast CT scan of patient 1, with no coronary calcium. (**b**) Coronal, shows coronal, transverse, and sagittal views from the non-contrast CT scan of patient 2, with substantial coronary calcium. The Agatston score for patent 2 was 1,306 and the percentile based on patient sex and gender was 97.

IMAGING CORONARY CALCIUM

Electron-beam CT: The reference standard for measurement of CAC, on the basis of substantial prognostic data, remains electron-beam CT (EBCT) [31]. EBCT (by General Electric, South San Francisco, CA) was first introduced in the early 1980s, specifically for cardiac imaging. In contrast with multi-slice CT (MSCT) scanner technology, the latest EBCT scanner utilizes four stationary tungsten "target" anode rings opposite a stationary arc of detectors, and a rotating electron beam; only the electron beam is moved and x-ray photons are produced at the target anode rings. In MSCT scanners, a specialized x-ray tube and the multislice detector array opposite the tube are mounted on a gantry, which moves about the patient; x-ray photons are generated within the x-ray tube. Table 1 summarizes the CT system components for coronary calcium scoring for EBCT and MSCT. Standardized methods for imaging and quantifying CAC using EBCT have been published [32]. Electrocardiographic (ECG) triggering is done during end-systole or early diastole at a time determined from the continuous ECG tracing recorded during the scan. ECG triggering is set prospectively (prospective triggering) to the early to mid-diastolic portion (40–60%) of the R–R interval, depending on the heart rate, since this is when there is the least cardiac motion for most heart rates [33, 34]. Typically the EBCT scan is acquired with 100 ms exposure time and 3 mm non-overlapping slices.

Multislice CT: Multislice CT technology is rapidly evolving. The current generation of MSCT systems, with gantry rotation times as low as 330 ms, is capable of acquiring 64–320 sections of the heart simultaneously with ECG-gating, either in prospective or retrospective mode. Several studies have compared coronary calcium scoring using EBCT and MSCT and found high correlation (r=0.96–0.99) and concordance between the two modalities [35–38]. Differences in CAC measurements using EBCT and MSCT have been shown to be similar to inter-scan differences in CAC measurements reported for EBCT or MSCT scanners individually [36]. It is now generally accepted that MSCT is equivalent to EBCT for quantification of coronary calcium [35–38], with low variability

Table 1
Summary of CT system components

	Electron-beam CT	*Multislice CT*
Electron source (cathode)	Electron gun	Tungsten filament
Gantry	Fixed: Electron beam rapidly sweeps across tungsten targets	Rotates: Tube and opposing detectors rotate within gantry
Image reconstruction	Filtered back-projection Sharp kernel	Filtered back-projection Standard kernel
Beam current, mA	Fixed	User selectable
Exposure time for coronary calcium	50 or 100 ms	≥167 ms for 64-slice CT, depending on gantry rotation speed 83 ms for dual-source CT
Exposure, mAs	Fixed mA × exposure time	User selectable mA × exposure time
Gating for Coronary Calcium Scoring	Prospective trigger	Prospective (recommended) or retrospective gating
Gating for CT Angiography	Prospective trigger	Retrospective gating with ECG-based tube current modulation or prospective gating
Minimum slice (z-axis) thickness	1.5 mm	0.5 mm

between the two modalities for higher coronary calcium scores (Agatston score>11) [37]. With MSCT, use of both prospective and retrospective gating has been reported. Retrospectively gated protocols are associated with a lower rescan variability, but also significantly higher radiation dose [39]. Therefore, it has been recommended that prospective ECG triggering, together with a slice collimation of 2.5–3 mm, be used for coronary calcium scoring [31]. With prospective ECG triggering, effective radiation doses range from 0.7–1 mSv for males and 0.9–1.3 mSv for females for EBCT systems [38, 40–43] and from 1–1.5 mSv for males and 1.1–1.9 mSv for females for MSCT systems [38, 41–43].

The recommended scan protocol for MSCT coronary calcium scoring utilizes prospective triggering at early to mid diastole, a tube voltage of 120 kVp, and axial scanning with 2.5 mm slice thickness. Whether originating from EBCT or MSCT scanner, the non-contrast CT study for coronary calcium scoring typically consists of 50–60 CT slices in 512×512 matrix reconstructed over a 350 mm field-of-view, with slice thickness of 2.5 or 3 mm.

QUANTIFICATION OF CORONARY CALCIUM

Agatston Score: The first group that used EBCT images for quantification of CAC was Agatston and colleagues in 1990 [44]. They introduced an overall CAC score, later called the Agatston score, which became the *de facto* standard [31]. In the Agatston method, calcified lesions are identified by applying a lower segmentation threshold of 130 Hounsfield Units (HU) and discarding structures with sizes less than 1 mm^2 to ignore the influence of image noise. A region-of-interest (ROI) is placed around each lesion in every slice, and the maximum CT number (CT_{max}) in the lesion is determined. The calcium score for each ROI is calculated by multiplying the area A_i of each lesion by a weighting factor that depends on the CT_{max} corresponding to the ROI:

$$CS_i = w_i \cdot A_i, \tag{28.1}$$

where i represents each ROI and the weight w_i is defined as follows:

$$w_i = \begin{bmatrix} 1 & \text{if } 130\,\text{HU} \leqslant CT_{max} \leqslant 200\,\text{HU} \\ 2 & \text{if } 200\,\text{HU} \leqslant CT_{max} \leqslant 300\,\text{HU} \\ 3 & \text{if } 300\,\text{HU} \leqslant CT_{max} \leqslant 400\,\text{HU} \\ 4 & \text{if } CT_{max} > 400\,\text{HU} \end{bmatrix}. \tag{28.2}$$

Agatston scores for each calcification, coronary artery, or for the entire heart (total coronary calcium score, TCS) are calculated by summing respective values for the regions of interest:

$$TCS = \sum_i CS_i . \tag{28.3}$$

The coronary artery corresponding to each lesion needs to be manually identified by the operator. The Agatston system was designed for a CT slice thickness of the scan of 3 mm. The Agatston score is influenced by partial volume effect, which results in higher maximum values for small lesions than for larger ones with the same calcium composition. Influence of partial volume effect as well as non-linear weighting with respect to the amount of calcium (28.2) results in high inter-scan variability [31]. Despite these limitations, the retention of the Agatston score has been predicated by the availability of databases and outcome data, which helps clinicians understand the significance of a certain score [31].

Volume Score: The volume score has been widely used since higher reproducibility compared to the Agatston score was reported in 1998 [45]. The volume score estimates the volume of the calcified lesion; it is calculated as the number of voxels which belong to the lesion (N), multiplied by the volume of one voxel (v_l):

$$V = N \cdot v_l \,. \tag{28.4}$$

The general approach to determine voxels belonging to the lesion is to use all connected voxels with an attenuation value above a certain threshold, typically 130 HU, similar to the Agatston score. However, this method is also sensitive to partial volume effect. In particular, for small calcified lesions with dimensions less than the slice thickness, this method overestimates the lesion volume [46].

Mass Score: The calcium mass score, which estimates the CAC mass, has been reported [46, 47]. To obtain the mass score, the mean number of each CT number (CT_i) of each voxel i in the calcified lesion is multiplied by the volume of the calcification (V_i). The product is directly proportional to the calcium mass for the lesion. To obtain absolute values for calcium mass, a calibration measurement with a known calcium hydroxyapatite mass is necessary; this yields a calibration factor c such that

$$c = \frac{\rho_{HA}}{\mathrm{CT}_c - \mathrm{CT}_w}, \tag{28.5}$$

where ρ_{HA} is the known density of the calcium hydroxyapatite mass, CT_c is the mean CT number for this calcification, and CT_w the mean CT number for water (0 for a well-calibrated scanner). The absolute mass for the calcification is then given by

$$m = \sum_i c \cdot \mathrm{CT}_i \cdot V_i \,. \tag{28.6}$$

Voxels included in the calcified lesion still need to be identified and typically a lower threshold is used. While this has traditionally been set to 130 HU, it has been recommended that a lower voxel calcium density (given by $c.\mathrm{CT}_i$) of 100 mg/cm^3 yields similar results with the added benefit of being less variable [46]. Although theoretically better for inter-scanner portability, the mass score has not yet been sufficiently validated (by autopsy, histology, or outcomes data) [31], and the requirement of the calcium phantom adds complexity and cost to the study. Rumberger et al. compared the Agatston, volume, and modified mass scores of 11,490 individuals and found the three scoring methods to be essentially equivalent [47].

Inter-scan variability: The inter-scan variability of CAC measurements has been shown to be fairly high. Mean inter-scan variability of 20–37% have been reported for Agatston scoring and 14–33% for volume scoring [48–50]. Inter-scan variability in a large cohort has been reported from the NIH-NHLBI funded Multi-Ethnic Study of Atherosclerosis (MESA) study. This is a population-based multi-ethnic multi-center study of 6,814 men and women, 45–84 years old, free of clinical apparent CAD, undergoing demographic, risk factor, and subclinical disease evaluations [51]. In this study, three study centers used EBCT, and three used MSCT. CAC was measured by using duplicate CT scans. In 3,355 participants with CAC, concordance for presence of calcium between duplicate scans was high and similar for both EBCT and MSCT (96%, k = 0.92). EBCT and MSCT also showed equivalent reproducibility for measuring CAC: mean absolute difference was 15.8 for EBCT and 16.9 for MSCT scanners ($P = .06$, not significant). Calcium volumes and interpolated volume scores were slightly but significantly more reproducible than the Agatston scores (mean relative difference 18.3 versus 20.1,

$p<0.01$). Reproducibility was significantly lower for scans with misregistrations or motion artifacts. To determine the smallest actual change in CAC, Sevrukov et al. have developed repeatability relationships for coronary calcium score on the basis of the baseline measurement [52]. Repeatability limits have also been derived from repeat non-contrast CT scans by Chung et al. from the MESA study [53]. These derived values can be used as a guide to evaluate whether an increase in CAC score exceeds that expected from measurement error alone.

PROGNOSTIC VALUE OF CORONARY CALCIUM SCORING

The majority of published studies have reported that the total amount of coronary calcium (quantified as the "Agatston Score") predicts coronary disease events beyond standard cardiovascular risk factors. Table 2 summarizes the prognostic studies, both retrospective and prospective, reported in asymptomatic populations using EBCT data. These studies have conclusively shown that CAC is both independent and incremental to standard cardiovascular risk factors in the prediction of cardiac events. These have also been discussed previously in [30, 31]. Results from the NIH-NHLBI MESA study have been reported. This report adds considerable strength to the recommendation for use of CCS as a risk stratification tool [28]. In this prospective study of 6,814 persons followed for over 3.5 years, the age, race/ethnicity, and sex-adjusted hazard ratios (95% CIs) for CAC scores of 0, 1–99,100–399, and ≥400 to predict cardiovascular events were 1.0, 4.7 (95% CI 2.5–8.7), 11.5 (95% CI 6.2–21.5), and 16.1 (95% CI 8.5–30.8), respectively, and outperformed measured carotid intima-media thickness and C-reactive protein in predicting future cardiovascular events in this cohort [54]. Becker et al. in a recent study demonstrated that among 1,726 asymptomatic individuals followed for a median of 40 months, the area under the ROC curve for CAC scores (0.81, 95% CI 0.78–0.84) was significantly larger than that of the Framingham risk score (0.63, 95% CI: 0.59–0.65), risk scores based on the *Pro*spective *Ca*rdiovascular *M*unster or PROCAM study (0.65, 95% CI: 0.6–0.68), and European Society of Cardiology scores (0.66, 95% CI: 0.62–0.6), respectively ($p=.03$) [55]. While continued progression of CAC appears to be an independent risk factor for future events [14], the expert consensus is that future studies are needed to justify the incremental population exposure to radiation and the cost associated with a repeat CT test to assess "change" [31]. Several ongoing prospective observational studies, such as MESA [56], EISNER (utilizing both EBCT and MSCT), and RECALL [57] (using EBCT), also aim to assess the prognostic value of increasing CAC burden in population-based samples.

OTHER MARKERS OF CARDIOVASCULAR RISK

As seen in Fig. 1, the coronary calcium scan, consisting of three-dimensional volume data, may contain additional information regarding the patient's cardiovascular risk, beyond the coronary calcium score. These include pericardial and thoracic fat, aortic calcification, aortic and left ventricular size, the presence of spotty calcification, and the number of calcified lesions. There is growing evidence regarding the clinical significance of these markers of cardiovascular risk. It has also been demonstrated that computer-aided fat quantitation in the coronary arteries in non-contrast CCS scans can potentially provide additional information regarding lipid-rich plaque [58, 59].

PERICARDIAL AND THORACIC FAT

There is growing evidence that adipose tissue surrounding coronary arteries may contribute to the development of coronary atherosclerosis, given its localization and potential for local production of inflammatory cytokines [60–62]. It has been shown that pericardial fat quantified from non-contrast

Table 2
Summary of Follow-up studies using EBCT in asymptomatic populations

Authors	*Number (N)*	*Mean age (y)*	*Mean follow-up duration (y)*	*Agatston score cutoff*	*Risk factor assessment*	*Relative Risk Ratio*
Arad et al. [17]	1,173	53	3.6	>160	Measured	20.2
Park et al. [19]	967	67	6.4	>142.1	Measured	4.9
Raggi et al. [18]	632	52	2.7	Top quartile	Self-reported	13
Shemesh et al. [20]	446	64	3.8	>0	Measured	2.8
Wong et al. [21]	926	54	3.3	Top quartile	Self-reported	8.8
Kondos et al. [22]	5,635	51	3.1	>0	Self-reported	3.86 men, 1.53 women*
Greenland et al. [23]	1,312	66	7.0	>300	Measured	3.9
Arad et al. [14] St Francis Heart Study+	4,613	59	4.3	≥100	Measured	9.2
LaMonte et al. [24] Cooper Clinic Study+	10,746	54	3.5	Top tertile	Measured	8.7 men, 6.3 women
Taylor et al. [25] Prospective Army Coronary Calcium Project+	2,000	43	3	>0	Measured	11.8
Vliegenthart et al. [26] The Rotterdam Heart Study+	1,795	71	3.3	>1000	Measured	8.1
Becker et al. [27]+	924	60	3	Top quartile	Measured	7.3
Detrano et al. [28] Multi-Ethnic Study of Atherosclerosis (MESA)++	6,722	62	3.8	>100	Measured	7.73 (Score 101–300), 9.67 (Score >300)
Budoff et al. [29]**	25,253	56	6.8	>0	Self-reported	2.2 (Score 11–100), 12.5 (Score >1,000)
Shaw et al. [15]**	10,377	53	5	401–1,000	Self-reported	6.2

+Prospective study
++Prospective, population-based study
*After multivariate analysis, $P<0.05$ for men, P=not significant for women
**End-point was all-cause mortality

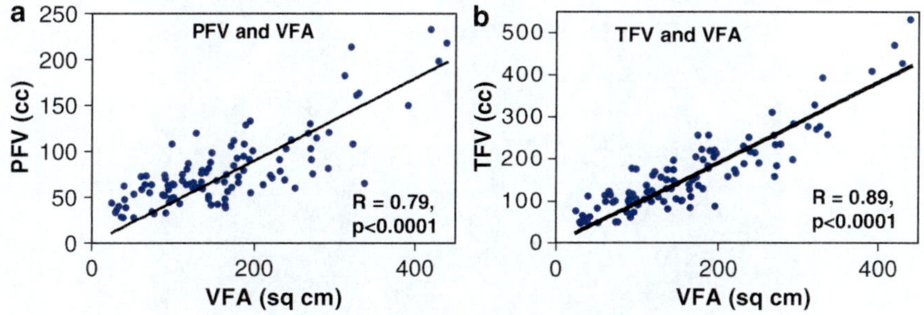

Fig. 2. Correlation of CT-measured pericardial fat volume (PFV) and thoracic fat volume (TFV) with abdominal visceral fat area (VFA) ($N=105$).

CT is associated with the presence of coronary calcium [60, 62] and with coronary artery disease assessed by invasive coronary angiography [63]. It has also been shown that total thoracic fat correlates with abdominal visceral fat, which is associated with the metabolic syndrome [64, 65] (Fig. 2). Rosito et al. found that pericardial and intra-thoracic fat volumes, quantified manually in 1,155 participants of the Framingham Heart Study, are associated with vascular calcification, suggesting that these fat depots may exert local toxic effects on the vasculature [60]. Very recently, the same group has reported that pericardial fat, and not intra-thoracic fat or abdominal visceral fat, is independently associated with cardiovascular events [66]. A study currently in press by Grief et al. have shown that increased total thoracic fat quantified from coronary CT angiography (CCTA) is associated with the presence of coronary plaques, low adiponectin levels, and inflammation measured by elevated hsCRP levels [67]. In particular, thoracic fat volumes >300 cc were strongly predictive of coronary atherosclerosis by CCTA.

To clarify the adipose tissue terminology, pericardial fat in these studies refers to all the adipose tissues enclosed by the pericardium, including the epicardial fat surrounding the coronary arteries. It is the fat deposit surrounding the coronary arteries. Total thoracic fat refers to the adipose tissue surrounding the heart enclosed by the rib-cage and above the diaphragm, and includes pericardial fat [66] (Fig. 3a). While pericardial fat is routinely imaged during CT for coronary calcium scoring, it is currently ignored in the analysis of CT images. The primary reasons for this are that there is currently no commercial software tool capable of automatic quantitation of pericardial fat, and data regarding the clinical significance of pericardial fat are recent. Software techniques for automated quantitation of total thoracic fat have been described by Dey et al. [65] and Bandekar et al. [68], which promise to add to existing practical clinical tools for cardiovascular risk assessment. Recently, we extended our previous algorithm for quantification of thoracic fat to also quantify pericardial fat volume (PFV), by computer-aided tracing of the pericardium; the algorithm "completes" the pericardium by spline interpolation between 5–7 user-defined control points, placed roughly on the pericardium (Fig. 3b,c) [69]. PFV and intra-thoracic fat volume correlate strongly with abdominal visceral fat measured from single-slice CT in 105 patients (Fig. 2). Figure 4 shows pericardial fat quantified from non-contrast CT images of a patient with this method. This patient also underwent a single-slice CT scan for measurement of abdominal fat (Fig. 4c,d).

AORTIC CALCIFICATION AND SIZE

Non-contrast CT scanning of the heart always includes imaging of the aortic valve, the ascending and descending aorta, and depending on the range of the scan it might also include information about the aortic arch. Assessment of these anatomical sites can provide details on the extent of the

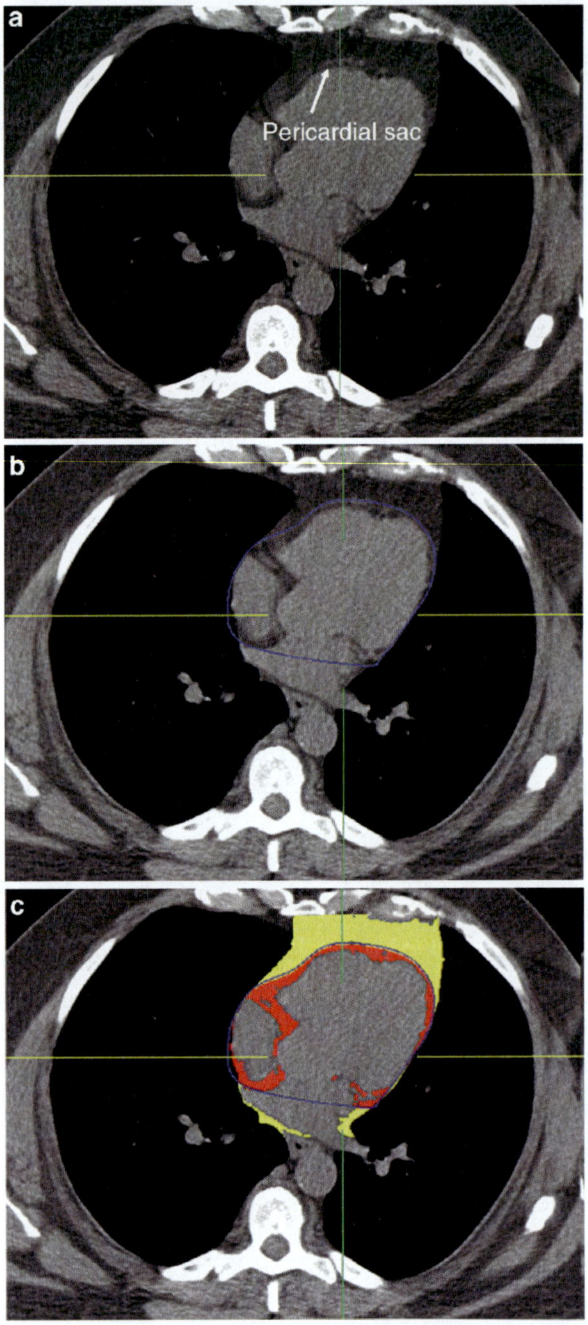

Fig. 3. Figure clarifying adipose tissue terminology. (**a**) Transverse non-contrast CT slice from a 65-year old asymptomatic male patient from the EISNER study is shown in (**a**). White arrow shows the pericardial sac as a thin band enveloping the heart. (**b**) The pericardial shows the pericardial sac (closed curve in blue) traced by an expert observer by placing 5–7 control points on the pericardium. (**c**) The result shows the result of fat quantification on the same transverse slice. Red overlay represents pericardial fat enclosed by the pericardium. Yellow overlay represents fat outside the pericardium. Color overlay (Red + Yellow) represents total thoracic fat.

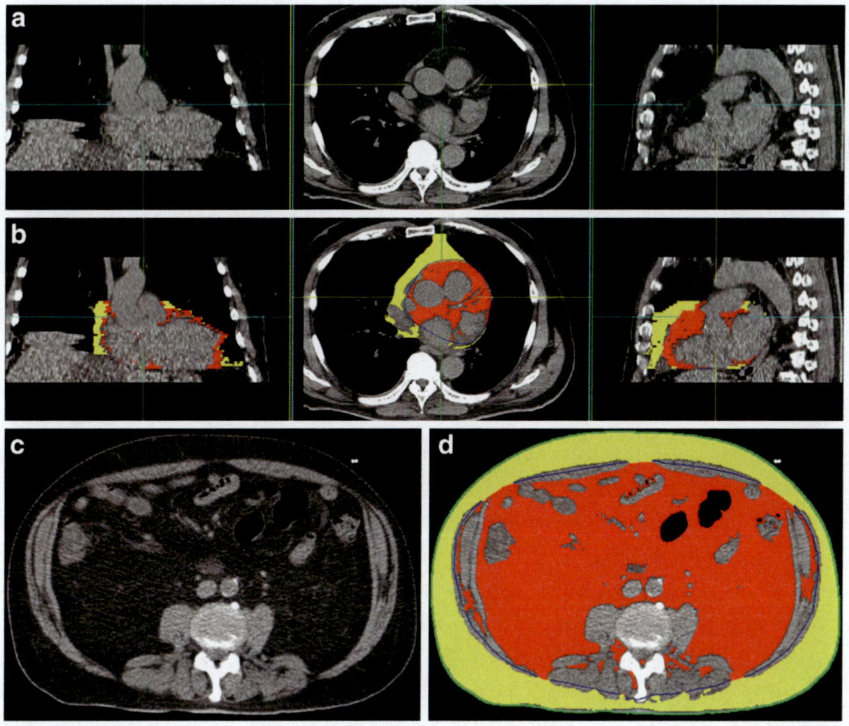

Fig. 4. Figure shows the CT study of a 71-year old male patient from our institution, without prior cardiovascular disease, but with a history of hypertension. This patient presented with mild chest pain upon heavy exertion. (**c**) Coronal, transverse, and sagittal slices from the non-contrast CT scan are shown in (**a**). (**b**) Results of pericardial fat quantitation are shown in (**b**). Red overlay represents pericardial fat enclosed by the pericardium. Yellow overlay represents thoracic fat outside the pericardium. Quantified pericardial fat volume was 224 cc and total thoracic fat volume was 470 cc. (**c**) Single abdominal CT slice through the L4-L5 region. (**d**) Same slice as in (**c**) with voxels quantified as visceral fat shown in red overlay, and voxels quantified as subcutaneous fat shown in yellow overlay.

atherosclerotic process as reflected by calcification as well as on the dimension of the thoracic aorta. The atherosclerotic process can engage one or more segments of the thoracic aorta (most frequently the arch, followed by the descending, and then ascending aorta) and/or the aortic valve [70, 71]. The presence of aortic valve and thoracic aortic calcifications was found to be associated with significant coronary arterial stenosis [72]. Moreover, repeated reports support the association between aortic calcification and cerebral ischemic events [71, 73–75].

Non-contrast CT can additionally be used as a relatively simple screening tool to detect dilation of the thoracic aorta in the patient who undergoes coronary calcium scoring. Recently, normal limits of ascending and descending aortic dimensions by non-contrast gated cardiac CT have been defined and it has been shown that assessment of aortic size is possible from CT scans obtained for calcium scoring measurements, thus providing a practical tool to point out suspected aortic dilation [76, 77].

A novel software method for the detection and delineation of ascending and descending aorta in non-contrast CT scans for CCS was recently described by Kurkure et al. [78], which can be used to compute the size of the aorta in different locations. Such potential software techniques can be incorporated within the existing practical clinical tools for improved cardiovascular risk assessment.

LEFT VENTRICULAR SIZE

Left ventricular size is a novel parameter that can be estimated from non-contrast CT scans by simply defining the mid-ventricular slice area and then multiplying it by the ventricular height. Historically, plain-film chest x-ray measurements were shown to provide useful information about left ventricular size [79] and the parameters provided by these studies were shown to be associated with cardiovascular prognosis [80, 81]. Recently, cardiac CT-calculated left ventricular size was shown to correlate well with cardiac MRI in a large cohort from the MESA study [82]. Such cardiac CT measurements can potentially add additional value to the diagnostic and prognostic capabilities of non-contrast enhanced CT imaging.

SPOTTY CALCIFICATION

Using gold-standard intravascular ultrasound (IVUS), Ehara et al. have shown that spotty calcification typifies the vulnerable plaque in patients with acute myocardial infarction [83]. IVUS studies have defined spotty calcifications as more than one calcification with length <3 mm within an IVUS arc of ≤90° [83, 84]. Using contrast-enhanced CT coronary angiography, Motoyama et al. have investigated the characteristics of culprit plaques in acute coronary syndrome (ACS), and found that positive remodeling and spotty calcification pattern (63% vs. 21%, $p=0.0005$) was significantly more frequent in the ACS culprit plaques, whereas extensive calcification (22% vs. 55%, $p=0.004$) was significantly more frequent in stable plaques [85]. While small calcifications are subject to partial volume effect (Fig. 5), Williams et al. recently reported that the number of calcified lesions provides valuable prognostic information; mortality rates increased proportionally with the number of calcified lesions in 14,759 asymptomatic patients undergoing coronary calcium scoring [86] (Fig. 6).

Recently, Kurkure et al. [87] presented a computer-assisted, coronary calcium detection method using machine learning techniques. They demonstrated that a classification-based coronary calcium detection method has potential to be used in calcium scoring software to reduce the manual interactions required by existing clinical tools and eventually eliminate them completely. Such a method can be further enhanced to produce additional calcium pattern information. Additionally, a heart-centered coordinate system was described by Brunner et al. [88] to identify different arterial zones and sec-

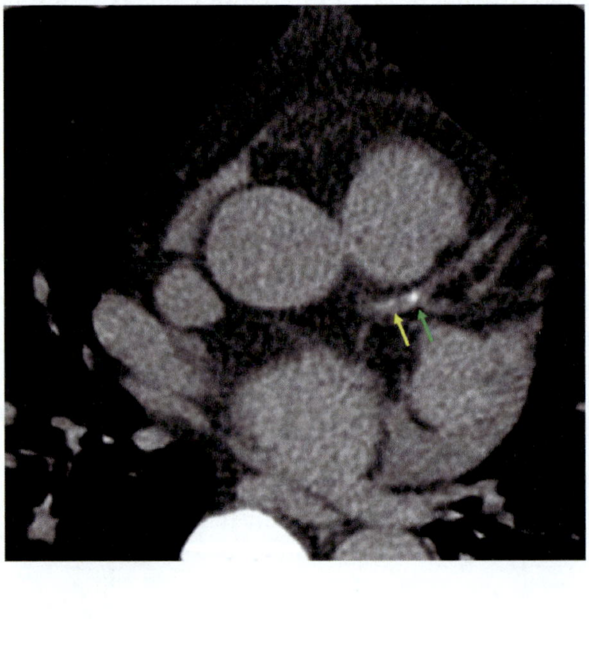

Fig. 5. Same patient as in Fig. 28.4 showing possible spotty calcification in the left main/proximal LAD artery. Mean Hounsfield Unit (HU) for blood/muscle in the aorta was 50 ± 22. The smaller proximal calcification (indicated with yellow arrow) cannot be visualized clearly because of partial volume effect; the maximum HU of this lesion was 128, below the 130-HU coronary calcium scoring threshold. Maximum HU of the larger distal calcified lesion (indicated with green arrow) was 276. Lengths of both lesions were <3 mm.

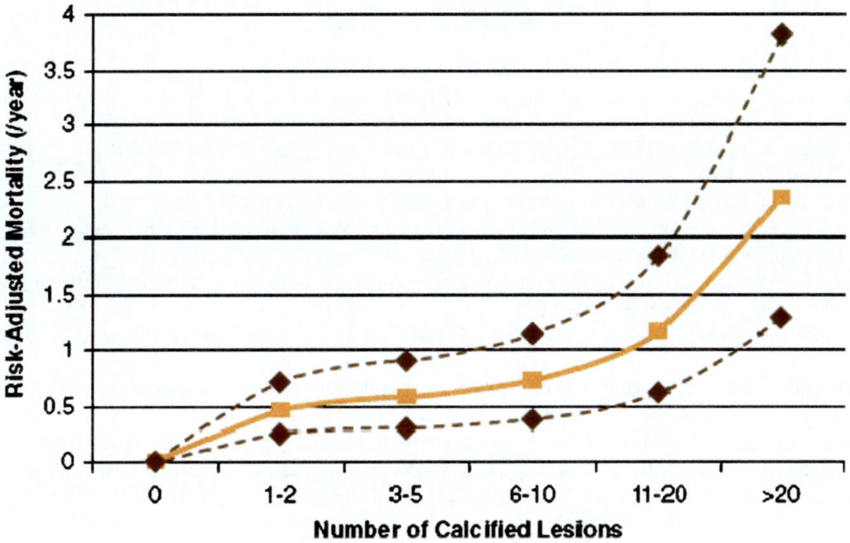

Fig. 6. Figure showing that mortality rate increases proportionally with number of calcified lesions in 14,759 asymptomatic individuals followed up for 6.8 years (adapted from [86]).

tions, which can potentially enhance the accuracy of the classification-based coronary calcium detection technique.

CASE EXAMPLE

Figures 4 and 5 present a case example from our institution showing the non-contrast CT study of a 71-year old male patient without prior cardiovascular disease, but with a history of hypertension. This patient presented with mild chest pain upon heavy exertion. The coronary calcium score was 11.6 and the patient was in the 12th percentile based on age and gender. The non-contrast CT scan workup also revealed increased pericardial and abdominal visceral fat (Fig. 4) and suggested the possible presence of spotty calcification (Fig. 5). Following non-contrast CT imaging, he underwent an exercise myocardial perfusion SPECT scan, which showed a large reversible anterior-apical-septal defect indicating the presence of hemodynamically significant stenosis in the left anterior descending (LAD) territory. Coronary catherization showed greater than 80% mid-LAD stenosis.

SUMMARY

To summarize, non-contrast cardiac CT is used worldwide to assess coronary artery calcium, a subclinical marker of coronary atherosclerosis. It is a screening test for the asymptomatic population due to its high prognostic value, low radiation burden, and simplicity. However, the non-contrast cardiac CT scan provides three-dimensional images of the heart and contains important additional information regarding the patient's cardiovascular risk beyond the coronary calcium score. These include pericardial and thoracic fat, aortic calcification, aortic and left ventricular size, spotty calcification pattern, and the number of calcified lesions. These markers are, however, not considered in routine clinical analysis. In this chapter, we summarize the methods to quantify these markers of cardiovascular risk and the growing evidence regarding their clinical and prognostic significance. Automated algorithms to identify and quantify these markers may help in identifying the vulnerable patient with silent heart disease.

REFERENCES

1. American Heart Association. Heart and Stroke Statistical Update. 2002.
2. Yusuf S, Reddy S, Ounpuu S, Anand S. Global burden of cardiovascular diseases: Part I: General considerations, the epidemiologic transition, risk factors, and impact of urbanization. Circulation 2001;104:2746–2753.
3. Myerburg RJ, Interian A, Jr., Mitrani RM, Kessler KM, Castellanos A. Frequency of sudden cardiac death and profiles of risk. Am J Cardiol 1997;80:10F–19F.
4. Virmani R, Burke AP, Farb A. Sudden cardiac death. Cardiovasc Pathol 2001;10:211–218.
5. Naghavi M, Libby P, Falk E, et al. From vulnerable plaque to vulnerable patient: A call for new definitions and risk assessment strategies: Part I. Circulation 2003;108:1664–1672.
6. Naghavi M, Libby P, Falk E, et al. From vulnerable plaque to vulnerable patient: A call for new definitions and risk assessment strategies: Part II. Circulation 2003;108:1772–1778.
7. Grundy SM. Primary prevention of coronary heart disease: Integrating risk assessment with intervention. Circulation 1999;100:988–998.
8. Wilson PW, D'Agostino RB, Levy D, Belanger AM, Silbershatz H, Kannel WB. Prediction of coronary heart disease using risk factor categories. Circulation 1998;97:1837–1847.
9. Executive Summary of The Third Report of The National Cholesterol Education Program (NCEP) Expert Panel on Detection, Evaluation, And Treatment of High Blood Cholesterol In Adults (Adult Treatment Panel III). Jama 2001;285:2486–2497.
10. Ridker PM, Cushman M, Stampfer MJ, Tracy RP, Hennekens CH. Inflammation, aspirin, and the risk of cardiovascular disease in apparently healthy men. N Engl J Med 1997;336:973–979.
11. Ridker PM, Hennekens CH, Buring JE, Rifai N. C-reactive protein and other markers of inflammation in the prediction of cardiovascular disease in women. N Engl J Med 2000;342:836–843.
12. Ridker PM, Rifai N, Rose L, Buring JE, Cook NR. Comparison of C-reactive protein and low-density lipoprotein cholesterol levels in the prediction of first cardiovascular events. N Engl J Med 2002;347:1557–1565.
13. Pasceri V, Willerson JT, Yeh ET. Direct proinflammatory effect of C-reactive protein on human endothelial cells. Circulation 2000;102:2165–2168.
14. Arad Y, Goodman KJ, Roth M, Newstein D, Guerci AD. Coronary calcification, coronary disease risk factors, C-reactive protein, and atherosclerotic cardiovascular disease events: The St. Francis Heart Study. J Am Coll Cardiol 2005;46:158–165.
15. Shaw L, Raggi P, Schisterman E, Berman D, Callister T. Prognostic value of cardiac risk factors and coronary artery calcium screening for all-cause mortality. Radiology 2003;228:826–833.
16. Berman DS, Hachamovitch R, Shaw LJ, et al. Roles of nuclear cardiology, cardiac computed tomography, and cardiac magnetic resonance: Noninvasive risk stratification and a conceptual framework for the selection of noninvasive imaging tests in patients with known or suspected coronary artery disease. J Nucl Med 2006;47:1107–1118.
17. Arad Y, Spadaro LA, Goodman K, Newstein D, Guerci AD. Prediction of coronary events with electron beam Computed Tomography. J Am Coll Cardiol 2000;36:1253–1260.
18. Raggi P, Callister TQ, Cooil B, et al. Identification of patients at increased risk of first unheralded acute myocardial infarction by electron-beam Computed Tomography. Circulation 2000;101:850–855.
19. Park R, Detrano R, Xiang M, et al. Combined use of Computed Tomography coronary calcium scores and C-reactive protein levels in predicting cardiovascular events in nondiabetic individuals. Circulation 2002;106:2073–2077.
20. Shemesh J, Morag-Koren N, Goldbourt U, et al. Coronary calcium by spiral computed tomography predicts cardiovascular events in high-risk hypertensive patients. J Hypertens 2004;22:605–610.
21. Wong ND, Hsu JC, Detrano RC, Diamond G, Eisenberg H, Gardin JM. Coronary artery calcium evaluation by electron beam Computed Tomography and its relation to new cardiovascular events. Am J Cardiol 2000;86:495–498.
22. Kondos GT, Hoff JA, Sevrukov A, et al. Electron-beam tomography coronary artery calcium and cardiac events: A 37-month follow-up of 5635 initially asymptomatic low- to intermediate-risk adults. Circulation 2003;107:2571–2576.
23. Greenland P, LaBree L, Azen SP, Doherty TM, Detrano RC. Coronary artery calcium score combined with Framingham score for risk prediction in asymptomatic individuals. J Am Med Assoc 2004;291:210–215.
24. LaMonte MJ, FitzGerald SJ, Church TS, et al. Coronary artery calcium score and coronary heart disease events in a large cohort of asymptomatic men and women. Am J Epidemiol 2005;162:421–429.
25. Taylor AJ, Bindeman J, Feuerstein I, Cao F, Brazaitis M, O'Malley PG. Coronary calcium independently predicts incident premature coronary heart disease over measured cardiovascular risk factors: mean three-year outcomes in the Prospective Army Coronary Calcium (PACC) project. J Am Coll Cardiol 2005;46:807–814.
26. Vliegenthart R, Oudkerk M, Hofman A, et al. Coronary calcification improves cardiovascular risk prediction in the elderly. Circulation 2005;112:572–577.
27. Becker A, Knez A, Becker C, et al. Prediction of serious cardiovascular events by determining coronary artery calcification measured by multi-slice computed tomography. Dtsch Med Wochenschr 2005;130:2433–2438.
28. Detrano R, Guerci AD, Carr JJ, et al. Coronary calcium as a predictor of coronary events in four racial or ethnic groups. N Engl J Med 2008;358:1336–1345.
29. Budoff MJ, Shaw LJ, Liu ST, et al. Long-term prognosis associated with coronary calcification: Observations from a registry of 25,253 patients. J Am Coll Cardiol 2007;49:1860–1870.
30. Budoff MJ, Gul KM. Expert review on coronary calcium. Vasc Health Risk Manag 2008;4:315–324.

31. Budoff MJ, Achenbach S, Blumenthal RS, et al. Assessment of coronary artery disease by cardiac computed tomography: A scientific statement from the American Heart Association Committee on Cardiovascular Imaging and Intervention, Council on Cardiovascular Radiology and Intervention, and Committee on Cardiac Imaging, Council on Clinical Cardiology. Circulation 2006;114:1761–1791.
32. O'Rourke RA, Brundage BH, Froelicher VF, et al. American College of Cardiology/American Heart Association expert consensus document on electron-beam Computed Tomography for the diagnosis and prognosis of coronary artery disease. J Am Coll Cardiol 2000;36:326–340.
33. Mao S, Lu B, Oudiz RJ, Bakhsheshi H, Liu SC, Budoff MJ. Coronary artery motion in electron beam tomography. J Comput Assist Tomogr 2000;24:253–258.
34. Mao S, Bakhsheshi H, Lu B, Liu SC, Oudiz RJ, Budoff MJ. Effect of electrocardiogram triggering on reproducibility of coronary artery calcium scoring. Radiology 2001;220:707–711.
35. Knez A, Becker C, Becker A, et al. Determination of coronary calcium with multi-slice spiral Computed Tomography: A comparative study with electron-beam CT. Int J Cardiovasc Imaging 2002;18:295–303.
36. Daniell AL, Wong ND, Friedman JD, et al. Concordance of coronary artery calcium estimates between MDCT and electron beam tomography. AJR Am J Roentgenol 2005;185:1542–1545.
37. Stanford W, Thompson BH, Burns TL, Heery SD, Burr MC. Coronary artery calcium quantification at multi-detector row helical CT versus electron-beam CT. Radiology 2004;230:397–402.
38. Carr JJ, Crouse JR, 3rd, Goff DC, Jr., D'Agostino RB, Jr., Peterson NP, Burke GL. Evaluation of subsecond gated helical CT for quantification of coronary artery calcium and comparison with electron beam CT. AJR Am J Roentgenol 2000; 174:915–921.
39. Ohnesorge B, Flohr T, Fischbach R, et al. Reproducibility of coronary calcium quantification in repeat examinations with retrospectively ECG-gated multisection spiral CT. Eur Radiol 2002;12:1532–1540.
40. Becker CR, Kleffel T, Crispin A, et al. Coronary artery calcium measurement: Agreement of multirow detector and electron beam CT. AJR Am J Roentgenol 2001;176:1295–1298.
41. Hunold P, Vogt F, Schmermund A, et al. Radiation exposure during cardiac CT: Effective doses at multi-detector row CT and electron-beam CT. Radiology 2003;226:145–152.
42. Morin RL, Gerber TC, McCollough CH. Radiation dose in computed tomography of the heart. Circulation 2003; 107:917–922.
43. Flohr T, Schoepf U, Kuettner A, et al. Advances in cardiac imaging with 16-section CT systems. Acad Radiol 2003;10: 386–401.
44. Agatston AS, Janowitz WR, Hildner FJ, Zusmer NR, Viamonte M, Jr., Detrano R. Quantification of coronary artery calcium using ultrafast Computed Tomography. J Am Coll Cardiol 1990;15:827–832.
45. Callister T, Cooil B, Raya S, Lippolis N, Russo D, Raggi P. Coronary artery disease: Improved reproducibility of calcium scoring with an electron-beam CT volumetric method. Radiology 1998;208:807–814.
46. McCollough CH, Ulzheimer S, Halliburton SS, Shanneik K, White RD, Kalender WA. Coronary artery calcium: A multi-institutional, multimanufacturer international standard for quantification at cardiac CT. Radiology 2007;243:527–538.
47. Rumberger JA, Kaufman L. A Rosetta Stone for Coronary Calcium Risk Stratification: Agatston, Volume, and Mass Scores in 11,490 Individuals. Am J Roentgentol 2003;181:743–748.
48. Hong C, Bae KT, Pilgram TK. Coronary artery calcium: accuracy and reproducibility of measurements with multi-detector row CT–assessment of effects of different thresholds and quantification methods. Radiology 2003;227:795–801.
49. Van Hoe LR, De Meerleer KG, Leyman PP, Vanhoenacker PK. Coronary artery calcium scoring using ECG-gated multidetector CT: Effect of individually optimized image-reconstruction windows on image quality and measurement reproducibility. AJR Am J Roentgenol 2003;181:1093–1100.
50. Takahashi N, Bae KT. Quantification of coronary artery calcium with multi-detector row CT: Assessing interscan variability with different tube currents pilot study. Radiology 2003;228:101–106.
51. Detrano RC, Anderson M, Nelson J, et al. Coronary calcium measurements: Effect of CT scanner type and calcium measure on rescan reproducibility–MESA study. Radiology 2005;236:477–484.
52. Sevrukov AB, Bland JM, Kondos GT. Serial electron beam CT measurements of coronary artery calcium: Has your patient's calcium score actually changed? AJR Am J Roentgenol 2005;185:1546–1553.
53. Chung H, McClelland RL, Katz R, Carr JJ, Budoff MJ. Repeatability limits for measurement of coronary artery calcified plaque with cardiac CT in The Multi-Ethnic Study of Atherosclerosis. AJR Am J Roentgenol 2008;190:W87–W92.
54. Folsom AR, Kronmal RA, Detrano RC, et al. Coronary artery calcification compared with carotid intima-media thickness in the prediction of cardiovascular disease incidence: The Multi-Ethnic Study of Atherosclerosis (MESA). Arch Intern Med 2008;168:1333–1339.
55. Becker A, Leber A, Becker C, Knez A. Predictive value of coronary calcifications for future cardiac events in asymptomatic individuals. Am Heart J 2008;155:154–160.
56. Bild DE, Bluemke DA, Burke GL, et al. Multi-Ethnic Study of Atherosclerosis: Objectives and design. Am J Epidemiol 2002;156:871–881.
57. Schmermund A, Mohlenkamp S, Stang A, et al. Assessment of clinically silent atherosclerotic disease and established and novel risk factors for predicting myocardial infarction and cardiac death in healthy middle-aged subjects: Rationale and design of the Heinz Nixdorf RECALL study. Risk factors, evaluation of coronary calcium and lifestyle. Am Heart J 2002;144:212–218.

58. Dey D, Callister TQ, Slomka PJ, Aboul-Enein F, Nishina H, Kang X, Gransar H, Wong ND, Miranda-Peats R, Hayes S, Friedman JD, Berman DS. Computer-aided detection and evaluation of lipid-rich plaque in non-contrast cardiac Computed Tomography. Am J Roentgenol 2006;186:S407–S413.
59. Teichholz LE, Petrillo S, Larson AJ, Klig V. Quantitative assessment of atherosclerosis by electron beam tomography. Am J Cardiol 2002;90:1416–1419.
60. Rosito GA, Massaro JM, Hoffmann U, et al. Pericardial fat, visceral abdominal fat, cardiovascular disease risk factors, and vascular calcification in a community-based sample: The Framingham Heart Study. Circulation 2008;117:605–613.
61. Gorter PM, van Lindert ASR, de Vos AM, et al. Quantification of epicardial and peri-coronary fat using cardiac Computed Tomography; reproducibility and relation with obesity and metabolic syndrome in patients suspected of coronary artery disease. Atherosclerosis 2008;197:896–903.
62. Ding J, Kritchevsky SB, Harris TB, et al. The association of pericardial fat with calcified coronary plaque. Obesity 2008;16:1914–1919.
63. Taguchi R, Takasu J, Itani Y, et al. Pericardial fat accumulation in men as a risk factor for coronary artery disease. Atherosclerosis 2001;157:203–209.
64. Wheeler GL, Shi R, Beck SR, et al. Pericardial and visceral adipose tissues measured volumetrically with Computed Tomography are highly associated in type 2 diabetic families. Invest Radiol 2005;40:97–101.
65. Dey D, Suzuki Y, Suzuki S, et al. Automated quantitation of pericardiac fat from noncontrast CT. Invest Radiol 2008;43:145–153.
66. Mahabadi AA, Massaro JM, Rosito GA, et al. Association of pericardial fat, intrathoracic fat, and visceral abdominal fat with cardiovascular disease burden: The Framingham Heart Study. Eur Heart J 2009;30(7):850–856.
67. Greif M, Becker A, von Ziegler F, Lebherz C, Lehrke M, Brödl U, Tittus J, Parhofer K, Becker C, Reiser M, Knez A, Leber AW. Pericardial adipose tissue determined by dual source CT is a risk factor for coronary atherosclerosis. Arterioscler Thromb Vasc Biol 2009;29(5):781–786.
68. Bandekar A, Naghavi M, Kakadiaris IA. Automated pericardial fat quantification in CT data. In: Proc. of the 28th Annual Intl. Conf. of the IEEE Engineering in Medical and Biology Society, (EMBS'06), New York, Aug 30 – Sep 3, 2006.
69. Dey D, Wong ND, Tamarappoo BK, Nakazato R, Shah A, Gransar H, Cheng VY, Ramesh A, Kakadiaris I, Germano G, Slomka PJ, Berman DS. Computer-aided non-contrast CT-based quantification of pericardial and thoracic fat and their associations with coronary calcium and metabolic syndrome. Atherosclerosis 2009: in press: doi:10.1016/j.atherosclerosis.2009.08.032.
70. Takasu J, Takanashi K, Naito S, et al. Evaluation of morphological changes of the atherosclerotic aorta by enhanced Computed Tomography. Atherosclerosis 1992;97:107–121.
71. Itani Y, Watanabe S, Masuda Y. Aortic calcification detected in a mass chest screening program using a mobile helical computed tomography unit. Relationship to risk factors and coronary artery disease. Circ J 2004;68:538–541.
72. Atak R, Ileri M, Yetkin O, et al. The role of valvular and thoracic aortic calcifications in distinction between ischemic and nonischemic cardiomyopathy. Angiology 2004;55:661–667.
73. Adler Y, Fisman EZ, Shemesh J, et al. Spiral computed tomography evidence of close correlation between coronary and thoracic aorta calcifications. Atherosclerosis 2004;176:133–138.
74. Tanne D, Tenenbaum A, Shemesh J, et al. Calcification of the thoracic aorta by spiral Computed Tomography among hypertensive patients: Associations and risk of ischemic cerebrovascular events. Int J Cardiol 2007;120:32–37.
75. Iribarren C, Sidney S, Sternfeld B, Browner WS. Calcification of the aortic arch: Risk factors and association with coronary heart disease, stroke, and peripheral vascular disease. J Am Med Assoc 2000;283:2810–2815.
76. Wolak A, Gransar H, Thomson LEJ, et al. Aortic size assessment by noncontrast cardiac Computed Tomography: Normal limits by age, gender, and body surface area. J Am Coll Cardiol Img 2008;1:200–209.
77. Mao SS, Ahmadi N, Shah B, et al. Normal thoracic aorta diameter on cardiac Computed Tomography in healthy asymptomatic adults impact of age and gender. Acad Radiol 2008;15:827–834.
78. Kurkure U, Avila-Montes OC, Kakadiaris IA. Automated localization and segmentation of thoracic aorta in non-contrast CT images. In: Proc. 5th IEEE International Symposium on Biomedical Imaging: From Nano to Macro. Paris, France, 2008.
79. Chikos PM, Figley MM, Fisher L. Correlation between chest film and angiographic assessment of left ventricular size. AJR Am J Roentgenol 1977;128:367–373.
80. Frishman WH, Nadelmann J, Ooi WL, et al. Cardiomegaly on chest X-ray: Prognostic implications from a ten-year cohort study of elderly subjects: a report from the Bronx Longitudinal Aging Study. Am Heart J 1992;124:1026–1030.
81. Sandvik L, Erikssen J, Thaulow E, Erikssen G, Mundal R, Aakhus T. Heart volume and cardiovascular mortality. A 16 year follow-up study of 1984 healthy middle-aged men. Eur Heart J 1993;14:592–596.
82. Nasir K, Katz R, Mao S, Takasu J, Bomma C, Lima J, Bluemke D, Kronmal R, Carr J, Budoff M. Comparison of left ventricular size by Computed Tomography with Magnetic Resonance Imaging measures of left ventricle mass and volumes: The Multi-Ethnic Study of Atherosclerosis. J Cardiovasc Comput Tomogr 2008;2:141–148.
83. Ehara S, Kobayashi Y, Yoshiyama M, et al. Spotty calcification typifies the culprit plaque in patients with acute myocardial infarction: An intravascular ultrasound study. Circulation 2004;110:3424–3429.
84. van der Hoeven BL, Liem SS, Oemrawsingh PV, et al. Role of calcified spots detected by intravascular ultrasound in patients with ST-segment elevation acute myocardial infarction. Am J Cardiol 2006;98:309–313.
85. Motoyama S, Kondo T, Sarai M, et al. Multislice Computed Tomographic characteristics of coronary lesions in acute coronary syndromes. J Am Coll Cardiol 2007;50:319–326.

86. Williams M, Shaw LJ, Raggi P, et al. Prognostic value of number and site of calcified coronary lesions compared with the total score. J Am Coll Cardiol Cardiovasc Imaging 2008;1:61–69.
87. Kurkure U, Chittajallu, D, Brunner, G, Yalamanchili, R, Kakadiaris IA. Detection of coronary calcifications using supervised hierarchical classification. In: Proc. 2nd MICCAI Workshop on Computer Vision for Intravascular and Intracardiac Imaging. New York, NY, 2008.
88. Brunner G, Chittajallu DR, Kurkure U, Kakadiaris IA. A heart-centered coordinate system for the detection of coronary artery zones in non-contrast Computed Tomography data. In: Proc. 2nd MICCAI Workshop on Computer Vision for Intravascular and Intracardiac Imaging. New York, NY, 2008.

IV

Non Invasive Functional Imaging of Asymptomatic Atherosclerotic Cardiovascular Disease

29 Ultrasound Assessment of Brachial Artery Reactivity

A. Rauoof Malik and Iftikhar J. Kullo

CONTENTS

Abstract

Conventional cardiovascular risk factors do not always provide sufficiently accurate estimates of cardiovascular risk. Detection of arterial abnormalities that antedate clinical cardiovascular disease could potentially help refine cardiovascular risk assessment. Brachial artery reactivity testing (BART) is a noninvasive modality to detect endothelial dysfunction, an early feature of atherogenesis. An increase in brachial artery blood flow is brought about through transient forearm occlusion, and high-resolution ultrasonography is used to measure the resulting flow-mediated dilatation (FMD) of the brachial artery, a vascular response that is believed to result at least in part from the hyperemia-induced release of nitric oxide from the endothelium in the upstream conduit artery. FMD is impaired in asymptomatic subjects with cardiovascular risk factors as well as in subjects with known cardiovascular disease. Several studies have shown impaired FMD to be associated with increased incidence of adverse cardiovascular events in select high-risk populations. Recent studies have also shown FMD to be predictive of future cardiovascular events in asymptomatic individuals. Furthermore, because endothelial dysfunction is involved in

From: *Asymptomatic Atherosclerosis: Pathophysiology, Detection and Treatment*
Edited by: M. Naghavi (ed.), DOI 10.1007/978-1-60327-179-0_29

the development of atherosclerosis and its sequelae, FMD could be used as an intermediate endpoint to monitor risk-reduction therapy. BART may also be used to assess forearm microcirculatory function that has been recently shown to provide insights into pathophysiology of cardiovascular disease and to correlate with cardiovascular risk factor burden. Thus, BART appears to be a promising adjunct in cardiovascular risk assessment. However, there is need to have more data about the incremental prognostic value of FMD in asymptomatic individuals and to establish its usefulness in treatment monitoring. There is also a need to establish consensus risk-defining cut-off values of FMD.

Key words: Arterial ultrasonography; Brachial artery reactivity; Cardiovascular risk, Endothelial dysfunction; Flow-mediated dilatation

TOPIC PEARLS

- Assessment of cardiovascular risk factor burden does not always provide sufficiently accurate estimates of future risk of adverse cardiovascular events such as myocardial infarction and stroke, particularly in asymptomatic individuals
- Detection of preclinical arterial dysfunction could help refine cardiovascular risk assessment in asymptomatic individuals
- Endothelial dysfunction is an early event during atherogenesis and is involved in its progression and complications
- High-resolution ultrasonography of the brachial artery is commonly used to assess flow-mediated dilatation (FMD) as a bioassay of systemic endothelial function.
- Impaired FMD has been shown to predict adverse cardiovascular events, particularly in high-risk individuals
- Further research is needed to demonstrate the incremental prognostic value of FMD in asymptomatic individuals

INTRODUCTION

Cardiovascular events such as myocardial infarction and stroke often occur in asymptomatic individuals, being the first manifestation of the underlying atherosclerotic arterial disease in up to half of the cases [1, 2]. Prevention of such events requires accurate estimation of risk in asymptomatic individuals. The sensitivity and specificity of contemporary risk prediction algorithms, which are based on conventional risk factors for atherosclerosis, have been found to be unsatisfactory [3, 4]. These risk factors are prevalent in the general population; however, individuals differ in their susceptibility to their proatherogenic effects. Screening for atherosclerotic cardiovascular disease (ACVD) using cardiac stress testing only detects hemodynamically significant lesions, whereas cardiovascular events typically complicate lesions that may not produce significant luminal stenosis. Conventional coronary angiography is invasive and produces only a "luminogram". Further, such tests rely on indirect inferences about the actual atherosclerotic changes in the arterial wall, do not identify "vulnerable" atherosclerotic plaque, and are not suitable for application in the general population.

Detection of changes in the arterial wall that precede clinical ACVD may help refine cardiovascular risk assessment. The predictive value of subclinical arterial abnormalities for future cardiovascular events has been demonstrated in several studies. Current guidelines include optional use of noninvasive testing modalities for detection of early structural and functional vascular abnormalities to improve risk stratification [3, 5–8]. Incorporation of such testing for cardiovascular risk assessment could aid in the primary prevention of adverse cardiovascular events. Assessment of endothelial function has attracted a lot of attention in this regard. Given its strategic location and function, the vascular endothelium is an important target of atherosclerotic risk factors. "Endothelial dysfunction" is an early event in atherogenesis and may reflect an integrated measure of the effects of various risk factors [9]. Endothelial dysfunction is a marker of early atherosclerosis and also mediates the progression of atherosclerotic lesions. The dysfunctional endothelium produces growth factors, expresses leukocyte adhesion molecules, and provides signals for adherent leukocytes to penetrate the endothelial barrier and migrate into the intima. In addition, endothelial dysfunction influences the dynamic behavior of atherosclerotic lesions, promoting plaque destabilization and rupture as well as the extent of subsequent thrombus formation [10]. Thus, the presence of endothelial dysfunction in an individual represents a high cardiovascular risk phenotype. Several studies have shown endothelial dysfunction to be associated with ACVD and adverse cardiovascular events [9, 11].

Currently, there is no "gold standard" test for the assessment of systemic endothelial function. Brachial artery reactivity testing (BART) is a noninvasive modality in which high-resolution ultrasound is used to assess endothelial function in the brachial artery as a measure of systemic endothelial function. It is the most studied among the host of tests that has been proposed for assessment of endothelial function and shows promise for clinical use. This chapter discusses the principles and technique of BART and summarizes the current scope of this technique in cardiovascular risk stratification in asymptomatic individuals.

PRINCIPLES OF BART

The use of BART as a test of arterial function is based on two important principles. The first is that reduction in the bioavailability of endothelium-derived vasodilators, in particular nitric oxide, is a key feature of endothelial dysfunction [12]. An increase in brachial artery blood flow is brought about by reactive hyperemia and the ensuing vasodilator response of the brachial artery is measured using high-resolution ultrasound. The increased blood flow stimulates the release of nitric oxide from the endothelium in the upstream conduit artery, resulting in dilatation of the conduit artery (Fig. 1) [13]. This FMD is considered an endothelium-dependent response and appears to be mediated in part by the endothelial release of nitric oxide [14, 15]. Thus BART can be viewed as an endothelial "stress test" – reduction in FMD of the brachial artery suggesting a limitation in the ability of endothelium to release nitric oxide under conditions of increased shear stress.

The other important principle behind BART is that endothelial dysfunction tends to be systemic in nature. The presence of abnormal endothelium-dependent vasodilatation in an arterial bed may be a marker of similar abnormalities in other arterial beds. Measures of endothelium-dependent vasomotion in the brachial circulation, including FMD of the brachial artery, have been found to correlate with coronary endothelial function [16–18]. Therefore, brachial artery FMD has been proposed as a bioassay of systemic endothelial function.

BART: THE TECHNIQUE

The brachial artery is scanned with a high-resolution ultrasound transducer, 4–10 cm above the antecubital fossa to obtain continuous 2-D images of the artery. Conventionally, a 3–5 cm longitudinal segment of the artery is studied, although recent evidence has shown that cross-sectional imaging may be superior to longitudinal imaging [19, 20]. Generally, both blood flow and diameter are measured and an average of two or three measurements is taken (Fig. 2). For blood flow measurement, angle-corrected pulsed Doppler is used with range gate in the centre of the artery lumen; blood flow is calculated from time velocity integral (TVI) as: *Flow, ml/min = TVI (cm) × CSA × heart rate (per min)*, where CSA is the cross sectional area of the brachial artery (0.785 × diameter [2]). Brachial artery

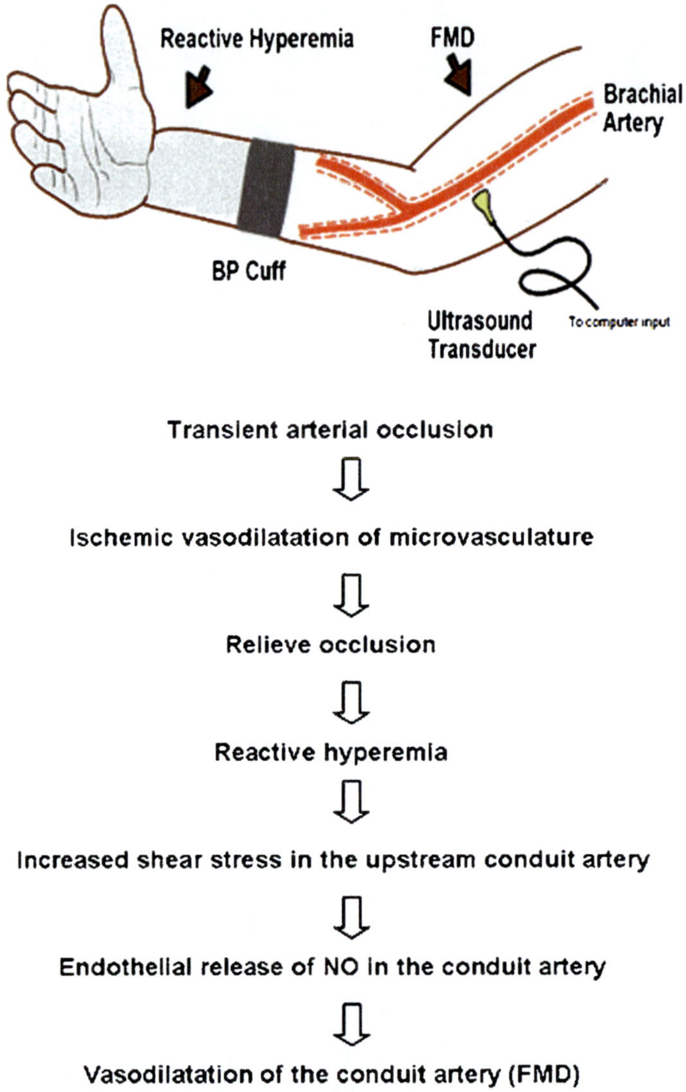

Fig. 1. The principle of brachial artery reactivity testing. A pediatric blood pressure (BP) cuff is inflated around the forearm to suprasystolic pressure for about 5 min. Ischemia of the forearm and hand during the occlusion causes vasodilatation in these tissues which brings about a marked increase in flow when the cuff is suddenly deflated. Increased blood flow during reactive hyperemia increases the shear stress acting on the endothelial surface of the upstream brachial artery that stimulates the release of vasodilators, particularly nitric oxide (NO) from the artery endothelium. The degree of reactive hyperemia obtained is a measure of functional and structural integrity of the microvasculature. The degree of vasodilation of the brachial artery (i.e. flow-mediated dilation, FMD) is a surrogate for the endothelial ability to release NO in response to increase in shear stress and is used as a bioassay for systemic endothelial function.

diameter is measured as the distance between anterior and posterior intima-lumen or media-adventitia interfaces.

After obtaining measurements of diameter and flow, forearm ischemia is induced by either upper arm or forearm occlusion. Arm occlusion produces greater degree of reactive hyperemia and FMD; [21] however, ischemia of the brachial artery wall could potentially confound the FMD measurement

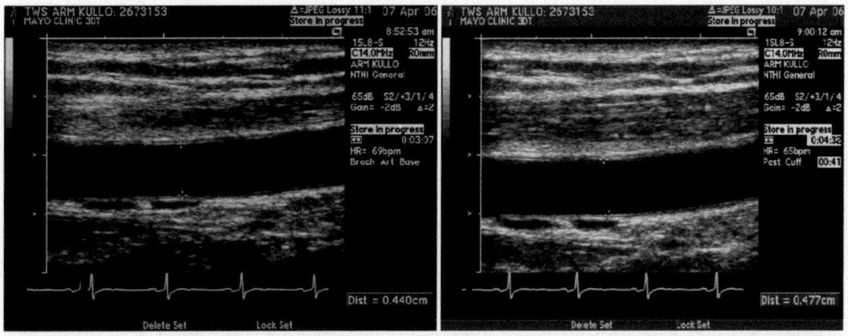

Fig. 2. Brachial artery reactivity testing – measurement of flow-mediated dilatation (FMD). Two-dimensional images of the artery before (*left*) and 45–90 s after (*right*) transient forearm ischemia are shown. The depth and gain settings are adjusted using a resolution box function to optimize the vessel wall-lumen interface and should be maintained constant throughout the procedure. Electronic calipers are used to measure brachial artery diameter at end diastole, coincident with the R wave of a simultaneously recorded electrocardiogram. Intima—lumen interface has been used to define the boundaries for diameter measurement at both near (anterior) and far (posterior) walls; alternatively, the diameter can be measured from the m-line (defined by the media-adventitia interface) at the near wall to that at the far wall. FMD in the postcuff image is calculated as percent increase in brachial artery from the baseline.

[22] and the repeatability of FMD measurement may not be as good as that for forearm occlusion [21]. A pediatric blood pressure cuff is placed well beyond the scanning site and inflated to supra-systolic pressure (50 mm Hg above systolic pressure or ~200 mmHg) for a period of 5 min at which time it is suddenly deflated. Electronic sphygmomanometer devices with timers may be helpful to maintain a constant inflation pressure and deflate automatically after a preselected time, obviating the need of a second operator. While blood flow increases 6- to 9-fold immediately after the release of cuff, the maximum increase in diameter is delayed for some time and is of the order of 10–20% in young healthy individuals. Generally, reactive hyperemia is calculated as the maximum flow during the first 15 s, while FMD is measured at 45–90 s after release of cuff; both responses (diameter and flow) are expressed as percent increase from the baseline. Recently, it has been shown that the peak vasodilator response may occur outside the conventional time points for FMD measurement; [23] thus continuous tracking of the artery diameter may be superior to visual assessment for determination of maximal FMD.

BART is generally performed using standard echo-Doppler equipment with a 7.0–13.0 MHz ultrasound scanning transducer [24]. Care should be taken to obtain high-quality images of the artery that clearly delineate the intima-media for reliable measurement of FMD. If synchronous B-mode images and Doppler recordings cannot be obtained, the diameter and flow data can be obtained by quickly alternating between the imaging modes. It is critical that the transducer position be maintained constant throughout the procedure; therefore, careful attention should be paid to the surrounding anatomical landmarks such as veins and fascial planes; use of a stereotactic clamp with micrometer movement capabilities may be helpful in this regard [25]. Further, a note should be made of the transducer position with respect to a fixed anatomical landmark like the olecranon process for future comparisons. A typical BART study takes 30 min for completion. The images can be recorded on a videotape or computer disk for subsequent off-line analysis. BART is generally well tolerated although slight, transient discomfort due to cuff occlusion may occur [26].

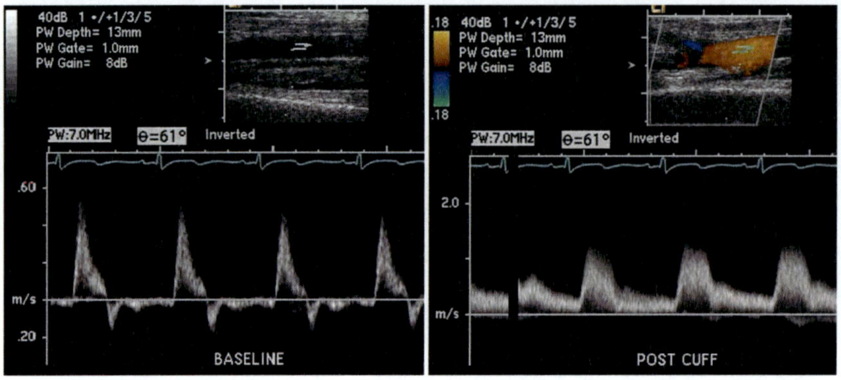

Fig. 3. Brachial artery reactivity testing – measurement of reactive hyperemia. The *left* panel shows pulsed Doppler of brachial artery with a Doppler angle of 60° and range gate in the centre of the lumen, before the inflation of a blood pressure cuff around forearm. Forward flow through the brachial artery is mostly systolic, with some flow reversal seen during diastole. The *right* panel shows marked increase in brachial artery blood flow immediately after the release of the forearm cuff and forward flow can be seen throughout the cardiac cycle. Volumic blood flow is calculated as the product of time-velocity integral, vessel cross sectional, area and heart rate. Reactive hyperemia is calculated as the ratio of maximum flow during the hyperemic phase to the baseline flow and expressed as percent increase from baseline.

In addition to brachial artery, other arterial sites like the carotid, radial, femoral, popliteal, and posterior tibial arteries have also been used to assess FMD. However, FMD measurements at these sites do not offer any operational advantage over those at the brachial artery and have not been adequately studied. Another variation concerns the method used to bring about the increase in blood flow to induce the FMD response. Stimuli like hand warming, intra-arterial infusion of vasodilators like adenosine or acetylcholine, and more prolonged ischemia have been used for this purpose. However, these methods have not been adequately standardized, may not be completely noninvasive, and may not reflect nitric oxide-dependent vasodilatation of the conduit artery [27].

PHYSIOLOGICAL VARIABILITY IN BRACHIAL ARTERY FMD

FMD is a physiological response and, like other such responses, shows variability with changing physiological conditions [28]. A study in apparently healthy young men found significant temporal variation in FMD but its measurement was more reproducible than blood pressure measurement [29]. FMD has been found to be inversely associated with plasma glucose and insulin levels [29, 30] and may be impaired after a fat-rich diet [31]; therefore, FMD is conventionally measured in the morning in a fasting state [24], although strict requirements for fasting may not be necessary [29]. Caffeine and smoking have acute effects on vascular physiology and should be avoided on the day of testing or for at least few hours prior to the test [25, 32, 33]. Even exposure to second-hand smoke may impair FMD [34, 35]. Regular physical activity improves endothelial function [36–38] and well-trained athletes tend to have higher FMD that correlates with maximum aerobic capacity [39]. FMD exhibits significant diurnal variations and is often attenuated during the early morning hours [40, 41], although a study found FMD to peak around 2.0 am in young women [42]. Endothelial function has significant interaction with autonomic nervous system activity [43, 44] and may be affected by mental stress [45–47]. Thus BART is best performed in the supine position in a warm temperature-controlled room after 10–15 min of rest with the arm placed in a comfortable position [24]. It is advisable to record any history of recent infections and the stage of menstrual cycle in women [25, 48].

FMD declines with age [38, 49] and is higher in women compared to men [49–51]. The age-related decline in FMD is delayed in women and generally occurs around menopause [52, 53], suggesting a protective role of estrogens on endothelial function. FMD is impaired under conditions of chronic stress [54], anxiety [55], and depression [56, 57]. Low levels of systemic inflammation associated with periodontitis may impair FMD which improves upon improvement in oral health [58]. While small amounts of alcohol may have neutral or even positive effects on FMD [59, 60], long-term heavy consumption of alcohol has been found to be associated with impaired FMD [61] that may not improve upon abstinence [62, 63]. The conventional guidelines for BART require the study to be performed 12–24 h off any vasoactive drugs [24], although withholding vasoactive antihypertensive medications may not be necessary [64].

THE VALUE OF BRACHIAL ARTERY FMD IN CARDIOVASCULAR RISK ASSESSMENT

BART has been extensively used to assess endothelial function in clinical investigations. Evidence gathered during past several years suggests that this testing modality could be potentially helpful in the assessment of subjects with or at risk of ACVD. Impaired brachial artery FMD has been found to correlate with the presence and severity of coronary artery disease [65, 66], although not consistently [67]. Brachial artery FMD has also been reported to predict ischemic episodes [68] and restenosis after percutaneous revascularization [69] in patients with known coronary artery disease. Several studies have shown brachial artery FMD to be predictive of incident cardiovascular events in high-risk individuals, even after accounting for conventional risk factors (Table 1) [70–72]. The independent predictive value of brachial artery FMD has been demonstrated in the setting of coronary artery disease [73], peripheral arterial disease [71, 72], and in patients undergoing evaluation for chest pain [70]. FMD was found to be predictive of increased mortality and the need for cardiac transplantation in patients with congestive heart failure [74, 75].

FMD has also been found to be impaired in asymptomatic subjects with cardiovascular risk factors [38, 49, 76]and several [38, 77, 78], though not all [79], studies have demonstrated FMD to be correlated with the risk factor burden, suggesting that impaired FMD represents the cumulative effects of risk factors on endothelial function. Whether brachial artery FMD can predict future cardiovascular events in asymptomatic individuals has been less clear. Shimbo et al found lower FMD to be predictive of incident cardiovascular event over a period of 3 years in community-based middle-age individuals who had no history of stroke or myocardial infarction. For every 1% decrease in FMD, the risk of experiencing an adverse event was 1.12, although the association of FMD with cardiovascular events was not statistically significant after adjustment for cardiovascular risk factors.

Larger, more recent studies have demonstrated the independent prognostic value of brachial FMD in asymptomatic individuals. In the Cardiovascular Health Study [80], 2729 population-based older adults (age 72–98 years) were followed for the development of cardiovascular events (cardiovascular death, myocardial infarction, stroke, congestive heart failure, claudication, angioplasty, or cardiac bypass graft surgery) after baseline measurement of brachial artery FMD. Five-year survival free of any incident or recurrent cardiovascular event was significantly better in subjects with brachial FMD greater than sex-specific median for the population compared to those with FMD equal to less than the sex-specific median value. FMD remained a significant predictor of cardiovascular events even after adjustment for risk factors and baseline presence of ACVD. However, FMD improved the accuracy of risk prediction by only ~1% over the prediction based on conventional risk factors and prevalent ACVD. Recently, Rossi et al [81] studied 2,264 asymptomatic postmenopausal women for the development of adverse cardiovascular events. Compared to women in the highest tertile of FMD,

Table 1
Studies investigating the association of brachial arterial FMD with cardiovascular events

No.	*Year*	*Study population*	*N*	*Mean age (follow-up)*	*Conclusions*
1	2000 [70]	Patients with chest pain	73	51 years (5 years)	Preserved FMD was predictive of low risk of CHD events
2	2002 [71]	Patients undergoing vascular surgery	187	65 years (1 month)	Impaired FMD was an independent predictor of postoperative CV events
3	2002 [98]	Hypertensive post-menopausal women	400	57 years (67 month)	Failure to improve FMD with 6 month of antihypertensive therapy was an independent predictor of CV events
4	2003 [72]	Patients undergoing vascular surgery	199	66 years (1.2 years)	Impaired FMD was an independent predictor of CV events
5	2003 [128]	Patients with PAD	131	64 years (23 month)	FMD and ankle-brachial index had additive prognostic value for prediction of CV events
6	2004 [129]	Patients at high risk of CHD	444	58 years (24 month)	FMD was lower for patients with CV events but not an independent predictor of events
7	2003 [73]	Patients with CHD	152	56 years (34 month)	Lower FMD and its deterioration over time were independently predictive of CV events
8	2005 [130]	Men with chest pain	398	54 years (39 month)	FMD was not independently predictive of CHD events
9	2005 [74]	CHF patients, UNOS status 2	75	56 years (3 years)	Impaired FMD was independent predictor of conversion to UNOS status 1 or death
10	2005 [75]	CHF patients, NYHA class II-III	149	54 years (28 month)	Lower FMD was associated with higher mortality risk after adjustment for known prognostic factors
11	2007 [78]	Asymptomatic subjects without h/o stroke or MI	842	67 years (36 month)	Impaired FMD at baseline was predictive of incident CV events; the predictive value for FMD was not independent of CV risk factors
12	2007 [105]	Patients undergoing vascular surgery	267	66 years (309 days)	Lower FMD and lower hyperemic flow velocity of the brachial artery were both associated with a higher risk of CV events, independent of each other and independent of CV risk factors.
13	2007 [80]	Population-based older adults	2792	78 years (5 years)	Impaired FMD was a predictor of incident CV events, independent of risk factors and baseline ACVD status; however, FMD added only 1% to the accuracy of the conventional risk prediction methods
14	2008 [81]	Asymptomatic postmenopausal women	2264	54 years (45 month)	FMD was an independent predictor of adverse cardiovascular events and contributed significantly to risk prediction beyond conventional risk factors

CHD Coronary heart disease, *CHF* Congestive heart failure, *CV* Cardiovascular, *FMD* Flow-mediated dilatation, *MI* Myocardial infarction, *NYHA* New York Heart Association, *PAD* Peripheral arterial disease, *UNOS* United Network of Organ Sharing. Follow-up is the mean duration unless indicated otherwise

women in the lowest tertile of FMD had relative risk for any cardiovascular event of 4.42, after adjustment for risk factors. Further, FMD significantly improved the predictive accuracy of the model based on cardiovascular risk factors.

FMD AS AN INTERMEDIATE END-POINT

Because endothelial dysfunction is in the causal pathway of atherosclerosis and its acute complications, restoration of endothelial function could slow or halt the progression of early atherosclerosis and stabilize established atherosclerotic lesions. The demonstration of the feasibility of reversing endothelial dysfunction with appropriate therapy [82, 83] has generated considerable interest in preventive cardiology. As a bioassay of systemic endothelial function, brachial artery FMD could be useful in assessing the effectiveness of therapies in this regard. Several interventions that are known to reduce the risk of ACVD (e.g. statins and renin-angiotensin system antagonists) have been shown to improve FMD of the brachial artery, [84–91] although some studies failed to demonstrate this effect [92, 93]. Even brief interventions with statins and renin-angiotensin system antagonists have been found to improve FMD [94–97]. A study of 400 hypertensive postmenopausal women followed for 67 months showed that lack of an improvement in FMD after 6 months of optimal antihypertensive therapy was associated with increased risk of nonfatal cardiovascular events [98]. However, the major clinical trials that demonstrated the reduction of ACVD endpoints with agents like statins and renin-angiotensin system antagonists did not include the measurement of FMD. Furthermore, some agents that have been shown to improve FMD (e.g. hormone replacement therapy [99, 100]) do not reduce the risk of cardiovascular events. Thus the clinical benefits of improved FMD are not presently clear. Prospective research is needed to establish whether interventions to improve FMD do indeed translate into a reduction in cardiovascular risk.

BART: BEYOND FMD

While brachial artery ultrasonography has typically focused on obtaining FMD, recently there has been increasing interest in characterizing other measures of arterial health that can be obtained with this technique. For example, forearm blood flow and flow response to ischemia are measures of microvascular function that are routinely obtained during FMD measurement. Several studies, including those from our laboratory, have demonstrated an association of conventional risk factors with higher resting forearm blood flow [49, 101] and an impaired flow reserve [49, 101, 102]. Microvascular dysfunction assessed using venous occlusion plethysmography has been associated with higher risk of cardiovascular events in patients with coronary artery disease [103] and in hypertensive patients [104]. In a recent study, impaired reactive hyperemia during BART was associated with increased risk of adverse cardiovascular events in patients with peripheral arterial disease [105]. Whether microvascular function measured during BART predicts cardiovascular events in asymptomatic subjects is not known.

In many laboratories, BART also includes assessment of vasodilator response of the brachial artery to nitroglycerin, an "endothelium-independent" response, as a control for FMD measurements. Nitroglycerin-mediated dilatation (NMD), a parameter that is believed to reflect arterial smooth muscle function [106], is assessed as the percent increase in brachial artery diameter 3–5 min after administration of sublingual nitroglycerin (~0.4 mg); the test being carried out 10–20 min after FMD test to allow for the brachial artery returning to its basal state. Impaired NMD has been reported in the presence of ACVD [107, 108] as well as in asymptomatic subjects with risk factors [68, 109, 110], and one study has found NMD to correlate with risk factor burden [111]. Impaired coronary artery NMD has been found to be predictive of adverse cardiovascular events [112]. However, the prognostic value of brachial artery NMD has not been investigated so far.

Baseline diameter of the brachial artery may also be a marker of cardiovascular risk. Positive remodeling of arteries is known to occur during atherosclerosis and some [113–115], though not all [116, 117], studies have shown increased brachial artery diameter in individuals with atherosclerotic risk factors. Increased brachial artery diameter has also been associated with quantity of coronary artery calcium on computed tomography scans [118] as well as with angiographic coronary artery disease [119]. Recently, brachial artery diameter was found to be predictive of incident ACVD, independently of conventional risk factors, and provided risk information comparable to that of FMD [80]. Resting brachial artery diameter measurement may be physiologically more stable [21, 29] and technically easier to obtain than FMD and its potential utility in cardiovascular risk stratification merits further exploration.

CURRENT LIMITATIONS IN ENDOTHELIAL FUNCTION ASSESSMENT

As a test, BART is technically challenging and requires a skilled ultrasonography technician, although recent technological advances have significantly reduced the dependence on operator skill [50, 120]. At least 100 supervised BART scans and at least 100 scans per year are recommended to be performed by an operator, respectively, to demonstrate and maintain competency in the use of BART [24]. Another important limitation is the significant test-to-test variability in FMD. Manual placement of the electronic calipers that is most often used for ultrasound measurement of the brachial artery diameter may be less accurate and difficult to reproduce, given that vessel diameters are generally small (3–5 mm) and the change in diameter even smaller (fraction of a mm even in healthy subjects). Edge-detection software that has been made available recently may improve the precision and reproducibility of FMD measurement [120, 121]. There is also a need for standardization of FMD measurement technique across laboratories and establishing consensus cut-off values that differentiate normal from abnormal. In addition to cardiovascular disease, endothelial function may be impaired in the presence of several inflammatory, metabolic, and other systemic disorders [122] and this should be considered while interpreting the results of BART in individual patients.

Several other testing modalities have also been proposed for "endothelial function testing [25, 123, 124]. For example, strain gauge venous plethysmography and laser digital Doppler may be used for the assessment of endothelium-dependent vasodilatation; however, the former is not entirely noninvasive while the latter is not sufficiently reproducible. Magnetic resonance imaging (MRI) is another modality that can be used to assess vasoreactivity in response to different stimuli and in different vascular beds with superior image resolution [125, 126]. However, MRI is limited in availability and is costly. Another test proposed for endothelial function assessment involves the use of peripheral arterial tonometry [127]. The change in augmentation index (a measure of peripheral arterial wave reflection) in response to inhalation of a beta-2 agonist has been proposed as a bioassay for systemic endothelial function [127]. However, arterial wave reflection is significantly affected by the structural properties of the arterial wall and the relative contribution of endothelial function is uncertain [124]. Finally, some circulatory biomarkers have also been used for the assessment of systemic endothelial function and reflect different aspects of endothelial activation involved in atherogenesis [25, 83, 124]. However, these markers are subject to modification by biological factors other than endothelial dysfunction and their use for the clinical assessment of endothelial function is not established as yet.

FUTURE PROSPECTS

Thus BART appears to be a promising tool for cardiovascular risk assessment in asymptomatic individuals. The technique for BART has been improving over past several years and several recent methodological advances have significantly refined the performance characteristics of the test. In particular, the availability of automatic edge-detection technique has improved the accuracy of FMD measurement and also made it possible to track the diameter changes continuously throughout the procedure, enabling measurement of true peak vasodilatation as well as the duration of the vasodilator response. With further refinements in technology, the impact of technical limitations on BART is expected to diminish even further.

Notwithstanding some limitations, BART has several advantages over other competing modalities that have been developed to aid in cardiovascular risk assessment. BART is noninvasive, safe, reproducible, and allows repeated measurements [124]. Brachial artery FMD is a physiological marker and can be measured even in young subjects in whom intima-media thickening or coronary calcification may not be demonstrable. Further, given that endothelial dysfunction is in the causative pathway of atherosclerosis and its complications, FMD could be useful as a biomarker at all stages of ACVD. In addition, FMD responds rapidly to interventions, making it suitable for early assessment of therapeutic interventions and for longitudinal assessment of disease course and stabilization.

Therefore, BART could be a valuable adjunct to cardiovascular risk stratification. The first Executive Summary of the Screening for Heart Attack Prevention and Education (SHAPE) Task Force [5] mentioned the assessment of systemic endothelial function as an emerging modality for cardiovascular risk assessment. Evidence published since then, including that from three prospectively conducted population-based studies, demonstrate that FMD is predictive of risk, independent of conventional risk factors for ACVD. However, the results of these studies are limited in their generalizability. Some ongoing studies are examining the prognostic utility of BART in younger subjects and in diverse ethnic groups as well as the relative merit of BART as compared to other noninvasive tools that are being proposed as adjuncts to risk factor-based assessment. Future studies should specifically investigate whether interventions to improve FMD result in reducing the risk of cardiovascular events.

SUMMARY

Screening for preclinical atherosclerotic disease may help refine cardiovascular risk assessment in asymptomatic individuals. Abnormalities in vasodilatation in response to endothelium-dependent and endothelium-independent stimuli as well as arterial remodeling may occur early during atherogenesis. BART using high-resolution ultrasonography provides a noninvasive method for the detection of such abnormalities and could potentially help identify individuals at high risk of future adverse cardiovascular events. The high-resolution ultrasound used for conventional BART provides real-time imaging at low cost, is easily available, and has no known safety concerns. Recently accumulated evidence suggests that vascular measures obtained using BART, in particular brachial artery FMD, may predict cardiovascular events independent of the risk factors for ACVD and might provide incremental prognostic information, although this needs to be proved more conclusively, particularly in younger asymptomatic individuals. Furthermore, FMD could be used as an intermediate endpoint to monitor risk-reduction therapy. However, prospective studies are needed to investigate whether interventions aimed at improving FMD are accompanied by a concomitant decrease in cardiovascular risk in asymptomatic individuals. Finally, some technological and interpretive limitations in the use of BART need to be addressed before the test can be recommended for routine clinical use.

REFERENCES

1. American Heart Association HDaSSUD, TX: American Heart Association, 2006http://www.americanheart.org/presenter.jhtml?identifier=3000090 Accessed June 11, 2006. American Heart Association, Heart Disease and Stroke Statistics – 2006 Update. Dallas, TX: American Heart Association
2. Zipes DP, Wellens HJ. Sudden cardiac death. *Circulation*. 1998;98:2334–2351.
3. Greenland P, Abrams J, Aurigemma GP, et al. Prevention Conference V: beyond secondary prevention: identifying the high-risk patient for primary prevention: noninvasive tests of atherosclerotic burden: Writing Group III. *Circulation*. 2000;101:E16–E22.
4. Kullo IJ, Ballantyne CM. Conditional risk factors for atherosclerosis. *Mayo Clin Proc*. 2005;80:219–230.
5. Naghavi M, Falk E, Hecht HS, et al. From vulnerable plaque to vulnerable patient--Part III: executive summary of the Screening for Heart Attack Prevention and Education (SHAPE) Task Force report. *Am J Cardiol*. 2006;98:2H–15H.
6. Fathi R, Marwick TH. Noninvasive tests of vascular function and structure: why and how to perform them. *Am Heart J*. 2001;141:694–703.
7. Jacoby DS, Mohler IE, Rader DJ. Noninvasive atherosclerosis imaging for predicting cardiovascular events and assessing therapeutic interventions. *Curr Atheroscler Rep*. 2004;6:20–26.
8. Patel SN, Rajaram V, Pandya S, et al. Emerging, noninvasive surrogate markers of atherosclerosis. *Curr Atheroscler Rep*. 2004;6:60–68.
9. Landmesser U, Hornig B, Drexler H. Endothelial function: a critical determinant in atherosclerosis? *Circulation*. 2004;109:II27–II33.
10. Schachinger V, Zeiher AM. Atherogenesis – recent insights into basic mechanisms and their clinical impact. *Nephrol Dial Transplant*. 2002;17:2055–2064.
11. Lerman A, Zeiher AM. Endothelial function: cardiac events. *Circulation*. 2005;111:363–368.
12. Ross R. Atherosclerosis – an inflammatory disease. *N Engl J Med*. 1999;340:115–126.
13. Anderson TJ. Assessment and treatment of endothelial dysfunction in humans. *J Am Coll Cardiol*. 1999;34:631–638.
14. Joannides R, Haefeli WE, Linder L, et al. Nitric oxide is responsible for flow-dependent dilatation of human peripheral conduit arteries in vivo. *Circulation*. 1995;91:1314–1319.
15. Dimmeler S, Fleming I, Fisslthaler B, Hermann C, Busse R, Zeiher AM. Activation of nitric oxide synthase in endothelial cells by Akt-dependent phosphorylation. *Nature*. 1999;399:601–605.
16. Anderson TJ, Uehata A, Gerhard MD, et al. Close relation of endothelial function in the human coronary and peripheral circulations. *J Am Coll Cardiol*. 1995;26:1235–1241.
17. Takase B, Hamabe A, Satomura K, et al. Close relationship between the vasodilator response to acetylcholine in the brachial and coronary artery in suspected coronary artery disease. *Int J Cardiol*. 2005;105:58–66.
18. Matsuo S, Matsumoto T, Takashima H, et al. The relationship between flow-mediated brachial artery vasodilation and coronary vasomotor responses to bradykinin: comparison with those to acetylcholine. *J Cardiovasc Pharmacol*. 2004;44:164–170.
19. Kao YH, Mohler ER, Arger PH, Sehgal CM. Brachial artery: measurement of flow-mediated dilatation with cross-sectional US – technical validation. *Radiology*. 2003;228:895–900.
20. Chaudhry FA, Bangalore S, Upadya S, et al. Cross-sectional imaging identifies flow-mediated vasodilatation more accurately compared with longitudinal imaging. *J Am Soc Echocardiogr*. 2007;20:1380–1385.
21. Peretz A, Leotta DF, Sullivan JH, et al. Flow mediated dilation of the brachial artery: an investigation of methods requiring further standardization. *BMC Cardiovasc Disord*. 2007;7:11.
22. Agewall S, Doughty RN, Bagg W, Whalley GA, Braatvedt G, Sharpe N. Comparison of ultrasound assessment of flow-mediated dilatation in the radial and brachial artery with upper and forearm cuff positions. *Clin Physiol*. 2001;21:9–14.
23. Black MA, Cable NT, Thijssen DH, Green DJ. Importance of measuring the time course of flow-mediated dilatation in humans. *Hypertension*. 2008;51:203–210.
24. Corretti MC, Anderson TJ, Benjamin EJ, et al. Guidelines for the ultrasound assessment of endothelial-dependent flow-mediated vasodilation of the brachial artery. A report of the International Brachial Artery Reactivity Task Force. *J Am Coll Cardiol*. 2002;39:257–265.
25. Deanfield J, Donald A, Ferri C, et al. Endothelial function and dysfunction. Part I: methodological issues for assessment in the different vascular beds: a statement by the Working Group on Endothelin and Endothelial Factors of the European Society of Hypertension. *J Hypertens*. 2005;23:7–17.
26. Mannion TC, Vita JA, Keaney JF, Jr., Benjamin EJ, Hunter L, Polak JF. Non-invasive assessment of brachial artery endothelial vasomotor function: the effect of cuff position on level of discomfort and vasomotor responses. *Vasc Med*. 1998;3:263–267.
27. Mullen MJ, Kharbanda RK, Cross J, et al. Heterogenous nature of flow-mediated dilatation in human conduit arteries in vivo: relevance to endothelial dysfunction in hypercholesterolemia. *Circ Res*. 2001;88:145–151.
28. Hijmering ML, Stroes ES, Pasterkamp G, Sierevogel M, Banga JD, Rabelink TJ. Variability of flow mediated dilation: consequences for clinical application. *Atherosclerosis*. 2001;157:369–373.
29. Jarvisalo MJ, Jartti L, Marniemi J, et al. Determinants of short-term variation in arterial flow-mediated dilatation in healthy young men. *Clin Sci (Lond)*. 2006;110:475–482.

30. Thomas GN, Chook P, Qiao M, et al. Deleterious impact of "high normal" glucose levels and other metabolic syndrome components on arterial endothelial function and intima-media thickness in apparently healthy Chinese subjects: the CATHAY study. *Arterioscler Thromb Vasc Biol.* 2004;24:739–743.
31. Giannattasio C, Zoppo A, Gentile G, et al. Acute effect of high-fat meal on endothelial function in moderately dyslipidemic subjects. *Arterioscler Thromb Vasc Biol.* 2005;25:406–410.
32. Papamichael CM, Aznaouridis KA, Karatzis EN, et al. Effect of coffee on endothelial function in healthy subjects: the role of caffeine. *Clin Sci (Lond).* 2005;109:55–60.
33. Lekakis J, Papamichael C, Vemmos C, et al. Effect of acute cigarette smoking on endothelium-dependent brachial artery dilatation in healthy individuals. *Am J Cardiol.* 1997;79:529–531.
34. Celermajer DS, Adams MR, et al. Passive smoking and impaired endothelium-dependent arterial dilatation in healthy young adults. *N Engl J Med.* 1996;334:150–154.
35. Woo KS, Chook P, Leong HC, Huang XS, Celermajer DS. The impact of heavy passive smoking on arterial endothelial function in modernized Chinese. *J Am Coll Cardiol.* 2000;36:1228–1232.
36. Abbott RA, Harkness MA, Davies PS. Correlation of habitual physical activity levels with flow-mediated dilation of the brachial artery in 5-10 year old children. *Atherosclerosis.* 2002;160:233–239.
37. Clarkson P, Montgomery HE, Mullen MJ, et al. Exercise training enhances endothelial function in young men. *J Am Coll Cardiol.* 1999;33:1379–1385.
38. Benjamin EJ, Larson MG, Keyes MJ, et al. Clinical correlates and heritability of flow-mediated dilation in the community: the Framingham Heart Study. *Circulation.* 2004;109:613–619.
39. Kasikcioglu E, Oflaz H, Kasikcioglu HA, Kayserilioglu A, Umman S, Meric M. Endothelial flow-mediated dilatation and exercise capacity in highly trained endurance athletes. *Tohoku J Exp Med.* 2005;205:45–51.
40. Otto ME, Svatikova A, Barretto RB, et al. Early morning attenuation of endothelial function in healthy humans. *Circulation.* 2004;109:2507–2510.
41. Etsuda H, Takase B, Uehata A, et al. Morning attenuation of endothelium-dependent, flow-mediated dilation in healthy young men: possible connection to morning peak of cardiac events? *Clin Cardiol.* 1999;22:417–421.
42. Ringqvist A, Caidahl K, Petersson AS, Wennmalm A. Diurnal variation of flow-mediated vasodilation in healthy premenopausal women. *Am J Physiol Heart Circ Physiol.* 2000;279:H2720–H2725.
43. Harris KF, Matthews KA. Interactions between autonomic nervous system activity and endothelial function: a model for the development of cardiovascular disease. *Psychosom Med.* 2004;66:153–164.
44. Hijmering ML, Stroes ES, Olijhoek J, Hutten BA, Blankestijn PJ, Rabelink TJ. Sympathetic activation markedly reduces endothelium-dependent, flow-mediated vasodilation. *J Am Coll Cardiol.* 2002;39:683–688.
45. Harris CW, Edwards JL, Baruch A, et al. Effects of mental stress on brachial artery flow-mediated vasodilation in healthy normal individuals. *Am Heart J.* 2000;139:405–411.
46. Lind L, Johansson K, Hall J. The effects of mental stress and the cold pressure test on flow-mediated vasodilation. *Blood Press.* 2002;11:22–27.
47. Gottdiener JS, Kop WJ, Hausner E, McCeney MK, Herrington D, Krantz DS. Effects of mental stress on flow-mediated brachial arterial dilation and influence of behavioral factors and hypercholesterolemia in subjects without cardiovascular disease. *Am J Cardiol.* 2003;92:687–691.
48. Hashimoto M, Akishita M, Eto M, et al. Modulation of endothelium-dependent flow-mediated dilatation of the brachial artery by sex and menstrual cycle. *Circulation.* 1995;92:3431–3435.
49. Kullo IJ, Malik AR, Santos S, Ehrsam JE, Turner ST. Association of cardiovascular risk factors with microvascular and conduit artery function in hypertensive subjects. *Am J Hypertens.* 2007;20:735–742.
50. Herrington DM, Fan L, Drum M, et al. Brachial flow-mediated vasodilator responses in population-based research: methods, reproducibility and effects of age, gender and baseline diameter. *J Cardiovasc Risk.* 2001;8:319–328.
51. Patel AR, Kuvin JT, Sliney KA, et al. Gender-based differences in brachial artery flow-mediated vasodilation as an indicator of significant coronary artery disease. *Am J Cardiol.* 2005;96:1223–1226.
52. Celermajer DS, Sorensen KE, et al. Aging is associated with endothelial dysfunction in healthy men years before the age-related decline in women. *J Am Coll Cardiol.* 1994;24:471–476.
53. Bush DE, Jones CE, Bass KM, Walters GK, Bruza JM, Ouyang P. Estrogen replacement reverses endothelial dysfunction in postmenopausal women. *Am J Med.* 1998;104:552–558.
54. Takase B, Akima T, Uehata A, Ohsuzu F, Kurita A. Effect of chronic stress and sleep deprivation on both flow-mediated dilation in the brachial artery and the intracellular magnesium level in humans. *Clin Cardiol.* 2004;27:223–227.
55. Harris KF, Matthews KA, Sutton-Tyrrell K, Kuller LH. Associations between psychological traits and endothelial function in postmenopausal women. *Psychosom Med.* 2003;65:402–409.
56. Rajagopalan S, Brook R, Rubenfire M, Pitt E, Young E, Pitt B. Abnormal brachial artery flow-mediated vasodilation in young adults with major depression. *Am J Cardiol.* 2001;88:196–198, A197.
57. Broadley AJ, Korszun A, Jones CJ, Frenneaux MP. Arterial endothelial function is impaired in treated depression. *Heart (British Cardiac Society).* 2002;88:521–523.
58. Tonetti MS, D'Aiuto F, Nibali L, et al. Treatment of periodontitis and endothelial function. *N Engl J Med.* 2007;356: 911–920.

59. Vlachopoulos C, Tsekoura D, Tsiamis E, Panagiotakos D, Stefanadis C. Effect of alcohol on endothelial function in healthy subjects. *Vasc Med.* 2003;8:263–265.
60. Puddey IB, Zilkens RR, Croft KD, Beilin LJ. Alcohol and endothelial function: a brief review. *Clin Exp Pharmacol Physiol.* 2001;28:1020–1024.
61. Maiorano G, Bartolomucci F, Contursi V, et al. Noninvasive detection of vascular dysfunction in alcoholic patients. *Am J Hypertens.* 1999;12:137–144.
62. Zilkens RR, Rich L, Burke V, Beilin LJ, Watts GF, Puddey IB. Effects of alcohol intake on endothelial function in men: a randomized controlled trial. *J Hypertens.* 2003;21:97–103.
63. Di Gennaro C, Biggi A, Barilli AL, et al. Endothelial dysfunction and cardiovascular risk profile in long-term withdrawing alcoholics. *J Hypertens.* 2007;25:367–373.
64. Gokce N, Holbrook M, Hunter LM, et al. Acute effects of vasoactive drug treatment on brachial artery reactivity. *J Am Coll Cardiol.* 2002;40:761–765.
65. Neunteufl T, Katzenschlager R, Hassan A, et al. Systemic endothelial dysfunction is related to the extent and severity of coronary artery disease. *Atherosclerosis.* 1997;129:111–118.
66. Kaku B, Mizuno S, Ohsato K, et al. The correlation between coronary stenosis index and flow-mediated dilation of the brachial artery. *Jpn Circ J.* 1998;62:425–430.
67. Schroeder S, Enderle MD, Ossen R, et al. Noninvasive determination of endothelium-mediated vasodilation as a screening test for coronary artery disease: pilot study to assess the predictive value in comparison with angina pectoris, exercise electrocardiography, and myocardial perfusion imaging. *Am Heart J.* 1999;138:731–739.
68. Sondergaard E, Moller JE, Egstrup K. Relationship between vascular dysfunction in peripheral arteries and ischemic episodes during daily life in patients with ischemic heart disease and hypercholesterolemia. *Am Heart J.* 2002;144:108–114.
69. Patti G, Pasceri V, Melfi R, et al. Impaired flow-mediated dilation and risk of restenosis in patients undergoing coronary stent implantation. *Circulation.* 2005;111:70–75.
70. Neunteufl T, Heher S, Katzenschlager R, et al. Late prognostic value of flow-mediated dilation in the brachial artery of patients with chest pain. *Am J Cardiol.* 2000;86:207–210.
71. Gokce N, Keaney JF, Jr., Hunter LM, Watkins MT, Menzoian JO, Vita JA. Risk stratification for postoperative cardiovascular events via noninvasive assessment of endothelial function: a prospective study. *Circulation.* 2002;105:1567–1572.
72. Gokce N, Keaney JF, Jr., Hunter LM, et al. Predictive value of noninvasively determined endothelial dysfunction for long-term cardiovascular events in patients with peripheral vascular disease. *J Am Coll Cardiol.* 2003;41:1769–1775.
73. Chan SY, Mancini GB, Kuramoto L, Schulzer M, Frohlich J, Ignaszewski A. The prognostic importance of endothelial dysfunction and carotid atheroma burden in patients with coronary artery disease. *J Am Coll Cardiol.* 2003;42:1037–1043.
74. Meyer B, Mortl D, Strecker K, et al. Flow-mediated vasodilation predicts outcome in patients with chronic heart failure comparison with B-type natriuretic Peptide. *J Am Coll Cardiol.* 2005;46:1011–1018.
75. Katz SD, Hryniewicz K, Hriljac I, et al. Vascular endothelial dysfunction and mortality risk in patients with chronic heart failure. *Circulation.* 2005;111:310–314.
76. Celermajer DS, Sorensen KE, Bull C, Robinson J, Deanfield JE. Endothelium-dependent dilation in the systemic arteries of asymptomatic subjects relates to coronary risk factors and their interaction. *J Am Coll Cardiol.* 1994;24:1468–1474.
77. Witte DR, Westerink J, de Koning EJ, van der Graaf Y, Grobbee DE, Bots ML. Is the association between flow-mediated dilation and cardiovascular risk limited to low-risk populations? *J Am Coll Cardiol.* 2005;45:1987–1993.
78. Shimbo D, Grahame-Clarke C, Miyake Y, et al. The association between endothelial dysfunction and cardiovascular outcomes in a population-based multi-ethnic cohort. *Atherosclerosis.* 2007;192:197–203.
79. Yan RT, Anderson TJ, Charbonneau F, Title L, Verma S, Lonn E. Relationship between carotid artery intima-media thickness and brachial artery flow-mediated dilation in middle-aged healthy men. *J Am Coll Cardiol.* 2005;45:1980–1986.
80. Yeboah J, Crouse JR, Hsu FC, Burke GL, Herrington DM. Brachial flow-mediated dilation predicts incident cardiovascular events in older adults: the Cardiovascular Health Study. *Circulation.* 2007;115:2390–2397.
81. Rossi R, Nuzzo A, Origliani G, Modena MG. Prognostic role of flow-mediated dilation and cardiac risk factors in post-menopausal women. *J Am Coll Cardiol.* 2008;51:997–1002.
82. Celermajer DS. Endothelial dysfunction: does it matter? Is it reversible? *J Am Coll Cardiol.* 1997;30:325–333.
83. Widlansky ME, Gokce N, Keaney JF, Jr., Vita JA. The clinical implications of endothelial dysfunction. *J Am Coll Cardiol.* 2003;42:1149–1160.
84. Dupuis J, Tardif JC, Rouleau JL, et al. Intensity of lipid lowering with statins and brachial artery vascular endothelium reactivity after acute coronary syndromes (from the BRAVER trial). *Am J Cardiol.* 2005;96:1207–1213.
85. Dogra GK, Watts GF, Chan DC, Stanton K. Statin therapy improves brachial artery vasodilator function in patients with Type 1 diabetes and microalbuminuria. *Diabet Med.* 2005;22:239–242.
86. Jensen LO, Thayssen P, Pedersen KE, Haghfelt T. Short- and long-term influence of diet and simvastatin on brachial artery endothelial function. *Int J Cardiol.* 2006;107:101–106.
87. Alber HF, Frick M, Sussenbacher A, et al. Effect of atorvastatin on peripheral endothelial function and systemic inflammatory markers in patients with stable coronary artery disease. *Wiener Medizinische Wochenschrift.* 2007;157:73–78.
88. Ferreira WP, Bertolami MC, Santos SN, et al. One-month therapy with simvastatin restores endothelial function in hypercholesterolemic children and adolescents. *Pediatr Cardiol.* 2007;28:8–13.

89. Agewall S, Hernberg A. Atorvastatin normalizes endothelial function in healthy smokers. *Clin Sci (Lond).* 2006;111: 87–91.
90. Mancini GB, Henry GC, Macaya C, et al. Angiotensin-converting enzyme inhibition with quinapril improves endothelial vasomotor dysfunction in patients with coronary artery disease. The TREND (Trial on Reversing ENdothelial Dysfunction) Study. *Circulation.* 1996;94:258–265
91. Anderson TJ, Elstein E, Haber H, Charbonneau F. Comparative study of ACE-inhibition, angiotensin II antagonism, and calcium channel blockade on flow-mediated vasodilation in patients with coronary disease (BANFF study). *J Am Coll Cardiol.* 2000;35:60–66.
92. Spring S, Simon R, van der Loo B, et al. High-dose atorvastatin in peripheral arterial disease (PAD): effect on endothelial function, intima-media-thickness and local progression of PAD. An open randomized controlled pilot trial. *Thromb Haemost.* 2008;99:182–189.
93. Asselbergs FW, van der Harst P, van Roon AM, et al. Long-term effects of pravastatin and fosinopril on peripheral endothelial function in albuminuric subjects. *Atherosclerosis.* 2008;196:349–355.
94. Vogel RA, Corretti MC, Plotnick GD. Changes in flow-mediated brachial artery vasoactivity with lowering of desirable cholesterol levels in healthy middle-aged men. *Am J Cardiol.* 1996;77:37–40.
95. Omori H, Nagashima H, Tsurumi Y, et al. Direct in vivo evidence of a vascular statin: a single dose of cerivastatin rapidly increases vascular endothelial responsiveness in healthy normocholesterolaemic subjects. *Br J Clin Pharmacol.* 2002;54:395–399.
96. Mercuro G, Zoncu S, Saiu F, Sarais C, Rosano GM. Effect of atorvastatin on endothelium-dependent vasodilation in postmenopausal women with average serum cholesterol levels. *Am J Cardiol.* 2002;90:747–750.
97. Koh KK, Bui MN, Hathaway L, et al. Mechanism by which quinapril improves vascular function in coronary artery disease. *Am J Cardiol.* 1999;83:327–331.
98. Modena MG, Bonetti L, Coppi F, Bursi F, Rossi R. Prognostic role of reversible endothelial dysfunction in hypertensive postmenopausal women. *J Am Coll Cardiol.* 2002;40:505–510.
99. Hashimoto M, Miyamoto Y, Matsuda Y, Akita H. New methods to evaluate endothelial function: non-invasive method of evaluating endothelial function in humans. *J Pharmacol Sci.* 2003;93:405–408.
100. Lieberman EH, Gerhard MD, Uehata A, et al. Estrogen improves endothelium-dependent, flow-mediated vasodilation in postmenopausal women. *Ann Intern Med.* 1994;121:936–941.
101. Mitchell GF, Parise H, Vita JA, et al. Local shear stress and brachial artery flow-mediated dilation: the Framingham Heart Study. *Hypertension.* 2004;44:134–139.
102. Dakak N, Husain S, Mulcahy D, et al. Contribution of nitric oxide to reactive hyperemia: impact of endothelial dysfunction. *Hypertension.* 1998;32:9–15.
103. Heitzer T, Schlinzig T, Krohn K, Meinertz T, Munzel T. Endothelial dysfunction, oxidative stress, and risk of cardiovascular events in patients with coronary artery disease. *Circulation.* 2001;104:2673–2678.
104. Perticone F, Ceravolo R, Pujia A, et al. Prognostic significance of endothelial dysfunction in hypertensive patients. *Circulation.* 2001;104:191–196.
105. Huang AL, Silver AE, Shvenke E, et al. Predictive value of reactive hyperemia for cardiovascular events in patients with peripheral arterial disease undergoing vascular surgery. *Arterioscler Thromb Vasc Biol.* 2007;27:2113–2119.
106. Mehta JL. Endothelium, coronary vasodilation, and organic nitrates. *Am Heart J.* 1995;129:382–391.
107. Adams MR, Robinson J, McCredie R, et al. Smooth muscle dysfunction occurs independently of impaired endothelium-dependent dilation in adults at risk of atherosclerosis. *J Am Coll Cardiol.* 1998;32:123–127.
108. Yugar-Toledo JC, Tanus-Santos JE, Sabha M, et al. Uncontrolled hypertension, uncompensated type II diabetes, and smoking have different patterns of vascular dysfunction. *Chest.* 2004;125:823–830.
109. Zhang X, Zhao SP, Li XP, Gao M, Zhou QC. Endothelium-dependent and -independent functions are impaired in patients with coronary heart disease. *Atherosclerosis.* 2000;149:19–24.
110. Raitakari OT, Seale JP, Celermajer DS. Impaired vascular responses to nitroglycerin in subjects with coronary atherosclerosis. *Am J Cardiol.* 2001;87:217–219, A218.
111. Jensen-Urstad K, Johansson J. Gender difference in age-related changes in vascular function. *J Intern Med.* 2001;250: 29–36.
112. Schachinger V, Britten MB, Zeiher AM. Prognostic impact of coronary vasodilator dysfunction on adverse long-term outcome of coronary heart disease. *Circulation.* 2000;101:1899–1906.
113. Jensen-Urstad K, Johansson J, Jensen-Urstad M. Vascular function correlates with risk factors for cardiovascular disease in a healthy population of 35-year-old subjects. *J Intern Med.* 1997;241:507–513.
114. Corretti MC, Plotnick GD, Vogel RA. Correlation of cold pressor and flow-mediated brachial artery diameter responses with the presence of coronary artery disease. *Am J Cardiol.* 1995;75:783–787.

115. Kuvin JT, Patel AR, Sidhu M, et al. Relation between high-density lipoprotein cholesterol and peripheral vasomotor function. *Am J Cardiol*. 2003;92:275–279.
116. Gaenzer H, Neumayr G, Marschang P, Sturm W, Kirchmair R, Patsch JR. Flow-mediated vasodilation of the femoral and brachial artery induced by exercise in healthy nonsmoking and smoking men. *J Am Coll Cardiol*. 2001;38:1313–1319.
117. Shechter M, Sharir M, Labrador MJ, Forrester J, Merz CN. Improvement in endothelium-dependent brachial artery flow-mediated vasodilation with low-density lipoprotein cholesterol levels <100 mg/dl. *Am J Cardiol*. 2000;86:1256–1259.
118. Kullo IJ, Malik AR, Bielak LF, Sheedy PF, Turner ST, Peyser PA. Brachial artery diameter and vasodilator response to nitroglycerin but not flow-mediated dilation are associated with presence and quantity of coronary artery calcium in asymptomatic adults. *Clin Sci (Lond)*. 2007;112:175–182.
119. Holubkov R, Karas RH, Pepine CJ, et al. Large brachial artery diameter is associated with angiographic coronary artery disease in women. *Am Heart J*. 2002;143:802–807.
120. Woodman RJ, Playford DA, Watts GF, et al. Improved analysis of brachial artery ultrasound using a novel edge-detection software system. *J Appl Physiol*. 2001;91:929–937.
121. Preik M, Lauer T, Heiss C, Tabery S, Strauer BE, Kelm M. Automated ultrasonic measurement of human arteries for the determination of endothelial function. *Ultraschall in der Medizin*. 2000;21:195–198.
122. Faulx MD, Wright AT, Hoit BD. Detection of endothelial dysfunction with brachial artery ultrasound scanning. *Am Heart J*. 2003;145:943–951.
123. Raitakari OT, Celermajer DS. Testing for endothelial dysfunction. *Ann Med*. 2000;32:293–304.
124. Deanfield JE, Halcox JP, Rabelink TJ. Endothelial function and dysfunction: testing and clinical relevance. *Circulation*. 2007;115:1285–1295.
125. Wiesmann F, Petersen SE, Leeson PM, et al. Global impairment of brachial, carotid, and aortic vascular function in young smokers: direct quantification by high-resolution magnetic resonance imaging. *J Am Coll Cardiol*. 2004;44: 2056–2064.
126. Silber HA, Ouyang P, Bluemke DA, Gupta SN, Foo TK, Lima JA. Why is flow-mediated dilation dependent on arterial size? Assessment of the shear stimulus using phase-contrast magnetic resonance imaging. *Am J Physiol Heart Circ Physiol*. 2005;288:H822–H828.
127. Hayward CS, Kraidly M, Webb CM, Collins P. Assessment of endothelial function using peripheral waveform analysis: a clinical application. *J Am Coll Cardiol*. 2002;40:521–528.
128. Brevetti G, Silvestro A, Schiano V, Chiariello M. Endothelial dysfunction and cardiovascular risk prediction in peripheral arterial disease: additive value of flow-mediated dilation to ankle-brachial pressure index. *Circulation*. 2003;108:2093–2098.
129. Fathi R, Haluska B, Isbel N, Short L, Marwick TH. The relative importance of vascular structure and function in predicting cardiovascular events. *J Am Coll Cardiol*. 2004;43:616–623.
130. Frick M, Suessenbacher A, Alber HF, et al. Prognostic value of brachial artery endothelial function and wall thickness. *J Am Coll Cardiol*. 2005;46:1006–1010.

30 Cardiac Imaging for Ischemia in Asymptomatic Patients: Use of Coronary Artery Calcium Scanning to Improve Patient Selection: Lessons from the EISNER Study

Alan Rozanski, Heidi Gransar, Nathan D. Wong, Leslee J. Shaw, Michael J. Zellweger, and Daniel S. Berman

CONTENTS

ABSTRACT

We review emerging data that identify how coronary artery calcium (CAC) scanning can complement radionuclide cardiac stress testing for ischemia in the work-up of patients with suspected coronary artery disease (CAD). First, among screening populations, i.e., patients with low (<15%) Bayesian likelihood of CAD, stress imaging is characterized by a high false-positive test rate for CAD prediction and inability to detect hemodynamically insignificant stenoses. Because CAC scanning does not have these limitations and is a specific measure for atherosclerosis, it is a better screening test for CAD. Second, with respect to diagnostic testing, typically applied to patients with intermediate (15–85%) CAD likelihood, radionuclide imaging for ischemia has been validated as an effective diagnostic procedure. However, CAC scanning might complement this process by permitting more effective triaging of diagnostic patients for stress testing. This is because studies have demonstrated a threshold relationship between CAC scores and the frequency of myocardial ischemia. This threshold is typically low for patients with CAC scores <400, but a lower

From: *Asymptomatic Atherosclerosis: Pathophysiology, Detection and Treatment*
Edited by: M. Naghavi (ed.), DOI 10.1007/978-1-60327-179-0_30

CAC threshold is observed among select risk factor subgroups, such as patients with diabetes and metabolic syndrome. Prospective work is thus needed to define the optimal CAC score criteria for triaging diagnostic patients for radionuclide stress testing on the basis of CAC scanning. Third, radionuclide stress testing is commonly used for risk stratification purposes in patients with both intermediate and high (>85%) pretest CAD likelihood. Of note, our data indicate when radionuclide stress testing is normal, a wide range of CAC scores is observed, including the presence of high CAC scores in approximately one-third of such patients. Thus, knowledge of CAC scores may represent important information for modifying projections of long-term risk and optimizing medical treatment when using stress tests for risk stratification purposes.

Key words: Atherosclerosis; Cardiac risk stratification; Coronary artery calcium; Coronary artery disease; Myocardial ischemia; Myocardial perfusion SPECT; Screening

KEY POINTS

- CAC scanning was initially introduced into medicine as a proposed screening test for CAD, whereas newer data not only validate this clinical use but also indicate that CAC scanning may now have a wider role in overall clinical management than was once perceived.
- CAC scanning is a more effective screening test for CAD than radionuclide cardiac stress imaging for ischemia, because it is a specific marker for atherosclerosis. Also, unlike stress testing, CAC scanning does not suffer from a high false positive rate, nor an inability to screen for hemodynamically insignificant coronary stenoses, for CAD detection imaging.
- The likelihood of observing inducible myocardial is generally very low among patients with CAC scores <400, but this ischemic threshold shifts to lower CAC scores among diabetics and metabolic syndrome and patients with more typical anginal symptoms.
- The threshold relationship between CAC scores and myocardial ischemia suggests that CAC scores may complement other clinical information in deciding which patients may benefit from radionuclide cardiac stress imaging among some diagnostic patient groups, such as patients with nonanginal chest pain.
- Among patients with normal radionuclide stress tests, a wide range of CAC scores are seen, with approximately one-third having CAC scores >400. These data suggest that in selected patients with normal cardiac stress tests, performance of CAC scanning may still be useful to aid in long-term clinical management.

Cardiac imaging during stress testing has long been used to evaluate patients with suspected coronary artery disease (CAD). This use is based on an extensive database that has validated the current applications of cardiac stress tests. The recent advent of newer technologies, such as coronary artery calcium (CAC) scanning, CT-coronary angiography (CCTA), and cardiac magnetic resonance imaging, has opened up new possibilities for evaluating patients with suspected CAD. One of the challenges that has emerged in this new arena of cardiac imaging is determining the optimal cost-effective means for combining the older established stress test modalities and newer imaging technologies for the common questions faced in the day-to-day evaluation of patients who present with signs or symptoms that suggest the presence of CAD.

To help address this issue, approximately 10 years ago, we initiated a study designed to assess the clinical utility of CAC scanning, with one of its chief aims being the assessment of the potential synergy between CAC scanning and stress-rest myocardial perfusion SPECT. This study, termed the Early Identification of Subclinical Atherosclerosis by Noninvasive Imaging Research (EISNER), enrolled >1,000 patients for research CAC scanning following the performance of SPECT imaging. Other patients within the EISNER study underwent a clinically ordered exercise SPECT study following physician or self-referral for CAC scanning. Both groups of patients have now been followed for a number of years. In this review, we summarize some of our data that have helped us to formulate principles regarding the synergistic use of CAC scanning and stress-rest myocardial SPECT relative for the evaluation of patients with suspected CAD. Stress testing within the EISNER study was limited to only SPECT imaging, whereas the results of our data are also applicable to all forms of cardiac stress testing.

CONVENTIONAL APPLICATIONS OF STRESS-REST MYOCARDIAL PERFUSION SPECT

In order to understand the synergistic applications of CAC scanning, we first review the current clinical applications of stress rest myocardial perfusion SPECT. Its uses are predicated on the ability of this technique to detect and size the magnitude of inducible myocardial ischemia and myocardial scar in reproducible manner. From a pathophysiological perspective, the induction of myocardial perfusion defects should be an early manifestation of myocardial ischemia, as it is the proximate cause for more "downstream" ischemic manifestations, including the induction of left ventricular (LV) dysfunction, ST-segment changes, and chest pain (Fig. 1). There are now multiple methods for assessing myocardial perfusion and LV dysfunction, each with its own advantages and disadvantages. Myocardial perfusion SPECT is considered an inherently sensitive means for evaluating myocardial ischemia with a low frequency of false positives when care is taken to avoid or account for imaging artifacts, such as patient motion during SPECT acquisition or soft tissue attenuation overlapping the myocardium. The induction of myocardial ischemia during SPECT imaging is related to the magnitude of underlying coronary stenoses, but many factors influence the potential induction of ischemia, including the number of stenoses, degree of coronary collaterization, and dynamic physiological factors, such as endothelial dysfunction which sensitizes the coronary media to the effects of circulating catecholamines [1].

The amount of ischemia as detected by myocardial perfusion imaging bears an exponential relationship to the occurrence of future adverse cardiac events (i.e., cardiac death or nonfatal myocardial infarction) [2]. Both the extent of myocardial ischemia – as measured by the number of stress induced perfusion defects, and the severity of ischemia – as measured by the degree of defect reversibility in a given myocardial zone, bear an *independent* exponential relationship to the occurrence of such events [2]. The former is predictive of extensive underlying CAD and the latter is predictive of the severity of

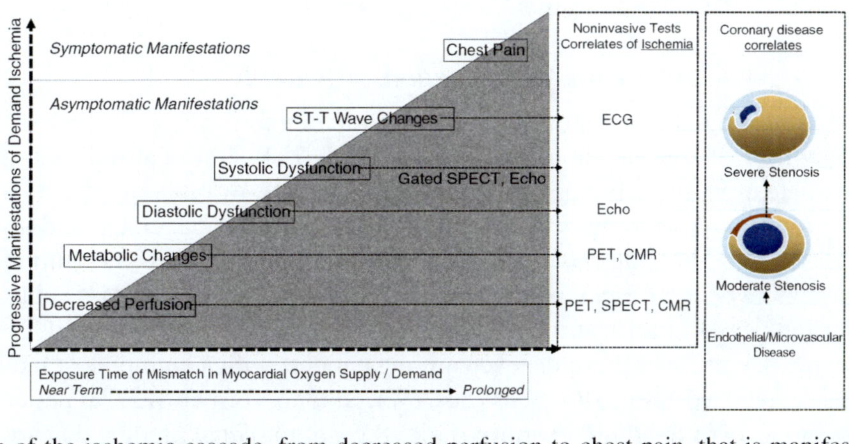

Fig. 1. Depiction of the ischemic cascade, from decreased perfusion to chest pain, that is manifest among patients with coronary artery disease (adapted from Shaw Hurst, The Manual, 2005).

stenosis within the coronary vessel that subtends a severely reversible myocardial perfusion defect. Patients having both extensive and severe ischemia manifest a cardiac event rate which is an order of magnitude higher compared to patients having just extensive ischemia or severe ischemia, but not both. In addition there are additional scintigraphic parameters which, when present, signify the presence of either extensive or severe underlying coronary disease, or both, including transient lung uptake (measurable on thallium-201 studies and less well seen on Tc-99m sestamibi or tetrofosmin studies) [3], and transient ischemic dilation of the LV poststress, which is usually a marker of both extensive and severe underlying CAD [4]. The performance of concomitant gated imaging to assess poststress wall motion following SPECT imaging allows one to also detect poststress ischemic "stunning" of LV function, by identifying transiently severe wall motion abnormality poststress within myocardial segments manifesting normal radiotracer uptake on rest sestamibi scanning.

The conventional uses of stress rest myocardial perfusion SPECT can be divided into three areas: (1) its diagnostic application; (2) risk stratification of patients with suspected or known CAD; and (3) screening purposes. Each of these applications will be discussed in sequence.

Diagnostic Application

Diagnosis of CAD is first predicated on determining patients' likelihood for having CAD. When discussing such likelihood, it is important to note that we are referring to the likelihood of having *angiographically significant* CAD (i.e., >50% or >70% luminal stenosis). A computer program that was developed by Diamond and Forrester years ago, based on pooled clinical and autopsy data, allows for the estimation of CAD likelihood based on the Bayesian analysis of patient age, sex, symptoms, and certain CAD risk factors [5]. Over time, it has become widely held that diagnostic stress testing is best reserved for those patients with an intermediate likelihood of CAD, defined broadly as having anywhere between a 15 and 85% pretest likelihood of CAD. A normal stress test will reclassify patients as having a low likelihood of CAD. Patients who are reclassified as having a high likelihood of CAD by virtue of having inducible myocardial ischemia may merit referral for cardiac catheterization if the magnitude of inducible ischemia on stress testing is substantial of if the combination of clinical and imaging factors suggests high risk. The greater the ischemic abnormality, the greater the increase that is observed in CAD likelihood post-testing. A commercial program may be used to assess pretest likelihood of CAD (CADENZA), but in clinical practice, post-test likelihood of CAD following SPECT imaging is only estimated, due to a lack of validated software for incorporating the SPECT results into CADENZA.

Risk Stratification of Patients

While *diagnostic* testing is best suited for patients with an intermediate likelihood of CAD, radionuclide stress testing is also used for *prognostic* purposes (risk stratification) among patients with either an intermediate or high likelihood of CAD (>85%) for risk stratification purposes. The issue in such patients is often that of deciding between aggressive medical management and invasive management. At the bedrock of addressing this issue is the understanding of the aforementioned exponential relationship between myocardial ischemia and the occurrence of cardiovascular events. A particularly important anchor in this risk stratification is the finding that a normal exercise SPECT study is associated with a very low risk of cardiac events, even among patients with a high pretest likelihood of CAD (Fig. 2) [6]. The annualized event risk rises, however, among normal SPECT patients who cannot achieve an adequate level of treadmill exercise (i.e., >85% of maximal predicted heart rate) due to an insensitivity of SPECT imaging for detecting ischemia at low workloads [7]. For this reason, among

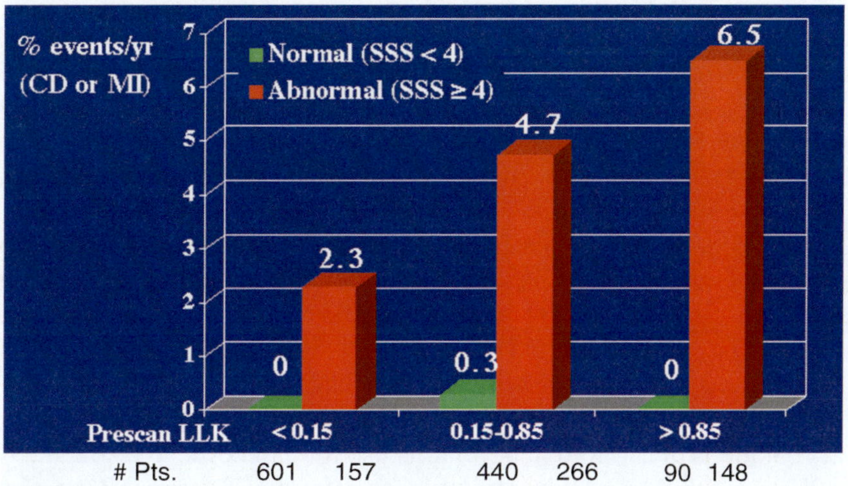

Fig. 2. The annualized frequency of cardiac events (cardiac death or myocardial infarction), for a normal SPECT study, defined as a summed stress score (SSS) <4, and an abnormal SPECT study (SSS >4), for patients divided into three prescanning CAD likelihood (LLK) groups: low (<0.15), intermediate (0.15–0.85), and high (>0.85). Note that regardless of prescanning likelihood level, the presence of a normal SPECT study was associated with a low likelihood of cardiac events (adapted from Berman et al. JACC 1995, [6]).

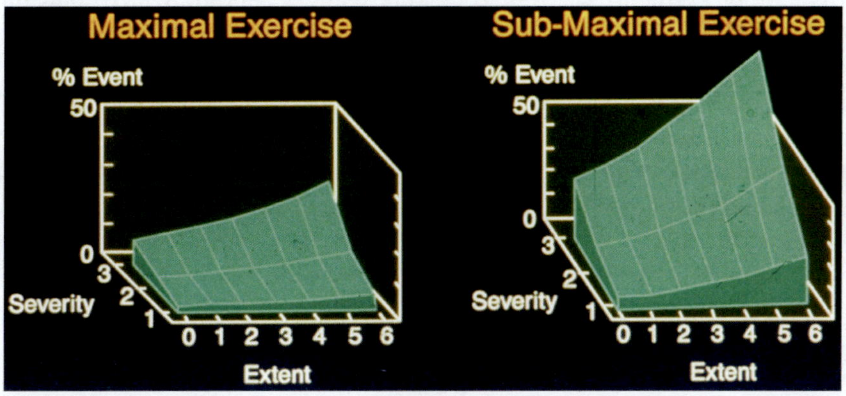

Fig. 3. Depiction on orthogonal axes of the relationship between extent of ischemia (divided into six regions) on the *x*-axis, the severity of ischemia on the *y*-axis (with scores ranging from 0 = no ischemia to 3 = severe ischemia), and cardiac event rate (*z*-axis) for patients exercising maximally (i.e., to >85% of maximal predicted heart rate) (*left graph*) and those not reaching this level of stress (*right graph*) during exercise thallium testing (*planar*). For any level of ischemia, the likelihood of cardiac events was approximately threefold higher if observed during submaximal exercise (from Ladenheim et al. JACC 1986, [2]).

those exercise patients failing to achieve adequate exercise stress, stopping the study before radionuclide injection is warranted, followed by restudy using pharmacological testing. Consistent with the exponential relationship between myocardial ischemia and cardiac events, the risk of cardiac events is only slightly elevated in those patients with mild SPECT abnormalities but increases up to tenfold for those patients with moderate to severe SPECT MPI findings [8]. The level of stress at which myocardial ischemia is induced is also an important predictor of clinical outcomes, with risk minified for those who have inducible ischemia at high workloads and risk augmented for those with inducible ischemia at low workloads (Fig. 3) [2].

Among patients who cannot adequately exercise, stress myocardial perfusion SPECT is performed using pharmacological "stress," usually using adenosine or dipyridamole. Among patients who have a contraindication to these vasodilators, such as patients with active wheezing due to chronic obstructive lung disease or asthma, SPECT imaging can be performed using dobutamine as a stressor agent. Of note, cardiac event rates are not as low with pharmacological stress compared to exercise SPECT, with a mean annualized event rate of between 1 and 2% in such patients, thus placing them into a low intermediate risk category for cardiac events [9, 10]. The increased event rate associated with pharmacological stress may be a potential function of many factors, including a much higher concentration of comorbidities in such patients [11] and the pathophysiological effects exerted by long-term sedentary behavior and physical disability [12].

Given the proven efficacy of stress rest myocardial perfusion SPECT in risk stratifying patients with suspected and known CAD, this test has been widely used for many years for the management of many medical conditions in cardiology beyond its use for diagnostic assessment. This includes its use for assessing the functional significance of stenoses noted on CTA or cardiac catheterization studies, evaluating the risk of future adverse events following recovery from acute myocardial infarction or resolution of acute ischemic syndrome, evaluating post-PCI or postbypass patients, or evaluating the efficacy of medical therapies (see Table 1).

To quantify the degree of ischemic or infarcted myocardium for each of these applications, we assess all SPECT studies according to a 17-segment myocardial model (previously we used a 20-segment model). Each myocardial segment is assigned a score using a 5-point system that ranges from 0 as normal perfusion, to 4 as absent perfusion. This scoring is applied to each of the 17 stress and rest segments and both sets of segmental scores are summed and then subtracted from each other to derive a summed difference score. The greater the summed difference score, the greater the amount of inducible myocardial ischemia. Since these summed scores have no intuitive meaning, we have recently provided for the normalization of these scores by dividing the scores by the maximum possible score, such that the summed difference score expressed as the % myocardium ischemic, and the summed rest score, representing the infarct or hibernating zone, is expressed as the % myocardium "fixed."

Table 1
Most common clinical uses of stress-rest myocardial perfusion SPECT

1. Assess patients with increased likelihood of CAD due to
   - chest pain symptoms
   - dyspnea
   - combination of significant CAD risk factors
2. Evaluate abnormal exercise electrocardiographic responses in low to intermediate CAD likelihood patients
3. Evaluate patients with high coronary calcium scores
4. Risk stratify patients following acute myocardial infarction
5. Assess patients who become asymptomatic following unstable angina
6. Evaluate clinical symptoms following PCI
7. Evaluate symptoms in post-CABG patients
8. Evaluate the functional significance of CCTA or coronary angiographic findings
9. Rule out ischemia in patients with left ventricular dysfunction
10. Preoperative evaluation of patients undergoing high risk surgery

Table 2
Indicators of significant ischemia on stress-rest myocardial perfusion SPECT

- Extensive stress-induced perfusion defects
- Perfusion defects in multiple coronary distributions
- Severe reversible perfusion defects
- Transient lung uptake of radiotracer (thallium studies)
- Transient ischemic dilation of the left ventricle
- Delayed defect reversibility or a resting perfusion defect with substantial reversibility on a subsequent 4-h redistribution thallium study or on a nitroglycerin segmented rest and study
- Increased right ventricular uptake
- Pattern of stunned myocardium following stress testing
- Substantially reduced exercise LVEF on poststress MPS or fall in LVEF between post stress and rest gated MPS study
- Myocardial perfusion defects induced at very low workloads associated with significant clinical signs of ischemia (e.g., prolonged chest pain)

In addition to having a large summed difference score, a number of SPECT findings are indicative of a high clinical risk (Table 2). These include large myocardial perfusion defects, those occurring in the distribution of multiple coronary vessels, transient ischemic dilation of the left ventricle post-stress, the occurrence of new or augmented wall motion abnormalities following stress (post-stress stunning), transiently increased lung uptake of radioactivity following stress (reflective of increased pulmonary capillary wedge pressure), and unusually prominent right ventricular visualization. Cardiac risk also rises as resting LV ejection fraction is progressively reduced. Of particular note, the % myocardium ischemic has been shown to be predictive not only of risk but of the likelihood of benefit with revascularization [13], across the range of ejection fractions [14].

Screening for CAD

Stress testing has also been used for many years for screening purposes. Screening implies the performance of testing for the purpose of detecting disease in a preclinical stage. It has long been recognized that stress testing for screening purposes is of limited use due to the fact that as CAD prevalence decreases to low levels, the likelihood of observing false-positive test results increases, even for tests with idealized test sensitivities and specificities for CAD detection (Fig. 4). The estimated prevalence of angiographically significant disease in the asymptomatic adult U.S. population is estimated to be around 5%. Thus, if stress ECG testing were employed in the population at large, given this prevalence of CAD and an estimated sensitivity of 60% for an ischemic exercise ECG test response and a specificity of 85% for a normal exercise ECG response, the likelihood that an abnormal exercise ECG would represent the presence of underlying CAD would be <20%. If stress SPECT imaging were employed in this population instead, and one assumed a sensitivity of 90% for SPECT, and a specificity of 85%, the likelihood of an abnormal SPECT scan representing the presence of underlying CAD would still be <25%.

Given this Bayesian understanding, screening through the use of ECG stress testing has not been recommended over the years, except for patients with at least two major CAD risk factors. When such screening is performed, a sequential Bayesian approach has been recommended. That is, when patients are first screened using exercise treadmill electrocardiography, if the test is positive, then the post-test likelihood for angiographically significant CAD increases to an intermediate range, and an exercise SPECT study can then be applied to resolve CAD status. If the stress SPECT study is normal,

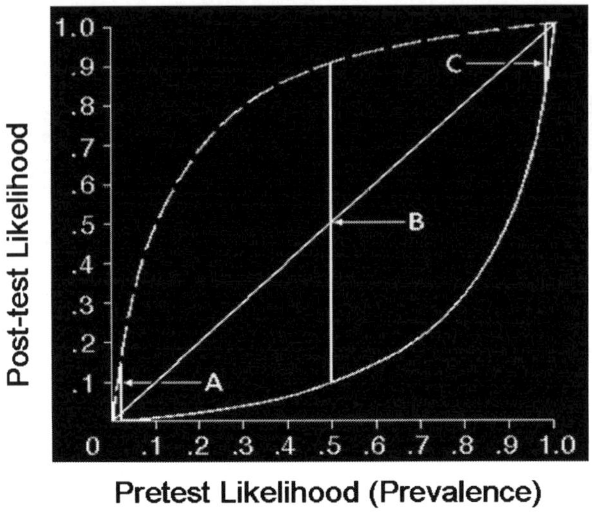

Fig. 4. Shown are the Bayesian curves relating pretest to post-test likelihood of CAD for an idealized test of 90% sensitivity and specificity. The Bayesian curve for a positive test is represented by the dotted curve and shows that the test yields a high false-positive rate (i.e., low post-test likelihood of CAD) for patients with a very low pretest likelihood of CAD (point *A*) and conversely, a high false negative rate for patients with a high pretest likelihood of CAD (point *C*). The test is most effective for patients with an intermediate likelihood of CAD (point *B*) [15].

the post-SPECT likelihood of CAD is now low, and the implication is that the exercise ECG response is a false-positive finding. By contrast, if both the stress ECG and the stress SPECT study are abnormal, then true ischemia is likely to be present, and the patient should then be managed according to the magnitude of ischemia on the SPECT study. Screening has also been applied to various population cohorts where testing has been mandated to serve a common community good, such as the mandatory screening of airline pilots, firemen, and policemen.

IMPACT OF CAC SCANNING ON THE CLINICAL USES OF STRESS-REST MYOCARDIAL PERFUSION SPECT

Impact on Diagnostic Testing

Conventional practice has been to select patients for cardiac stress testing, whether by using SPECT or other stress testing modality, based on Bayesian analysis of clinical factors, such as age, gender, chest pain symptoms, and CAD risk factors. Data from our EISNER study as well as that from other centers suggest that CAC scanning may be used to modify the selection of patients for cardiac stress testing. This is due to a strong threshold relationship that has been noted between the magnitude of absolute CAC and the likelihood of observing inducible myocardial ischemia on SPECT. In our initial work, we evaluated 1,195 patients who underwent both exercise SPECT testing and CAC scanning [16]. After stratifying our patients according to the magnitude of ischemia, we noted that an ischemic SPECT study was observed in <5% of patient with CAC scores <400, with an increasing frequency of ischemia for CAC scores above this threshold (Fig. 5). When results were compared according to the CAC score expressed as a percentile in age and gender, the results were not nearly as strong. This indicates that it is the magnitude of underlying atherosclerosis within the coronary arterial bed, rather than the amount of CAC that is adjusted for age and sex, which governs the relationship between CAC and ischemia.

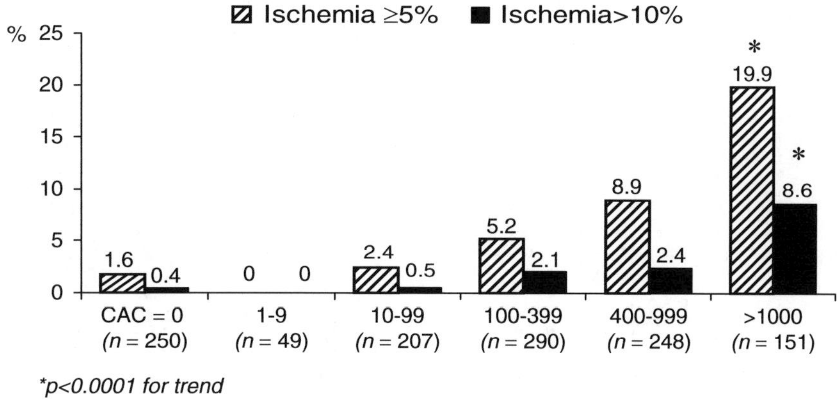

Fig. 5. Frequency of observed myocardial ischemia during exercise SPECT testing (*y*-axis) for patients divided into six categories of CAC scores, ranging from zero scores to scores >1,000. Shown is the frequency for ischemia that is >5% of the myocardium (hatched bars) and >10% of the myocardium (black bars) (from Berman et al. JACC 2004, [16]).

Preceding our study, He et al. also reported on the relationship between the frequency of inducible ischemia by SPECT MPI and the CAC scores [17]. These authors noted the same threshold relationship between ischemia and CAC scores among 411 patients, but noted a much higher frequency of ischemia than we did among those with CAC scores >400. Other studies have failed to replicate their high rate of ischemic findings among patients with CAC scores >400, but importantly, the studies to date have consistently noted a threshold relationship whereby the frequency of inducible ischemia on SPECT MPI increases substantially for a CAC score >400 [16–18].

This relationship between CAC scores and inducible myocardial ischemia considers grouped patients who have not been stratified relative to cardiac risk factors. In subsequent work, however, we examined whether the threshold for myocardial ischemia among patients undergoing CAC scanning was potentially modified, among 1,043 patients divided into 140 diabetic patients, 173 who had metabolic syndrome without diabetes, and 730 patients without either risk factor [19]. As noted in Fig. 6, the threshold for myocardial ischemia was lower among patients who had either diabetes or metabolic syndrome. While the frequency of inducible myocardial ischemia remained low among patients with CAC scores<400 if there were neither risk factor, among patients with either metabolic syndrome or diabetes, there was a significant increase in the observed frequency of ischemia among patients with CAC scores between 100 and 400. Other data indicate a lower CAC score threshold for myocardial ischemia among men compared to women [16]. The work of Anand et al. [20]. further illustrated the importance of a reduced threshold for considering stress imaging in patients with diabetes. Based on these various studies, several investigators have suggested that for diabetic patients an effective manner of "screening" might be to perform CAC testing, followed by stress imaging in those with CAC >100 [20, 21, 22].

In other work, we compared the relationship between CAC scores and myocardial ischemia according to patients' chest pain symptoms [23]. Our results indicate a marked influence on this threshold relationship according to the pattern of patients' chest pain (Fig. 7). Patients with nonanginal chest pain showed the same CAC threshold for myocardial ischemia as did asymptomatic patients: a CAC score >400. At the other end of the spectrum, patients with typical angina showed a frequency of ischemia that was 11% among those with CAC scores <10, although these data must be viewed as very preliminary as they were examined in only a small cohort of patients with typical angina. By contrast, we had a large cohort of patients with atypical angina, a group that is commonly referred for

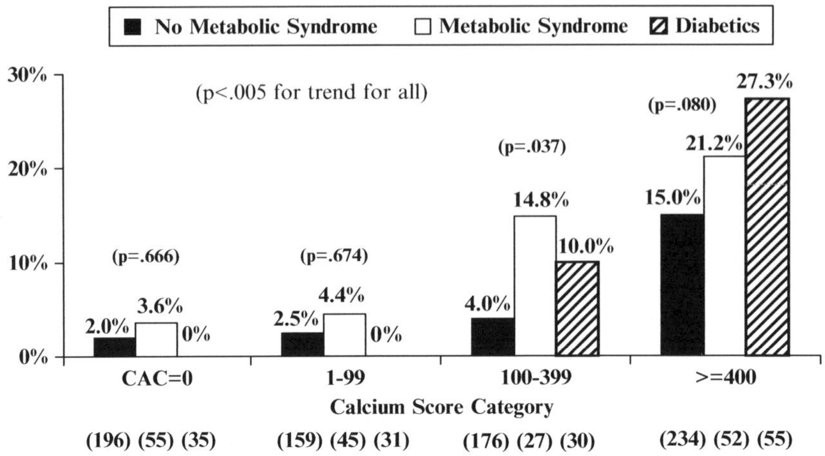

Fig. 6. Relationship between CAC scores and the observed frequency of observed myocardial ischemia during exercise SPECT testing according to the absence or presence of either diabetes or metabolic syndrome (from Wong et al. Diabetes Care 2005, [20]).

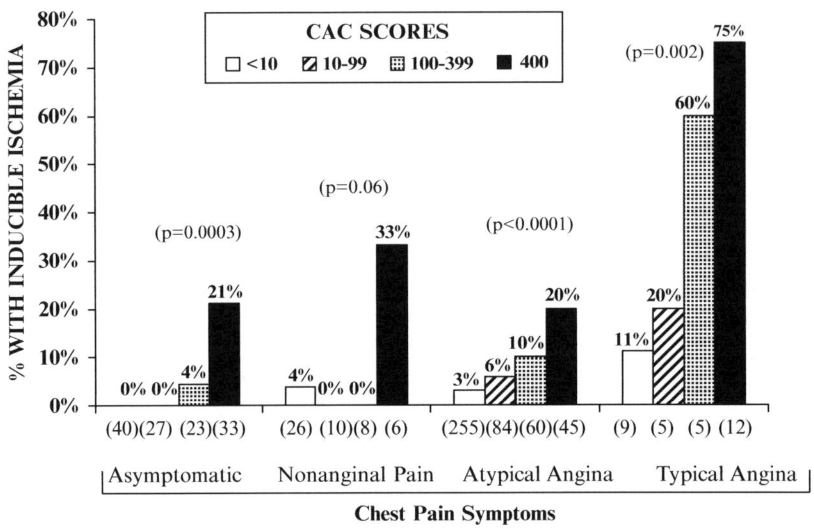

Fig. 7. Relationship between CAC scores and the observed frequency of observed myocardial ischemia during exercise SPECT testing following the grouping of patients according to the presence and type of anginal chest pain symptoms (from Rozanski et al. J Nucl Cardiol 2007, [23]).

cardiac stress testing; in this group, the frequency of myocardial ischemia was 10% among patients with a CAC score between 100 and 400.

Ideally, ascertaining the appropriate threshold relationship between myocardial ischemia and CAC scores would include consideration of chest pain symptoms, sex, and CAD risk factors, but assessment of even a larger database will be necessary to allow us to assess the relationship between CAC scores and ischemia according to the simultaneous consideration of all these factors. Still, it is sufficiently evident from our data that CAC scanning can aid in the appropriate selection of patients for cardiac stress testing according to the following general paradigm: among patients who are asymptomatic or have nonanginal chest pain, a CAC score ≥400 appears to be a reasonable indication for pursuing cardiac stress testing, with the threshold score reduced among diabetic patients and those with metabolic syndrome. Future work needs to determine if and what other cardiac risk factors may also reduce the CAC score associated with ischemia among asymptomatic patients and those with nonanginal chest pain. Among patients with atypical angina, it may also be more appropriate to lower the threshold value for stress testing to a CAC score of 100. It must be strongly emphasized, however, that these initial suggestions are based on data coming primarily from a single medical center. More study, hopefully pooling the experience of multiple centers, would be desirable to further study this issue.

Impact on Risk Stratification

The prognostic significance of SPECT studies is based on observations obtained during more than 25 years of medical experience. The fundamental underpinning of this prognostic application is the reproducible finding, as discussed earlier, that a normal perfusion during exercise myocardial perfusion SPECT reliably predicts that patients who have an <1% annualized risk of sustaining a cardiovascular event (cardiac death or myocardial infarction) over at least the following 2–3 years. Notably, however, within various clinical cohorts with a normal exercise SPECT study, cardiac event rates average between 1 and 2% per year, thus placing such patients into an intermediate risk category for future cardiac events. This includes patients with atrial fibrillation [24], those whom complained of dyspnea [25], and diabetic patients [26].

We became interested in determining whether high CAC scores serve as another factor that would place patients with normal SPECT studies into an intermediate risk for future cardiac events. Notably, sequential longitudinal studies [27–34] have reproducibly demonstrated that measurement of CAC predicts the likelihood of future cardiac events (Fig. 8), as does the distribution of CAC within vessels

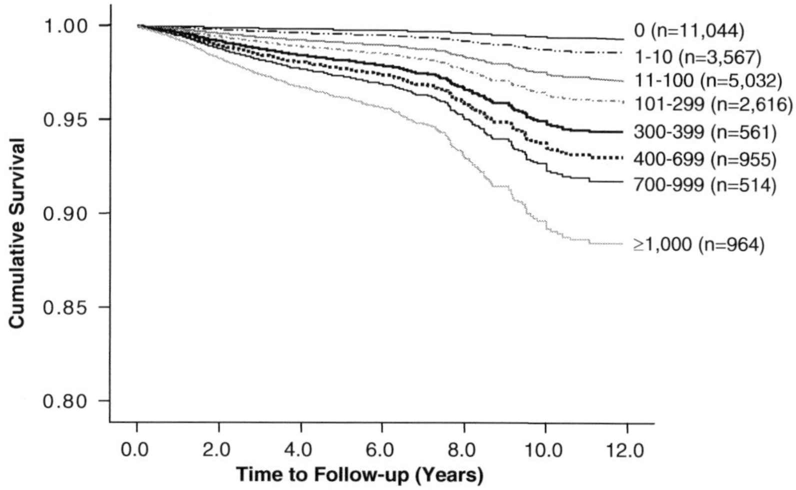

Risk-adjustment included the following variables: age, hypercholesterolemia, diabetes, smoking, hypertension, and a family history of premature coronary heart disease, Model $\chi2$=2,017, p<0.0001 and $\chi2$ =274 for variable (p<0.0001 overall and for each category subset). Note: Scale on this survival curve is from 0.80 to 1.00 while the remaining curves are plotted within a range of 0.90 to 1.00.

Fig. 8. Cumulative survival among 25,253 subjects undergoing CAC scanning after grouping according to the magnitude of the CAC score. There was a significantly increased risk for all-cause mortality for each increment in CAC scoring (from Budoff et al. JACC 2007, [33]).

(Fig. 9) [33], but these studies had not, prior to our EISNER study, considered the prognostic information that could be obtained when SPECT imaging and CAC scanning are *both* performed. Therefore, we followed 1,089 patients with a normal SPECT study for a mean of approximately 32 months [35]. In these patients, the frequency of early coronary revascularization was extremely low, occurring in only 3 (0.3%) of the patients. Thus, referral to early myocardial revascularization was not a factor influencing the results of our study. Our principal finding upon analyzing the results of our follow-up was that the annualized cardiac event rate remained <1% in all CAC subgroups, including those with CAC scores ≥1,000 (Fig. 10). Superficially, these findings seemingly contrast with the widely reported findings that an elevated CAC score is associated with an increased risk of cardiac events [33, 36]. However, the difference in these prior findings and our results is likely related to the high proportion of high CAC scores among ischemic patients, all of whom were excluded from our analysis of patients with CAC scanning and normal SPECT studies. Moreover, there was a likely strong influence

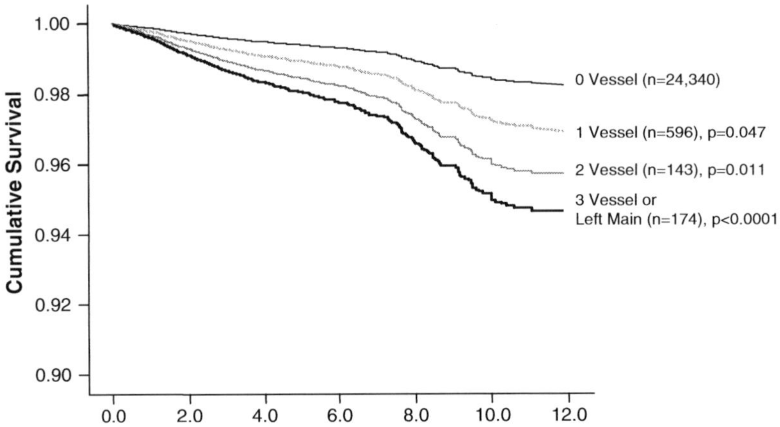

Risk-adjustment included the following variables: age, hypercholesterolemia, diabetes, smoking, hypertension, and a family history of premature coronary heart disease, Model $\chi 2$=1,290, p<0.0001 and$\chi 2$ =27 for variable (p<0.0001 overall and p value for each category subset is stated above). The survival curve for 3 vessel (n=28) was superimposed on the Left Main subset and, for that reason, the two were combined to form 1 category.

Fig. 9. Cumulative survival in the same population after stratifying patients according to the number of vessels manifesting coronary calcium scores ≥100 (from Budoff et al. JACC 2007, [28]).

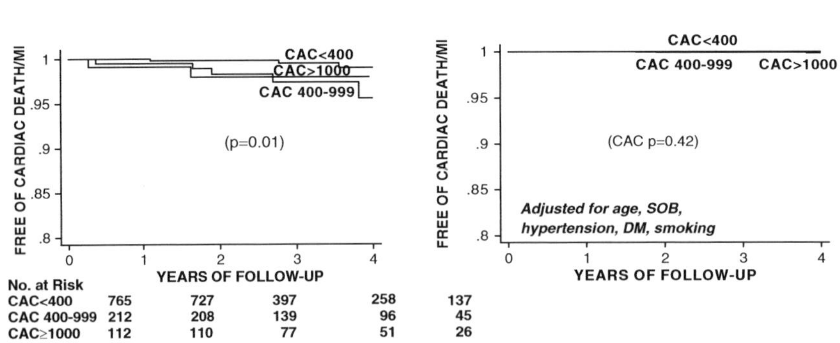

Fig. 10. Kaplan Meier survival curves for the occurrence of cardiac events (death or myocardial infarction) among patients with normal exercise SPECT studies grouped according to the magnitude of CAC on the left and adjusted for clinical factors on the right. Even the presence of high CAC scores (>1,000) did not impair 3-year outcome among these patients with normal exercise SPECT studies (from Rozanski et al. JACC 2007, [35]).

that the elevated CAC score had on subsequent medical management in our physician community, such that the patients with extensive CAC and normal exercise SPECT were treated with secondary prevention guidelines.

These clinical results are highly relevant to justifying emerging management strategies that call for the performance of CAC scanning as an initial test in selected patient cohorts or, for that matter, wide screening, as suggested by the SHAPE guidelines [37]. Whatever strategy is employed, if SPECT imaging were not able to identify which patients with high CAC scores are at low risk for cardiac events, than fears that CAC scanning could lead to increased cardiac catheterizations and invasive interventions would be justified. Of note, in our experience, only approximately 20% of patients with very high CAC scores (≥1,000) will manifest inducible myocardial ischemia (see Fig. 5), indicating that the vast majority of patients with high CAC scores undergoing stress-rest myocardial perfusion SPECT will not need to undergo cardiac catheterization according to our results. Also, our findings show that about 10% of patients screened would have a CAC score > 400, requires randomized stress testing.

In fact, the distribution of CAC scores is markedly heterogeneous among patients who have demonstrated normal exercise SPECT studies in our laboratory (Fig. 11). This observation points to an obvious limitation of stress testing: while it may be sensitive for the detection of hemodynamically significant, flow-limiting, coronary stenoses, it is not an accurate means for assessing the extent of atherosclerosis in the coronary arterial bed. Accordingly, we have previously suggested that the strength of SPECT imaging may be its use in predicting relatively *shorter-term* risk [25]. By contrast, CAC scanning may be a better predictor of relatively *long-term* risk. If so, it may be expected that as our cohort of patients with both normal SPECT studies and CAC scans is followed for longer duration, eventually those with higher CAC scores may demonstrate a higher event rate compared to those with low CAC scores or its absence. Practically, it is our contention (while not yet medically evaluated for efficacy) that the combined presence of a normal SPECT but high CAC score should lead to very aggressive medical treatment, including lowering serum LDL levels to the range of 60–70 mg/dl, which is the LDL target when employing so-called secondary prevention.

Interestingly, based on recent Framingham results that define the role of even >1 suboptimal coronary risk factor in increasing the lifetime risk of cardiac events [38], there is an increasing recognition that aggressive patient management is probably crucial for maintaining a low long-term event rate among patients with normal SPECT studies. Along these lines, finding more successful means for promoting long-term patient adherence to medical management is highly desirable.

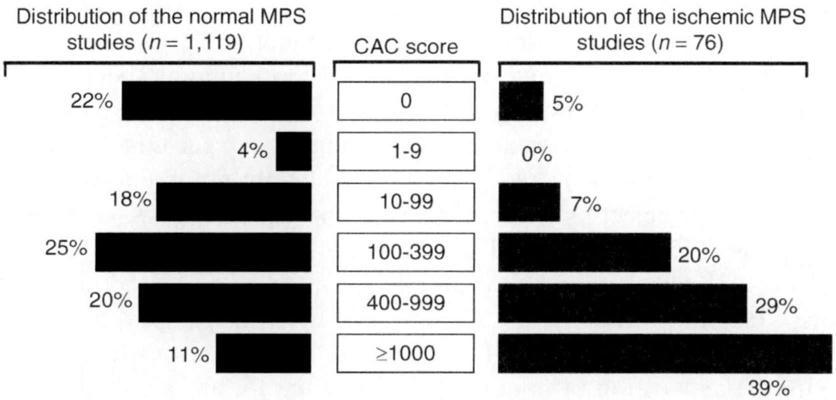

Fig. 11. The frequency of CAC scores among patients with normal exercise myocardial perfusion scinigraphy (MPS) studies on the left and ischemic MPS studies on the right. A wide distribution of CAC scores is noted among the patients with normal MPS studies (from Berman et al. JACC 2004, [16]).

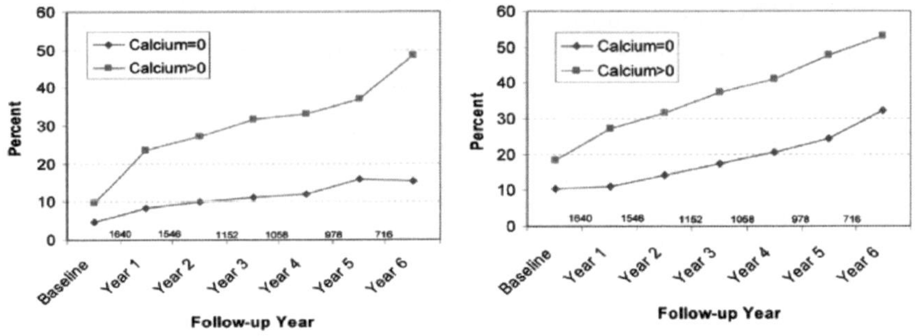

Fig. 12. The incidence of statin use (*left*) and aspirin use (*right*) according to the presence or absence of calcium on CAC scanning during a 6-year actuarial follow-up following the CAC scanning (from Taylor et al. JACC 2008, [39]).

Data from the PACC study suggest that an added benefit to CAC scanning may be its ability to promote patient adherence (Fig. 12) [39]. Conceivably, the use of CAC scanning may thus also be useful among selected patients who have normal SPECT studies but difficult-to-manage coronary risk factors, as a means of incentivizing these patients and/or their physicians to participate in more aggressive medical management.

In patients who have undergone rest/stress SPECT, CAC testing can be of additional value. As noted earlier, if patients have a normal exercise SPECT, their prognosis is excellent, regardless of their CAC score, provided they and their referring physician are aware of the need for secondary prevention guidelines. Observations by Schenker et al. [40]. raise the question, however, as to whether these observations may be relevant to higher risk populations. In their work, they observed a higher event rate among patients with normal vasodilator PET/CT and CAC scores above ≥1,000, but their patient population had a higher risk profile and underwent pharmacologic stress as opposed to exercise stress. It is also not known if patients in their cohort may have been as aggressively medically managed. More study is thus needed to assess the prognostic significance of patients presenting with high CAC scores but normal stress perfusion studies as both a function of medical acuity and the aggressiveness of medical management.

Impact on Screening for CAD

CAC scanning affords the opportunity to create a revolutionary approach to screening for CAD, and should, based on our review of the recent data, replace stress testing as an initial test for screening purposes. As aforementioned, cardiac stress testing is associated with a high false-positive rate in screening populations. Moreover, reliance on stress testing can only detect disease that is sufficiently advanced to produce sufficient ischemia-producing flow limitation during stress. By contrast, CAC scanning does not suffer these twin limitations. Rather, CAC scanning is specific for the presence of atherosclerotic disease and it offers physicians the ability to detect CAD at an early phase of the disease process, even decades prior to when clinical symptoms might be expected to manifest themselves.

Currently, there is considerable debate as to which populations deserve to undergo CAC scanning as a screening technique for detecting atherosclerosis. Some investigators have suggested using the Framingham Risk Score (FRS) as a litmus for CAC scanning, reserving its use for patients with an intermediate FRS [41–43]. Others are critical of this notion since the FRS does not include some of the major CAD risk factors, such as family history and degree of physical activity, nor necessarily predicts CAC with accuracy according to other results [44–47]. A competing concept, the SHAPE guidelines, calls for the application of routine CAC screening for all middle-aged adults with CAD risk factors [37]. However, the future use of CAC scanning as a screening technique for CAD is likely to be shaped by various dynamic factors. One of these factors will be the degree of future third-party coverage for CAC scanning. In general, there is a current reluctance to add new coverage for screening techniques, per se, but CAC scanning has now gained coverage by Medicare in some states and is slowly gaining coverage among other third-party carriers as well. As appreciation of the other clinical utilities of CAC scanning become more recognized, such as its ability to aid in the triage of patients for cardiac stress testing, third-party coverage for CAC scanning may accelerate. A second factor which may govern the future use of CAC scanning is the future pricing for CAC scanning. Whereas CAC scanning was first introduced into Medicine using expensive electron beam technology, there is current widespread ability to assess CAC using multislice detectors which can also be used to perform CCTA and many other imaging procedures. This and various market forces are likely to result in a progressive decrease in the cost for CAC scanning, thus making it more affordable within the healthcare structure. A third important factor regarding the future use of CAC scanning will be the emerging uses of CCTA, which offers a more powerful means for sizing atherosclerotic burden by virtue of its ability to noninvasively image the coronary vascular tree and assess both soft plaque as well as the calcified plaque that is assessed by dedicated CAC scanning. While we have reviewed the now substantial evidence base regarding how CAC scanning can impact the use of stress testing, to date, the synergistic use of CCTA scanning and stress testing is now just emerging and is not reviewed here. In the future, patient management paradigms for diagnosis, risk management, and screening are all likely to consider the best sequence of three technologies – CAC scanning, CCTA imaging, and cardiac stress testing – for providing cardiac care in the most cost-effective manner possible.

In the interim, CAC scanning stands to replace cardiac stress testing as the preferred first means for screening purposes as well as for evaluating most patients with a low (<15%) likelihood of CAD, with stress testing then reserved for those screened or low likelihood patients manifesting high CAC scores (i.e., ≥400) or in those with clinical factors that increase their risk (e.g., diabetes, metabolic syndrome), in whom the threshold for recommending stress imaging may be lower (e.g., ≥100).

SUMMARY

In this review, we have assessed new data that indicate that the future use of CAC scanning is likely to be much more widespread than previously recognized and that used judiciously, CAC scanning offers the promise of making cardiac stress testing more efficient and effective, as summarized in Fig. 13. Specifically, CAC scanning has the ability to overcome the considerable limitations of stress testing as a screening method for CAD and result in the much earlier detection of CAD, many years before the potential advent of clinical symptoms or cardiac events. Second, we have reviewed new data

Clinical Indication	Purpose of Stress Cardiac Imaging	Utility of CAC Scanning
Screening	Detect clinically silent but significant coronary stenosis	Detect subclinical atherosclerosis
Diagnosis	↑ or ↓ likelihood estimate for CAD	Improve selection for diagnostic testing
Prognosis	Predict *short-term* risk for cardiac events	Aid in *long-term* risk prediction.

Fig. 13. Projected means in which CAC scanning can either aid or replace cardiac stress testing for the three current principal uses of cardiac stress testing: screening, diagnosis, and prognosis.

which suggests that CAC scanning can also improve diagnostic management by aiding in a more appropriate selection of patients for cardiac stress imaging. Third, our data also suggest that CAC scanning can aid in patient risk assessment and management by using this test to determine the extent of underlying atherosclerosis in patients with normal SPECT studies. Given these considerations, we believe that CAC scanning may play an important world-wide role in the prevention of events related to subclinical atherosclerotic disease, and that in the stress imaging for ischemia will come to be reserved for those asymptomatic patients with extensive atherosclerosis according to CAC testing.

REFERENCES

1. Berman DS, Hachamovitch R, Shaw LJ, Hayes SW, Germano G. Nuclear Cardiology. In: Fuster V, O'Rourke RA, Walsh RA, Poole-Wilson P, King III SB, Roberts R, Nash IS, Prystowsky EN, eds. Hurst's The Heart. 12th Edition. McGraw-Hill Companies, Inc. New York, NY. 2008;544–76.
2. Ladenheim ML, Pollack BH, Rozanski A, Berman DS, Staniloff HM, Forrester JS, Diamond GA. Extent and severity of myocardial hypoperfusion as orthogonal indices of prognosis in patients with suspected coronary artery disease. J Am Coll Cardiol 1986;7:464-71.
3. Levy R, Rozanski A, Berman DS, Garcia E, Van Train K, Maddahi J, Swan HJC. Analyses of the degree of pulmonary thallium "washout" following exercise. J Am Coll Cardiol 1983;2:719-28.
4. Abidov A, Bax JJ, Hayes SW, Cohen I, Nishina H, Yoda S, et al. Integration of automatically measured transient ischemic dilation ratio into interpretation of adenosine stress myocardial perfusion SPECT for detection of severe and extensive CAD. J Nuc Med 2004;45:1999–2007.
5. Diamond GA, Forrester JS. Analysis of probability as an aid in the clinical diagnosis of coronary-artery disease. N Engl J Med 1979;300(24):1350–8.
6. Berman DS. Hockhamovitch R, Kiat H, et al. Incremental value of prognostic testing in patients with known or suspected heart disease: a basis for optimal utilization of exercise technetium-99m sestamibi myocardial perfusion single-photon emission computed tomography. J Am Coll Cardiol 1995;26:639–47.
7. Bairey CN, Rozanski A, Maddahi A, Resser KJ, Berman DS. Exercise thallium – 201 scintigraphy and prognosis in patients with typical angina and negative exercise electrocardiography. Am J Cardiol 1989;64:282–8.
8. Berman DS, Shaw LJ, Hachamovitch R, Friedman JD, Polk DM, Hayes SW, et al. Comparative use of radionuclide stress testing, coronary artery calcium scanning, and noninvasive coronary angiography for diagnostic and prognostic cardiac assessment. Semin Nucl Med 2007;37(1):2–16.
9. Navare SM, Mather JF, Shaw LJ, Fowler MS, Heller GV. Comparison if risk stratification with pharmacologic and exercise stress myocardial perfusion imaging: a meta-analysis. J Nucl Cardiol 2004;11:551–6.
10. Calnon DA, McGrath PD, Doss AL, Harrell FE, Watson DD, Beller GA. Prognostic value of dobutamine stress technetium-99m-sestamibi single-photon emission computed tomography myocardial perfusion imaging: stratification of a high-risk population. J Am Coll Cardiol 2001;38:1151–517.
11. Shaw LJ, Iskandrian AE. Prognostic value of gated myocardial perfusion SPECT. J Nucl Cardiol 2004;11:171–85.
12. Booth FW, Chakravarthy MV, Gordon SE, Spangenburg EE. Waging war on physical inactivity: using modern molecular ammunition against an ancient enemy. J Appl Physiol 2002;93:3–30.
13. Hachamovitch R, Hayes SW, Friedman JD, Cohen I, Berman DS. Comparison of the short-term survival benefit associated with revascularization compared with medical therapy in patients with no prior coronary artery disease undergoing stress myocardial perfusion single photon emission computed tomography. Circulation 2003;107:2900–7.
14. Hachamovitch R, Rozanski A, Hayes SW, et al. Predicting therapeutic benefit from myocardial revascularization procedures: are measurements of both resting left ventricular ejection fraction and stress-induced myocardial ischemia necessary? J Nucl Cardiol 2006;13:742–6.
15. Berman DS, Garcia EV, Maddahi J. Thallium-201 myocardial scintigraphy in the detection and evaluation of coronary artery disease. (Chapter 3) In: Clinical Nuclear Cardiology (Berman DS, Mason DT, eds), Grune & Stratton, New York, 1981; 49–106.
16. Berman DS, Wong ND, Gransar H, Miranda-Peats R, Dahlbeck J, Arad Y, et al. Relationship between stress-induced myocardial ischemia and atherosclerosis measured by coronary calcium tomography. J Am Coll Cardiol 2004;44:923–30.
17. He ZX, Hedrick TD, Pratt CM, Verani MS, Aquino V, Roberts R, et al. Severity of coronary artery calcification by electron beam computed tomography predicts silent myocardial ischemia. Circulation 2000;101(3):244–51.
18. Moser KW, O'Keefe JH, Bateman TM, McGhie IA. Coronary calcium screening in asymptomatic patients as a guide to risk factor modification and stress myocardial perfusion imaging. J Nucl Cardiol 2003;10:590–8.
19. Anand DV, Lim E, Hopkins D, Corder R, Shaw LJ, Sharp P, et al. Risk stratification in uncomplicated type 2 diabetes: prospective evaluation of the combined use of coronary artery calcium imaging and selective myocardial perfusion scintigraphy. Eur Heart J 2006;27(6):713–21.
20. Wong ND, Rozanski A, Gransar H, Miranda-Peats R, Kang X, Hayes S, et al. Metabolic syndrome and diabetes are associated with an increased likelihood of inducible myocardial ischemia among patients with subclinical atherosclerosis. Diabetes Care 2005;28:1445–50.

21. Beller GA. Noninvasive screening for coronary atherosclerosis and silent ischemia in asymptomatic type 2 diabetes mellitus patients: is it appropriate and cost-effective? J Am Coll Cardiol 2007;49:1918–23.
22. Yerramasu A, Maggae SV, Lahiri A, Anand DV. Cardiac computed tomography and myocardial perfusion imaging for risk stratification in asymptomatic diabetic patients: a critical review. J Nucl Cardiol 2008;15:13–22.
23. Rozanski A, Gransar H, Wong ND, et al. Use of coronary calcium scanning for predicting inducible myocardial ischemia: influence of patients' clinical presentation. J Nucl Cardiol 2007;14:669–79.
24. Abidov A, Hachamovitch R, Rozanski A, et al. Prognostic implications of atrial fibrillation in patients undergoing myocardial perfusion single-photon emission computed tomography. J Am Coll Cardiol 2004;44:1062–70.
25. Abidov A, Rozanski A, Hachamovitch R, Hayes SW, Aboul-Enein F, Cohen I, et al. Complaints of dyspnea among patients referred for cardiac stress testing. New Eng J Med 2005;353:1889–98.
26. Shaw LJ, Berman DS, Hendel RC, Alazraki N, Krawczynska E, Borges-Neto S, et al. Cardiovascular disease risk stratification with stress single-photon emission computed tomography technetium-99m tetrofosmin imaging in patients with thc metabolic syndrome and diabetes mellitus. Am J Cardiol 2006;97:1538–44.
27. Arad Y, Sparado LA, Goodman K, et al. Prediction of coronary events with electron beam computed tomography. J Am Coll Cardiol 2000;36:1253–60.
28. Wong ND, Hsu JC, Detrano RC, et al. Coronary artery calcium evaluation by electron beam computed tomography and its relation to new cardiovascular events. Am J Cardiol 2000;86:495–8.
29. Raggi P, Callister TQ, Cooil B, et al. Identification of patients at increased risk of first unheralded acute myocardial infarction by electron beam computed tomography. Circulation 2000;101:850–5.
30. Park R, Detrano R, Xiang M, et al. Combined use of computed tomography coronary calcium scores and C-reactive protein levels in predicting cardiovascular events in nondiabetic individuals. Circulation 2002;106:2073–7.
31. Kondos GT, Hoff JA, Sevrukov A, et al. Coronary artery calcium and cardiac events electron-beam tomography coronary artery calcium and cardiac events: a 37-month follow-up of 5,635 initially asymptomatic low to intermediate risk adults. Circulation 2003;107:2571–6.
32. Arad Y, Goodman KJ, Roth M, et al. Coronary calcification, coronary disease risk factors, C-reactive protein, and atherosclerotic cardiovascular disease events. J Am Coll Cardiol 2005;46:158–65.
33. Budoff MJ, Shaw LJ, Liu ST. Long-term prognosis associated with coronary calcification: observations from a registry of 25,253 patients. J Am Coll Cardiol 2007;49:1860–70.
34. Kronmal RA, McClelland RL, Detrano R, et al. Risk factors for the progression of coronary artery calcification in asymptomatic subjects. Results from the Multi-Ethnic Study of Atherosclerosis (MESA). Circulation 2007;115:2722–30.
35. Rozanski A, Gransar H, Wong ND, Shaw LJ, Miranda-Peats R, Polk D, Hayes SW, Friedman JD, Berman DS. Clinical outcomes after both coronary calcium scanning and exercise myocardial perfusion scinitigraphy. J Am Coll Cardiol 2007;49:1352–61.
36. Detrano R, Guerci AD, Car JJ, et al. Coronary calcium as a predictor of coronary events in four racial or ethnic groups. N Engl J Med 2008;358:1336–45.
37. Naghavi M, Falk E, Hecht HS, Jamieson MJ, Berman D, Budoff MJ, et al. From vulnerable plaque to vulnerable patient – Part III: executive summary of the Screening for Heart Attack Prevention and Education (SHAPE) Task Force report. Am J Cardiol 2006;98:2H–15.
38. Lloyd-Jones DM, Leip EP, Larson MG, et al. Prediction of lifetime risk for cardiovascular disease by risk factor burden at 50 years of age. Circulation 2006;113:791–8.
39. Taylor AJ, Binderman J, Feuerstein I, et al. Community-based provision of statin and aspirin after the detection of coronary artery calcium within a community-based screening cohort. J Am Coll Cardiol 2008;51:1337–41.
40. Schenker MP, Dorbala S, Hong EC, et al. Interrelation of coronary calcification, myocardial ischemia, and outcomes in patients with intermediate threshold of coronary artery disease: a combined positron emission tomography/computed tomography study. Circulation 2008;117:1693–700.
41. Greenland P, Bonow RO, Brundage BH, Bundoff MJ. Eisenberg MJ, Grundy SM, et al. ACCF/AHA 2007 clinical expert consensus document on coronary artery calcium scoring by computed tomography in global cardiovascular risk assessment and in evaluation of patients with chest pain: a report of the American College of Cardiology Foundation Clinical Expert Consensus Task Force (ACCF/AHA Writing Committee to Update the 2000 Expert Consensus Document on Electron Beam Computed Tomography). Circulation 2007;115(3):402–26.
42. O'Rourke RA, Brudage BH, Froelicher VF, et al. American college of Cardiology/American heart association expert consensus document on electron-beam computed tomography for the diagnosis and prognosis of coronary artery disease. Circulation 2000;102:126–40.
43. Mieres JH, Shaw LJ, Arai A, et al. The role of non-invasive testing in the clinical evaluation of women with suspected coronary artery disease: American Heart Association consensus statement. Circulation 2005;111:682–96.
44. Taylor AJ, Feurstein I, Wong H, et al. Do conventional risk factors predict subclinical coronary artery disease? Results from the prospective army coronary calcium project. Am Heart J 2001;141:463–8.
45. Hecht HS, Superko HR, Smith LK, McColgan BP. Relation of coronary artery calcium identified by electron beam tomography to serum lipoprotein levels and implications for treatment. Am J Cardiol 2001;87(4):406–12.
46. Mahoney LT, Burns TL, Stanford W, Thompson BH, Witt JD, Rost CA, Lauer RM. Usefulness of the Framingham risk score and body mass index to predict early coronary artery calcium in young adults (Muscatine Study). Am J Cardiol 2001;88(5):509–15.
47. Michos ED, Vasamreddy CR, Becker DM, et al. Women with a low Framingham risk score and a family history of premature coronary heart disease have a high prevalence of subclinical coronary atherosclerosis. Am Heart J 2005;150:1276–81.

31 Targeted MRI of Molecular Components in Atherosclerotic Plaque

Zahi A. Fayad

CONTENTS

ABSTRACT

Traditionally, diagnosis of atherosclerosis was possible only at advanced stages of disease, either by directly revealing the narrowing of the arterial lumen (stenosis) or by evaluating the effect of arterial stenosis on organ perfusion. However, new imaging approaches such as targeted magnetic resonance imaging (MRI) allow the assessment not only of the morphology of blood vessels but also of the composition of the vessel walls, enabling atherosclerosis-associated abnormalities in the arteries (including the coronary arteries) to be observed, down to the cellular and molecular level.

Key words: Atherosclerosis; Magnetic resonance imaging; Molecular imaging; Noninvasive imaging

KEY POINTS

- Atherosclerosis disease of the vessel wall that manifest itself at the molecular and cellular levels.
- New imaging methods are needed to better characterization molecular and cellular disregulation of atherosclerosis.
- Molecular imaging by magnetic resonance using novel and targeted contrast agents and nanoparticles may allow improved patient care in the future.

The ability to target specific molecules of plaques may greatly enhance detection and characterization of atherosclerotic and atherothrombotic lesions using MRI [1]. Contrast agents linked to antibodies [2–5] or peptides [6, 7] that target specific plaque components or molecules that localize to specific regions of atherosclerotic plaque [8–11] are examples of strategies that have been employed to image atherosclerosis with MR. The ability to target mononuclear cells such as monocytes, macrophages,

From: *Asymptomatic Atherosclerosis: Pathophysiology, Detection and Treatment*
Edited by: M. Naghavi (ed.), DOI 10.1007/978-1-60327-179-0_31

and foam cells is an attractive means of identifying atherosclerosis since these cells have been shown to play a pivotal role in the progression of atherosclerosis to symptomatic disease [12, 13]. While current research is underway to target macrophages with gadolinium-based contrast agents that target the macrophage scavenger receptor, macrophages have only been imaged with iron oxide compounds (USPIOs, SPIOs) that are removed from the circulation by macrophages and other cells of the reticuloendothelial system [14–16]. In a study by Kooi et al. on 11 symptomatic patients scheduled for carotid endarterectomy, 75% of ruptured or rupture-prone lesions demonstrated uptake of USPIOs compared with only 7% of stable lesions and a decrease in signal intensity of 24% on T2* [17].

Neovascularization has been shown to play an important role in atherosclerosis, and the integrin $\alpha_v\beta_3$ has been targeted to identify regions in the vessel wall undergoing neovascularization [3–5]. Winter et al. demonstrated in a rabbit model of atherosclerosis that regions of neovascularization in plaque had a 47% increase in signal intensity following treatment with $\alpha_v\beta_3$-targeted nanoparticles [5].

Additional targets of interest for imaging of atherosclerotic plaque with molecular specific MR contrast agents are oxidized low-density lipoprotein (oxLDL), tissue factor, endothelial integrins, matrix metalloproteinases, and extracellular matrix proteins such as tenascin-C. These targets are also highlighted in a recent study by Choudhury et al. [14]. While targeted nuclear imaging through the use of antibodies specific to oxLDL has been demonstrated promises at detecting atherosclerosis [15], estimating plaque volume [16], and following progression/regression of atherosclerosis [17], we are unaware of any studies evaluating oxLDL as a target for molecular MRI of atherosclerosis. Additionally, molecules such as tissue factor [18] and endothelial integrins [18–20] such as E-selectin, P-selectin, intracellular adhesion molecule-1, or vascular cell adhesion molecule-1 have been targeted with antibodies linked to echogenic contrast agents. While these agents utilize echocardiography or nuclear imaging, the echogenic or nuclear contrast agent could easily be replaced by linking an MR contrast agent to the monoclonal antibody to target the molecule of interest. However, the identification of molecules found only in atherosclerotic plaque will ultimately enable improved detection of atherosclerotic plaque assuming that the target is expressed in adequate quantity for detection by molecular MRI.

Gadofluorine M is a lipophilic, macrocyclic (1,528 Da), water-soluble, gadolinium chelate complex (Gd-DO3A-derivative) with a perfluorinated side chain. Sirol et al. [8] and others [21] demonstrated that Gadofluorine M enhanced aortic wall imaging in Watanabe heritable hyperlipidemic rabbits but did not enhance the aorta of control rabbits.

Another recently developed imaging agent is a recombinant high-density lipoprotein (rHDL) molecule that incorporates gadolinium-DTPA phospholipids [22]. This imaging agent has a small diameter of 7–12 nm, is endogenous, does not trigger an immune reaction, and is easy to reconstitute [22]. This agent was tested in vivo in ApoE knockout mice and demonstrated a 35% mean normalized enhancement ratio 24 h following intravascular injection and significant uptake of fluorescent rHDL was demonstrated by confocal microscopy [22].

The ability to identify components of thrombus with molecular MRI may enable enhanced detection and characterization of both luminal thrombus and components of thrombus organized in an old atherothrombotic lesion. Therefore, selection of targets pivotal in the coagulation cascade, such as fibrin, factor XIII, integrins on the surface of platelets, and tissue factor, is necessary to identify the areas of old or active thrombus formation. The attachment of MR contrast agents to both monoclonal antibodies and peptide ligands that specifically bind components of thrombus has been performed in animal models [7, 23–25] and humans [26, 27]. Additionally, thrombus resulting from plaque rupture has been identified using fibrin-specific MR contrast agents in a rabbit carotid crush injury model [6, 28]. In the 25 arterial thrombi induced by carotid crush injury, Botnar et al. demonstrated a sensitivity and specificity of 100% for in vivo thrombus detection using MRI [6]. Sirol et al. [28] investigated a similar fibrin-specific MR contrast agent in 12 guinea pigs demonstrating that thrombus signal intensity was increased by over fourfold after intravascular delivery of contrast agent, and thrombus was detected in 100% of animals postcontrast compared with 42% identification of thrombus precontrast [28].

Advances in research and technologies in noninvasive MRI are coming to fruition in clinical practice. For other reviews, see [29–33]. The targeting of plaque components as well as the conjugation of ligands (antibodies, small peptides, antibody fragments etc.) that specifically target these components might enable assessment of the progress of therapy to reduce plaque volume and inflammation. With the merging of exciting research in the fields of molecular biology and MRI, major advances in the imaging of atherosclerosis may soon translate to the clinical setting.

REFERENCES

1. Lipinski MJ, Fuster V, Fisher EA, Fayad ZA. Targeting of biological molecules for evaluation of high-risk atherosclerotic plaques with magnetic resonance imaging. Nat Clin Pract Cardiovasc Med. 2004;1:48–55.
2. Kang HW, Josephson L, Petrovsky A, Weissleder R, Bogdanov A, Jr. Magnetic resonance imaging of inducible E-selectin expression in human endothelial cell culture. Bioconjug Chem. 2002;13:122–7.
3. Kerwin W, Hooker A, Spilker M, Vicini P, Ferguson M, Hatsukami T, Yuan C. Quantitative magnetic resonance imaging analysis of neovasculature volume in carotid atherosclerotic plaque. Circulation. 2003;107:851–6.
4. Anderson SA, Rader RK, Westlin WF, Null C, Jackson D, Lanza GM, Wickline SA, Kotyk JJ. Magnetic resonance contrast enhancement of neovasculature with alpha(v)beta(3)-targeted nanoparticles. Magn Reson Med. 2000;44:433–9.
5. Winter PM, Morawski AM, Caruthers SD, Fuhrhop RW, Zhang H, Williams TA, Allen JS, Lacy EK, Robertson JD, Lanza GM, Wickline SA. Molecular imaging of angiogenesis in early-stage atherosclerosis with alpha(v)beta3-integrin-targeted nanoparticles. Circulation. 2003;108:2270–4.
6. Botnar RM, Perez AS, Witte S, Wiethoff AJ, Laredo J, Hamilton J, Quist W, Parsons EC, Jr., Vaidya A, Kolodziej A, Barrett JA, Graham PB, Weisskoff RM, Manning WJ, Johnstone MT. In vivo molecular imaging of acute and subacute thrombosis using a fibrin-binding magnetic resonance imaging contrast agent. Circulation. 2004;109:2023–9.
7. Johansson LO, Bjornerud A, Ahlstrom HK, Ladd DL, Fujii DK. A targeted contrast agent for magnetic resonance imaging of thrombus: implications of spatial resolution. J Magn Reson Imaging. 2001;13:615–8.
8. Sirol M, Itskovich VV, Mani V, Aguinaldo JG, Fallon JT, Misselwitz B, Weinmann HJ, Fuster V, Toussaint JF, Fayad ZA. Lipid-rich atherosclerotic plaques detected by gadofluorine-enhanced in vivo magnetic resonance imaging. Circulation. 2004;109:2890–6.
9. Ruehm SG, Corot C, Vogt P, Kolb S, Debatin JF. Magnetic resonance imaging of atherosclerotic plaque with ultrasmall superparamagnetic particles of iron oxide in hyperlipidemic rabbits. Circulation. 2001;103:415–22.
10. Kooi ME, Cappendijk VC, Cleutjens KB, Kessels AG, Kitslaar PJ, Borgers M, Frederik PM, Daemen MJ, van Engelshoven JM. Accumulation of ultrasmall superparamagnetic particles of iron oxide in human atherosclerotic plaques can be detected by in vivo magnetic resonance imaging. Circulation. 2003;107:2453–8.
11. Trivedi RA, JM UK-I, Graves MJ, Cross JJ, Horsley J, Goddard MJ, Skepper JN, Quartey G, Warburton E, Joubert I, Wang L, Kirkpatrick PJ, Brown J, Gillard JH. In vivo detection of macrophages in human carotid atheroma: temporal dependence of ultrasmall superparamagnetic particles of iron oxide-enhanced MRI. Stroke. 2004;35:1631–5.
12. Falk E. Plaque rupture with severe pre-existing stenosis precipitating coronary thrombosis. Characteristics of coronary atherosclerotic plaques underlying fatal occlusive thrombi. Br Heart J. 1983;50:127–34.
13. Ross R. Atherosclerosis – an inflammatory disease. N Engl J Med. 1999;340:115–26.
14. Choudhury RP, Fuster V, Fayad ZA. Molecular, cellular and functional imaging of atherothrombosis. Nat Rev Drug Discov. 2004;3:913–25.
15. Tsimikas S, Palinski W, Halpern SE, Yeung DW, Curtiss LK, Witztum JL. Radiolabeled MDA2, an oxidation-specific, monoclonal antibody, identifies native atherosclerotic lesions in vivo. J Nucl Cardiol. 1999;6:41–53.
16. Tsimikas S. Noninvasive imaging of oxidized low-density lipoprotein in atherosclerotic plaques with tagged oxidation-specific antibodies. Am J Cardiol. 2002;90:22L–7.
17. Tsimikas S, Shortal BP, Witztum JL, Palinski W. In vivo uptake of radiolabeled MDA2, an oxidation-specific monoclonal antibody, provides an accurate measure of atherosclerotic lesions rich in oxidized ldl and is highly sensitive to their regression. Arterioscler Thromb Vasc Biol. 2000;20:689–97.
18. Hamilton AJ, Huang SL, Warnick D, Rabbat M, Kane B, Nagaraj A, Klegerman M, McPherson DD. Intravascular ultrasound molecular imaging of atheroma components in vivo. J Am Coll Cardiol. 2004;43:453–60.
19. Villanueva FS, Jankowski RJ, Klibanov S, Pina ML, Alber SM, Watkins SC, Brandenburger GH, Wagner WR. Microbubbles targeted to intercellular adhesion molecule-1 bind to activated coronary artery endothelial cells. Circulation. 1998;98:1–5.

20. Lindner JR, Song J, Christiansen J, Klibanov AL, Xu F, Ley K. Ultrasound assessment of inflammation and renal tissue injury with microbubbles targeted to P-selectin. Circulation. 2001;104:2107–12.
21. Barkhausen J, Ebert W, Heyer C, Debatin JF, Weinmann HJ. Detection of atherosclerotic plaque with Gadofluorine-enhanced magnetic resonance imaging. Circulation. 2003;108:605–9.
22. Frias JC, Williams KJ, Fisher EA, Fayad ZA. Recombinant HDL-like nanoparticles: a specific contrast agent for MRI of atherosclerotic plaques. J Am Chem Soc. 2004;126:16316–7.
23. Schmitz SA, Winterhalter S, Schiffler S, Gust R, Wagner S, Kresse M, Coupland SE, Semmler W, Wolf KJ. USPIO-enhanced direct MR imaging of thrombus: preclinical evaluation in rabbits. Radiology. 2001;221:237–43.
24. Johnstone MT, Botnar RM, Perez AS, Stewart R, Quist WC, Hamilton JA, Manning WJ. In vivo magnetic resonance imaging of experimental thrombosis in a rabbit model. Arterioscler Thromb Vasc Biol. 2001;21:1556–60.
25. Flacke S, Fischer S, Scott MJ, Fuhrhop RJ, Allen JS, McLean M, Winter P, Sicard GA, Gaffney PJ, Wickline SA, Lanza GM. Novel MRI contrast agent for molecular imaging of fibrin: implications for detecting vulnerable plaques. Circulation. 2001;104:1280–5.
26. Yu X, Song SK, Chen J, Scott MJ, Fuhrhop RJ, Hall CS, Gaffney PJ, Wickline SA, Lanza GM. High-resolution MRI characterization of human thrombus using a novel fibrin-targeted paramagnetic nanoparticle contrast agent. Magn Reson Med. 2000;44:867–72.
27. Winter PM, Caruthers SD, Yu X, Song SK, Chen J, Miller B, Bulte JW, Robertson JD, Gaffney PJ, Wickline SA, Lanza GM. Improved molecular imaging contrast agent for detection of human thrombus. Magn Reson Med. 2003;50:411–6.
28. Sirol M, Aguinaldo JGS, Graham G, Weisskoff R, Mizsei G, Lauffer R, Chereshnev I, Fallon JT, Reis ED, Fuster V, Toussaint JF, Fayad ZA. Fibrin-targeted contrast agent for improvement of in vivo acute thrombus detection with magnetic resonance imaging. Atherosclerosis. 2005;182:79–85.
29. Cormode DP, Skajaa T, Fayad ZA, Mulder WJ. Nanotechnology in medical imaging: probe design and applications. Arterioscler Thromb Vasc Biol. 2009;29:992–1000.
30. Mulder WJ, Cormode DP, Hak S, Lobatto ME, Silvera S, Fayad ZA. Multimodality nanotracers for cardiovascular applications. Nat Clin Pract Cardiovasc Med. 2008;5(Suppl 2):S103–11.
31. Fayad ZA, Fuster V. Prologue: relevance of molecular imaging in clinical medicine. Nat Clin Pract Cardiovasc Med. 2008;5(Suppl 2):S1.
32. Mulder WJ, Fayad ZA. Nanomedicine captures cardiovascular disease. Arterioscler Thromb Vasc Biol. 2008;28(5):801–2.
33. Sanz J, Fayad ZA. Imaging of atherosclerotic cardiovascular disease. Nature. 2008;451(7181):953–7.

32 Noninvasive Imaging of the Vulnerable Myocardium: Cardiac MRI and CT Based

Ricardo C. Cury, Anand Soni, and Ron Blankstein

CONTENTS

ABSTRACT

Multiple noninvasive imaging modalities can be used for the evaluation of the vulnerable myocardium. In this chapter, the applications of advanced cardiac imaging with cardiac MRI and cardiac CT are reviewed for the assessment of myocardial perfusion, viability, infarct size, and myocardium at risk. The accurate characterization of the vulnerable myocardium can provide important information that can guide therapeutics by detection of myocardial ischemia under stress conditions, the detection and characterization of myocardial infarct (size, transmural and circumferential extent), or the assessment of myocardium at risk (myocardial edema, microvascular obstruction, "grey zone"). Modalities with high spatial resolution and excellent tissue characterization, such as cardiac MRI and CT, will permit to obtain this type of information. Animal and human data will be reviewed and will be placed in clinical perspective, taking into account the limitations of each modality. Finally, we aim to demonstrate that the search and characterization of the vulnerable myocardium can help and provide important information in the overall characterization and management of the vulnerable patient.

Key words: Angina; Computed tomography; Diagnosis; Magnetic resonance imaging; Myocardial infarction

KEY POINTS

- Comprehensive stress perfusion (SP) cardiac MR protocol can obtain information on myocardial ischemia under coronary vasodilation; rest perfusion MRI can assess for "reversibility" of perfusion defects, cine MRI for left ventricular morphology, function, and wall motion, and delayed enhanced MRI for infarct detection.

From: *Asymptomatic Atherosclerosis: Pathophysiology, Detection and Treatment*
Edited by: M. Naghavi (ed.), DOI 10.1007/978-1-60327-179-0_32

- Cardiac MRI has the potential to identify myocardium at risk by combining T2W images to detect myocardial edema and delayed enhancement for detection of myocardial necrosis.
- Cardiac MR can detect another marker for vulnerable myocardium – the "grey zone", which is the peri-infarct zone with intermediate signal intensity which corresponds to increased potentials for ventricular arrhythmogenicity.
- Cardiac CT has also the capability for detection of myocardial infarct using rest perfusion and delayed-enhancement techniques. Stress perfusion (SP) cardiac CT under pharmacological stress is in the experimental phase with initial animal and human studies presented.

CLINICAL CASE

A 48 year old obese female patient presents to her physician with chest pain. She has metabolic syndrome and is being treated for her glucose intolerance, hypertriglyceridemia, hypertension, and obesity with aggressive diet and lifestyle intervention and a single antihypertensive agent. She is a nonsmoker and has no family history of CAD. Her chest pain has atypical features, occurs at rest, and is provoked by low level activities.

Given her body habitus and the high likelihood of diaphragmatic and breast tissue attenuation on nuclear imaging, her physician opted for an exercise echocardiogram to assess for ischemia. At peak exercise, she had minimal chest pain with 1–2 mm horizontal ST segment depression. The echocardiogram was limited because of poor acoustic windows but showed normal LV systolic function and wall motion at rest and exercise.

Given the ischemic ECG changes and symptoms at exercise with discordant echocardiographic findings, her physician opted for SP MRI because the patient was reluctant to undergo invasive coronary angiography. She underwent adenosine SP MRI (Fig. 1) without complications, and the findings conclusively demonstrated inferior wall ischemia in the RCA territory, which was later confirmed by invasive angiography showing a significant stenosis in the mid RCA.

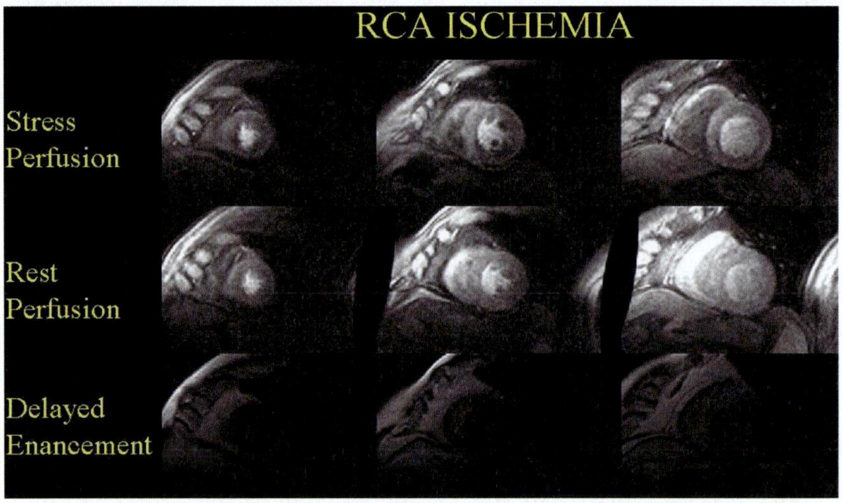

Fig. 1. Clinical example of RCA ischemia and stress perfusion MR (see text for details).

IMAGING THE VULNERABLE MYOCARDIUM WITH CARDIAC MRI

Stress Perfusion MRI

SP MRI has emerged as a useful modality in the assessment of patients with chest pain syndromes [1]. However, once a research tool, cardiac MRI is now a useful clinical imaging modality with multiple advantages over conventional stress tests such as nuclear imaging and echocardiography. Our clinical case demonstrates this point very nicely. MRI operates with superior spatial and temporal resolution and offers no ionizing radiation. Over the past 20 years, evaluation of cardiac function with cardiac magnetic resonance imaging (CMR) has improved because of the advances in gradient echo pulse sequences [2]. Short repetition times (TR) and smaller flip angles enable imaging of the heart during various phases of the cardiac cycle. Moreover, the superb tissue contrast and signal—noise ratio allows for excellent depiction of endocardial and epicardial borders as well as the blood pool. Furthermore, new techniques have been developed to optimally display nonviable myocardium as areas of delayed hyperenhancement and normal myocardium being nulled by a inversion pulse resulting in dark signal [3]. In high volume cardiac MRI centers, SP testing is becoming a popular exam as its diagnostic accuracy is proving to be superior to radionuclide myocardial perfusion imaging.

The goal of SP MRI is to visualize the first pass of gadolinium contrast agent within the LV blood pool into the myocardium during rest and stress. Stress is achieved with pharmacological vasodilation, either with adenosine or with dipyridamole. Under vasodilatory stress, myocardial blood flow (MBF) should increase 4–5 times, except in areas of obstructive epicardial coronary artery disease where downstream vascular beds are already maximally vasodilated. These coronary territories obtain lower peak myocardial signal intensity upon contrast administration compared to resting conditions. Note in our clinical case of RCA ischemia, the inferior wall subendocardium is hypointense under stress and is completely normal at rest. This would be termed a reversible perfusion defect and is diagnostic for a physiologically significant coronary stenosis. The diagnosis of coronary artery disease in this patient is critical as her current management for metabolic syndrome would change to include more aggressive drug therapy and possible percutaneous revascularization if her angina persists despite medical therapy.

Preclinical and Clinical Evaluation

There have been numerous animal studies that have demonstrated good correlation of MRI perfusion with tissue perfusion as measured by radioactive microspheres [4–6]. Notable studies included work by Wilke et al. and Klocke et al. wherein porcine and canine models of LCX stenosis were created, respectively, that showed that MRI can detect different degrees of myocardial perfusion under adenosine stress.

Following this, Lee et al. used a canine model of LCX stenosis and compared perfusion MRI to technetium-99m sestamibi and 201-thallium. They showed that MRI could detect perfusion defects with a LCX stenosis of ≥50% whereas SPECT perfusion defects were only detected with LCX stenosis of ≥85%.

Multiple clinical human studies testing the diagnostic accuracy and performance of SP MRI were performed as compared to nuclear imaging and conventional coronary angiography. Table 1 is a summary of published data with x-ray angiography as the reference standard [7–23]. Nandular et al. [24] performed a meta-analysis of all stress MRI studies with 2 main techniques in use: (1) perfusion imaging; and (2) stress-induced wall motion abnormalities imaging from January 1990 to January 2007 with a total of 37 studies involving 2191 patients. All studies used catheter x-ray angiography as the reference standard. Fourteen studies (754 patients) using stress-induced wall motion

Table 1
Diagnostic accuracy of stress perfusion MRI studies since 2000, having invasive coronary angiography as the reference standard

Author	*Year*	*Journal*	*Patients (N)*	*Stenosis definition (%)*	*Sensitivity*	*Specificity*
Al-Saadi	2000	Circulation	34	≥75	90	83
Bertschinger	2001	JMRI	14	≥50	85	81
Schwitter	2001	Circulation	48	≥50	87	85
Panting	2001	JMRI	22	>50	79	83
Ibrahim	2002	JACC	25	>75	69	89
Chiu	2003	Radiology	13	>50	92	92
Ishida	2003	Radiology	104	≥70	90	85
Nagel	2003	Circulation	84	≥75	88	90
Wolff	2004	Circulation	75	≥70	93	75
Giang	2004	EHJ	80	≥50	93	75
Paetsch	2004	Circulation	79	>50	91	62
Plein	2004	JACC	68	≥70	88	83
Plein	2005	Radiology	92	≥70	88	82
Klem	2006	JACC	100	≥70	89	87
Cury	2006	Radiology	47	≥70	87	89
Rieber	2006	EHJ	43	≥50	88	90
Cheng	2007	JACC	61	≥50	3.0 T=98 1.5 T=90	3.0 T=76 1.5 T=67

abnormalities imaging demonstrated 83% sensitivity and 86% specificity on a patient level. Perfusion imaging demonstrated a sensitivity of 91% and specificity of 81% on a patient level (disease prevalence=57.4%).

Two recent studies in Table 1 by Klem et al. and Cury et al. [20, 21] sought to improve the diagnostic accuracy of SP MRI by using a comprehensive imaging approach of first pass contrast for myocardial perfusion at rest and stress with delayed enhancement imaging for infarct detection. Cury showed that the combined approach yields 87% sensitivity, 89% specificity, and 88% accuracy and was superior to a rest/SP MR imaging alone that has 81% sensitivity, 87% specificity, and 85% accuracy, having invasive coronary angiography as the reference standard. Similar results were demonstrated by Klem et al. that SP and delayed-enhancement better detect inducible ischemia and fixed defects as compared to stress/rest perfusion MRI.

The conclusion from these various studies is that we should endorse a comprehensive SP CMR protocol that includes SP MRI for myocardial ischemia under coronary vasodilation, rest perfusion MRI to assess for "reversibility" of perfusion defects, cine MRI for left ventricular morphology, function, and wall motion, and delayed enhanced MRI for infarct detection. Given the high volume of stress imaging studies performed in the US each year, it is imperative that a noninvasive imaging modality for CAD has high diagnostic accuracy such as cardiac MRI [25].

Stress Perfusion Protocol

After the initial localizing images, the patient is removed from the scanner bore and a vasodilator, typically adenosine, is infused under continuous ECG and blood pressure monitoring. The patient is recentered in the magnet and after 5 min a dynamic first pass perfusion pulse sequence is performed with gadolinium administration. Multiphase multislice cardiac gated breath hold images are obtained

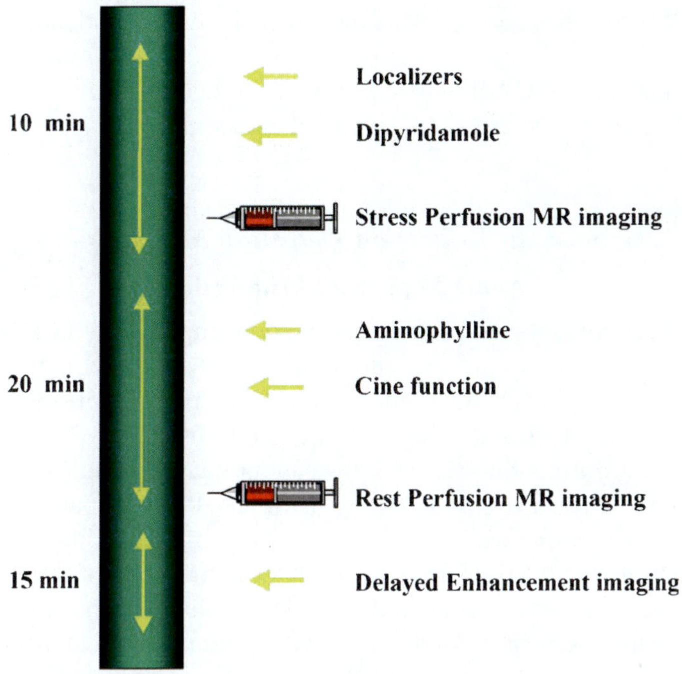

Fig. 2. Stress perfusion MR protocol.

in the short axis as the gadolinium bolus arrives into the right ventricle and has perfused the LV myocardium. Total imaging time is approximately 40–50 s and includes 8–10 short axis slices from base to the apex at 8 mm thickness with a 2 mm gap.

Next, a balanced steady-state free procession cine MRI sequence is used to obtain left ventricular functional images throughout the cardiac cycle. Eight to ten short axis images are prescribed to cover from base to apex with a slice thickness of 8 mm and a gap of 2 mm. Ideally, the prescription should be identical to the perfusion sequence to allow for coregistration of all slices. Image analysis is performed off line and includes LV systolic function and wall motion under stress. Total imaging time takes approximately 5 min.

Afterwards, a second dynamic perfusion scan is obtained after a repeated injection of gadolinum. These images represent resting myocardial perfusion and are essential for data analysis and artifact detection, and aid in the diagnosis for "reversible" defects.

Lastly, after approximately 10 min delayed enhancement imaging is performed using the same short axis slice prescription from the perfusion sequences and cine-MRI.

The schema for this protocol is nicely depicted in Fig. 2.

Stress Perfusion Image Analysis

Comprehensive image analysis needs to first assess perfusion defects at stress. Comparison with resting perfusion is mandatory to assess reversibility, similar to nuclear imaging. A perfusion defect under vasodilator stress in a coronary territory that appears normal at rest indicates a significant epicardial coronary artery stenosis. A SP defect that remains "fixed" at rest may indicate a chronic infarction or artifact. Delayed enhancement images then become vital because a fixed perfusion defect due to infarction will have a matched area of hyperenhancement on delayed images. Lastly, an assessment of left ventricular systolic function and wall motion is made under stress. A wall motion abnormality in a coronary territory that matches with a perfusion defects is further evidence of ischemic, vulnerable myocardium.

In conclusion, the diagnosis of CAD is made in the presence of a stress induced perfusion defect or if a myocardial infarction is detected on delayed enhanced images.

Myocardial Infarction Detection and Viability

Acute Myocardial Infarction

Cardiac MRI has a well defined role in the assessment of myocardial infarction, both in the acute and chronic setting [3, 26–32]. Using a short but comprehensive protocol, MRI has the capability to provide left and right ventricular volumes and systolic function (ejection fraction), regional wall motion, and evaluation of infarct size and degree of transmurality [2]. All of the aforementioned provide important prognostic information and can alter patient management [33].

Gerber et al. [34] performed an important study using CMR on 20 patients 4 days and 7 months after an acute MI. The question being studied is what MRI imaging finding could best predict LV functional recovery after an acute MI. Gerber found that the presence of delayed hyperenhancement had a better diagnostic accuracy than the lack of early hypoenhancement in predicting functional LV recovery. Early hypoenhancement in this setting likely represents a smaller portion of the infarction resulting from microvascular obstruction (MVO) and thus underestimates final infarct size when compared to delayed enhancement. This study also concluded that the degree of transmurality has to be <75% to signify myocardial recovery in the acute setting.

This is not to say that the presence of MVO after an acute myocardial infarction holds no prognostic information [35] Baks et al. [27] assessed early and late infarct size and LV function in 22 patients using a comprehensive CMR protocol including cine, first pass resting perfusion, and delayed enhanced MRI at 5 days and 5 months after primary PCI for an acute MI. The authors concluded that myocardial segments with MVO were more likely to have late thinning and hypokinesia/akinesia at 5 months compared to segments without MVO. Finally, the study also showed that total infarct size decreased by 31% over time. This final conclusion raises the observation that in the acute setting there are portions of the myocardium "at risk" for irreversible damage and the goal for therapy should be to minimize final infarct size.

Myocardium at Risk

Cardiac MRI has proven to be a useful experimental tool at identifying myocardium at risk following reperfused acute MI. Aletras et al. [36] utilized T2 weighted cardiac MRI to quantify myocardial edema at 2 days in a 90 min canine coronary artery occlusion model. The authors showed that by subtracting final infarct size determined by delayed enhanced MRI from the area of signal hyperintensity on T2-weighted images (i.e. myocardial edema), an area of "myocardium at risk" can be determined. This proved to correlate well with radioactive microsphere data.

Our group demonstrated that a concise and comprehensive cardiac MRI protocol including T2W images can detect patients with acute coronary syndrome in the Emergency Department [37]. What it is most intriguing in this data is that myocardial edema as detected by T2W images can precede the appearance of delayed hyperenhancement (myocardial necrosis) and can be visualized in patients with unstable angina. This is the in vivo validation that cardiac MRI can detect vulnerable myocardium or "myocardium at risk" in a time where intervention can still be performed. Further studies will be needed to confirm this data in a larger population and also if this information will be able to guide reperfusion therapies.

Other area of interest is the assessment of myocardial infarct border zone using the high spatial resolution and contrast-to-noise (CNR) ratio of delayed-enhancement MR imaging to further evaluate the physiologic basis of peri-infarct tissue heterogeneity. Using semiautomated signal intensity thresholding criteria on delayed-enhancement imaging, Schmidt et al. assessed 47 patients with clinical indications for automated internal cardioverter defibrillator and found a significant association of inducible sustained monomorphic ventricular tachycardia during electrophysiological testing and tissue heterogeneity [38]. This finding supports the notion that CMR can detect a peri-infarct zone with intermediate signal intensity "grey zone" which corresponds to increased potentials for ventricular arrhythmogenicity. There has been growing clinical evidence that tissue characteristics of delayed-enhancement imaging provide information valuable to patient outcome. Two separate clinical reports demonstrated the unique and important prognostic value of MVO identified on delayed-enhancement imaging in patients who suffered from a recent myocardial infarction [33, 35]. In a clinical cohort of 144 post-MI patients followed for up to 4.5 years, Yan et al. found that assessment of infarct heterogeneity, using an algorithm similar to that of Schmidt et al. to be the strongest predictor of post-MI mortality, complementary to the robust prognostic value of LV end-systolic volume [39].

Chronic Myocardial Infarction and Viability

Delayed enhancement MRI is a very sensitive technique for the detection of chronic myocardial infarction. Fieno et al. [40] compared infarct sizes determined by in vivo and ex vivo contrast MRI with histopathologic tissue sections of the entire LV in a dog model of myocardial infarction. The authors showed that the spatial extents of hyperenhancement for both in vivo and ex vivo MRI were the same as the histopathologic extent of infarction at every stage of healing.

Wu et al. [41] showed that in 44 patients with proven myocardial necrosis by cardiac enzymes imaged at either 3 or 14 months, MRI was able to detect the infarct by hyperenhancement in the same coronary territory as initially identified by coronary angiography.

The ability of CMR to accurately identify and quantify infarct size in the setting of chronic infarction has been instrumental in myocardial viability assessment. Multiple studies have shown that the degree of transmurality of scar on delayed enhancement MRI has important prognostic information. Kim et al. [42] studied delayed enhancement MRI in animal models and found it occur only in regions of nonviable myocardium when compared to histopathology. This important data led the same authors to evaluate a group of patients with chronic ischemic heart disease prior to surgical revascularization – cardiac MRI was performed before and after bypass surgery [43]. The study concluded that most segments with <50% infarct transmurality were viable and recovered function after revascularization. Segments with infarct transmurality of >50% were less likely to have improvements in regional LV function and not benefit from high risk cardiac surgery, and hence were deemed nonviable.

Imaging the Vulnerable Myocardium with Cardiac CT

While multiple recent single and multicenter [44] studies have established the diagnostic accuracy of cardiac CT for the detection of coronary artery stenosis, the functional significance of many coronary artery lesions identified by such techniques (or by invasive coronary angiography) is often unknown [45, 46]. To that end, myocardial perfusion imaging and angiography have the potential to provide complementary information by imaging both ischemia and atherosclerosis, respectively. Naturally, it follows that the potential of obtaining this information from a single imaging modality would be very attractive.

Recent recognition that cardiac MDCT may emerge as a modality capable of assessing myocardial perfusion has generated much excitement. Indeed, for a certain subset of patients, it would be desirable and useful to have a single modality which could provide a comprehensive assessment of anatomy, function, and perfusion. In addition, for patients who have obstructive coronary artery disease and left ventricular dysfunction, the presence or absence of viable myocardium is extremely useful in guiding therapy. As some of these patients have contra-indications to cardiac MRI, it remains advantageous to have alternative diagnostic tests, which can assess for the presence of viability.

At present, multiple noninvasive imaging modalities are used in evaluating myocardial perfusion and viability, including single-photon emission computed tomography (SPECT), positron emission tomography (PET), echocardiography, and cardiac MRI. While SPECT has been well shown to accurately assess rest and SP and provides useful prognostic data based on a patient's burden of ischemia and infarct [47–49], it is limited by its low spatial resolution and attenuation artifacts which can lead to equivocal studies. Similarly, assessment of viability with SPECT, while commonly used, is subject to limitations [50, 51]. FDG-PET has the ability to reliably evaluate myocardial viability; however, due to its superior spatial resolution, MRI is currently the most rigorous modality used in evaluating infarct size and transmurality. As CT has the best spatial resolution of any imaging modality, many emerging studies suggests that it may have an important role for the future evaluation of myocardial perfusion, infarct size, and myocardial viability.

In this section, a brief overview of the animal and human studies demonstrating the use of CT perfusion and delayed hyperenhancement will be presented. As most of the initial animal studies employed an infarct model to assess perfusion defects, they demonstrated the use of CT in accurately characterizing rest perfusion defects, which are found in infarcted myocardium. In the process of further characterizing such resting perfusion defects, the use of delayed enhancement was found to be useful in distinguishing nonviable (i.e. typically infarcted) from viable myocardium. As a natural extension of the ability to assess perfusion, recent human and animal studies have used adenosine based SP in order to identify ischemia. Current animal studies in this field utilize a "stenosis-model" in order to identify lesions which are nonflow-limiting at rest but are significant during stress. Only recently have small human studies been conducted demonstrating the feasibility of using MDCT to characterize perfusion during adenosine stress.

Although not a focus of this chapter, it is noteworthy that rapidly evolving industry-driven technological advances in CT such as improving spatial resolution [52], reducing beam hardening artifacts, and using dual energy acquisition techniques all stand to advance the capabilities of MDCT in evaluating the vulnerable myocardium.

Animal Studies: Rest Perfusion and Delayed Hyperenhancement

The ability of CT to detect acute MI in explanted hearts and experimental animal models dates back to the late 1970s [53, 54]. More recently, MDCT has been utilized to assess myocardial perfusion in animal models of total coronary occlusion [55, 56]. Table 2 lists some of the main studies which characterized perfusion and delayed hyperenhancement in animal models.

The study by Hoffmann et al. used 4-slice MDCT and performed a quantitative analysis of CT attenuation and compared that to microsphere-determined blood flow and TTC-stained tissue samples. The quantitative analysis by MDCT showed significant differences in the mean CT attenuation of infarct and reference areas (32.1 HU ± 8.5 vs. 75.6 HU ± 16.7; $p<0.001$) and this correlated with changes in microsphere-determined blood flow. The volume of perfusion defect (infarct) was similar to volume of tissue that lacked TTC staining (17% ± 6.4 vs. 13.6% ± 6.0), with slight overestimation of infarct size by MDCT.

Mahnken et al. utilized a similar porcine model to assess the ability of MDCT to evaluate rest myocardial perfusion vs. first pass perfusion (FP) MRI with TTC staining serving as the gold standard [56]. In their protocol they utilized dynamic MDCT imaging by acquiring 64 scans at the apical level with

Table 2
MDCT rest perfusion and delayed enhancement: animal studies

Study	*Model*	*Imaging*	*Results*	*Conclusions*
Hoffmann [55]	• 7 pigs • Acute MI via LAD balloon occlusion	MDCT vs. TTC and microsphere blood flow	Area: CT (ED): 16.1 ± 4.8% CT (ES): 17.0 ± 6.4% TTC: 13.6 ± 6.0% (One animal had non-evaluable images due to high HR)	MDCT permits detection and further characterization of AMI
Mahnken [56]	• 5 pigs • Acute MI via LAD balloon occlusion	MDCT vs. FP-MRI vs. TTC	Area: MDCT: 19.3 ± 4.5% MR: 17.2 ± 4% TTC: 18.7 ± 5.7%	Demonstrated potential for semi-quantitative evaluation of myocardial perfusion using MDCT
Lardo [57]	• Acute canine reperfusion model (N = 10) • Chronic porcine reperfusion model (N = 8)	DE-MDCT vs. TTC and thioflavin S (infarcts were characterized by hyperenhancement, whereas regions of microvascular obstruction were characterized by hypoenhancement)	Infarct volume: Acute infarcts 21.1+/−7.2% vs. 20.4+/−7.4%, mean difference 0.7% Chronic infarcts 4.15+/−1.93% vs. 4.92+/−2.06%, mean difference −0.76%	Extent of acute and healed myocardial infarction can be determined and quantified accurately with contrast-enhanced MDCT
Baks [69]	• 10 pigs • Balloon occlusion of circumflex coronary artery × 2 h. followed by reperfusion	DE-MSCT vs. DE-MRI vs. ex vivo TTC staining	DE-MSCT and DE-MRI showed a good correlation with infarct size assessed with TTC pathology (R^2 = 0.96 [p < 0.001] and R^2 = 0.93 [p < 0.001], respectively)	DE-MSCT can assess acute reperfused myocardial infarction in good agreement with in vivo DE-MRI and TTC pathology
Nahrendorf [70]	• 20 mice coronary ligation induced MI	DE cine micro CT vs. ex vivo TCT staining: 5 and 35 days post MI	5 d post-MI: r^2 = 0.86, p < 0.01; 35 d post-MI: r^2 = 0.92, p < 0.01	Despite the small size and fast movement of the mouse heart, cine microCT reliably and rapidly quantifies infarct size

DE Delayed enhancement, *MI* Myocardial infarction, *TTC* Triphenyltetrazoline-chloride stain

a prospectively acquired ECG triggered exam protocol. Hypoenhanced regions on MDCT corresponded directly to perfusion defects visualized on MRI and areas of MI seen on TTC-staining. The hypoenhanced regions detected by MDCT were again slightly larger than areas of acute MI as detected by MRI and TTC-staining.

These aforementioned studies exploited the ability of MDCT to visualize areas of myocardial hypoattenuation, indicative of decreased myocardial perfusion. However, it is known that areas of decreased myocardial perfusion in the setting of myocardial infarction can represent (a) ischemia, (b) infarction with MVO, or (c) areas of infarction with preserved MVO. CMR studies have demonstrated that delayed hyperenhacement correlates well with infarct size and that these are inversely correlated with recovery of myocardial dysfunction after revascularization [43].

To determine whether MDCT based delayed hyperenhancement can be used in a similar manner, Lardo et al. studied 10 dogs that underwent 90 min balloon occlusion of the proximal left anterior descending coronary artery [57]. Postinfarct DE-MDCT identified myocardial lesions characterized by well-delineated hyperenhanced myocardial segments 5 min after contrast administration. The mean attenuations for infarcted and remote myocardium 5 min after contrast were 260.5±56.5 and 133.8±10.8 HU, respectively ($p=0.018$). Direct comparisons of MDCT-DE to TTC showed excellent correlation with infarct morphology, transmurality, and infarct volume ratios. Additionally, analogous to MRI, MDCT hypoenhanced regions identified regions of MVO at 5 min after contrast injection in 3 of 7 animals, which compared well with thioflavin-S derived measurements.

As part of the same study, the investigators also performed experiments to evaluate a chronic MI model. Seven pigs underwent proximal LAD balloon occlusion for 60 min followed by reperfusion, and 8 weeks after MI, the animals were imaged by MDCT and sectioned for TTC-staining. Similar to acute infarcts, myocardial scar by MDCT was characterized by subendocardial regions of hyper-enhancement in the LAD territory that also reached maximum intensity approximately 5 min after contrast injection. Chronic infarct volume by MDCT also compared well with TTC staining with a trend toward underestimation by MDCT (4.15±1.93% vs. 4.91±2.06%, mean difference –0.763%). It is important to emphasize that these animal experiments benefited from the ability to use ideal conditions with high amount of iodine contrast and high radiation dose.

Human Studies of Rest Perfusion

Nikolaou et al. attempted to correlate rest MDCT to SP CMR and delayed enhancement (DE) MRI among 30 patients with chronic infarcts and /or suspected CAD.[58] In this retrospective study, all patient previously underwent MDCT (16 detectors) and MRI within 10±16 days. MDCT was able to detect 13/17 perfusion defects correctly (sensitivity 76%, specificity 92%, accuracy 83%); however, when considering only the six perfusion defects not associated with chronic MI, the sensitivity dropped to 50% – not surprising given that MDCT was performed under resting conditions while SP-MRI imaging utilized vasodilator induced hyperemic blood flow. On the other hand comparing MDCT vs. DE-CMR for detection of infarct resulted in a sensitivity of 91%, specificity of 79%, and accuracy of 83%. The attenuation values in the 10 infarcted areas correctly detected by MDCT were significantly lower than in noninfarcted areas of myocardium (53.7±33.5 vs. 122.3±25.5 HU; $p<0.01$). In the volumetric assessment of infarct size, a strong correlation between the volumes of 16-MDCT and DE-CMR was found ($r=0.98$), but 16-MDCT tended to underestimate the infarct volume as assessed by CMR by 19% ($p<0.01$) (Table 3).

Nieman et al. retrospectively tested the hypothesis that 64-MDCT can differentiate recent (<7 days) vs. old (>12 months) MI [59]. They found significantly lower CT attenuation values in patients with long-standing MI (–13±37 HU) than those with acute MI (26±26 HU) and normal controls (73±14 HU, $p<0.001$). The attenuation difference between infarcted and remote myocardium was larger in patients with long-standing MI than in patients with recent MI (89±41 and 55±33 HU, respectively, $p<0.001$). As anticipated, long-standing MI was associated with wall thinning and ventricular dilation whereas recent MI was not ($p>0.05$).

Table 3
MDCT rest perfusion and delayed enhancement: human studies

Study	*Population*	*Imaging*	*Results*	*Conclusion*
Nikolaou [58]	• 30 patients • 11 chronic MI, 19 known or suspected CAD • Retrospective	• CE-MDCT (rest) • SP-CMR DE-CMR	• CT vs. DE-CMR: 10/11 infarcts identified (SN=91%, SP=79%) • CT vs. SP-CMR: 13/17 perfusion defects identified (SN=76%, SP=92%)	Rest CT can detect chronic infarctions but has a poor sensitivity for detecting perfusion defects in noninfarcted regions
Nieman [59]	CE-MDCT retrospectively evaluated for patients with: • recent MI (<7 days, $n=16$) • long-standing MI (>12 months, $n=13$) • no MI ($n=13$)	• MDCT measurement of attenuation (HU) at consecutive transmural locations of injured and normal remote myocardium	• Significantly lower CT attenuation with long-standing MI (−13 +/− 37 HU) vs. acute MI (26 +/− 26 HU) vs. normal controls (73 +/− 14 HU, p <0.001) • Attenuation difference between infarcted and remote myocardia was larger in patients with long-standing MI than in patients with recent MI (89 +/− 41 and 55 +/− 33 HU, respectively, p<0.001)	Recent and long-standing MIs may be differentiated by computed tomography based on myocardial CT attenuation values and ventricular dimensions
Mahnken [62]	• 28 patients with reperfused STEMI	• 16-MDCT early and DE (15 min) • DE-MRI	• Infarct size on MRI 31.2 +/− 22.5% compared with 33.3 +/− 23.8% for DE- MSCT and 24.5 +/− 18.3% early-perfusion-deficit MSCT	Late-enhancement MSCT appears to be as reliable as delayed contrast-enhanced MRI in assessing infarct size and myocardial viability in acute MI
Gerber [61]	• 16 patients with acute MI • 21 patients with chronic LV dysfunction	• CE-MDCT (rest) • Delayed MDCT (10 min post contrast) • FP-MRI • DE-MRI	• Concordance of early hypoenhanced regions (92%, kappa=0.54, p<0.001) and late hyperenhanced regions (82%, kappa=0.61, p<0.001)	CE-MDCT can characterize acute and chronic MI with contrast patterns similar to CE-MR, thus providing important information on infarct size and viability

(continued)

Table 3
(continued)

Study	*Population*	*Imaging*	*Results*	*Conclusion*
Lessick [71]	26 patients post AMI; 11 underwent PCI pre CT	• 16-MDCT: (a) ED: gated CT 120–130 mL nonionic contrast (b) DE: second scan 6 min later; no contrast • TTE: 3 months post MI to assess for recovery	For patent arteries (*n*=21): DE had SN=73% and SP=85% for predicting follow-up segment dysfunction, compared with SN=57% and SP=90% for ED	The presence and size of ED and DE post AMI are related to follow-up myocardial functional recovery
Habis [63]	36 patients with first acute MI	• 64CT (without contrast) gated mid-diastole, 24±11 min post PCI. Segment analysis: no, subendocardial, or transmural hyperenhancement • Rest TTE/Low-dose DSE 2–4 weeks post CT	• Per segment: SN 98%, SP 94%, AC 97%, PPV 99%, NPV 79% for detecting viable myocardial segments • Per-patient analysis SN 92%, SP 100%, AC 94%, PPV 100% and NPV 85%	A 64-slice CT after coronary angiography for an acute myocardial infarction is a promising method for early evaluation of viable myocardium

CMR Cardiac magnetic resonance imaging, *SP* Stress perfusion, *CE* Contrast enhanced, *DE* Delayed enhancement, *MI* Myocardial infarction, *CAD* Coronary artery disease, *SN* Sensitivity, *SP* Specificity, *HU* Hounsfield unit, *AMI* Acute myocardial infarction, *ED* Early perfusion defects, *PCI* Percutaneous coronary intervention, *TTE* Trans-thoracic echocardiography, *DSE* Dobutamine stress echocardiography

MDCT Imaging of Viability: Can MDCT be Used to Predict Recovery after Coronary Revascularization?

An accurate noninvasive determination of myocardial viability that is capable of distinguishing irreversible myocardial cellular injury from hibernation is critically important in appropriately selecting patients with CAD and left ventricular dysfunction that will benefit most from revascularization procedures [60]. As an area of reduced enhancement on arterial phase contrast CT can represent infarct, resting perfusion abnormality, or scar, there is a need to further differentiate the mechanism underlying such patterns.

MDCT allows assessment of myocardial viability by studying late enhancement in a fashion similar to magnetic resonance imaging. Analogous to DE-MRI, the mechanism of hyperenhancement is based on regional differences in contrast agent wash-in and washout time constants. In both acute and chronic myocardial infarction, there is an increased extracellular space which has slow wash in and slow washout of low molecular weight contrast agents.

In order to validate this concept in humans, Gerber et al. studied 37 patients with either acute MI or chronic LV dysfunction and compared resting MDCT perfusion with first pass MRI perfusion as well as delayed (10 min post contrast administration) MDCT with DE-MRI [61]. After showing a reasonable correlation between the two modalities, they concluded that MDCT can characterize acute and chronic MI with contrast patterns similar to FP-MR and DE-MRI.

In a similar study, Mahnken et al. evaluated 28 patients with reperfused acute ST-elevation MI who underwent 16-MDCT with first-pass and delayed (15 min) imaging as well as MRI [62]. Mean infarct size by DHE-CMR was 31.2±22.5% per slice compared with 33.3±23.8% per slice for DHE-MDCT, with excellent agreement between these two techniques (κ=0.878). Mean size of early perfusion-defect MDCT was only 24.5±18.3% per slice. That is, DHE-MDCT slightly overestimated MI size as compared to DHE-CMR and first-pass MDCT underestimated infarct size as compared to DHE-CMR. This latter finding may be explained by the fact that the part of the reperfused necrotic area with patent microvasculature enhances normally on first pass perfusion but is included in the region of delayed hyperenhancement. This same concept is also illustrated in the clinical example provided in Fig. 3. As a result of these findings, we speculate that the early hypoenhanced regions, which represent only the fraction of infarcted tissue with concomitant MVO, underestimate the amount of irreversibly injured myocardium present after acute MI.

The ability of CT to predict viability in the early stages of myocardial infarction was demonstrated by Habis et al. [63] who performed noncontrast enhanced cardiac CT in 36 patients immediately following percutaneous intervention. In this study the majority of the patients had a ST ***elevation*** myocardial infarction. During delayed imaging with CT, no or subendocardial (<50% of left ventricle thickness) hyperenhancement was expected to reflect viability. When compared to a follow up echo exam 2–4 weeks later, DE-CT was highly accurate in predicting recovery.

It is important to appreciate the limitations of DHE-MDCT. DHE-MDCT requires a second CT examination within 5–15 min after the first scan. By virtue of this fact, the patient is exposed to

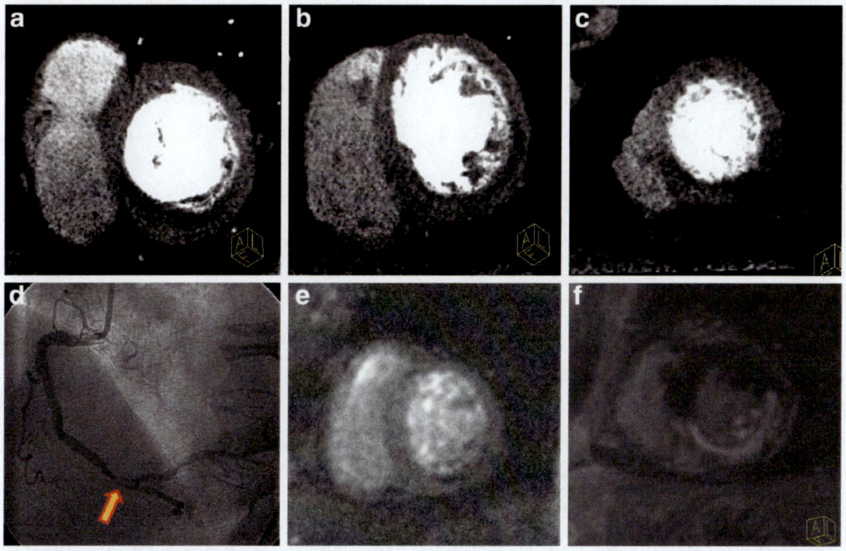

Fig. 3. 70-year-old male patient with history of dyslipidemia was admitted with inferior ST elevation myocardial infarction. He underwent a percutaneous intervention to the RCA and PDA. Cardiac CT 2 days later demonstrated resting perfusion defects in the basal inferior segment (**a**); mid inferior and inferolateral segments (**b**); and apical inferior, inferolateral, and inferoseptal segments (**c**). Cardiac MRI was performed on the same day. First pass perfusion revealed an inferior subendocardial perfusion defect (**e**). Delayed hyperenhancement (**f**) was prominent in the sub and mid-myocardial regions of the inferoseptal, inferior, and inferolateral segments consistent with nonviable infracted myocardium.

additional radiation. Furthermore, more iodinated contrast is necessary to achieve a reasonable CNR ratio between the normal and infarcted myocardium. To justify the additional radiation and contrast exposure, future studies will need to address the clinical utility of the DHE-MDCT technique. One particular group of patients who may benefit are those who have previously implanted pacemakers or defibrillators that would preclude evaluation by MRI.

The above studies provide data validating the ability of cardiac CT to identify perfusion defects and delayed hyperenhancement and also to further differentiate perfusion defects into acute and chronic MI. These findings set the stage for further clinical applications of this technology such as the use SP to identify ischemic myocardium.

Stress MDCT: Can CT Identify Ischemia?

Table 4 lists animal and human studies of stress CT. George et al. [64] performed rest and adenosine-mediated stress MDCT on a canine model of LAD stenosis and were able to achieve lesions which were nonflow limiting at rest but flow limiting during pharmacologic stress. Thus, they were able to identify perfusion defects in noninfarcted myocardium. By using microspheres to measure MBF, they were able to elegantly demonstrate that the myocardial signal density (SD) ratio (myocardial SD/LV blood pool SD) corresponded well with microsphere derived MBF.

Preliminary human studies investigating the feasibility and accuracy of MDCT stress myocardial perfusion have been only recently presented [65]. In 19 patients with an abnormal SPECT, George et al. used a 256 row MDCT to assess for subendocardial perfusion defects during rest and adenosine infusion. When compared to ≥50% stenosis by CT angiography, the sensitivity and specificity MDCT was 85% and 77% compared to 69% and 74% by SPECT. When compared to a gold standard combining ≥50% stenosis by CTA with a SPECT perfusion defect, the 256 row MDCT was 78% sensitive and 90% specific. Although these findings represent preliminary work, they suggest that ischemia can be detected with a modest sensitivity and reasonably high specificity.

Imaging the Vulnerable Myocardium: Technical Considerations and Perils

Most of the MDCT studies reviewed in this section are small and given that many of these imaging approaches are new and are continuously being enhanced, there are no current established protocols on how to best image the myocardium.

While a discussion of the different technical parameters utilized in these studies is beyond the scope of this chapter, it is useful to acknowledge a few studies which have evaluated the use of different technical parameters. Using a porcine infarct model, Mahnken et al. [66] showed that when comparing images obtained from 3 different kV settings (80, 100, and 120 kV; all with 550 $mAs^{effective}$, 16×0.75 mm) and comparing them to ex vivo staining and MRI, use of 80 kV resulted in the highest CNR ratio as well as the highest signal difference between normal and infracted myocardium. These findings have important implications and when combined with other advances in CT such as prospective gating [67], suggest that perfusion imaging can be achieved with reasonably low levels of radiation exposure to patients.

Future studies to determine the ideal contrast agent for MDCT coronary anatomy and perfusion imaging are needed. A recent study (Tsai et. al. [68]) randomized 72 patients to receive either iohexol (Omnipaque) or iodixanol (Visipaque). While there was no significant difference in the arterial phase enhancement in the right heart, left heart, coronary arteries, and LV myocardium; interestingly, the agent with the lower iodine content – iodixanol – resulted in higher enhancement in the LV myocardium in the delayed phase, possibly because of its large dimeric molecular structure resulting in a slower wash out phase.

Table 4
MDCT stress perfusion: animal and human studies

Study	*Subjects*	*Imaging*	*Results*	*Conclusions*
George [64]	8 dogsCanine model of LAD stenosis (nonflow limiting at rest but flow limiting during stress)	64×0.5 MDCT rest and stress perfusion vs. ex vivo staining	• Myocardial SD was 92.3+/−39.5 HU in stenosed vs. 180.4+/−41.9 HU in remote territories ($p<0.001$) • There was a significant linear association of the SD ratio with MBF in the stenosed territory ($R=0.98$, $p=0.001$)	Adenosine-augmented MDCT myocardial perfusion imaging provides semiquantitative measurements of myocardial perfusion during first-pass MDCT imaging in a canine model of LAD stenosis
George [72][a]	17 patients with (+) MPI and chest pain referred for invasive angiography	64×0.5 MDCT: • Rest perfusion • Stress perfusion – using Adenosine (140 µg/kg/min) infusion	• For identifying stenosis ≥50% stenosis by CTA and ICA, MDCT SN=83%, SP=100% (vs. 67% and 80% for MPI)	Adenosine stress CT can accurately assess coronary atherosclerosis and its physiological significance in patients with chest pain
George [65][a]	19 patients with (+) SPECT	256×0.5 mm MDCT: • Rest perfusion • Stress perfusion – using adenosine (140 µg/kg/min) infusion	• Compared to ≥50% stenosis by CTA, MDCT SN=85%, SP=77% (vs. 69% and 74% for SPECT) Compared to a gold standard combining ≥50% stenosis by CTA and SPECT perfusion defect, SN=78%, SP=90%	256 MDCT enables combination of noninvasive CT angiography and perfusion with high accuracy and at radiation levels similar to currently used dual isotope nuclear techniques
George [73]	6 dogs with moderate to severe LAD stenosis	64×0.5 dynamic MDCT stress perfusion (adenosine 140 µg/kg/min) vs. microsphere derived MBF	• The myocardial upslope-to-LV-upslope and myocardial upslope-to-LV-max ratio strongly correlated with MBF ($R^2=0.92$, $p<0.0001$ and $R^2=0.87$, $p<0.0001$, respectively) • Absolute MBF derived by model-based deconvolution analysis modestly overestimated MBF • Overall, MDCT-derived MBF strongly correlated with microspheres ($R=0.91$, $p<0.0001$)	d-MDCT MBF measurements using upslope and model-based deconvolution methods correlate well with microsphere MBF

[a]Abstract

CTA CT angiography, *SN* Sensitivity, *SP* Specificity, *MPI* Radionuclide myocardial perfusion imaging, *CTA* CT angiography, *ICA* Invasive coronary angiography, *MBF* Myocardial blood flow

Cardiac MRI and CT Assessing the Vulnerable Myocardium: Summary and Recommendations

Current data favor cardiac MRI for the assessment of myocardial perfusion, viability, infarct size, and ultimately detection and characterization of the vulnerable myocardium. Cardiac MRI has the possibility of detecting inducible ischemia under stress imaging with high diagnostic accuracy. Also, cardiac MRI provides accurate information of infarct size, MVO, transmural and circumferential extent, and characteristics of the border zone ("grey zone") that are fundamental to identify high-risk patients who are prone to ventricular arrhythmias. Furthermore, new techniques to detect myocardial edema open the possibility to identify myocardium at risk. While clinical data are currently too limited to advocate use of CT as a primary modality to assess perfusion and viability, in patients already undergoing rest cardiac CT for evaluation of coronary anatomy and function, rest perfusion defects – when present – can be very helpful in identifying areas of infarcted myocardium. Within such areas, levels of attenuation values, in combination with other morphological features such as wall thinning, dilation, and/or wall motion abnormalities, can be helpful in distinguishing between acute and chronic infarcts and suggest whether viable myocardium is present. Current CT research involving SP and delayed enhancement will further define the future role of these developing techniques.

Factors including physician comfort level and experience with different modalities, future research, and published guidelines as well as economic and political factors will ultimately determine how these new techniques get adopted into clinical practice.

REFERENCES

1. Hendel RC, Patel MR, Kramer CM, et al. ACCF/ACR/SCCT/SCMR/ASNC/NASCI/SCAI/SIR 2006 appropriateness criteria for cardiac computed tomography and cardiac magnetic resonance imaging: a report of the American College of Cardiology Foundation Quality Strategic Directions Committee Appropriateness Criteria Working Group, American College of Radiology, Society of Cardiovascular Computed Tomography, Society for Cardiovascular Magnetic Resonance, American Society of Nuclear Cardiology, North American Society for Cardiac Imaging, Society for Cardiovascular Angiography and Interventions, and Society of Interventional Radiology. J Am Coll Cardiol 2006;48(7):1475–97.
2. Barkhausen J, Ruehm SG, Goyen M, Buck T, Laub G, Debatin JF. MR evaluation of ventricular function: true fast imaging with steady-state precession versus fast low-angle shot cine MR imaging: feasibility study. Radiology 2001;219(1):264–9.
3. Simonetti OP, Kim RJ, Fieno DS, et al. An improved MR imaging technique for the visualization of myocardial infarction. Radiology 2001;218(1):215–23.
4. Klocke FJ, Simonetti OP, Judd RM, et al. Limits of detection of regional differences in vasodilated flow in viable myocardium by first-pass magnetic resonance perfusion imaging. Circulation 2001;104(20):2412–6.
5. Lee DC, Simonetti OP, Harris KR, et al. Magnetic resonance versus radionuclide pharmacological stress perfusion imaging for flow-limiting stenoses of varying severity. Circulation 2004;110(1):58–65.
6. Wilke N, Jerosch-Herold M, Wang Y, et al. Myocardial perfusion reserve: assessment with multisection, quantitative, first-pass MR imaging. Radiology 1997;204(2):373–84.
7. Al-Saadi N, Nagel E, Gross M, et al. Noninvasive detection of myocardial ischemia from perfusion reserve based on cardiovascular magnetic resonance. Circulation 2000;101(12):1379–83.
8. Bertschinger KM, Nanz D, Buechi M, et al. Magnetic resonance myocardial first-pass perfusion imaging: parameter optimization for signal response and cardiac coverage. J Magn Reson Imaging 2001;14(5):556 62.
9. Panting JR, Gatehouse PD, Yang GZ, et al. Echo-planar magnetic resonance myocardial perfusion imaging: parametric map analysis and comparison with thallium SPECT. J Magn Reson Imaging 2001;13(2):192–200.
10. Schwitter J, Nanz D, Kneifel S, et al. Assessment of myocardial perfusion in coronary artery disease by magnetic resonance: a comparison with positron emission tomography and coronary angiography. Circulation 2001;103(18):2230–5.
11. Ibrahim T, Nekolla SG, Schreiber K, et al. Assessment of coronary flow reserve: comparison between contrast-enhanced magnetic resonance imaging and positron emission tomography. J Am Coll Cardiol 2002;39(5):864–70.
12. Chiu CW, So NM, Lam WW, Chan KY, Sanderson JE. Combined first-pass perfusion and viability study at MR imaging in patients with non-ST segment-elevation acute coronary syndromes: feasibility study. Radiology 2003;226(3):717–22.
13. Ishida N, Sakuma H, Motoyasu M, et al. Noninfarcted myocardium: correlation between dynamic first-pass contrast-enhanced myocardial MR imaging and quantitative coronary angiography. Radiology 2003;229(1):209–16.

14. Nagel E, Thouet T, Klein C, et al. Noninvasive determination of coronary blood flow velocity with cardiovascular magnetic resonance in patients after stent deployment. Circulation 2003;107(13):1738–43.
15. Giang TH, Nanz D, Coulden R, et al. Detection of coronary artery disease by magnetic resonance myocardial perfusion imaging with various contrast medium doses: first European multi-centre experience. Eur Heart J 2004;25(18):1657–65.
16. Paetsch I, Jahnke C, Wahl A, et al. Comparison of dobutamine stress magnetic resonance, adenosine stress magnetic resonance, and adenosine stress magnetic resonance perfusion. Circulation 2004;110(7):835–42.
17. Plein S, Greenwood JP, Ridgway JP, Cranny G, Ball SG, Sivananthan MU. Assessment of non-ST-segment elevation acute coronary syndromes with cardiac magnetic resonance imaging. J Am Coll Cardiol 2004;44(11):2173–81.
18. Wolff SD, Schwitter J, Coulden R, et al. Myocardial first-pass perfusion magnetic resonance imaging: a multicenter dose-ranging study. Circulation 2004;110(6):732–7.
19. Plein S, Radjenovic A, Ridgway JP, et al. Coronary artery disease: myocardial perfusion MR imaging with sensitivity encoding versus conventional angiography. Radiology 2005;235(2):423–30.
20. Cury RC, Cattani CA, Gabure LA, et al. Diagnostic performance of stress perfusion and delayed-enhancement MR imaging in patients with coronary artery disease. Radiology 2006;240(1):39–45.
21. Klem I, Heitner JF, Shah DJ, et al. Improved detection of coronary artery disease by stress perfusion cardiovascular magnetic resonance with the use of delayed enhancement infarction imaging. J Am Coll Cardiol 2006;47(8):1630–8.
22. Rieber J, Huber A, Erhard I, et al. Cardiac magnetic resonance perfusion imaging for the functional assessment of coronary artery disease: a comparison with coronary angiography and fractional flow reserve. Eur Heart J 2006;27(12):1465–71.
23. Cheng AS, Pegg TJ, Karamitsos TD, et al. Cardiovascular magnetic resonance perfusion imaging at 3-tesla for the detection of coronary artery disease: a comparison with 1.5-tesla. J Am Coll Cardiol 2007;49(25):2440–9.
24. Nandalur KR, Dwamena BA, Choudhri AF, Nandalur MR, Carlos RC. Diagnostic performance of stress cardiac magnetic resonance imaging in the detection of coronary artery disease: a meta-analysis. J Am Coll Cardiol 2007;50(14):1343–53.
25. Ingkanisorn WP, Kwong RY, Bohme NS, et al. Prognosis of negative adenosine stress magnetic resonance in patients presenting to an emergency department with chest pain. J Am Coll Cardiol 2006;47(7):1427–32.
26. Amado LC, Gerber BL, Gupta SN, et al. Accurate and objective infarct sizing by contrast-enhanced magnetic resonance imaging in a canine myocardial infarction model. J Am Coll Cardiol 2004;44(12):2383–9.
27. Baks T, van Geuns RJ, Biagini E, et al. Effects of primary angioplasty for acute myocardial infarction on early and late infarct size and left ventricular wall characteristics. J Am Coll Cardiol 2006;47(1):40–4.
28. Ibrahim T, Bulow HP, Hackl T, et al. Diagnostic value of contrast-enhanced magnetic resonance imaging and single-photon emission computed tomography for detection of myocardial necrosis early after acute myocardial infarction. J Am Coll Cardiol 2007;49(2):208–16.
29. Kim RJ, Chen EL, Lima JA, Judd RM. Myocardial Gd-DTPA kinetics determine MRI contrast enhancement and reflect the extent and severity of myocardial injury after acute reperfused infarction. Circulation 1996;94(12):3318–26.
30. Mahrholdt H, Wagner A, Holly TA, et al. Reproducibility of chronic infarct size measurement by contrast-enhanced magnetic resonance imaging. Circulation 2002;106(18):2322–7.
31. Wagner A, Mahrholdt H, Thomson L, et al. Effects of time, dose, and inversion time for acute myocardial infarct size measurements based on magnetic resonance imaging-delayed contrast enhancement. J Am Coll Cardiol 2006;47(10):2027–33.
32. Yang Z, Berr SS, Gilson WD, Toufektsian MC, French BA. Simultaneous evaluation of infarct size and cardiac function in intact mice by contrast-enhanced cardiac magnetic resonance imaging reveals contractile dysfunction in noninfarcted regions early after myocardial infarction. Circulation 2004;109(9):1161–7.
33. Hombach V, Grebe O, Merkle N, et al. Sequelae of acute myocardial infarction regarding cardiac structure and function and their prognostic significance as assessed by magnetic resonance imaging. Eur Heart J 2005;26(6):549–57.
34. Gerber BL, Rochitte CE, Melin JA, et al. Microvascular obstruction and left ventricular remodeling early after acute myocardial infarction. Circulation 2000;101(23):2734–41.
35. Wu KC, Zerhouni EA, Judd RM, et al. Prognostic significance of microvascular obstruction by magnetic resonance imaging in patients with acute myocardial infarction. Circulation 1998;97(8):765–72.
36. Aletras AH, Tilak GS, Natanzon A, et al. Retrospective determination of the area at risk for reperfused acute myocardial infarction with T2-weighted cardiac magnetic resonance imaging: histopathological and displacement encoding with stimulated echoes (DENSE) functional validations. Circulation 2006;113(15):1865–70.
37. Cury RC NJ, Shash K, et al. Comprehensive cardiac magnetic resonance imaging protocol in the emergency department: T2W imaging improves diagnostic accuracy for detection of patients with acute coronary syndrome. Circulation 2006; 114(18:II):542.
38. Schmidt A, Azevedo CF, Cheng A, et al. Infarct tissue heterogeneity by magnetic resonance imaging identifies enhanced cardiac arrhythmia susceptibility in patients with left ventricular dysfunction. Circulation 2007;115(15):2006–14.
39. Yan AT, Shayne AJ, Brown KA, et al. Characterization of the peri-infarct zone by contrast-enhanced cardiac magnetic resonance imaging is a powerful predictor of post-myocardial infarction mortality. Circulation 2006;114(1):32–9.
40. Fieno DS, Kim RJ, Chen EL, Lomasney JW, Klocke FJ, Judd RM. Contrast-enhanced magnetic resonance imaging of myocardium at risk: distinction between reversible and irreversible injury throughout infarct healing. J Am Coll Cardiol 2000;36(6):1985–91.
41. Wu E, Judd RM, Vargas JD, Klocke FJ, Bonow RO, Kim RJ. Visualisation of presence, location, and transmural extent of healed Q-wave and non-Q-wave myocardial infarction. Lancet 2001;357(9249):21–8.

42. Kim RJ, Fieno DS, Parrish TB, et al. Relationship of MRI delayed contrast enhancement to irreversible injury, infarct age, and contractile function. Circulation 1999;100(19):1992–2002.
43. Kim RJ, Wu E, Rafael A, et al. The use of contrast-enhanced magnetic resonance imaging to identify reversible myocardial dysfunction. N Engl J Med 2000;343(20):1445–53.
44. Miller J RC, Dewey M, et al. Coronary artery evaluation using 64-row multidetector computed tomography angiography (CORE-64): results of a multicenter, international trial to assess diagnostic accuracy compared with conventional coronary angiography. #PS-03. Presented at American Heart Association 30th Annual Scientific Sessions, Orlando, Nov 3–7, 2007.
45. Schuijf JD, Wijns W, Jukema JW, et al. Relationship between noninvasive coronary angiography with multi-slice computed tomography and myocardial perfusion imaging. J Am Coll Cardiol 2006;48(12):2508–14.
46. Hacker M, Jakobs T, Matthiesen F, et al. Comparison of spiral multidetector CT angiography and myocardial perfusion imaging in the noninvasive detection of functionally relevant coronary artery lesions: first clinical experiences. J Nucl Med 2005;46(8):1294–300.
47. Berman DS, Hachamovitch R. Risk assessment in patients with stable coronary artery disease: incremental value of nuclear imaging. J Nucl Cardiol 1996;3(6 Pt 2):S41–9.
48. Hachamovitch R, Berman DS, Shaw LJ, et al. Incremental prognostic value of myocardial perfusion single photon emission computed tomography for the prediction of cardiac death: differential stratification for risk of cardiac death and myocardial infarction. Circulation 1998;97(6):535–43.
49. Hachamovitch R, Hayes SW, Friedman JD, Cohen I, Berman DS. A prognostic score for prediction of cardiac mortality risk after adenosine stress myocardial perfusion scintigraphy. J Am Coll Cardiol 2005;45(5):722–9.
50. Lee VS, Resnick D, Tiu SS, et al. MR imaging evaluation of myocardial viability in the setting of equivocal SPECT results with (99m)Tc sestamibi. Radiology 2004;230(1):191–7.
51. Patel RA, Beller GA. Prognostic role of single-photon emission computed tomography (SPECT) imaging in myocardial viability. Curr Opin Cardiol 2006;21(5):457–63.
52. GE unveils clinician-driven future of CT; HD technologies. (Accessed 1/13/2008, at http://www.genewscenter.com/content/Detail.asp?ReleaseID=2846&NewsAreaID=2.)
53. Higgins CB, Sovak M, Schmidt W, Siemers PT. Uptake of contrast materials by experimental acute myocardial infarctions: a preliminary report. Invest Radiol 1978;13(4):337–9.
54. Higgins CB, Sovak M, Schmidt W, Siemers PT. Differential accumulation of radiopaque contrast material in acute myocardial infarction. Am J Cardiol 1979;43(1):47–51.
55. Hoffmann U, Millea R, Enzweiler C, et al. Acute myocardial infarction: contrast-enhanced multi-detector row CT in a porcine model. Radiology 2004;231(3):697–701.
56. Mahnken AH, Bruners P, Katoh M, Wildberger JE, Gunther RW, Buecker A. Dynamic multi-section CT imaging in acute myocardial infarction: preliminary animal experience. Eur Radiol 2006;16(3):746–52.
57. Lardo AC, Cordeiro MA, Silva C, et al. Contrast-enhanced multidetector computed tomography viability imaging after myocardial infarction: characterization of myocyte death, microvascular obstruction, and chronic scar. Circulation 2006;113(3):394–404.
58. Nikolaou K, Sanz J, Poon M, et al. Assessment of myocardial perfusion and viability from routine contrast-enhanced 16-detector-row computed tomography of the heart: preliminary results. Eur Radiol 2005;15(5):864–71.
59. Nieman K, Cury RC, Ferencik M, et al. Differentiation of recent and chronic myocardial infarction by cardiac computed tomography. Am J Cardiol 2006;98(3):303–8.
60. Zipes DP, Braunwald E. Braunwald's heart disease: a textbook of cardiovascular medicine, 7th edn. Philadelphia, Pa: Elsevier Saunders, 2005.
61. Gerber BL, Belge B, Legros GJ, et al. Characterization of acute and chronic myocardial infarcts by multidetector computed tomography: comparison with contrast-enhanced magnetic resonance. Circulation 2006;113(6):823–33.
62. Mahnken AH, Koos R, Katoh M, et al. Assessment of myocardial viability in reperfused acute myocardial infarction using 16-slice computed tomography in comparison to magnetic resonance imaging. J Am Coll Cardiol 2005;45(12):2042–7.
63. Habis M, Capderou A, Ghostine S, et al. Acute myocardial infarction early viability assessment by 64-slice computed tomography immediately after coronary angiography: comparison with low-dose dobutamine echocardiography. J Am Coll Cardiol 2007; 49(11):1178–85.
64. George RT, Silva C, Cordeiro MA, et al. Multidetector computed tomography myocardial perfusion imaging during adenosine stress. J Am Coll Cardiol 2006;48(1):153–60.
65. George RT, Yousuf O, Kitagawa K, et al. Abstract 2547: quantification of myocardial perfusion in patients using 256-row multidetector computed tomography: evaluation of endocardial vs. epicardial blood flow. Circulation 2007;116(16_Meeting Abstracts):II_563.
66. Mahnken AH, Bruners P, Muhlenbruch G, et al. Low tube voltage improves computed tomography imaging of delayed myocardial contrast enhancement in an experimental acute myocardial infarction model. Invest Radiol 2007;42(2):123–9.
67. Husmann L, Valenta I, Gaemperli O, et al. Feasibility of low-dose coronary CT angiography: first experience with prospective ECG-gating. Eur Heart J 2008;29:191–7.
68. Tsai IC, Lee T, Tsai WL, et al. Contrast enhancement in cardiac MDCT: comparison of iodixanol 320 versus iohexol 350. AJR 2008;190(1):W47–53.
69. Baks T, Cademartiri F, Moelker AD, et al. Multislice computed tomography and magnetic resonance imaging for the assessment of reperfused acute myocardial infarction. J Am Coll Cardiol 2006;48(1):144–52.

70. Nahrendorf M, Badea C, Hedlund LW, et al. High-resolution imaging of murine myocardial infarction with delayed-enhancement cine micro-CT. Am J Physiol 2007;292(6):H3172–8.
71. Lessick J, Dragu R, Mutlak D, et al. Is functional improvement after myocardial infarction predicted with myocardial enhancement patterns at multidetector CT? Radiology 2007;244(3):736–44.
72. George RT SK, Bluemke DA, et al. Prospectively ECG-gated multidetector computed tomography viability imaging accurately quantifies infarct size while lowering the radiation dose by an order of magnitude. Circulation. 2006;114(suppl II):818.
73. George RT, Jerosch-Herold M, Silva C, et al. Quantification of myocardial perfusion using dynamic 64-detector computed tomography. Invest Radiol 2007;42(12):815–22.

V

Invasive (Intravascular) Risk Stratification for Detection of Vulnerable (High-Risk) Asymptomatic Atherosclerotic Plaques

33 Angiography for Detection of Complex and Vulnerable Atherosclerotic Plaque

James A. Goldstein

CONTENTS

ABSTRACT

Selective coronary angiography is the "gold standard" for detection of atherosclerosis and quantitation of the magnitude of obstructive disease. Unfortunately, angiography has intrinsic limitations in that it provides a two-dimensional "lumenogram" that at best delineates the effects of plaque in the vessel wall that encroaches on the lumen. While these images delineate the gross presence of disease and can quantify percent stenosis, angiography consistently underestimates the magnitude of atherosclerotic burden. Angiography is very accurate in the detection of complex unstable plaques in patients with acute coronary syndromes. Unfortunately, it has substantial limitations in delineating whether a noncomplex lesion is stable, vulnerable, or in transition to complex-unstable pathology. Furthermore, angiography is also limited in that this data can only be obtained as a "snapshot" in time in the tiny fraction of athersosclerotic patients who end up in the catheterization laboratory. This chapter elucidates the clinical data regarding the following: (1) strengths and limits of angiography for quantification of coronary plaque, (2) angiographic patterns of complex unstable plaque, (3) evidence of pancoronary inflammation and its relationship to multifocal plaque instability, (4) natural history of angiographically complex lesions, and (5) limitations of angiography in detection of unstable and vulnerable plaques.

Key words: Angiography; Vulnerable plaque; Complex plaque

From: *Asymptomatic Atherosclerosis: Pathophysiology, Detection and Treatment*
Edited by: M. Naghavi (ed.), DOI 10.1007/978-1-60327-179-0_33

OVERVIEW

This chapter discusses the strengths and limitations of angiography in detecting vulnerable and complex coronary plaques. Selective coronary angiography is the "gold standard" for detection of atherosclerosis and quantitation of the magnitude of obstructive disease. Unfortunately, angiography has intrinsic limitations in that it provides a two-dimensional "lumenogram" that at best delineates the effects of plaque in the vessel wall that encroaches on the lumen. While these images delineate the gross presence of disease and can quantify percent stenosis, angiography consistently underestimates the magnitude of atherosclerotic burden, particularly in earlier stage disease in which positive vascular remodeling may allow "normal" lumen caliber despite substantial vascular wall plaque. Angiography is very accurate in the detection of complex unstable plaques in patients with acute coronary syndromes. Unfortunately, it has substantial limitations in delineating whether a noncomplex lesion is stable, vulnerable, or in transition to complex-unstable pathology. Furthermore, angiography is also limited in that this data can only be obtained as a "snapshot" in time in the tiny fraction of athersosclerotic patients who end up in the catheterization laboratory.

ANGIOGRAPHIC PATTERNS OF PLAQUE INSTABILITY: THE COMPLEX PLAQUE

Acute coronary syndromes result from rupture of an inflamed plaque with superimposed thrombus formation. Complex coronary plaque morphology (fissuring, ulceration, haziness, and filling defect) is the angiographic hallmark of unstable coronary syndromes and correlates with pathological plaque rupture and thrombus [1–9]. Traditionally, the acute coronary syndromes have been considered as distinct entities, the conditions of ST elevation myocardial infarction, nontransmural infarction, and unstable angina differentiated primarily on the basis of electrocardiographic manifestations and myocardial enzyme elevations, rather than coronary anatomy and left ventricular function. It is important to ask the question whether these syndromes represent distinct entities or overlapping conditions. All three conditions share common pathophysiology, characterized by acute coronary insufficiency typically attributable to coronary plaque disruption with superimposed thrombus that may range from superficially adherent to occlusive. Angiographic studies document that the vast majority of all patients with acute coronary syndromes harbor a complex culprit lesion. Patients with ST-elevation transmural injury characteristically manifest a complex plaque with superimposed thrombus leading to total or subtotal occlusion and compromised flow. In contrast, whereas those with nontransmural infarcts and unstable angina similarly have complex unstable culprit lesions, the presence of angiographic thrombus is variable and antegrade flow is often intact, at least in part. These disparate presentations and angiographic patterns are explained in part by the fact that plaque rupture induces a dynamic process of clot formation and dissolution that may evolve over minutes or days, a time frame in which resting coronary flow may be intermittently or persistently compromised. Plaque rupture does not inevitably lead to myocardial infarction, with the clinical expression in an individual patient a function of the interplay between the severity of atheromatous plaque stenosis, magnitude of superimposed thrombus, degree of local coronary vasoconstriction, development of distal plaque-clot embolization, and extent of collateral flow. Plaque erosions and ruptures commonly occur in previously nonflow limiting lesions and, if minimal superimposed thrombus is generated, may not compromise resting coronary flow sufficiently to induce ischemia; such erosions are initially clinically silent, but do appear to accelerate plaque growth. On the catastrophic end of the spectrum, plaque rupture results in abrupt thrombotic occlusion, and unless there are extensive pre-existing collaterals, acute transmural ischemia manifest as ST elevation MI and/or sudden death; at angiography, such patients manifest thrombotically occluded vessels. Unstable angina and nontransmural infarction constitute intermediate steps in the clinical spectrum of plaque rupture, with both conditions representing acute compromise of coronary blood flow sufficient to provoke unstable symptoms, often with ischemic ECG changes. At angiography, these conditions overlap with both conditions sharing in common complex culprit plaques, but differentiated clinically on the basis of biochemical evidence of myocyte necrosis, a function of the interplay of multiple factors including severity of flow compromise, collaterals, duration of ischemia, distal microembolization, and myocardial oxygen demand.

In some patients with acute coronary syndromes, angiography fails to identify a complex culprit lesion, likely attributable at least in part to the inherent imaging resolution limitations of angiography. It is also recognized that performance of angiography 3–7 days after the acute event likely further contributes to an underestimation of the prevalence of complex unstable plaques, as the effects of aspirin and heparin together with the "tincture of time" may allow some complex plaques to heal sufficiently, such that they appeared angiographically "benign." This healing effect of time is seen in patients with ST elevation myocardial infarction, in whom angiography performed acutely identifies a culprit occlusion in nearly all cases, whereas patients studied later may have a greater frequency of patent although diseased arteries.

MULTIFOCAL PLAQUE INSTABILITY

A significant proportion of patients with acute coronary syndromes harbor multiple complex coronary plaques, the presence of which is associated with angiographic progression and adverse clinical outcome [10–17]. The clinical importance of multifocal plaque instability was first documented in a study of patients with acute transmural myocardial infarction, with nearly 40% manifesting angiographic evidence of multiple complex coronary plaques [10]. Compared to those with single complex plaques, patients with multiple unstable lesions had a less favorable in-hospital course as they more frequently required early coronary artery bypass surgery or staged multivessel percutaneous interventions, and had greater depression of left ventricular function. The presence of multiple complex plaques was also independently predictive of future adverse clinical events over 1 year, including an increased incidence of recurrent angina and acute coronary syndromes, higher rates of repeat percutaneous revascularization not only in the initial culprit vessel but also in noninfarct-related lesions previously documented as complex, and greater likelihood of requiring coronary artery bypass surgery.

A review of pathological, angiographic, angioscopic, and intravascular ultrasound studies now document that multifocal plaque instability is common in patients with acute coronary syndromes [8, 10–15]. Multifocal plaque ruptures and multiple coronary thrombi are evident in autopsy studies of fatal acute ischemic heart disease. In fact, extensive multifocal coronary ulceration and multicentric clot formation may be the rule rather than the exception [8]. Multifocal plaque instability is also evident in prior angiographic studies of patients with unstable angina, with one study documenting an average of 2.6 complex lesions per patient [15]. Similar findings are evident patients with nontransmural infarction [16, 17]. Recent angioscopic and intravascular ultrasound observations [12–14] in patients with acute coronary syndromes not only provide morphological confirmation of multiple unstable plaques but also emphasize the many subtler plaque ruptures that are not yet angiographically complex and thus beneath the angiographic "radar screen."

These observations support the concept that plaque instability is not merely a local vascular accident, but likely reflects more systemic pathophysiological processes with potential to destabilize atherosclerotic plaques throughout the coronary tree. Until recently, plaque rupture was thought to reflect local plaque instability attributable to spontaneous or triggered disruption of a lone vulnerable plaque, manifest angiographically or pathologically as a solitary complex unstable lesion. However, the pathophysiological factors proposed to precipitate plaque instability, whether due to primary weakening of the fibrous cap attributable to inflammation [18, 19] or the extrinsic influences of intraluminal mechanical forces modulated by sympathic tone and catecholamines, would be expected to exert their effects in a widespread pattern throughout the coronary vasculature. Given the potential "pancoronary" impact of these factors adversely influencing plaques, together with the typically diffuse nature of coronary atherosclerosis, it would not be unexpected that plaque instability might develop in a multifocal pattern, resulting in multiple anatomically remote complex unstable plaques, one of which may progress to total occlusion and emerge as the culprit infarct related lesion.

NATURAL HISTORY OF ANGIOGRAPHICALLY COMPLEX LESIONS

Stenosis progression and clinical instability are characteristics of complex lesions [10, 20–27].

Studies in patients with acute myocardial infarction have demonstrated striking rapid multifocal progression of both infarct related and nonculprit complex lesions over 1 month [10]. The presence of multiple complex plaques was also independently predictive of future adverse clinical events over 1 year, including an increased incidence of recurrent angina and acute coronary syndromes, higher rates of repeat percutaneous revascularization not only in the initial culprit vessel but also in noninfarct-related lesions previously documented as complex, and greater likelihood of requiring coronary artery bypass surgery. Angiographic natural history studies in patients with unstable angina document that complex lesions are at great risk for worsening stenoses, recurrent unstable ischemia and death [20–24]. The prognosis is particularly foreboding in patients with multiple unstable plaques, in whom rapid progression of culprit and nonculprit complex lesions is common. These findings emphasize that the angiographic documentation of multiple unstable plaques identifies a subset of patients particularly predisposed to rapid plaque progression associated with greater risk for recurrent ischemia, findings that may influence revascularization strategies.

LIMITATIONS OF ANGIOGRAPHY IN DETECTION OF UNSTABLE AND VULNERABLE PLAQUES

Although a crucial tool for assessment of patients with coronary artery disease, angiography is well known to underestimate the presence and severity of coronary artery disease in general and has significant limitations in the precise delineation of plaque architecture and biology. It is important to emphasize the qualitative nature of angiographic evaluation, for complexity may be in the "eye of the beholder." Although complex morphology by angiography correlates closely with plaque instability pathologically and complex plaques are associated with angiographic progression and clinical instability, some complex plaques may remain stable over time [28]. Furthermore, complex lesion morphology may in some cases reflect more chronic occlusions. Therefore, angiographic complexity does not by itself necessarily determine plaque destiny.

Angiography is an insensitive tool that is only able to detect those plaques that have relatively gross plaque disruption. Observations from intravascular ultrasound, angioscopic and pathological studies clearly document that the majority of ulcerated plaques are not sufficiently disrupted anatomically to be detected angiographically. Furthermore, it is certain that patients with unstable (and silent) coronary artery disease harbor lipid-rich inflamed "vulnerable" plaques that have not yet ulcerated and ruptured. Angiography fails to detect the many plaques with subtler but pathologically manifest ulceration and rupture, reflecting only a subset of those coronary lesions that are truly unstable and revealing virtually no insight regarding the many vulnerable but not yet ruptured plaques that serve as the substrate for subsequent coronary events. Therefore, angiographic confirmation of complex plaque undoubtedly represents only the "Tip of the Iceberg" of plaque instability [29]. Clearly, there is a need for invasive and noninvasive techniques that are sufficiently sensitive and accurate to detect lipid-rich plaques with thin inflamed fibrous caps that represent vulnerable but not yet ruptured plaques.

REFERENCES

1. Falk E. Plaque rupture with severe pre-existing stenosis precipitating coronary thrombosis. Characteristics of coronary atherosclerotic plaques underlying fatal occlusive thrombi. Br Heart J 1983;50:127–134.
2. Davies MJ, Thomas A. Thrombosis and acute coronary artery lesions in sudden cardiac ischemic death. N Engl J Med 1984;310:1137–1140.
3. Levin DC, Fallon JT. Significance of the angiographic morphology of localized coronary stenoses: Histopathologic correlations. Circulation 1982;66:316–320.
4. Ambrose JA, Winters SL, Stern A, et al. Angiographic morphology and the pathogenesis of unstable angina pectoris. J Am Coll Cardiol 1985;5:609–616.
5. Falk E. Unstable angina with fatal outcome: Dynamic coronary thrombosis leading to infarction and/or sudden death. Circulation 1985;71(4):699–708.
6. Rehr R, Disciascio G, Vetrovec G, Cowley M. Angiographic morphology of coronary artery stenoses in prolonged rest angina: Evidence of intracoronary thrombosis. J Am Coll Cardiol 1989;14:1429–1437.
7. Warnes CA, Roberts WC. Sudden coronary death: Relation of amount and distribution of coronary narrowing at necropsy to previous symptoms of myocardial ischemia, left ventricular scarring and heart weight. Am J Cardiol 1984;54:65–73.
8. Frink RJ. Chronic ulcerated plaques: New insights into the pathogenesis of acute coronary disease. J Invasive Cardiol 1994;6:173–185.
9. DeWood MA, Spores J, Notske R, et al. Prevalence of total coronary occlusion during the early hours of transmural myocardial infarction. N Engl J Med 1980;303:897–902.
10. Goldstein JA, Demetriou D, Grines CL, et al. Multiple complex coronary plaques in patients with acute myocardial infarction. N Engl J Med 2000;343:915–922.
11. Guazzi MD, Bussotti M, Grancini L, et al. Evidence of multifocal activity of coronary disease in patients with acute myocardial infarction. Circulation 1997;96:1145–1151.
12. Asakura M, Ueda Y, Yamaguchi O, et al. Extensive development of vulnerable plaques as a pan-coronary process in patients with myocardial infarction: An angioscopic study. J Am Coll Cardiol 2001;37:1284–1288.
13. Maehara A, Mintz G, Bui A, et al. Morphologic and angiographic features of coronary plaque rupture detected by intravascular ultrasound. J Am Coll Cardiol 2002;40:904–910.
14. Rioful G, Finet G, Ginon I, et al. Multiple atherosclerotic plaque rupture in acute coronary syndrome: A three-vessel intravascular ultrasound study. Circulation 2002;106:804–808.
15. Garcia-Moll X, Coccolo F, Cole D, et al. Serum neopterin and complex stenosis morphology in patients with unstable angina. J Am Coll Cardiol 2000;35:956–962.
16. DeWood MA, Stifter WF, Simpson CS, et al. Coronary arteriographic findings soon after non-Q-wave myocardial infarction. N Engl J Med 1986;315:417–423.
17. Kerensky RA, Wade M, Deedwania P, et al. Non-Q-Wave infarction strategies in-hospital (VANQWISH) trial investigators. J Am Coll Cardiol 2002;39:1456–1463.
18. Van der Wal AC, Becker AE, Van der Loos CM, et al. Site of intimal rupture or erosion of thrombosed coronary atherosclerotic plaques is characterized by an inflammatory process irrespective of the dominant plaque morphology. Circulation 1994;89:36–44.
19. Moreno PR, Falk E, Palacios IF, Newell JB, et al. Macrophage infiltration in acute coronary syndromes. Implications for plaque rupture. Circulation 1994;90:775–778.
20. Theroux P. Angiographic and clinical progression in unstable angina. Circulation 1995;91:2295–2298.
21. Moise A, Theroux P, Taeymans Y, et al. Unstable angina and progression of coronary atherosclerosis. N Engl J Med 1983;309:685–689.
22. Chen L, Chester MR, Redwood S, et al. Angiographic stenosis progression and coronary events in patients with 'stabilized' unstable angina. Circulation 1995;91:2319–2324.
23. Chester MR, Chen L, Kaski JC. The natural history of unheralded complex coronary plaques. J Am Coll Cardiol 1996; 28:604–608.
24. Chen L, Chester MR, Crook R, et al. Differential progression of complex culprit stenoses in patients with stable and unstable angina pectoris. J Am Coll Cardiol 1996;28:597–603.
25. Ambrose JA. Prognostic implications of lesion irregularity on coronary angiography. J Am Coll Cardiol 1991;18:675–676.
26. Freeman MR, Williams AE, Chisholm RJ, et al. Intracoronary thrombus and complex morphology in unstable angina. Relation to timing of angiography and in-hospital cardiac events. Circulation 1989;80:17–23.
27. Davies SW, Marchant B, Lyons JP, et al. Irregular coronary lesion morphology after thrombolysis predicts early clinical instability. J Am Coll Cardiol 1991;18:669–674.
28. Haft JI, Al-Zarka AM. The origin and fate of complex coronary lesions. Am Heart J 1991;121:1050.
29. Goldstein J. Angiographic plaque complexity: The tip of the unstable plaque iceberg. J Am Coll Cardiol 2002;39:1456–1463.

34 Intravascular Characterization of Vulnerable Coronary Plaque

James A. Goldstein and James E. Muller

CONTENTS

ABSTRACT

Acute coronary syndromes result from rupture of macrophage-rich, inflamed thin-capped fibroatheroma with superimposed thrombus formation. Ruptured plaques are felt to arise from precursor "vulnerable" lesions that are presumed to be at high risk of disruption. Observations now document that many patients with ACS harbor multiple complex unstable plaques, supporting the concept that plaque instability is not merely a local vascular accident, but instead reflects more systemic pathophysiologic processes. The recognition of the ubiquity of substantial but nonflow limiting lesions that may serve as the fodder for subsequent plaque rupture has resulted in a paradigm shift in thinking about the pathophysiology of coronary artery disease, with the focus no longer solely on the degree of arterial luminal narrowing. This chapter will review: (1) Definitions of vulnerable plaque; (2) Limitations of conventional angiography for detection of vulnerable plaque; (3) Nonangiographic invasive methods to image vulnerable plaques; (4) Invasive technologies to characterize plaque including IVUS, angioscopy, NIR spectroscopy, optical coherence tomography (OCT), catheter-based MRI and thermography.

Key words: Ruptured plaque; Vulnerable plaque; IVUS; Near-infrared spectroscopy

"PEARLS"

- Unstable coronary artery plaques are not simply local phenomena but reflect widespread cardiovascular pathophysiology.

From: *Asymptomatic Atherosclerosis: Pathophysiology, Detection and Treatment*
Edited by: M. Naghavi (ed.), DOI 10.1007/978-1-60327-179-0_34

- The focus is now on the nature of the plaque and the role of inflammation in addition to the extent of arterial narrowing.
- New tools to identify and characterize coronary artery plaques promise to transform their intravascular treatment.
- Lesion-specific data can now be obtained using a variety of imaging modalities, including IVUS, OCT, NIRS, and MRI.

Most acute coronary syndromes (ACS) result from rupture of macrophage-rich, inflamed, thin-capped fibroatheromas (TCFAs) leading to superimposed thrombus formation [1–3]. The resulting focal coronary obstructions limit blood flow and are the targets of revascularization procedures to relieve myocardial ischemia [4]. Since the atherosclerotic process is widespread, many patients with coronary artery disease harbor multiple complex precursor lesions, putting them at high risk for sudden plaque disruption and consequent ACS [5–7]. This finding supports the concept that plaque instability is not merely a local vascular phenomenon but rather reflects potentially destabilizing pathophysiologic processes occurring throughout the cardiovascular system [5,8].

Pancoronary plaque inflammation probably accounts, at least in part, for the clinical instability that lasts for weeks to months after the index event resolves in patients with ACS. Such patients typically have additional foci of vulnerable or frankly complex plaques that are prone to rupture, providing substrates for subsequent coronary events. Recognition that these ubiquitous nonflow-limiting yet substantially dangerous lesions may lead to life-threatening plaque rupture has led to a paradigm shift in our understanding of the pathophysiology of coronary artery disease – i.e., the focus is no longer solely on the degree of arterial luminal narrowing but now includes both the nature of the plaques that are present and the role of inflammation [5,8–11].

WHAT IS A VULNERABLE PLAQUE?

Disruption of a coronary plaque seems to depend on the interplay between intrinsic factors that influence lesion vulnerability (e.g., presence of a lipid core, a thin fibrous cap) and extrinsic forces that may destabilize the plaque and precipitate rupture (e.g., presence of proteases, high shear stress) [3,5,6,8–11] Although prospective evidence from natural history studies is lacking, retrospective autopsy studies suggest that plaques of certain histologic types may be more prone to rupture. The most common "precursor" lesion is believed to be the inflamed, thin-capped fibroatheroma (TCFA) (Fig. 1), thought to account for 60–70% of coronary events [11–14]; another 30–40% may be attributed to plaque erosion, especially in younger women [15].

TCFAs are focal structures. If, as suspected, they represent precursors of culprit lesions, risk for a coronary event depends on local conditions. In their study of patients with sudden cardiac death, Kolodgie et al. [16] found that the incidence of TCFAs was only 1.3 ± 1.4 per heart even though less advanced – and presumably lower-risk – atherosclerotic lesions were widespread. Moreover, an autopsy study by Cheruvu et al. [17] showed that the distribution of TCFAs was limited and focal, typically in the proximal third of the coronary vessels.

Most of the devices being developed to detect vulnerable plaques are designed to identify TCFAs. However, because these devices are unable to detect sites of erosion, their sensitivity for predicting cardiac events is limited. The specificity of a TCFA detector for predicting plaque rupture is also limited because not all these lesions will rupture nor will all ruptures lead to a cardiac event. In this review, we describe and evaluate the various invasive tools that are available or under development for coronary plaque detection and characterization. Ultimately, however, the clinician needs to know whether the features identified indicate a greater likelihood of plaque rupture and a subsequent coronary event.

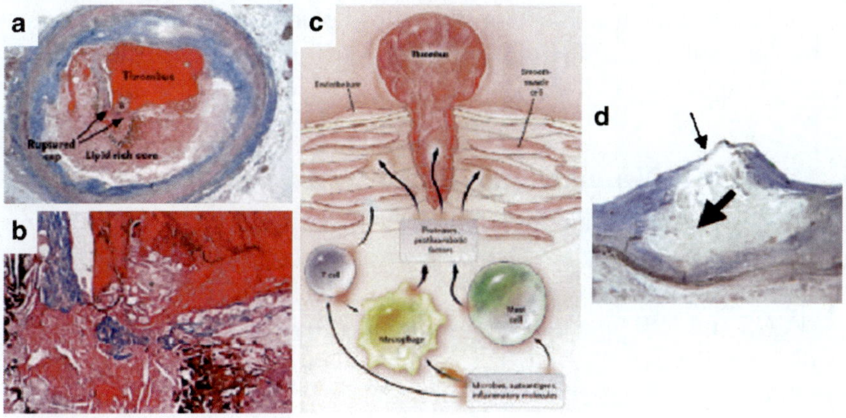

Fig. 1. Culprit and suspected vulnerable atherosclerotic lesions. (**a**) Cross-section of coronary artery after fatal infarction. An occlusive thrombus overlies a ruptured thin-capped fibroatheroma (TCFA). (**b**) High-power magnification of Panel A. The erupted contents of the atheromatous plaque have led to thrombosis. (Courtesy of Dr. Erling Falk.) (**c**) Molecular and cellular inflammatory processes contributing to TCFA formation and rupture. T lymphocytes, macrophages, and mast cells all contribute to the inflammatory reaction associated with accumulation of oxidized LDL and microvascular hemorrhage. Proteases may weaken the cap, leading to rupture and thrombosis. (Modified from Hansson [11], with permission from the Massachusetts Medical Society. Copyright 2005.) (**d**) TCFA detected in longitudinal section of human coronary artery autopsy specimen. A thin fibrous cap (*small arrow*) covers a relatively large lipid pool and necrotic core (*large arrow*) (Courtesy of InfraReDx, Inc.).

TOOLS FOR PLAQUE DETECTION AND CHARACTERIZATION

The ideal invasive tool for characterizing coronary plaques would provide a roadmap of the total atherosclerotic burden throughout the coronary tree as well as lesion-specific data regarding the architecture, composition, physiology, and dynamic biologic properties of each individual plaque. Specific features of interest should include (1) extent of luminal stenosis; (2) lesion length; (3) coronary blood flow reserve through any given stenosis; (4) intramural plaque architecture, including atheroma burden, eccentricity, and local vascular remodeling; (5) plaque composition, specifically lipid content; (6) fibrous cap thickness; and (7) presence of inflammation.

Conventional Coronary Angiography

Selective coronary angiography provides a "lumenogram" delineating the effects of an arterial wall plaque that encroaches on the vessel lumen. Although this imaging technique can detect gross disease and quantify the degree of stenosis, it is an insensitive tool in that it consistently underestimates the magnitude of atherosclerotic burden. This is true, particularly in the early stages of the disease, when positive vascular remodeling may demonstrate a "normal" lumen caliber despite the presence of substantial plaque. The limitations of angiography are significant in that it cannot precisely delineate plaque architecture and provides little or no information regarding a plaque's composition or biologic activity [9].

Patients with unstable (and silent) coronary artery disease are known to harbor lipid-rich, inflamed vulnerable plaques that have not yet ulcerated and ruptured. Yet angiography fails to detect such plaques, which are the precursors of subsequent coronary events. In addition, studies using intravascular ultrasound (IVUS), angioscopy, and histopathology clearly indicate that many ulcerated plaques are not sufficiently disrupted anatomically to be detected by angiography.

Because angiographic assessment can detect only gross plaque ruptures, it reveals only a subset of coronary lesions that are truly unstable [9]. Clearly, imaging techniques sufficiently sensitive to detect vulnerable but intact lesions are needed.

Nonangiographic Invasive Methods

Invasive technologies other than angiography are now being used to characterize plaques. These include IVUS, angioscopy, near-infrared (NIR) spectroscopy, optical coherence tomography (OCT), thermography, and catheter-based magnetic resonance imaging (MRI) [18]. The most versatile of these techniques (IVUS and NIR spectroscopy) can obtain images through intervening blood and can scan the interior of the artery rapidly, whereas other modalities require the absence of arterial blood and/or can interrogate only a specific location (i.e., OCT).

Intravascular Ultrasound (IVUS)

IVUS provides images of the arterial wall and delineates the effects of any existing lesions, such as luminal narrowing and vessel remodeling [19,20]. Clinically, this imaging technique is used to quantify the degree of stenosis and the extent of lesion calcification as well as to assist in optimal stent deployment. On IVUS, unstable plaques typically appear bulky, eccentric, and positively remodeled [21,22]. IVUS can identify many features of complex unstable plaques, such as the presence of ulceration, intimal flaps, and thrombus.

Also, IVUS has shown that culprit lesions are associated with more expansive remodeling in patients with ACS than in those with stable angina, suggesting that such changes might be associated with plaque vulnerability [23,24]. Histologic findings support this linkage because sites with expansive remodeling have plaques with larger lipid cores and more macrophages than do sites with constrictive remodeling [25]. Hence, expansive remodeling, once thought to be beneficial because it reduced luminal narrowing, could indicate a predisposition to plaque rupture [26,27]. Overall, features visualized on IVUS correlate with plaque complexity as determined by angiography and at necropsy (Fig. 2).

IVUS is currently being investigated as a means of identifying vulnerable plaques [28]. TCFAs, which are believed to represent vulnerable but still intact plaques, tend to exhibit a multifocal pattern in patients with ACS compared with stable patients. In contrast, plaque rupture is less commonly seen in those with stable angina. By definition, a ruptured plaque would be considered "vulnerable"

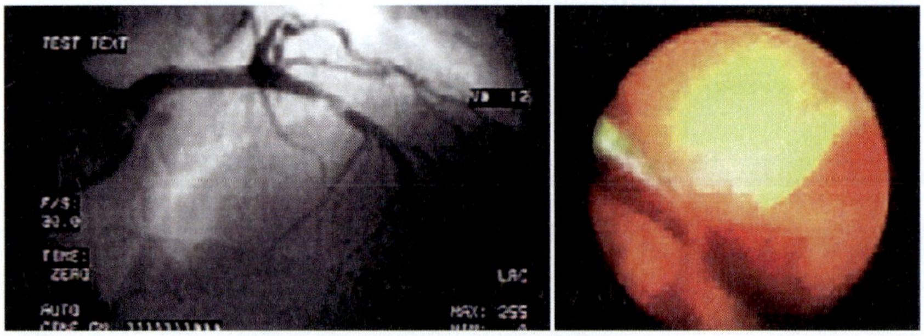

Fig. 2. *Left panel*, Angiogram revealing type II eccentric stenosis with filling defect in left anterior descending artery. Such complex morphology is a marker of high-risk lesions. *Right panel*, Angioscopic image revealing deep-yellow, intensely colored plaque with intimal disruption and a mural thrombus, indicating that the "complex" appearance on angiography correctly identified a disrupted plaque with thrombus. (Modified from Ishibashi et al. [46] with permission from Blackwell Publishing, copyright 2006. Images courtesy of Dr. Richard Nesto and Dr. SergioWaxman).

even before it ruptures, yet it is also suspected to remain prone to subsequent episodes of rupture and thrombosis. Hence, a ruptured plaque identified on IVUS might indicate a certain type of vulnerable plaque. To date, this issue has not been resolved. One IVUS-based study reported that ruptured plaques causing mild stenosis were not associated with progressive narrowing or recurrent ACS after infarction in patients receiving adequate medical therapy [21]; however, a second study demonstrated increases in stenosis at rupture sites in the absence of statin therapy [22].

Novel IVUS methods have been developed to characterize the stiffness of plaques and to detect the presence of necrotic cores or fibrofatty tissue. Standard IVUS is an excellent tool to determine whether plaques contain calcium, which produces a bright ultrasonic reflection. However, the association of calcification with plaque vulnerability is complex. Although calcification is associated with atherosclerosis, the plaques causing ACS contain less calcium than those causing stable angina [29–31]. Furthermore, stress analysis in autopsy specimens has revealed that the presence of calcium does not increase fibrous cap stress and is less likely than a lipid pool to decrease mechanical stability of an atheroma [29]. A spotty pattern of calcification, which is more likely to be found in culprit lesions of patients with MI than in those with stable angina, may be an indicator of vulnerability [30,31].

IVUS has also been employed to identify other plaque components. Studies in autopsy specimens have shown that hypoechoic areas represent plaques with an increased lipid content, low-intensity or "soft" echoes represent fibromuscular lesions, and moderately hyperechoic areas are associated with fibrous plaques [19]. A prospective study in a small number of patients found an increased risk of rupture and ACS caused by echolucent (presumably lipid-rich) plaques [32].

Recent efforts have focused on improving IVUS signal processing to enhance the analysis of plaque composition. Novel techniques to analyze the integrated backscatter of the radiofrequency (RF) signal may improve our ability to characterize plaques [33–35]. This approach, termed *Virtual Histology* (Volcano, Inc., Rancho Cordova, CA), categorizes plaques as fibrotic, fibrofatty, calcific, and those with a necrotic core (Fig. 3). In one study involving patients with stable angina, 6 months of statin therapy induced changes in the RF IVUS signal consistent with a reduced lipid component, indicating plaque stabilization [36]. Other Virtual Histology studies have reported that (a) positive (expansive) remodeling is more common with fibrofatty plaques found on IVUS [37]; (b) sites found to

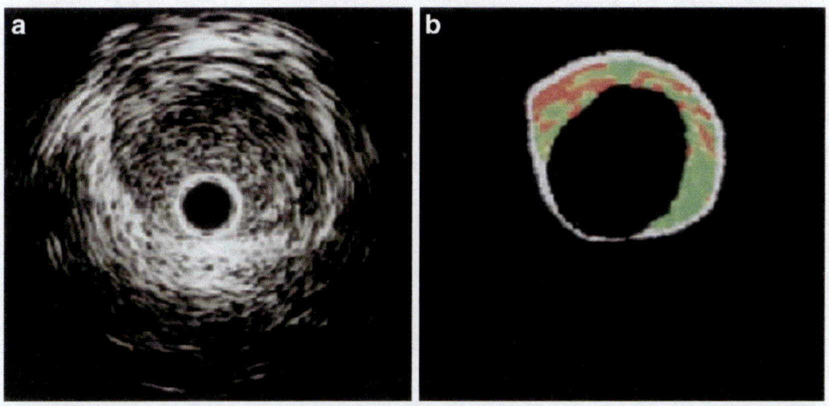

Fig. 3. Plaque characterization on IVUS imaging. (**a**) Traditional gray-scale cross-sectional IVUS image showing plaque in left anterior descending artery. (**b**) Corresponding image using Virtual Histology (Volcano, Inc.) to characterize tissue based on spectral analysis of backscatter data. White = calcification; green = fibrotic tissue; greenish-yellow = fibrolipidic tissue; red = necrotic core. (Modified from Rodriguez-Granillo GA, et al. In vivo intravascular ultrasound-derived thin-cap fibroatheroma detection using ultrasound radiofrequency data analysis. J Am Coll Cardiol 2005;46:2038–2042, with permission from The American College of Cardiology Foundation, copyright 2005).

have larger lipid cores are more likely to be associated with expansive remodeling [38]; and (c) patients with ACS are more likely than those with stable angina to have signs of a TCFA on Virtual Histology [39]. Long-term, large-scale studies designed to determine whether IVUS signals can prospectively identify plaques and/or patients prone to coronary events are under way [40].

Elastography

Elastography, an IVUS-based technique, assesses plaque deformation during changes in intracoronary pressure that occur during the cardiac cycle [41]. It has been used to characterize the softness of plaques, which might be a sign of vulnerability. In postmortem coronary artery specimens, elastography has a high sensitivity and specificity for detecting TCFAs (Fig. 4) [42]. Deformable plaques are more frequent in patients with acute MI and unstable angina than in patients with stable angina and are associated with higher levels of high-sensitivity C-reactive protein [43].

Optical Methods to Detect Vulnerable Plaque

Angioscopy. Coronary angioscopy is the most precise clinical method available for detecting thrombus, plaque disruption, and color variations in arterial wall tissue that reflect its lipid composition (Fig. 5) [44–48]. A ruptured plaque appears as an irregular area on angioscopy, and thrombus appears as a red, pink, or whitish mass. Nondisrupted plaques may be white, indicating a fibrotic composition, or yellow, owing to a lipid content rich in carotenoid pigments [44–46]. The more intense the yellow color, the thinner the fibrous cap; a glistening yellow appearance indicates a TCFA [47,48].

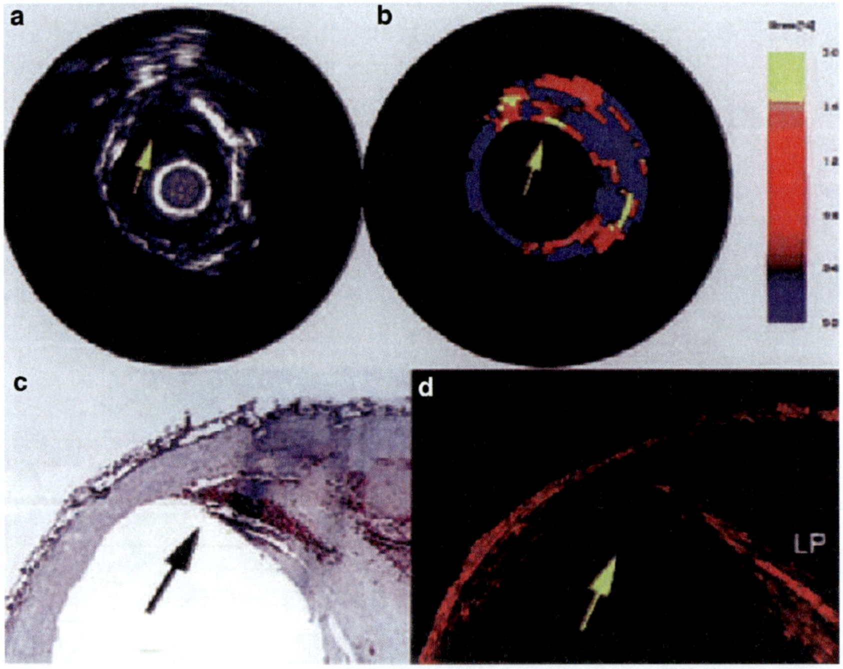

Fig. 4. Ex vivo images of a coronary artery TCFA obtained by IVUS (**a**) and elastography (**b**), followed by macrophage (**c**) and collagen staining (**d**). In the elastogram, a soft plaque is indicated by deformability with higher pressure (*small yellow arrow*). Macrophage presence is increased (*black arrow*) and collagen is decreased over a lipid pool (*large yellow arrow*). (Modified from Schaar et al. [42] with permission from the American Heart Association, copyright 2003).

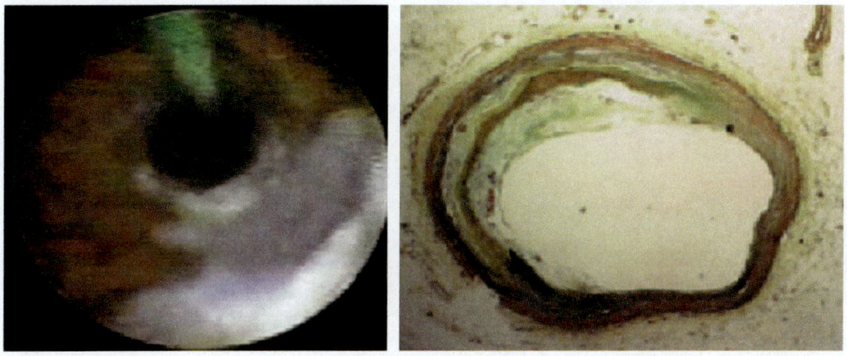

Fig. 5. (**a**) Angioscopic image of yellow plaque in human coronary autopsy specimen. (**b**) Histology reveals a TCFA. (Image courtesy of Dr. Fumiyuki Ishibashi and Dr. Sergio Waxman).

Angioscopic signs of both thrombus and disruption of the culprit lesion are more frequent in patients with unstable angina and MI than in those with stable angina [49–51]. Angioscopy has also confirmed that disrupted and thrombotic plaques can be present at sites other than the site of the culprit lesion. Because ruptured plaques with thrombi may be prone to recurrent thrombosis, it is possible that these ruptured plaques detected by angioscopy may be a type of vulnerable plaque [52–54]. Nonculprit lesions with disruption or thrombus detected by angioscopy tend to heal but may cause progression of angiographically detected stenosis. Angioscopic studies have documented multiple, frankly ruptured, thrombus-laden plaques as well as the frequent presence of presumably "vulnerable" yellow plaques distant from the culprit lesion [55].

Yellow plaques, which may be associated with vulnerability, are five times more likely to be associated with thrombus than are white plaques, and the culprit lesions in patients with MI are often yellow [56,57]. Because visual assessment of yellow is subjective and can be affected by multiple variables, efforts are being made to develop quantitative colorimetric systems [56–59]. Importantly, yellow plaques are frequently found at nonculprit sites in patients with acute MI, and yellow plaques not associated with thrombosis occur in 50–60% of patients with stable angina. Although these findings indicate the diffuse nature of atherosclerosis, the more locally occurring TCFAs, which are a subset of yellow plaques, might represent focal sites of vulnerability. Uchida et al. [47] employed angioscopy in patients with stable angina to study the natural history of "yellow" lesions suspected to be vulnerable; over a one-year period, about 33% of patients with glistening yellow plaques experienced a coronary event versus only 8% of those with nonglistening yellow plaque and 3% of those with white plaques alone. This important finding could represent the prospective identification of vulnerable plaque.

Recent studies suggest that the angioscopic characterization of plaques may be useful in predicting vascular healing responses to stent implantation [60]. Ideally, following their insertion, stents completely endothelialize over time, thereby providing a smooth, nonthrombogenic surface. Although drug-eluting stents beneficially minimize in-stent stenosis by inhibiting this expected and necessary vascular growth response, they may delay endothelialization, leaving patients at risk for subacute stent thrombosis. Angioscopically yellow (lipid-laden) plaques appear to endothelialize less effectively than white fibrous lesions. If these findings can be substantiated, they may have implications for stent selection based on lesion characteristics. Despite its capabilities, angioscopy is rarely used in clinical practice because it requires a blood-free field of view. Still, the technique is valuable for research, with most such studies being conducted in Japan.

Optical coherence tomography (OCT). OCT uses the back-reflection of NIR light from optical interfaces in tissue to create cross-sectional images with a higher resolution (10 microns).

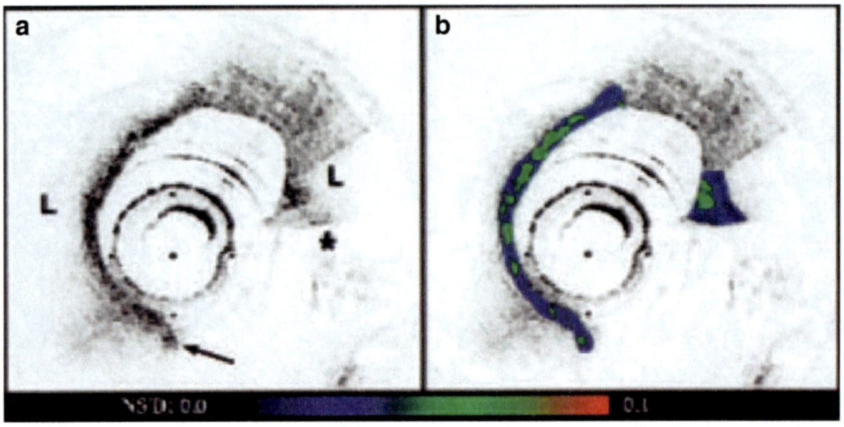

Fig. 6. (**a**) OCT image of ruptured TCFA in patient with acute MI. Evident are a lipid pool (*L*), intimal disruption (*arrow*) and guidewire artifact (*). (**b**) Macrophage density data are superimposed on the image. (Modified from Tearney et al. [61] with permission from the International Society for Optical Engineering, copyright 2006).

Compared with IVUS, which has a resolution of 100 microns, OCT provides high-resolution views of cap thickness and plaque microarchitecture and may be able to image macrophage infiltration [61–67]. Autopsy studies have documented that OCT can accurately identify fibrous, fibrocalcific, and lipid-rich plaques and macrophages and is the best technique for measuring cap thickness (Fig. 6) [63,64]. OCT can provide striking images of cap rupture not visible on conventional angiography or even IVUS.

The promising features of OCT, as documented in ex vivo studies, can also be valuable in the clinical setting. In 57 patients undergoing percutaneous coronary interventions, signs of lipid-rich plaques on OCT were observed in 90% of MI patients, 75% of ACS patients, and 59% of stable angina patients. The frequency of fibrous caps 65 microns or less in thickness was 72%, 50%, and 20% in the MI, ACS, and stable angina patients, respectively [66]. The presence of macrophages on OCT was found to be greater in patients with ACS than in those with stable angina [67].

OCT is limited by signal attenuation attributable to luminal blood, which reduces imaging time and complicates its use. A modification of OCT, *optical frequency domain imaging*, has been designed to permit more rapid signal acquisition and will facilitate scanning of a greater portion of the artery during a single flush [67].

Intracoronary near-infrared spectroscopy (NIRS). NIRS is a promising technique to identify lipid-laden plaques. *Diffuse reflectance NIRS* is widely used in many fields to identify the chemical composition of unknown substances [18,68,69]. Because this type of spectroscopy appeared to be well suited to determining the composition of atherosclerotic plaques, several investigators tested its ability to identify lipids in ex vivo studies of coronary autopsy or endarterectomy specimens [70–72]. TCFAs and ruptured plaques could be readily identified by spectroscopy even in preparations containing up to 2 mm of intervening blood. Initially there was doubt as to whether NIRS would prove useful in vivo because of interference from cardiac motion and blood flow and the need to scan entire arteries [69], but technologic innovations have now overcome these obstacles.

Recently a catheter-based NIRS device (InfraReDx, Burlington, Massachusetts) has proved to be an accurate detector of lipid-rich plaque (LRP) in human coronary autopsy histologic specimens [69,73]. The device is similar in size and use to an IVUS catheter. Calibration and validation studies have been performed in intact, perfused human coronary artery autopsy specimens [73].

To create an advanced algorithm ultimately applicable to interpretation of NIR signals obtained in patients, NIR spectrographic data were compared to the gold standard of histology in 33 donor hearts, with calibration accomplished by acquiring coregistered spectroscopic and histologic data. The calibrated algorithm was then validated in a prospective, double-blind study in 51 additional hearts. The NIR system was found to be accurate for localized detection of LRP, a suspected precursor of plaque rupture, as well as for determining the overall lipid burden of a scanned artery [73].

Studies of this catheter system in patients have documented NIR signals similar to those obtained in the autopsy studies. NIRS involving motorized pullback scanning was performed in patients undergoing PCI for stable angina or ACS [74]. Initially, unblinded studies were carried out in 30 of the patients to test system calibration; data were then prospectively obtained in 59 other patients and compared with autopsy NIR signals in blinded studies. The primary endpoint was "spectral similarity" – i.e., over two-third of spectra shapes were similar to those of autopsy spectra. The device was well tolerated, was easy to use, and provided a full scan of the area of interest. High-quality spectra were obtained in the unblinded study [74]; an analysis of the full data set is in progress. These results indicate the feasibility of obtaining reliable NIRS data from the coronary arteries of patients undergoing cardiac catheterization.

Raman NIRS has also used to assess coronary plaque composition [75–77]. Raman differs from diffuse reflectance NIRS in that it is based on the shift of photons to a different wavelength by the tissue being imaged. Although the Raman shift is more specific for individual chemicals than is diffuse reflectance NIR, its signal is much weaker and therefore more difficult to detect in vivo. Raman spectroscopy has been shown to be capable of differentiating atherosclerotic plaque from diffuse intimal thickening ex vivo in carotid endarterectomy specimens. If the problems attending in vivo measurement can be overcome, a compact fiberoptic-based Raman spectroscopy system has the potential to characterize plaques in patients [78].

Thermography

Increased temperature of inflamed human atherosclerotic plaques obtained at carotid endarterectomy has been documented in an ex vivo setting using thermography [79,80]. These findings prompted several groups of researchers to measure the temperature of plaques in patients undergoing cardiac catheterization [81–83]. However, coronary blood flow and catheter design complicate in vivo measurement. Since the contracting heart generates heat, coronary blood flow acts as a coolant and makes it difficult to measure relatively small increases in plaque temperature without interrupting flow [80]. In addition, measuring the relatively small thermal signals will require catheters with increased sensitivity.

Intravascular Magnetic Resonance Imaging (MRI)

MRI can be used invasively to detect lipid within coronary plaques [84–86]. A system has been developed that combines all the MRI components–magnets, RF coil, and detectors–in a single coronary catheter [87]. This system has been validated in aortic and coronary tissue ex vivo (Fig. 7) and has revealed significant differences in apparent diffusion coefficients among fibrous tissue, fatty streak, and lipid-rich necrotic cores. A catheter has been developed and utilized successfully in patients to identify lipid-rich plaque in coronary arteries, with the following limitations: only a few arterial sites are interrogated, it takes over a minute to complete the measurement, and coronary occlusion is required.

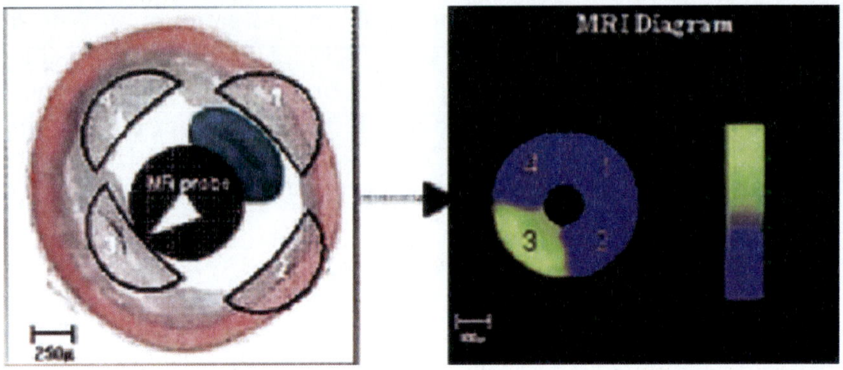

Fig. 7. *Left*, Self-contained intravascular MRI system with imaging areas superimposed on human coronary artery, showing one of four fields of view (*arrowhead*). *Right*, Lipid fraction in each quadrant of ex vivo autopsy specimen. An increased lipid concentration is displayed in yellow. (From Schneiderman et al. [87] with permission from The American College of Cardiology Foundation, copyright 2005).

SUMMARY

These novel diagnostic tools are likely to transform the intravascular treatment of coronary artery plaques. Today, clinical decisions are typically made based on selective angiography, which provides data limited to the effects of atherosclerosis on the vessel lumen. The future holds a more sophisticated and comprehensive approach to plaque characterization, including more detailed lesion-specific data regarding plaque architecture (with IVUS, OCT, and possibly MRI), chemical composition (with NIRS, OCT, and perhaps IVUS), and biologic activity (with molecular imaging agents). Both singly and together, these promising new modalities offer a more informed approach to plaque evaluation and therapy. Further research is needed to determine whether the application of these tools will provide diagnostic, prognostic, and therapeutic data that will improve outcomes for patients with coronary atherosclerosis.

ACKNOWLEDGMENT

We are grateful for the excellent editorial assistance of Diane Q. Forti in the preparation of this manuscript.

REFERENCES

1. Davies MJ, Thomas A. Thrombosis and acute coronary artery lesions in sudden cardiac ischemic death. N Engl J Med 1984;310:1137–1140.
2. Falk E, Shah PK, Fuster V. Coronary plaque disruption. Circulation 1995;92:657–671.
3. Libby P. Molecular bases of the acute coronary syndromes. Circulation 1995:91:2844–2850.
4. Cutlip DE, Chhabra AG, Baim DS, Chauhan MS, Marulkar S, Massaro J, Bakhai A, Cohen DJ, Kuntz RE, Ho KK. Beyond restenosis: five-year clinical outcomes from second-generation coronary stent trials. Circulation 2004;110:1226–1230.
5. Goldstein JA, Demetriou D, Grines CL, et al. Multiple complex coronary plaques in patients with acute myocardial infarction. N Engl J Med 2000;343:915–922.
6. Muller JE, Abela GS, Nesto RW, Tofler GH. Triggers, acute risk factors and vulnerable plaques: the lexicon of a new frontier. J Am Coll Cardiol 1994;23:809–813.
7. Glaser R, Selzer F, Faxon DP, Laskey WK, Cohen HA, Slater J, Detre KM, Wilensky RL. Clinical progression of incidental, asymptomatic lesions discovered during culprit vessel coronary intervention. Circulation 2005;111:143–149.
8. Libby P. Act local, act global: inflammation and the multiplicity of "vulnerable" coronary plaques. J Am Coll Cardiol 2005;45: 1600–1602.

9. Goldstein JA. Angiographic plaque complexity: the tip of the unstable plaque iceberg. J Am Coll Cardiol 2002;39(9): 1456–1463.
10. Lutgens E, van Suylen RJ, Faber BC, Gijbels MJ, Eurlings PM, Bijnens AP, Cleutjens KB, Heeneman S, Daemen MJ. Atherosclerotic plaque rupture: local or systemic process? Arterioscler Thromb Vasc Biol 2003;23:2123–2130.
11. Hansson GK. Inflammation, atherosclerosis, and coronary artery disease. N Engl J Med 2005;352:1685–1695.
12. Virmani R, Kolodgie FD, Burke AP, Farb A, Schwartz SM. Lessons from sudden coronary death: a comprehensive morphological classification scheme for atherosclerotic lesions. Arterioscler Thromb Vasc Biol 2000;20:1262–1275.
13. Schaar JA, Muller JE, Falk E, Virmani R, Fuster V, Serruys PW, Colombo A, Stefanadis C, Casscells W, Moreno PR, Maseri A, van der Steen AF. Terminology for high-risk and vulnerable coronary artery plaques: report of a meeting on the vulnerable plaque, June 17 and 18, 2003, Santorini, Italy. Eur Heart J 2004;25:1077–1082.
14. Fuster V, Moreno PR, Fayad ZA, Corti R, Badimon JJ. Atherothrombosis and high-risk plaque. Part I: Evolving concepts. J Am Coll Cardiol 2005;20:46:937–954.
15. Farb A, Burke AP, Tang AL, Liang TY, Mannan P, Smialek J, Virmani R. Coronary plaque erosion without rupture into a lipid core: a frequent cause of coronary thrombosis in sudden coronary death. Circulation 1996;93:1354–1363.
16. Kolodgie FD, Burke AP, Farb A, Gold HK, Yuan J, Narula J, Finn AV, Virmani R. The thin-cap fibroatheroma: a type of vulnerable plaque: the major precursor lesion to acute coronary syndromes. Curr Opin Cardiol 2001;16:285–292.
17. Cheruvu P, Finn A, Gardner C, Caplan J, Goldstein JA, Stone GW, Virmani R, Muller JE. Frequency and distribution of thin-cap fibroatheroma and ruptured plaques in human coronary arteries – a pathologic study. J Am Coll Cardiol 2007;50: 940–949.
18. Waxman S, Ishibashi F, Muller JE. Detection and treatment of vulnerable plaques and vulnerable patients: novel approaches to prevention of coronary events. Circulation 2006;114:2390–2411.
19. Nishimura RA, Edwards WD, Warnes CA, Reeder GS, Holmes DR Jr, Tajik AJ, Yock PG. Intravascular ultrasound imaging: in vitro validation and pathologic correlation. J Am Coll Cardiol 1990;16:145–154.
20. DeMaria AN, Narula J, Mahmud E, Tsimikas S. Imaging vulnerable plaque by ultrasound. J Am Coll Cardiol 2006;47: C32–C39.
21. Rioufol G, Gilard M, Finet G, Ginon I, Boschat J, Andre-Fouet X. Evolution of spontaneous atherosclerotic plaque rupture with medical therapy: long-term follow-up with intravascular ultrasound. Circulation 2004;110:2875–2880.
22. Hong MK, Mintz GS, Lee CW, Suh IW, Hwang ES, Jeong YH, Park DW, Kim YH, Han KH, Cheong SS, Kim JJ, Park SW, Park SJ. Serial intravascular ultrasound evidence of both plaque stabilization and lesion progression in patients with ruptured coronary plaques: effects of statin therapy on ruptured coronary plaque. Atherosclerosis April 3, 2006.DOI:10.1016/j. atherosclerosis.2006.02.040. Available at: http://www.sciencedirect.com. Accessed September 19, 2006.
23. Smits PC, Pasterkamp G, Quarles van Ufford MA, Eefting FD, Stella PR, de Jaegere PP, Borst C. Coronary artery disease: arterial remodeling and clinical presentation. Heart 1999;82:461–464.
24. Schoenhagen P, Ziada KM, Kapadia SR, Crowe TD, Nissen SE, Tuzcu EM. Extent and direction of arterial remodeling in stable versus unstable coronary syndromes: an intravascular ultrasound study. Circulation 2000;101:598–603.
25. Pasterkamp G, Schoneveld AH, Hijnen DJ, de Kleijn DP, Teepen H, van der Wal AC, Borst C. Atherosclerotic arterial remodeling and the localization of macrophages and matrix metalloproteases 1, 2, and 9 in the human coronary artery. Atherosclerosis 2000;150:245–253.
26. Varnava AM, Mills PG, Davies MJ. Relationship between coronary artery remodeling and plaque vulnerability. Circulation 2002;105:939–943.
27. Pasterkamp G, Galis ZS, de Kleijn DP. Expansive arterial remodeling: location, location, location. Arterioscler Thromb Vasc Biol 2004;24:650–657.
28. Guedes A, Tardif JC. Intravascular ultrasound assessment of atherosclerosis. Curr Atheroscler Rep 2004;6:219–224.
29. Huang H, Virmani R, Younis H, Burke AP, Kamm RD, Lee RT. The impact of calcification on the biomechanical stability of atherosclerotic plaques. Circulation 2001;103:1051–1056.
30. Ehara S, Kobayashi Y, Yoshiyama M, Shimada K, Shimada Y, Fukuda D, Nakamura Y, Yamashita H, Yamagishi H, Takeuchi K, Naruko T, Haze K, Becker AE, Yoshikawa J, Ueda M. Spotty calcification typifies the culprit plaque in patients with acute myocardial infarction: an intravascular ultrasound study. Circulation 2004;110:3424–3429.
31. Burke AP, Weber DK, Kolodgie FD, Farb A, Taylor AJ, Virmani R. Pathophysiology of calcium deposition in coronary arteries. Herz 2001;26:239–244.
32. Yamagishi M, Terashima M, Awano K, Kijima M, Nakatani S, Daikoku S, Ito K, Yasumura Y, Miyatake K. Morphology of vulnerable coronary plaque: insights from follow-up of patients examined by intravascular ultrasound before an acute coronary syndrome. J Am Coll Cardiol 2000;35:106–111.
33. Kawasaki M, Takatsu H, Noda T, Ito Y, Kunishima A, Arai M, Nishigaki K, Takemura G, Morita N, Minatoguchi S, Fujiwara H. Noninvasive quantitative tissue characterization and two-dimensional color-coded map of human atherosclerotic lesions using ultrasound integrated backscatter: comparison between histology and integrated backscatter images. J Am Coll Cardiol 2001;38:486–492.
34. Murashige A, Hiro T, Fujii T, Imoto K, Murata T, Fukumoto Y, Matsuzaki M. Detection of lipid-laden atherosclerotic plaque by wavelet analysis of radiofrequency intravascular ultrasound signals: in vitro validation and preliminary in vivo application. J Am Coll Cardiol 2005;45:1954–1960.
35. Nair A, Kuban BD, Tuzcu EM, Schoenhagen P, Nissen SE, Vince DG. Coronary plaque classification with intravascular ultrasound radiofrequency data analysis. Circulation 2002;106:2200–2206.

36. Kawasaki M, Sano K, Okubo M, Yokoyama H, Ito Y, Murata I, Tsuchiya K, Minatoguchi S, Zhou X, Fujita H, Fujiwara H. Volumetric quantitative analysis of tissue characteristics of coronary plaques after statin therapy using three-dimensional integrated backscatter intravascular ultrasound. J Am Coll Cardiol 2005;45:1946–1953.
37. Fujii K, Carlier SG, Mintz GS, Wijns W, Colombo A, Bose D, Erbel R, de Ribamar Costa J Jr, Kimura M, Sano K, Costa RA, Lui J, Stone GW, Moses JW, Leon MB. Association of plaque characterization by intravascular ultrasound virtual histology and arterial remodeling. Am J Cardiol 2005;96:1476–1483.
38. Rodriguez-Granillo GA, Serruys PW, Garcia-Garcia HM, Aoki J, Valgimigli M, van Mieghem CA, McFadden E, de Jaegere PP, de Feyter P. Coronary artery remodelling is related to plaque composition. Heart 2006;92:388–391.
39. Valgimigli M, Rodriguez-Granillo GA, Garcia-Garcia HM, Malagutti P, Regar E, de Jaegere P, de Feyter P, Serruys PW. Distance from the ostium as an independent determinant of coronary plaque composition in vivo: an intravascular ultrasound study based radiofrequency data analysis in humans. Eur Heart J 2006;27:655–663.
40. Carlier SG, Mintz GS, Stone GW. Imaging of atherosclerotic plaque using radiofrequency ultrasound signal processing. J Nucl Cardiol 2006;13(6):831–840.
41. de Korte CL, van der Steen AF, Cespedes EI, Pasterkamp G. Intravascular ultrasound elastography in human arteries: initial experience in vitro. Ultrasound Med Biol 1998;24:401–408.
42. Schaar JA, de Korte CL, Mastik F, Strijder C, Pasterkamp G, Boersma E, Serruys PW, van der Steen AF. Characterizing vulnerable plaque features with intravascular elastography. Circulation 2003;108:2636–2641.
43. Schaar JA, Regar E, Mastik F, McFadden EP, Saia F, Disco C, de Korte CL, de Feyter PJ, van der Steen AF, Serruys PW. Incidence of high strain patterns in human coronary arteries: assessment with three dimensional intravascular palpography and correlation with clinical presentation. Circulation 2004;109:2716–2719.
44. Thieme T, Wernecke KD, Meyer R, Brandenstein E, Habedank D, Hinz A, Felix SB, Baumann G, Kleber FX. Angioscopic evaluation of atherosclerotic plaques: validation by histomorphologic analysis and association with stable and unstable coronary syndromes. J Am Coll Cardiol 1996;28:1–6.
45. Blankenhorn DH. The infiltration of carotenoids into human atheromas and xanthomas. Ann Intern Med 1960;53:944–954.
46. Ishibashi F, Aziz K, Abela GS, Waxman S. Update on coronary angioscopy: review of a 20-year experience and potential application for detection of vulnerable plaque. J Intervent Cardiol 2006;19:17–25.
47. Uchida Y, Nakamura F, Tomaru T, Morita T, Oshima T, Sasaki T, Morizuki S, Hirose J. Prediction of acute coronary syndromes by percutaneous coronary angioscopy in patients with stable angina. Am Heart J 1995;130:195–203.
48. Miyamoto A, Prieto AR, Friedl SE, Lin FC, Muller JE, Nesto RW, Abela GS. Atheromatous plaque cap thickness can be determined by quantitative color analysis during angioscopy: implications for identifying the vulnerable plaque. Clin Cardiol 2004;27:9–15.
49. Waxman S, Sassower MA, Mittleman MA, Zarich S, Miyamoto A, Manzo KS, Muller JE, Abela GS, Nesto RW. Angioscopic predictors of early adverse outcome after coronary angioplasty in patients with unstable angina and non-Q-wave myocardial infarction. Circulation 1996;93:2106–2113.
50. Mizuno K, Satomura K, Miyamoto A, Arakawa K, Shibuya T, Arai T, Kurita A, Nakamura H, Ambrose JA. Angioscopic evaluation of coronary-artery thrombi in acute coronary syndromes. N Engl J Med 1992;326:287–291.
51. de Feyter PJ, Ozaki Y, Baptista J, Escaned J, Di Mario C, de Jaegere PP, Serruys PW, Roelandt JR. Ischemia-related lesion characteristics in patients with stable or unstable angina: a study with intracoronary angioscopy and ultrasound. Circulation 1995;92:1408–1413.
52. Nissen SE. Pathobiology, not angiography, should guide management in acute coronary syndrome/non-ST-segment elevation myocardial infarction: the non-interventionist's perspective. J Am Coll Cardiol 2003;41:103S–112S.
53. Takano M, Inami S, Ishibashi F, Okamatsu K, Seimiya K, Ohba T, Sakai S, Mizuno K. Angioscopic follow-up study of coronary ruptured plaques in nonculprit lesions. J Am Coll Cardiol 2005;45:652–658.
54. Rentrop KP. Thrombi in acute coronary syndromes: revisited and revised. Circulation 2000;101:1619–1626.
55. Asakura M, Ueda Y, Yamaguchi O, Adachi T, Hirayama A, Hori M, Kodama K. Extensive development of vulnerable plaques as a pancoronary process in patients with myocardial infarction: an angioscopic study. J Am Coll Cardiol 2001;37: 1284–1288.
56. Waxman S, Mittleman MA, Zarich SW, Fitzpatrick PJ, Lewis SM, Leeman DE, Shubrooks SJ Jr, Snyder JT, Muller JE, Nesto RW. Angioscopic assessment of coronary lesions underlying thrombus. Am J Cardiol 1997;79:1106–1109.
57. Mizuno K, Miyamoto A, Satomura K, Kurita A, Arai T, Sakurada M, Yanagida S, Nakamura H. Angioscopic coronary macromorphology in patients with acute coronary disorders. Lancet 1991;337:809–812.
58. Lehmann KG, Oomen JA, Slager CJ, de Feyter PJ, Serruys PW. Chromatic distortion during angioscopy: assessment and correction by quantitative colorimetric angioscopic analysis. Cathet Cardiovasc Diagn 1998;45:191–201.
59. Ueda Y, Ohtani T, Shimizu M, Hirayama A, Kodama K. Assessment of plaque vulnerability by angioscopic classification of plaque color. Am Heart J 2004;148:333–335.
60. Oyabu J, Ueda Y, Ogasawara N, Okada K, Hirayama A, Kodama K. Angioscopic evaluation of neointima coverage: sirolimus drug-eluting stent versus bare metal stent. Am Heart J 2006;152(6):1168–1174.
61. Tearney GJ, Jang IK, Bouma BE. Optical coherence tomography for imaging vulnerable plaque. J Biomed Opt 2006;11:021002.
62. Jang IK, Bouma BE, Kang DH, Park SJ, Park SW, Seung KB, Choi KB, Shishkov M, Schlendorf KH, Pomerantsev E, Houser SL, Aretz HT, Tearney GJ. Visualization of coronary atherosclerotic plaques in patients using optical coherence tomography: comparison with intravascular ultrasound. J Am Coll Cardiol 2002;39:604–609.

63. Yabushita H, Bouma BE, Houser SL, Aretz HT, Jang IK, Schlendorf KH, Kauffman CR, Shishkov M, Kang DH, Halpern EF, Tearney GJ. Characterization of human atherosclerosis by optical coherence tomography. Circulation 2002;106:1640–1645.
64. Tearney GJ, Yabushita H, Houser SL, Aretz HT, Jang IK, Schlendorf KH, Kauffman CR, Shishkov M, Halpern EF, Bouma BE. Quantification of macrophage content in atherosclerotic plaques by optical coherence tomography. Circulation 2003;107:113–119.
65. Stamper D, Weissman NJ, Brezinski M. Plaque characterization with optical coherence tomography. J Am Coll Cardiol 2006; 47:C69–C79.
66. Jang IK, Tearney GJ, MacNeill B, Takano M, Moselewski F, Iftima N, Shishkov M, Houser S, Aretz HT, Halpern EF, Bouma BE. In vivo characterization of coronary atherosclerotic plaque by use of optical coherence tomography. Circulation 2005;111:1551–1555.
67. Yun SH, Tearney GJ, de Boer JF, Iftima N, Bouma BE. High-speed optical frequency-domain imaging. Optics Express 2003; 11:2953–2963.
68. MacNeill BD, Jang IK, Bouma BE, Iftima N, Takano M, Yabushita H, Shishkov M, Kauffman CR, Houser SL, Aretz HT, DeJoseph D, Halpern EF, Tearney GJ. Focal and multi-focal plaque macrophage distributions in patients with acute and stable presentations of coronary artery disease. J Am Coll Cardiol 2004;44:972–979.
69. Caplan JD, Waxman S, Nesto RW, Muller JE. Near-infrared spectroscopy for the detection of vulnerable coronary artery plaques. J Am Coll Cardiol 2006;47:C92–C96.
70. Jaross W, Neumeister V, Lattke P, Schuh D. Determination of cholesterol in atherosclerotic plaques using near infrared diffuse reflection spectroscopy. Atherosclerosis 1999;147:327–337.
71. Moreno PR, Lodder RA, Purushothaman KR, Charash WE, O'Connor WN, Muller JE. Detection of lipid pool, thin fibrous cap, and inflammatory cells in human aortic atherosclerotic plaques by near-infrared spectroscopy. Circulation 2002;105:923–927.
72. Wang J, Geng YJ, Guo B, Klima T, Lal BN, Willerson JT, Casscells W. Near-infrared spectroscopic characterization of human advanced atherosclerotic plaques. J Am Coll Cardiol 2002;39:1305–1313.
73. Gardner C, Tan H, DeJesus S, Caplan J, Muller JE. Identification of thin-capped fibroatheroma through blood with probe-based near infrared spectroscopy in human coronary autopsy specimens . Abstract, TCT Meeting, 2007.
74. Waxman S, L'Allier P, Goldstein J, Krucoff MW, Tardif J-C, Dixon S, Petersen J, Nesto RW, Sum S, Hendricks M, Caplan J, Muller JE. Detection of lipid rich plaque by near-infrared spectroscopy (NIRS) in patients undergoing coronary intervention: results in an unblended cohort of the SPECTroscopic Assessment of Coronary Lipid (SPECTACL) Study. Abstract, TCT Meeting, 2007.
75. Brennan JF 3rd, Romer TJ, Lees RS, Tercyak AM, Kramer JR Jr, Feld MS. Determination of human coronary artery composition by Raman spectroscopy. Circulation 1997;96:99105.
76. Romer TJ, Brennan JF 3rd, Fitzmaurice M, Feldstein ML, Deinum G, Myles JL, Kramer JR, Lees RS, Feld MS. Histopathology of human coronary atherosclerosis by quantifying its chemical composition with Raman spectroscopy. Circulation 1998;97: 878–885.
77. Romer TJ, Brennan JF 3rd, Puppels GJ, Zwinderman AH, van Duinen SG, van der Laarse A, van der Steen AF, Bom NA, Bruschke AV. Intravascular ultrasound combined with Raman spectroscopy to localize and quantify cholesterol and calcium salts in atherosclerotic coronary arteries. Arterioscler Thromb Vasc Biol 2000;20:478–483.
78. Nogueira GV, Silveira L, Martin AA, Zangaro RA, Pacheco MT, Chavantes MC, Pasqualucci CA. Raman spectroscopy study of atherosclerosis in human carotid artery. J Biomed Opt 2005;10:031117.
79. Casscells W, Hathorn B, David M, Krabach T, Vaughn WK, McAllister HA, Bearman G, Willerson JT. Thermal detection of cellular infiltrates in living atherosclerotic plaques: possible implications for plaque rupture and thrombosis. Lancet 1996;347: 1447–1451.
80. Diamantopoulos L. Arterial wall thermography. J Interv Cardiol 2003;16:261–266.
81. Stefanadis C, Diamantopoulos L, Vlachopoulos C, Tsiamis E, Dernellis J, Toutouzas K, Stefanadi E, Toutouzas P. Thermal heterogeneity within human atherosclerotic coronary arteries detected in vivo: a new method of detection by application of a special thermography catheter. Circulation 1999;99:1965–1971.
82. Stefanadis C, Toutouzas K, Tsiamis E, Stratos C, Vavuranakis M, Kallikazaros I, Panagiotakos D, Toutouzas P. Increased local temperature in human coronary atherosclerotic plaques: an independent predictor of clinical outcome in patients undergoing a percutaneous coronary intervention. J Am Coll Cardiol 2001;37:1277–1283.
83. Ten Have AG, Draaijers EB, Gijsen FJ, Wentzel JJ, Slager CJ, Serruys PW, van der Steen AF. Influence of catheter design on lumen wall temperature distribution in intracoronary thermography. J Biomech Published online before print, April 5, 2006.
84. Wilensky RL, Song HK, Ferrari VA. Role of magnetic resonance and intravascular magnetic resonance in the detection of vulnerable plaques. J Am Coll Cardiol 2006;47:C48–C56.
85. Larose E, Yeghiazarians Y, Libby P, Yucel EK, Aikawa M, Kacher DF, Aikawa E, Kinlay S, Schoen FJ, Selwyn AP, Ganz P. Characterization of human atherosclerotic plaques by intravascular magnetic resonance imaging. Circulation 2005;112: 2324–2331.
86. Correia LC, Atalar E, Kelemen MD, Ocali O, Hutchins GM, Fleg JL, Gerstenblith G, Zerhouni EA, Lima JA. Intravascular magnetic resonance imaging of aortic atherosclerotic plaque composition. Arterioscler Thromb Vasc Biol 1997;17: 3626–3632.
87. Schneiderman J, Wilensky RL, Weiss A, Samouha E, Muchnik L, Chen-Zion M, Ilovitch M, Golan E, Blank A, Flugelman M, Rozenman Y, Virmani R. Diagnosis of thin-cap fibroatheromas by a self-contained intravascular magnetic resonance imaging probe in ex vivo human aortas and in situ coronary arteries. J Am Coll Cardiol 2005;45:1961–1969.

35 Detecting Vulnerable Plaque Using Invasive Methods

Robert S. Schwartz and Arturo G. Touchard

CONTENTS

ABSTRACT

Identifying plaque morphology and surface characteristics, especially for the carotid arteries, has proven important for revealing stroke pathogenesis. Imaging modalities that provide such information now exist and can monitor the progression of the diseased vessel, along with the effects of drugs on atherosclerotic plaque. This chapter summarizes the imaging tools to visualize and characterize vulnerable and stable atherosclerotic carotid plaque.

Key words: Carotid artery; CTA, MRI, Radionuclide imaging; Plaque Inflammation

KEY POINTS

- Carotid Vulnerable Plaque is highly analogous to Coronary Vulnerable Plaque
- Imaging methods include Radionuclide Imaging, Color Doppler Ultrasonograpy, Transcranial Doppler, CTA, and MRI
- Improvements in Imaging will involve cell and physiologic Imaging to monitor inflammation and cell traffic

From: *Asymptomatic Atherosclerosis: Pathophysiology, Detection and Treatment*
Edited by: M. Naghavi (ed.), DOI 10.1007/978-1-60327-179-0_35

INTRODUCTION

Cardiovascular mortality remains the number one cause of death in adults 65 years and older in Western societies. Of all cardiac-related deaths, half are sudden and unexpected. Thrombus is found obstructing the coronary artery in 60% of sudden cardiac death, and the remaining patients have severe anatomic coronary artery disease without thrombus [1]. As noted from other chapters in this text, most thrombus results from either coronary plaque rupture or erosion. Ruptured or eroded plaques are histopathologically distinct and cluster in different patient subsets, each with substantially different risk factors [2–5]. Multiple strategies for noninvasive detection have either been devised, or are validated. These noninvasive risk assessment methods have limited success to date, but are rapidly improving. Given the limitations of noninvasive detection, a next logical step is invasive verification or detection.

The inherent advantage of using invasive methods for detecting and characterizing vulnerable regions of coronary artery is that the detecting transducer can be placed in close proximity to the plaque. The disadvantages are obvious, in that the technique requires invasive methods. The invasive technologies emerging for detecting vulnerable coronary artery regions are based either on anatomy through imaging (lipid-necrotic regions, thin cap, calcium spicules) or on physiology (cells, inflammation, hemorrhage).

INVASIVE CORONARY ANGIOGRAPHY

Invasive coronary angiography is a well-known method for establishing lumen stenosis severity. It is, however, limited to determining lumen size and cannot well visualize the artery wall except to detect large calcific deposits. X-rays are typically used, with digital analysis and recording. This technique provides spatial resolution of 0.3–0.4 mm with temporal resolution of 15 ms or less. It can detect plaque vulnerability when secondary to severe stenosis are present, but this is of limited application since, when mody acute coronary occlusions arise from nonobstructive lesions its predictive power of occurrence of ACS is rather low. Coronary angiograms frequently fail to identify culprit lesions in clinical syndromes of non-ST elevation myocardial infarction [6]. It is for this reason that other invasive methods are being developed.

CORONARY ANGIOSCOPY

Coronary angioscopy achieves direct images of the coronary artery surface from the lumen, using a bundle of microscopic fibers to create and image array. The images from this technique appear to show color differences depending on lipid content, and may also characterize plaque composition and reveal thrombus, endoluminal ulcerations, fissures, or tears all suggestive of vulnerable plaque. The normal coronary artery appears angioscopically as glistening white, whereas atherosclerotic plaque can be categorized on the basis of its angioscopic color as yellow or white. Yellow plaques appear to show increased susceptibility to rupture and thrombosis [2,7] and are seen more commonly as culprit lesions being predictive of ischemic events. In patients with stable angina (SA), ACS occur more frequently in patients with yellow plaques than in those with white plaques [2,7]. Increased intensity of yellow color appears associated with increased susceptibility to rupture and thrombosis. Platelet-rich thrombus can also be imaged, often at the site of plaque rupture which is characterized as white granular material, and fibrin/erythrocyte-rich thrombus, as an irregular, red structure protruding into the lumen [8,9].

INTRAVASCULAR ULTRASOUND

Intravascular ultrasound (IVUS) images are produced by acoustic energy from piezoelectric (pressure-electric) crystals that vibrate at a frequency and magnitude in proportion to their physical size. The sound wave is reflected in proportion to density, reflected from the tissue, with the return wave detected by the transducer. An image is reconstructed by displaying intensity versus time for reflections. IVUS provide subsecond temporal resolution and cross-sectional information of the lumen and vessel wall.

IVUS allows measuring lumen area to obtain stenosis severity but can also measure plaque remodeling and detect features of the plaque such as calcification and hypoechoic regions. Vascular remodeling assessment by IVUS may help to classify plaques with the highest probability of spontaneous rupture [2,10,11]. IVUS can also image plaque rupture (identified as cavities, or echolucent areas within the plaque) and thrombus (usually echolucent with speckling or scintillation). IVUS is not as sensitive as angioscopy. Often, an echolucent zone within the atheroma is covered by a distinct "cap" of greater echogenicity, presumably representing the classic fibrous cap described by histology. However, one important IVUS limitation to detect vulnerable plaque features is its 100–200 μm axial resolution and 250 μm of lateral resolution. IVUS cannot thus easily distinguish caps of 0.15 mm in thickness from those that are 0.1 mm or less in thickness nor can it detect small tears on plaque cap.

IVUS discriminates different atherosclerotic plaque types, as high lipid-content plaques (soft plaques or echolucent) commonly show low echogenicity. Calcified plaques typically show highly echogenic zones with acoustic shadowing. Fibrous plaques commonly show intermediate echogenicity. However, due to its low contrast to noise ratio, different plaque features may exhibit comparable acoustic properties (echogenicity and texture) and therefore, appear quite similar on IVUS. Thus, distinguishing lipid plaques from fibrous plaques (which are more stable plaques) is sometimes difficult. Similarly, due to the low contrast to noise ratio and IVUS resolution limitations, IVUS is not a good tool to provide plaque composition information. IVUS cannot distinguish, for example, whether a zone represents an area of lipid deposition or a necrotic degeneration (both of which can appear as zones of low density) or detecting intraplaque microcalcification.

Despite these limitations IVUS can be a powerful tool to detect vulnerable plaques. Large eccentric plaques containing an echolucent zone have been shown by IVUS to be at increased risk for instability after 24 months of follow up even though the lumen area is preserved at the time of initial study. In addition, IVUS is a powerful tool to detect plaque macrocalcification, yielding a higher detection rate compared with angiography, with a sensitivity and a specificity of 89 and 97%, respectively [2,10,11]. However, because of the inability of the ultrasound to penetrate intralesional calcium, IVUS underestimates the total calcium amount.

IVUS BASED "VIRTUAL HISTOLOGY"

IVUS shows gray-scale images, so that calcified regions and dense fibrous components are generally brighter since they reflect energy well. By contrast, low echo-reflectance echogenicity in IVUS images are typically shown as "soft" or "mixed" plaque. Since gray-scale visual interpretation is limited and does not allow real time assessment of quantitative plaque composition, a frequency processing technique called Virtual Histology was developed which measures and color-code regions of the display within plaque into four distinct types [12–15].

The radiofrequency (RF) ultrasound backscatter signal can be analyzed for frequency content, a method that seems to correlate with histopathologic details of plaque composition. Previous studies have demonstrated the potential of spectral analysis for discerning plaque components in real time.

Virtual Histology by IVUS was developed from data where analytical determination of plaque components, using easily accessible IVUS backscattered signals, was compared with matched histology results of autopsy specimens. Using a combination of backscatter spectral parameters, a classification scheme has been developed for the analysis of IVUS RF data.

Virtual histology has been shown to have 80–92% accuracy to identify the four possible basic tissue types in an atherosclerotic plaque: fibrosis, fibro-lipidic, calcified, and lipid necrotic using in vitro analyses. Clinical trials are currently underway to validate carefully the histologic findings.

INTRAVASCULAR ELASTOGRAPHY

Intravascular elastography measures radial plaque deformation using conventional IVUS catheters. The underlying concept is then with uniform loading, deformation (strain) of a tissue is related to the local mechanical properties of that tissue. Theoretically, in coronary plaques, at a given blood pressure, soft plaque components will deform more than hard components. Thus, with this method theoretically, it is possible to identify vulnerable plaques through the detection of high strain regions. For intravascular purposes, the intraluminal pressure is used as the excitation force (circumferential stress), using typically pressure differences in the order of 5 mmHg. The strain induced by this pressure differential in vascular tissue is in the order or 1%. The strain is color coded and plotted as a complementary image to the IVUS echogram [16–22].

Using human coronary and femoral arteries, elastography in vitro shows that different strain values are found between fibrous, fibro-fatty, and fatty plaque components. Particularly between fibrous and fatty tissue, a highly significant difference is found [23]. Elastography can detect vulnerable plaque with high sensitivity and specificity in coronary artery specimens acquired from patients after death. Interestingly, using Yucatan minipigs this technique showed that high-strain spots are associated with the presence of macrophages. The presence of a high-strain spot (strain >1%) has 92% sensitivity and 92% specificity to identify macrophages [24]. Thus, elastography may relate indirectly to the histopathological composition of the atherosclerotic plaque.

Human IVUS elastography in vivo is feasible since it is done with conventional IVUS catheters, making this technique a powerful clinical tool. Although its clinical value is currently under investigation, data acquired in patients referred for PTCA show the elastogram may identify the weak spots in an artery in the future. . In vivo soft plaques (identified from the deformation during the pressure cycle) reveal strain values of 1% with increased strain up to 2% at the shoulders of the plaque. Calcified material, as identified from the echogram, shows low strain values of 0–0.2%. The elastogram of stented plaques reveals very low strain values, except for two regions: these are between the stent struts and at the shoulders of the plaque.

THERMOGRAPHY

Inflammation is a major component of plaque vulnerability. Macrophages are metabolically active and have high turnover rate of total ATP. This high metabolic rate theoretically increases heat production in areas of macrophage accumulation. Casscells et al. [25] demonstrated, in living carotid artery plaques, that thermal heterogeneity exist in this plaque, with temperature significantly correlated positively with cell density (r=0.68) where most cells are macrophages, and inversely with the distance of the cell clusters from the luminal surface (r=–0.38). It appears that blood flow and other physical features can change the apparent temperature, a finding that may limit thermographic observations.

Regardless, temperature differences between atherosclerotic plaque and healthy vessel wall increase progressively from SA to unstable angina (UA) and to AMI patients (difference of plaque temperature from background, SA: 0.106±0.110°C, UA: 0.683±0.347°C, and AMI: 1.472±0.691°C in) [26]. Heterogeneity within the plaque was shown in 20, 40, and 67% of the patients with SA, UA, and AMI, respectively, whereas no heterogeneity was shown in the control subjects. This heterogeneity may suggest that intraplaque temperature may be related to the pathogenesis. Local heat at the site of lesion increased in patients with ACS, may arise from an aggressive inflammatory response occurring in these situations [27,28]. In addition a strong correlation has been documented between reactants of the acute phase of inflammation (C-reactive protein and serum amyloid A) and the temperature ($r=0.796$, $P=0.01$ and $r=0.848$, $P=0.01$, respectively) in patients with CAD (SA, UA, AMI) which may relate the systemic inflammation with plaque composition. Temperature difference also has prognostic significance. Increased local temperature in atherosclerotic plaques more than 0.50°C is a strong predictor of an unfavorable clinical outcome in patients with coronary artery disease undergoing percutaneous interventions [29,30]. Although the clinical implication of this technique needs to be proven with additional studies, these studies of heat detection on atherosclerotic plaques support the potential clinical use of this tool to predict plaque rupture and thrombosis.

OPTICAL COHERENCE TOMOGRAPHY

Optical Coherence Tomography (OCT) is a novel technology using infrared wavelength light to create high-resolution images, about 10 microns. The light needs a blood-free field to function optimally since blood artificially reflects the incident beam infrared light. Excellent images are emerging with this high-resolution technique, visualizing lipid-rich regions and fibrous tissue as well [31–35].

OTHER TECHNIQUES

Many other techniques such as intravascular, Magnetic Resonance Imaging, RF, and Raman infrared spectroscopy are now under development. To date, however, these technologies have not been investigated in sufficient detail to assess its accuracy for characterizing vulnerable atherosclerotic plaques in the clinical settings and can be reviewed elsewhere. Of these techniques, the RF deserves special mention due to its potential use. RF can be done with most IVUS systems since they have an external connector that provides access to the RF signal. The RF signal is the unprocessed ultrasound signal (not subject to machine-dependent processing or operator-dependent settings). Spectral analysis of the RF ultrasound signals is emerging to improve the IVUS detection of plaque vulnerability. This technique is promising as it allows detailed assessment of plaque composition (a limitation of conventional grayscale IVUS densitometric analysis). Ex vivo studies with histological validation have revealed that spectral analysis of IVUS RF can reveal information regarding plaque characteristics [36–38]. In addition, RF is capable of visualizing lipid cores, fibrous caps, intimal hyperplasia, fibrous tissue, mixed lesions, and calcification in the plaque of human coronary arteries in vivo.

CONCLUSIONS

There is a pressing need to develop methods for invasive determination of atherosclerotic coronary artery regions that are at risk of thrombosis. The field of detecting such sites, whether invasive or noninvasive, remains uncertain. The likely solutions will entail anatomic imaging to detect high-risk plaque morphology. However, these anatomic images must be combined with functional and molecular imaging that will permit observation of high-risk physiology, as we understand further that cellular components are a major factor in rendering a coronary artery at risk. The future is bright, as these methods are under accelerated development.

REFERENCES

1. Virmani R, Kolodgie FD, Burke AP, Farb A, Schwartz SM. Lessons from sudden coronary death: a comprehensive morphological classification scheme for atherosclerotic lesions. Arterioscler Thromb Vasc Biol. 2000;20:1262–1275.
2. Madjid M, Zarrabi A, Litovsky S, Willerson JT, Casscells W. Finding vulnerable atherosclerotic plaques: is it worth the effort? Arterioscler Thromb Vasc Biol. 2004;24:1775–1782.
3. Lund J, Qin QP, Ilva T, Pettersson K, Voipio-Pulkki LM, Porela P, Pulkki K. Circulating pregnancy-associated plasma protein a predicts outcome in patients with acute coronary syndrome but no troponin I elevation. Circulation. 2003;108:1924–1926.
4. Burke AP, Tracy RP, Kolodgie F, Malcom GT, Zieske A, Kutys R, Pestaner J, Smialek J, Virmani R. Elevated C-reactive protein values and atherosclerosis in sudden coronary death: association with different pathologies. Circulation. 2002;105: 2019–2023.
5. Smith DA, Irving SD, Sheldon J, Cole D, Kaski JC. Serum levels of the antiinflammatory cytokine interleukin-10 are decreased in patients with unstable angina. Circulation. 2001;104:746–749.
6. Kerensky RA, Wade M, Deedwania P, Boden WE, Pepine CJ. Revisiting the culprit lesion in non-Q-wave myocardial infarction. Results from the VANQWISH trial angiographic core laboratory. J Am Coll Cardiol. 2002;39:1456–1463.
7. MacNeill BD, Lowe HC, Takano M, Fuster V, Jang IK. Intravascular modalities for detection of vulnerable plaque: current status. Arterioscler Thromb Vasc Biol. 2003;23:1333–1342.
8. Naghavi M, Madjid M, Khan MR, Mohammadi RM, Willerson JT, Casscells SW. New developments in the detection of vulnerable plaque. Curr Atheroscler Rep. 2001;3:125–135.
9. Fayad ZA, Fuster V. Clinical imaging of the high-risk or vulnerable atherosclerotic plaque. Circ Res. 2001;89:305–316.
10. Nissen SE. Application of intravascular ultrasound to characterize coronary artery disease and assess the progression or regression of atherosclerosis. Am J Cardiol. 2002;89:24B–31B.
11. Nair A, Kuban BD, Tuzcu EM, Schoenhagen P, Nissen SE, Vince DG. Coronary plaque classification with intravascular ultrasound radiofrequency data analysis. Circulation. 2002;106:2200–2206.
12. Hernandez JM, de Prada JA, Burgos V, Sainz Laso F, Valls MF, Vilchez FG, Llano M, Ruano J, Zueco J, Colman T, Duran RM. Virtual histology intravascular ultrasound assessment of cardiac allograft vasculopathy from 1 to 20 years after heart transplantation. J Heart Lung Transplant. 2009;28:156–162.
13. Sawada T, Shite J, Garcia-Garcia HM, Shinke T, Watanabe S, Otake H, Matsumoto D, Tanino Y, Ogasawara D, Kawamori H, Kato H, Miyoshi N, Yokoyama M, Serruys PW, Hirata K. Feasibility of combined use of intravascular ultrasound radiofrequency data analysis and optical coherence tomography for detecting thin-cap fibroatheroma. Eur Heart J. 2008;29:1136–1146.
14. Missel E, Mintz GS, Carlier SG, Sano K, Qian J, Kaple RK, Castellanos C, Dangas G, Mehran R, Moses JW, Stone GW, Leon MB. Necrotic core and its ratio to dense calcium are predictors of high-risk non-ST-elevation acute coronary syndrome. Am J Cardiol. 2008;101:573–578.
15. Missel E, Mintz GS, Carlier SG, Qian J, Shan S, Castellanos C, Kaple R, Biro S, Fahy M, Moses JW, Stone GW, Leon MB. In vivo virtual histology intravascular ultrasound correlates of risk factors for sudden coronary death in men: results from the prospective, multi-centre virtual histology intravascular ultrasound registry. Eur Heart J. 2008;29:2141–2147.
16. Sipahi I, Nicholls SJ, Tuzcu EM. Recent trends in coronary intravascular ultrasound: tracking atherosclerosis, pursuit of vulnerable plaques, and beyond. J Nucl Cardiol. 2006;13:91–96.
17. Zheng J, El Naqa I, Rowold FE, Pilgram TK, Woodard PK, Saffitz JE, Tang D. Quantitative assessment of coronary artery plaque vulnerability by high-resolution magnetic resonance imaging and computational biomechanics: a pilot study ex vivo. Magn Reson Med. 2005;54:1360–1368.
18. Baldewsing RA, Schaar JA, de Korte CL, Mastik F, Serruys PW, van der Steen AF. Intravascular ultrasound elastography: A clinician's tool for assessing vulnerability and material composition of plaques. Stud Health Technol Inform. 2005; 113:75–96.
19. Baldewsing RA, Schaar JA, Mastik F, Oomens CW, van der Steen AF. Assessment of vulnerable plaque composition by matching the deformation of a parametric plaque model to measured plaque deformation. IEEE Trans Med Imaging. 2005;24:514–528.
20. Baldewsing RA, de Korte CL, Schaar JA, Mastik F, van der Steen AF. Finite element modeling and intravascular ultrasound elastography of vulnerable plaques: parameter variation. Ultrasonics. 2004;42:723–729.
21. Schaar JA, De Korte CL, Mastik F, Strijder C, Pasterkamp G, Boersma E, Serruys PW, Van Der Steen AF. Characterizing vulnerable plaque features with intravascular elastography. Circulation. 2003;108:2636–2641.
22. Perrey C, Braeker G, Bojara W, Lindstaedt M, Holt S, Ermert H. Strain imaging with intravascular ultrasound array scanners: validation with phantom experiments. Biomed Tech (Berl). 2003;48:135–140.
23. de Korte CL, Pasterkamp G, van der Steen AF, Woutman HA, Bom N. Characterization of plaque components with intravascular ultrasound elastography in human femoral and coronary arteries in vitro. Circulation. 2000;102:617–623.
24. de Korte CL, Sierevogel MJ, Mastik F, Strijder C, Schaar JA, Velema E, Pasterkamp G, Serruys PW, van der Steen AF. Identification of atherosclerotic plaque components with intravascular ultrasound elastography in vivo: a Yucatan pig study. Circulation. 2002;105:1627–1630.
25. Casscells W, Hathorn B, David M, Krabach T, Vaughn WK, McAllister HA, Bearman G, Willerson JT. Thermal detection of cellular infiltrates in living atherosclerotic plaques: possible implications for plaque rupture and thrombosis. Lancet. 1996;347: 1447–1451.

26. Stefanadis C, Diamantopoulos L, Vlachopoulos C, Tsiamis E, Dernellis J, Toutouzas K, Stefanadi E, Toutouzas P. Thermal heterogeneity within human atherosclerotic coronary arteries detected in vivo: A new method of detection by application of a special thermography catheter. Circulation. 1999;99:1965–1971.
27. Toutouzas K, Drakopoulou M, Mitropoulos J, Tsiamis E, Vaina S, Vavuranakis M, Markou V, Bosinakou E, Stefanadis C. Elevated plaque temperature in non-culprit de novo atheromatous lesions of patients with acute coronary syndromes. J Am Coll Cardiol. 2006;47:301–306.
28. Toutouzas K, Drakopoulou M, Stefanadi E, Siasos G, Stefanadis C. Intracoronary thermography: does it help us in clinical decision making? J Interv Cardiol. 2005;18:485–489.
29. Stefanadis C, Toutouzas K, Tsiamis E, Vavuranakis M, Tsioufis C, Stefanadi E, Boudoulas H. Relation between local temperature and C-reactive protein levels in patients with coronary artery disease: effects of atorvastatin treatment. Atherosclerosis. 2007;192:396–400.
30. Saia F, Schaar J, Regar E, Rodriguez G, De Feyter PJ, Mastik F, Marzocchi A, Marrozzini C, Ortolani P, Palmerini T, Branzi A, van der Steen AF, Serruys PW. Clinical imaging of the vulnerable plaque in the coronary arteries: new intracoronary diagnostic methods. J Cardiovasc Med (Hagerstown). 2006;7:21–28.
31. Tanimoto T, Imanishi T, Tanaka A, Yamano T, Kitabata H, Takarada S, Kubo T, Nakamura N, Hirata K, Mizukoshi M, Akasaka T. Various types of plaque disruption in culprit coronary artery visualized by optical coherence tomography in a patient with unstable angina. Circ J. 2009;73:187–189.
32. Takano M, Yamamoto M, Murakami D, Takano H, Asai K, Yasutake M, Seino Y, Mizuno K. Optical coherence tomography after new scoring balloon angioplasty for in-stent restenosis and de novo coronary lesions. Int J Cardiol. 2009; [Epub ahead of print].
33. Yamaguchi T, Terashima M, Akasaka T, Hayashi T, Mizuno K, Muramatsu T, Nakamura M, Nakamura S, Saito S, Takano M, Takayama T, Yoshikawa J, Suzuki T. Safety and feasibility of an intravascular optical coherence tomography image wire system in the clinical setting. Am J Cardiol. 2008;101:562–567.
34. Xu C, Schmitt JM, Carlier SG, Virmani R. Characterization of atherosclerosis plaques by measuring both backscattering and attenuation coefficients in optical coherence tomography. J Biomed Opt. 2008;13:034003.
35. Takano M, Jang IK, Inami S, Yamamoto M, Murakami D, Okamatsu K, Seimiya K, Ohba T, Mizuno K. In vivo comparison of optical coherence tomography and angioscopy for the evaluation of coronary plaque characteristics. Am J Cardiol. 2008;101:471–476.
36. Choi SH, Chae A, Chen CH, Merki E, Shaw PX, Tsimikas S. Emerging approaches for imaging vulnerable plaques in patients. Curr Opin Biotechnol. 2007;18:73–82.
37. Toussaint JF, LaMuraglia GM, Southern JF, Fuster V, Kantor HL. Magnetic resonance images lipid, fibrous, calcified, hemorrhagic, and thrombotic components of human atherosclerosis in vivo. Circulation. 1996;94:932–938.
38. Farb A, Burke AP, Tang AL, Liang TY, Mannan P, Smialek J, Virmani R. Coronary plaque erosion without rupture into a lipid core. A frequent cause of coronary thrombosis in sudden coronary death. Circulation. 1996;93:1354–1363.

36 Assessment of Plaque Burden and Plaque Composition Using Intravascular Ultrasound

Paul Schoenhagen, Anuja Nair, Stephen Nicholls, and Geoffrey Vince

CONTENTS

ABSTRACT

Intravascular ultrasound (IVUS) allows reliable identification, quantification, and characterization of coronary atherosclerotic plaque and has been validated as a precise atherosclerosis imaging modality. The knowledge accumulated with IVUS already has a major influence on treatment and prevention of coronary artery disease (CAD) and its risk factors. As a tool in clinical trials examining atherosclerotic disease progression, it is an integral part of antiatherosclerotic drug development. The primary endpoint in these trials is progression/regression of plaque burden and changes in plaque characteristics in long segments of the coronary tree, rather than focal assessment of individual "vulnerable plaques." While definitive confirmation in combined imaging and clinical endpoint trials is incomplete, these results strongly suggest that global assessment of plaque burden and plaque characteristics can predict risk of future events or "patient vulnerability."

Key words: Atherosclerosis; Plaque burden; Plaque composition; Intravascular ultrasound; Radiofrequency analysis

From: *Asymptomatic Atherosclerosis: Pathophysiology, Detection and Treatment*
Edited by: M. Naghavi (ed.), DOI 10.1007/978-1-60327-179-0_36

KEY POINTS

- Post mortem studies demonstrate that rupture of nonstenotic coronary plaques and subsequent thrombosis are the main cause of acute coronary syndromes.
- Reproducing findings of post mortem studies, echolucent plaque appearance, and expansive (positive) remodeling by intravascular ultrasound have been associated with plaque instability.
- Advanced tissue characterization with IVUS-derived radiofrequency analysis (virtual histology, VH-IVUS) allows display of plaque composition as color-coded tissue maps on top of standard gray-scale cross-sectional IVUS images.
- Monitoring of progression of coronary atherosclerosis by IVUS is an established endpoint in clinical trials. Multicenter, randomized IVUS trials have collectively demonstrated a beneficial impact of intensive lowering of LDL cholesterol on plaque burden progression.

INTRODUCTION

Intravascular ultrasound (IVUS) allows reliable identification, quantification, and characterization of coronary atherosclerotic plaque and has been validated as a precise atherosclerosis imaging modality. The knowledge accumulated with IVUS already has a major influence on treatment and prevention of coronary artery disease (CAD) and its risk factors. As a tool in clinical trials examining atherosclerotic disease progression, it is an integral part of antiatherosclerotic drug development. The primary endpoint in these trials is progression/regression of plaque burden and changes in plaque characteristics in long segments of the coronary tree, rather than focal assessment of individual "vulnerable plaques." While definitive confirmation in combined imaging and clinical endpoint trials is incomplete, these results strongly suggest that global assessment of plaque burden and plaque characteristics can predict risk of future events or "patient vulnerability."

POST MORTEM OBSERVATIONS AND THE CONCEPT OF PLAQUE VULNERABILITY

Post mortem studies demonstrate that rupture of nonstenotic coronary plaques and subsequent thrombosis are the main cause of acute coronary syndromes (ACS) [1–3]. Plaques at risk of rupture are called vulnerable plaques and are characterized by typical histological features, summarized in the term thin cap fibroatheroma (TCFA) [3]. The plaque structure of a TCFA is characterized by a large necrotic core, which is separated from the coronary lumen by a thin fibrous cap. The size of the necrotic core and the thickness of the fibrous cap are critical for the stability of the plaque. Other characteristics of a vulnerable lesion are expansive enlargement of the vessel wall (positive remodeling), microcalcification, hemorrhage within the lesion, and macrophage accumulation [4–7].

It is important to consider the frequency and distribution of these focal findings in the entire coronary tree [8]. It is obvious that the location of a vulnerable lesion, the length of a lesion, and the number of such lesions are important parameters for the evaluation of vulnerability on a patient-based scale. In fact, histological studies suggest that episodes of plaque destabilization and rupture are common, and are most frequently not associated with clinical symptoms [9,10]. Presumably, after episode of rupture the local balance between thrombosis and spontaneous thrombolysis prevents the occlusion in most vessel segments, and nonocclusive clot formation is then followed by a "healing" process, which is characterized by fibrosis. On the other hand, studies in patients at the time of an acute coronary event suggest that multiple ruptured plaques can be found distant from the "culprit" lesion throughout the coronary tree. Presumably, such patients have an underlying milieu conducive to the development of multifocal plaque ulceration [11]. This systemic vulnerability at the time of acute MI is associated with evidence of systemic inflammation and may explain the high propensity for recurrent acute coronary events in the months following the initial event. Disease/patient vulnerability therefore describes a temporary, systemic biochemical stage of plaque activation with increased risk to rupture at several sites.

The challenge of translating these histologic observations into atherosclerosis imaging is the need to simultaneously observe focal plaque and overall plaque burden, which is a paradigm change from the typical culprit-lesion focused approach with angiography [12].

FROM BENCH TO BEDSIDE: STANDARD GRAY-SCALE IVUS AND LIMITATIONS OF THE TECHNOLOGY

The development of intravascular ultrasound (IVUS) in the 1990s allowed in vivo assessment of the vessel wall [13, 14]. The strong signal reflected from the intima and external elastic membrane (EEM), and the weaker internal ultrasound reflection from the vessels wall/plaque allow identification, characterization, and quantification of atheroma. As a clinical tool in the catheterization laboratory, IVUS complemented the angiographic lumen-based view of CAD [15, 16].

There was early interest in its use to understand the atherosclerotic disease process in vivo, in parallel to the earlier-described histologic findings. IVUS confirmed in vivo that coronary atherosclerosis is commonly present at an early stage and progresses silently over long periods of time. Subclinical progression of accumulating atherosclerotic plaque is associated with outward, expansive remodeling of the arterial wall, initially maintaining luminal dimensions [17]. Similar to post mortem observations, further description of plaque morphology focused on culprit lesions identified by angiography in patients presenting with acute or stable coronary syndromes [18–20]. Reproducing the earlier-described findings of post mortem studies, echolucent appearance and expansive (positive) remodeling by intravascular ultrasound have been associated with the clinical presentation of unstable angina. However, the initial experience demonstrated a number of limitations and challenges:

1. It became obvious that standard gray-scale IVUS imaging is limited for the analysis of the plaque composition. For example, both calcified and densely fibrotic tissues have strong echoreflections. Similarly, areas of low echoreflections can represent necrotic core, fibrotic tissue, intraplaque hemorrhage, or intraluminal thrombus.
2. It became obvious that a better understanding of CAD would require observing temporal changes of coronary anatomy. Most of the post mortem and early imaging observations *retrospectively* describe anatomical characteristics of highly stenotic lesions that had already caused clinical symptoms. However, plaque vulnerability is a *prospective* definition of a plaque at risk to rupture in the future. While it has been inferred that the characteristics present in symptomatic lesion are identical to those of vulnerable lesions before rupture, supporting prospective data are limited. Imaging studies, both with angiography and IVUS, have provided limited insight into the temporal changes. Angiographic studies have relied on retrospective review of prior angiograms of patients later presenting with ACS [21, 22]. A prospective intravascular ultrasound study examined morphologic features in mild-to-moderately stenotic plaques at baseline and hypothesized that certain features would be associated with the development of acute coronary syndromes during follow-up [23]. During 2-year follow-up period, 12 patients had an acute coronary event at a previously examined coronary site. The pre-existing plaques, related to the subsequent acute events, demonstrated an eccentric pattern and the mean percent plaque area was greater than in the patients without acute events. However, there was no statistically significant difference in lumen area between two patient groups. These results suggest that imaging equivalents of the necrotic core could in fact identify lesions at increased risk for future instability. The study also confirms prospectively that, despite significant plaque accumulation, lumen area is preserved at the time of initial study, secondary to expansive remodeling of the vessel wall. Subsequent serial IVUS studies confirmed the hypothesis that plaque-stabilizing therapy is associated with constrictive remodeling [24].
3. It became obvious that despite the critical importance of focal morphological characteristic of vulnerable plaques, an understanding of the distribution and frequency of lesions in the entire coronary tree would be

necessary. Similar to histology, atherosclerosis imaging has challenged the paradigm of individual culprit lesions (the vulnerable plaque) and had demonstrated the diffuse, systemic nature of CAD (the vulnerable patient). Angiographic studies in patients presenting with ACS have demonstrated lesions with characteristics of plaque rupture at multiple sites other than the culprit lesion in patients [25, 26]. Recent IVUS studies also demonstrate the presence of diffuse destabilization throughout the coronary tree in an early time period after an acute coronary syndrome but also in patient with stable clinical presentation [27, 28].

In summary, the initial experience with gray-scale IVUS has allowed to translate and extend histologic findings into in vivo atherosclerosis imaging and identified a number of challenges for the further evaluation, including more precise focal assessment of plaque composition, the volumetric assessment of plaque burden and composition, and the serial assessment of changes over time. In response to these limitations two approaches have developed, which were initially considered competing strategies. In the following we will describe both radiofrequency analysis (RFA) assessment of plaque composition and serial volumetric assessment of plaque burden individually, but then argue that these need to be combined into composite endpoints of disease progression and regression.

BEYOND VISUAL GRAY-SCALE ANALYSIS: RADIOFREQUENCY ANALYSIS OF PLAQUE COMPONENTS

The reflected ultrasound signal contains more information than displayed in the standard gray-scale display. The additional information can be analyzed by advanced mathematical algorithms, including radiofrequency analysis (RFA) and elastography [29, 30].

Advanced tissue characterization with IVUS-derived virtual histology (VH-IVUS) is based on RFA of reflected ultrasound signals and displays the reconstructed data as a color-coded tissue map of plaque composition on top of standard gray-scale cross-sectional IVUS images (Fig. 1) [29]. Initial evaluation was based on the evaluation of cross-sectional images in comparison to histology [31–34].

VH-IVUS classifies plaque components into four basic tissue types (Fig. 2): fibrous (dark-green), fibro-fatty (light-green), necrotic core (red), and dense calcium (white). Fibrous tissue is represented as dark green pixels. In histologic comparison, this tissue is characterized by bundles of collagen fibers with little to no lipid accumulation [35]. Fibro-fatty tissue is represented in VH-IVUS as light green pixels. Histology demonstrates loosely packed collagen fibers and proteoglycan, with interspersed foam cell accumulation [35]. There is no necrotic core, and cholesterol clefts are either absent or rare. Macrophages may be present and indicate an initial or ongoing inflammatory response. Necrotic core tissue is represented in VH-IVUS as red pixels. In histologic comparison there is significant presence of extracellular lipid and remnants of dead lipid filled smooth muscle cells, macrophage foam cells, trapped red cells, and fibrin [35]. There is little to no collagen, and there is

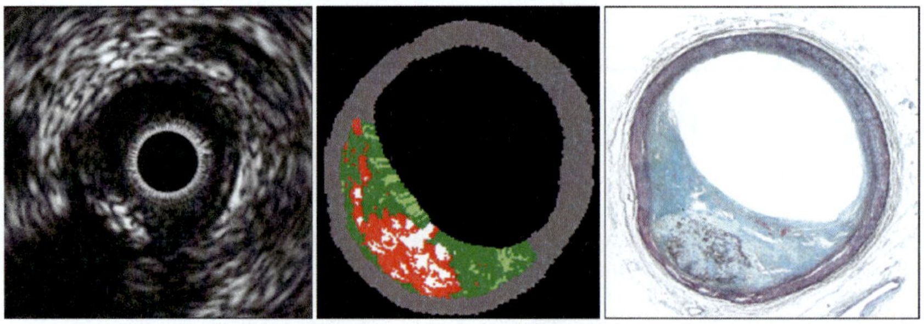

Fig. 1. This figure shows an IVUS gray-scale image (*left*), VH-IVUS cross-sectional image (*middle*), and a histologic cross-section of a fibrocalcific plaque.

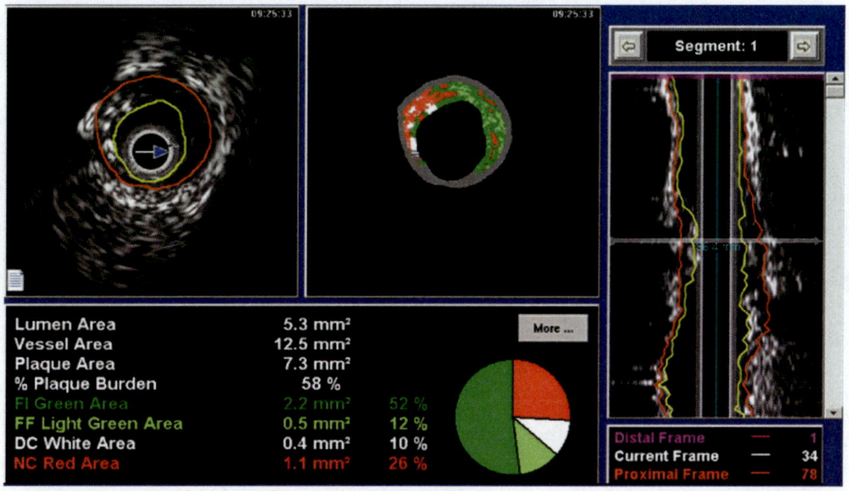

Fig. 2. This figure shows VH-IVUS analysis of a vessel segment. A longitudinal view (*right*) allows localization of the analyzed cross-section. In the analyzed cross-section, planimetry of the lumen and EEM area allows assessment of plaque burden. VH-IVUS analysis provides quantitative assessment of plaque components.

absence of a matrix. Microcalcification or areas of solid calcification are often observed. Dense calcium is represented in VH-IVUS as a white pixel, and compact calcium deposits.

In a recent study IVUS backscatter data from 51 left anterior descending coronary arteries were tested ex vivo and compared to the histological interpretation of the matched site. The overall predictive accuracies were 93.5% for fibrotic tissue, 94.1% for fibro-fatty tissue, 95.8% for necrotic core, and 96.7% for dense calcium [35].

While these postprocessing techniques provide additional information about plaque composition, it is important to remember that they are derived from the same IVUS data and are therefore subject to the same limitation, in particular in regard to spatial resolution. The axial resolution of VH-IVUS (100–200 mm) is too low to detect critical fibrous cap thickness, which by histology is defined as 65 mm. Despite better differentiation of low echogenic reflexes with VH-IVUS a differential diagnosis between soft plaque material and intraluminal organizing thrombus is currently not possible by RF analysis. The inflammatory activity of the plaque representing the actual vulnerability of the interrogated lesion cannot be directly visualized by VH-IVUS imaging.

Further analysis of this compositional data allows cross-sectional classification of plaque types and volumetric analysis of plaque components. For focal, cross-sectional plaque classification with VH-IVUS discrete lesion types is defined by their tissue composition, in analogy to recent histopathological classification [3]. These types include pathologic intimal thickening, fibroatheromas, and fibrotic-calcific plaques. Pathologic intimal thickening is a mixture of fibrous and fibrofatty plaque with absence or small amount of necrotic core (<10% confluent necrotic core) and absent or small amount of microcalcification <10% [36]. Fibroatheroma (FA) is a plaque with a true necrotic core. A fibrous cap separates the coronary lumen from the necrotic core and consists of smooth muscle cells in a proteoglycan-rich collagen matrix. The amount of inflammatory cells within the fibrous cap is variable. As lesions progress, the fibrous cap overlying the necrotic core is assumed to become thinner, and when the thickness is <65 mm, the lesion is classified as a thin cap fibroatheroma (TCFA) by histology. As described earlier several of these characteristics are below the resolution of IVUS. Therefore, VH-IVUS defines a FA as a confluent necrotic core >10% of the total plaque volume in a mainly fibrous and/or fibro-fatty tissue. The amount of calcium is variable. The longitudinal distribution of the necrotic core can be either focal or diffuse.

The IVUS-derived fibroatheroma (ID TCFA) is assumed to be the precursor of vulnerable plaques. There is ongoing research in the further classification of ID-TCFA, based on size and confluence of the necrotic core, absence of evidence of a visible fibrous cap, presence of minor amount of calcium, length of the necrotic core against the lumen surface, occurrence of multiple, confluent necrotic cores and positive remodeling [37–39]. Based on current data, the most vulnerable plaque type is a TCFA with a confluent necrotic core >20%, no evidence of a fibrous cap, an amount of calcium >10% with a speckled appearance. In vivo studies using VH-IVUS have shown that presumed vulnerable plaques (ID TCFAs) occur more often in patients with acute coronary syndrome than in patients with stable angina. In the Carotid Artery Plaque Virtual Histology Evaluation (CAPITAL) study a strong correlation between VH-IVUS plaque characterization and the true histological examination of the plaque following endarterectomy was found. Specifically, there was a high predictive accuracy for the identification of TCFA [40]. However, prospective validation is currently limited.

Fibrocalcific plaques are predominantly fibrous plaques with dense calcium (>10% of confluent plaque volume) (Fig. 1). There can be a minor amount of confluent necrotic core (<10% of the plaque volume). The role of fibrocalcific plaques in the evolutionary process of native coronary atherosclerosis is incompletely understood. However, densely calcified tissue as the predominant plaque component is frequently found in advanced stages of atherosclerosis.

While focal description of plaque composition is important, there is increasing interest in reconstruction of VH-IVUS images in a longitudinal view, thus allowing a more comprehensive analysis of the total length of the plaque, and its location in relation to the rest of the coronary tree (Figs. 2 and 3). The importance of location has been described in angiographic studies showing that acute

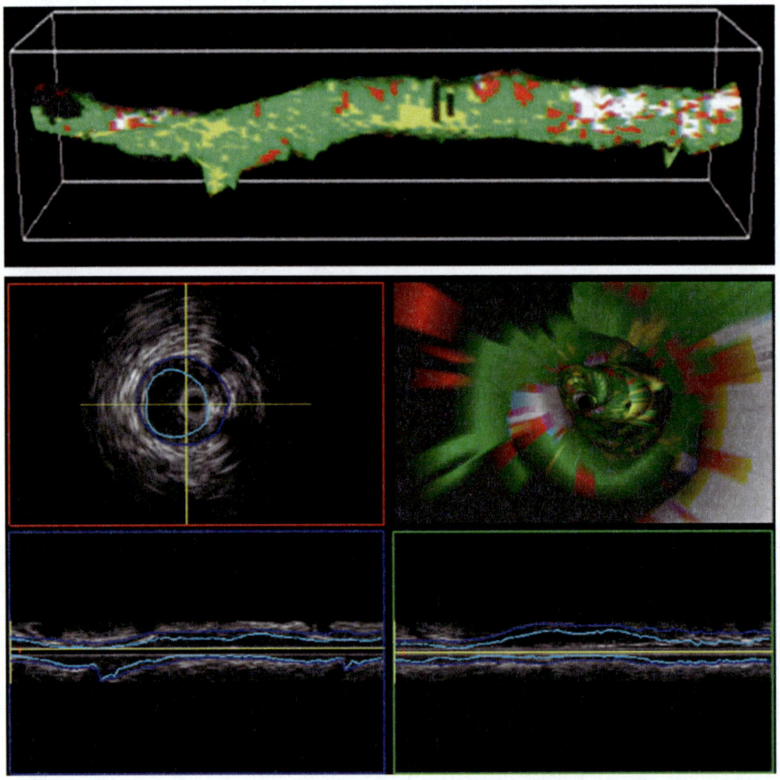

Fig. 3. Advanced 3-D reconstruction of entire coronary artery segments can show localization and distribution of plaque components and will allow volumetric analysis of plaque components as en endpoint in progression/regression trials.

coronary occlusions leading to STEMI tend to cluster in predictable "hot spots," especially in the proximal third of the coronary arteries [41]. Recent in vivo studies with VH-IVUS demonstrate that plaque composition has a nonuniform longitudinal distribution along the coronary arteries, with higher incidence of ID TCFAs closer to the ostium [42].

The emerging results with VH-IVUS are encouraging. Similar to IVUS plaque burden, confirmation of its usefulness as an endpoint in clinical trials will be necessary in large multicenter progression/ regression trials. The ongoing PROSPECT trial (Providing Regional Observations to Study Predictors of Events in the Coronary Tree; ClinicalTrials.gov identifier: NCT00180466) is a natural history study to assess the relationship of unexpected acute coronary events and plaque burden, composition, and type in intermediate lesions. It is the first prospective study that is aimed detecting high-risk lesions using both gray-scale and VH IVUS technologies.

PLAQUE BURDEN AS THE PRIMARY ENDPOINT IN SERIAL PROGRESSION REGRESSION TRIALS

A number of imaging modalities are used to evaluate the impact of medical therapies on progression and regression of atherosclerosis [43]. IVUS permits precise determination of the lumen and EEM borders. Given the negligible thickness of the medial layer of the artery wall, consensus guidelines consider the area between the intima and EEM borders to represent atherosclerotic plaque (intima-media area) [15, 16]. While early serial studies attempted to compare the plaque area at a specific site at different time points, the difficulty matching individual slices suggested that comparing plaque volume in segments defined by the fixed anatomic location of side branches would be the preferred approach.

Monitoring of progression of coronary atherosclerosis by IVUS has subsequently been employed in a large number of clinical trials. Volumetric analysis approaches integrate consecutive plaque area measurements at 0.5–1 mm intervals along long vessel segments, which are typically defined by the fixed anatomic location of side branches to ensure precise matching. The change in plaque volume from baseline to the end of study in a long segment of coronary artery is the primary endpoint. Monitoring volume over a large segment of vessel provides more statistical power to detect small changes in plaque burden than an approach, which compares the plaque area at one specific location in the vessel [43, 44]. Total atheroma volume (TAV) within the segment of interest is determined by summation of the plaque areas from each image (n) using the equation:

$$\text{TAV} = \Sigma_n\,(\text{EEM}_{\text{area}} - \text{Lume}_{\text{area}}).$$

In order to account for variability in arterial segment length evaluated in different subjects, TAV is "normalized" to the median number of images in the entire study population using the equation:

$$\text{TAV}_{\text{normalized}} = \frac{\sum(\text{EEM}_{\text{area}} - \text{Lumen}_{\text{area}})}{\text{Number of images in pullback}} \times \text{Median number of images in cohort.}$$

In addition, the percent atheroma volume (PAV) expresses plaque volume as a proportion of the EEM:

$$\text{PAV} = \frac{\sum(\text{EEM}_{\text{area}} - \text{Lumen}_{\text{area}})}{\sum(\text{EEM}_{\text{area}})} \times 100.$$

Results of Volumetric Progression/Regression Trials

Multicenter, randomized IVUS trials have collectively demonstrated a beneficial impact of intensive lowering of LDL cholesterol on plaque progression with statins [44–48]. In an early report the GAIN investigators demonstrated a change in the hyperechogenicity index, a surrogate marker of plaque composition, based on visual gray-scale analysis [45]. This marker of fibrous tissue of the plaque increased to a larger extent for the atorvastatin group than for the usual care group. The REVERSAL trial [44] showed arrest of progression with intensive lowering of LDL cholesterol to 79 mg/dL. The additional findings that C-reactive protein (CRP) was lowered 36.4% by atorvastatin and that changes in CRP correlated with the rate of plaque progression and remodeling [24,46], suggested a central role of inflammation in plaque progression and remodeling. The ESTABLISH trial demonstrated early regression in a small arterial segment with early statin treatment in 70 patients with acute coronary syndrome [47]. Finally, in the ASTEROID trial intensive the combination of lowering LDL cholesterol and raising HDL cholesterol with rosuvastatin was associated with plaque regression [48].

The independent role of HDL [49] has been demonstrated in studies in which synthetic forms of HDL were administered to patients with a recent ACS. In the first proof-of-concept study patients within 2 weeks of an acute coronary syndrome received five weekly infusions of reconstituted HDL particles containing recombinant apoA-I Milano and phospholipid or placebo. Plaque regression was observed in patients who received infusions of HDL [50]. In a more recent study, a similar benefit was observed with infusions of reconstituted HDL, which contained wild-type apoA-I [51].

However, other lipid-modifying treatments with potential shown in animal and preclinical studies, including inhibition of acyl-coenzyme A:cholesterol acyltransferase (ACAT) and cholesteryl ester transfer protein (CETP) did not demonstrate benefit in clinical IVUS trials [52–54]. For these medications, it remains unclear if the lack of effect on plaque burden is a class effect or results from molecule-specific toxicities.

Extending beyond the management of lipids, IVUS imaging demonstrated the effect of amlodipine and enalapril on plaque burden in the CAMELOT trial and its relationship to blood pressure control [55,56]. More recently, a pooled analysis of 1,515 patients from four IVUS trials supported the hypothesis that beta-blocker therapy is associated with reduced atheroma progression in adults with known coronary artery disease, a finding which remained significant after controlling for heart rate and blood pressure [57]. Ongoing IVUS studies evaluate the effect of the PPAR-agonist, pioglitazone, in patients with diabetes mellitus and of the endocannibanoid receptor antagonist rimonabant on plaque progression in patients with obesity and coronary artery disease [58].

Serial volumetric IVUS progression/regression trials have already become an integral part of antiatherosclerotic drug development and have already changed treatment approaches for patients with CAD. The validity of this approach as an intermediate endpoint in progression/regression trials is best documented for carotid ultrasound (CIMT) and coronary intravascular ultrasound (IVUS) [44,52–54, 59]. In these studies the change in plaque burden has been concordant with clinical endpoint in similar designed studies [60, 61]. However, evidence of large combined imaging and clinical endpoint trials is incomplete.

CONCLUSION: VOLUMETRIC PLAQUE BURDEN AND PLAQUE COMPOSITION. TOWARDS A COMBINED ENDPOINT IN PROGRESSION/REGRESSION TRIALS

As described above, the development of IVUS has extended our understanding of the natural history of atherosclerosis including plaque burden, plaque composition, arterial remodeling, and plaque vulnerability. Atherosclerosis imaging with IVUS in the context of serial progression/regression trials allows applying these observations as imaging endpoints. The ability to evaluate the same arterial segment at different time points provides a unique opportunity to define the impact of a wide range of antiatherosclerotic strategies on the progression of atherosclerotic plaque. Demonstrating a beneficial or detrimental impact of experimental agents on plaque progression rates has become a powerful tool in the development of new pharmacological compounds.

As described earlier, serial volumetric assessment of plaque burden and RFA assessment of plaque composition have developed simultaneously and often in parallel but have initially been considered as competing approaches. Interestingly, an early progression/regression trial [45] found changes in plaque burden, associated with changes in the hyperechogenicity index, a marker of fibrous tissue content of the plaque.

The reviewed data support the notion that RFA assessment of plaque composition and serial volumetric assessment of plaque burden together, as a composite endpoint of disease progression and regression, would provide further insight into disease progression/regression and in particular vulnerability. However, further validation of the individual approaches and eventual correlation with clinical endpoints in combined imaging and clinical endpoint studies will be necessary.

REFERENCES

1. Libby P, Theroux P. Pathophysiology of coronary artery disease. Circulation 2005;111:3481–3488.
2. Burke AP, Farb A, Malcom GT, et al. Coronary risk factors and plaque morphology in men with coronary disease who died suddenly. N Engl J Med 1997;336:1276–1282.
3. Virmani R, Kolodgie FD, Burke AP, et al. Lessons from sudden coronary death: A comprehensive morphological classification scheme for atherosclerotic lesions. Arterioscler Thromb Vasc Biol 2000;20:1262–1275.
4. Pasterkamp G, Schoneveld AH, van der Wal AC, et al. Relation of arterial geometry to luminal narrowing and histologic markers for plaque vulnerability: The remodeling paradox. J Am Coll Cardiol 1998;32:655–662.
5. Varnava AM, Mills PG, Davies MJ. Relationship between coronary artery remodeling and plaque vulnerability. Circulation 2002;105:939–943.
6. Kolodgie FD, Gold HK, Burke AP, et al. Intraplaque hemorrhage and progression of coronary atheroma. N Engl J Med 2003;349:2316–2325.
7. Moreno PR, Falk E, Palacios IF, et al. Macrophage infiltration in acute coronary syndromes: Implications for plaque rupture. Circulation 1994;90:775–777.
8. Cheruvu PK, Finn AV, Gardner C, et al. Frequency and distribution of thin-cap fibroatheroma and ruptured plaques in human coronary arteries: A pathologic study. J Am Coll Cardiol 2007;50:940–949.
9. Mann J, Davies MJ. Mechanisms of progression in native coronary artery disease: Role of healed plaque disruption. Heart 1999;82:265–268.
10. Burke AP, Kolodgie FD, Farb A, et al. Healed plaque ruptures and sudden coronary death: Evidence that subclinical rupture has a role in plaque progression. Circulation 2001;103:934–940.
11. Buffon A, Biasucci LM, Liuzzo G, et al. Widespread coronary inflammation in unstable angina. N Engl J Med 2002;347:5–12.
12. Topol EJ, Nissen SE. Our preoccupation with coronary luminology. The dissociation between clinical and angiographic findings in ischemic heart disease. Circulation 1995;92:2333–2334.
13. Gussenhoven EJ, Essed CE, Lancee CT, et al. Arterial wall characteristics determined by intravascular ultrasound imaging: An in vitro study. J Am Coll Cardiol 1989;14:947–952.
14. Nissen SE, Grines CL, Gurley JC, et al. Application of a new phased-array ultrasound imaging catheter in the assessment of vascular dimensions. In vivo comparison to cineangiography. Circulation 1990;81:660–666.
15. Mintz GS, Nissen SE, Anderson WD, et al. American college of cardiology clinical expert consensus document on standards for acquisition, measurement and reporting of intravascular ultrasound studies (IVUS). J Am Coll Cardiol 2001;37:1478–1492.
16. Di Mario C, Gorge G, Peters R, et al. Clinical application and image interpretation in intracoronary ultrasound. Study group on intracoronary imaging of the working group of coronary circulation and of the subgroup on intravascular ultrasound of the working group of echocardiography of the European society of cardiology. Eur Heart J 1998;19:207–229.
17. Glagov S, Weisenberg E, Zarins CK, et al. Compensatory enlargement of human atherosclerotic coronary arteries. N Engl J Med 1987;316:1371–1375.
18. Hodgson JMcB, Reddy KG, Suneja R, et al. Intracoronary ultrasound imaging: Correlation of plaque morphology with angiography, clinical syndrome and procedural results in patients undergoing coronary angioplasty. J Am Coll Cardiol 1993;21:35–44.
19. Schoenhagen P, Ziada KM, Kapadia SR, et al. Extent and direction of arterial remodeling in stable and unstable coronary syndromes. Circulation 2000;101:598–603.

20. Nakamura M, Nishikawa H, Mukai S, et al. Impact of coronary artery remodeling on clinical presentation of coronary artery disease: An intravascular ultrasound study. J Am Coll Cardiol 2001;37:63–69.
21. Ambrose JA, Tannenbaum MA, Alexopoulos D, et al. Angiographic progression of coronary artery disease and the development of myocardial infarction. J Am Coll Cardiol 1988;12:56–62.
22. Ojio S, Takatsu H, Tanaka T, et al. Considerable time from the onset of plaque rupture and/or thrombi until the onset of acute myocardial infarction in humans: Coronary angiographic findings within 1 week before the onset of infarction. Circulation 2000;102:2063–2069.
23. Yamagishi M, Terashima M, Awano K, et al. Morphology of vulnerable coronary plaque: Insights from follow-up of patients examined by intravascular ultrasound before and acute coronary syndrome. J Am Coll Cardiol 2000;35:106–111.
24. Schoenhagen P, Tuzcu EM, Apperson-Hansen C, et al. Determinants of arterial wall remodeling during lipid-lowering therapy: Serial intravascular ultrasound observations from the reversal of atherosclerosis with aggressive lipid lowering therapy (REVERSAL) trial. Circulation 2006;113:2826–2834.
25. Goldstein JA, Demetriou D, Grines CL, et al. Multiple complex coronary plaques in patients with acute myocardial infarction. N Engl J Med 2000;343:915–922.
26. Guazzi MD, Bussotti M, Grancini L, et al. Evidence of multifocal activity of coronary disease in patients with acute myocardial infarction. Circulation 1997;96:1145–1151.
27. Rioufol G, Finet G, Ginon I, et al. Multiple atherosclerotic plaque rupture in acute coronary syndrome: A three-vessel intravascular ultrasound study. Circulation 2002;106:804–808.
28. Schoenhagen P, Stone GW, Nissen SE, et al. Coronary plaque morphology and frequency of ulceration distant from culprit lesions in patients with unstable and stable presentation. Arterioscler Thromb Vasc Biol 2003;23:1895–1900.
29. König A, Klauss V. Virtual histology. Heart 2007;93:977–982.
30. de Korte CL, Pasterkamp G, van der Steen AF, et al. Characterization of plaque components with intravascular ultrasound elastography in human femoral and coronary arteries in vitro. Circulation 2000;102:617–623.
31. Nair A, Kuban BD, Tuzcu EM, et al. Coronary plaque classification with intravascular ultrasound radiofrequency data analysis. Circulation 2002;106:2200–2206.
32. Kawasaki M, Takatsu H, Noda T, et al. Noninvasive quantitative tissue characterization and two-dimensional color-coded map of human atherosclerotic lesions using ultrasound integrated backscatter: Comparison between histology and integrated backscatter images. J Am Coll Cardiol 2001;38:486–492.
33. Takiuchi S, Rakugi H, Honda K, et al. Quantitative ultrasonic tissue characterization can identify high-risk atherosclerotic alteration in human carotid arteries. Circulation 2000;102:766–770.
34. Stahr PM, Hofflinghaus T, Voigtlander T, et al. Discrimination of early/intermediate and advanced/complicated coronary plaque types by radiofrequency intravascular ultrasound analysis. Am J Cardiol 2002;90:19–23.
35. Nair A, et al. Automated coronary plaque characterisation with intravascular ultrasound backscatter: Ex vivo validation. EuroInterv 2007;3:113–120.
36. Nakashima Y, Fujii H, Sumiyoshi S, et al. Early human atherosclerosis: Accumulation of lipid and proteoglycans in intimal thickenings followed by macrophage infiltration. Arterioscler Thromb Vasc Biol 2007;27:1159–1165.
37. Rodriguez-Granillo GA, García-García HM, Mc Fadden EP, et al. In vivo intravascular ultrasound-derived thin cap fibroatheroma detection using ultrasound radiofrequency data analysis. J Am Coll Cardiol 2005;46:2038–2042.
38. Rodriguez-Granillo GA, Vaina S, García-García HM, et al. Reproducibility of intravascular ultrasound radiofrequency data analysis: Implications for the design of longitudinal studies. Int J Cardiovasc Imaging 2006;22:621–631.
39. Rodriguez-Granillo GA, Serruys PW, Garcia-Garcia HM, et al. Coronary artery remodelling is related to plaque composition. Heart 2006;92:388–391.
40. Diethrich EB, Margolis PM, Reid DB, et al. Virtual histology intravascular ultrasound assessment of carotid artery disease: The carotid artery plaque virtual histology evaluation (CAPITAL) study. J Endovasc Ther 2007;14:676–686.
41. Wang JC, Normand SL, Mauri L, et al. Coronary artery spatial distribution of acute myocardial infarction occlusions. Circulation 2004;110:278–284.
42. Valgimigli M, Rodriguez-Granillo GA, Garcia-Garcia HM, et al. Distance from the ostium as an independent determinant of coronary plaque composition in vivo: An intravascular ultrasound study based radiofrequency data analysis in humans. Eur Heart J 2006;27:655–666.
43. Sankatsing RR, de Groot E, Jukema JW, et al. Surrogate markers for atherosclerotic disease. Curr Opin Lipidol 2005;16:434–441.
44. Nissen SE, Tuzcu EM, Schoenhagen P, et al. REVERSAL investigators. Effect of intensive compared with moderate lipid-lowering therapy on progression of coronary atherosclerosis: A randomized controlled trial. JAMA 2004;291:1071–1080.
45. Schartl M, Bocksch W, Koschyk DH, et al. Use of intravascular ultrasound to compare effects of different strategies of lipid-lowering therapy on plaque volume and composition in patients with coronary artery disease. Circulation 2001;104:387–392.
46. Nissen SE, Tuzcu EM, Schoenhagen P, et al. Reversal of atherosclerosis with aggressive lipid lowering (REVERSAL) investigators. Statin therapy, LDL cholesterol, C-reactive protein, and coronary artery disease. N Engl J Med 2005;352:29–38.
47. Okazaki S, Yokoyama T, Miyauchi K, et al. Early statin treatment in patients with acute coronary syndrome: Demonstration of the beneficial effect on atherosclerotic lesions by serial volumetric intravascular ultrasound analysis during half a year after coronary event: The ESTABLISH study. Circulation 2004;110:1061–1068.

48. Nissen SE, Nicholls SJ, Sipahi I, et al. Effect of very high-intensity statin therapy on regression of coronary atherosclerosis: The ASTEROID trial. JAMA 2006;295:1556–1565.
49. Nicholls SJ, Tuzcu EM, Sipahi I, et al. Statins, high-density lipoprotein cholesterol, and regression of coronary atherosclerosis. JAMA 2007;297:499–508.
50. Nissen SE, Tsunoda T, Tuzcu EM, et al. Effect of recombinant ApoA-I Milano on coronary atherosclerosis in patients with acute coronary syndromes: A randomized controlled trial. JAMA 2003;290:2292–2300.
51. Tardif JC, Gregoire J, L'Allier PL, et al. Effects of reconstituted high-density lipoprotein infusions on coronary atherosclerosis: A randomized controlled trial. JAMA 2007;297:1675–1682.
52. Tardif JC, Gregoire J, L'Allier PL, et al. Effects of the acyl coenzyme A:cholesterol acyltransferase inhibitor avasimibe on human atherosclerotic lesions. Circulation 2004;110:3372–3377.
53. Nissen SE, Tuzcu EM, Brewer HB, et al. ACTIVATE investigators. Effect of ACAT inhibition on the progression of coronary atherosclerosis. N Engl J Med 2006;354:1253–1263.
54. Nissen SE, Tardif JC, Nicholls SJ, et al. ILLUSTRATE investigators. Effect of torcetrapib on the progression of coronary atherosclerosis. N Engl J Med 2007;356:1304–1316.
55. Nissen SE, Tuzcu EM, Libby P, et al. Effect of antihypertensive agents on cardiovascular events in patients with coronary disease and normal blood pressure: The CAMELOT study: A randomized controlled trial. JAMA 2004;292:2217–2225.
56. Sipahi I, Tuzcu EM, Schoenhagen P, et al. Effects of normal, pre-hypertensive, and hypertensive blood pressure levels on progression of coronary atherosclerosis. J Am Coll Cardiol 2006;48:833–838.
57. Sipahi I, Tuzcu EM, Wolski KE, et al. Beta-blockers and progression of coronary atherosclerosis: Pooled analysis of 4 intravascular ultrasonography trials. Ann Intern Med 2007;147:10–18.
58. Schoenhagen P, Nissen SE. Coronary atherosclerotic disease burden: An emerging endpoint in progression/regression studies using intravascular ultrasound. Curr Drug Targets Cardiovasc Haematol Disord 2003;3:218–226.
59. Taylor AJ, Kent SM, Flaherty PJ, et al. ARBITER: Arterial biology for the investigation of the treatment effects of reducing cholesterol: A randomized trial comparing the effects of atorvastatin and pravastatin on carotid intima medial thickness. Circulation 2002;106:2055–2060.
60. Cannon CP, Braunwald E, McCabe CH, et al. Intensive versus moderate lipid lowering with statins after acute coronary syndromes. N Engl J Med 2004;350:1495–1504.
61. Barter PJ, Caulfield M, Eriksson M, Grundy SM, Kastelein JJ, Komajda M, Lopez-Sendon J, Mosca L, Tardif JC, Waters DD, Shear CL, Revkin JH, Buhr KA, Fisher MR, Tall AR, Brewer B. ILLUMINATE investigators. Effects of torcetrapib in patients at high risk for coronary events. N Engl J Med 2007;357:2109–2122.

37

Vulnerable Anatomy; The Role of Coronary Anatomy and Endothelial Shear Stress in the Progression and Vulnerability of Coronary Artery Lesions: *Is Anatomy Destiny?*

Charles L. Feldman, Yiannis S. Chatzizisis, Ahmet U. Coskun, Konstantinos C. Koskinas, Morteza Naghavi, and Peter H. Stone

Contents

Abstract

It is well recognized for that anatomic variations play a key role in the localization of atherosclerosis in the coronary arterial system as well as in other susceptible arteries. Several decades of in vitro research as well as in vivo studies in noncoronary arteries such as carotid arteries, first established that the factor responsible for local atherosclerosis formation and progression was low endothelial shear stress (ESS), caused by irregularities in arterial geometry and the resulting variations in local blood flow patterns.

Recent in vivo studies in humans and diabetic, hypercholesterolemic swine have shown unequivocally that low ESS promotes the development of early fibroatheromas, which subsequently follow an individualized natural history of progression. This individual natural history is critically dependent on the magnitude

From: *Asymptomatic Atherosclerosis: Pathophysiology, Detection and Treatment*
Edited by: M. Naghavi (ed.), DOI 10.1007/978-1-60327-179-0_37

of low ESS, which subsequently regulates the severity of inflammation within the wall and ultimately the vascular remodeling response. High-risk plaques develop in arterial areas with the lowest values of ESS, which enhance plaque inflammation leading to excessive expansive remodeling. Excessive expansive remodeling leads to perpetuation, or even exacerbation, of the local low ESS environment, thereby setting up a self-perpetuating vicious cycle among low local ESS, inflammation, and excessive expansive remodeling, which transforms an early fibroatheroma to a high-risk plaque. In view of this is seems reasonable to talk of vulnerable anatomy, with the understanding that local coronary anatomy is dynamic, ever changing with the growth and regression of individual plaques and that the mediating factor, connecting anatomy to disease, is ESS.

Key words: Atherosclerosis; Endothelial Shear Stress; Vulnerable Plaque; Periadventitial Fat; Pericardial Fat; Vascular Profiling; Intravascular Ultrasound (IVUS)

INTRODUCTION

Atherosclerosis is a chronic inflammatory, fibroproliferative disease primarily of large and medium-sized conduit arteries, whose clinical manifestations constitute the primary cause of morbidity and mortality in the industrialized world [1]. Despite the systemic nature of atherosclerosis, its distribution is multifocal and heterogeneous, such that multiple atherosclerotic lesions at a different stage of progression coexist in the same individual indeed, in the same artery at a single point in time [2, 3].

Although the entire coronary artery system is exposed to identical, systemic risk factors, lesions form preferentially at branch points and on the inner surfaces of curved arterial segments. Other anatomic variations that seem to confer increased risk on "vulnerable" portions of the arterial tree are variations in the geometry of the aortic bifurcation [4] and the length of the left main coronary artery [5].

The first evidence implicating endothelial shear stress (ESS) in the localization of atherosclerosis was described over 40-years ago by Caro et al. [6]. Later, sophisticated computational fluid dynamic simulations in autopsy-based models of coronary arteries [7], carotid bifurcations [8], and distal abdominal aortas [9] showed that areas with low ESS correlated with the localization of atherosclerosis found at autopsy. Further support of the atherogenic role of low ESS was also derived from in vivo experiments in animal models [10–13]. In vivo investigations in humans, utilizing a combination of intravascular ultrasound (IVUS), or magnetic resonance imaging, and computational fluid dynamics confirmed the mechanistic role of low ESS in the development and progression of atherosclerosis [14–16].

When atherosclerotic lesions form, each presents its own potential for progression and risk. A portion of atherosclerotic lesions are thin cap fibroatheromas (i.e., TCFAs) prone to acute disruption, and consequent acute coronary syndrome; a second portion progress to lumen narrowing fibro-calcific lesions with the potential to cause stable angina pectoris; by far the largest portion become quiescent with no clinical consequences [17]. Furthermore, certain arterial segments, such as myocardial bridges, seem to be immune to the development of atherosclerosis.

The purpose of this brief review will be to present the evidence linking ESS to coronary artery disease, explain how ESS is measured in vivo, connect the magnitude of low ESS to plaque morphology and discuss how this information might be used clinically.

DEFINITION OF ESS AND THE ROLE OF ESS IN THE DEVELOPMENT OF CORONARY ATHEROSCLEROSIS

ESS is the tangential stress derived from the friction of the flowing blood on the endothelial surface of the arterial wall [18, 19] (Fig. 1a). The pulsatile nature of the coronary blood flow in combination with the blood's rheological properties and the complex geometric configuration of the coronary

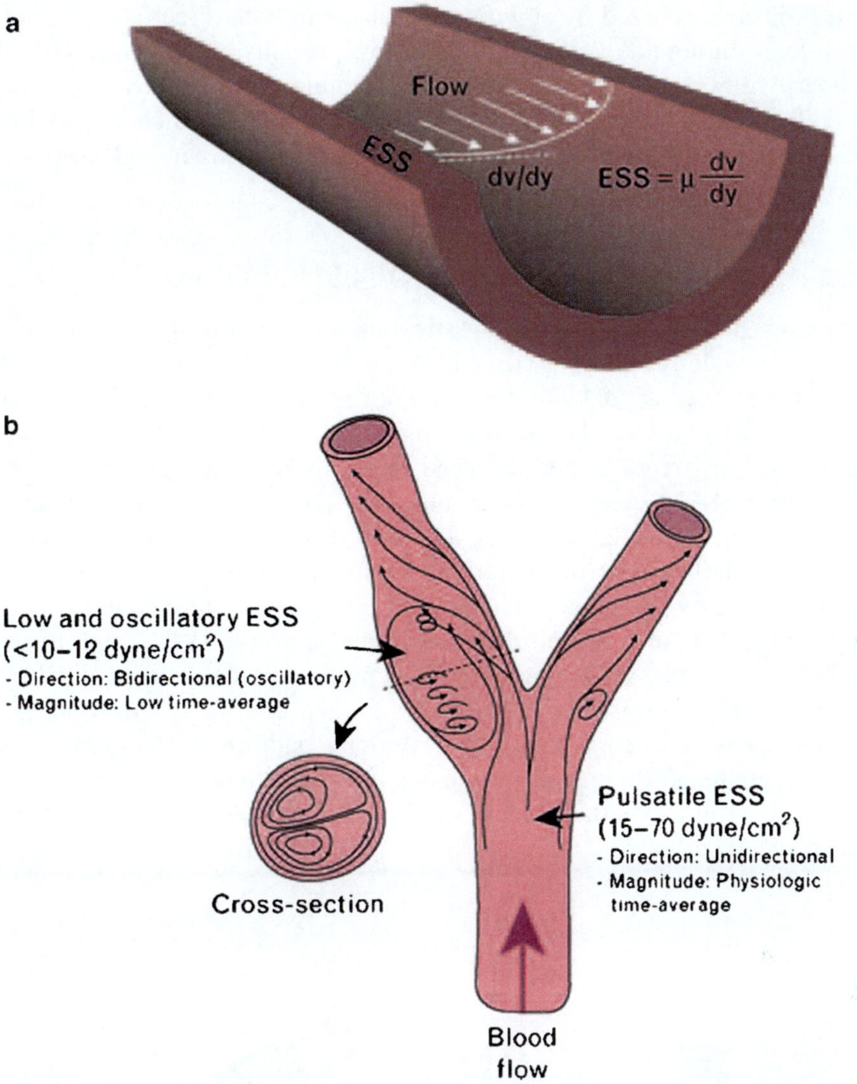

Fig. 1. (**a**) Endothelial shear stress (ESS) is proportional to the product of blood viscosity (μ) and the spatial gradient of blood velocity at the wall (dv/dy). It is expressed in units of force per unit area [N/m^2 or Pascal (Pa) or $dyne/cm^2$; $1\ N/m^2 = 1\ Pa = 10\ dyne/cm^2$]. Reprinted from [18]. (**b**) Definition of ESS patterns. Reprinted from [8].

arteries determines the ESS patterns, which are characterized by direction and magnitude [18, 20, 21] (Fig. 1b). In relatively straight arterial segments, ESS is pulsatile and unidirectional with a magnitude that varies within a range of 1.5–7.0 Pa over the cardiac cycle and yields a positive time-average.

In contrast, in geometrically irregular regions, where disturbed laminar flow occurs, pulsatile flow generates low and/or oscillatory ESS. Low ESS refers to ESS which is unidirectional at any given point with a fluctuating magnitude during the cardiac cycle that results in a significantly low time-average (<1.0–1.2 Pa) [14] (Fig. 1b). Low ESS typically occurs at the inner areas of curvatures, as well as upstream of stenoses.

Oscillatory ESS is characterized by significant changes in both direction and magnitude between systole and diastole, resulting in a very low time-average, usually close to zero (Fig. 1b). Oscillatory ESS occurs primarily downstream of stenoses, at the lateral walls of bifurcations and in the vicinity of branch points. Beside the temporal oscillations, ESS exhibits significant spatial oscillations over short distances, especially in geometrically irregular regions, resulting in high spatial gradients, which are also involved in atherosclerosis [22, 23].

MEASUREMENT OF ESS IN VIVO

The most comprehensive technique for investigating the relationship between ESS and vascular pathobiology is a methodology known as *vascular profiling,* which utilizes routine IVUS and coronary angiography to create an accurate 3D representation of the coronary artery, and this forms the basis of identifying both local ESS and vascular remodeling behavior [14, 24] (Fig. 2). Vascular profiling is accurate [25–27] and highly reproducible [28], and can be used to track changes in lumen, wall thickness and ESS in periods as short as 6–9 months in human [14, 29] or in experimental animals [13].

In brief, the 3D anatomy of the coronary artery is reconstructed from IVUS images and two planes of angiography. IVUS is performed with a controlled pullback, typically 0.5 mm/s and the ECG is recorded with the IVUS images. The arterial lumen and outer vessel wall are reconstructed by locating digitized and segmented end-diastolic frames onto the IVUS core, the path of which is determined from the two planes of angiography. Flow rate is typically determined by measuring the time required for injected contrast medium to fill a known arterial volume and blood viscosity is estimated from the measured hematocrit. Local velocity patterns are determined by numerically solving the basic equations of fluid mechanics, using any one of a number of commercially available solvers and ESS is determined as the product of blood viscosity and velocity gradient evaluated at the endothelial surface.

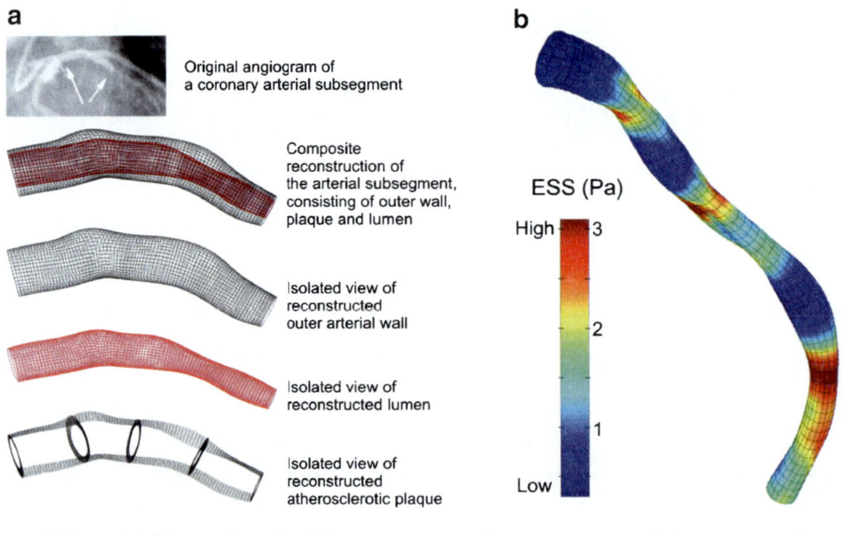

Fig. 2. Vascular profiling: (**a**) Example of a 3D reconstructed coronary arterial segment. Reprinted from [13]. (**b**) Example of endothelial shear stress (ESS) profiling along the 3D reconstructed lumen of a left anterior descending artery. Blue denotes regions with low ESS; *Pa* Pascal. Reprinted from [18].

LOW ESS MODULATES THE NATURAL HISTORY OF ATHEROSCLEROTIC PLAQUES

Following their formation in regions of low ESS early fibroatheromata follow an individualized natural history, which is critically dependent on the balance of two competing processes: inflammation with concomitant ECM degradation versus fibroproliferation with ECM synthesis. Experimental histopathology studies in a diabetic, hyperlipidemic swine model of native atherosclerosis showed that the *magnitude* of low ESS is a key regulator of the balance between inflammation/ECM degradation and fibroproliferation/ECM synthesis, thereby determining the remodeling response of the vascular wall to the growing plaque [13] (Fig. 3). A portion of early fibroatheromas will evolve into *high-risk plaques*, whereas others will remain *quiescent* and still others will evolve to *flow-limiting fibro-calcific* plaques [18] (Fig. 4).

High-Risk Plaques

High-risk plaques are typically TCFAs, characterized by a thin, highly inflamed fibrous cap overlying a large necrotic lipid core, rich in neovessels [30] (Figs. 4 and 5). These plaques are usually minimally stenotic lesions associated with expansive vascular remodeling, and an increased risk of sudden rupture that precipitates 60–70% of acute coronary syndromes [30–33]. Experimental studies showed that TCFAs develop in arterial areas with the lowest values of ESS, which enhance plaque inflammation, especially at the base of the plaque [13]. In this setting, the underlying IEL undergoes severe degradation, the media becomes severely inflamed and acquires the enzymatic products that shift the ECM balance toward intensive degradation, thereby promoting excessive (aneurysm-like) wall expansion and accommodation of the enlarging plaque [34]. Excessive expansive remodeling leads to perpetuation, or even exacerbation, of the local low ESS environment, thereby fostering continued lipid accumulation and inflammation, which lead to additional matrix protease expression, intensive matrix degradation within the inflamed vascular wall and the fibrous cap shoulders, additional wall expansion, and fibrous cap thinning. This self-perpetuating vicious cycle among low local ESS, inflammation, and excessive expansive remodeling, exacerbates the inflammatory status of the plaque and may rapidly transform an early fibroatheroma to a TCFA.

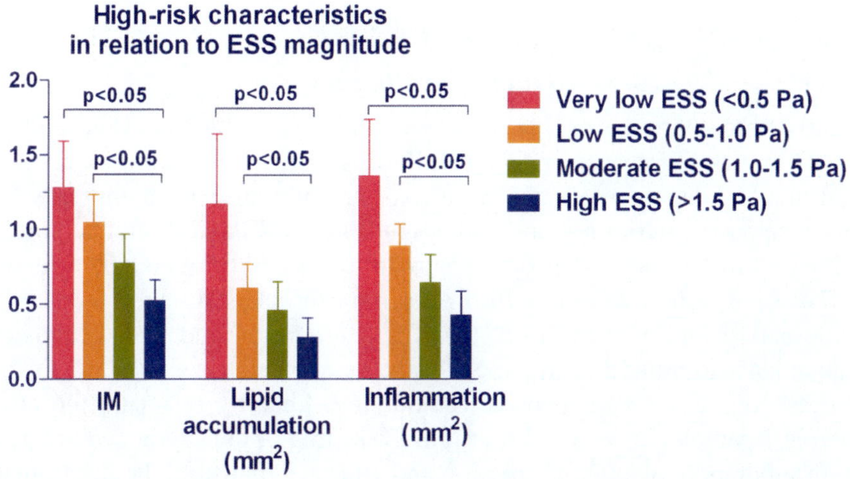

Fig. 3. Correlation between magnitude of Low ESS and high-risk characteristics of coronary artery lesions.

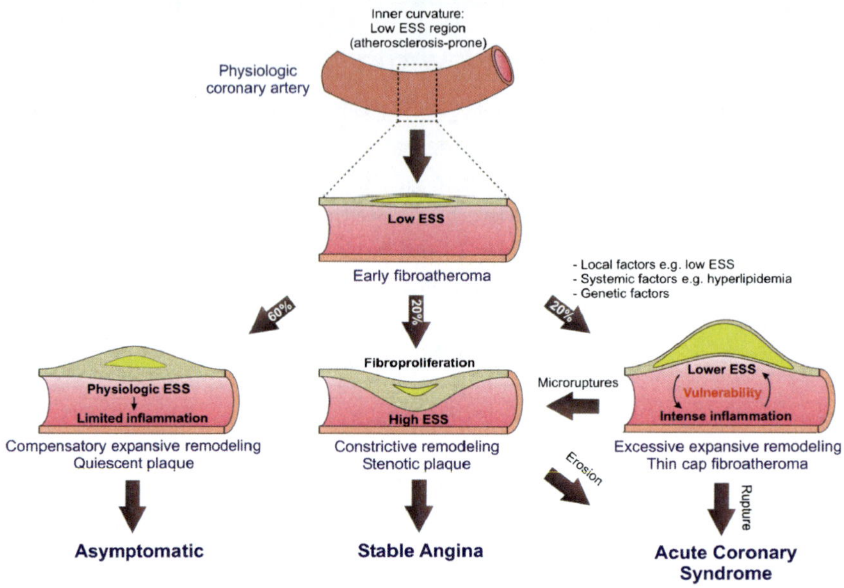

Fig. 4. Proposed natural history of coronary atherosclerosis: **1**. Early fibroatheroma forms in a region of low ESS. **2a**. In regions with very low ESS plaque inflammation is exacerbated, shifting the extracellular matrix balance toward intensive degradation and promoting excessive (aneurysm-like) wall and lumen expansion. Excessive expansive remodeling leads to a self-perpetuating vicious cycle among low local ESS, inflammation, rapid plaque formation, and excessive expansive remodeling, which may rapidly transform an early fibroatheroma to a thin cap fibroatheroma. **2b.** In arterial regions with slightly low ESS the severity of lipid accumulation, inflammation, and wall expansion are limited. In this setting, the growing plaque slightly narrows the lumen (i.e., compensatory expansive remodeling), thereby restoring the adverse ESS stimulus to less pathologic levels and establishing quiescence. **2c**. Fibrous stenotic plaques with constrictive remodeling may either directly evolve with a phenotype promoting fibroproliferation or represent an end-stage of scarring in the setting of prior inflamed thin cap fibroatheromas through repetitive micro-ruptures and subsequent healing. Reprinted from [18].

The presence and severity of systemic factors (e.g., magnitude of hyperlipidemia, hyperglycemia, hypertension), as well as genetic factors also interplay with the low ESS microenvironment and modulate the excessive expansion of the arterial wall.

Quiescent Plaques

A portion of early fibroatheromas evolve to quiescent plaques, which are nonstenotic or minimally stenotic lesions with a thick fibrous cap and a small lipid core (Fig. 4). These plaques are characterized by limited inflammation, remain biologically quiescent, and cause no symptoms [35]. Quiescent lesions appear to develop in arterial regions with slightly low ESS and do not acquire the severity of lipid accumulation and inflammation, as do areas with lower ESS in which TCFAs develop; hence, a stable balance between inflammation and fibroproliferation is established [13, 18]. As a result of the limited inflammation that is stimulated, the IEL degradation and wall expansion are limited. The growing plaque leads to limited enlargement of the vessel wall and then starts to slightly protrude into the lumen (i.e., compensatory expansive remodeling), thereby restoring the adverse low ESS stimulus to higher, less pathologic, levels [13, 36]. In the setting of the attenuated low ESS stimulus for exacerbation of inflammation, plaque progression and arterial expansion, the inflammatory process is limited and quiescence is established.

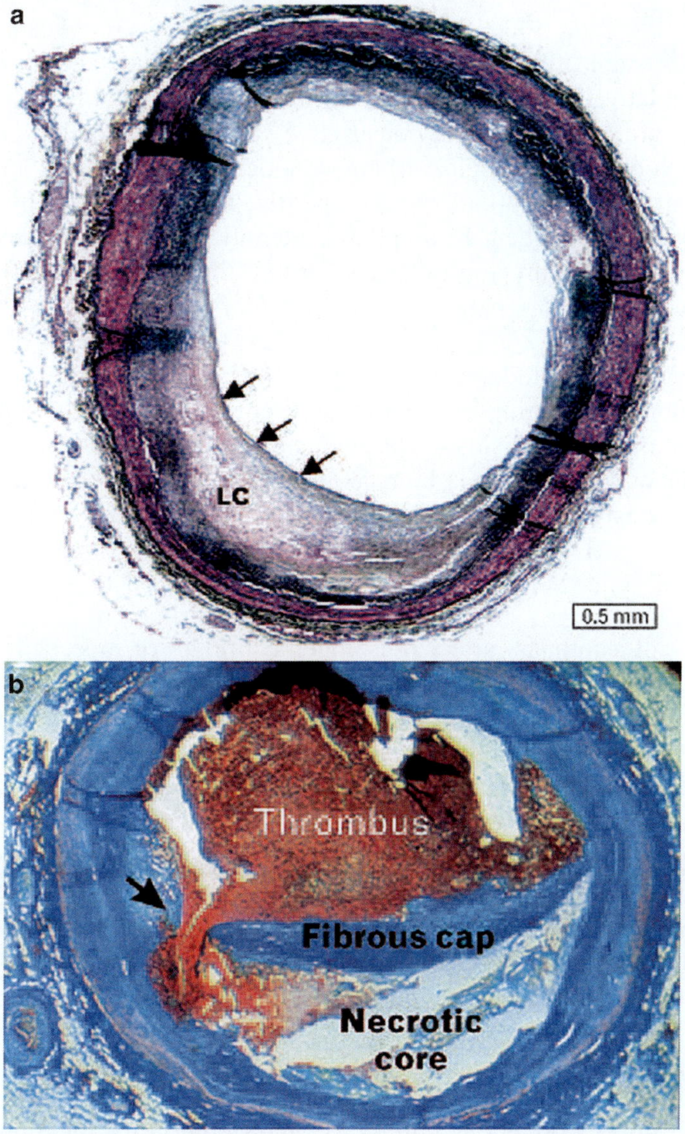

Fig. 5. (**a**) Histologic appearance of an eccentric thin cap fibroatheroma (TCFA); *arrows* denote the thin cap, *LC* lipid core. The lumen is preserved because of the expansive remodeling accommodating the enlarging plaque. Reprinted from MacNeill BD et al. Intravascular modalities for detection of vulnerable plaque: current status. Arterioscler Thromb Vasc Biol 2003; 23:1333-42. (**b**) Histologic appearance of a ruptured plaque (*arrow* indicates the site of rupture) implicated with acute luminal thrombus formation and obstruction. Reprinted from Constantinides P. Plaque fissures in human coronary thrombosis. J Atheroscler Res. Published by Elsevier, 1966.

However, the long-term stability or quiescence of these plaques is unknown. If local vascular conditions later change, such that a low ESS microenvironment is recreated, or the systemic atherosclerotic stimuli are enhanced (e.g., increased magnitude of hyperlipidemia), then the process of inflammation, progressive atherosclerosis, and excessive expansive remodeling may again re-emerge, and may transform the quiescent lesion to a TCFA.

Fibrous Plaques

Stenotic plaques are stable fibroproliferative lesions with limited inflammation, characterized morphologically by a relatively thick, collagen-rich fibrous cap, overlying a small lipid core [30, 32] (Fig. 4). These lesions are associated with constrictive vascular remodeling, and over time become occlusive resulting in chronic stable angina. Many stenotic lesions represent an end-stage of scarring in the setting of prior inflamed TCFA undergoing repetitive microruptures, VSMC proliferation, local deposition of collagen and subsequent healing [37]. Stenotic lesions may also directly evolve from early fibroatheromas with a phenotype promoting fibroproliferation versus inflammation throughout its natural history course [38]. The pathophysiologic factors involved in this process are currently unknown.

Stenotic plaques infrequently undergo local erosion or develop calcified nodules, which lead to local thrombus formation precipitating 20–40% of acute coronary syndromes [30]. Low ESS does not appear to play a role in the pathophysiology of plaque erosion. However, high ESS, which occurs at the throat of highly stenotic plaques, may be responsible for local endothelial erosion and induction of acute coronary thrombosis.

Myocardial Bridges

Sometimes a portion of a coronary artery runs under a "bridge" of superficial myocardial fibers for a short distance. The reported incidence of myocardial bridging varies widely, from 0.5 to 2.5% in angiographic series and from 15 to 85% in autopsy series. Although the discovery of bridging is often an incidental finding during angiography, it can result in a variety of clinical syndromes including unstable angina, acute myocardial infarction and life-threatening arrhythmias. Detailed angiographic, hemodynamic, and IVUS studies have shown that the bridged segment is typically narrower than the adjoining arterial segments and narrows substantially during systole. Flow during systole is typically minimal but the velocity during diastole is substantially elevated. The bridge segment is typically free of atherosclerotic disease, but the segment immediately proximal to the bridge is severely diseased. In all likelihood, the absence of atherosclerotic disease in the bridge segment is the result of increased velocity and, hence, increased ESS within the bridged segment [39].

Effect of Periadventitial and Pericardial Fat

It has become increasingly evident that adipose tissue is a multifunctional organ that produces and secretes multiple paracrine and endocrine factors. Research into obesity, insulin resistance, and diabetes has identified a proinflammatory state associated with obesity. Substantial differences between subcutaneous and omental fat have been noted, including the fact that omental fat produces relatively more inflammatory cytokines. It is unknown whether autonomic stimulation affects periadventitial fat. Interesting data from several studies suggest a possible association between a lack of periadventitial fat and protection against atherosclerosis [40]. For reasons that are still not clear, atherosclerosis appears to be suppressed in intramyocardial segments of coronary arteries (Fig. 6). Hemodynamic factors are usually implicated. Likewise, the intramural aortic segments of anomalous coronary arteries arising from a wrong sinus of Valsalva also appear to resist atherosclerosis. In both instances, it seems plausible to attribute the absence of atherosclerosis to the lack of periadventitial fat. The potential involvement of periadventitial fat in atherosclerosis has certain implications for therapeutic delivery methods. Pericardial drug delivery is most promising because the entire coronary tree and its surrounding fat are in direct contact with the overlying pericardial fluid. Perivascular intrapericardial

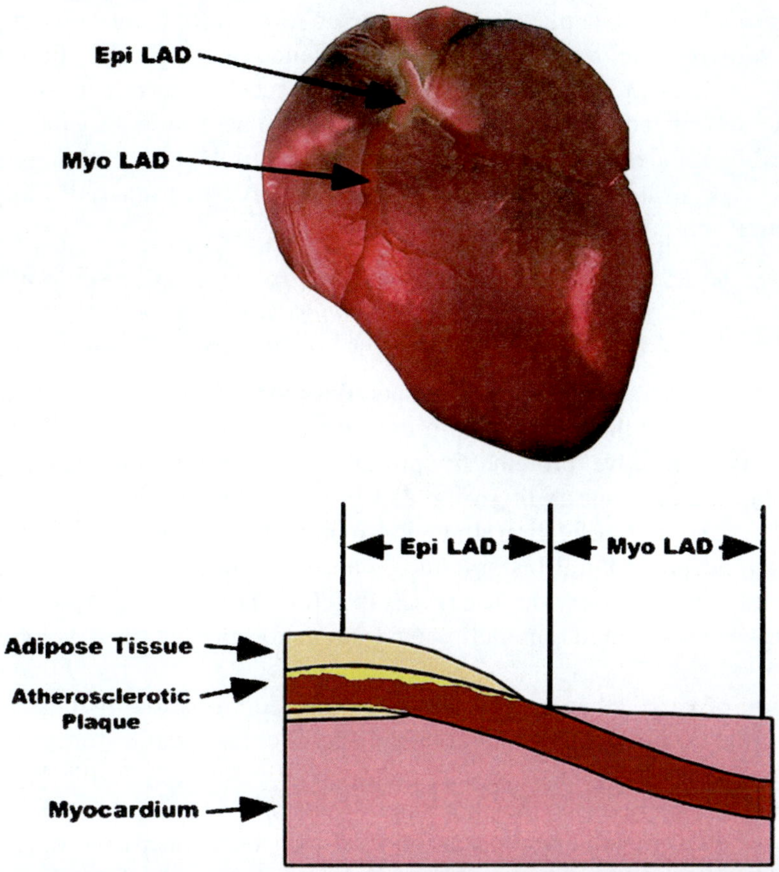

Fig. 6. Schematic representation of tissue sampling from rabbit heart. Epi LAD is the intraepicardial segment of the left anterior descending coronary artery covered by adipose tissue. Myo LAD is the intramyocardial segment of the left anterior descending coronary artery covered by myocardium. From Vela et al. [40] with permission from Springer Science and Business Media.

delivery of nitric oxide donors has been successfully used in experimental animals to prevent restenosis after vessel injury. It is unknown, however, whether such therapy primarily affects the periadventitial fat, the adventitia, or both. New developments in molecular imaging as well as positron emission tomography, magnetic resonance imaging, and computed tomography should allow investigators to distinguish quiescent periadventitial and pericardial fat from inflammatory and metabolically active adipose tissue that contribute to the development and progression of atherosclerotic plaques [40].

RISK STRATIFICATION OF INDIVIDUAL ATHEROSCLEROTIC LESIONS

Given the marked heterogeneity of natural history trajectories of coronary atherosclerosis, development of a comprehensive approach for risk stratification of each individual plaque at an early stage would be invaluable. The major characteristics of individual atherosclerotic plaques contributing to the ongoing process of the respective natural history trajectories include [1] the *magnitude of ESS*, which constitutes the stimulus for ongoing inflammation and plaque progression, [2] the *severity of inflammation* that plaque acquires over its development and progression, and [3] the nature of *vascular remodeling response* to the presence of the plaque; both the magnitude of inflammation and the vascular remodeling response are directly determined by the local ESS environment. Measurement of local ESS, complemented by the assessment of the severity of inflammation and vascular remodeling at early stages of the natural history of a given lesion, would allow for detailed risk stratification of that lesion to evolve to high-risk plaque based on the following conceptual scheme:

- High-risk with *very low ESS, intense inflammation,* and *excessive expansive remodeling*
- Medium risk with *low/moderate ESS, moderate inflammation,* and *less excessive expansive remodeling*
- Low risk with *physiologic ESS, limited inflammation,* and *compensatory expansive remodeling*

Integration into the above scheme of patient-specific systemic characteristics (e.g., magnitude of hyperlipidemia), as well as of the information provided by traditional and novel systemic biomarkers (e.g., high sensitivity C-reactive protein, lipoprotein-associated phospholipase A_2) [41, 42] and genomics [43] would increase our ability to predict the future natural history of individual plaques. The ability, however, of such stratification strategies to predict the clinical outcomes needs to be tested in the clinical arena. Several natural history studies are now underway [44]; a large natural history study in patients with coronary artery disease (PREDICTION Trial) investigates the incremental value of characterizing the local ESS and remodeling environment to predict the development of new acute cardiac events.

Risk stratification of early atherosclerotic lesions and identification of their subsequent natural history may permit the development of novel lesion-specific therapeutic strategies. Identification of a high-risk plaque at its early stages of development would potentially justify highly selective, prophylactic local interventions, such as implantation of stents or targeted nanoparticle-based delivery of anti-inflammatory drugs, supplemented by an intensive systemic pharmacologic approach to limit the severity of inflammation, stabilize the plaque, and therefore avert a future acute coronary event. The clinical and economic implications of identifying and treating high-risk individual coronary lesions before an adverse cardiac event can occur are anticipated to be enormous.

CONCLUSION

The magnitude of low ESS – primarily determined by variations in coronary artery anatomy – is a critical factor that determines the severity of inflammation within a given early atherosclerotic plaque, the lesion's rate of progression, the nature of plaque's remodeling response and the individual natural history of that plaque. In the setting of very low ESS, plaque inflammation is intense, progression is rapid, the artery undergoes local excessive expansive remodeling, and the lesion evolves to high-risk plaque. In the setting of only slightly low ESS, the inflammation is limited, the artery undergoes compensatory expansive remodeling, which restores the local ESS to less pathologic levels, and the plaque remains quiescent. In vivo assessment of the local ESS environment, the severity of inflammation, and the vascular remodeling response in combination with the information provided by systemic biomarkers of vulnerability, may allow for detailed risk stratification of individual early coronary plaques, thereby guiding pre-emptive, lesion-specific therapeutic strategies. Current imaging techniques make it possible to determine coronary artery anatomy and coronary artery flow rates. Knowing coronary artery anatomy, blood flow rate, and hematocrit is all that is required to calculate ESS, thus enabling risk stratification of early plaque and prediction of which lesions are likely to progress to high-risk plaque. Future natural history studies based on detailed measurement of coronary artery anatomy as well as peri-adventitial fat will clarify whether prediction of progression of vulnerability, culminating in plaque rupture, can be accomplished.

REFERENCES

1. Libby P. Inflammation in atherosclerosis. Nature 2002; 420:868-74.
2. VanderLaan PA, Reardon CA, Getz GS. Site specificity of atherosclerosis: site-selective responses to atherosclerotic modulators. Arterioscler Thromb Vasc Biol 2004; 24:12-22.
3. Rioufol G, Finet G, Ginon I, André-Fouët X, Rossi R, Vialle E, Desjoyaux E, Convert G, Huret JF, Tabib A. Multiple atherosclerotic plaque rupture in acute coronary syndrome: a three-vessel intravascular ultrasound study. Circulation 2002; 106:804-8
4. Friedman MH, Deters OJ, Mark FF, Bargeron CB, Hutchins GM. Arterial geometry affects hemodynamics – a potential risk factor for atherosclerosis. Atherosclerosis 1983; 46:225-31.
5. Gazetopoulos N, Ionnidis PJ, Karydis C, Lolas C, Kiriakou K, Tountas C. Short left coronary trunk as a risk factor in the development of coronary atherosclerosis – pathological study. Br Heart J 1976; 38:1160-5.
6. Caro CG, Fitz-Gerald JM, Schroter RC. Arterial wall shear and distribution of early atheroma in man. Nature 1969; 223:1159-60.
7. Asakura T, Karino T. Flow patterns and spatial distribution of atherosclerotic lesions in human coronary arteries. Circ Res 1990; 66:1045-66.
8. Ku DN, Giddens DP, Zarins CK, Glagov S. Pulsatile flow and atherosclerosis in the human carotid bifurcation. Positive correlation between plaque location and low oscillating shear stress. Arteriosclerosis 1985; 5:293-302.
9. Moore JE, Jr., Xu C, Glagov S, Zarins CK, Ku DN. Fluid wall shear stress measurements in a model of the human abdominal aorta: oscillatory behavior and relationship to atherosclerosis. Atherosclerosis 1994; 110:225-40.
10. Gambillara V, Chambaz C, Montorzi G, Roy S, Stergiopulos N, Silacci P. Plaque-prone hemodynamics impair endothelial function in pig carotid arteries. Am J Physiol Heart Circ Physiol 2006; 290:H2320-8.
11. Cheng C, van Haperen R, de Waard M, van Damme LC, Tempel D, Hanemaaijer L, van Cappellen GW, Bos J, Slager CJ, Duncker DJ, van der Steen AF, de Crom R, Krams R. Shear stress affects the intracellular distribution of eNOS: direct demonstration by a novel in vivo technique. Blood 2005; 106:3691-8.
12. Buchanan JR, Jr., Kleinstreuer C, Truskey GA, Lei M. Relation between non-uniform hemodynamics and sites of altered permeability and lesion growth at the rabbit aorto-celiac junction. Atherosclerosis 1999; 143:27-40.
13. Chatzizisis YS, Jonas M, Coskun AU, Beigel R, Stone BV, Maynard C, Gerrity RG, Daley W, Rogers C, Edelman ER, Feldman CL, Stone PH. Prediction of the localization of high-risk coronary atherosclerotic plaques based on low endothelial shear stress: A serial intravascular ultrasound and histopathology natural history study. Circulation 2008; 117:993-1002.
14. Stone PH, Coskun AU, Kinlay S, Clark ME, Sonka M, Wahle A, Ilegbusi OJ, Yeghiazarians Y, Popma JJ, Orav J, Kuntz RE, Feldman CL. Effect of endothelial shear stress on the progression of coronary artery disease, vascular remodeling, and in-stent restenosis in humans: in vivo 6-month follow-up study. Circulation 2003; 108:438-44.
15. Wentzel JJ, Krams R, Schuurbiers JC, Oomen JA, Kloet J, van Der Giessen WJ, Serruys PW, Slager CJ. Relationship between neointimal thickness and shear stress after Wallstent implantation in human coronary arteries. Circulation 2001; 103:1740-5.
16. Wentzel JJ, Corti R, Fayad ZA, Wisdom P, Macaluso F, Winkelman MO, Fuster V, Badimon JJ. Does shear stress modulate both plaque progression and regression in the thoracic aorta? Human study using serial magnetic resonance imaging. J Am Coll Cardiol 2005; 45:846-54.
17. Chatzizisis YS, Coskun AU, Jonas M, Edelman ER, Stone PH, Feldman CL. Risk stratification of individual coronary lesions using local endothelial shear stress: a new paradigm for managing coronary artery disease. Curr Opin Cardiol 2007; 22:552-64.
18. Chatzizisis YS, Coskun AU, Jonas M, Edelman ER, Feldman CL, Stone PH. Role of endothelial shear stress in the natural history of coronary atherosclerosis and vascular remodeling: molecular, cellular, and vascular behavior. J Am Coll Cardiol 2007; 49:2379-93.
19. Slager CJ, Wentzel JJ, Gijsen FJ, Schuurbiers JC, van der Wal AC, van der Steen AF, Serruys PW. The role of shear stress in the generation of rupture-prone vulnerable plaques. Nat Clin Pract Cardiovasc Med 2005; 2:401-7.
20. Feldman CL, Stone PH. Intravascular hemodynamic factors responsible for progression of coronary atherosclerosis and development of vulnerable plaque. Curr Opin Cardiol 2000; 15:430-40.
21. Chatzizisis YS, Giannoglou GD. Pulsatile flow: a critical modulator of the natural history of atherosclerosis. Med Hypotheses 2006; 67:338-40.
22. Giannoglou GD, Soulis JV, Farmakis TM, Farmakis DM, Louridas GE. Haemodynamic factors and the important role of local low static pressure in coronary wall thickening. Int J Cardiol 2002; 86:27-40.
23. Soulis JV, Giannoglou GD, Chatzizisis YS, Farmakis TM, Giannakoulas GA, Parcharidis GE, Louridas GE. Spatial and phasic oscillation of non-Newtonian wall shear stress in human left coronary artery bifurcation: an insight to atherogenesis. Coron Artery Dis 2006; 17:351-8.
24. Stone PH, Coskun AU, Yeghiazarians Y, Kinlay S, Popma JJ, Kuntz RE, Feldman CL. Prediction of sites of coronary atherosclerosis progression: in vivo profiling of endothelial shear stress, lumen, and outer vessel wall characteristics to predict vascular behavior. Curr Opin Cardiol 2003; 18:458-70.
25. Slager CJ, Wentzel JJ, Schuurbiers JC, Oomen JA, Kloet J, Krams R, von Birgelen C, van der Giessen WJ, Serruys PW, de Feyter PJ. True 3-dimensional reconstruction of coronary arteries in patients by fusion of angiography and IVUS (ANGUS) and its quantitative validation. Circulation 2000; 102:511-6.
26. Giannoglou GD, Chatzizisis YS, Sianos G, Tsikaderis D, Matakos A, Koutkias V, Diamantopoulos P, Maglaveras N, Parcharidis GE, Louridas GE. In-vivo validation of spatially correct three-dimensional reconstruction of human coronary arteries by integrating intravascular ultrasound and biplane angiography. Coron Artery Dis 2006; 17:533-43.

27. Chatzizisis YS, Giannoglou GD, Matakos A, Basdekidou C, Sianos G, Panagiotou A, Dimakis C, Parcharidis GE, Louridas GE. In-vivo accuracy of geometrically correct three-dimensional reconstruction of human coronary arteries: is it influenced by certain parameters? Coron Artery Dis 2006; 17:545-51.
28. Coskun AU, Yeghiazarians Y, Kinlay S, Clark ME, Ilegbusi OJ, Wahle A, Sonka M, Popma JJ, Kuntz RE, Feldman CL, Stone PH. Reproducibility of coronary lumen, plaque, and vessel wall reconstruction and of endothelial shear stress measurements in vivo in humans. Catheter Cardiovasc Interv 2003; 60:67-78.
29. Stone PH, Coskun AU, Kinlay S, Popma JJ, Sonka M, Wahle A, Yeghiazarians Y, Maynard C, Kuntz RE, Feldman CL. Regions of low endothelial shear stress are sites where coronary plaque progress and vascular remodeling occurs in humans: An in-vivo serial study. Eur Heart J 2007; 28:705-10.
30. Virmani R, Kolodgie FD, Burke, Farb A, Schwartz SM. Lessons from sudden coronary death: a comprehensive morphological classification scheme for atherosclerotic lesions. Arterioscler Thromb Vasc Biol 2000; 20:1262-75.
31. Burke AP, Kolodgie FD, Farb A, Weber D, Virmani R. Morphological predictors of arterial remodeling in coronary atherosclerosis. Circulation 2002; 105:297-303.
32. Varnava AM, Mills PG, Davies MJ. Relationship between coronary artery remodeling and plaque vulnerability. Circulation 2002; 105:939-43.
33. Schoenhagen P, Ziada KM, Kapadia SR, Crowe TD, Nissen SE, Tuzcu EM. Extent and direction of arterial remodeling in stable versus unstable coronary syndromes: an intravascular ultrasound study. Circulation 2000; 101:598-603.
34. Sipahi I, Tuzcu EM, Schoenhagen P, Nicholls SJ, Chen MS, Crowe T, Loyd AB, Kapadia S, Nissen SE. Paradoxical increase in lumen size during progression of coronary atherosclerosis: Observations from the REVERSAL trial. Atherosclerosis 2006; 189:229-35.
35. MacIsaac AI, Thomas JD, Topol EJ. Toward the quiescent coronary plaque. J Am Coll Cardiol 1993; 22:1228-41.
36. Wentzel JJ, Janssen E, Vos J, Schuurbiers JC, Krams R, Serruys PW, de Feyter PJ, Slager CJ. Extension of increased atherosclerotic wall thickness into high shear stress regions is associated with loss of compensatory remodeling. Circulation 2003; 108:17-23.
37. Burke AP, Kolodgie FD, Farb A, Weber DK, Malcom GT, Smialek J, Virmani R. Healed plaque ruptures and sudden coronary death: evidence that subclinical rupture has a role in plaque progression. Circulation 2001; 103:934-40.
38. Feldman CL, Coskun AU, Yeghiazarians Y, Kinlay S, Wahle A, Olszewski ME, Rossen JD, Sonka M, Popma JJ, Orav J, Kuntz RE, Stone PH. Remodeling characteristics of minimally diseased coronary arteries are consistent along the length of the artery. Am J Cardiol 2006; 97:13-6.
39. Bourassa MG, Butnaru A, Lesperance J, Tardif J-C. Symptomatic myocardial bridges: Overview of ischemic mechanisms and current diagnostic and treatment strategies. J Am Coll Cardiol 2003; 41:351-59.
40. Vela D, Buja LM, Madjid M, Burke A, Naghavi M, Willerson JT, Casscells SW, Litovsky S. The role of periadventitial fat in atherosclerosis. Arch Pathol Lab Med. 2007; 131(3):481-7.
41. Lavi S, McConnell JP, Rihal CS, Prasad A, Mathew V, Lerman LO, Lerman A. Local production of lipoproteinassociated phospholipase A2 and lysophosphatidylcholine in the coronary circulation: association with early coronary atherosclerosis and endothelial dysfunction in humans. Circulation 2007; 115:2715-21.
42. Ridker PM. C-reactive protein and the prediction of cardiovascular events among those at intermediate risk: moving an inflammatory hypothesis toward consensus. J Am Coll Cardiol 2007; 49:2129-38.
43. Miller DT, Ridker PM, Libby P, Kwiatkowski DJ. Atherosclerosis: the path from genomics to therapeutics. J Am Coll Cardiol 2007; 49:1589-99.
44. Waxman S, Ishibashi F, Muller JE. Detection and treatment of vulnerable plaques and vulnerable patients: novel approaches to prevention of coronary events. Circulation 2006; 114:2390-411.

38 Vasa Vasorum Imaging

Ioannis A. Kakadiaris, Sean O'Malley, Manolis Vavuranakis, Ralph Metcalfe, Craig J. Hartley, Erling Falk, and Morteza Naghavi

Contents

Abstract

The majority of acute coronary syndromes are the result of coronary plaque rupture. Recent studies have revealed the presence of neovascularization in and around the plaque to be a common feature of presumed rupture-prone (vulnerable) plaques. Intravascular ultrasound combined with contrast enhancement agents has been shown to be useful for the detection and quantification of vasa vasorum (VV) and angiogenesis within the vessel wall. In this chapter, the two state-of-the-art techniques for VV imaging are reviewed.

Key words: ACES; Cardiovascular disease; Contrast-enhanced intravascular ultrasound; Image analysis; IVUS; Microbubbles; Neoangiogenesis; Neovascularization; Plaque rupture; Vasa vasorum; Vulnerable plaque; VV

KEY POINTS

- Acute coronary syndromes are to a great extent the result of coronary plaque rupture. Studies indicate that increased vasa vasorum neovascularization in the adventitia and within the atherosclerotic plaque is related to the development and progression of coronary atherosclerosis, and may be used as a marker of plaque inflammation and risk of plaque rupture.
- Contrast-enhanced intravascular imaging can be used to trace perfusion because of vasa vasorum. Specifically, there exist two main approaches: (1) fundamental imaging combined with computational image analysis and (2) harmonic ultrasound imaging.

From: *Asymptomatic Atherosclerosis: Pathophysiology, Detection and Treatment*
Edited by: M. Naghavi (ed.), DOI 10.1007/978-1-60327-179-0_38

- The fist approach relies on detection of local echogenicity changes in stationary intravascular ultrasound sequences, using differential imaging techniques (ACES™; Computational Biomedicine Laboratory, University of Houston, Houston, TX, USA).
- In the second approach, harmonic oscillations are induced on the contrast agent and detected by a specially designed intravascular ultrasound system.
- Contrast-enhanced intravascular ultrasound methods have been applied in vivo with promising results for the assessment of blood perfusion, plaque VV revealing, and plaque inflammation.

INTRODUCTION

Cardiovascular Disease

Atherosclerotic cardiovascular disease (CVD) and its complications are a leading cause of death worldwide [1]. For a significant percentage of these patients, the first symptom of atherosclerotic CVD is sudden death without previous warnings. It has been shown that for up to 75% of the acute coronary syndromes, atherosclerotic plaque rupture is the underlying pathological mechanism [2, 3]. Although atherosclerotic plaques are widespread in the coronary artery tree of CAD patients, only a small portion of these plaques present a particularly high risk of rupture (vulnerable plaques), and an even smaller number of them will rupture.

The risk of plaque rupture depends on the plaque type (e.g., morphology, composition) more than the degree of luminal stenosis. Most ruptures occur in plaques containing a soft, lipid-rich core that is covered by an inflamed thin cap of fibrous tissue [3]. These ruptures manifest positive remodeling and cell infiltration of the fibrous cap and adventitia, and they exhibit increased neovascularization within the plaque [4, 5]. Since the ruptured caps are thinner (usually less than 65 mm) than intact caps, the term "thin-cap fibroatheroma" (TCFA) has being proposed for presumed rupture-prone plaques [6].

Detection of rupture-prone plaques is one of the most active areas of research in both the cardiology and the biomedical imaging communities. While several invasive and noninvasive techniques such as thermography, magnetic resonance imaging (MRI), optical coherence tomography, IVUS-based virtual histology, elastography, and others have been used for the assessment of plaque vulnerability [7], none of them can completely identify a vulnerable plaque and accurately predict its further development.

Vasa Vasorum

Vasa vasorum (VV) constitute a network of microvessels that nourish the wall of larger vessels [8]. In normal conditions, VV are present in the adventitial layer of larger arteries such as the aorta, and play an important role in the functional and structural characteristics of the vessel wall [9]. Recent studies in human and animal coronary arteries have indicated that adventitial VV are related to the development and progression of coronary atherosclerosis [10]. In several investigations [11–14], VV have been implicated in the pathogenesis of atherosclerotic plaques. An increase in the density of the VV has been associated with the advancement of a plaque from being stable, to TCFA, and finally to rupture [5, 12].

In addition, intraplaque hemorrhage has been documented to be present in atherosclerotic plaques in many cases of sudden coronary death [15]. The hemorrhage is believed to occur from the disruption of thin-walled immature microvessels that are lined by the discontinuous endothelium without supporting smooth muscle cells [6]. This may also contribute to the progression of atherosclerotic plaques by allowing the accumulation of large amounts of cholesterol-rich red cell membranes which may become oxidized and provide the stimulus for macrophage accumulation and atherogenic cytokine secretion.

These microvessels are associated with extensive VV proliferation and represent a form of neoangiogenesis within the plaque confines.

This evidence suggests VV proliferation as a marker of plaque inflammation and a preceding or concomitant factor associated with plaque rupture and instability [15, 16]. It is thus quite demanding to develop tools that allow for the detection and measurement of plaque neovascularization and the detection of leakage and entrapment of blood within atherosclerotic plaques in order to obtain a quantitative index of plaque vulnerability.

Intravascular Ultrasound

Intravascular ultrasound (IVUS) is an invasive medical imaging technique that is capable of providing high-resolution real-time cross-sectional images of the arterial wall and has therefore become an important clinical tool for the detection and evaluation of coronary artery diseases as well as for therapy guidance and clinical research.

IVUS consists of a specially designed catheter with a miniaturized ultrasound probe attached to the distal end of the catheter. The IVUS catheter is advanced percutaneously within the examined vessel. High-frequency sound signals are emitted and received radially by a solid-state or mechanically rotated ultrasound transducer at a discrete set of angles (commonly 240–360). The ultrasound signals are partially reflected and transmitted differently depending on the acoustic impedance of the tissues within the blood vessel at each particular angle. The received signals are then processed and converted to a gray-scale image known as B-mode (Fig. 1).

Contrast Agents

Although IVUS provides reliable cross-section images of the coronary arteries, the in vivo imaging of the coronary VV remains a great challenge because of their small size, their echo transparency, and the different IVUS artifacts. To overcome these limitations, IVUS has been used in combination with contrast agents. Most modern ultrasound contrast agents consist of solutions of echogenic microbubbles that are introduced into the systemic circulation, resulting in enhanced backscatter from microbubble-infused free blood or from microbubble-perfused tissue. These microbubbles are gas-filled spheres surrounded by a shell designed to aid their longevity in the bloodstream. The size of these

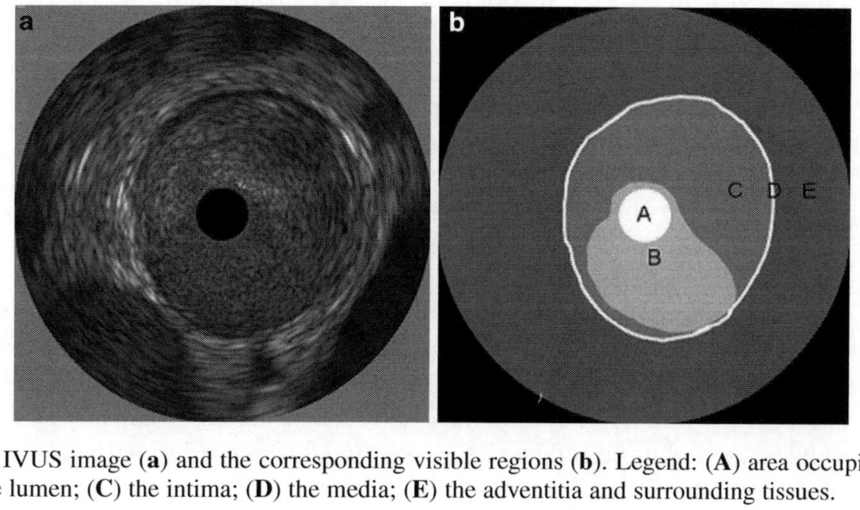

Fig. 1. B-Mode IVUS image (**a**) and the corresponding visible regions (**b**). Legend: (**A**) area occupied by the IVUS catheter; (**B**) the lumen; (**C**) the intima; (**D**) the media; (**E**) the adventitia and surrounding tissues.

microbubbles (diameter: 1–10 μm) is similar to the size of red blood cells (diameter: ~8 μm), and hence they are used as tracer of blood flow.

Microbubbles resonate as a response to pressure changes induced by an ultrasound wave. This makes them several times more echogenic than normal body tissues, and consequently they appear extremely bright in the B-mode ultrasound images. Depending on the energy and frequency of the ultrasound beam, the microbubbles will present linear or nonlinear oscillations.

Linear oscillation means that the contraction and the relaxation of the microbubbles induced by the ultrasound signal are equal in amplitude. On the other hand, nonlinear oscillation means that the microbubbles expand above their baseline diameter at a greater scale than they are able to compress below it.

In the first case (fundamental mode), the microbubbles produce echo signals with the same frequency as that to which they are exposed. In the nonlinear case, the microbubbles will produce the fundamental frequency and multiples of this frequency called harmonics [17].

Imaging of the coronary VV is a great challenge. Until now only contrast-enhanced IVUS has been applied in vivo with promising results. In this scope, there exist two main different approaches for the imaging of VV by contrast-enhanced IVUS: (1) fundamental imaging combined with computational image analysis [18–20, 26] and (2) harmonic ultrasound imaging [21–25].

FUNDAMENTAL IMAGING WITH COMPUTATIONAL IMAGE ANALYSIS FOR VASA VASORUM IMAGING

O'Malley et al. have proposed a protocol and an automatic algorithm (Analysis of Contrast Enhanced Sequences, ACES™) for quantification and visualization of VV in contrast-enhanced IVUS image sequences [18]. This method relies on detection of local echogenicity changes in stationary IVUS sequences due to microbubble perfusion into the vessel wall. According to the proposed protocol, an IVUS catheter is first placed at the maximally-stenotic point of a suspect plaque or of any other plaque of interest. The catheter is held steady and images are acquired for a period of time (10–30 s). Then a bolus injection of contrast agent is made through the guiding catheter and proximal to the imaging catheter. After the contrast agent disappears, more images are continuously acquired for another period of time (10–20 s) with the catheter kept at steady position.

Enhancement detection is accomplished as follows. First, it is necessary to eliminate the motion artifact from the IVUS sequence that is resulting from the heart beating while the catheter is inside the coronary arteries. When an electrocardiogram (ECG) is available in addition to the IVUS analysis, the sequence stabilization is made by synchronizing the sequence with the ECG. Then, only frames corresponding to the same phase on the cardiac cycle are selected. This method is known as ECG-based sequence gating. However, sometimes an ECG is not available. In such cases, the proposed algorithm introduces a sequence-gating algorithm based on the analysis of the interframe correlations with a standard registration metric. These frames are clustered and then selected to build a new gated sequence eliminating cardiac motion.

Next, the region of interest (ROI) is defined manually by a human operator tracing its inner and outer borders (luminal and media/adventitia contours in the case of plaque monitoring) in the first frame of the gated set of images. The ROI corresponding to each frame in the gated sequence is located and "unwrapped" into a rectangular domain. These images are aligned and superimposed to obtain a pixel-wise correspondence. A precontrast baseline image is computed by averaging the subset of gated frames corresponding to the period before the microbubble injection. The precontrast baseline image is subtracted from all frames in the gated sequence. As a result, any change that occurs due to contrast enhancement will be reflected as a positive difference in the intensities in particular regions of the difference image. To quantify the enhancement of a particular frame, the average of the gray intensity levels in the difference image is obtained within the ROI to produce a mean enhancement in ROI (MEIR) statistic. This statistic is obtained for all the frames in the gated sequence. If a perfusion within the ROI (e.g., plaque area) occurs during the injection, the MEIR level will increase in the frames corresponding to the postcontrast injection period (Fig. 2). If no perfusion occurs, the MEIR will return to its precontrast value almost immediately after contrast agent flows through the vessel lumen. Finally, the difference images corresponding to the postinjection period are summed and filtered with a threshold in order to image the perfusion in the ROI (Fig. 3).

Animal studies have been carried out verifying the feasibility of imaging intracoronary-injected microbubbles using an intracoronary ultrasound system (central frequency: 20 MHz, peak pressure: 100 KPa Invision; Volcano Therapeutics, Rancho Cordova, CA), employing injections of SonoVue™ (Bracco Diagnostics Inc., Italy) or Optison™ (GE Healthcare, US) as contrast agent [7]. In these studies it was demonstrated that contrast-enhanced intravascular ultrasound in combination with appropriate image analysis (ACES™) can detect intracoronary and perivascular flow of microbubbles. In a preliminary study, contrast-enhanced IVUS and ACES™ were used in seven nonconsecutive human patients (6 males, 1 female) with unstable angina due to coronary artery disease. These patients were undergoing percutaneous coronary interventions (PCI) and intravascular ultrasound evaluation.

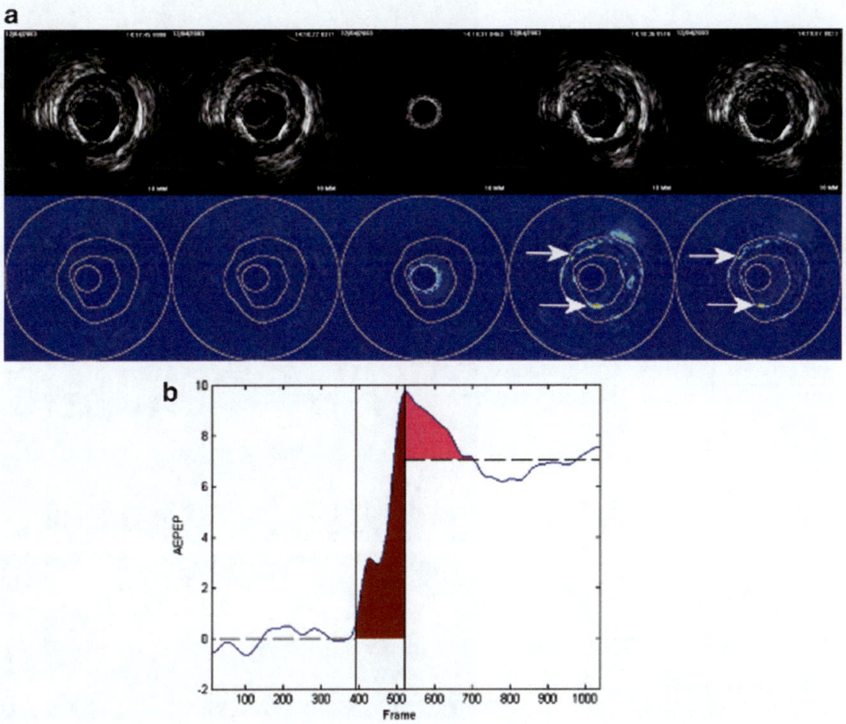

Fig. 2. IVUS contrast study depicting pronounced plaque perfusion. (**a**) *Top panel* illustrates original IVUS sequence over time; *bottom panel* illustrates corresponding analysis frames. IVUS regions have been outlined in the *bottom panel* for reference (from the center outward: the catheter blank, the lumen, the intima-medial region, and the adventitia and surrounding tissues). *Middle* frames indicate the peak of injection and consequent luminal echo-opacity. *Arrows* indicate prominent enhancement. From 10 to 12 o'clock, we observe small features at the media-intima boundary indicative of vasa vasorum perfusion. At 6 o'clock, we observe evidence of direct microbubble entry into an existing plaque. Note eventual diminution of enhancement (time from fourth frame to fifth frame is 31 s), as reflected in the perfusion plot. (**b**) Perfusion curve for intima-medial region of study, quantifying enhancement levels following injection of contrast agent.

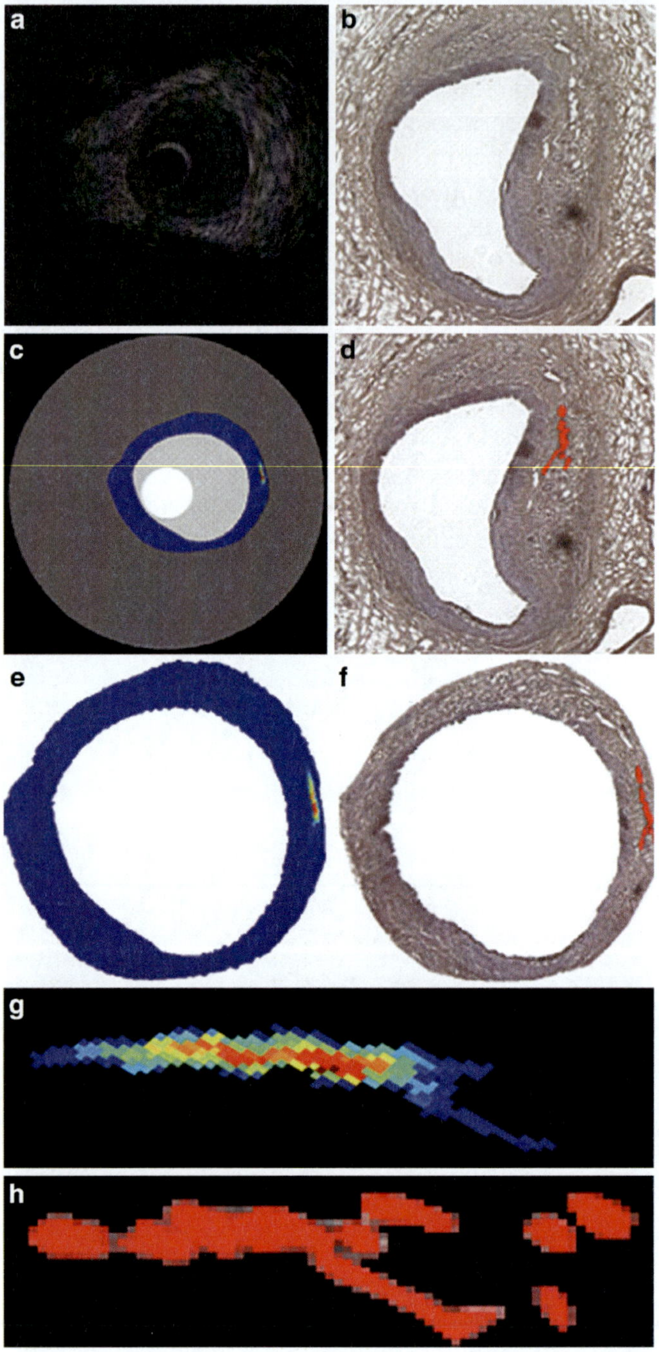

Fig. 3. (**a**) B-mode IVUS image of a lesion identified in the proximal left circumflex artery of a pig and (**b**) corresponding histology; (**c**) in vivo appearance of the enhancement after injection of microbubbles; (**d**) Manual annotation of wall perfusion, (**e**) and (**f**) Coregistration of the histology with the analysis result demonstrates the agreement of the result. (**g**) and (**h**) Zoomed region of interest of the enhanced and histology images, respectively. (We thank Dr. Granada for the preclinical data and the histology annotation).

In this study, a solid-state, synthetic aperture, 20-MHz IVUS scanner (Invision; Volcano Therapeutics, Rancho Cordova, CA) was employed. The image sequences were recorded using DICOM format at a rate of 10 frames per second while the catheter was left stationary at nonobstructive (<75%) coronary lesions proximal to the treated segment which showed positive remodeling and low echogenicity areas within the plaque. Baseline recording was performed for 10 s and then a bolus injection of 2 mL of Sonovue™ was made through the guiding catheter, followed by 5 mL of normal saline to flush out remaining microbubbles. The recording was stopped after 2 min of the contrast agent injection. Off-line analysis of the recorded sequences with ACES™ showed a significant enhancement in adventitial echogenicity. For this study, the average enhancement of the adventitial plaque echogenicity was 1.2%±0.8%, with ranges from 0.3% to 2.5%. No side effects were reported on the patients [19, 20].

More recently, a study in 16 human patients with acute coronary syndrome using ACES™ has been presented [26]. Here, a qualitative analysis of the areas of enhancement was observed in distinct areas within the intima-media area and adventitia. After quantitative analysis, a statistically significant postcontrast enhancement was demonstrated in the echogenicity of the intima-media, adventitia, and combined intima-media and adventitia. MEIR increased significantly after the injection of microbubbles (from 6.01±2.46 to 7.88±3.28, $p=0.006$) in the intima-media region. A significant increase, though in a lesser degree, was also observed in MEIR for the adventitia region (from 7.10±2.20 to 7.60±2.50, $p=0.035$). All patients manifested an increase in the mean gray level of all examined regions as expressed by MEIR from pre- to postinjection of microbubbles, although to a different degree. Specifically, in the intima-media region the percentage increase of MEIR after the injection of microbubbles was <20% in 5 pts, 20–50% in 7 pts and >50% in 4 pts. In the adventitia region the percentage increase of MEIR was <20% in 13 pts, 20–50% in 2 pts and >50% in 1 pt.

Due to the inherent limitation of in vivo human coronary IVUS studies, in these studies it was not possible to correlate the described clinical findings with histopathology. However, since all blood perfusion in plaques comes from coronary branches through the VV and their extension into the atherosclerotic plaques, the investigators of this clinical study concluded that the observed enhancement reflects VV density and flow.

Contrast Harmonic IVUS for Vasa Vasorum Imaging

Goertz et al. have investigated the feasibility of harmonic and subharmonic IVUS for detection of microbubbles using a prototype nonlinear IVUS system and commercially available contrast agents [21–23]. This method is able to provide microbubble-specific imaging by detecting nonlinear signals. With this method, the background signal from tissues is minimal compared with the microbubbles signal, making them easier to detect (Fig. 4).

The prototype nonlinear IVUS system consists of a custom-built, single-element transducer that is mechanically rotated, and specially designed signal filters for processing the received signal. In this method, the transducer emits a fundamental frequency with certain intensity (usually stronger than the one used in baseline IVUS) that stimulates the microbubbles to resonate at frequencies different from the frequencies to which it was exposed. The reflected signal is then filtered to isolate the frequencies corresponding to the nonlinear response of the microbubbles. In the harmonic imaging method, the microbubbles are expected to resonate at frequencies higher than the base frequency, while in the subharmonic method, lower frequencies are expected.

Animal studies were carried out to investigate the use of microbubble contrast agent in combination with prototype nonlinear IVUS systems as a means of imaging vasa vasorum [21, 22]. First, the IVUS catheter was situated in an ROI in an atherosclerotic rabbit aorta. The transducer transmits pulses at 20 MHz (fundamental frequency) and registers pulses with frequencies centered at 40 MHz (second harmonic). Then, a bolus injection of contrast agent (Definity™, Bristol-Myers Squibb Inc., New York, NY) is made through a delivery catheter. The microbubbles were first detected within the main lumen, and then (after 5–10 s) within the adventitia surrounding the plaque. A quantification of the enhancement was found to be statistically significant. In addition, the general spatial pattern of the agent presence within the adventitia and not the plaque itself was consistent with the microvascular distribution revealed by histological sections taken in the vicinity of the imaging planes.

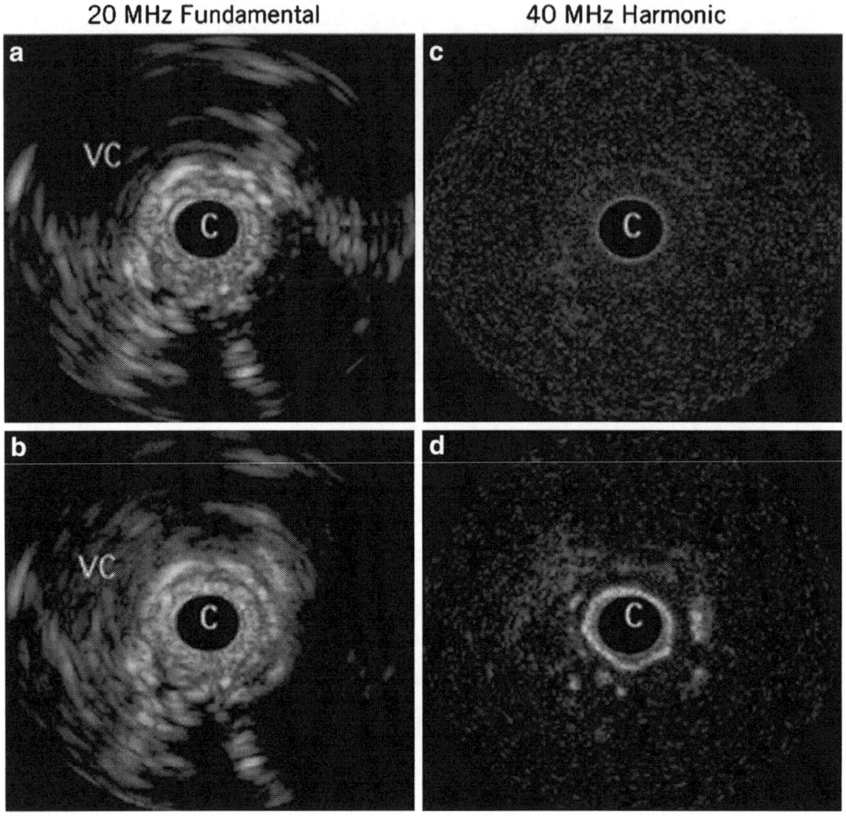

Fig. 4. (**a**, **b**) Fundamental mode before and after the injection of microbubbles, respectively; (**c**, **d**) harmonic mode before and after the injection of microbubbles, respectively. Legend: C: catheter, VC: vena cava. (Reprinted from [22]).

In vivo phantom experiments were carried out to investigate the feasibility of subharmonic IVUS imaging using an atherosclerotic rabbit aorta model [23]. In this study, a frequency of 30 MHz is used as fundamental while the system is focused on registering the microbubble response at frequencies of 15 MHz (subharmonic). The results provide evidence of the potential use of this technique for the imaging of vasa vasorum.

Tissue harmonic imaging (THI) is investigated in [24, 25]. Here, a dual-frequency transducer element was mounted in an IVUS catheter. As a result, this prototype IVUS system can operate in both fundamental frequency and second harmonic imaging modes. This system uses a conventional, continuously rotating, single-element IVUS catheter and was operated in fundamental 20 MHz, fundamental 40 MHz, and harmonic 40 MHz modes (transmit 20 MHz, receive 40 MHz). Imaging experiments were conducted in both a tissue-mimicking phantom and in an atherosclerotic rabbit model in vivo. The harmonic results of the imaging experiments show the feasibility of this system for improving the IVUS image quality. In addition, this system has the potential to be used with contrast agents for VV imaging.

The advantage of the use of nonlinear IVUS techniques is that it overcomes the limitation of fundamental imaging to detect microvessels, which is related to its susceptibility to motion effects. Moreover, harmonic imaging is capable of using the resonant bubble oscillations from commercial contrast agents, using pressure levels that are within the range of current commercial catheters. However, despite the effectiveness of the harmonic imaging methods, contrast-enhanced fundamental IVUS with proper image analysis has the potential for large-scale clinical application due to the fact that commercial harmonic IVUS catheters are not currently available.

CONCLUSIONS

The identification of patients with a high risk for developing an acute coronary syndrome remains a challenge because of the limited knowledge on vulnerable coronary atherosclerotic plaques, the mechanisms that trigger their rupture, and the lack of reliable techniques for detecting them. However, since the presence of neovascularization has been documented to be highly related to plaque inflammation, intraplaque hemorrhage, and plaque rupture and thus has been identified as a major characteristic of plaque vulnerability, it is desirable to test with techniques that can provide reliable assessment of the VV density in vivo. Contrast-enhanced intravascular ultrasound techniques such as those described here have been shown to be useful for the assessment of luminal and plaque characteristics, plaque VV revealing, and plaque inflammation. These techniques may contribute significantly to the detection of neovascularization within the coronary atherosclerotic plaques. Future developments as improvement in resolution, signal-to-noise ratio, and robustness to IVUS artifacts as well as histological validation are necessary in order to augment the reliability of the detection of vulnerable plaque. However, since VV are not the only feature of plaque vulnerability, the combination of this and other invasive and noninvasive existing modalities would be necessary in order to provide an effective way to determine and study the causes that lead to plaque rupture and the consequent thrombotic complications.

ACKNOWLEDGMENTS

We would like to thank S. Carlier, J. Granada, N. Dib, C. Stefanadis, T. Papaioannou, S. Vaina, M. Drakopoulou, and I. Mitropoulos for their contributions and assistance on the UIVUS project. Vasa Vasorum detection and quantification using differential imaging was supported in part by NSF Grant IIS-0431144 and an NSF Graduate Research Fellowship (SMO). Any opinions, findings, and conclusions or recommendations expressed in this material are those of the authors and do not necessarily reflect the views of the NSF.

REFERENCES

1. M. Naghavi, P. Libby, E. Falk, S. W. Casscells, S. Litovsky, J. Rumberger, J. J. Badimon, C. Stefanadis, P. Moreno, G. Pasterkamp, Z. Fayad, P. H. Stone, S. Waxman, P. Raggi, M. Madjid, A. Zarrabi, A. Burke, C. Yuan, P. J. Fitzgerald, D. S. Siscovick, C. L. de Korte, M. Aikawa, K. E. Airaksinen, G. Assmann, C. R. Becker, J. H. Chesebro, A. Farb, Z. S. Galis, C. Jackson, I. K. Jang, W. Koenig, R. A. Lodder, K. March, J. Demirovic, M. Navab, S. G. Priori, M. D. Rekhter, R. Bahr, S. M. Grundy, R. Mehran, A. Colombo, E. Boerwinkle, C. Ballantyne, W. Insull, Jr., R. S. Schwartz, R. Vogel, P. W. Serruys, G. K. Hansson, D. P. Faxon, S. Kaul, H. Drexler, P. Greenland, J. E. Muller, R. Virmani, P. M. Ridker, D. P. Zipes, P. K. Shah, and J. T. Willerson, "From vulnerable plaque to vulnerable patient: A call for new definitions and risk assessment strategies: Part I," Circulation, vol. 108, pp. 1664–1672, 2003.
2. A. P. Burke, A. Farb, G. T. Malcom, Y. Liang, J. Smialek, and R. Virmani, "Coronary risk factors and plaque morphology in men with coronary disease who died suddenly," N Engl J Med, vol. 336, pp. 1276–1282, 1997.
3. P. Constantinides, "Cause of thrombosis in human atherosclerotic arteries," Am J Cardiol, vol. 66, pp. 37G–40G, 1990.
4. F. D. Kolodgie, A. P. Burke, A. Farb, H. K. Gold, J. Yuan, J. Narula, A. V. Finn, and R. Virmani, "The thin-cap fibroatheroma: A type of vulnerable plaque: The major precursor lesion to acute coronary syndromes," Curr Opin Cardiol, vol. 16, pp. 285–292, 2001.
5. R. Virmani, F. D. Kolodgie, A. P. Burke, A. V. Finn, H. K. Gold, T. N. Tulenko, S. P. Wrenn, and J. Narula, "Atherosclerotic plaque progression and vulnerability to rupture: Angiogenesis as a source of intraplaque hemorrhage," Arterioscler Thromb Vasc Biol, vol. 25, pp. 2054–2061, 2005.
6. R. Virmani, F. D. Kolodgie, A. P. Burke, A. Farb, and S. M. Schwartz, "Lessons from sudden coronary death a comprehensive morphological classification scheme for atherosclerotic lesions," Arterioscler Thromb Vasc Biol, vol. 20, pp. 1262–1275, 2000.
7. M. Vavuranakis, T. G. Papaioannou, I. A. Kakadiaris, S. M. O'Malley, M. Naghavi, K. Filis, E. A. Sanidas, A. Papalois, I. Stamatopoulos, and C. Stefanadis, "Detection of perivascular blood flow in vivo by contrast-enhanced intracoronary ultrasonography and image analysis: An animal study," Clin Exp Pharmacol Physiol, vol. 34, pp. 1319–1323, 2007.
8. D. D. Heistad and M. L. Marcus, "Role of vasa vasorum in nourishment of the aorta," Blood Vessels, vol. 16, pp. 225–238, 1979.
9. C. Stefanadis, C. Vlachopoulos, P. Karayannacos, H. Boudoulas, C. Stratos, T. Filippides, M. Agapitos, and P. Toutouzas, "Effect of vasa vasorum flow on structure and function of the aorta in experimental animals," Circulation, vol. 91, pp. 2669–2678, 1995.

10. H. M. Kwon, G. Sangiorgi, E. L. Ritman, C. McKenna, D. R. Holmes Jr, R. S. Schwartz, and A. Lerman, "Enhanced coronary vasa vasorum neovascularization in experimental hypercholesterolemia," J Clin Invest, vol. 101, p. 1551–6, 1998.
11. P. R. Moreno, K. R. Purushothaman, V. Fuster, and W. N. O'Connor, "Intimomedial interface damage and adventitial inflammation is increased beneath disrupted atherosclerosis in the aorta: Implications for plaque vulnerability," Circulation, vol. 105, pp. 2504–2511, 2002.
12. K. S. Moulton, K. Vakili, D. Zurakowski, M. Soliman, C. Butterfield, E. Sylvin, K. M. Lo, S. Gillies, K. Javaherian, and J. Folkman, "Inhibition of plaque neovascularization reduces macrophage accumulation and progression of advanced atherosclerosis," Proc Natl Acad Sci USA, 2003, vol. 100, pp. 4736–4741.
13. M. Fleiner, M. Kummer, M. Mirlacher, G. Sauter, G. Cathomas, R. Krapf, and B. C. Biedermann, "Arterial neovascularization and inflammation in vulnerable patients: Early and late signs of symptomatic atherosclerosis," Circulation, vol. 110, pp. 2843–2850, 2004.
14. P. R. Moreno, K. R. Purushothaman, V. Fuster, D. Echeverri, H. Truszczynska, S. K. Sharma, J. J. Badimon, and W. N. O'Connor, "Plaque neovascularization is increased in ruptured atherosclerotic lesions of human aorta: Implications for plaque vulnerability," Circulation, vol. 110, pp. 2032–2038, 2004.
15. F. D. Kolodgie, H. K. Gold, A. P. Burke, D. R. Fowler, H. S. Kruth, D. K. Weber, A. Farb, L. J. Guerrero, M. Hayase, R. Kutys, J. Narula, A. V. Finn, and R. Virmani, "Intraplaque hemorrhage and progression of coronary atheroma," N Engl J Med, vol. 349, pp. 2316–2325, 2003.
16. M. R. Hayden and S. C. Tyagi, "Vasa vasorum in plaque angiogenesis, metabolic syndrome, type 2 diabetes mellitus, and atheroscleropathy: A malignant transformation," Cardiovasc Diabetol, vol. 3, 1, 2004.
17. N. de Jong, A. Bouakaz, and F. J. T. Cate, "Contrast harmonic imaging," Ultrasonics, vol. 40, pp. 567–573, 2002.
18. S. M. O'Malley, M. Vavuranakis, M. Naghavi, and I. A. Kakadiaris, "Intravascular ultrasound-based imaging of vasa vasorum for the detection of vulnerable atherosclerotic plaque," Int Conf Med Image Comput Comput Assist Interv, 2005 vol. 8, pp. 343–351.
19. M. Vavuranakis, I. A. Kakadiaris, S. M. O'Malley, C. Stefanadis, S. Vaina, M. Drakopoulou, I. Mitropoulos, S. Carlier, and M. Naghavi, "Detection of luminal-intimal border and coronary wall enhancement in intravascular ultrasound imaging after injection of microbubbles and simultaneous sonication with transthoracic echocardiography," Circulation, vol. 112, pp. e1–e2, 2005.
20. S. Carlier, I. A. Kakadiaris, N. Dib, M. Vavuranakis, C. Stefanadis, S. M. O'Malley, C. J. Hartley, R. W. Metcalfe, R. Mehran, E. Falk, K. Gul, and M. Naghavi, "Vasa vasorum imaging: A new window to the clinical detection of vulnerable atherosclerotic plaques," Curr Atheroscler Rep, vol. 7, pp. 164–169, 2005.
21. D. E. Goertz, M. E. Frijlink, N. de Jong, and A. F. van der Steen, "Nonlinear intravascular ultrasound contrast imaging," Ultrasound Med Biol, vol. 32, pp. 491–502, 2006.
22. D. E. Goertz, M. E. Frijlink, D. Tempel, L. C. A. van Damme, R. Krams, J. A. Schaar, F. J. ten Cate, P. W. Serruys, N. de Jong, and A. F. W. van der Steen, "Contrast harmonic intravascular ultrasound: A feasibility study for vasa vasorum imaging," Invest Radiol, vol. 41, pp. 631–638, 2006.
23. D. E. Goertz, M. E. Frijlink, D. Tempel, V. Bhagwandas, A. Gisolf, R. Krams, N. de Jong, and A. F. van der Steen, "Subharmonic contrast intravascular ultrasound for vasa vasorum imaging," Ultrasound Med Biol, vol. 33, pp. 1859–1872, 2007.
24. M. E. Frijlink, D. E. Goertz, L. C. A. van Damme, R. Krams, and A. F. van der Steen, "Intravascular ultrasound tissue harmonic imaging in vivo," Ultrasonics Symposium, 2004 IEEE, vol. 2, pp. 1118–1121, 2004.
25. M. E. Frijlink, D. E. Goertz, H. J. Vos, E. Tesselaar, G. Blacquicre, A. Gisolf, R. Krams, and A. F. W. van der Steen, "Harmonic intravascular ultrasound imaging with a dual-frequency catheter," Ultrasound Med Biol, vol. 32, pp. 1649–1654, 2006.
26. M. Vavuranakis, I. A. Kakadiaris, S. M. O'Malley, T. G. Papaioannou, E. A. Sanidas, M. Naghavi, S. Carlier, D. Tousoulis, and C. Stefanadis, "A new method for assessment of plaque vulnerability based on vasa vasorum imaging, by using contrast-enhanced intravascular ultrasound and differential image analysis," Int J Cardiol, vol. 130, pp. 23–29, 2008.

39

From Vulnerable Plaque to Vulnerable Patient – Part III

The SHAPE Paradigm – Screening for Detection and Treatment of Asymptomatic Atherosclerosis

Task Force Report Executive Summary

Morteza Naghavi, Erling Falk, Harvey S. Hecht, Michael J. Jamieson, Sanjay Kaul, Daniel S. Berman, Zahi Fayad, Matthew J. Budoff, John Rumberger, Tasneem Z. Naqvi, Leslee J. Shaw, Jay N. Cohn, Ole Faergeman, Raymond D. Bahr, Wolfgang Koenig, Jasenka Demirovic, Dan Arking, Victoria L.M. Herrera, Juan Jose Badimon, James A. Goldstein, Arturo G.Touchard, Yoram Rudy, K.E. Juhani Airaksinen, Robert S. Schwartz, Ward A. Riley, Robert A. Mendes, Pamela S. Douglas, and Prediman K. Shah

From: *Asymptomatic Atherosclerosis: Pathophysiology, Detection and Treatment*
Edited by: M. Naghavi (ed.), DOI 10.1007/978-1-60327-179-0_39

Contents

Abstract

Screening for early-stage asymptomatic cancers (e.g., breast and colon) to prevent late-stage malignancies has been widely accepted. However, although atherosclerotic cardiovascular disease (e.g., heart attack and stroke) accounts for more death and disability than all cancers combined, there are no national screening guidelines for asymptomatic (subclinical) atherosclerosis, and there is no government or healthcare-sponsored reimbursement for atherosclerosis screening. Parts I and II of this consensus statement elaborated on new discoveries in the field of atherosclerosis that led to the concept of the vulnerable patient. These landmark discoveries, along with the new diagnostic and therapeutic options, have set the stage for the next step: translation of this knowledge into a new practice of preventive cardiology. *The identification and the treatment of the vulnerable patient are the focus of this consensus statement.*

In this report, the Screening for Heart Attack Prevention and Education (SHAPE) Task Force presents a new practice guideline for cardiovascular screening in the asymptomatic at-risk population. In summary, the SHAPE Guideline calls for noninvasive screening of all asymptomatic men 45–75 years of age and asymptomatic women 55–75 years of age (except those defined as very low risk) to detect and treat those with subclinical atherosclerosis. A variety of screening tests are available, and the cost effectiveness of their use in a comprehensive strategy must be validated. Some of these screening tests, such as measurement of coronary artery calcification (CAC) by computed tomography (CT) scanning and carotid artery intima-media thickness and plaque by ultrasonography, have been available longer than others and are capable of providing direct evidence for the presence and extent of atherosclerosis. Both these imaging methods provide prognostic information of proven value regarding the future risk of heart attack and stroke. Careful and responsible implementation of these tests as part of a comprehensive risk assessment and reduction approach is warranted and outlined by this report. Other tests for the detection of atherosclerosis and abnormal arterial structure and function, such as magnetic resonance imaging (MRI) of the great arteries, studies of small and large artery stiffness, and assessment of systemic endothelial dysfunction, are emerging and need to be further validated. The screening results (severity of subclinical arterial disease) combined with risk factor assessment are used for risk stratification to identify the vulnerable patient and secure appropriate therapy. The higher the risk, the more vulnerable an individual is to a near-term adverse event. Since less than 10% of the population who test positive for atherosclerosis will experience a near-term event, additional risk stratification based on reliable markers of disease activity is needed and is expected to further focus the search for the vulnerable patient in the future.

All individuals with asymptomatic atherosclerosis should be counseled and treated to prevent progression to overt clinical disease. The aggressiveness of the treatment should be proportional to the level of risk. Individuals with no evidence of subclinical disease may be reassured of the low risk of a future near-term event, yet encouraged to adhere to a healthy lifestyle and maintain appropriate risk factor levels. Early heart attack care education is urged for all individuals with a positive test for atherosclerosis.

The SHAPE Task Force reinforces existing guidelines for the screening and treatment of risk factors in younger populations.

Cardiovascular healthcare professionals and policymakers are urged to adopt the SHAPE proposal and its attendant cost effectiveness as a new strategy to contain the epidemic of atherosclerotic cardiovascular disease and the rising cost of therapies associated with this epidemic.

Key words: Cardiovascular Screening; Atherosclerosis; Asymptomatic Atherosclerosis; Subclinical Atherosclerosis; Noninvasive Imaging; Coronary Artery Calcium Score; Carotid Intima Media Thickness; CAC; IMT; Vascular Function; Primary Prevention; Vulnerable Plaque; Vulnerable Patient; Acute Coronary Syndromes; Sudden Cardiac Death; Preventive Cardiology

KEY POINTS

- Screening for risk factors of cardiovascular disease is not sufficient for identification of asymptomatic patients with subclinical atherosclerosis who are at risk of a near future adverse event.
- Direct assessment of vascular structure and function is needed, in addition to measuring risk factors.
- The SHAPE Task Force thoroughly evaluated the available evidence until 2005, and recommended noninvasive imaging of coronary artery calcium and carotid intima-media thickness for screening asymptomatic populations (male: 45–75 and female: 55–75).
- The SHAPE Task will revise its recommendations in 2010 in light of new evidence.

INTRODUCTION

Atherosclerosis is a common and dangerous disease of the arteries of the heart, brain, and periphery. It is by far the most frequent underlying cause of angina, heart attack, and peripheral arterial disease and is responsible for many cases of stroke. Thus, atherosclerosis and its thrombotic complications are the most deadly and disabling diseases in affluent countries, and, in the near future, will be so in the entire world [1, 2]. Yet many individuals, even those with severe atherosclerosis, are unaware, because they have no symptoms. In 30–50% of these individuals, the first indicator of atherosclerosis is an acute heart attack, which often is fatal [3–5].

Although easily measured, potentially modifiable risk factors account for over 90% of the risk of an initial acute myocardial infarction (MI) [1, 6, 7] and effective risk-lowering therapies exist, MI or sudden unexpected death remain all too common first manifestations of coronary atherosclerosis. These attacks often occur in patients who are not receiving the benefits of preventive therapies of proven efficacy because their arterial disease was unrecognized (asymptomatic) and/or they had been misclassified by conventional risk factors and assigned a treatment goal at odds with their individual burden of atherosclerosis.

Many pharmacologic and nonpharmacologic therapies have been shown to prevent atherosclerotic events and prolong survival. Therefore, early detection of atherosclerosis itself before symptoms occur can provide a major opportunity to prevent many cardiovascular events. Since screening to identify subclinical or asymptomatic atherosclerosis could confer great public health benefit, it may seem surprising that it has not yet been incorporated into national and international clinical guidelines. Therapeutic strategies targeting at-risk vulnerable patients can reduce the heavy economic burden of symptomatic and end-stage care for cardiovascular disease (CVD).

There have been two primary reasons for this conservative strategy. First, there has been a presumed lack of data demonstrating that screening for subclinical atherosclerosis improves the risk assessment beyond that provided by traditional risk factors such as smoking, hypertension, hypercholesterolemia, and diabetes. Second, the appropriate tools for the detection of subclinical atherosclerosis have not been widely available to clinicians. However, recent developments have provided us with both the requisite data and the necessary technology, as well as highly effective and safe therapies.

Burden of Atherosclerotic Cardiovascular Disease

Atherosclerosis is responsible for nearly all cases of coronary heart disease (CHD), intermittent claudication and critical limb ischemia, and many cases of strokes. CHD alone is the single largest killer of American males and females (479,300 in 2003), causing more than 1 of every 5 deaths [3]. This year, an estimated 875,000 Americans will have a first heart attack, and 500,000 will have a recurrent attack [3]. Because the risk of CHD increases markedly with age, and women live longer than men, almost as many women ultimately die of CHD as men [3].

About 700,000 Americans will have a stroke this year. Stroke is the number 3 killer and a leading cause of severe, long-term disability [3]. In 2002, 657,054 people succumbed in the United States to heart attacks and stroke compared to 557,264 deaths to cancers [8, 9]. Despite the greater magnitude of CVD, screening for occult breast and colorectal cancer has become a widely adopted public policy strategy, while screening for subclinical atherosclerosis in at-risk adults to prevent heart attack and stroke is not currently recommended [10].

The cost of clinical care during and after an acute heart attack is growing rapidly, and the number of patients with heart failure after heart attack has been escalating in the past two decades [11, 12]. There is, therefore, an imperative to develop a new paradigm to screen for subclinical atherosclerosis and circumvent its transition to deadly and costly clinical and symptomatic stages.

Risk Factors, Susceptibility, and Vulnerability

Atherosclerosis begins to develop early in life and progresses with time, but the speed of progression is to a large extent unpredictable and differs markedly among seemingly comparable individuals. At every level of risk factor exposure, the amount of established atherosclerosis and the vulnerability to acute events vary greatly, probably because of genetic variability in an individual's susceptibility to atherosclerosis and propensity to arterial thrombosis (vulnerable blood) and ventricular arrhythmias (vulnerable myocardium). Comparative studies of prospective trials with clinical follow-up have revealed that the observed event rate may differ several fold among populations predicted to have similar risk by risk factor scoring [13–19].

The prevalence of one or more major risk factors (beyond age) is very high among Americans aged 40 years and above who develop CHD [20]. However, it is also high among those who do not develop CHD, illustrating that when risk factors are almost universally present in a population, they do not predict the development of disease very well in individuals [21–24]. Based on data recently published from three influential prospective epidemiological studies [20], Weissler highlighted this failure by using likelihood ratio (LR) analysis [25]. An LR of 2.0 or less denotes low predictive power and an LR of 9.0 or more denotes high predictive power. Remarkably low predictive power (LR < 1.4) was found for one or more risk factors in predicting CHD death and/or nonfatal MI, despite the high frequency of this risk profile in the population with CHD events. The relationship between cigarette smoking and lung cancer provides a reasonable analogy: when almost everyone in a given population smokes, smoking itself fails to predict the risk of cancer.

The limitations of the traditional risk factors to identify at-risk individuals constitute the foundation behind the "*Polypill*" strategy in which people with known CVD or over a specified age would be treated with a single daily pill containing 6 components to reduce events and prolong survival, regardless of what current risk assessment algorithms predict [26]. Age is the most discriminatory screening factor in apparently healthy individuals; 96% of deaths from CHD or stroke occur in people aged 55 and over [26].

CURRENT GUIDELINES IN PRIMARY PREVENTION

The current guidelines in primary prevention recommend initial assessment and risk stratification based on traditional risk factors (e.g., the Framingham Risk Score in the United States and the SCORE in Europe), followed by goal-directed therapy when necessary [19, 27–29]. Although this approach may identify persons at very low or very high risk of a heart attack or stroke within the next 10 years, the majority of the population belongs to an intermediate risk group in which the predictive power of risk factors is low. Most heart attacks occur in this group. Consequently, many individuals at-risk will not be properly identified and will not be treated to appropriate "individualized" goals. Others will be erroneously classified as high risk and will be unnecessarily treated with drug therapy for the rest of their lives. This strategy is neither cost effective nor good medicine.

The limitations of current guidelines are recognized by the American Heart Association (AHA), the National Cholesterol Education Program (NCEP) expert panel, and by the European Third Joint Task Force [19, 27, 29]. Therefore, these organizations recommended the use of noninvasive screening tests that identify abnormal arterial structure and function as an option for advanced risk assessment in appropriately selected persons, particularly in those with multiple risk factors who are judged to be at intermediate (or indeterminate) risk. These tests include carotid intima-media thickness (CIMT) measured by ultrasound, coronary artery calcification (CAC) determined by computed tomography (CT), endothelial vasomotor dysfunction evaluated by ultrasound, ankle/brachial blood pressure ratio (ABI), and magnetic resonance imaging (MRI) techniques [19, 27, 29].

CHD Risk Equivalents

Patients who already have developed clinical atherosclerotic disease, whether cerebral (transient ischemic attack or stroke of carotid origin) or peripheral (claudication or abdominal aortic aneurysm), have declared themselves to be at continued high risk (vulnerable) [30]. Current American and European guidelines also recognize groups of asymptomatic patients who are at similar high risk [19,27,29]. They include patients with diabetes, as well as asymptomatic patients in whom atherosclerosis and/or its consequences have been demonstrated by noninvasive testing. For example, the presence of myocardial ischemia appropriately identified by stress testing qualifies as a diagnosis of CHD. Moreover, carotid or ilio-femoral atherosclerosis is considered a CHD risk equivalent and should be treated aggressively; atherosclerosis in one vascular bed predicts atherosclerosis in other vascular beds. In addition, patients with two or more risk factors with a 10-year risk for CHD > 20% are consider a CHD risk equivalent. *However, existing guidelines do not recognize severe nonobstructive coronary atherosclerosis as a CHD risk equivalent even though most heart attacks originate from nonobstructive coronary plaques.*

Screening for Subclinical Atherosclerosis

In a recent scientific statement, the American Cancer Society (ACS), the AHA, and the American Diabetes Association announced a new collaborative initiative to create a national commitment to the prevention and early detection of cancer, CVD, and diabetes [31]. The ACS recommends the following screening ages: 20 for breast cancer with mammography from age 40 (at least annually), 21 for cervical cancer (Pap test), 50 for colorectal cancer (several options), and 50 for prostate cancer (prostate-specific antigen test and digital rectal examination annually) [31].

The AHA recommends that assessment of cardiovascular risk begin at age 20, to be repeated at regular intervals, preferentially by calculating the Framingham Risk Score [31]. In contrast to cancer, early detection of CVD by screening with the best available technology is not mentioned, despite, the more than 500,000 deaths per year from atherosclerosis, compared to ~57,000 from colorectoanal cancer, ~42,000 from breast cancer, and ~31,000 from prostate cancer [8, 9]. The current focus on breast cancer overlooks the much greater threat to young and middle-aged women posed by CVD.

At this juncture, it is imperative that the traditional, imprecise risk factor approach to individual risk assessment in primary prevention be revamped, with implementation of a paradigm largely based on noninvasive screening for the disease itself (subclinical atherosclerosis). The Screening for Heart Attack Prevention and Education (SHAPE) Task Force has developed such a model to identify those who are susceptible to atherosclerosis and its thrombotic and arrhythmogenic complications (vulnerable patients) and initiate appropriate care to prevent the sequelae of CVD, and to avoid unnecessarily intensive treatment.

NEW PARADIGM FOR THE PREVENTION OF HEART ATTACK

In Search of the Vulnerable Patient

Parts I and II of this consensus statement elaborated on new discoveries in the field of atherosclerosis that led to the concept of the vulnerable patient [32,33]. This, in turn, focused on the identification and aggressive treatment of the previously unrecognized very-high-risk population, neglecting the majority of the population who are not in the very-high-risk category. To rectify this major omission, the SHAPE report introduces a new paradigm to stratify the entire US population at risk and to tailor recommendations accordingly. Almost all vulnerable individuals have detectable subclinical atherosclerosis, and we now possess the tools to identify it with sufficient predictive power. It is therefore proposed that all apparently healthy men 45–75 years of age, and women 55–75 years of age, with no known CHD and who are considered *not* to be at very low risk (footnoted under Figure 4) – undergo screening for atherosclerosis. Of the 61,163,000 US populations in the SHAPE age range, 3,951,000 have known CHD. The size of the very-low-risk population is difficult to ascertain but is probably around 5–10% based on data from large US cohort studies [7]. This population, and those who have already undergone CACS or CIMT assessment, is excluded from the SHAPE eligible population. Since exact number is not available, 50 million has been chosen as the approximate number who will require SHAPE evaluation. Based on a 50% compliance rate for SHAPE screening over 10 years, and a 5-year re-examination cycle, the number of people required to annual screening after a decade will decrease to 5–6 million per year.

An estimated 875,000 Americans annually experience a first heart attack of which 175,000 are silent heart attacks [3]. Since approximately 500,000 of the total will occur in the 50 million SHAPE eligible population (the peak of the pyramid in Fig. 1), a screening ratio of 1/100 (500,000/50,000,000) is anticipated. Almost all the events will occur in the ~50% of the eligible population who have a positive atherosclerosis test. They, therefore, have ~2% annual risk, consistent with the high-risk classification used in the existing US guidelines. However, according to the SHAPE classification in those with positive tests, the annual risk escalates as the burden of atherosclerosis increases, as demonstrated in Fig. 1. Those with the highest burden of atherosclerosis are the most vulnerable patients. A major advantage of the SHAPE guideline over the existing guidelines is that in the existing guidelines the low-risk and intermediate-risk population account for the majority of heart attacks, and only less than

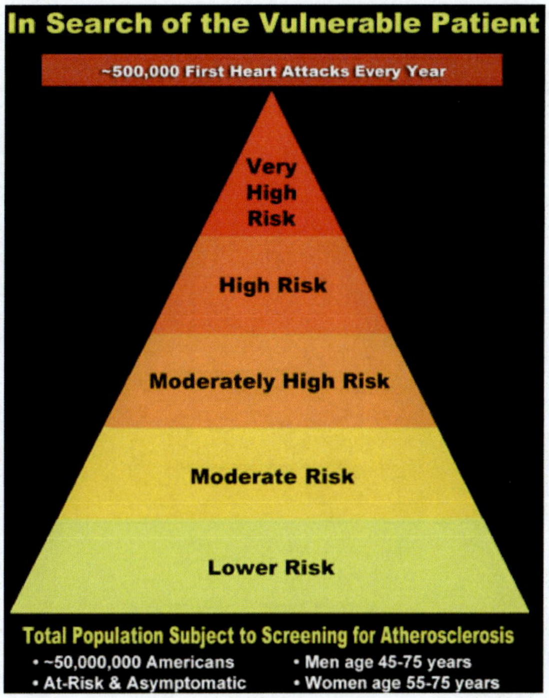

Fig. 1. The SHAPE paradigm calls for screening all apparently healthy (with no prior diagnosis of CHD) men 45–75 years of age and women 55–75 years of age who are not considered very low risk. This population accounts for approximately 50 million people in the US.

20% of the total number of the events results from the high-risk population, whereas in the SHAPE guideline, the majority of heart attacks happens in the high-risk population.

Criteria for Recommended Screening Tests

Several factors are used in selecting individual tests as part of a screening program. These factors include (1) the abundance of evidence for the predictive value of the test in the recommended population over and above that available from standard office-based risk assessment tools (incremental value), (2) availability, (3) reproducibility, (4) complementary value with respect to the concept of the vulnerable patient, and/or (5) cost effectiveness relative to the status quo.

Figure 2 illustrates the array of available diagnostic tests, including traditional risk factor based and tests that more directly evaluate the presence or effect of atherosclerosis.

The following atherosclerosis screening methods were selected by virtue of best fulfilling the aforementioned criteria:

- Coronary artery calcium (CAC) determined by CT
- Carotid intima-media thickness (CIMT) and plaque determined by ultrasonography

The evidence behind this selection and the suggested threshold values in the 1st SHAPE Guideline have accumulated in recent years [34–69], and further support can be found in the full SHAPE Report (www.aeha.org).

The 1st SHAPE Guideline

A conceptual flow chart illustrating the principles of the new paradigm is shown in Fig. 3.

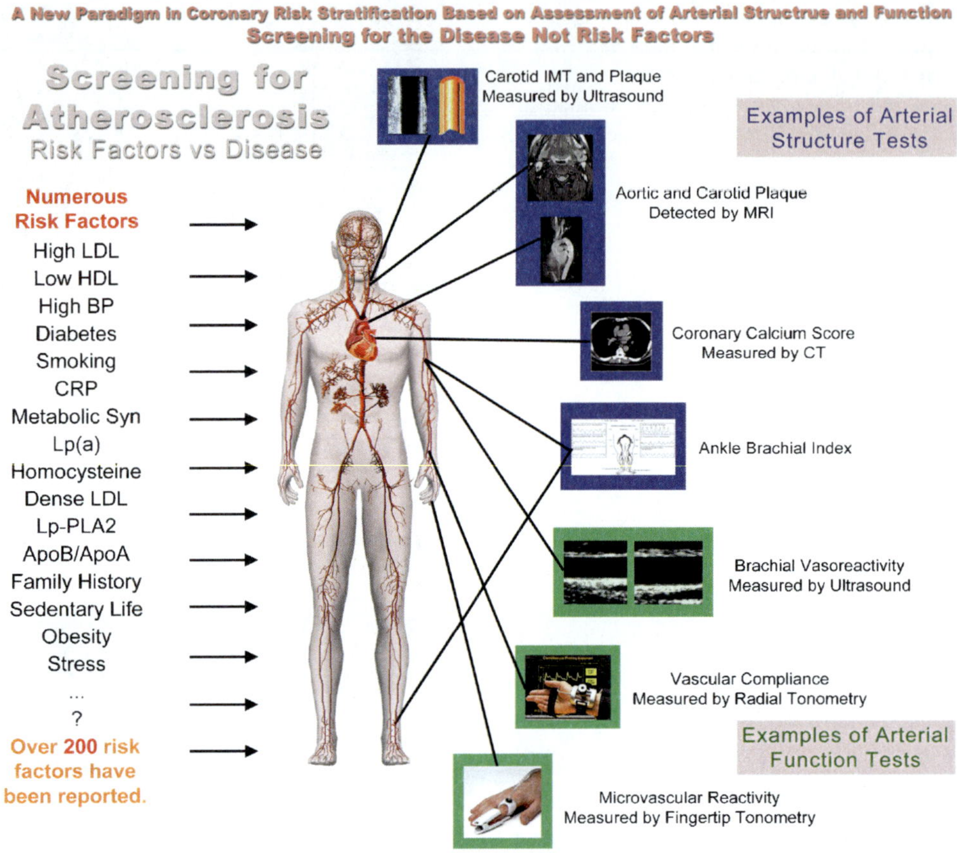

Fig. 2. The new SHAPE paradigm: screening *directly* for the presence and severity of atherosclerosis by structure and function testing (*right*), versus the traditional approach in which the likelihood of atherosclerotic disease is estimated *indirectly* by evaluating risk factors for the disease (*left*).

In contrast to the existing traditional risk-factor-based guidelines, this new strategy is primarily based on noninvasive screening for subclinical atherosclerosis using two well-established noninvasive imaging modalities – CT for measurement of CACS and B mode ultrasound for measurement of CIMT and carotid plaque [34–69]. This strategy is driven by the data-supported principle that the major determinant of risk for atherosclerotic CVD in asymptomatic adults is the presence of the underlying disease itself, i.e., subclinical atherosclerosis. Early detection of atherosclerosis will permit more widespread and effective prevention strategies to be implemented through accurate risk stratification and tailoring the intensity of therapy to the underlying CHD risk in a cost-effective manner.

The screening strategy for risk assessment and the associated treatment algorithm of the 1st SHAPE Guideline are summarized in Fig. 4.

Briefly, all asymptomatic men 45–75 years of age and women 55–75 years of age who do not have very-low-risk characteristics or a documented history of CVD are encouraged to undergo screening for atherosclerosis. The *very-low-risk* group is characterized by the absence of any traditional cardiovascular risk factors (footnoted under Fig. 4).

Individuals with negative tests for atherosclerosis (defined as CACS = 0, or CIMT < 50th percentile without carotid plaque) are classified as *Lower Risk* (those without conventional risk factors)

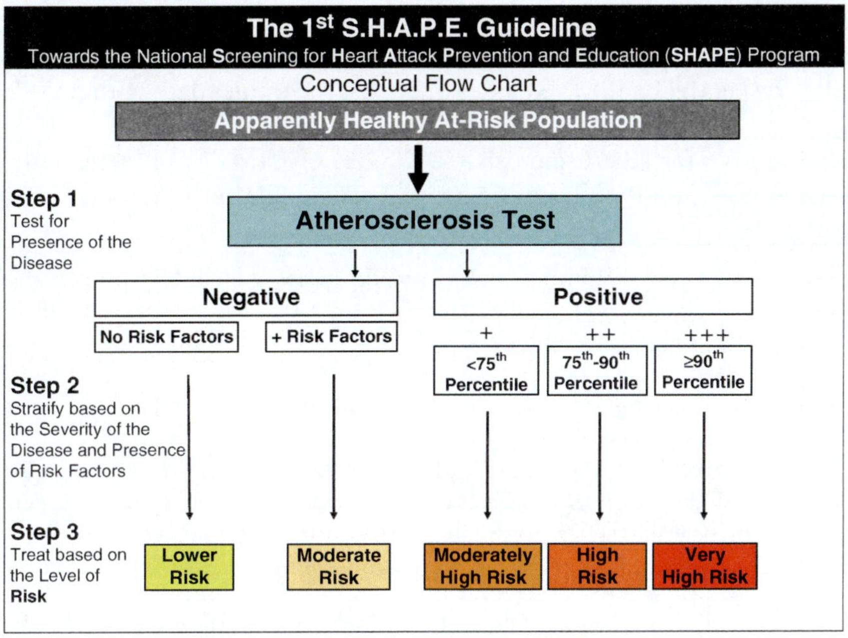

Fig. 3. Conceptual flow chart illustrating the principles of the new algorithm.

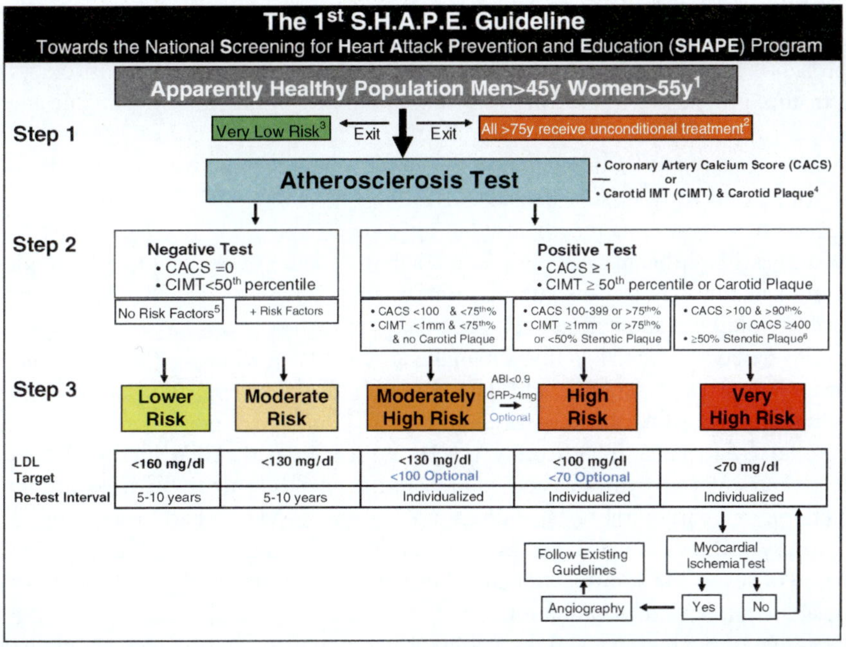

Fig. 4. The SHAPE Guideline Flow Chart. **1**: No history of angina, heart attack, stroke, or peripheral arterial disease. **2**: Population over age 75 years is considered high risk and must receive therapy without testing for atherosclerosis. **3**: Must not have any of the following: Chol>200 mg/dl, blood pressure>120/80 mmHg, diabetes, smoking, family history, metabolic syndrome. **4**: Pending the development of standard practice guidelines. **5**: High cholesterol, high blood pressure, diabetes, smoking, family history, metabolic syndrome. **6**: For stroke prevention, follow existing guidelines.

or *Moderate Risk* (those with established risk factors), and treated as recommended in the NCEP ATP III guidelines with low-density lipoprotein cholesterol (LDL-C) targets of <160 mg/dL and <130 mg/dL, respectively [28]. Reassessment is recommended within 5–10 years unless otherwise indicated.

Those who test positive for atherosclerosis (CACS ≥ 1, or CIMT ≥ 50th percentile or presence of carotid plaque) are further stratified according to the magnitude of atherosclerotic burden into the following risk categories:

- *Moderately High Risk*: CACS <100 (but >0) and <75th percentile, or a CIMT <1 mm and <75th (but ≥50th) percentile without discernable carotid plaque. Treatment includes lifestyle modifications and an LDL-C target of <130 mg/dL; <100 mg/dL is optional.
- *High Risk*: CACS 100–399 or >75th percentile, or a CIMT ≥1 mm or >75th percentile or a carotid plaque causing <50% stenosis. Treatment calls for aggressive lifestyle modifications and an LDL-C target of <100 mg/dL; <70 mg/dL is optional.
- *Very High Risk*: CACS >100 and >90th percentile or a CACS ≥400, or carotid plaque causing ≥ 50% stenosis. Treatment includes aggressive lifestyle modification and an LDL-C target of <70 mg/dL. Additional testing for myocardial ischemia is recommended for this group, and those who test positive for ischemia should be considered for angiography depending on the extent of the ischemia.

Thus, the 1st SHAPE Guideline emphasizes titrating the intensity of risk factor modification and treatment goals proportional to the risk.

Important Considerations

- The importance of lifestyle modifications recommended by existing guidelines applies to all categories of SHAPE [19,27–29].
- Although arguments could be made for applying the paradigm to those above 75 years, the cost effectiveness of such an approach is questionable [26]. Consequently, the most reasonable path is to apply high risk treatment to those in this group, in view of the high likelihood of significant subclinical atherosclerosis with increasing age.
- Other tests may be considered for optional use. For example, a high C-reactive protein (CRP) value may confer higher risk than lower values [70–72], as does an ABI <0.6 versus 0.6–0.9 [27, 73, 74]. The SHAPE Guideline Flow Chart suggests how these tests may be used to upgrade an individual to a higher risk category.
- ABI below 0.9 suggests significant peripheral atherosclerosis and is associated with a high heart attack risk because of the high likelihood of co-existing coronary atherosclerosis [27, 28]. Aggressive therapy against atherothrombosis should be mandated in such patients.
- Diabetes is not considered a CHD risk equivalent in the absence of subclinical atherosclerosis [75]. If, however, subclinical atherosclerosis is present, diabetes is accorded high-risk status; an increased propensity to arterial thrombosis (vulnerable blood) may be contributory [76, 77].
- The presence of left ventricular hypertrophy (LVH) is also considered a high-risk state because of the increased risk of ventricular arrhythmias and sudden cardiac death (vulnerable myocardium) [78].
- Additional functional and structural tests, such as MRI of the aorta and carotid arteries [79–82], studies of small and large artery stiffness [83, 84], and assessment of endothelial dysfunction [85–87], have been shown to predict events. However, the additive value of these tests to the sensitivity and specificity of detection of subclinical disease requires further validation.
- With the advancement of noninvasive and intravascular imaging techniques aimed at detailed characterization of coronary atherosclerotic plaque, screening for identification of vulnerable plaques might be realized [88–94]. However, it is the *search for the vulnerable patients* and their aggressive treatment that remain the focus of the SHAPE guidelines.
- Reassessment in those with negative atherosclerosis is recommended every 5–10 years. In those with a positive atherosclerosis test, reassessment is recommended within 5 years unless otherwise indicated. In this

context, one may consider factors associated with a higher rate of progression of the disease in individuals within the same level of risk (burden of the disease). For example, patients with diabetes, autoimmune disorders such as rheumatoid arteritis, lupus, and those with renal failure may be on a faster trajectory [95, 96].
- All individuals in the high-risk categories (the atherosclerosis positive SHAPE subpopulation) and their closest relatives should be offered Early Heart Attack Care (EHAC) education, focusing on early warning signs and reducing delay time in seeking medical assistance after the onset of symptoms [97, 98].

Compliance with Treatment

Despite significant and consistent data on the benefits of lipid-lowering agents to reduce cardiovascular events, adherence and utilization of these agents remain low. A recent study demonstrated that statin compliance increased from 44% over 3 years to over 90% in those with baseline calcium scores in the top 75th percentile for age and gender ($p<0.001$) [99]. In multivariable analysis, after adjusting for cardiovascular risk factors, age and gender, higher baseline CAC scores were strongly associated with adherence to statin therapy. In addition to risk stratification for the asymptomatic person, patients visualizing coronary artery calcium may improve utilization and adherence to lipid-lowering therapy.

Cost Effectiveness of SHAPE Guideline vs. Existing Preventive Guideline

In this era of limited health care resources, proof of cost effectiveness is a prerequisite for inclusion of CACS and CIMT in national guidelines on screening to prevent CHD. The SHAPE guideline maintains that shifting of CHD care to subclinical arterial disease (atherosclerosis), particularly to the most vulnerable individuals who bear the highest risk for a near future heart attack, has the potential to circumvent the downstream economic burden of symptomatic CHD and to alleviate the heavy and rising cost of CHD patients in this country.

The cost-effectiveness analysis in this report is based on comparing among competing choices for screening to prevent CHD, with the result being the incremental price of an additional outcome for one strategy as compared with an alternative approach.

The initial economic models examined the cost effectiveness of treating selective at-risk adults (i.e., men 45–75 years and women 55–75 years) with evidence of subclinical atherosclerosis compared to the existing guideline (based on screening for risk factors using the Framingham risk score).

We have also compared the SHAPE guideline with the usual preventive screening care using exercise EKG test.

For our cost-effectiveness analysis, we devised a model comparing:

$$\frac{\text{Costs of Screening} - \text{Costs Averted}}{\text{Net Effectiveness}}$$

We devised our decision models to examine the burden of CHD including the prevalence of CHD, years of life lost prematurely to CHD, disability or changes in quality of life, and the current economic burden of CHD [100]. This, in total, comprised the burden of the disease and incorporated into a single measure both mortality and morbidity of CHD.

From the SHAPE model, when compared with the existing guideline (screening based on risk factors), the use of screening for subclinical atherosclerosis is cost effective, consistently resulting in cost-effectiveness ratios <$50,000 per life year saved.

Based upon evidence that a high percentage of patients are missed by Framingham risk scores [101, 102], approximately 25 million men and 20 million women would be treated with statins based upon evidence of high-risk subclinical atherosclerosis, resulting in 50–65% increase. Treatment of patients with high-risk subclinical disease resulted in an average of 0.58 life year saved given a relative risk reduction with treatment of 35%.

As our economic model attempted to identify costs that may be averted with treatment, we utilized the current costs of CHD burden and used sensitivity analyses to evaluate potential costs averted in our SHAPE analysis. The following table details the results of this analysis including an estimated $21.5 billion dollars each year in care for CHD patients that may be offset by the use of subclinical disease screening with CACS or CIMT.

	Number (per year)	*Estimated Impact of SHAPE (Sensitivity Analysis Range)*	*Estimated Change in Cost*
CVD Deaths	910,600	↓10% (5–25%)	($1.2 b)
MI (prevalence)	7,200,000	↓ 25% (5–35%)	($18.0 b)
Chest Pain Symptoms (ER visits)	6,500,000	↓ 5% (2.5–25%)	($4.1 b)
Hospital Discharge for Primary Diagnosis of CVD	6,373,000	↑ 10% (5–25%)	$3.8 b
Hospital Discharge for Primary Diagnosis of CHD	970,000	↓ 10% (5–25%)	($9.9 b)
Cholesterol Lowering Therapy		↑ 50% (50–65%)	8.00 b
CV Imaging	8,700,000	↑ 10% (5–25%)	$358 m
Angiography	6,800,000	↑ 15% – CTA (2.5–25%)	$600 m
PCI (percutaneous coronary interventions per year)	657,000	↓ 10% (5–50%)	($580 m)
CABS (coronary artery bypass surgeries per year)	515,000	↓ 5% (2.5–50%)	($672 m)
Total Δ in Cost			($21.5 b)

Costs in parentheses are negative costs or reductions in cost. m=Millions, b=Billions
Source: http://www.americanheart.org/presenter.jhtml?identifier=3000090
http://www.acc.org/advocacy/word_files/2005ProposedPhysicianPmtRulev3%20web.xls

It should be noted that decision models do not replace evidence gathered from randomized clinical trials comparing screening for subclinical atherosclerosis to usual care or other strategies. However, given the high cost of such a clinical trial on screening to prevent CHD and that no such study is planned during the next 3–5 years, the current evidence based upon the SHAPE cost models should be considered as state-of-the-economic evidence. Thus, we believe that the application of the SHAPE model, using high-quality prognostic and economic evidence, can aid in the targeting of preventive screening strategies that may result in more dramatic declines in CHD mortality and avert the presentation of symptomatic CHD for thousands of patients every year.

FUTURE DIRECTIONS

Genetic, Structural, and Functional Assessment

Serum markers that can accurately identify the vulnerable individual with both high sensitivity and specificity might be derived from a thorough proteomic survey of blood samples collected from heart attack victims within a few months prior to the event [103]. The incremental predictive value of genes over existing and emerging nongene predictors will need careful scientific and economic evaluation

[104,105]. Noninvasive screening tests for subclinical atherosclerosis are rapidly advancing, and include MRI detection of plaque inflammation, contrast-enhanced CT for assessment of noncalcified plaques, PET-CT for combined assessment of plaque burden and activity of the plaques [106–113]. Other innovative tests for the assessment of vascular structure and function are under development and clinical testing. These include noninvasive molecular imaging tests and noninvasive nonimaging tests such as molecular pulsewave analysis and endothelial function assessment [83–87, 114]. In addition, new serum biomarkers of inflammation and oxidative stress in the arterial wall, e.g., LP-PLA2 and myeloperoxidase, are being actively researched [115, 116]. These emerging tools have the potential to advance the SHAPE guideline and may significantly change the further updates of the Guidelines. Combinations of tests may offer great promise. An ideal scenario would be a combination of a very low-cost, noninvasive, nonimaging test or serum marker (such as endothelial function tests and serum markers of arterial inflammation/oxidation) with an accurate, inexpensive, and widely available imaging tool capable of imaging plaque burden and activity. Such molecular imaging techniques may enable us to accurately identify the site of *vulnerable plaques* based on markers of inflammation, oxidation, angiogenesis, apoptosis, and matrix degradation. The future direction of screening will also be greatly influenced by new developments in therapeutic modalities. The balance between new noninvasive systemic drug therapies capable of rapid stabilization of vulnerable plaques, and new invasive focal therapies without long-term adverse effects, will impact the future of diagnostic screening. Needless to say, in this outcome-oriented era, analysis of the cost effectiveness of the SHAPE guideline will be crucial to its continued implementation.

MISSION

Eradicating Heart Attack

In view of the widespread epidemic of heart attack inherited from the twentieth century, it is difficult for most people to imagine a future in which heart attack is no longer a threat.

However, this goal may achieve reality by the end of the twenty first century [117]. The following illustrates the potential path:

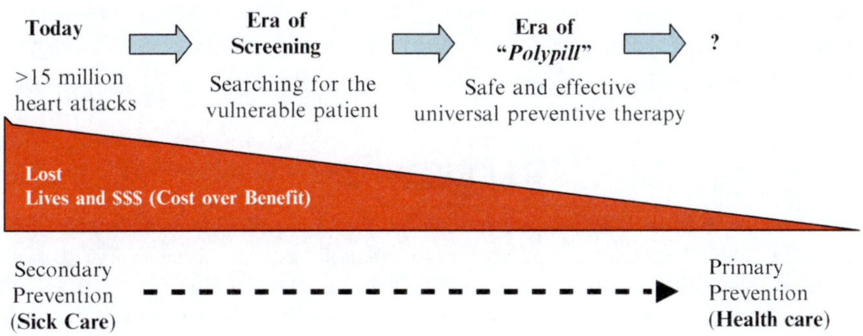

CONCLUSION

The SHAPE Task Force strongly recommends screening of the at-risk asymptomatic population (men 45–75 years of age and women 55–75 years of age) for subclinical atherosclerosis to more accurately identify, and allocate treatment resources to the patients at high risk for acute ischemic events, as well as to identify those at lower risk who may be treated more conservatively. The Task Force reinforces the existing guidelines for screening and treatment of atherosclerosis risk factors in the younger, very low-risk population.

THE SHAPE TASK FORCE

Chairman: Morteza Naghavi, M.D.

Editorial Committee: Prediman K. Shah, M.D. (Chief); (alphabetic order): Raymond Bahr, M.D., Daniel Berman, M.D., Roger Blumenthal, M.D., Matthew J. Budoff, M.D., Jay Cohn, M.D., Erling Falk, M.D., Ph.D., Ole Faergeman, M.D., Zahi Fayad, Ph.D., Harvey S. Hecht, M.D., Michael J Jamieson, M.D., Wolfgang Koenig, M.D., Ph.D., Daniel Lane, M.D., Ph.D., Morteza Naghavi, M.D., John Rumberger, M.D., Ph.D., Allen J. Taylor, M.D.

Writing Group: Erling Falk, M.D., Ph.D. (Coordinator); (alphabetic order): Juhani Airaksinen, M.D., Dan Arking, Ph.D., Juan Badimon, Ph.D., Raymond Bahr, M.D., Daniel Berman, M.D., Matthew J. Budoff, M.D., Jay Cohn, M.D., Jasenka Demirovic, M.D., Ph.D., George A. Diamond, M.D., Pamela Douglas, M.D., Ole Faergeman, M.D., Zahi Fayad, Ph.D., James A. Goldstein, M.D., Harvey S. Hecht, M.D., Victoria L.M. Herrera, M.D., Michael J Jamieson, M.D., Sanjay Kaul, M.D., M.P.H., Wolfgang Koenig, M.D., Ph.D., Robert A. Mendes, M.D., Morteza Naghavi, M.D.; Tasneem Z. Naqvi, M.D., Ward A. Riley, Ph.D., Yoram Rudy, PhD, John Rumberger, M.D., Ph.D., Leslee Shaw, Ph.D., Robert S. Schwartz, M.D., Arturo G. Touchard, M.D.

Advisors (alphabetic order): Arthur Agagston, M.D., Stephane Carlier, M.D., Ph.D., Raimund Erbel, M.D., Chris deKorte, Ph.D., Craig Hartley, Ph.D., Ioannis Kakadiaris, Ph.D., Roxana Mehran, M.D., Daniel O'Leary, M.D., Jan Nilsson, M.D., Gerard Pasterkamp, M.D., Ph.D., Paul Schoenhagen, M.D., Henrik Sillesen, M.D., Ph.D.

Guest Editor: Valentin Fuster, M.D., Ph.D.

ACKNOWLEDGMENTS

The SHAPE organization would like to thank the following for their administrative support to the SHAPE Task Force: (alphabetic order): Asif Ali, M.D., Lori Cantu, Suzanne Ekblad, M.P.H., Uzma Gul, and Daniel Jamieson. *Special Thanks to*: Khawar Gul, M.D., Lisa Brown, Craig Jamieson, Bryan Jenkins, Mark Johnson, Daniel Keeney, and Kelly Papinchak.

REFERENCES

1. Mackay J, Mensah G. The Atlas of Heart Disease and Stroke. World Health Organization and US Centers for Disease Control and Prevention, 2004. Available at http://www.who.int/cardiovascular_diseases/resources/atlas/en/
2. A Race Against Time. The Challenge of Cardiovascular Disease in Developing Economies. Columbia University, New York, 2004. Available at http://www.earth.columbia.edu/news/2004/images/raceagainsttime_FINAL_0410404.pdf
3. American Heart Association. Heart Disease and Stroke Statistics – 2006 Update. Dallas, TX: AHA, 2006. Available at: http://www.americanheart.org/presenter.jhtml?identifier=3000090
4. Zipes DP, Wellnes HJJ. Sudden cardiac death. Circulation 1998;98:2334–2351.
5. Zheng ZJ, Croft JB, Giles WH, Ayala CI, Greenlund KJ, Keenan NL, Neff L, Wattigney WA, Mensah GA. State-specific mortality from sudden cardiac death–United States, 1999. Morb Mortal Wkly Rep 2002;51:123–126. Available at http://www.cdc.gov/mmwr/preview/mmwrhtml/mm5106a3.htm.
6. Yusuf S, Hawken S, Ounpuu S, Dans T, Avezum A, Lanas F, McQueen M, Budaj A, Pais P, Varigos J, Lisheng L; INTERHEART Study Investigators. Effect of potentially modifiable risk factors associated with myocardial infarction in 52 countries (the INTERHEART study): case-control study. Lancet 2004;364:937–952.

7. Stamler J, Stamler R, Neaton JD, Wentworth D, Daviglus ML, Garside D, Dyer AR, Liu K, Greenland P. Low risk-factor profile and long-term cardiovascular and noncardiovascular mortality and life expectancy: findings for 5 large cohorts of young adult and middle-aged men and women. J Am Med Assoc 1999;282:2012–2018.
8. American Heart Association. Heart Disease and Stroke Statistics – 2005 Update. Dallas, TX: AHA, 2005.
9. United States Cancer Statistics. 2002 Incidence and Mortality. US Department of Health and Human Services. Available at: http://www.cdc.gov/cancer/npcr/uscs/
10. US Preventive Services Task Force. Screening for Coronary Heart Disease, 2004. Available at http://www.ahcpr.gov/clinic/uspstf/uspsacad.htm
11. Lloyd-Jones DM, Larson MG, Leip EP, Beiser A, D'Agostino RB, Kannel WB, Murabito JM, Vasan RS, Benjamin EJ, Levy D; Framingham Heart Study. Lifetime risk for developing congestive heart failure: the Framingham Heart Study. Circulation 2002;106:3068–72.
12. Young JB. The global epidemiology of heart failure. Med Clin North Am 2004;88:1135–43, ix.
13. D'Agostino RB Sr, Grundy S, Sullivan LM, Wilson P; CHD Risk Prediction Group. Validation of the Framingham coronary heart disease prediction scores: results of a multiple ethnic groups investigation. J Am Med Assoc 2001;286: 180–187.
14. Danesh J, Wheeler JG, Hirschfield GM, Eda S, Eiriksdottir G, Rumley A, Lowe GD, Pepys MB, Gudnason V. C-reactive protein and other circulating markers of inflammation in the prediction of coronary heart disease. N Engl J Med 2004;350:1387–1397.
15. Cooper JA, Miller GJ, Humphries SE. A comparison of the PROCAM and Framingham point-scoring systems for estimation of individual risk of coronary heart disease in the Second Northwick Park Heart Study. Atherosclerosis 2005;181:93–100.
16. Liu J, Hong Y, D'Agostino RB Sr, Wu Z, Wang W, Sun J, Wilson PW, Kannel WB, Zhao D. Predictive value for the Chinese population of the Framingham CHD risk assessment tool compared with the Chinese Multi-Provincial Cohort Study. J Am Med Assoc 2004;291:2591–2599.
17. Arad Y, Goodman KJ, Roth M, Newstein D, Guerci AD. Coronary calcification, coronary disease risk factors, C-reactive protein, and atherosclerotic cardiovascular disease events: the St. Francis Heart Study. J Am Coll Cardiol 2005;46: 158–165.
18. Grundy SM. The changing face of cardiovascular risk. J Am Coll Cardiol 2005;46:173–175. Editorial.
19. De Backer G, Ambrosioni E, Borch-Johnsen K, Brotons C, Cifkova R, Dallongeville J, Ebrahim S, Faergeman O, Graham I, Mancia G, Manger Cats V, Orth-Gomer K, Perk J, Pyorala K, Rodicio JL, Sans S, Sansoy V, Sechtem U, Silber S, Thomsen T, Wood D; Third Joint Task Force of European and Other Societies on Cardiovascular Disease Prevention in Clinical Practice. European guidelines on cardiovascular disease prevention in clinical practice. Third Joint Task Force of European and Other Societies on Cardiovascular Disease Prevention in Clinical Practice. Eur Heart J 2003;24:1601–1610. Full text available at: http://www.escardio.org/NR/rdonlyres/A0EF5CA5-421B-45EF-A65C-19B9EC411261/0/CVD_Prevention_03_full.pdf
20. Greenland P, Knoll MD, Stamler J, Neaton JD, Dyer AR, Garside DB, Wilson PW. Major risk factors as antecedents of fatal and nonfatal coronary heart disease events. J Am Med Assoc 2003;290:891–897.
21. Wald NJ, Law M, Watt HC, Wu T, Bailey A, Johnson AM, Craig WY, Ledue TB, Haddow JE. Apolipoproteins and ischaemic heart disease: implications for screening. Lancet 1994;343:75–79.
22. Wald NJ, Hackshaw AK, Frost CD. When can a risk factor be used as a worthwhile screening test? Br Med J 1999;319: 1562–1565.
23. Law MR, Wald NJ. Risk factor thresholds: their existence under scrutiny. Br Med J 2002;324:1570–1576.
24. Law MR, Wald NJ, Morris JK. The performance of blood pressure and other cardiovascular risk factors as screening tests for ischaemic heart disease and stroke. J Med Screen 2004;11:3–7.
25. Weissler AM. Traditional risk factors for coronary heart disease. J Am Med Assoc 2004;291:299–300. Letter.
26. Wald NJ, Law MR. A strategy to reduce cardiovascular disease by more than 80%. Br Med J 2003;326:1419
27. National Cholesterol Education Program (NCEP) Expert Panel on Detection, Evaluation, and Treatment of High Blood Cholesterol in Adults (Adult Treatment Panel III). Third Report of the National Cholesterol Education Program (NCEP) Expert Panel on Detection, Evaluation, and Treatment of High Blood Cholesterol in Adults (Adult Treatment Panel III) final report. Circulation 2002;106:3143–421. Available at http://circ.ahajournals.org/cgi/reprint/106/25/3143
28. Grundy SM, Cleeman JI, Merz CN, Brewer HB Jr, Clark LT, Hunninghake DB, Pasternak RC, Smith SC Jr, Stone NJ. Implications of recent clinical trials for the national cholesterol education program adult treatment panel III guidelines. Circulation 2004;110:227–239.
29. Smith SC Jr, Greenland P, Grundy SM. AHA Conference proceedings. prevention conference V: beyond secondary prevention: identifying the high-risk patient for primary prevention: executive summary. Circulation 2000;101:111–116.

30. Law MR, Watt HC, Wald NJ. The underlying risk of death after myocardial infarction in the absence of treatment. Arch Intern Med 2002;162:2405–2410.
31. Eyre H, Kahn R, Robertson RM, Clark NG, Doyle C, Hong Y, Gansler T, Glynn T, Smith RA, Taubert K, Thun MJ. Preventing cancer, cardiovascular disease, and diabetes: a common agenda for the American Cancer Society, the American Diabetes Association, and the American Heart Association. Circulation 2004;109:3244–3255.
32. Naghavi M, Libby P, Falk E, Casscells SW, Litovsky S, Rumberger J, Badimon JJ, Stefanadis C, Moreno P, Pasterkamp G, Fayad Z, Stone PH, Waxman S, Raggi P, Madjid M, Zarrabi A, Burke A, Yuan C, Fitzgerald PJ, Siscovick DS, de Korte CL, Aikawa M, Airaksinen KE, Assmann G, Becker CR, Chesebro JH, Farb A, Galis ZS, Jackson C, Jang IK, Koenig W, Lodder RA, March K, Demirovic J, Navab M, Priori SG, Rekhter MD, Bahr R, Grundy SM, Mehran R, Colombo A, Boerwinkle E, Ballantyne C, Insull W Jr, Schwartz RS, Vogel R, Serruys PW, Hansson GK, Faxon DP, Kaul S, Drexler H, Greenland P, Muller JE, Virmani R, Ridker PM, Zipes DP, Shah PK, Willerson JT. From vulnerable plaque to vulnerable patient: a call for new definitions and risk assessment strategies: Part I. Circulation 2003;108:1664–1672. Review.
33. Naghavi M, Libby P, Falk E, Casscells SW, Litovsky S, Rumberger J, Badimon JJ, Stefanadis C, Moreno P, Pasterkamp G, Fayad Z, Stone PH, Waxman S, Raggi P, Madjid M, Zarrabi A, Burke A, Yuan C, Fitzgerald PJ, Siscovick DS, de Korte CL, Aikawa M, Airaksinen KE, Assmann G, Becker CR, Chesebro JH, Farb A, Galis ZS, Jackson C, Jang IK, Koenig W, Lodder RA, March K, Demirovic J, Navab M, Priori SG, Rekhter MD, Bahr R, Grundy SM, Mehran R, Colombo A, Boerwinkle E, Ballantyne C, Insull W Jr, Schwartz RS, Vogel R, Serruys PW, Hansson GK, Faxon DP, Kaul S, Drexler H, Greenland P, Muller JE, Virmani R, Ridker PM, Zipes DP, Shah PK, Willerson JT. From vulnerable plaque to vulnerable patient: a call for new definitions and risk assessment strategies: Part II. Circulation 2003;108:1772–1778. Review.
34. Hoff JA, Chomka EV, Krainik AJ, et al. Age and gender distributions of coronary artery calcium detected by electron beam tomography in 35,246 adults. Am J Cardiol 2001;87:1335.
35. Arad Y, Spadaro L, Goodman K, et al.: Prediction of coronary events with electron beam computed tomography. J Am Coll Cardiol 2000;36:1253–1260.
36. Park, R, Detrano R, Xiang M, et al. Combined use of computed tomography coronary calcium scores and C-reactive protein levels in predicting cardiovascular events in non-diabetic individuals. Circulation 2002;106:2073–2077.
37. Raggi P, Callister TQ, Cooil B, et al.: Identification of patients at increased risk of first unheralded acute myocardial infarction by electron beam computed tomography. Circulation 2000;101:850–885.
38. Wong ND, Hsu JC, Detrano RC, et al. Coronary artery calcium evaluation by electron beam computed tomography and its relation to new cardiovascular events. Am J Cardiol 2000;86:495–498.
39. Third Report of the National Cholesterol Education Program (NCEP) Expert Panel on Detection, Evaluation, and Treatment of High Blood Cholesterol in Adults (Adult Treatment Panel III). Final Report. NIH Publication No. 02-5215. September 2002.
40. Vliegenthart R, Oudkerk M, Song B. The Rotterdam Coronary Calcification Study. Coronary calcification detected by electron-beam computed tomography and myocardial infarction. Eur Heart J 2002;23:1596–1603.
41. Kondos GT, Hoff JA, Sevrukov A, et al. Coronary Artery calcium and cardiac events electron-beam tomography coronary artery calcium and cardiac events: a 37-month follow-up of 5,635 initially asymptomatic low to intermediate risk adults. Circulation 2003;107:2571–2576.
42. DeBacker G, Ambrosioni E, Borch-Johnson K, et al. European guidelines on cardiovascular disease prevention in clinical practice. Third joint task force of European and other countries in cardiovascular disease in clinical practice. Eur J Rehab Prev 2003;10(suppl 1):S1–S78.
43. Greenland P, Gaziano JM. Clinical practice. Selecting asymptomatic patients for coronary computed tomography or electrocardiographic exercise testing. N Engl J Med 2003;349:465–73. Review.
44. Shaw LJ, Raggi P, Schisterman E, et al. Prognostic Value of Cardiac Risk Factors and Coronary Artery Calcium Screening for All-Cause Mortality. Radiology 2003;28:826–833.
45. Pletcher MJ, Tice JA, Pignone M, Browner WS. Using the coronary artery calcium score to predict coronary heart disease events: a systematic review and meta-analysis. Arch Intern Med 2004;164:1285–1292.
46. Greenland P, LaBree L, Azen SP, et al. Coronary artery calcium score combined with Framingham score for risk prediction in asymptomatic individuals. J Am Med Assoc 2004;291:210–215.
47. Mosca L, Appel LJ, Benjamin EJ, et al. Evidence-based guidelines for cardiovascular disease prevention in women expert panel/writing group. Circulation 2004;109:672–693.
48. Arad Y, Roth M, Newstein D, et al. Coronary calcification, coronary risk factors, and atherosclerotic cardiovascular disease events. The St. Francis Heart Study. J Am Coll Cardiol 2005;46:158–165.
49. Vliegenthart R, Oudkerk M, Hofman A, et al. Coronary Calcification Improves Cardiovascular Risk Prediction in the Elderly. Circulation 2005;112:572–577.

50. Taylor AJ, Bindeman J, Feuerstein I, et al. Coronary calcium independently predicts incident premature coronary heart disease over measured cardiovascular risk factors mean three-year outcomes in the Prospective army coronary calcium (PACC) project. J Am Coll Cardiol 2005;46:807–14.
51. Berman DS, Wong ND, Gransar H, Miranda-Peats R, Dahlbeck J, Hayes SW, Friedman JD, Kang X, Polk D, Hachamovitch R, Shaw L, Rozanski A. Relationship between stress-induced myocardial ischemia and atherosclerosis measured by coronary calcium tomography. J Am Coll Cardiol 2004;44:923–930.
52. Simons DB, Schwartz RS, Edwards WD, Sheedy PF, Breen JF, Rumberger JA: Non-invasive definition of anatomic coronary artery disease by ultrafast CT: a quantitative pathologic study. J Am Coll Cardiol 1992;20:1118–1126.
53. Rumberger JA, Simons DB, Fitzpatrick LA, Sheedy PF, Schwartz RS. Coronary artery calcium areas by electron beam computed tomography and coronary atherosclerotic plaque area: a histopathologic correlative study. Circulation 1995;92:2157–2162.
54. Sangiorgi G, Rumberger JA, Severson A, Edwards WD, Gregoire J, Fitzpatrick LA, Schwartz RS. Arterial calcification and not lumen stenosis is highly correlated with atherosclerotic plaque burden in humans: a histologic study of 723 coronary artery segments using non-decalcifying methodology. J Am Coll Cardiol 1998;31:126–133.
55. Chambless LE, Heiss G, Folsom AR, et al. Association of coronary heart disease incidence with carotid arterial wall thickness and major risk factors: the atherosclerosis risk in communities (ARIC) study. 1987–1993. Am J Epidemiol 1997;146:483–494.
56. Chambless LE, Folsom AR, Clegg LX, et al. Carotid wall thickness is predictive of incident clinical stroke: the Atherosclerosis risk in communities (ARIC) study. Am J Epidemiol 2000;151:478–487.
57. Bonithon-Kopp C, Scarabin P, Taquet A, Touboul P, Malmejac A, Guize L. Risk factors for early carotid atherosclerosis in middle-aged French women. Arterioscler Thromb 1991;11:966–972.
58. Prevention Conference V. Beyond secondary prevention: identifying the high-risk patient for primary prevention: non-invasive tests of atherosclerosis burden: Writing Group III. Circulation 2000;101:e16.
59. Belcaro G, Nicolaides AN, Laurora G, Cesarone MR, De Sanctis M, Incandela L, Barsotti A. Ultrasound morphology classification of the arterial wall and cardiovascular events in a 6-year follow-up study. Arterioscler Thromb Vasc Biol 1996;16:851–856.
60. Touboul PJ, Hennerici MG, Meairs S, Adams H, Amarenco P, Desvarieux M, Ebrahim S, Fatar M, Hernandez Hernandez R, Kownator S, Prati P, Rundek T, Taylor A, Bornstein N, Csiba L, Vicaut E, Woo KS, Zannad F; Advisory Board of the 3rd Watching the Risk Symposium 2004, 13th European Stroke Conference. Mannheim intima-media thickness consensus. Cerebrovasc Dis 2004;18:346–349.
61. Stork S, van den Beld AW, von Schacky C, Angermann CE, Lamberts SW, Grobbee DE, Bots ML. Carotid artery plaque burden, stiffness, and mortality risk in elderly men: a prospective, population-based cohort study. Circulation 2004;110:344–348.
62. O'Leary DH, Polak JF, Kronmal RA, Manolio TA, Burke GL, Wolfson SK Jr. Carotid-artery intima and media thickness as a risk factor for myocardial infarction and stroke in older adults. N Engl J Med 1999;340:14–22.
63. Hodis HN, Mack WJ, LaBree L, Selzer RH, Liu CR, Liu CH, Azen SP. The role of carotid arterial intima-media thickness in predicting clinical coronary events. Ann Intern Med 1998;128:262–269.
64. Bots ML, Hoes AW, Koudstaal PJ, Hofman A, Grobbee DE. Common carotid intima-media thickness and risk of stroke and myocardial infarction: the Rotterdam Study. Circulation 1997;96:1432–1437.
65. Hollander M, Hak AE, Koudstaal PJ, Bots ML, Grobbee DE, Hofman A, Witteman JC, Breteler MM. Comparison between measures of atherosclerosis and risk of stroke: the Rotterdam Study. Stroke 2003;34:2367–2372.
66. van der Meer IM, Bots ML, Hofman A, del Sol AI, van der Kuip DA, Witteman JC. Predictive value of non-invasive measures of atherosclerosis for incident myocardial infarction: the Rotterdam Study. Circulation 2004;109:1089–1094.
67. Brook RD, Bard RL, Patel S, Rubenfire M, Clarke NS, Kazerooni EA, Wakefield TW, Henke PK, Eagle KA. A negative carotid plaque area test is superior to other non-invasive atherosclerosis studies for reducing the likelihood of having underlying significant coronary artery disease. Arterioscler Thromb Vasc Biol. 2005 Dec 15; [Epub ahead of print]
68. Riley WA. Cardiovascular risk assessment in individual patients from carotid intimal-medial thickness measurements. Curr Athero Reports 2004;6:225–231.
69. Bots ML, Evans GW, Riley WA, Grobbee DE. Carotid intimal-medial thickness measurements in intervention studies: design options, progression rates, and sample size considerations: a point of view. Stroke 2003;34:2985–2994.
70. Van Der Meer IM, De Maat MP, Hak AE, Kiliaan AJ, Del Sol AI, Van Der Kuip DA, Nijhuis RL, Hofman A, Witteman JC. C-reactive protein predicts progression of atherosclerosis measured at various sites in the arterial tree: the Rotterdam Study. Stroke 2002;33:2750–2755.
71. Khera A, de Lemos JA, Peshock RM, Lo HS, Stanek HG, Murphy SA, Wians FH Jr, Grundy SM, McGuire DK. Relationship between C-reactive protein and subclinical atherosclerosis: the Dallas Heart Study. Circulation 2006;113: 38–43.
72. Koenig W. Predicting risk and treatment benefit in atherosclerosis: the role of C-reactive protein. Int J Cardiol 2005;98:199–206.

73. Murabito JM, Evans JC, Larson MG, Nieto K, Levy D, Wilson PW; Framingham Study. The ankle-brachial index in the elderly and risk of stroke, coronary disease, and death: the Framingham Study. Arch Intern Med 2003;163:1939–1942.
74. Ostergren J, Sleight P, Dagenais G, Danisa K, Bosch J, Qilong Y, Yusuf S; HOPE study investigators. Impact of ramipril in patients with evidence of clinical or subclinical peripheral arterial disease. Eur Heart J 2004;25:17–24.
75. Raggi P, Shaw LJ, Berman DS, Callister TQ. Prognostic value of coronary artery calcium screening in subjects with and without diabetes. J Am Coll Cardiol 2004;43:1663–1669.
76. Sobel BE, Schneider DJ. Cardiovascular complications in diabetes mellitus. Curr Opin Pharmacol 2005;5:143–148.
77. Schneider DJ. Abnormalities of coagulation, platelet function, and fibrinolysis associated with syndromes of insulin resistance. Coron Artery Dis 2005;16:473–476.
78. Tin LL, Beevers DG, Lip GY. Hypertension, left ventricular hypertrophy, and sudden death. Curr Cardiol Rep 2002;4:449–457.
79. Lipinski MJ, Fuster V, Fisher EA, Fayad ZA. Technology insight: targeting of biological molecules for evaluation of high-risk atherosclerotic plaques with magnetic resonance imaging. Nat Clin Pract Cardiovasc Med 2004;1:48–55.
80. Fuster V, Fayad ZA, Moreno PR, Poon M, Corti R, Badimon JJ. Atherothrombosis and high-risk plaque: Part II: approaches by non-invasive computed tomographic/magnetic resonance imaging. J Am Coll Cardiol 2005;46:1209–1218.
81. Takaya N, Yuan C, Chu B, Saam T, Polissar NL, Jarvik GP, Isaac C, McDonough J, Natiello C, Small R, Ferguson MS, Hatsukami TS. Presence of intraplaque hemorrhage stimulates progression of carotid atherosclerotic plaques: a high-resolution magnetic resonance imaging study. Circulation 2005;111:2768–2775.
82. Yuan C, Hatsukami TS, Cai J. MRI plaque tissue characterization and assessment of plaque stability. Stud Health Technol Inform 2005;113:55–74.
83. Cohn JN, Quyyumi AA, Hollenberg NK, Jamerson KA. Surrogate markers for cardiovascular disease: Functional markers. Circulation 2004;109(suppl IV):IV31–IV46. Review.
84. Zieman SJ, Melenovsky V, Kass DA. Mechanisms, pathophysiology, and therapy of arterial stiffness. Arterioscler Thromb Vasc Biol 2005;25:932–943.
85. Bonetti PO, Lerman LO, Lerman A. Endothelial dysfunction: a marker of atherosclerotic risk. Arterioscler Thromb Vasc Biol 2003;23:168–175. Review.
86. Ganz P, Vita JA. Testing endothelial vasomotor function: nitric oxide, a multipotent molecule. Circulation 2003;108:2049–2053. Review.
87. Widlansky ME, Gokce N, Keaney JF Jr, Vita JA. The clinical implications of endothelial dysfunction. J Am Coll Cardiol 2003;42:1149–1160. Review
88. Madjid M, Zarrabi A, Litovsky S, Willerson JT, Casscells W. Finding vulnerable atherosclerotic plaques: is it worth the effort? Arterioscler Thromb Vasc Biol 2004;24:1775–1782.
89. MacNeill BD, Bouma BE, Yabushita H, Jang IK, Tearney GJ. Intravascular optical coherence tomography: cellular imaging. J Nucl Cardiol 2005;12:460–465.
90. Carlier S, Kakadiaris IA, Dib N, Vavuranakis M, O'Malley SM, Gul K, Hartley CJ, Metcalfe R, Mehran R, Stefanadis C, Falk E, Stone G, Leon M, Naghavi M. Vasa vasorum imaging: a new window to the clinical detection of vulnerable atherosclerotic plaques. Curr Atheroscler Rep 2005;7:164–169.
91. Fujii K, Carlier SG, Mintz GS, Wijns W, Colombo A, Bose D, Erbel R, de Ribamar Costa J Jr, Kimura M, Sano K, Costa RA, Lui J, Stone GW, Moses JW, Leon MB. Association of plaque characterization by intravascular ultrasound virtual histology and arterial remodeling. Am J Cardiol 2005;96:1476–1483.
92. Chen JW, Wasserman BA. Vulnerable plaque imaging. Neuroimaging Clin N Am 2005;15:609–621.
93. Baldewsing RA, Schaar JA, Mastik F, Oomens CW, van der Steen AF. Assessment of vulnerable plaque composition by matching the deformation of a parametric plaque model to measured plaque deformation. IEEE Trans Med Imaging 2005;24:514–528.
94. Schoenhagen P, Nissen SE. Assessing coronary plaque burden and plaque vulnerability: atherosclerosis imaging with IVUS and emerging non-invasive modalities. Am Heart Hosp J 2003;1:164–169.
95. Sattar N, McCarey DW, Capell H, McInnes IB. Explaining how "high-grade" systemic inflammation accelerates vascular risk in rheumatoid arthritis. Circulation 2003;108:2957–2963.
96. Gonzalez-Gay MA, Gonzalez-Juanatey C, Martin J. Rheumatoid arthritis: a disease associated with accelerated atherogenesis. Semin Arthritis Rheum 2005;35:8–17.
97. Joseph AJ, Cohen AG, Bahr RD. A formal, standardized and evidence-based approach to Chest pain center development and process improvement: the society of chest pain centers and providers accreditation process. J Cardiovasc Manag 2003;14:11–14.
98. Luepker RV, Raczynski JM, Osganian S, Goldberg RJ, Finnegan JR Jr, Hedges JR, Goff DC Jr, Eisenberg MS, Zapka JG, Feldman HA, Labarthe DR, McGovern PG, Cornell CE, Proschan MA, Simons-Morton DG. Effect of a community intervention on patient delay and emergency medical service use in acute coronary heart disease: The Rapid Early Action for Coronary Treatment (REACT) Trial. J Am Med Assoc 2000;284:60–67.

99. Kalia NK, Miller LG, Nasir K, Blumenthal RS, Agrawal N, Budoff MJ. Visualizing coronary calcium is associated with improvements in adherence to statin therapy. Atherosclerosis. 2005 Jul 25; [Epub ahead of print]
100. Mark DB, Shaw LJ, Lauer MS, O'Malley P, Heidenreich P. 34th Bethesda conference: task force #5 – Is atherosclerotic imaging cost effective? from the 34th bethesda conference on atherosclerotic imaging. J Am Coll Cardiol 2003;41: 1906–1917.
101. Fedder DO, Koro CE, L'Italien GJ. New National cholesterol education program III guidelines for primary prevention lipid-lowering drug therapy: projected impact on the size, sex, and age distribution of the treatment-eligible population. Circulation 2002;105:152–156.
102. Nasir K, Michos ED, Blumenthal RS, Raggi P. Detection of high-risk young adults and women by coronary calcium and National cholesterol education program panel III guidelines. J Am Coll Cardiol 2005;46:1931–1936.
103. Vivanco F, Martin-Ventura JL, Duran MC, Barderas MG, Blanco-Colio L, Darde VM, Mas S, Meilhac O, Michel JB, Tunon J, Egido J. Quest for novel cardiovascular biomarkers by proteomic analysis. J Proteome Res 2005;4:1181–1191.
104. Humphries SE, Ridker PM, Talmud PJ. Genetic testing for cardiovascular disease susceptibility: a useful clinical management tool or possible misinformation? Arterioscler Thromb Vasc Biol 2004;24:628–636.
105. Topol EJ. Simon Dack Lecture. The genomic basis of myocardial infarction. J Am Coll Cardiol 2005;46:1456–1465.
106. Kooi ME, Cappendijk VC, Cleutjens KBJM, Kessels AGH, Kitslaar PJEHM, Borgers M, Frederik PM, Daemen MJAP, van Engelshoven JMA. Accumulation of ultrasmall superparamagnetic particles of iron oxide in human atherosclerotic plaques can be detected by in vivo magnetic resonance imaging. Circulation 2003;107:2453–2458.
107. Trivedi RA, U-King-Im JM, Graves MJ, Cross JJ, Horsley J, Goddard MJ, Skepper JN, Quartey G, Warburton E, Joubert I, Wang L, Kirkpatrick PJ, Brown J, Gillard JH. In vivo detection of macrophages in human carotid atheroma: temporal dependence of ultrasmall superparamagnetic particles of iron oxide-enhanced MRI. Stroke 2004;35: 1631–1635.
108. Cyrus T, Winter PM, Caruthers SD, Wickline SA, Lanza GM. Magnetic resonance nanoparticles for cardiovascular molecular imaging and therapy. Expert Rev Cardiovasc Ther 2005;3:705–715.
109. Davies JR, Rudd JH, Weissberg PL. Molecular and metabolic imaging of atherosclerosis. J Nucl Med 2004;45: 1898–1907. Review.
110. Kietselaer BLJH, Reutelingsperger CPM, Heidendal GAK, Daemen MJAP, Mess WH, Hofstra L, Narula J. Non-invasive detection of plaque instability with use of radiolabeled annexin A5 in patients with carotid-artery atherosclerosis. New Engl J Med 2004;350:1472–1473.
111. Davies JR, Rudd JH, Fryer TD, Graves MJ, Clark JC, Kirkpatrick PJ, Gillard JH, Warburton EA, Weissberg PL. Identification of culprit lesions after transient ischemic attack by combined 18F fluorodeoxyglucose positron-emission tomography and high-resolution magnetic resonance imaging. Stroke 2005;36:2642–2647.
112. Dunphy MP, Freiman A, Larson SM, Strauss HW. Association of vascular 18F-FDG uptake with vascular calcification. J Nucl Med 2005;46:1278–1284.
113. Leber AW, Knez A, Becker A, Becker C, Reiser M, Steinbeck G, Boekstegers P. Visualising noncalcified coronary plaques by CT. Int J Cardiovasc Imaging 2005;21:55–61.
114. Bonetti PO, Pumper GM, Higano ST, Holmes DR Jr, Kuvin JT, Lerman A. Non-invasive identification of patients with early coronary atherosclerosis by assessment of digital reactive hyperemia. J Am Coll Cardiol 2004;44:2137–2141.
115. Zalewski A, Macphee C. Role of lipoprotein-associated phospholipase A2 in atherosclerosis: biology, epidemiology, and possible therapeutic target. Arterioscler Thromb Vasc Biol 2005;25:923–931.
116. Schwartz RS, Bayes-Genis A, Lesser JR, Sangiorgi M, Henry TD, Conover CA. Detecting vulnerable plaque using peripheral blood: inflammatory and cellular markers. J Interv Cardiol 2003;16:231–242.
117. Shah PK, Chyu KY, Fredrikson GN, Nilsson J. Immunomodulation of atherosclerosis with a vaccine. Nat Clin Pract Cardiovasc Med 2005;2:639–646.

40 Cost Effectiveness of Screening Atherosclerosis

Leslee J. Shaw and Ron Blankenstein

CONTENTS

ABSTRACT

There remains a significant detection gap for cardiovascular disease that could be reduced provided that screening programs are employed, directed toward at-risk patient populations. However, given the current state of the healthcare system and the spiraling healthcare costs, expansion of current coverage decisions to include screening beyond cancer is incomprehensible.

From: *Asymptomatic Atherosclerosis: Pathophysiology, Detection and Treatment*
Edited by: M. Naghavi (ed.), DOI 10.1007/978-1-60327-179-0_40

Data are unfolding that current tests are highly accurate at detecting risk and provide significant improvements in our global risk scores, such as the Framingham risk score. This chapter reviews the methods applied toward evaluating the economics of screening including cost-effectiveness principles. In addition to the presentation of screening cost models, this chapter introduces the concept of an early intervention model as a means to avert the enormous burden of symptomatic care in this country. Ongoing dialog about the importance of cost considerations and focused evaluations to consider the benefits and the risks of cardiovascular screening are important steps toward devising a platform for reducing the burden of atherosclerosis in this country.

Key words: Atherosclerosis; Cost effectiveness; Screening

KEY POINTS

- The economic burden of cardiovascular disease is enormous in this country and worldwide.
- There are available effective tools to screening for subclinical atherosclerosis.
- Cost-effectiveness analyses are a valuable method to examine the benefits of any screening program.
- Preliminary cost models suggest that an early intervention approach may alleviate the significant economic burden of symptomatic disease.
- The US healthcare system ranks with that of the world's most advanced, with an abundance of high technology care. A recent report noted that the US spends twice as much per capita on health care as other nations ($6,102 vs. $2,571) [1]. Of the most expensive health conditions, the US spent $21.5 billion in Medicare in 2004 on ischemic heart disease [2]. With the addition of diabetes, hypertension, peripheral arterial disease, heart failure, and arrhythmias, the total economic burden increases to more than $70 billion for Medicare alone. The investment in high cost diseases, such as coronary artery disease (CAD), has had dramatic results on our healthcare system. Within the past two decades, there has been a 35–50% decline in cardiovascular mortality [3]. However, there remains a tremendous detection gap with sizeable proportions of the adult population still at risk, as pointed out during a recent Bethesda Conference on atherosclerotic imaging [4]. In 2004, a total of 870,000 deaths related to cardiovascular diseases were reported with nearly half of all incident events, including sudden cardiac death, occurring in asymptomatic, apparently healthy individuals [3]. As noted by Murabito and et al. [5], the initial CAD presentation is acute myocardial infarction or sudden cardiac death in nearly two thirds of men and 42% of women. Thus, despite our "high tech" and high cost care, further improvements remain necessary for detection and treatment of a sizeable at-risk population.
- It is for this reason that many have proposed an expansion of our current paradigm of caring for symptomatic CAD to detection of subclinical atherosclerosis. It seems logical that an early detection and treatment screening program could serve to define patients and avert catastrophic loss of life and morbid complications that are observed today. Yet, within our current healthcare system, the lone screening test approved by Medicare (for patients without a prior diagnosis of CAD) is a lipid panel that may be performed every 5 years. From the burden of morbid and fatal complications, the evidence remains as strong for CAD screening as for that of other accepted programs such as breast or lung cancer [6]. However, the healthcare policy experts often point to the current burden of costs for CAD and that further expansion would exhaust our limited healthcare resources. Within the current chapter, we will highlight the available evidence on the costs of screening and evaluate relevant evidence on the cost effectiveness of screening for atherosclerosis.

ESTIMATED DIRECT AND INDIRECT COSTS OF CAD CARE

Each year, the American Heart Association [7] releases estimates of the total direct and indirect costs of care combined from both the public and private healthcare sectors. The most recent estimate revealed that, in 2007, a total of $448.5 billion was spent on coronary heart disease, stroke, hypertension, and heart failure. What this estimate fails to categorize is the total costs associated with symptomatic care. In a recent NIH-NHLBI-sponsored project, Shaw and colleagues [8] estimated lifetime costs of care for symptomatic women with nonobstructive, single, multivessel CAD. These results reveal a heavy burden of cardiac symptoms exceeding $1 million in lifetime costs for patient with chronic CAD. Even for those with chest pain and nonobstructive CAD, lifetime costs of care were estimated at $767,000. Factors that added considerably to the costs of care included diabetes ($302,000), hyperlipidemia ($177,000), disability ($172,000), and unstable angina presentation ($220–$447,000). This report highlights the toll of symptomatic care if one realizes that nearly 19 million patients are living in the US with chronic stable angina, the economic burden for chest pain in this country is enormous.

CURRENT STATE OF OUR HEALTHCARE SYSTEM

A more comprehensive review of our healthcare system reveals that nearly 50% of costs are spent on hospital-based or end-of-life care [9]. If one reviews the gamut of hospital-based care in 2004, this would include $412 billion, of which Medicare pays 31%. An additional $571 billion is spent on related physician, drug, nursing home, and home healthcare costs. The potential exist that shifting care that is now based on a disease or sickness model to wellness care could provide a means to identify less economically, catastrophic pathways.

EARLY INTERVENTION MODEL

The early intervention model is just such a proposal to define low-cost, effective pathways for identifying subclinical or presymptomatic at-risk patients while offsetting expenses associated with high-cost symptom care. For CAD, the early intervention model can be viewed if one considers an investment in a screening test for a broad range of at-risk patients, sufficient to significantly impact our national statistics for morbid and fatal disease complications. The screening test would have to have a positive risk:benefit ratio. That is, the test should be effective at identifying patients with a high risk of CAD events and has only modest upfront costs. Should we propose such a paradigm shift within our healthcare system, the potential exists that we could shift the balance in expenditures to care for healthier people with the result being an offset in the current outlay for hospital or disease-based care.

COST IMPLICATIONS OF THE EARLY INTERVENTION MODEL: SHAPE TASKFORCE ANALYSIS

We devised a decision analytic model to estimate the potential cost implications of an early intervention model for CAD [10]. In this model (Table 1), we propose to employ a screening test, either carotid intima-media thickness (C-IMT) or coronary artery calcification (CAC), in the evaluation of a wide segment of the adult at-risk population. Recent data from the National Centers for Health Statistics reveal that only 11% of adults are at low CAD risk with more than 80% of women and men having one or more cardiac risk factor [11]. Given that such a broad scope of the adult population is at risk, our model examined the cost implications of screening men aged 45–75 years and women aged 55–75 years. Based on expert guidance within the SHAPE taskforce, we estimated that a screening program would decrease cardiovascular mortality and incident myocardial infarction (MI) by 10–25% resulting in reduced costs of care approaching $19 billion, when compared to our current cost outlays. Other declines in CAD costs would be for emergency department visits and hospitalizations for

Table 1
Cost implications of an early intervention proposal to screen 45–75-year-old adult men and 55–75-year-old adult women. The costs listed on this table are estimates based on decision model to screen for atherosclerosis using a modestly expensive carotid intima media thickness or coronary calcium scan

	No. (/year)	*Estimated impact*	*Δ Cost*
CVD death	910.6k	10% (5–25%)	$1.2 b
MI	7.2 m	25% (5–35%)	$18.0 b
ED visits	6.5 m	5% (2.5–25%)	$4.1 b
CVD hospitalization	6.4 m	10% (5–25%)	$3.8 b
CHD hospitalization	970k	10% (5–25%)	$9.9 b
Cholesterol-↓ Rx	–	50% (50–65%)	$8.00 b
CV imaging	8.7 m	10% (5–25%)	$358 m
Angiography	6.8 m	15%–CTA (2.5–25%)	$600 m
PCI	657k	10% (5–50%)	$580 m
CABG	515k	5% (2.5–50%)	$672 m
Total cost Δ			$21.5 b

CVD Cardiovascular Disease, *MI* Myocardial Infarction, *ED* Emergency Department, *Cholesterol-↓ Rx* Cholesterol Reducing Therapy, *PCI* Percutaneous Coronary Intervention, *CABG* Coronary Artery Bypass Graft Surgery

acute coronary syndromes as well as surgical intervention for obstructive CAD including percutaneous coronary intervention and coronary artery bypass surgery. If one calculates all the inputs within our economic model, the final result is an estimated decline in costs of care for CAD expected to exceed $20 billion in savings. This latter estimate does include an increase in costs of care, in particular, for more follow-up testing and treatment for patients with abnormal C-IMT and CAC. However, we believe that the targeting of those with disease markers such as C-IMT and CAC could result in an effective reduction in morbid and fatal downstream complications.

REALITY OF CV IMAGING IN TODAY'S HEALTH CARE

Although the early intervention model provides a pathway and hope for future generations, there is another reality in today's healthcare system. This reality is the current heavy burden for costs of imaging procedures in the US. A recent evaluation from the Medicare Payment Advisory Commission reveals that, on average, there is a 22% annual growth for all physician services, as detailed in the physician's fee schedule [12]. However, annual growth for all of medical imaging procedures exceeds 40%. Additionally, temporal trends in CAD procedures reveal dramatic growth in stress testing where, in 1993, Medicare utilization rates were 60 patients/1,000 but grew to more than 100/1,000 of Medicare beneficiaries by 2001 [13]. If one examines a commonly performed cardiovascular procedure, stress myocardial perfusion single-photon emission computed tomography, in 2003, Medicare payments exceeded $1 billion, representing 2% of the total CMS budget [14]. As a result, cardiovascular imaging procedures now represent a "big ticket" item in health care with most health plans instituting numerous efforts aimed at constraining growth and curtailing further investments in any CAD procedures.

The recent approaches by health plans to target imaging include a focus on managing resource utilization, programs to maintain quality, and ensuring patient safety. Current programs for managing imaging utilization include control efforts through prior notification or authorization, often using external companies or benefits managers with very effective results at reducing costs [15]. Efforts aimed at maintaining imaging quality include mandatory physician credentialing, laboratory certification, and guidance documents on appropriate use or clinical indications for a given procedure. Finally, there has been recent interest in reducing radiation exposure to the patient, and these efforts on the part of health plans will have an impact on advanced imaging procedures such as computed tomography.

The result for our proposal of an early intervention model is that it will be very difficult in today's healthcare environment with limited resources to consider proposals to expand coverage for screening for atherosclerosis in asymptomatic adults. Given this somber appraisal of healthcare, we would like to examine deficiencies in our current (accepted) approaches to risk assessment and to evaluate our current evidence base on cost-effectiveness analysis (CEA). Both these may provide a more reasoned pathway to devising selected strategies for screening presymptomatic patients.

LIMITATIONS TO GLOBAL RISK SCORES: MAGNITUDE OF THE DETECTION GAP

Current guidelines and expert consensus statements support selected screening of patients with an intermediate Framingham risk score (FRS) [4,16]. This would include approximately 40% of the US adult population. The rationale for restricting screening to only those intermediate risk patients is that imaging within this sizeable proportion of the adult population could have a dramatic impact on cardiovascular morbidity and mortality, with nearly half of CAD events occurring in this patient subset. However, use of the FRS as a guide to screening will disproportionately include men over the age of 60 [17] and, in particular, miss many at-risk patients (including women and young men, those outside the US, and of diverse ethnicity). In one recent report of 222 patients presenting with acute MI, 70% had a low FRS [18]. A number of reports present a consistent message that the FRS underestimates risk in women and younger men (i.e., <60 years) [17,19]. In a recent report from Michos et al. [19] in 2,447 asymptomatic, nondiabetic women, 84% with significant CAC were classified as having a low FRS. Other patients that are also at-risk include patients with a family history of premature coronary heart disease; a risk factor not included in the scoring for the FRS [20].

Given that our current primary prevention treatments are based on the FRS, where more intensive management of hypertension and hyperlipidemia is guided by this scoring system, the resulting care pathway result in undertreatment of key at-risk patients. Thus, we need to devise a strategy to focus care for those at-risk segments of the adult population, strategies that remain effective for women and men of diverse ethnicity. It is for this reason that many have proposed using imaging markers that directly visualize subcomponents of atherosclerosis, such as C-IMT and CAC.

PROCEDURAL AND LABORATORY DIRECT COSTS

A compilation of direct cost estimates has been published on an array of CAD diagnostic tests (Fig. 1) [6]. Figure 1 provides a detail of direct costs including production costs for any given test; higher dollar values will be reported for charges for these procedures. For those not familiar with looking at direct costs, these estimates would represent the economic requirements to do one procedure where generally higher dollar values would be expected for reimbursement and even higher values for charges. Note that this figure puts forth (direct) cost estimates for 2008, where specific data are unavailable throughout many different healthcare sectors and the inclusion of these results may alter the current findings. However, the pattern of low to high cost tests should remain valid for most sectors of the healthcare marketplace. In general, the costs of available tests can be categorized

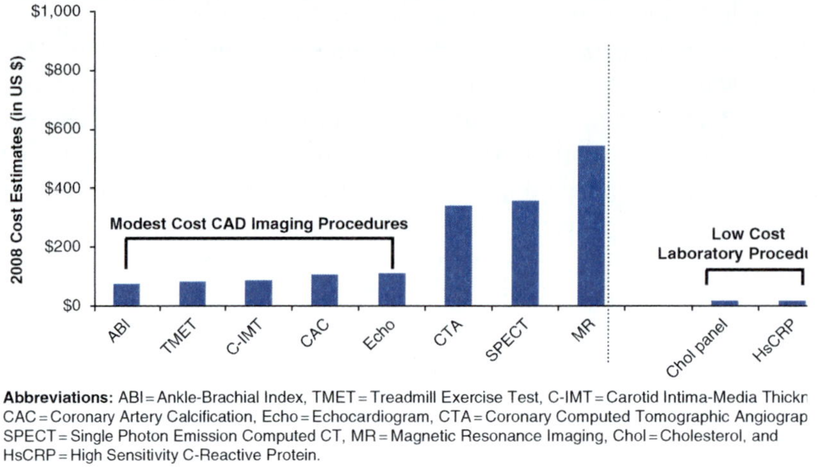

Fig. 1. Direct procedural costs for many cardiovascular imaging and laboratory procedures; based on 2003 cost estimates.

from low to moderate cost. In this way, low-cost tests are those such as high sensitivity C-reactive protein (CRP) or a cholesterol panel; direct cost <\$20. Modest costs are noted from >\$50 to ~\$100 for ankle-brachial index, C-IMT, CAC, treadmill exercise test, and echocardiographic screening for left ventricular hypertrophy. Moderate cost tests, including computed tomographic coronary angiography, would not be prudent for screening large segments of the population, with direct costs that are, on average, \$412.

COST MODELS FOR SCREENING

In the 34th Bethesda Conference on atherosclerotic imaging, cost models were proposed that may aid in focusing screening strategies for this review. In one model (Fig. 39.2), the cost inputs for screening are identified. Although we have highlighted the direct procedural costs, the induced costs are of foremost concern, on the part of public and private payers. These are highlighted in Fig. 2 including downstream costs for treatment, procedures, as well as that for incidental findings. In one report, it was noted that the induced or downstream costs following screening may be as much as 10–20 times greater than the initial test costs [21]. In this latter series of nearly 700 patients, induced costs were estimated through 3–5 years of follow-up. Higher costs would be expected when considering lifetime expenditures for patients with subclinical atherosclerosis. Based on this model, the Bethesda Conference committee estimated 1–2 year procedural costs for testing a cohort of 300,000 patients could approach \$50 million [6]. Applying this number to the 40% of the US population that are at intermediate FRS, this cost estimate could exceed \$10 billion.

COST-EFFECTIVENESS ANALYSIS

Within our discussion, there remains a method that may prove helpful in devising a reasoned path forward on screening for subclinical atherosclerosis. This includes calculation of marginal CEA where the added benefit, in terms of improved outcome, is considered along with the upfront

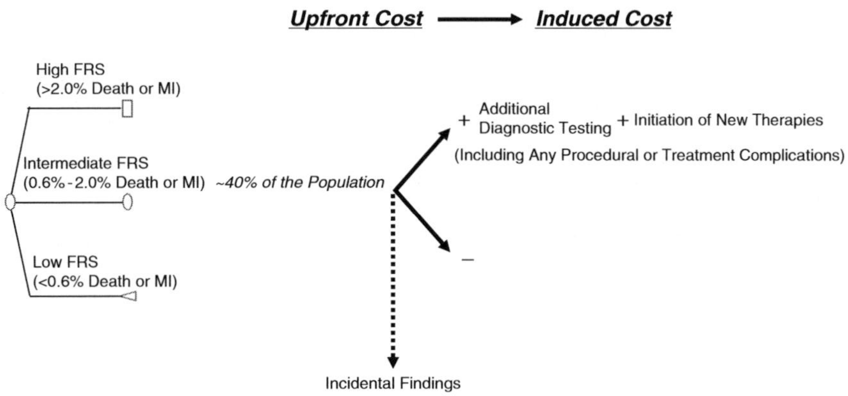

Fig. 2. Simplistic model for identifying cost inputs for atherosclerotic screening.

and induced costs associated with a proposed screening program. CEA is a technique that allows evaluation of several comparable testing choices (including a decision not to test) [22]. It has been defined as a measure of a test's "value for money" [6]. A recent review of the methods has been published and defines CEA as the price of an additional outcome by switching from current practice to a new strategy [22]. If the price is low enough, then the decision to undertake a given novel approach, such as screening for atherosclerosis, may be considered favorable. In general, the CEA threshold for economic attractiveness has been set at <\$50,000 per life year saved. This figure represents an incremental or marginal cost-effectiveness ratio (ICER) as based on the calculation noted in Table 1.

As can be seen in this table, there are several approaches to evaluate this interaction between cost and quality. First, a test can be less effective at defining at-risk patients but still remain favorable due to its lower cost. Many would propose that our current methods relying on the FRS or lipid panel for screening represent such a low-cost effort. Certainly, a screening test that is both ineffective and costly would not be favored. However, a dominant strategy is one where costs are reduced and effectiveness is improved, with the result being a negative ICER. As is likely the case for our current tests that we discuss in this chapter, they will add to current costs of care yet provide more effective means to define at-risk individuals. And, as such, it remains possible that CEA strategies could be identified.

CURRENT ICER EVIDENCE ON SCREENING FOR ATHEROSCLEROSIS

There are now a number of published reports that have evaluated the ICER of screening using a variety of tests for diagnosis of obstructive CAD and identification of subclinical atherosclerosis [23–29]. This final section will highlight many of the relevant reports and detail the ICER evidence.

EXERCISE TREADMILL TESTING

The US Preventive Services Taskforce (USPSTF) performed a systematic review of the evidence for screening with a treadmill exercise test to identify patients with silent ischemia and obstructive CAD [23]. Although our prior discussion have focused on detection of subclinical atherosclerosis, the focus of the USPSTF report was on detection of latent or silent obstructive CAD with the results from their CEA models being informative to our current discussion. The authors noted that the evidence for using treadmill exercise testing supports its utility as a cost-effective modality with favorable ICER similar to that of other screening modalities, such as mammography. In particular, the authors highlighted the evidence for women and men of varying ages. Their results reveal that it is largely cost ineffective to use a treadmill exercise test for women and men in their 40s (ICER in the range of \$80–\$217,000). However, if one considers the base case of screening patients in their 60s, the ICERs are \$25,000 and \$48,000 for men and women, respectively. Thus, by identifying patients at slightly higher risk (i.e., of advancing age), the ICERs become more favorable and support the utility of exercise testing to screen for CAD. This result would be translatable to the use of C-IMT or CAC where screening low-risk, younger patients would largely be cost ineffective.

CAC

There have been several recent reports that have evaluated the ICER of screening using CAC [21,24,25]. Two decision models were published evaluating the ICER of the FRS versus CAC scanning [21,24]. Both these reports revealed that the use of CAC is cost ineffective in patients with a low FRS with cost per life year saved up to \$504,000 [21]. By comparison, the ICER of CAC scanning in patients with an intermediate FRS was favorable at approximately \$42,000 per life year saved [21].

In a follow-up analysis from the Prospective Army Coronary Calcium (PACC) Project, the authors evaluated the interactive relationship between therapeutic relative risk reduction and the proportion of at-risk patients [25]. This report revealed, using data from nearly 2,000 middle-aged patients enrolled in the PACC study, that ICER could be favorable under two conditions: (1) the relative risk reduction with therapeutic intervention was at least 30% and (2) the proportion of at-risk patients was at least 25% based on a combined estimate from the FRS and CAC. Thus, these data revealed that should a given therapy reduce cardiovascular risk by at least 30% for the nearly 5% of high-risk patients identified by CAC screening, then the ICER would be <\$50,000 per life year saved.

ABI

In a recent report, Treesak and colleagues [26] evaluated the use of ABI as a screening tool and compared the ICER of three treatments: (a) no therapy, (b) percutaneous transluminal angioplasty (PTA), and (c) exercise rehabilitation. For this analysis, the ICER was a disease specific measure of the cost per \$ an additional meter walked. In this report, ABI was used as the entry criteria where <0.9 was considered abnormal and diagnostic for peripheral arterial disease. In this report, PTA exhibited a more favorable ICER with a cost of \$177 per additional meter walked. By comparison, at 6 months, the ICER was negative for exercise rehabilitation, revealing a dominant strategy, at –\$61 per additional meter walked.

CAROTID ULTRASOUND

In a decision model evaluating screening of 1,000 asymptomatic men with a high prevalence of carotid stenosis (i.e., 20% prevalence) using Doppler ultrasound [27], the cost of one time screen was \$35,130 per life year saved. However, annual screening was excessive at \$457,773 per life year saved. One factor that was most influential in their decision model was the long-term stroke risk reduction following surgical intervention. This study also highlights the economic disadvantages of repeat screening.

OTHER ICER MODELS

There are several decision models that evaluate the role of laboratory measurements that are also relevant to the current discussion [28,29]. The first of which evaluated the ICER for treating patients based on evidence of a high-risk CRP. This report detailed a strategy of evaluating the cost of treating a high-risk CRP with targeted statin therapy as compared to usual care alone [28], using the base cases of nonhyperlipidemic patients age 45–65 years. The ICER for screening with CRP was $48,100 per life year saved for 58-year-old men as compared to $94,400 per life year saved for 58-year-old women. Based on this report, screening was most cost effective for 65-year-old men ($42,600/life year saved) and least effective for 35-year-old women ($207,300/life year saved). Importantly, the results from this model were most sensitive to several factors, including baseline CAD risk, the cost of statin therapy, and the efficacy of statin therapy in patients with high CRP levels. Thus, they add more components to our understanding of how we can achieve enhanced cost effectiveness for screening tests. For example, should we provide the cost of statins at $1/day, then the ICER for 58-year-old men and women would be $4,900 and $19,600 per life year saved.

Heidenreich et al. [29] devised a similar decision model to screen 1,000 asymptomatic patients with B-Natriuretic Peptide, a marker of left ventricular stretch and ventricular dysfunction, followed by echocardiography in those with elevated measurements. The results are rather intriguing in that, although the overall lifetime costs of care were excessive ($176,000 for men, $101,000 for women), the results reveal a dramatic improvement in outcome within the range of 1.3–7.9 added life years (adjusted for the patient's quality of life). This tremendous improvement in patient life expectancy resulted in an ICER of $22,300 for men and $77,700 for women. This study illustrates that should the prevalence of a condition, such as depressed left ventricular ejection fraction, be such that testing would identify enough at-risk patients, then ICER thresholds would be favorably influenced. Moreover, another factor that is notable from this study is that should we define patients whose lifetime costs of care are devastatingly high, such as that associated with heart failure, then screening (even the added cost of BNP plus an echocardiogram) can result in favorable ICER.

Given the dramatic increase in the prevalence of obesity, there have been explorations of the value for screening for diabetes. Hoerger et al. [30] devised a Markov simulation model to estimate the ICER of no screening versus fasting glucose measurement followed by lifestyle intervention for those with impairment. These data revealed a very dramatic result noting an ICER of $8,181 per cost per life year saved. These data show promise for screening for atherosclerosis that if the "appropriate" at risk patients are targeted, then dramatic ICER can be achieved enough, so that it may be seen as favorable to the payer community (Table 2).

CONCLUSIONS

Throughout this chapter, we have attempted to provide a realistic view of the "value for money" for atherosclerotic screening approaches. Importantly, the evidence does support that these tests are highly effective at defining risk in asymptomatic individuals. However, we are constrained within our current healthcare environment such that any expansion of cardiovascular services is unlikely to be supported by healthcare payers. What does seem likely are approaches that define clearly at-risk patients whose near-term and long-term costs of care can be quite excessive including obese patients or those with a family history of premature coronary heart disease.

Table 2
Defining cost-effective screening for atherosclerosis
Cost effective screening is defined:

$$\frac{\Delta \text{Cost}}{\Delta \text{Life years saved}}$$

	Decreased effectiveness	*Improved effectiveness*
Decreased cost	Need to determine whether cost savings are worth decreased effectiveness	Cost effective
Increased cost	Not cost effective	Need to determine whether increased effectiveness worth increased cost

Standard: <$50,000/LYS

Another approach introduced within an information statement from the American Society of Nuclear Cardiology this concept of bringing the discussion of screening out of the population arena and back into the clinical setting [31]. So, we are not discussing widespread "screening" of the adult population but we are focusing on "testing patients evaluated in the outpatient setting. By defining high-risk patients who may be defined as presymptomatic yet at high risk for CAD, it is possible that an expansion of testing may be slowly unraveled. By defining selected high-risk patients including diabetics or obese patients, it may be possible for payers to see that the near-term costs exceed that of C-IMT or CAC scan (including induced costs).

It is clear that universal screening will "break the bank" of our healthcare system. As such, we now have to devise more reasoned steps forward to define those who clearly benefit from screening in terms of a cost and effectiveness advantage during a time horizon that is meaningful to healthcare payers. It should also be noted that much of our evidence on cost effectiveness is based on decision models. A decision analysis does not replace evidence derived from randomized controlled trials that would be favorable in today's healthcare marketplace that is demanding higher and higher quality evidence to improve care for our patients. We look forward to further developments in the field where additional evidence can start to devise strategies for identifying asymptomatic patients with subclinical atherosclerosis who may clearly benefit from more intensive management and that the ensuing strategy of care would be established to be a cost-effective pattern of care.

REFERENCES

1. http://www.commonwealthfund.org/publications/publications_show.htm?doc_id=482678. Access date: April 11, 2008.
2. http://www.meps.ahrq.gov/mepsweb/. Access date: March 29, 2008.
3. http://www.cdc.gov/nchs/data/nvsr/nvsr56/nvsr56_10.pdf. Access date: April 11, 2008.
4. Pasternak RC, Abrams J, Greenland P, Smaha LA, Wilson PW, Houston-Miller N. 34th Bethesda Conference: Task force #1-Identification of coronary heart disease risk: Is there a detection gap? J Am Coll Cardiol 2003;41(11):1863–74.
5. Murabito JM, Evans JC, Larson MG, Levy D. Prognosis after the onset of coronary heart disease. An investigation of differences in outcome between the sexes according to initial coronary disease presentation. Circulation 1993;88(6):2548–55.
6. Mark DB, Shaw LJ, Lauer MS, O'Malley P, Heidenreich P. 34th Bethesda Conference: Task force #5 – is atherosclerotic imaging cost effective? From the 34th Bethesda Conference on Atherosclerotic Imaging. J Am Coll Cardiol 2003;41(11):1906–17.
7. http://circ.ahajournals.org/cgi/reprint/CIRCULATIONAHA.107.187998. Access date: April 11, 2008.
8. Shaw LJ, Bairey Merz CN, Pepine CJ, Reis SE, Bittner V, Kip K, Kelsey SF, Olson M, Johnson BD, Mankad S, Sharaf BL, Rogers WJ, Pohost GM, Sopko G, for the WISE Investigators. The economic burden of angina in women with suspected ischemic heart disease: Results from the National Institutes of Hevalth – National Heart, Lung, and Blood Institute – sponsored Women's Ischemia Syndrome Evaluation. Circulation 2006;114:894–904.
9. Center for Medicaid and Medicare Services, Office of the Actuary, National Health Statistics Group. Access date: March 2, 2004.

10. Naghavi M, Falk E, Hecht H, Jamieson MJ, Kaul S, Berman D, Fayad Z, Budoff MJ, Rumberger J, Naqvu TZ, Shaw LJ, Faergeman O, Cohn J, Bahr R, Koenig W, Demirovic J, Arking D, Herrera VL, Badimon J, Goldstein JA, Rudy Y, Airaksinen J, Schwartz RS, Riley WA, Mendes RA, Douglas P, Shah PK, for the SHAPE Task Force. From vulnerable plaque to vulnerable patient – Part III: Executive summary of the Screening for Heart Attack and Prevention and Education (SHAPE) Task Force Report. Am J Cardiol 2006;98(2 Suppl 1):2–15.
11. Mokdad AH, Ford ES, Bowman BA, Dietz WH, Vinicor F, Bales VS, Marks JS. Prevalence of obesity, diabetes, and obesity-related health risk factors, 2001. JAMA 2003;289(1):76–9.
12. MEDPAC Analysis of Medicare Claims Data, March 17, 2005, Executive Director, Medicare Payment Advisory Commission, Mark Miller.htm.
13. Lucas FL, DeLorenzo MA, Siewers AE, Wennberg DE. Temporal trends in the utilization of diagnostic testing and treatments for cardiovascular disease in the United States, 1993–2001. Circulation 2006;113(3):374–9.
14. Personal communications, AMA/Specialty Society Relative Value Scale Update Committee (RUC).
15. http://www.rwjf.org/files/research/022008ib118final.pdf. Access date: March 28, 2008.
16. Greenland P, Bonow RO, Brundage BH, Budoff MJ, Eisenberg MJ, Grundy SM, Lauer MS, Post WS, Raggi P, Redberg RF, Rodgers GP, Shaw LJ, Taylor AJ, Weintraub WS, Harrington RA, Abrams J, Anderson JL, Bates ER, Eisenberg MJ, Grines CL, Hlatky MA, Lichtenberg RC, Lindner JR, Pohost GM, Schofield RS, Shubrooks SJ Jr, Stein JH, Tracy CM, Vogel RA, Wesley DJ; American College of Cardiology Foundation Clinical Expert Consensus Task Force (ACCF/AHA Writing Committee to Update the 2000 Expert Consensus Document on Electron Beam Computed Tomography); Society of Atherosclerosis Imaging and Prevention; Society of Cardiovascular Computed Tomography. ACCF/AHA 2007 clinical expert consensus document on coronary artery calcium scoring by computed tomography in global cardiovascular risk assessment and in evaluation of patients with chest pain: A report of the American College of Cardiology Foundation Clinical Expert Consensus Task Force (ACCF/AHA Writing Committee to Update the 2000 Expert Consensus Document on Electron Beam Computed Tomography) developed in collaboration with the Society of Atherosclerosis Imaging and Prevention and the Society of Cardiovascular Computed Tomography. J Am Coll Cardiol 2007;49(3):378–402.
17. Nasir K, Michos ED, Blumenthal RS, Raggi P. Detection of high-risk young adults and women by coronary calcium and National Cholesterol Education Program Panel III guidelines. J Am Coll Cardiol 2005;46(10):1931–6.
18. Akosah KO, Schaper A, Cogbill C, Schoenfeld P. Preventing myocardial infarction in the young adult in the first place: How do the National Cholesterol Education Panel III guidelines perform? J Am Coll Cardiol 2003;41(9):1475-9.
19. Michos ED, Nasir K, Braunstein JB, Rumberger JA, Budoff MJ, Post WS, Blumenthal RS. Framingham risk equation underestimates subclinical atherosclerosis risk in asymptomatic women. Atherosclerosis 2006;184(1):201-6.
20. Nasir K, Budoff MJ, Wong ND, Scheuner M, Herrington D, Arnett DK, Szklo M, Greenland P, Blumenthal RS. Family history of premature coronary heart disease and coronary artery calcification: Multi-Ethnic Study of Atherosclerosis (MESA). Circulation 2007;116(6):619-26.
21. Shaw LJ, Raggi P, Berman DS. Cost effectiveness of screening for CVD with measures of coronary calcium. Prog Cardiov Dis 2003;46:171-84.
22. http://www.acponline.org/journals/ecp/sepoct00/primer.htm. Access date: July 15, 2006.
23. Fowler-Brown A, Pignone M, Pletcher M, Tice JA, Sutton SF, Lohr KN; U.S. Preventive Services Task Force. Exercise tolerance testing to screen for coronary heart disease: A systematic review for the technical support for the U.S. Preventive Services Task Force. Ann Intern Med 2004;140(7):W9-24.
24. O'Malley PG, Greenberg BA, Taylor AJ. Cost-effectiveness of using electron beam computed tomography to identify patients at risk for clinical coronary artery disease. Am Heart J 2004;148(1):106–13.
25. Taylor AJ, Bindeman J, Feurerstein I, Cao F, Brazaitis M, O'Malley PG. The independent prognostic value of coronary calcium over measured cardiovascular risk factors in an asymptomatic male screening population: 6-year outcomes in the prospective army coronary calcium project. J Am Coll Cardiol 2005;46(5):807-14.
26. Treesak C, Kasemsup V, Treat-Jacobson D, Nyman JA, Hirsch AT. Cost-effectiveness of exercise training to improve claudication symptoms in patients with peripheral arterial disease. Vasc Med 2004;9(4):279–85.
27. Derdeyn CP, Powers WJ. Cost-effectiveness of screening for asymptomatic carotid atherosclerotic disease. Stroke 1996;27:1944-50.
28. Blake GJ, Ridker PM, Kuntz KM. Potential cost-effectiveness of C-reactive protein screening followed by targeted statin therapy for the primary prevention of cardiovascular disease among patients without overt hyperlipidemia. Am J Med 2003;114:485–494.
29. Heidenreich PA, Gubens MA, Fonarow GC, Konstam MA, Stevenson LW, Shekelle PG. Cost-effectiveness of screening with B-type natriuretic peptide to identify patients with reduced LVEF. J Am Coll Cardiol 2004;43(6):1019–26.
30. Hoerger TJ, Hicks KA, Sorensen SW, Herman WH, Ratner RE, Ackermann RT, Zhang P, Engelgau MM. Cost-effectiveness of screening for pre-diabetes among overweight and obese U.S. adults. Diabetes Care 2007;30:2874–79.
31. Shaw LJ, Berman DS, Blumenthal RS, Budoff MJ, Faber TL, Goraya T, Halliburton SS, Hecht H, Kiat H, Koenig W, Malik S, Merhige M, Nasir K, Min JK, O'Keefe J, Polk DM, Raggi P, Rosenblatt JA, Schwartz RG, Taylor AJ, Thomas GS, Wijns W. Clinical imaging for prevention: Directed strategies for improved detection of presymptomatic patients with undetected atherosclerosis-Part I: Clinical imaging for prevention. J Nucl Cardiol 2008;15(1):e6–19.

41 Monitoring of Subclinical Atherosclerotic Disease

Daming Zhu, Allen J. Taylor, and Todd C. Villines

CONTENTS

Abstract

Direct assessment of the vascular wall provides the capability to monitor atherosclerosis progression and assess the response to pharmacotherapy as a surrogate to clinical outcomes. Carotid intima-media thickness (IMT) using high-frequency ultrasound (10 MHz) accurately measures arterial wall thickness, with the recommendation that the far wall of the common carotid artery is the optimal site for serial assessment. A 15–18% increase in relative risk for myocardial infarction and stroke is observed for each 0.10 mm increase in carotid IMT. Inter-test reproducibility is high, but the application to individual patients is limited by generally slow progression of IMT. Coronary artery calcium correlates to overall atherosclerosis burden and independently predicts incident cardiovascular events up to tenfold over standard risk factors. Progression of coronary calcium is rapid, and a rate ≥15% per year clinically identifies individuals with increased cardiovascular risk. A complicated relationship exists between cardiovascular risk factor modification and coronary calcium progression, such that its use in pharmacotherapy evaluation is limited. Contrast enhanced CT angiography provides the ability to image both calcified and non-calcified coronary atherosclerosis, but requires careful attention to image quality. Nuclear imaging of the vascular wall, with positron emission tomography, targets inflammation within the vascular wall of larger vessels. Pharmacotherapies with anti-inflammatory properties may be studied with FDG-PET, but these findings have not yet been related to cardiovascular outcomes.

Key words: Atherosclerosis; Carotid artery; Coronary calcium; Inflammation; Risk factors; Computed tomography; Clinical trials

From: *Asymptomatic Atherosclerosis: Pathophysiology, Detection and Treatment*
Edited by: M. Naghavi (ed.), DOI 10.1007/978-1-60327-179-0_41

KEY POINTS

- Carotid IMT imaging of the far wall of the common carotid using high frequency ultrasound identifies atherosclerosis and its response to therapy.
- A 15–18% increase in relative risk for myocardial infarction and stroke is observed for each 0.10 mm increase in carotid IMT.
- Coronary artery calcium utilizes low levels of radiation to identify calcified atherosclerosis, which predicts incident cardiovascular events up to tenfold over standard risk factors.
- Progression of coronary calcium ≥15% per year clinically identifies individuals with increased cardiovascular risk; however, the complex relationship of therapies to atherosclerosis calcification limits application to pharmacotherapy assessment.
- Non-calcified atherosclerosis of the coronary arteries can be quantified with contrast-enhanced CT angiography. However, this requires high levels of image quality, and a relationship to cardiovascular outcomes has not yet been demonstrated.
- Positron-emission tomography, using FDG-PET, detects inflammatory changes in larger arteries, which may enable serial testing although a relationship to cardiovascular outcomes has not yet been demonstrated.

The availability of accurate coronary and vascular imaging procedures has permitted the serial evaluation of atherosclerosis, and led to a direct understanding of the relationship between atherosclerosis progression, coronary risk, and its management. Early work utilized invasive angiography with quantitative vessel analysis, which, despite its accuracy, is nonetheless an invasive and indirect assessment of atherosclerosis from the perspective of the coronary lumen. However, until recently, this was the standard modality used in the imaging evaluation of atherosclerosis. For example, work by Waters and colleagues showed that a greater than 15% increase in atherosclerosis progression on quantitative coronary angiography was associated with a 50% increase in coronary events [1]. Subsequent advancements in vascular imaging have permitted a more direct assessment of the arterial wall using carotid ultrasound [2], cardiac computed tomography [3], and intravascular ultrasound [4] and strengthened the clinical understanding of atherosclerosis progression as a marker of cardiovascular risk. Representative data are summarized in Table 1 and are consistent in supporting the concept that atherosclerosis progression is a marker of heightened risk from ischemic heart disease.

As an extension of this concept, these imaging surrogates, such as B-mode ultrasound to measure carotid intima-media thickness (CIMT), coronary computed tomography (CT) and cardiovascular magnetic resonance imaging (CMR), have been extensively utilized in clinical trials to detect and monitor atherosclerosis longitudinally, specifically its response (regression, progression or stabilization) to combination or novel lipid management therapies. Use of these technologies as surrogates for clinical cardiovascular endpoints is based on the fact that atherosclerosis progression is a well-validated marker of an increased risk of cardiovascular events. In the absence of large clinical outcomes trials, the use of validated atherosclerosis imaging modalities to assess response to lipid modifying therapies is advantageous as it allows for reduced sample size and a shortened trial duration, thus providing potentially useful clinical information prior to the results of larger randomized clinical outcomes trials. Additionally, use of these non-invasive surrogates may have inherent value as clinical endpoints as they may provide insight into pathophysiologic mechanisms and plaque composition, and are able to detect clinically relevant changes in the atherosclerotic disease process prior to clinical outcomes.

When considering use of atherosclerosis imaging tests as surrogates for cardiovascular outcomes, it is important to consider if the proposed modality is valid for clinical study. Boissel proposed three criteria for the validity of surrogate markers as a substitute for clinical end points [5]. Specifically, the surrogate marker should be more sensitive and more readily available than the clinical end point, and convenient to measure. Secondly, there should be a well-established causal relationship between the surrogate marker and the clinical end point, based on epidemiological, pathophysiological and clinical

Table 1
Representative clinical studies examining atherosclerosis progression by different modalities and its association with clinical cardiovascular outcomes

Modality	*Study*	*Progression endpoint*	*Association with clinical outcomes*
Quantitative coronary angiography	Canadian Coronary Atherosclerosis Intervention Trial [1]	>15% worsening in diameter stenosis associated with significant increase in coronary event rate over 5 years	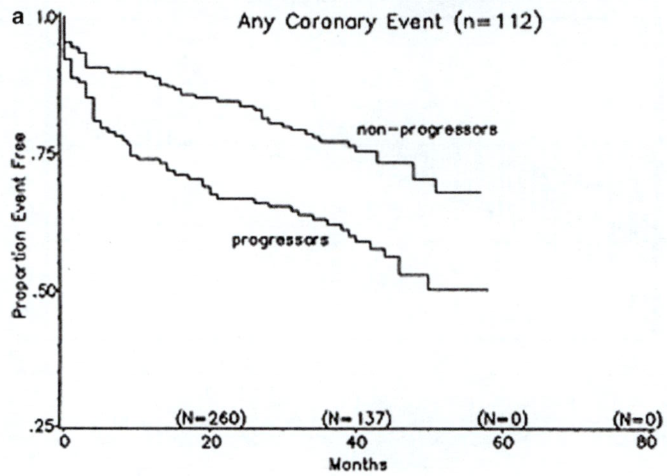
Carotid intima-media thickness	Cholesterol Lowering Atherosclerosis Study [78]	Annualized progression of CIMT>0.033 mm/y associated with 2.8-fold increased CHD event rate over 7 years	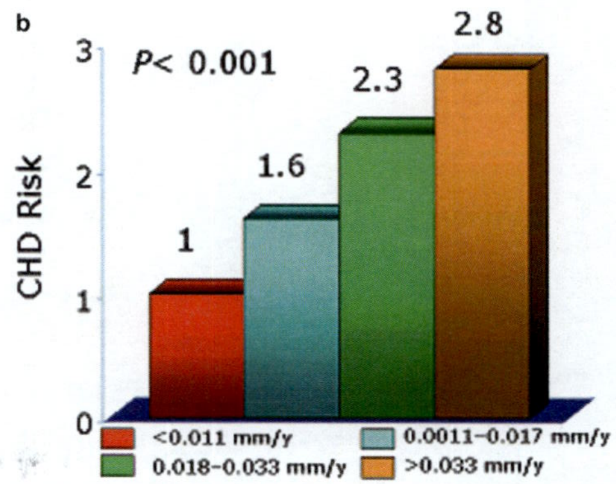

(continued)

Table 1
(continued)

Modality	*Study*	*Progression endpoint*	*Association with clinical outcomes*
Coronary computed tomography	Raggi [44]	≥15% annualized change in coronary calcium score associated with 17.2-fold increased relative risk of events over 6 years	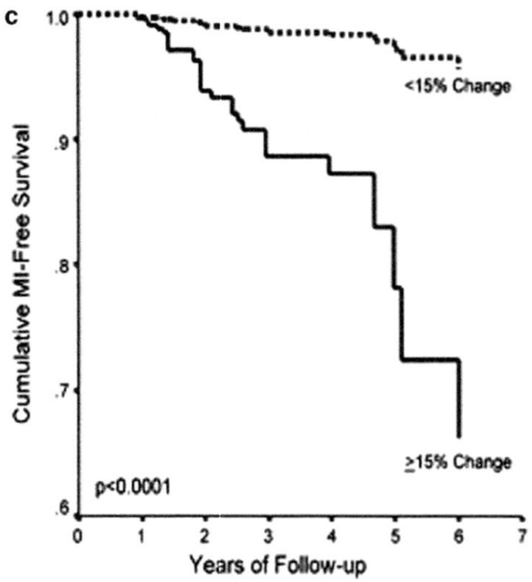
Intravascular ultrasound	Von Birgelen [79]	Change in left main plaque plus media cross sectional area associated with LDL, inversely associated with HDL and future events.	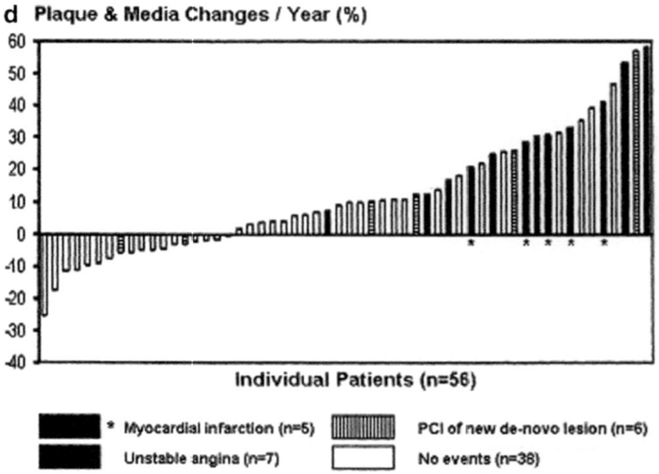

studies. Finally, in intervention studies, anticipated clinical benefits should be deducible from changes in the surrogate marker. We will review several non-invasive imaging modalities currently used to detect and monitor atherosclerosis and its response to lipid modifying agents.

CAROTID INTIMA-MEDIA THICKNESS

Use as a Surrogate for Cardiovascular Risk

B-mode, high-frequency (7–10 MHz) ultrasound has been shown to accurately identify and quantify atherosclerosis. Pioli et al. [6] showed that measurement of the thickness of the combined intima and medial layers of aortic and/or carotid arteries using B-mode ultrasound was extremely accurate as compared to histologic examination. In the absence of atherosclerotic plaque, the intima-media layers are easily identified on ultrasound as tissue residing between a "double-line" pattern in the longitudinal plane of a relatively straight arterial segment, with the lines representing the lumen-intima and media-adventitia interfaces (Fig. 1). Clearly delineated using modern, B-mode high-resolution ultrasound, measurements of the carotid artery intima-media thickness (CIMT) can be made with precision to the degree of hundredths of millimeters, with the inter-test variability improved using computer-aided edge-detection and measurements, and based upon the anatomic site evaluated. Recently, the Mannheim Intima-Media Thickness Consensus document was published that proposed standardization of CIMT measurements as used to assess atherosclerosis [7]. This expert panel recommended that although various sites may be used, the common carotid artery is the most easily and reliably assessable site in nearly all patients. Successful examination of the internal carotid artery or of the carotid bulb is more variable and related to patient anatomical tomography and sonographer

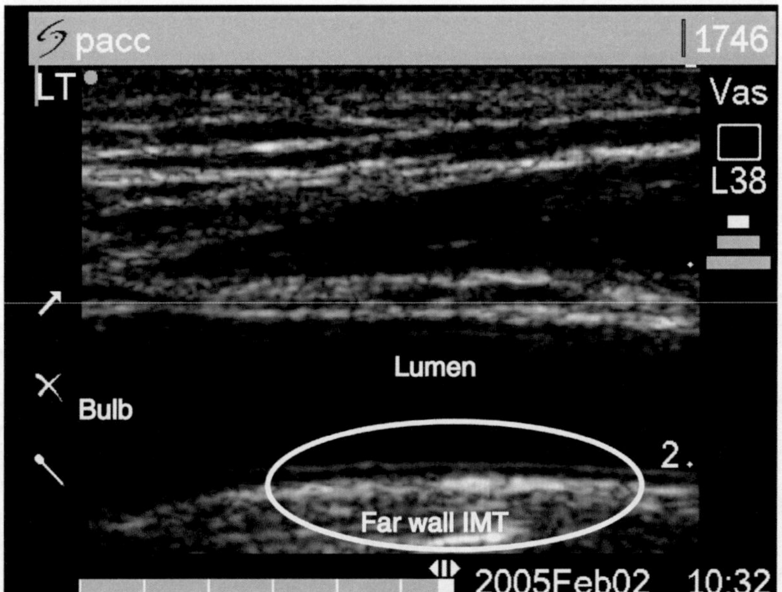

Fig. 1. Serial mean CIMT measurement from the far wall of the bilateral common carotid arteries at baseline and 12 months during treatment with either placebo or extended release niacin (Niaspan) added to stable statin therapy in the ARBITER-2 study. Sample carotid intima media thickness image identifying the far wall of the common carotid artery.

expertise. Additionally, CIMT should be assessed on the far wall of the artery (Fig. 2) as images of the near wall are less reliable and more dependent on ultrasound gain settings, and that CIMT should be measured in areas free of plaque. Standards for measurement of CIMT have also been published under the auspices of the American Society of Echocardiography, including a comprehensive discussion of technical aspects of image quality and population estimates for CIMT values [8].

The two implicit assumptions that underlie the use of ultrasound-measured CIMT as a surrogate marker of CVD are (a) atherosclerosis is a systemic vascular disorder where disease in superficial arteries (e.g., carotid) indicates disease in other vascular beds (coronary arteries), and (b) vessel wall thickness is associated with clinical events. Multiple prospective studies have shown that increased carotid artery intima-media thickness (CIMT) is associated with increased risk of myocardial infarction and stroke in adults without a history of CVD and is an independent risk factor for cardiovascular events after adjustment for traditional cardiovascular risk factors. The Atherosclerosis Risk in Communities (ARIC) Study [9, 10] completed baseline carotid B-mode ultrasound examinations on over 15,800 subjects, 45–64 years of age, and without prior CVD. The ARIC protocol focused on obtaining measurement of the far wall of the right and left common carotid artery (CCA), the carotid bulb and the internal carotid artery (ICA). Their CIMT index was defined as the mean of CIMT measurements at these 6 sites and showed a high level of reproducibility. Over a 4–7 year follow-up period, a strong and graded relationship was shown between coronary heart disease (CHD) incidence and CIMT. Hazard ratios comparing extreme mean CIMT (≥1 mm) to below extreme values (<1 mm) were 5.07 for women and 1.85 for men. Similarly, in the Cardiovascular Health Study (CHS) [11] of 5,858 patients over 65 years of age, individuals in the highest quintile of CIMT were over threefold more likely to have a CV event. After adjustment for conventional CV risk factors, carotid IMT was the variable most strongly predictive of future CV risk. In this study, measurements were made of the

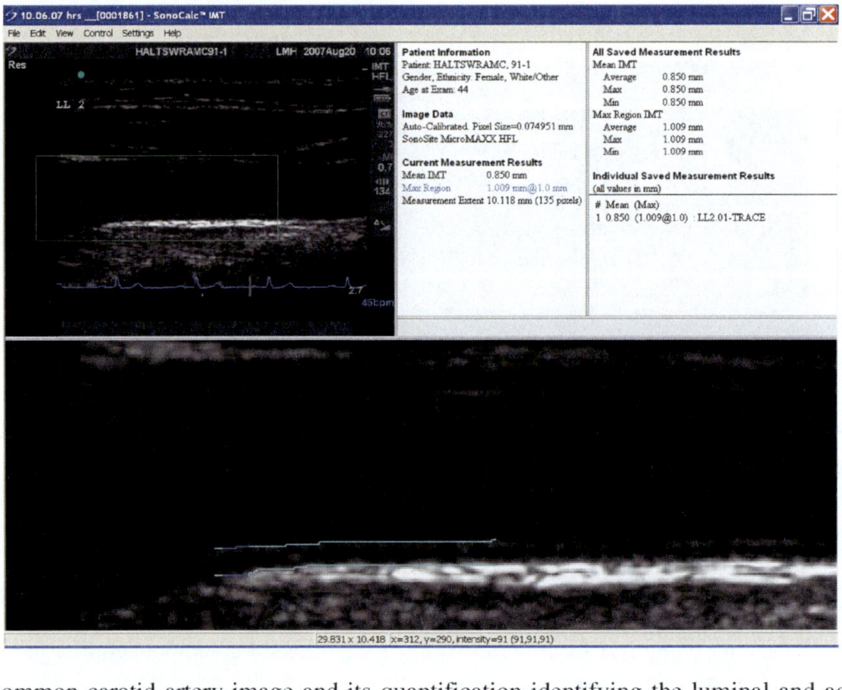

Fig. 2. Sample common carotid artery image and its quantification identifying the luminal and adventitial borders using automated border detection software.

near and far wall of the left and right CCA and ICA and were combined into a summary mean CIMT value. These data have been summarized in a recent meta-analysis showing that the age- and sex-adjusted estimates of the relative risk of myocardial infarction was 1.15 (95% CI, 1.12–1.17), and the relative risks of stroke was 1.18 (95% CI, 1.16–1.21) per 0.10-mm common carotid artery IMT difference [12]. Beyond CIMT, the identification of plaque (defined as a raised lesion that is 1.5× in thickness relative to the surround CIMT) is incrementally predictive of outcomes; however, further work and standardization of the assessment of plaque vs. CIMT is needed [13].

Carotid IMT has been the subject of clinical guidelines [14]. Guidelines for the use of CIMT in clinical medicine include the American Heart Association Prevention V statement [15] and the recent iteration of the National Cholesterol Education Program which suggested that high CIMT values formulate a rationale to more aggressively treat lipid risk factors [16]. In contrast, the utility of CIMT in clinical management has been the subject of only limited clinical trials. In one study, smokers randomized to view images of their carotid artery ultrasound study had a higher 6-month rate of quitting smoking.

CIMT to Monitor Atherosclerosis and Therapeutic Efficacy

Carotid ultrasound is proven to be a valuable marker for therapeutic benefit in multiple clinical trials. It is safe, noninvasive, relatively inexpensive, and provides continuous and quantitative indices of atherosclerosis. Serial evaluations of CIMT have been used as a marker of benefit for virtually all cardiovascular therapies including lifestyle changes, and agents for the management of lipids, blood pressure and blood glucose. A major focus area for this application of CIMT has been lipid lowering therapies. The Cholesterol Lowering Atherosclerosis Study (CLAS) showed that the risk of an adverse cardiovascular event was increased >2-fold for each 0.03-mm increase per year in CIMT, as measured in the distal common carotid artery [2]. This trial further demonstrated that reduced progression of atherosclerosis, as measured by CIMT, using combination niacin and colestipol, resulted in reduced cardiovascular events. The Arterial Biology for the Investigation of the Treatment Effects of Reducing Cholesterol (ARBITER 1) trial evaluated the effects of marked LDL-C reduction to a level well below 100 mg/dL using a high-potency statin (atorvastatin 80 mg/day, mean LDL-C 76±23 mg/dL), as compared to moderate intensity lipid-lowering with pravastatin (40 mg/day, mean LDL-C 110±30 mg/dL) in 161 patients (46% with known cardiovascular disease), using serial assessments of the far wall of the distal CCA [17]. In the atorvastatin group there was a significant CIMT regression over 12 months (change in CIMT −0.034±0.021 mm, $P=0.03$), as compared to the pravastatin group where the CIMT was stable (change of 0.025±0.017 mm). This study was the first to demonstrate a potential clinical benefit of marked LDL-C reduction using B-mode ultrasound as a surrogate marker for clinical cardiovascular events. Subsequently, similarly designed, large randomized clinical trials evaluating the efficacy of marked LDL-C reduction, using both intravascular ultrasound [18] and clinical events [19, 20] as the primary outcome, have confirmed the benefit of intensive LDL-C reduction in patients with known CVD, confirming that short term changes in CIMT are a useful surrogate for changes in coronary atherosclerosis and clinical CV endpoints.

The Arterial Biology for the Investigation of the Treatment Effect of Reducing Cholesterol (ARBITER) 2 trial [21] was a double-blind randomized placebo-controlled study of once daily extended-release niacin (1,000 mg) added to adequate background, stable statin therapy (mean LDL-C 89±20 mg/dL) in 167 patients (mean age 67 years) with known coronary heart disease and low levels of high-density lipoprotein cholesterol (HDL-C <45 mg/dL). The primary endpoint was the change in common carotid IMT. After 12 months, HDL-C rose significantly in the niacin group, from 39±7 to 47±16 mg/dL ($P=0.002$), and was unchanged in the placebo group. Triglycerides also decreased significantly in the niacin group, from 164±83 to 134±87 mg/dL. There were no differences in elevations of liver-associated enzymes, myositis or compliance in the placebo and niacin groups. Over 12 months, mean CIMT increased significantly in the placebo group (0.044±0.100 mm; $P<0.001$) and was unchanged in the niacin group (0.014±0.104 mm; $P=0.23$), Fig. 1. This data extended our understanding of the potential benefit of combination therapy with statin and niacin and was the first study to demonstrate the incremental effect of niacin added to background statin therapy on cardiovascular outcomes or their surrogates. Slowed progression of atherosclerosis in the setting of increased HDL-C is consistent with the current paradigm in which HDL-C participates in reverse cholesterol transport, and is further supported by the small clinical trial that showed regression of atherosclerosis during treatment with a man-made nascent HDL-C particle with apoA1 Milano [22]. Further clinical trials confirming the benefit of combination therapy using clinical endpoints are indicated. However, this study offers convincing preliminary evidence of the benefit of combination niacin and statin in patients with known cardiovascular disease and low HDL-C, as compared to adequate statin monotherapy alone.

Compared to the use of CIMT in clinical trials, its role in individual patients as a serial method of atherosclerosis evaluation is limited. This is due to the minor degree of expected annual CIMT progression (~0.01–0.015 mm/y or greater) relative to the inter-test variability unless there is a long time horizon between studies. Thus, discriminating true change from imaging noise is too technically challenging to confidently direct individual patient management decisions across short time intervals.

Future directions of CIMT include more focused and standards of measurement. Presently, effort is primarily directed at the detection of common carotid CIMT; however, a more broad survey for plaque in other carotid segments may enhance the cardiovascular risk assessment [13]. Volumetric assessment of carotid plaque through external ultrasound imaging performed to reconstruct 3-dimensional plaque volume is actively in methodologic development [23]. In addition, higher frequency imaging with specialized software tools may enable the discrimination of intima and media, arterial wall elements that may respond differently under different therapeutic interventions [24]. Plaque characterization with grey scale assessments [25] or assessment of neovascularization [26, 27] with contrast are possible, although their role as tools in the assessment of cardiovascular risk or therapeutic benefit is uncertain. Lastly, the integration of CIMT measurement within clinical risk prediction algorithms, and its role in clinical management (e.g., as a factor in behavioral management) requires additional investigation.

In summary, CIMT measurements can accurately assess arterial wall changes with atherosclerosis as a continuous, in-vivo variable and can provide information on future cardiovascular risk in a broad spectrum of at-risk individuals. Serial CIMT measurements can also provide longitudinal data on the efficacy of lipid-modifying medications. Considering the above, CIMT measurements using B-mode ultrasound imaging meet all validity criteria of a surrogate marker and have been accepted by the American Heart Association (AHA) and the United States Food and Drug Administration (FDA) as a validated noninvasive measure of the atherosclerotic process.

CORONARY COMPUTED TOMOGRAPHY

Coronary Calcium Assessment

Coronary calcium can be detected using non-contrast coronary computed tomography (CT) imaging. Although classically performed using electron beam CT (EBCT), today most exams are performed with multidetector-row CT (MDCT) (Fig. 3). Both methods generate prospectively triggered, axial images generally 2.5–3 mm in thickness across the heart using a low-energy CT technique. In general, EBCT and MDCT provide comparable data on the presence and extent of coronary calcium.

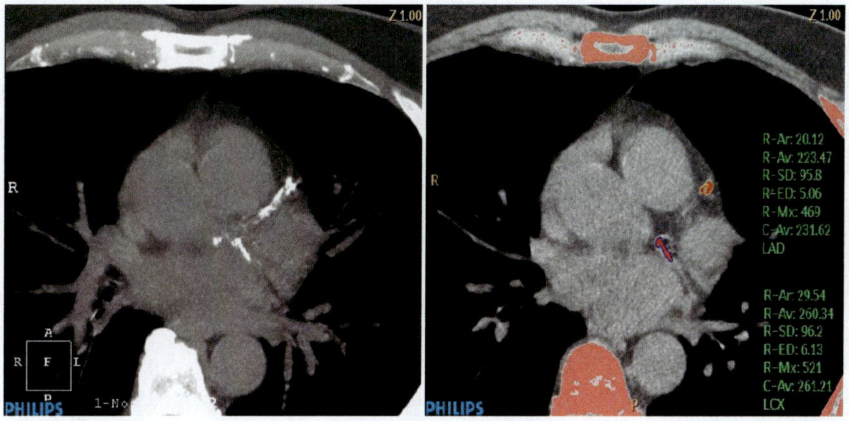

Fig. 3. Thick maximum intensity projection of calcified coronary arterial plaque identified on multidetector computed tomography.

The extent of detected coronary calcium deposits broadly correlates to atherosclerosis burden [28, 29]. As a consequence, numerous studies have demonstrated that individuals with coronary calcium deposits are approximately 4–10-fold more likely to have a future cardiovascular event, independent of standard cardiovascular risk factors [30–33]. However, calcium accumulation within atherosclerotic lesions is dependent on age, gender, genetic variability, and other non-lipid parameters. As such, early atherosclerosis can exist without coexisting calcification, as the majority of men younger than age 50 and women younger than age 60 have normal scans [34].

The use of coronary calcium as a monitoring tool for atherosclerosis is contingent upon the reproducibility of the calcium score data. Early data using EBCT showed high inter-test variability using the area-density score (also known as the Agatston score). Calculation of the total calcium score from a single EBCT has excellent inter-observer and intra-observer reliability [35]. Interscan variability, however, has been wide-ranging [36, 37], but when performed in skilled laboratories using adequate ECG-gating, is generally below 15% and varies mostly at lower total calcium scores [37–39]. The variability in total calcium scoring algorithms may be improved by use of volumetric calcified plaque scoring systems [40]. Callister and colleagues performed 52 paired EBCT scans taken 5 min apart and calculated a total calcium volume score (CVS). They found that this score had better reproducibility than the traditional Agatston calcium score and its variability was smaller in untreated patients at the end of 1 year [41]. In the present era of MDCT, particularly when utilized only for calcium scoring and without beta blocker use for heart rate slowing, inter-test variability is likely lower than EBCT, given the lower temporal resolution of the method. Inter-test variability on MDCT can exceed 50% particularly at low calcium score values.

One advantageous feature of coronary calcium is that its natural progression tends to be rapid, thus, across modest time horizons, discriminating true change from measurement error is possible. Thus, coronary calcium has been proposed as a surrogate marker of atherosclerosis in randomized clinical trials and within prospective cohorts as a marker of cardiovascular risk. Paradoxically, despite our present understanding of statin therapy and reductions in cardiovascular risk, two large, prospective, randomized controlled trials evaluating coronary calcium score progression to predict the benefit of statin therapy were negative. In the St. Francis Heart Study, which studied atorvastatin 20 mg/d vs. placebo, and in the BELLES trial, which studied high dose atorvastatin vs. moderate dose pravastatin, statin therapy did not slow coronary calcium progression across modest time horizons (years). However, it is important to note that progression of coronary calcification is a complex process that is not solely predicted by lipid reduction and the potential exists for the non-calcified component of plaques to respond and not reflect the calcified component. Interestingly, it has been recently shown that statin drugs may affect calcification in a diverse way, paradoxically stimulating calcification in some tissue types that may be involved in the atherosclerotic process [42]. One compound that has been shown to reduce coronary calcium progression is sevelamer. In a study of hemodialysis patients, the phosphorous binder sevelamer significantly reduced progression of vascular and valvular calcification as compared to calcium-based phosphorous binders. This reduced progression of vascular and valvular calcification in the sevelamer group was independent of the LDL-C lowering effect seen with sevelamer therapy [43]. At this time, the use of serial coronary calcium scores as a surrogate of cardiovascular disease risk in clinical trials has fallen out of favor.

However, the use of serial calcium scanning as a method of refining cardiovascular risk in patients remains under active investigation. Typical calcium score progression rates exceed 20% per year, thus, within modest time horizons the "rate" of calcium score progression can be estimated. The calculation of calcium score progression is complex, but the most studied method simply reports the change in calcium score as a percent of the baseline score on an annual basis. For example, a calcium score that increased from 100 to 200 in 5 years would represent an increase of 20% per year. Two studies have examined serial calcium score progression as a marker of cardiovascular risk. In work by Raggi and colleagues, calcium volume score progression of ≥15% per year was associated with a relative risk for MI of 17.9 among asymptomatic, statin-treated patients initially referred for calcium score testing. Overall, event-free survival was 97% versus 66% for patients without or with a yearly CVS change ≥15% [44]. These data suggest the dynamic nature of coronary calcium may indeed be more important than the actual value, and provide a hypothesis for future studies to pursue.

At this time, coronary calcium imaging is best validated as an indicator for cardiovascular risk in intermediate risk populations, as suggested by the statements of the American Heart Association [45] and the American College of Cardiology [46]. Present guidelines do not recommend serial calcium testing. Using calcium imaging alone to follow disease progression and response to lipid modifying therapy is limited by the fact that non-calcified atherosclerosis will not be detected and that factors that promote calcification of atherosclerosis are diverse. However, the use of serial testing in patients to further discriminate individuals whose risk is presumably not well controlled by risk factor treatments is an area of active study. Although initial data suggest this to be the case, additional studies are needed, including studies of the impact of serial testing on medical therapy for cardiovascular risk.

Coronary CT Imaging of Non-calcified Atherosclerosis: Beyond the Calcium Score

Rapid technical advances in cardiac CT have improved the temporal and spatial resolution of contrast-enhanced MDCT to such a degree that this technique is now a reasonable alternative to invasive coronary angiography in selected clinical situations. Additionally, MDCT is now increasingly several recent reports have also emphasized the potential of MDCT for the noninvasive detection and characterization of noncalcified, atherosclerotic coronary lesions (Fig. 4) [47, 48]. Preliminary experience using MDCT scanners has shown modest correlation between coronary plaque characteristics as compared to intravascular ultrasound (the invasive, non-histological gold-standard) [47, 49–51] and histology [52, 53]. Non-calcified coronary artery plaques can be quantified for their size (Fig. 5) and morphology based upon tissue density and vessel remodeling characteristics. These concepts are being applied in algorithms to provide "virtual histology" images. However, the technical requirements for the CT acquisition and data quality are high, requiring optimal signal to noise characteristics (at the expense of increased radiation exposure), motion free imaging, and use of intravenous contrast media.

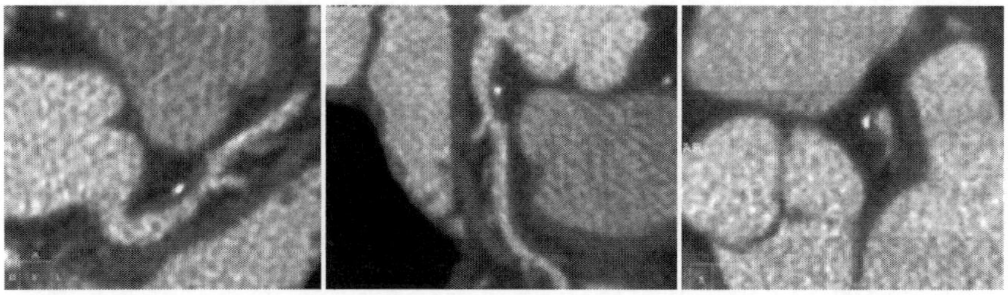

Fig. 4. Coronary CT angiogram (left anterior descending artery; curved multiplanar reformat) showing predominately noncalcified plaque with a central area of calcification.

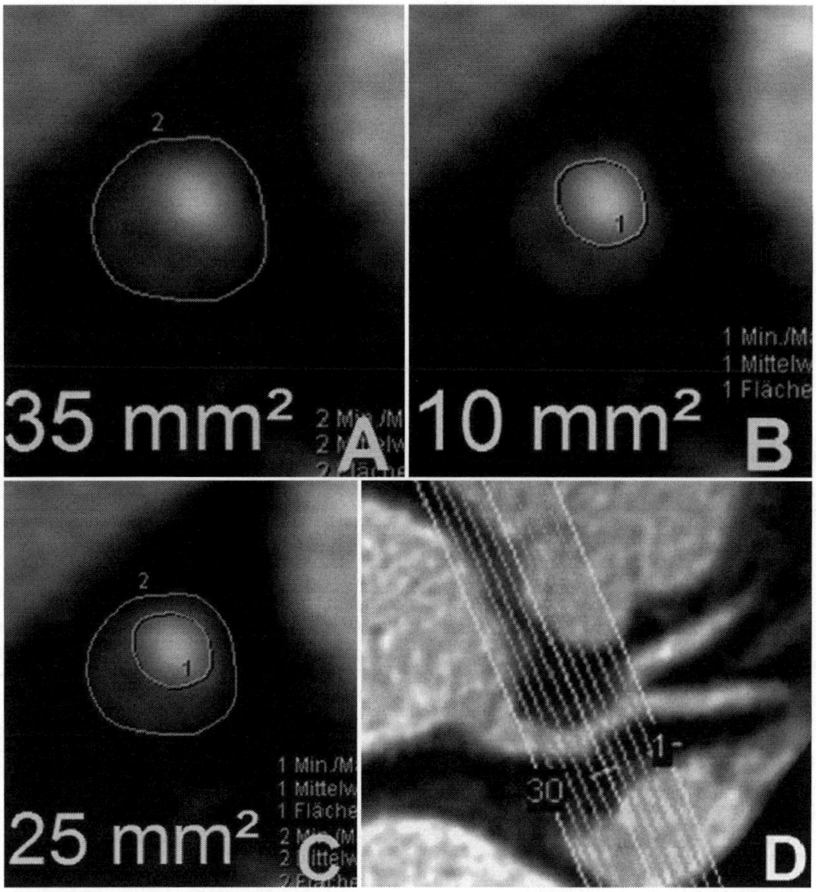

Fig. 5. Example of cross sectional coronary artery analysis for quantification of plaque (arterial wall area) in the proximal coronary arteries [76].

Non-calcified plaque as the sole finding on coronary CTA is relatively uncommon compared to calcified plaque. Cheng and associates studied the presence and severity of non-calcified coronary artery plaque (NCP) on 64-slice CT in patients with zero and low coronary artery calcium (CAC) in a retrospective study. Prevalence of detectable NCP was 6.5% in patients with zero CAC and 65.2% in those with low CAC. In outpatients with a low to intermediate risk clinical presentation and no known coronary artery disease, the absence of coronary artery calcium predicted a low prevalence of any NCP and very low prevalence of significantly occlusive NCP. Furthermore, low but detectable CAC scores were significantly less reliable in predicting plaque burden due to their association with high overall NCP prevalence and nearly a 10% rate of significantly occlusive NCP. Thus, the detection of NCP may provide an opportunity to refine the risk assessment beyond that provided by detecting only calcified plaque; however, well-controlled data from screening cohorts examining the incremental value of this data are required.

Detection of NCP is also being explored as a possible surrogate marker in treatment studies. For example, a recent pilot study suggested that the effect of statins on atherosclerosis burden could be detected using MDCT [54]. At the present time, further study and better standardization of the quantification of NCP is needed.

CARDIOVASCULAR MRI AND ATHEROSCLEROTIC PLAQUE IMAGING

CMR has emerged as a promising non-invasive plaque imaging modality. High-resolution "black blood" spin echo sequences, in which the signal from flowing blood is rendered black by preparatory pulses, allow accurate identification and quantification of the vessel wall and atherosclerotic plaque thickness and size [55, 56]. Additionally, bright blood imaging can be used to assess fibrous cap thickness and intra-plaque lipid and calcium content [56–58]. Modern magnetic resonance imaging (MRI) is attractive as it is now capable of providing images with high spatial resolution and high reproducibility, without the use of ionizing radiation.

Non-coronary Plaque Imaging

Using a multi-contrast approach for full plaque assessment by combining black blood spin-echo and fast spin echo based MR sequences (Fig. 6), CMR imaging of the thoracic aorta and carotid artery has been shown to be comparable to histological [59] and transesophageal echocardiography (TEE) imaging (for thoracic aortic plaque) for assessment of plaque thickness, extent and composition [56]. Additionally, CMR is now being utilized to assess plaque burden and morphology longitudinally. In a study of 21 asymptomatic hypercholesterolemic patients, black blood CMR imaging was used to examine 44 aortic and 32 carotid arteries at baseline and again every 6 months for a total of 24 months while on statin therapy [60]. The effect of statin therapy on atherosclerotic lesions was evaluated as changes in lumen area, vessel wall thickness and vessel wall area. After a sustained mean LDL-C reduction of 38%, CMR at 12 and 24 months demonstrated significant reductions in vessel wall thickness and vessel wall area (20% at 24 months) in both the aorta and carotid arteries, with a minimal (4–6%) increase in luminal area. This study and similar studies have begun to demonstrate the ability of CMR to visualize longitudinal vessel remodeling and plaque regression. Additionally, high-resolution CMR has been shown to accurately distinguish intact thick fibrous caps from intact thin and disrupted caps in human carotid arteries [59], and to distinguish intra-plaque from extra-plaque hemorrhage and thrombus [61], highlighting the potential for CMR to identify and examine longitudinal plaque composition changes and potential plaque stability, in response to lipid modifying therapies.

Coronary Plaque Imaging

CMR imaging of the coronary arteries must overcome several inherent technical challenges that include cardiac and respiratory motion, the small caliber and tortuosity of coronary vessels, surrounding epicardial fat and MRI artifacts caused by intracoronary stents and sternal wires in patients with prior interventional procedures. Recent advances in MRI imaging technology and protocols have started

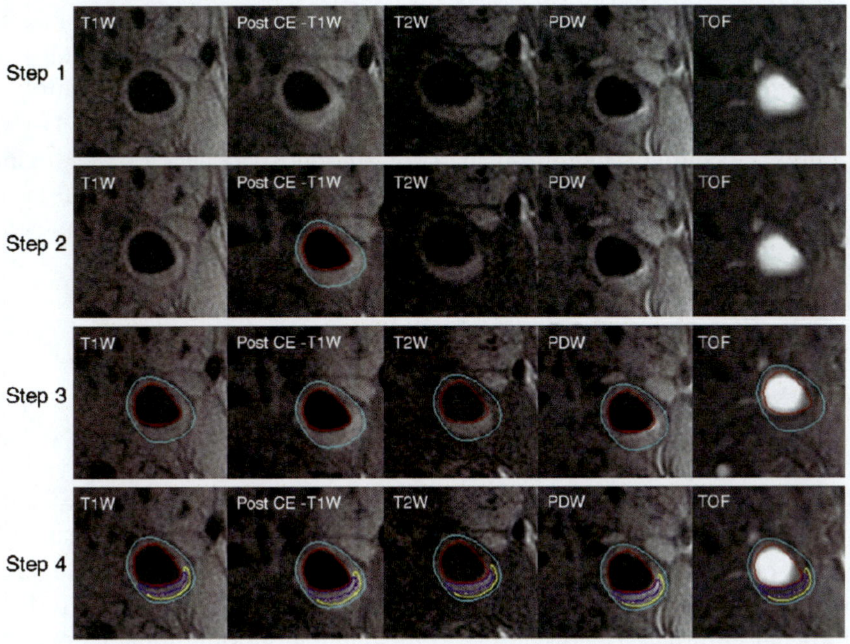

Fig. 6. Sample of measurement of quantity and components of atherosclerosis using magnetic resonance imaging [77].

to overcome these obstacles, however, experience in coronary imaging using CMR is still limited and evolving. Fayad et al. [55] utilized high-resolution (down to 0.46 mm in-plane resolution and 3 mm slice thickness) black-blood CMR imaging to assess 13 subjects, 5 of which had known coronary artery disease (≥40% stenosis by x-ray angiography). Those with known coronary disease had significantly increased mean cross-sectional coronary vessel wall thickness (4.38 ± 0.71 mm) as compared to normals (0.75 ± 0.17 mm). Further experience in MRI coronary plaque imaging is needed, specifically in standardization of pulse sequences and imaging protocols, before use of this promising technique becomes widespread.

In summary, CMR imaging is a promising tool with low interscan variability to assess and follow atherosclerosis longitudinally. Currently, multi-contrast imaging of non-coronary atherosclerosis is the most mature application, but standardization of imaging sequences and protocols is still needed. With further refinement of sophisticated pulse sequences and newer 3-tesla (T) MR systems, atherosclerosis imaging will only continue to improve towards being a valuable non-invasive tool for assessing plaque regression in response to lipid modifying therapies. Additionally, research is ongoing in the development of newer intravascular MR contrast agents or molecular imaging agents [62, 63] that are specific to imaging atherosclerotic plaque components, and that may allow for more detailed plaque characterization.

FDG-PET Plaque Imaging

Technical Performance

Positron emission tomography (PET) is a nuclear medicine diagnostic technique which produces a three-dimensional image and accurately images the cellular function of the human body. It is a major diagnostic imaging modality in oncology, neurological conditions, and cardiovascular diseases. PET scanning is non-invasive, but it does involve exposure to ionizing radiation, although the radiation exposure is low because of the short half-life and small amount of the radionuclide used. A PET scanner detects pairs of gamma ray signals emitted by the injected radionuclide, and measures the amount of metabolic activity at a site in the body, and then a computer reassembles the signals into images. Radionuclides used in PET scanning are typically isotopes with short half lives such as carbon-11 (around 20 min), nitrogen-13 (around 10 min), oxygen-15 (around 2 min), and fluorine-18 (around 110 min). The molecule most commonly used is 2-[^{18}F] fluoro-2-deoxy-D-glucose (FDG), a glucose analog that is taken up by glucose-using cells and phosphorylated by hexokinase. FDG-PET is a mainstay of nuclear medicine diagnosis, not only because of its utility in cancer imaging; but also of its promising role in cardiovascular diseases to identify metabolically active and potentially vulnerable atherosclerotic plaque.

Atherosclerotic plaque and inflammation and FDG-PET

Following from the paradigm of plaque rupture as a consequence of plaque composition vs. size, the inflammatory component of plaques is thus a target of PET imaging. Macrophages and smooth muscle cells are activated by inflammatory mediators to release degradative enzymes which weaken the connective tissue framework of the plaque's fibrous cap. In an atherosclerotic rabbit model, FDG accumulated in macrophage-rich atherosclerotic plaques and the data demonstrated that vascular macrophage activity could be quantified noninvasively with FDG-PET [64]. The uptake of FDG-PET in human atherosclerosis has been related to macrophage infiltration. In a study by Tawakol [65], there was a significant correlation between the PET signal from the human carotid plaques and the macrophage staining from the corresponding histological sections ($r=0.70$; $p<0.0001$) in 17 patients who subsequently underwent carotid endarterectomy. When mean FDG uptake was compared with mean inflammation (mean percentage of cells positive for CD68 staining- a inflammatory cell stain), the correlation was even stronger ($r=0.85$; $p<0.0001$). Wu studied the relationship between FDG-PET and matrix metalloproteinase (MMP) activity in patients with significant carotid stenosis and showed that subjects with higher FDG uptake in target lesions had higher baseline and post-stenting MMP-1 levels [66]. Since high tissue matrix metalloproteinase (MMP) activity has been associated with advanced atherosclerosis and plaque rupture, the link between FDG uptake and circulating MMP-1 indicated the potential of FDG-PET to be used as an adjunct to the clinical management of high-risk atherosclerosis and an in-vivo tool to study plaque biology.

Prevalence of Inflammation in Atherosclerosis

Increasing evidence has shown that FDG-PET imaging can be useful for non-invasive measurement of atherosclerotic plaque inflammation in humans; however, there is a paucity of data regarding how often atherosclerosis has caused inflammation in humans. Rudd [67] successfully imaged atherosclerotic plaque inflammation with FDG-PET in atherosclerotic carotid arteries, finding no measurable FDG uptake into normal carotid arteries. In addition, symptomatic, unstable plaques were shown to accumulate more FDG than asymptomatic lesions. Tahara showed that inflammation was visualized by FDG-PET imaging in approximately 30% of patients with documented carotid atherosclerosis, in 100 consecutive patients who underwent carotid artery ultra-sonography for screening of carotid atherosclerosis (Fig. 7) [68]. Although more studies are needed to accurately quantify the prevalence of inflammation in atherosclerosis in humans, this study provides some preliminary information that inflammation detected by FDG-PET is prevalent enough to be used as a marker to assess atherosclerosis clinically. Coronary risk factors are also related to FDG-PET imaging results. A further study by the same group performed in 216 consecutive patients undergoing cancer screening with FDG-PET imaging, the age- and gender-adjusted standardized uptake value of FDG was significantly higher ($p<0.0001$) in proportion to the accumulation of the number of the components of the metabolic syndrome including waist circumference, hypertensive medication, carotid intima-media thickness

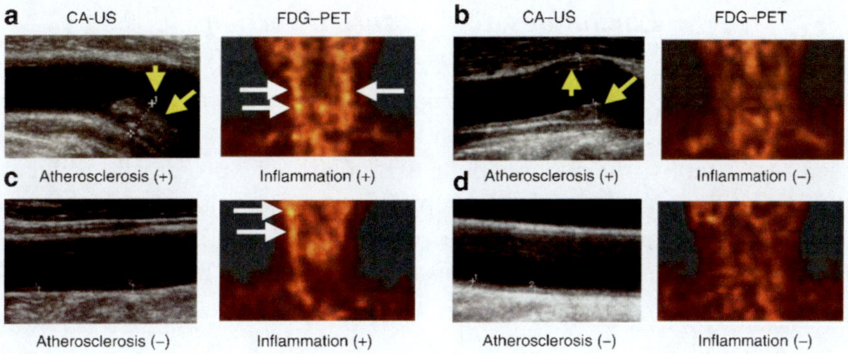

Fig. 7. Example of FDG-PET imaging of carotid atherosclerosis [68].

(CIMT), high-density lipoprotein cholesterol, homeostasis model assessment of insulin resistance, or high sensitivity C-reactive protein [69]. These data suggest that metabolic syndrome is associated with inflammation in carotid atherosclerosis.

Quantification of Atherosclerotic Plaque by FDG-PET

The standardized uptake value (SUV), which is commonly employed for assessing disease activity with FDG-PET imaging, can provide quantitative information about the severity of the inflammatory process in the arterial wall. Tatsumi used a grading score system to semi-quantitatively evaluate aortic wall FDG uptake: Grade 1: slightly higher than blood pool and mediastinal uptake; Grade 2: clearly visible and greater than Grade 1 uptake but lower than liver uptake; and Grade 3: equal to or greater than liver uptake [70]. The longitudinal spread of the abnormal FDG uptake was recorded as focal, linear, or bandlike according to the shape on coronal PET images. Bural developed a novel quantitative method to measure the extent of atherosclerosis in the aorta by multiplying SUV from FDG-PET with wall volume from CT volumetric data [71]. The end product is called the atherosclerotic burden, which can be used as an indicator of the extent of the atherosclerotic process in the aorta through the use of both metabolic and morphologic data provided by FDG-PET and CT, respectively.

FDG-PET as a tool to Assess Response to Therapy

As a potential marker for use in serial studies, inter-test reproducibility is a key test characteristic. Rudd measured serial carotid arterial and aortic FDG-PET/computed tomography uptake on consecutive studies performed 14 days apart [72, 73]. The results showed that the spontaneous change in plaque FDG uptake was low over 2 weeks, with favorable inter- and intra-observer agreement. These data set the stage for future work using this imaging modality to serially assess atherosclerosis. In an animal model using myocardial infarction-prone Watanabe heritable hyper-lipidemic rabbits [74], probucol treatment for 6 months resulted in a significant reduction of macrophage infiltration as shown by FDG-PET and histologic staining. Similarly, in a study of the effect of statins on arterial inflammation, Tahara and colleagues studied 43 consecutive subjects who underwent FDG-PET for cancer screening and had FDG uptake evaluated in the thoracic aorta and/or the carotid arteries [75]. Following three months treatment with simvastatin, but not with diet alone, plaque FDG uptake was significantly attenuated ($p<0.01$). Interestingly, in the statin group, the decrease in the SUV was well correlated with the HDL-C elevation ($p<0.01$) but not with the LDL-C reduction. Thus, beyond measuring the effect of drug on atherosclerosis, FDG-PET imaging of atherosclerosis may extend our understanding of the mechanisms of benefit of therapies with pleiotropic actions.

Limitations, and Future Directions

At the present time, in-plane resolution with FDG-PET is limited; thus this modality cannot easily image small structures such as coronary arteries. Furthermore, prospective studies and long-term follow up are warranted to study the correlation between FDG-PET activity in atherosclerosis carotid artery and clinical events to establish its independent diagnostic and prognostic value above standard cardiovascular risk factors, and serum measurements of inflammation (e.g., C-reactive protein). Additional investigation is needed on the role of FDG-PET as a surrogate imaging technique, potentially complementary to anatomic assessments of atherosclerosis burden, to assess the effectiveness of antiatherosclerosis therapies.

CONCLUSIONS

Due to continued cardiovascular risk and persistent atherogenic lipid abnormalities in patients on single-agent lipid modifying therapies, combination antilipidemic regimens are a clinical reality. As we await randomized clinical outcomes, trials evaluating combination therapies, the use of atherosclerosis imaging in trials such as the ARBITER-2 trial, has provided us with valuable clinical and pathophysiological insights. As new lipid modifying therapies arise, the desire for studying their effects on atherosclerosis longitudinally will intensify. However, it is important to note that atherosclerosis imaging, even with the most well-validated surrogate tests, is not a replacement for well-conducted clinical outcomes trials. Further data is also needed regarding the comparative performance of these different imaging modalities. This is often a difficult task in an age where the pace of technological advances, as seen currently with 3T MRI scanners and 128-slice MDCT scanners, outpaces the rate of clinical studies. Finally, the use of atherosclerosis imaging in the trial setting to evaluate drug effects on atherosclerosis is not an endorsement for widespread clinical use of the studied imaging procedure. In the setting of limited healthcare resources, the clinical utility and cost-effectiveness of atherosclerosis imaging to assess and monitor individual cardiovascular risk, above and beyond current global risk assessments and newer serologic risk markers, should be demonstrated.

REFERENCES

1. Waters D, Higginson L, Gladstone P et al. Effects of monotherapy with an HMG-CoA reductase inhibitor on the progression of coronary atherosclerosis as assessed by serial quantitative arteriography. The canadian coronary atherosclerosis intervention trial. Circulation 1994;89(3):959–68.
2. Hodis HN, Mack WJ, LaBree L et al. The role of carotid arterial intima-media thickness in predicting clinical coronary events. Ann Intern Med 1998;128(4):262–269.
3. Raggi P, Cooil B, Shaw LJ et al. Progression of coronary calcium on serial electron beam tomographic scanning is greater in patients with future myocardial infarction. Am J Cardiol 2003;92(7):827–829.
4. von Birgelen C, Hartmann M, Mintz GS et al. Relationship between cardiovascular risk as predicted by established risk scores versus plaque progression as measured by serial intravascular ultrasound in left main coronary arteries. Circulation 2004;110(12):1579–1585.
5. Boissel JP, Collet JP, Moleur P, Haugh M. Surrogate endpoints: a basis for a rational approach. Eur J Clin Pharmacol 1992;43(3):235–244.
6. Pignoli P, Tremoli E, Poli A, Oreste P, Paoletti R. Intimal plus medial thickness of the arterial wall: a direct measurement with ultrasound imaging. Circulation 1986;74(6):1399–1406.
7. Touboul PJ, Hennerici MG, Meairs S et al. Mannheim intima-media thickness consensus. Cerebrovasc Dis 2004; 18(4):346–349.
8. Stein JH, Korcarz CE, Hurst RT et al. Use of carotid ultrasound to identify subclinical vascular disease and evaluate cardiovascular disease risk: a consensus statement from the American Society of Echocardiography Carotid Intima-Media Thickness Task Force. Endorsed by the Society for Vascular Medicine. J Am Soc Echocardiogr 2008;21(2):93–111.

9. Chambless LE, Heiss G, Folsom AR et al. Association of coronary heart disease incidence with carotid arterial wall thickness and major risk factors: the Atherosclerosis Risk in Communities (ARIC) Study, 1987-1993. Am J Epidemiol 1997;146(6):483–494.
10. Howard G, Sharrett AR, Heiss G et al. Carotid artery intimal-medial thickness distribution in general populations as evaluated by B-mode ultrasound. ARIC Investigators. Stroke 1993;24(9):1297–1304.
11. O'Leary DH, Polak JF, Kronmal RA, Manolio TA, Burke GL, Wolfson SK, Jr. Carotid-artery intima and media thickness as a risk factor for myocardial infarction and stroke in older adults. Cardiovascular Health Study Collaborative Research Group. N Engl J Med 1999;340(1):14–22.
12. Lorenz MW, Markus HS, Bots ML, Rosvall M, Sitzer M. Prediction of clinical cardiovascular events with carotid intima-media thickness: a systematic review and meta-analysis. Circulation 2007;115(4):459–467.
13. Belcaro G, Nicolaides AN, Laurora G et al. Ultrasound morphology classification of the arterial wall and cardiovascular events in a 6-year follow-up study. Arterioscler Thromb Vasc Biol 1996;16(7):851–856.
14. Shahab L, Hall S, Marteau T. Showing smokers with vascular disease images of their arteries to motivate cessation: a pilot study. Br J Health Psychol 2007;12(Pt 2):275–283.
15. Greenland P, Abrams J, Aurigemma GP et al. Prevention Conference V: Beyond secondary prevention: identifying the high-risk patient for primary prevention: noninvasive tests of atherosclerotic burden: Writing Group III. Circulation 2000;101(1):E16–E22.
16. Grundy SM, Cleeman JI, Merz CN et al. Implications of recent clinical trials for the National Cholesterol Education Program Adult Treatment Panel III Guidelines. J Am Coll Cardiol 2004;44(3):720–732.
17. Taylor AJ, Kent SM, Flaherty PJ, Coyle LC, Markwood TT, Vernalis MN. ARBITER: Arterial Biology for the Investigation of the Treatment Effects of Reducing Cholesterol: a randomized trial comparing the effects of atorvastatin and pravastatin on carotid intima medial thickness. Circulation 2002;106(16):2055–2060.
18. Nissen SE, Tuzcu EM, Schoenhagen P et al. Effect of intensive compared with moderate lipid-lowering therapy on progression of coronary atherosclerosis: a randomized controlled trial. J Am Med Assoc 2004;291(9):1071–1080.
19. Cannon CP, Braunwald E, McCabe CH et al. Intensive versus moderate lipid lowering with statins after acute coronary syndromes. N Engl J Med 2004;350(15):1495–1504.
20. Larosa JC, Grundy SM, Waters DD et al. Intensive Lipid Lowering with Atorvastatin in Patients with Stable Coronary Disease. N Engl J Med 2005:352(14):1425–1435.
21. Taylor AJ, Sullenberger LE, Lee HJ, Lee JK, Grace KA. Arterial Biology for the Investigation of the Treatment Effects of Reducing Cholesterol (ARBITER) 2: a double-blind, placebo-controlled study of extended-release niacin on atherosclerosis progression in secondary prevention patients treated with statins. Circulation 2004;110(23):3512–3517.
22. Nissen SE, Tsunoda T, Tuzcu EM et al. Effect of recombinant ApoA-I Milano on coronary atherosclerosis in patients with acute coronary syndromes: a randomized controlled trial. J Am Med Assoc 2003;290(17):2292–2300.
23. Al-Shali K, House AA, Hanley AJ et al. Differences between carotid wall morphological phenotypes measured by ultrasound in one, two and three dimensions. Atherosclerosis 2005;178(2):319–325.
24. Bae JH, Kim WS, Rihal CS, Lerman A. Individual measurement and significance of carotid intima, media, and intima-media thickness by B-mode ultrasonographic image processing. Arterioscler Thromb Vasc Biol 2006;26(10):2380–2385.
25. Gronholdt ML, Nordestgaard BG, Wiebe BM, Wilhjelm JE, Sillesen H. Echo-lucency of computerized ultrasound images of carotid atherosclerotic plaques are associated with increased levels of triglyceride-rich lipoproteins as well as increased plaque lipid content. Circulation 1998;97(1):34-40.
26. Shah F, Balan P, Weinberg M et al. Contrast-enhanced ultrasound imaging of atherosclerotic carotid plaque neovascularization: a new surrogate marker of atherosclerosis? Vasc Med 2007;12(4):291–297.
27. Feinstein SB. Contrast ultrasound imaging of the carotid artery vasa vasorum and atherosclerotic plaque neovascularization. J Am Coll Cardiol 2006;48(2):236–243.
28. Rumberger JA, Simons DB, Fitzpatrick LA, Sheedy PF, Schwartz RS. Coronary artery calcium area by electron-beam computed tomography and coronary atherosclerotic plaque area. A histopathologic correlative study. Circulation 1995;92(8):2157–2162.
29. Sangiorgi G, Rumberger JA, Severson A et al. Arterial calcification and not lumen stenosis is highly correlated with atherosclerotic plaque burden in humans: a histologic study of 723 coronary artery segments using nondecalcifying methodology. J Am Coll Cardiol 1998;31(1):126–133.
30. O'Malley PG, Taylor AJ, Jackson JL, Doherty TM, Detrano RC. Prognostic value of coronary electron-beam computed tomography for coronary heart disease events in asymptomatic populations. Am J Cardiol 2000;85(8):945–948.
31. Arad Y, Spadaro LA, Goodman K, Newstein D, Guerci AD. Prediction of coronary events with electron beam computed tomography. J Am Coll Cardiol 2000;36(4):1253–1260.
32. Kondos GT, Hoff JA, Sevrukov A et al. Electron-beam tomography coronary artery calcium and cardiac events: a 37-month follow-up of 5635 initially asymptomatic low- to intermediate-risk adults. Circulation 2003;107(20):2571–2576.

33. Shaw LJ, Raggi P, Schisterman E, Berman DS, Callister TQ. Prognostic value of cardiac risk factors and coronary artery calcium screening for all-cause mortality. Radiology 2003;228(3):826–833.
34. Hoff JA, Chomka EV, Krainik AJ, Daviglus M, Rich S, Kondos GT. Age and gender distributions of coronary artery calcium detected by electron beam tomography in 35,246 adults. Am J Cardiol 2001;87(12):1335–1339.
35. Kaufmann RB, Sheedy PF, Breen JF et al. Detection of heart calcification with electron beam CT: interobserver and intraobserver reliability for scoring quantification. Radiology 1994;190(2):347–352.
36. Devries S, Wolfkiel C, Shah V, Chomka E, Rich S. Reproducibility of the measurement of coronary calcium with ultrafast computed tomography. Am J Cardiol 1995;75(14):973–975.
37. Lu B, Budoff MJ, Zhuang N et al. Causes of interscan variability of coronary artery calcium measurements at electron-beam CT. Acad Radiol 2002;9(6):654–661.
38. Shields JP, Mielke CH, Jr., Rockwood TH, Short RA, Viren FK. Reliability of electron beam computed tomography to detect coronary artery calcification. Am J Card Imaging 1995;9(2):62–66.
39. Kopp AF, Ohnesorge B, Becker C et al. Reproducibility and accuracy of coronary calcium measurements with multi-detector row versus electron-beam CT. Radiology 2002;225(1):113–119.
40. Knez A, Becker A, Becker C et al. Detection of coronary calcinosis with multislice spiral computerized tomography: an alternative to electron beam tomography. Z Kardiol 2002;91(8):642–649.
41. Callister TQ, Cooil B, Raya SP, Lippolis NJ, Russo DJ, Raggi P. Coronary artery disease: improved reproducibility of calcium scoring with an electron-beam CT volumetric method. Radiology 1998;208(3):807–814.
42. Wu B, Elmariah S, Kaplan FS, Cheng G, Mohler ER, III. Paradoxical effects of statins on aortic valve myofibroblasts and osteoblasts: implications for end-stage valvular heart disease. Arterioscler Thromb Vasc Biol 2005;25(3): 592–597.
43. Raggi P, Bommer J, Chertow GM. Valvular calcification in hemodialysis patients randomized to calcium-based phosphorus binders or sevelamer. J Heart Valve Dis 2004;13(1):134–141.
44. Raggi P, Callister TQ, Shaw LJ. Progression of coronary artery calcium and risk of first myocardial infarction in patients receiving cholesterol-lowering therapy. Arterioscler Thromb Vasc Biol 2004;24(7):1272–1277.
45. Budoff MJ, Achenbach S, Blumenthal RS et al. Assessment of Coronary artery disease by cardiac computed tomography: a scientific statement from the American heart association committee on cardiovascular imaging and intervention, council on cardiovascular radiology and intervention, and committee on cardiac imaging, council on clinical cardiology. Circulation 2006;114(16):1761–1791.
46. Greenland P, Bonow RO, Brundage BH et al. ACCF/AHA 2007 clinical expert consensus document on coronary artery calcium scoring by computed tomography in global cardiovascular risk assessment and in evaluation of patients with chest pain: a report of the American College of Cardiology Foundation Clinical Expert Consensus Task Force (ACCF/AHA Writing Committee to Update the 2000 Expert Consensus Document on Electron Beam Computed Tomography) developed in collaboration with the Society of Atherosclerosis Imaging and Prevention and the Society of Cardiovascular Computed Tomography. J Am Coll Cardiol 2007 January 23;49(3):378–402.
47. Leber AW, Knez A, Becker A et al. Accuracy of multidetector spiral computed tomography in identifying and differentiating the composition of coronary atherosclerotic plaques: a comparative study with intracoronary ultrasound. J Am Coll Cardiol 2004;43(7):1241–1247.
48. Nikolaou K, Sagmeister S, Knez A et al. Multidetector-row computed tomography of the coronary arteries: predictive value and quantitative assessment of non-calcified vessel-wall changes. Eur Radiol 2003;13(11):2505–2512.
49. Kopp AF, Schroeder S, Baumbach A et al. Non-invasive characterisation of coronary lesion morphology and composition by multislice CT: first results in comparison with intracoronary ultrasound. Eur Radiol 2001;11(9):1607–1611.
50. Schoenhagen P, Tuzcu EM, Stillman AE et al. Non-invasive assessment of plaque morphology and remodeling in mildly stenotic coronary segments: comparison of 16-slice computed tomography and intravascular ultrasound. Coron Artery Dis 2003;14(6):459–462.
51. Achenbach S, Moselewski F, Ropers D et al. Detection of calcified and noncalcified coronary atherosclerotic plaque by contrast-enhanced, submillimeter multidetector spiral computed tomography: a segment-based comparison with intravascular ultrasound. Circulation 2004;109(1):14–17.
52. Schroeder S, Kuettner A, Leitritz M et al. Reliability of differentiating human coronary plaque morphology using contrast-enhanced multislice spiral computed tomography: a comparison with histology. J Comput Assist Tomogr 2004; 28(4):449–454.
53. Nikolaou K, Becker CR, Muders M et al. Multidetector-row computed tomography and magnetic resonance imaging of atherosclerotic lesions in human ex vivo coronary arteries. Atherosclerosis 2004;174(2):243–252.
54. Burgstahler C, Reimann A, Beck T et al. Influence of a lipid-lowering therapy on calcified and noncalcified coronary plaques monitored by multislice detector computed tomography: results of the New Age II Pilot Study. Invest Radiol 2007;42(3):189–195.

55. Fayad ZA, Fuster V, Fallon JT et al. Noninvasive in vivo human coronary artery lumen and wall imaging using black-blood magnetic resonance imaging. Circulation 2000;102(5):506–510.
56. Fayad ZA, Nahar T, Fallon JT et al. In vivo magnetic resonance evaluation of atherosclerotic plaques in the human thoracic aorta: a comparison with transesophageal echocardiography. Circulation 2000;101(21):2503–2309.
57. Itskovich VV, Samber DD, Mani V et al. Quantification of human atherosclerotic plaques using spatially enhanced cluster analysis of multicontrast-weighted magnetic resonance images. Magn Reson Med 2004;52(3):515–523.
58. Sirol M, Itskovich VV, Mani V et al. Lipid-rich atherosclerotic plaques detected by gadofluorine-enhanced in vivo magnetic resonance imaging. Circulation 2004;109(23):2890–2896.
59. Hatsukami TS, Ross R, Polissar NL, Yuan C. Visualization of fibrous cap thickness and rupture in human atherosclerotic carotid plaque in vivo with high-resolution magnetic resonance imaging. Circulation 2000;102(9):959–964.
60. Corti R, Fayad ZA, Fuster V et al. Effects of lipid-lowering by simvastatin on human atherosclerotic lesions: a longitudinal study by high-resolution, noninvasive magnetic resonance imaging. Circulation 2001;104(3):249–252.
61. Kampschulte A, Ferguson MS, Kerwin WS et al. Differentiation of intraplaque versus juxtaluminal hemorrhage/thrombus in advanced human carotid atherosclerotic lesions by in vivo magnetic resonance imaging. Circulation 2004;110(20): 3239–3244.
62. Flacke S, Fischer S, Scott MJ et al. Novel MRI contrast agent for molecular imaging of fibrin: implications for detecting vulnerable plaques. Circulation 2001;104(11):1280–1285.
63. Kooi ME, Cappendijk VC, Cleutjens KB et al. Accumulation of ultrasmall superparamagnetic particles of iron oxide in human atherosclerotic plaques can be detected by in vivo magnetic resonance imaging. Circulation 2003;107(19): 2453–2458.
64. Tawakol A, Castano AP, Gad F et al. Intravascular detection of inflamed atherosclerotic plaques using a fluorescent photosensitizer targeted to the scavenger receptor. Photochem Photobiol Sci 2008;7(1):33–39.
65. Tawakol A, Migrino RQ, Bashian GG et al. In vivo 18F-fluorodeoxyglucose positron emission tomography imaging provides a noninvasive measure of carotid plaque inflammation in patients. J Am Coll Cardiol 2006;48(9):1818–1824.
66. Wu YW, Kao HL, Chen MF et al. Characterization of plaques using 18F-FDG PET/CT in patients with carotid atherosclerosis and correlation with matrix metalloproteinase-1. J Nucl Med 2007;48(2):227–233.
67. Rudd JH, Warburton EA, Fryer TD et al. Imaging atherosclerotic plaque inflammation with [18F]-fluorodeoxyglucose positron emission tomography. Circulation 2002;105(23):2708–2711.
68. Tahara N, Kai H, Nakaura H et al. The prevalence of inflammation in carotid atherosclerosis: analysis with fluorodeoxyglucose-positron emission tomography. Eur Heart J 2007;28(18):2243–2248.
69. Tahara N, Kai H, Yamagishi S et al. Vascular inflammation evaluated by [18F]-fluorodeoxyglucose positron emission tomography is associated with the metabolic syndrome. J Am Coll Cardiol 2007;49(14):1533–1539.
70. Tatsumi M, Cohade C, Nakamoto Y, Wahl RL. Fluorodeoxyglucose uptake in the aortic wall at PET/CT: possible finding for active atherosclerosis. Radiology 2003;229(3):831–837.
71. Bural GG, Torigian DA, Chamroonrat W et al. Quantitative assessment of the atherosclerotic burden of the aorta by combined FDG-PET and CT image analysis: a new concept. Nucl Med Biol 2006;33(8):1037–1043.
72. Rudd JH, Myers KS, Bansilal S et al. Atherosclerosis Inflammation Imaging with 18F-FDG PET: Carotid, Iliac, and Femoral Uptake Reproducibility, Quantification Methods, and Recommendations. J Nucl Med 2008;49(6):871–878.
73. Rudd JH, Myers KS, Bansilal S et al. (18)Fluorodeoxyglucose positron emission tomography imaging of atherosclerotic plaque inflammation is highly reproducible: implications for atherosclerosis therapy trials. J Am Coll Cardiol 2007; 50(9):892–896.
74. Ogawa M, Magata Y, Kato T et al. Application of 18F-FDG PET for monitoring the therapeutic effect of antiinflammatory drugs on stabilization of vulnerable atherosclerotic plaques. J Nucl Med 2006;47(11):1845–1850.
75. Tahara N, Kai H, Ishibashi M et al. Simvastatin attenuates plaque inflammation: evaluation by fluorodeoxyglucose positron emission tomography. J Am Coll Cardiol 2006;48(9):1825–1831.
76. Schmid M, Achenbach S, Ropers D et al. Assessment of changes in non-calcified atherosclerotic plaque volume in the left main and left anterior descending coronary arteries over time by 64-slice computed tomography. Am J Cardiol 2008;101(5):579–584.
77. Zhao XQ, Phan BA, Chu B et al. Testing the hypothesis of atherosclerotic plaque lipid depletion during lipid therapy by magnetic resonance imaging: study design of carotid plaque composition study. Am Heart J 2007;154(2):239–246.
78. Azen SP, Mack WJ, Cashin-Hemphill L et al. Progression of coronary artery disease predicts clinical coronary events. long-term follow-up from the cholesterol lowering atherosclerosis study. Circulation 1996;93(1):34–41.
79. von Birgelen C, Hartmann M, Mintz GS, Baumgart D, Schmermund A, Erbel R. Relation between progression and regression of atherosclerotic left main coronary artery disease and serum cholesterol levels as assessed with serial long-term (> or =12 months) follow-up intravascular ultrasound. Circulation 2003;108(22):2757–2762.

42 Implications of SHAPE Guideline for Improving Patient Compliance

Matthew J. Budoff

CONTENTS

ABSTRACT

While excellent therapies exist for prevention of coronary artery disease, one of the biggest problems is adherence to these therapies. Multiple prospective observational studies have shown that coronary artery calcium (CAC) is an independent marker of cardiovascular risk providing incremental prognostic value over traditional and emerging risk markers. Several studies have been done to evaluate the potential for adherence/compliance of visualizing CAC. Theoretically, visualizing CAC provides tangible evidence of the disease and would be associated with improvements in adherence to statin therapy. Several studies have now shown that measuring and reporting of CAC leads to changes in cardiovascular risk management. Multiple studies, including the Multi-Ethnic Study of Atherosclerosis, have shown that initiation and persistence of lipid-lowering medications, blood-pressure-lowering medications, and aspirin were greater in those with higher CAC. These studies support the notion that subclinical atherosclerosis testing may lead to greater use of evidence-based, cardiovascular preventive medications.

Key words: Cardiac CT; Multidetector CT; Electron Beam CT; Compliance; Adherence; Statin therapy; Carotid intimal medial thickness

KEY POINTS

- Compliance is one of the major public health issues facing preventive medicine today.
- Coronary artery calcium scores are associated with increased cardiovascular risk.

From: *Asymptomatic Atherosclerosis: Pathophysiology, Detection and Treatment*
Edited by: M. Naghavi (ed.), DOI 10.1007/978-1-60327-179-0_42

- Higher calcium scores are associated with increased initiation and adherence to statin therapy.
- Studies have shown that interventions including carotid intimal-media thickness and biomarkers fail to improve adherence.

INTRODUCTION

Low adherence rates lead to increased adverse health outcomes, including increased ambulatory care visits, emergency department visits, and hospitalizations. In a claims database analysis, patients who were adherent experienced up to 50% lower all-cause hospitalization risks. This problem may be magnified in the treatment of cardiovascular conditions, in which up to 50% of cardiovascular admissions may be attributable to nonadherence. Furthermore, although drug costs for adherent patients are higher, overall health care costs related to fewer hospital admissions are substantially lower in patients who are adherent [1]. Poor medication adherence can cost an extra $2,000 a year for each patient in extra doctor visits alone, and its associated with as many as 40% of nursing home admissions [2–4]. Reports estimate that poor medication adherence could be costing the country $177 billion in medical bills and lost productivity. In a recent study assessing drug-dispensing and hospital discharge records, Penning-van Beest [5] assessed 59,094 who started statin therapy in a three-year period. In a two-year follow-up, a total of 31 557 patients (53%) discontinued statin use within two years. Overall a 30% reduction in risk of hospitalization for acute myocardial infarction (AMI) with persistent statin use was observed. Despite significant and consistent data on the benefits of lipid-lowering agents to reduce cardiovascular events, adherence and utilization of these agents remains low. In a recent study a 2-year adherence rate following statin initiation was only 40% for acute coronary syndrome, 36% for chronic CAD, and only 25% for primary prevention cohorts perhaps signifying a relationship between awareness of disease and adherence to therapy [5].

CORONARY ARTERY CALCIUM SCANNING

Coronary artery calcification (CAC) is rapidly gaining prominence as a risk marker for adverse cardiovascular events in an asymptomatic population. Studies clearly show the risk associated with increasing CAC score, which signifies a higher plaque burden and significant cardiovascular risk [6]. Multiple prospective observational studies have shown that CAC is an independent marker of cardiovascular risk providing incremental prognostic value over traditional and emerging risk markers [6]. The incremental value of CAC testing for the detection of CHD risk has led the National Cholesterol Education Panel [7], American Heart Association [6], and American College of Cardiology [8] to include CAC as a candidate component of the coronary risk assessment within published guidelines and expert consensus statements. While its relevance as a risk marker for asymptomatic patients has been established, the implications on compliance have just started to be demonstrated.

Calcium Scanning and Compliance

Willpower lasts about two weeks...And is usually soluble in alcohol – Sam Clemens

Several studies have been done to evaluate the potential for adherence/compliance of visualizing CAC. Theoretically, visualizing CAC provides tangible evidence of the disease and would be associated with improvements in adherence to statin therapy. An early observation study indicated that certain potentially beneficial behavioral changes, such as new aspirin usage, new cholesterol medication, decreasing dietary fat, and losing weight, may be motivated by the knowledge of a positive coronary artery (CAC) score [9]. This initially positive data were followed by a more neutral study.

In the study by O'Malley et al. [10], a very well-designed study fell prey to a significant problem, patient selection. The authors carefully evaluated the ability of CAC by Electron Beam Tomography (EBT) and Intensive Case Management (ICM) to modify cardiovascular risk in 450 persons. The authors showed the patients their EBT scans, describing that calcification is a marker of underlying atherosclerosis. The authors describe, "The counseling was coupled with risk factor identification and advice with the intent of capturing the "teachable moment" in those who had coronary calcification." Unfortunately, this low-intermediate risk population of active military personnel (ages 39–45) had very few persons with coronary calcification, only 18% (59 of 230) were ultimately shown arteries with atherosclerosis, while 82% were shown normal studies (no detectable plaque). The authors further acknowledge that of those with calcification, most had trivial amounts (mean score <10). It seems implausible that given a "clean bill of health" (i.e., no or minimal coronary calcification) would be a strong motivator of lifestyle change. Despite only having a minimal amount of atherosclerosis, subgroup analysis in those persons with EBT-defined coronary calcium ($n=59$) showed a trend toward a smaller increase in risk associated with receiving the EBT information as compared to those from whom EBT information was withheld (0.21% vs. 1.52%, $p=0.13$), and more participants who received the information had stable or reduced cardiovascular risk (41.7% vs. 26.1%, $p=0.27$). We know this army study does not represent the general population. The prevalence of calcification is significantly lower than what is observed in large population-based studies, such as the Multi-Ethnic Study of Atherosclerosis, where 46% of participants were found to have coronary calcification [11].

A larger and longer observational study evaluated the potential association between EBT and adherence to lipid-lowering therapy and lifestyle modifications among consecutive patients physician-referred for evaluation of coronary atherosclerosis [12]. The patient population studied had a much higher cardiovascular risk than that studied by O'Malley, with an average age of 60.4 ± 10.1 years with an average Framingham risk of 13.4%. This study hypothesized that increasing CAC burden will be associated with improved patient adherence to coronary risk reducing behaviors, such as lipid-lowering therapy, exercise, diet, and smoking cessation. The study population consisted of 505 individuals on statin therapy on baseline who were followed for a mean of 3 ± 2 years. Overall the statin compliance was lowest (44%) among those with CAC score in the first quartile (0–30), whereas 91% of individuals with baseline CAC score in the fourth quartile (≥526) adhered to statin therapy (Fig. 1). In multivariable analysis, after adjusting for cardiovascular risk factors, age, and gender, higher baseline CAC scores were strongly associated with adherence to statin therapy.

Studies then assessed whether higher CAC scores were associated with aspirin (ASA) utilization as well beneficial lifestyle behaviors in physician referred asymptomatic individuals [13]. A total of 980 asymptomatic patients referred for CAC risk assessment were surveyed regarding health behaviors in 3 years. This study evaluated long-term ASA utilization, exercise, and dietary changes based on CAC using multivariable analysis. Overall ASA initiation was lowest (29%) among those with CAC = 0 and gradually increased with higher CAC (1–99: 55%, 100–399: 61%, ≥400:63%, $p<0.001$ for trend). Similarly, dietary changes and exercise were lowest (33% and 44%, respectively) among those with CAC = 0 and gradually increased with higher CAC (1–99: 40%, 100–399: 58%, ≥400:56%, $p<0.001$ for trend for dietary changes; and 1–99: 62%, 100–399: 63%, ≥400:67%, $p<0.001$ for trend for exercise). In multivariable analysis, higher baseline CAC was strongly associated with initiation of ASA therapy, dietary changes and increased exercise (Table 1).

Population-based study data also demonstrate that baseline coronary artery calcium is associated with improvements in adherence to statin therapy and ASA in a population-based study [14].

MESA is a prospective cohort study of 6,814 participants free of clinical cardiovascular disease who underwent CAC testing at baseline examination [5]. Information on LLT as well ASA usage was obtained at baseline, and at 1.6 and 3.2 years after baseline. LLT initiation increasing with higher

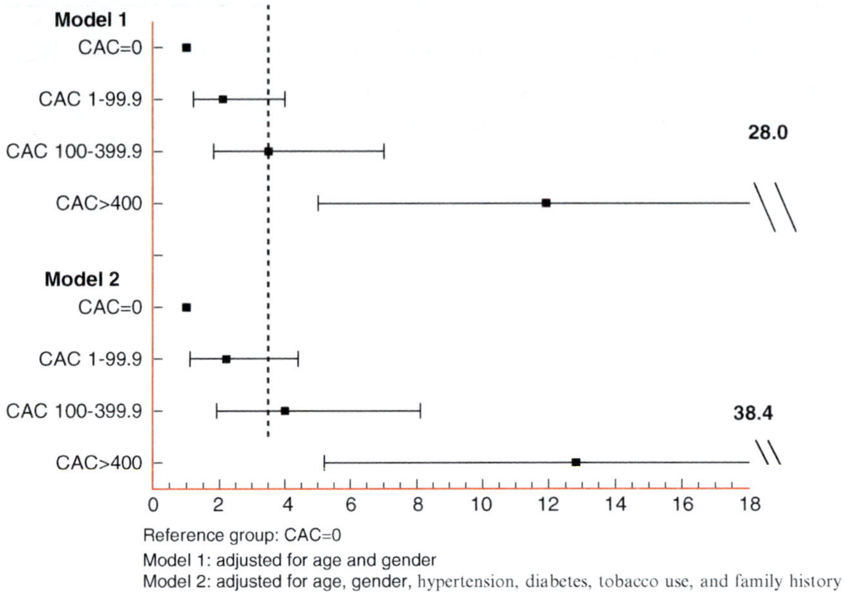

Fig. 1. Odds ratio (95% CI) of maintaining statin therapy with increasing absolute CAC scores.

Table 1
Odds ratio for initiation of lifestyle measures after adjustment of cardiovascular risk factors

Odds ratio	*CAC=0*	*CAC 1–99*	*CAC 100–399*	*CAC≥400*	*P value(trend)*
Aspirin initiation	1 (ref)	2.61 (1.78–3.84)	2.99 (1.91–4.65)	2.98 (1.83–4.83)	<0.0001
Changed Diet	1 (ref)	1.33 (0.91–1.96)	2.94 (1.88–4.57)	2.66 (1.63–4.32)	<0.0001
Increased Exercise	1 (ref)	1.88 (1.30–2.73)	1.79 (1.15–2.73)	2.03 (1.26–3.27)	<0.0001

[a]Adjusted for age, sex, FH of CHD, hypertension, hyperlipidemia, DM, and smoking status

Table 2
Relative risk regression for continuation of lipid-lowering therapy and aspirin with increasing CAC

	Initiation of LLT		
	NCEP recommends drug therapy?		*Initiation of Aspirin*
CAC Group:	No – RR (95% CI)	Yes – RR (95% CI)	RR (95% CI)
Score 0	Reference Group		
1–100	1.31 (1.00, 1.71)	1.04 (0.75, 1.44)	1.22 (1.15, 1.55)
101–400	2.20 (1.67, 2.91)	1.18 (0.81, 1.72)	1.87 (1.59, 2.21)
>400	2.78 (2.06, 3.75)	1.70 (1.21, 2.39)	2.24 (1.88, 2.68)

CAC regardless of whether drug therapy would be recommended based on NCEP ATP III or not (Yes: 0=21%, 1–100=22%, 101–400=25% and >400=36%, p=0.02; No: 0=6%, 1–100=8%, 101–400=13% and >400=16%, p=<0.001). An increasing rate of new ASA initiation with higher CAC was observed (0=14%, 1–100=19%, 101–400=26% and >400=32%, $p<0.001$). The relative risks for initiation of LLT and ASA were significantly higher with increasing CAC burden. The relationship was observed in all ethnic groups (Table 2).

The Prospective Army Coronary Calcium (PACC) Project evaluated whether the detection of CAC leads to changes in cardiovascular risk management. The finding of CAC in PACC participants has been shown to be associated with an 11.8-fold increased risk for CHD events during mean 3-year follow-up [15]. The authors then examined if CAC, a marker of increased CHD risk, was independently associated with greater use of these preventive therapies. 1,640 asymptomatic men, aged 40–50 years, were screened for CHD risk factors and CAC using Electron Beam Tomography (EBT). During 6 years of prospective annual structured telephone contacts, the authors observed subsequent "ever use" and "consistent use" of daily ASA and statins using logistic regression to control for CAC, baseline medication use, and NCEP risk variables [16]. Over six years of follow-up, both statin and ASA use increased to a greater degree in patients found to have CAC, with the curves for both drugs diverging clearly after the baseline scan. During follow-up the use of both ASA and statins increased progressively, but by 6 years statin use was 3× more likely among those with CAC (48.5% vs. 15.5%, $P<0.001$) and ASA use was nearly twice as likely (53.0% vs. 32.3% $P<0.01$). Multiple logistic regression controlling for NCEP risk variables showed that CAC was independently associated with a significantly higher likelihood of statin use, ASA use, or use of both medications (OR: 6.97; 95% CI: 4.81–10.10). The odds ratio for drug use based on NCEP risk factors alone was dramatically lower (OR: 1.52; CI: 1.27–1.82). Odds ratios were unchanged after controlling for depression, somatization, fitness, diet, income, or education.

Adherence and Progression of Coronary Artery Calcium

Recent studies have suggested that in addition to risk stratification for the asymptomatic person, individuals with higher CAC scores are more likely to maintain adherence to lipid-lowering medication (LLM). However whether adherence to LLM will be associated with less progression of atherosclerosis is not clear. A study compared the progression on CACS according to LLM adherence status across increasing baseline CACS.

The study population consisted of 505 individuals on statin therapy at baseline who were followed for a mean of 3 ± 2 years. Overall the LLM continuation was lowest (40%) among those with CACS = 0, score in the first quartile (0–30), whereas 90% of those with CACS > 400) adhered to LLM. Overall , the annualized as well as percentage change in CACS was significantly less with LLM adherence only among those with baseline CACS > 400 (Table 1). In quantile multivariate regression (adjusting for age, sex, hypercholesteremia; hypertension, diabetes mellitus, smoking; and family history of heart disease), LLM adherence also was significantly associated with a lower median progression of annualized absolute CACS (regression coefficient, –42.0; $P=0.05$) annualized percentage CACS (regression coefficient, –9%; $P=0.005$) among those with scores >400. Higher baseline CACS, especially >400, is associated with both increased LLM adherence and slower progression of atherosclerosis. This study shows that in this subset of patients, therapeutic intervention with statins coupled with increased compliance did result in a slowed progression of coronary calcium. The results of this study also underscore the role of coronary calcium measurement as a means of monitoring progress in patients being treated for subclinical atherosclerotic disease. The results of identification and monitoring also appear to garner more compliance (especially in the population which is at higher risk for a cardiac event) with treatment strategies initiated. It remains to be seen whether this approach results in higher rates of adherence and compliance with the ultimate goal of reduced progression and hence lower incidence of clinical events.

CAROTID INTIMAL MEDIAL THICKNESS (IMT)

One small study suggested that screening for carotid plaque and presenting the patients with pictures of plaques improved smoking cessation rates [17]; there is scant evidence that screening for atherosclerosis affects physician management, patient motivation, or long-term health-related outcomes [18].

A more recent study was reported to address this issue of whether detection of carotid plaque affects physician behavior or motivates patients [19]. Subjects included asymptomatic patients without known vascular disease who had two or more cardiac risk factors underwent IMT scanning. Subjects completed a survey to assess motivation to make lifestyle changes before and after the results of the scan were provided. Fifty subjects were enrolled over 9 months. Their mean (SD) age was 54.0 (10.4) years and their mean Framingham 10-year cardiovascular risk was 7.8% (7.9%). More than half (58%) of the subjects had at least one carotid plaque. When carotid plaque was identified, physicians were more likely to prescribe aspirin ($P=0.031$) and lipid-lowering therapy ($P=0.004$). Although subjects with carotid plaque reported an increase in their perceived likelihood of developing heart disease ($P=0.013$), they did not report increased motivation to make lifestyle changes. Ultrasound screening for carotid plaque in an office setting can alter physician treatment plans. This study shows that carotid IMT plaque increased patient perception of cardiovascular risk, but did not motivate patients to make lifestyle changes, as was demonstrated by CAC testing. Further studies with IMT are underway.

CONCLUSIONS

Atherosclerosis imaging has been shown in multiple studies to have a motivating impact on patient behavior. These studies show that an image of atherosclerosis can motivate behavioral change. Studies to date suggest a long-term, durable, motivational effect of atherosclerosis imaging. Several survey studies using either cardiac computed tomography for the detection of coronary calcium or carotid ultrasonography for the detection of intima-media thickness, or plaque have suggested that survey respondents among primarily referred populations report being motivated for healthy behavioral change with a common theme of increased perception of risk.

In multiple studies, the presence of coronary calcification was associated with an independent greater likelihood of statin and aspirin usage and more appropriate use of statins with studies reporting up to 6-year follow-up. These findings support the concept that the identification of coronary calcium in a screening population leads to shifts in clinical patient management reflected in the provision of preventive cardiovascular pharmacotherapies. Thus, the SHAPE Guidelines, utilizing imaging (CAC or IMT testing) to assess cardiovascular risk, will not only improve risk stratification, but should be associated with improved adherence to therapies that positively impact coronary artery disease outcomes (aspirin, medication use, diet, and exercise).

REFERENCES

1. Balkrishnan R, Rajagopalan R, Camacho FT, Huston SA, Murray FT, Anderson RT. Predictors of medication adherence and associated health care costs in an older population with type 2 diabetes mellitus: a longitudinal cohort study. Clin Ther 2003;25:2958–2971.
2. Abughosh SM, Kogut SJ, Andrade SE, Larrat P, Gurwitz JH. Persistence with lipid-lowering therapy: influence of the type of lipid-lowering agent and drug benefit plan option in elderly patients. J Manag Care Pharm 2004;10:404–411.
3. Blackburn DF, Dobson RT, Blackburn JL, Wilson TW. Cardiovascular morbidity associated with nonadherence to statin therapy. Pharmacotherapy 2005;25:1035–1043.
4. Jackevicius CA, Mamdani M, Tu JV. Adherence with statin therapy in elderly patients with and without acute coronary syndromes. J Am Med Assoc 2002;288:462–467.
5. Penning-van Beest FJA, Termorshuizen F, Goettsch WG, Klungel OH, Kastelein JJP, Herings RMC. Adherence to evidence-based statin guidelines reduces the risk of hospitalizations for acute myocardial infarction by 40%: a cohort study. Eur Heart J 2007;28:154–159.
6. Budoff MJ, Achenbach S, Blumenthal RS, Carr JJ, Goldin JG, Greenland P, Guerci AD, Lima JA, Rader DJ, Rubin GD, Shaw LJ, Wiegers SE. Assessment of coronary artery disease by cardiac computed tomography: a scientific statement from the American heart association committee on cardiovascular imaging and intervention, council on cardiovascular radiology and intervention, and committee on cardiac imaging, council on clinical cardiology. Circulation 2006;114:1761–1791.

7. Grundy SM, Cleeman JI, Merz CN, et al. Implications of recent clinical trials for the national cholesterol education program adult treatment panel III guidelines. J Am Coll Cardiol 2004;44:720–732.
8. Greenland P, Bonow RO, Brundage BH, et al. ACCF/AHA 2007 clinical expert consensus document on coronary artery calcium scoring by computed tomography in global cardiovascular risk assessment and in evaluation of patients with chest pain: a report of the American college of cardiology foundation clinical expert consensus task force (ACCF/AHA writing committee to update the 2000 expert consensus document on electron beam computed tomography) developed in collaboration with the society of atherosclerosis imaging and prevention and the society of cardiovascular computed tomography. J Am Coll Cardiol 2007;49:378–402.
9. Wong ND, Detrano RC. Does Coronary artery screening by electron beam computed tomography motivate potentially beneficial lifestyle behavior? Am J Cardiol 1996;78:1220–1223.
10. O'Malley PG, Feuerstein IM, Taylor AJ. Impact of Electron Beam Tomography, with or without case management, on motivation, behavioral change and cardiovascular risk profile. A randomized controlled trial. J Am Med Assoc 2003;289: 2215–2223.
11. Detrano R, Anderson M, Nelson J, et al. Effect of Scanner Type and Calcium Measure on the Re-Scan Variability of Calcium Quantity by Computed Tomography.
12. Kalia NK, Miller LG, Nasir K, Blumenthal RS, Agrawal N, Budoff MJ. Visualizing coronary calcium is associated with improvements in adherence to statin therapy. Atherosclerosis 2006;185:394–349.
13. Orakzai RH, Nasir K, Orakzai SH, Kalia N, Gopal A, Blumenthal RS, Budoff MJ. Increased Coronary artery calcium scores on electron beam computed tomography is associated with increased utilization of aspirin therapy. J Am Coll Cardiol 2008;51:A152.
14. Nasir K, McClelland R, Hoffmann U, Blumenthal RS, Greenland P, Kronmal R, Budoff MJ. Coronary artery calcification testing and adherence/initiation of cholesterol lowering medications. Circulation 2008 (submitted).
15. Taylor AJ, Bindeman J, Feuerstein I, Cao F, Brazaitis M, O'Malley PG. Coronary calcium independently predicts incident premature coronary heart disease over measured cardiovascular risk factors: mean three-year outcomes in the prospective army coronary calcium (PACC) project. J Am Coll Cardiol 2005;46:807–814.
16. Taylor A, Bindeman J, Le T, Bauer K, Byrd C, Feuerstein I, Lee JK, Grace KA, O'Malley PG. Community-Based provision of statin and aspirin after the detection of coronary artery calcium within a community-based screening cohort. J Am Coll Cardiol 2008;51:1337–1341.
17. Bovet P, Perret F, Cornuz J, et al. Improved smoking cessation in smokers given ultrasound photographs of their own atherosclerotic plaques. Prev Med 2002;34:215–220.
18. O'Malley PG. Atherosclerosis imaging of asymptomatic individuals: is the sales cart before the evidence horse? Arch Intern Med 2006;166:1065–1068.
19. Wyman RA, Gimelli G, McBride PE, Korcarz CE, Stein JH. Does detection of carotid plaque affect physician behavior or motivate patients? Am Heart J 2008: in press.
20. Corretti MC, Anderson TJ, Benjamin EJ, Celermajer D, Charbonneau F, Creager MA, Deanfield J, Drexler H, Gerhard-Herman M, Herrington D, Vallance P, Vita J, Vogel R; International Brachial Artery Reactivity Task Force. Guidelines for the ultrasound assessment of endothelial-dependent flow-mediated vasodilation of the brachial artery: a report of the International Brachial Artery Reactivity Task Force. J Am Coll Cardiol 2002 Jan 16;39(2):257–65

43 The SHAPE Guideline: Why Primary Care Physicians Should Embrace It

Robert A. Mendes

CONTENTS

ABSTRACT

The vast majority of patients who have traditional cardiovascular disease risk factors but lack overt evidence of atherosclerotic disease (i.e., "primary prevention" patients) are managed by primary care physicians. A relatively small percentage of these patients currently achieve their JNC-VII and/or NCEP ATP-III goals, a reflection of both patient-specific and physician-related barriers. Many patients have unrealistic expectations of what can be achieved through diet alone, lack an appreciation of the potential benefit of pharmaceuticals, and/or have an inappropriate fear of medication side effects, all of which contribute to resistance to medication initiation and poor long-term adherence. This perspective is not easily changed as primary care physicians have difficulty in persuasively communicating long-term cardiovascular risks and the benefit of intervention. Most primary care physicians do not use Framingham Risk Scores to stratify higher risk patients. As time constraints make the scoring system impractical to utilize consistently, it provides an incomplete assessment of risk, and the derived 10 year-risk of having an event is difficult to interpret meaningfully for patients. Furthermore, many primary care physicians perceive current guidelines as being too complicated and find "optional" goals confusing. Thus, a more efficient means of identifying high-risk patients, coupled with simplified guidelines containing succinct, clear recommendations for LDL-C target levels and therapeutic interventions, would likely improve the CVD prevention goal attainment rates in these at-risk patients. The SHAPE Guideline addresses many of the barriers primary care physicians face in striving to optimally manage their dyslipidemic patients. Positive screening tests will help physicians to identify those patients who need more aggressive treatment, and likewise help to

From: *Asymptomatic Atherosclerosis: Pathophysiology, Detection and Treatment*
Edited by: M. Naghavi (ed.), DOI 10.1007/978-1-60327-179-0_43

motivate at-risk patients to comply with their physician's treatment recommendations. The heightened risk awareness afforded by a positive screening test will thereby enhance patient compliance and clearly improve the treatment of this high-risk population.

Key words: Adherence; Compliance; Guidelines; NCEP ATP-III; Goal attainment; Barriers; Dyslipidemia; Framingham risk score

KEY POINTS

- Patients who have cardiovascular disease risk factors but lack overt evidence of atherosclerotic disease are typically managed by primary care physicians.
- A relatively low percent of these primary prevention patients achieve their JNC-VII and/or NCEP ATP-III goals, which reflects patient perspectives on medication utilization as well as physician inability to effectively communicate the risk of having a cardiovascular event and the potential benefit of a medical intervention versus the likelihood of experiencing an adverse effect from that medication.
- Many primary care physicians find current guidelines to be too complicated and/or too time consuming to fully integrate into their practice. A more efficient means of identifying high-risk patients, coupled with simplified guidelines containing succinct, clear recommendations for LDL-C target levels and therapeutic interventions, would likely improve the CVD prevention goal attainment rates in these at-risk patients.
- The SHAPE Guideline addresses many of the barriers primary care physicians face in striving to optimally manage their dyslipidemic patients. Positive screening tests will help physicians to easily identify those patients who need more aggressive treatment, and likewise help to motivate at-risk patients to comply with their physician's treatment recommendations, thereby enhancing patient compliance and improving the overall treatment of this high-risk population.

The vast majority of patients who have traditional cardiovascular disease risk factors (e.g., hypertension, dyslipidemia, tobacco use, etc.) but lack overt evidence of atherosclerotic disease are managed by primary care physicians. In the 1999–2000 NHANES survey only 22% of hypertensive patients had achieved their BP goal, while only 5% of dyslipidemic patients had achieved their LDL-C treatment goal [1]. The revised JNC-VII and NCEP ATP-III guidelines indicate that higher risk populations should be treated even more aggressively than previous versions advised. The fact that only a small percentage of these patients are currently reaching their JNC-VII and/or NCEP ATP-III goals reflect multifactorial barriers that primary care physicians face in striving to achieve them. Acceptance of the SHAPE Guideline by primary care physicians would address many of these barriers, thereby enhancing their ability to achieve these goals in a greater percentage of their patients.

PATIENT-RELATED BARRIERS TO NCEP ATP-III GOAL ATTAINMENT

Many patients have unrealistic expectations for dieting as a solution, lack an appreciation of the benefit of medication, and/or have an inappropriate fear of medication side effects, all of which contribute to resistance to medication initiation and poor long-term adherence. Predictors of poor adherence to medication include the treatment of an asymptomatic condition, patient's lack of insight into the illness being treated, and patient's lack of belief in the benefit of treatment [2]. These factors help to explain why 1-year adherence rates for statins in primary prevention are typically only 40% or less [3]. Furthermore, many older adults have multiple comorbidities. In 1999, 48% of Medicare beneficiaries aged 65 years or older had at least three chronic medical conditions and 21% had five or more [4]. These comorbid conditions necessitate complex treatment regimens involving multiple medications which adversely influence compliance with physician recommendations, with obvious implications for goal attainment. Failure to achieve goals in older patients with multiple comorbidities is easily understood. However, even in less complicated patients primary care physicians have difficulty persuasively communicating long-term cardiovascular risks and the benefit of intervention. While a 20% 10-year risk of having a cardiovascular event is alarming to physicians, it does not resonate with patients and the need for risk factor modification is not perceived as "urgent." Furthermore, recommending a trial of Therapeutic Lifestyle Changes ("TLC") before advising pharmaceutical intervention, as guidelines suggest, conveys a lack of urgency to patients. As a result, after failing to reach their target LDL-C level with an "appropriate" trial of TLC, many patients remain reluctant to initiating lipid-lowering medication.

PHYSICIAN-RELATED BARRIERS TO NCEP ATP-III GOAL ATTAINMENT

These patient barriers only partially explain the relatively poor rate of NCEP ATP-III and JNC-VII goal attainment. A study of 300 primary care physicians and 100 cardiologists evaluated their awareness and utilization of cardiovascular disease prevention guidelines and revealed that less than 60% of those familiar with these guidelines actually incorporate them into their practice [5]. This study also suggests that recommendations for CVD prevention are driven by risk level assessment. Patients identified as having intermediate or high cardiovascular risk were significantly more likely to receive recommendations for preventive interventions, including lifestyle changes, blood pressure control, lipid management, and aspirin therapy. Unfortunately, when these physician's perceptions of patients' risk levels were compared with the calculated ATP III Framingham Risk Scores, only about 50% of the intermediate-risk and 60% of the high-risk patients were correctly identified by either cardiologists or primary care physicians. Additionally, women were more likely than men to be assigned a lower-risk category despite having a similar calculated risk [5]. Consistent utilization of Framingham Risk Scores would likely help to identify a greater percentage of higher risk patients. However, most primary care physicians don't use Framingham Risk Scores to stratify higher risk patients, as time constraints make the scoring system impractical to utilize consistently, it provides an incomplete assessment of risk, and the derived 10-year risk of having an event is difficult to interpret meaningfully for patients. Furthermore, many primary care physicians perceive current guidelines as being too complicated and find "optional" goals confusing. Thus, a more efficient means of identifying high-risk patients, coupled with simplified guidelines containing succinct, clear recommendations for LDL-C target levels and therapeutic interventions would likely improve the CVD prevention goal attainment rates in these at-risk patients.

PRACTICAL CONSIDERATIONS OF THE SHAPE GUIDELINE

Given this perspective and the relatively small percentage of high-risk patients who are currently achieving their lipid goals, the SHAPE Guideline is timely and appropriate. It simplifies the process of identifying patients who need to be screened (e.g., all men > 45 years of age and women > 55 years of age except those clearly at very low risk, those older than 75 years of age, and those with established cardiovascular disease). Thus, the vast majority of adults managed by primary care physicians would qualify for a screening procedure. The noninvasive tests reflected in the SHAPE Guideline will likely have high patient acceptance, although the degree to which health insurance helps to defray the cost will directly influence patient compliance with these screening recommendations.

IMPLICATIONS OF THE SHAPE GUIDELINE ON NCEP GOAL ATTAINMENT

The SHAPE Guideline addresses many of the barriers primary care physicians face in striving to optimally manage their dyslipidemic patients. Positive screening tests will help physicians to identify those patients who need more aggressive treatment, and likewise help to motivate at-risk patients to comply with their physician's treatment recommendations. Perhaps more importantly, since many at-risk patients are reluctant to take a medication chronically for an asymptomatic condition like dyslipidemia, identifying the presence of previously undetected coronary and/or carotid atherosclerosis will likely provide a "teachable moment," creating an urgent desire for intervention in that particular patient, leading to enhanced compliance. Note that several studies have documented higher long-term statin and antihypertensive therapy adherence rates in secondary prevention populations [3,6]. Thus, if implemented, the SHAPE Guideline will clearly simplify the recognition of the "vulnerable patient" and in doing so will substantially change the physician-patient dialog. Instead of simply emphasizing the need to optimize management of cardiovascular disease risk factors in their patients, physicians can focus on the importance of preventing asymptomatic atherosclerosis from progressing into a heart attack or stroke. The heightened risk awareness afforded by a positive screening test will thereby enhance patient compliance and clearly improve the treatment of this high-risk population.

COST EFFECTIVENESS OF THE SHAPE GUIDELINE

Despite the obvious beneficial impact this approach would have on the number one cause of death in the U.S., some will likely view the SHAPE Guideline as controversial. Using noninvasive vascular tests to screen the vast majority of US adults may be perceived by some members of the medical community as being too aggressive, impractical, and/or expensive to support. A cost-effectiveness analysis reflecting the quality adjusted life years saved by the implementation of the SHAPE Guideline, as compared to current practice trends, will likely enhance its acceptance by primary care physicians and the medical community at large.

REFERENCES

1. Ford ES, Mokdad AH, Giles WH, Mensah GA. Serum Total Cholesterol Concentrations and Awareness, Treatment, and Control of Hypercholesterolemia Among US Adults: Findings From the National Health and Nutrition Examination Survey, 1999 to 2000. Circulation. 2003;107:2185–2189
2. Osterberg L, Blaschke T. Drug Therapy: Adherence to Medication. N Engl J Med 2005;353(5):487–497
3. Jackevicius CA, Mamdani M, Tu JV. Adherence with Statin Therapy in Elderly Patients with and without Acute Coronary Syndromes. JAMA. 2002;288:462–467
4. Anderson G, Horvath J. Chronic Conditions: Making the Case for Ongoing Care. Princeton, NJ: Robert Wood Johnson Foundation's Partnership for Solutions; 2002
5. Mosca L, Linfante A, Benjamin E, Berra K, Hayes S, Walsh B, Fabunmi R, Kwan J, Mills T, Simpson SL. National Study of Physician Awareness and Adherence to Cardiovascular Disease Prevention Guidelines. Circulation. 2005;111:499–510
6. Monane M, Bohn RL, Gurwitz JH, Glynn RJ, Levin R, Avorn J. The Effects of Initial Drug Choice and Comorbidity on Antihypertensive Therapy Compliance: Results From a Population-Based Study in the Elderly. Am J Hypertens. 1997;10:697–704

44 Should We Treat According to the SHAPE Guidelines?

Paolo Raggi and Stamatios Lerakis

CONTENTS

ABSTRACT

We were asked to address this simple question: should we treat according to the SHAPE (Naghavi Am J Cardiol 98:2H–15H, 2006) guidelines? It sounds like a simple and direct question and yet there are no direct answers. None that would satisfy every reader, at least. SHAPE sounds like a grandiose attempt at rephrasing priorities, and the approach to the diagnosis and therapy of cardiovascular disease; does it not? Or is it a first honest effort at differing from structured and aligned thinkers? The "*evidence seized medicine*" of the past several decades may have overlooked a lot of common sense, good indirect evidence and a lot of self evident truth that may need to be readdressed. Among the common things one may have forgotten, is the simple tenet that not all humans are born the same (from the genetic point of view, that is); not all diabetic patients have the same risk of coronary artery disease, not all 60-year old black men have the same degree of renal damage after 10 years of systolic hypertension, not everyone suffers the same degree of complications from various ailments or risk factors. So, it may be worth taking an "*outside of the box*" look while reviewing the SHAPE guidelines (Am J Cardiol 98:2H–15H, 2006), with an open mind toward alternative values inherent in the proposed approach. That is what we set out to do in this brief chapter.

Key words: Atherosclerosis; Atherosclerosis imaging; Carotid intima-media thickness; Coronary artery calcium; Risk factors

KEY POINTS

- Although the majority of patients who suffered a cardiovascular event have at least one risk factor, only a minority of individuals in the population with one risk factor will suffer a cardiovascular event.

From: *Asymptomatic Atherosclerosis: Pathophysiology, Detection and Treatment*
Edited by: M. Naghavi (ed.), DOI 10.1007/978-1-60327-179-0_44

- The majority of adults in the US population is classifiable as being at intermediate risk for cardiovascular events, hence, this is the segment of the population on whom preventive efforts should be concentrated to lower the cost of future care;
- Risk factors affect individuals of different race and sex, differently.
- Age carries a heavy weight in the currently utilized risk estimation tools. However, though atherosclerosis progresses with advancing age, there is substantial heterogeneity among adult individuals.
- An alternative approach could be to use the vascular age of an individual instead of his chronological age, based on the extent of coronary artery calcium or thickness of the carotid artery wall.
- Since subclinical atherosclerosis reflects the life-time impact of all known and unknown risk factors on the arterial wall, an approach that combines clinical and imaging information may substantially improve management of the individual patient.

WHAT IS THE EVIDENCE?

The publication of the SHAPE guidelines [1] was followed by an editorial by Diamond and Kaul [2] that left little room for doubt: imaging for atherosclerosis is expensive and does not save as many lives as an approach based on "*treatment for all*", independent of baseline risk. Interestingly, Dr. Kaul coauthored the SHAPE position statement [1] and proceeded to write a "cons" editorial about it [2] (this is a truly unusual conflict of interest!). Sadly, the argument proposed by Diamond and Kaul was based on some incorrect assumptions. The first and most noticeable is the assumed cost of a chest CT for calcium screening of $400. In our institution calcium screening is offered along with a lipid panel, fasting glucose and blood pressure check (to allow the calculation of a Framingham risk score) for the total cost of $150; at other academic institutions around the country the cost for a chest CT for calcium alone is priced at about $100, although a few private imaging centers still price it ~$400. If we redo the calculations performed by Diamond and Kaul, assuming a cost for a CT of $150, we assess a total cost of screening 50 million adult Americans at $7.5 billion, not $20 billion; a very sizeable saving compared to any other approach discussed in the editorial. Another dissonant piece of information often put forward by various experts, and suggested by the editorial as well, is the well-known tenet that the majority of patients suffering a cardiovascular event have at least one cardiovascular risk factor [3]. It would follow that all is needed is to find and treat risk factors and the risk (and attendant cost) is reduced. Unfortunately, the tenet gives erroneous information to the reader and listener; in fact, although the majority of patients with events have at least one risk factor (fact), only a minority of individuals in the population with one or two risk factors will suffer a cardiovascular event (fact!). The majority of adults in the US population is classifiable as being at intermediate risk for cardiovascular events in the intermediate to long-term [4]; although the absolute risk for events is greater in subjects at high-risk, intermediate risk patients make up for 40–45% of the population over the age of 20 [4] and the majority of events will therefore take place in this segment of society. Hence, this is the group on whom most efforts should be concentrated to discriminate those in greater need of preventive efforts from those with less of a need. The approach suggested by SHAPE is the most reasonable, at this time, to pursue the "venue of discovery". Indeed, the proportion of intermediate risk subjects is even larger than 40–45%, if one takes into consideration men above the age of 45 and women above age 55 as the SHAPE opinion leaders suggested doing. In this case, the intermediate risk group probably makes up 50–55% of the population and the burden of events is therefore proportionally higher than in the >20 year-old group. That is the group of subjects that the SHAPE writing group members would like us to screen with imaging for atherosclerosis, and the advice is sound and extremely logical. At the time of this writing (as discussed in other chapters of this book) there is a wealth of information proving that coronary artery calcium is an excellent marker of risk for future events, and the evidence is both epidemiological as well as prospective, randomized, involving different segments of the adult population and different races [5–10]. Evidence surrounding carotid intima-media thickness is strong and shows the value of this marker as independent of other risk factors for prediction of events [11]. A large epidemiological body of evidence that supports the utility of highly sensitive C-reactive protein (hCRP) as a marker of risk [12, 13] and a large clinical trial, in which patients were randomized to either a statin or placebo based on hCRP levels, was prematurely terminated, due to the benefit of active therapy [14].

Where is, then, the evidence that treating the population at large (the *blanket* approach proposed by Diamond and Kaul [2]) helps? Do initial cost savings translate into late costs? What are the risks inherent in treating the population at large? Are there costs to be considered inherent in the potential complications and side effects of medications?

Furthermore, where is the evidence that treating subjects "at risk" but without evidence of atherosclerosis helps in reducing risk? Indeed the best risk reduction obtainable with statin therapy is in the order of 30–35%? Should we not look past, therefore, the initial "cost" of screening proposed by SHAPE?

A DIFFERENT LOOK AT THINGS

The currently utilized risk estimation tools are heavily influenced by age as a surrogate marker of atherosclerosis burden [15, 16]. However, though atherosclerosis progresses with advancing age, there is substantial heterogeneity among adult individuals of the same age and a clear trend to underestimate risk in younger patients. That age alone should not be given excessive weight was demonstrated by two recent publications. Akosah et al. [17] addressed a very interesting question in a retrospective analysis of patients presenting to the emergency department with an acute coronary syndrome: according to the NCEP-III guidelines how many young men (<55 years old) and women (<65 years old) would have qualified for preventive interventions the day before the event? In Akosah's study, only 25% of patients would have met criteria for pharmacotherapy. The tendency for the guidelines to underestimate risk was even more pronounced in women, with only 18% of women qualifying for pharmacotherapy for primary prevention; 58% of these patients had LDL-C <130mg/dl and 40% had LDL-C <100mg/dl. A similar notion was addressed by Nasir et al. [18]. The investigators performed CT imaging for coronary artery calcium in 1,611 asymptomatic individuals (67% men, mean age: 53 ± 10 years) and divided the participants as low-risk (n=738, 46%), intermediate-risk (n=583, 36%), moderately high-risk (n=263, 16%), and high-risk (n=27, 2%) according to NCEP guidelines. Overall, 59 and 78% of participants with a calcium score ≥400 and ≥75th percentile were not identified as high risk and candidates for pharmacotherapy on the basis of NCEP categories. Furthermore, women and young individuals were less likely to be considered candidates for pharmacotherapy compared with men and older individuals in each calcium score category. Hence, both Akosah's [17] and Nasir's [18] study show that current guidelines underestimate cardiovascular risk in asymptomatic individuals, especially if young and female. For these individuals, assessment of plaque burden might provide incremental value to global risk assessment. Along these lines, it has been suggested that since plaque burden is an accurate estimate of risk, it could be substituted for age in risk calculations [19]. In essence, "vascular age" could be substituted for chronological age to improve risk assessment when using predictive scores such as the Framingham risk equations. The best way to apply this notion is to use normative ranges for a specific age, sex and race; such tables are available for coronary artery calcium scores as described by McLellan et al. [20]. In this light, the vessels of a 50 year old individual with an elevated calcium score resemble those of an average, older individual of the same sex and race [21], and this subject would receive a larger number of points for age in the calculation of his Framingham score. Indeed coronary calcium helps reclassify risk in all age groups and both sexes as shown recently in a population sample of 35,388 subjects submitted to calcium screening, and followed for several years for the occurrence of all-cause death [22]. Among women, 43% of the subjects were reclassified to either higher or lower categories of risk and the same was seen for 45% of men [22].

Similar to age, other conditions affect atherosclerosis development and its attendant consequences differently in different individuals. A prominent example of this is diabetes mellitus. Because patients with diabetes mellitus have a very high lifetime risk of developing cardiovascular disease, diabetes is considered a *cardiovascular disease equivalent*. Not surprisingly, several clinical studies have shown that glucose intolerance and insulin resistance are associated with increased prevalence of coronary calcium [23, 24]. In addition to the greater prevalence, the extent of coronary calcium is also greater in the diabetic population compared to a non-diabetic population [25]. Furthermore, there is no longer a gender advantage for women with diabetes over men; indeed, patients of both sexes show a similar disease burden when affected by diabetes mellitus, unlike subjects from the general population. The question is, therefore, whether atherosclerosis imaging may help to better discriminate risk among diabetic patients. Anand et al. [26], demonstrated an increasing incidence of inducible myocardial ischemia on stress myocardial perfusion imaging in diabetic patients with increasing amounts of coronary calcium. In that report, type-2 diabetic patients with a calcium score of 0, 11–100, 101–400, 401–1,000, and >1,000, had an incidence of myocardial ischemia of 0, 18, 23, 48, and 71%, respectively. During follow-up, morbidity and mortality increased proportional to the calcium score and ischemic burden, with extremely low event rates in patients with low burden of disease. In an observational registry, Raggi et al. [27] showed a higher rate of all-cause mortality in diabetic patients for any extent of coronary calcium compared with non-diabetic subjects ($P>0.001$); however, the 5-year mortality of diabetic patients with little or no calcium (approximately 30% of a cohort of 903 diabetic patients) was as low as that of non-diabetic subjects without coronary calcium (about 1% at the end of follow-up). Hence the question: are all diabetic patients really "a risk equivalent" or is there a difference between individuals that cannot be determined on the basis of risk factors alone?

What about race? Are all races responding to exposure to risk factors the same way? And what is the impact of atherosclerosis on outcome in different races? The proponents of the Framingham risk score would have us believe that the algorithm works as well in Caucasians as in African American individuals, but it may not be so. It has been conclusively shown by the *Multi Ethnic Study of Atherosclerosis* (MESA) investigators that there is a noticeable difference in extent of atherosclerosis accumulation between Caucasians, African Americans, Hispanic and Chinese subjects living in the US [28]. In a recent study, Santos et al. [29] compared the prevalence and extent of coronary calcium in three large population samples from Portugal, Brazil and the United States. North American Caucasian subjects had more coronary calcium than Caucasian subjects from Brazil and Portugal, despite the higher prevalence of risk factors in the latter two ethnic groups [29]. Interestingly, despite a substantial genetic similarity between Brazilian and Portuguese Caucasians, and the presence of more smokers among the latter, Brazilians had a greater extent of coronary calcium than Portuguese subjects. These findings mirrored the national mortality and morbidity statistics indicating a greater cardiovascular event rate in the North American, followed by the Brazilian and finally the Portuguese population. Thus, it would appear that risk factors *do not affect* different races and individuals from the same race on different continents the same way. And is the outcome different in subjects of different race but with subclinical atherosclerosis? Detrano et al. [9] recently reported that coronary calcium is a strong predictor of cardiovascular death, nonfatal myocardial infarction, angina and revascularization (total events = 162) in all 6722 MESA patients, independent of race, and that coronary calcium added incremental prognostic value to traditional risk factors for the prediction of events. However, whether atherosclerosis is more "damaging" in one race compared to another was not addressed in Detrano's paper [9]. This is what Nasir et al. did in a large observational study [10]. In 14,812 patients belonging to the same four races (Caucasian, African American, Hispanic and Chinese) considered in MESA, the investigators assessed the occurrence of all-cause death (505 deaths total) during a 10 year follow-up period. As demonstrated by Bild et al. [28], the prevalence of

CAC was highest in Whites, although Blacks and Hispanics had a greater clustering of risk factors for atherosclerosis. Surprisingly, despite a lower prevalence of calcium and lower scores compared to the other races, black patients had the highest mortality rates even after multivariable adjustment for clinical risk factors and baseline calcium scores ($p<0.0001$). Compared with Whites, the relative risk of death was 2.97 (CI:1.87–4.72) in Blacks, 1.58 (CI: 0.92–2.71) in Hispanics and 0.85 (CI: 0.47–1.54) in Chinese individuals. A 50 year old black patient with a CAC score >400 had an estimated loss of 7 years of life, as opposed to 2.5 years of life for a white patient with the same score. Here then is the demonstration, once again, that we were not all born the same (genetically, of course!). The question therefore recurs: why treat all with the same approach?

WHAT SHOULD WE DO NOW?

In the preceding paragraphs we discussed the evidence that supports the use of a different approach to diagnosis and prevention of cardiovascular disease; we are convinced that an approach that combines clinical and imaging information may substantially improve management of the individual patient. Subclinical atherosclerosis reflects the life-time impact on the arterial wall of all known and unknown risk factors for a particular patient. Thus, noninvasive measurements of plaque burden must provide a more accurate estimate of risk for events than the mere exposure to factors that may induce the disease. The strength of this statement is not only demonstrated by all evidence collected during many years of research on atherosclerosis imaging, but it is also hidden behind "*the power of nothing*" [30, 31]. In fact, nothing appears to be as safe as the absence of atherosclerosis, independent of underlying risk factors. Patients with diabetes, advanced renal failure, elderly, or smokers [27, 32–34] appear to have an extremely low risk of events in the short to intermediate term in the absence of subclinical atherosclerosis. Of course we are concerned with the cost of care and would not want to increase the national debt any further. Hence, we support firstly and above all the avoidance of risky behaviors that favor development of disease while we support the promotion of life styles that will help maintain long-term health. However, as seen all too often, a low risk-factor load may not be sufficient to guarantee freedom from atherosclerosis and its consequences. We are left with no choice but to *re-SHAPE* our approach to diagnosis and treatment of the most prevalent ailment in human kind.

REFERENCES

1. Naghavi M, Falk E, Hecht HS, et al. From vulnerable plaque to vulnerable patient – Part III: Executive summary of the Screening for Heart Attack Prevention and Education (SHAPE) Task Force report. Am J Cardiol 2006;98(2A):2H–15H
2. Diamond GA, Kaul S. The things to come of SHAPE: cost and effectiveness of cardiovascular prevention. Am J Cardiol 2007;99(7):1013–5.
3. Greenland P, Knoll MD, Stamler J, et al. Major risk factors as antecedents of fatal and nonfatal coronary heart disease events. JAMA 2003;290(7):891–7.
4. Greenland P, Smith SC, Jr., Grundy SM. Improving coronary heart disease risk assessment in asymptomatic people: role of traditional risk factors and noninvasive cardiovascular tests. Circulation 2001;104(15):1863–7.
5. Arad Y, Goodman KJ, Roth M, Newstein D, Guerci AD. Coronary calcification, coronary disease risk factors, C-reactive protein, and atherosclerotic cardiovascular disease events: the St. Francis Heart Study. J Am Coll Cardiol 2005;46(1):158–65
6. Kondos GT, Hoff JA, Sevrukov A, et al. Electron-beam tomography coronary artery calcium and cardiac events: a 37-month follow-up of 5635 initially asymptomatic low- to intermediate-risk adults. Circulation 2003;107(20):2571–6.
7. LaMonte MJ, FitzGerald SJ, Church TS, et al. Coronary artery calcium score and coronary heart disease events in a large cohort of asymptomatic men and women. Am J Epidemiol 2005;162(5):421–9.
8. Shaw LJ, Raggi P, Schisterman E, Berman DS, Callister TQ. Prognostic value of cardiac risk factors and coronary artery calcium screening for all-cause mortality. Radiology 2003;228(3):826–33.
9. Detrano R, Guerci AD, Carr JJ, et al. Coronary calcium as a predictor of coronary events in four racial or ethnic groups. N Engl J Med 2008;358(13):1336–45.

10. Nasir K, Shaw LJ, Liu ST, et al. Ethnic differences in the prognostic value of coronary artery calcification for all-cause mortality. J Am Coll Cardiol 2007;50(10):953–60.
11. Lorenz MW, Markus HS, Bots ML, Rosvall M, Sitzer M. Prediction of clinical cardiovascular events with carotid intima-media thickness: a systematic review and meta-analysis. Circulation 2007;115(4):459–67.
12. Ridker PM. Inflammatory biomarkers and risks of myocardial infarction, stroke, diabetes, and total mortality: implications for longevity. Nutr Rev 2007;65(12 Pt 2):S253–9.
13. Abi-Saleh B, Iskandar SB, Elgharib N, Cohen MV. C-reactive protein: the harbinger of cardiovascular diseases. South Med J 2008;101(5):525–33.
14. Ridker PM, Danielson E, Fonseca FA, Genest J, Gotto AM Jr, Kastelein JJ, Koenig W, Libby P, Lorenzatti AJ, MacFadyen JG, Nordestgaard BG, Shepherd J, Willerson JT, Glynn RJ; JUPITER Study Group. Rosuvastatin to prevent vascular events in men and women with elevated C-reactive protein. N Engl J Med. 2008 Nov 20;359(21):2195-207. Epub 2008 Nov 9.
15. Third Report of the National Cholesterol Education Program (NCEP) Expert panel on detection, evaluation, and treatment of high blood cholesterol in adults (Adult Treatment Panel III) final report. Circulation 2002;106(25):3143–421.
16. De Backer G, Ambrosioni E, Borch-Johnsen K, et al. European guidelines on cardiovascular disease prevention in clinical practice. Third Joint Task Force of European and other Societies on Cardiovascular Disease Prevention in Clinical Practice (constituted by representatives of eight societies and by invited experts). Atherosclerosis 2004;173(2):381–91
17. Akosah KO, Schaper A, Cogbill C, Schoenfeld P. Preventing myocardial infarction in the young adult in the first place: how do the National Cholesterol Education Panel III guidelines perform? J Am Coll Cardiol 2003;41(9):1475–9.
18. Nasir K, Michos ED, Blumenthal RS, Raggi P. Detection of high-risk young adults and women by coronary calcium and National Cholesterol Education Program Panel III guidelines. J Am Coll Cardiol 2005;46(10):1931–6.
19. Grundy SM. Coronary plaque as a replacement for age as a risk factor in global risk assessment. Am J Cardiol 2001;88(2A):8E–11.
20. McClelland RL, Chung H, Detrano R, Post W, Kronmal RA. Distribution of coronary artery calcium by race, gender, and age: results from the Multi-Ethnic Study of Atherosclerosis (MESA). Circulation 2006;113(1):30–7.
21. Sirineni GK, Raggi P, Shaw LJ, Stillman AE. Calculation of coronary age using calcium scores in multiple ethnicities. Int J Cardiovasc Imaging 2008;24(1):107–11.
22. Raggi P, Gongara MC, Gopal A, Callister TQ, Budoff MP, Shaw LJ. Coronary artery calcium to predict all-cause mortality in elderly men and women. J Am Coll Cardiol 2008;52:17–23.
23. Dabelea D, Kinney G, Snell-Bergeon JK, et al. Effect of type 1 diabetes on the gender difference in coronary artery calcification: a role for insulin resistance? The Coronary Artery Calcification in Type 1 Diabetes (CACTI) Study. Diabetes 2003;52(11):2833–9.
24. Meigs JB, Larson MG, D'Agostino RB, et al. Coronary artery calcification in type 2 diabetes and insulin resistance: the framingham offspring study. Diabetes Care 2002;25(8):1313–9.
25. Wong ND, Sciammarella MG, Polk D, et al. The metabolic syndrome, diabetes, and subclinical atherosclerosis assessed by coronary calcium. J Am Coll Cardiol 2003;41(9):1547–53.
26. Anand DV, Lim E, Hopkins D, et al. Risk stratification in uncomplicated type 2 diabetes: prospective evaluation of the combined use of coronary artery calcium imaging and selective myocardial perfusion scintigraphy. Eur Heart J 2006;27(6):713–21.
27. Raggi P, Shaw LJ, Berman DS, Callister TQ. Prognostic value of coronary artery calcium screening in subjects with and without diabetes. J Am Coll Cardiol 2004;43(9):1663–9.
28. Bild DE, Detrano R, Peterson D, et al. Ethnic differences in coronary calcification: the Multi-Ethnic Study of Atherosclerosis (MESA). Circulation 2005;111(10):1313–20.
29. Santos RD, Nasir K, Rumberger JA, et al. Difference in atherosclerosis burden in different nations and continents assessed by coronary artery calcium. Atherosclerosis 2006;187(2):378–84.
30. Oudkerk M, Stillman AE, Halliburton SS, et al. Coronary artery calcium screening: current status and recommendations from the European Society of Cardiac Radiology and North American Society for Cardiovascular Imaging. Int J Cardiovasc Imaging 2008;24(6):645–71.
31. Taylor AJ, Raggi J, Raggi P. The power of nothing: the zero calcium score. J Cardiovasc Comp Tomogr 2007;1:160–1.
32. Block GA, Raggi P, Bellasi A, Kooienga L, Spiegel DM. Mortality effect of coronary calcification and phosphate binder choice in incident hemodialysis patients. Kidney Int 2007:71:438–41.
33. Shaw LJ, Raggi P, Callister TQ, Berman DS. Prognostic value of coronary artery calcium screening in asymptomatic smokers and non-smokers. Eur Heart J 2006;27(8):968–75.
34. Vliegenthart R, Oudkerk M, Hofman A, et al. Coronary calcification improves cardiovascular risk prediction in the elderly. Circulation 2005;112(4):572–7.

45 Duty-Bound: Rational Foundations of Clinical Strategies for Prevention of Cardiovascular Events

George A. Diamond and Sanjay Kaul

CONTENTS

Abstract

Cardiovascular screening involves numerous philosophic, epidemiologic, and economic assumptions that often go unstated. In this study, we discuss several of these assumptions and illustrate their impact on the accuracy and practicality of screening. We thereby conclude that these assumptions and their consequences should be made explicit by advocates of particular operative strategies.

Key Words: Cardiovascular screening; Cardiovascular prevention; Cost effectiveness; Decision analysis; Risk stratification

KEY POINTS

- The utility of clinical prevention strategies depends on a variety of assumptions that are often unstated and unexamined.
- Violation of these assumptions can have material clinical and epidemiological consequences.

From: *Asymptomatic Atherosclerosis: Pathophysiology, Detection and Treatment*
Edited by: M. Naghavi (ed.), DOI 10.1007/978-1-60327-179-0_45

- The influence of these assumptions on cost and effectiveness should be understood before any clinical prevention strategy is implemented.

DUTY, *n*. That which sternly impels us in the direction of profit, along the line of desire.

Ambrose Bierce

Clinical prevention strategies are founded on a variety of subtle philosophical assumptions. For example, much of our medical knowledge derives from the statistical analysis of groups, while medical care is directed largely at individuals. Is what is good for the group good for each *member* of the group? Obviously not. National vaccination policy clearly saves lives [1], but every so often someone dies as a consequence [2]. How then do we decide if this (or any other) clinical strategy is *good*?

DEONTOLOGY

One answer to this question is based on the "deontological principle" of moral law (from the Greek root, *dein*, meaning *duty*). According to its most influential proponent, Immanuel Kant, what makes an act good is not the outcome (which is often a matter of chance), but one's sense of obligation to act out of respect for an underlying moral principle – his famed "categorical imperative." [3] This duty-bound standard is expressly presaged in the Hippocratic Oath, by which the physician vows to act

according to my ability and my judgment... only for the good of my patients, keeping myself far from all intentional ill-doing.

In other words, one's actions are good – regardless of their consequences – if their *intentions* are honorable. Kant's deontology thereby serves as the putative ethical justification for most individual clinical decisions.

UTILITARIANISM

An alternative answer to our question is based on the "utilitarian principle" first enunciated in 1729 by Francis Hutcheson [4], and later refined by Jeremy Bentham [5] and John Stuart Mill: [6]

In comparing .... actions,...judge thus; that in equal degrees of happiness...the virtue is in proportion to the number of persons to whom the happiness shall extend;... and in equal numbers, the virtue is as the quantity of the happiness...so that, that action is best, which procures the greatest happiness for the greatest numbers... [4]

Here, the focus is on the *outcomes* and not the intentions. According to this principle, one's actions are good if the positive consequences outweigh the negative consequences. The utilitarian perspective is commonly applied to strategic decisions regarding health care policy. The current emphasis on clinical outcomes research is a clear reflection of the influence of utilitarianism on modern medical practice.

Unfortunately, the philosophy of utilitarianism is logically inconsistent, because its guiding principle – *the greatest happiness for the greatest numbers* – requires us to maximize two variables simultaneously (a mathematical impossibility). This inconsistency causes some troubling dilemmas with direct relevance to medical decision making.

Suppose, for example, that two mutually exclusive management strategies are available for some disease. If you prescribe Strategy 1, 90% of patients will benefit by an average of 20%, and the remaining 10% will be unaffected. If you prescribe Strategy 2, 60% of patients will benefit by an average of 30%, and the remaining 40% will be unaffected. The axioms of decision theory define the *expected value* of each strategy as the summed product of the individual probabilities and outcomes:

Expected Value of Strategy $1 = 0.9 \times 0.2 + 0.1 \times 0 = 0.18$

Expected Value of Strategy $2 = 0.6 \times 0.3 + 0.4 \times 0 = 0.18$

According to this analysis, the two strategies are equivalent. Based on the Hutcheson–Bentham–Mill utilitarian principle, however, Strategy 2 should be preferred to Strategy 1 because it provides the "greatest happiness" (30% versus 20%), while Strategy 1 should be preferred to Strategy 2 because it serves the "greatest numbers" (90% versus 60%)!

One can avoid being crushed between these opposing Mill-stones only by recognizing that the ultimate choice actually depends on one's intentions [7–9]. For example, a health care *planner* might opt for the strategy that produces the greatest *average* benefit (without regard for the number of individuals who benefit), while a health care *provider* might opt for the strategy that benefits the greatest *number* of individuals (without regard for the magnitude of benefit). Accordingly, an epidemiological perspective emphasizes the average benefit in a group of individuals, while a clinical perspective emphasizes the likelihood that an individual member of the group will derive benefit. In this way, utilitarianism can be molded to accommodate either the individual or the group by placing the outcomes in a particular intentional context.

DIVERSIFICATION

Asch believes that the duty-bound, deontological perspective serves to explain – and even justify – much of the current variability in clinical practice [10]. Consequently, efforts to reduce this variability (through practice guidelines, for example) might do more harm than good. He argues instead that we should be encouraging "diversification" in health care (the application of a common strategy to a diversity of individuals, or the application of a diversity of strategies to a common group on a case-by-case basis) rather than trying to eliminate it.

The conjecture that diversification is good has major implications for the quality and cost of health care (Fig. 1). If it's true, current disease management efforts are inadvertently undermining the quality of care by impeding independent decision making. If it's false, it unwittingly provides a specious

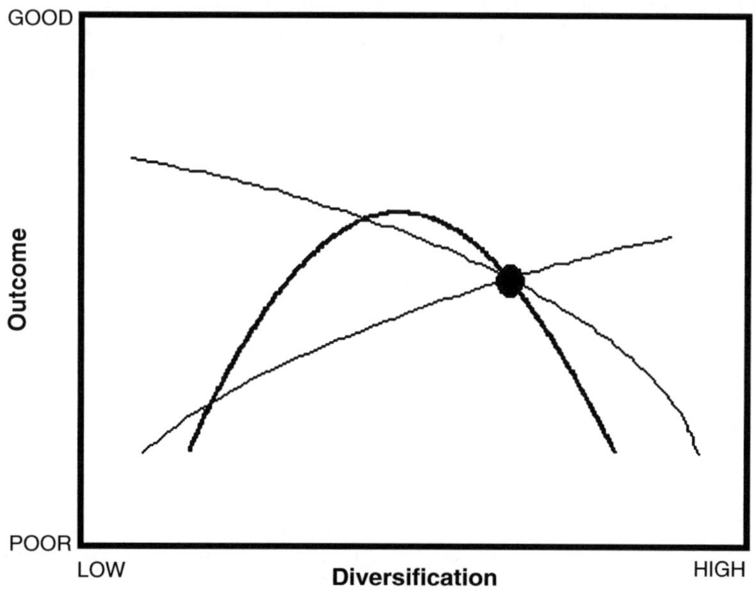

Fig. 1. Relationship between outcome and diversification. Three possibilities are illustrated, each of which passes through a common point (•) representing the status quo. Deontological fee-for-service advocates assume that outcomes improve when physicians are free to make choices on a case-by-case basis (thereby increasing diversity). Utilitarian managed care advocates assume that outcomes improve when physicians are limited to a few "optimal" choices (thereby decreasing diversity). In contrast, the parabolic curve implies that better outcomes might result from some combination of these two extremes (thereby causing a nonlinear change in diversity).

justification for bad decisions, "... in the direction of profit along the line of desire." This conjecture therefore deserves a thorough and thoughtful analysis. We hope to stimulate the conduct of that analysis by raising a few issues with relevance to the underlying philosophic principles discussed earlier.

INDIVIDUAL VERSUS GROUP OUTCOMES

It goes without saying that physicians *ought* to care about individual outcomes rather than group outcomes. Care as we might, however, Kantian deontology altogether rejects the relevance of outcomes (whether of the group or of the individual) to moral judgments. It is *never* the consequent outcomes of an action that determine its moral worth, but *always* the intentions and principles by which we are obliged to act. On the other hand, although these outcomes are indeed central to the utilitarian perspective, it is obvious that they cannot be known beforehand. Instead, only the probability distribution of the aggregate outcome – not the individual outcomes themselves – can be known at the time the decision is made. We can care about the individual in principle, but we can only deal with the aggregate in practice. Moreover, whenever individual physicians and patients must *compete* for limited resources, the choice ceases to be a problem in utility theory and becomes instead a problem in game theory [11].

COST-EFFECTIVENESS

Conflicts can indeed arise as a consequence of the individual and group perspectives. Thus, when decision makers were offered a choice between two hypothetical test strategies with equivalent expected value, they often preferred using the less costly Test 1 in the whole population (at a total cost of \$200,000 versus \$400,000), rather than the more effective Test 2 (with the potential of saving 2,200 versus 1,000 lives) in a portion of that population [12]. The authors' explanation for this finding focused on the perceived *fairness* of a general strategy to reduce group risk over that of a targeted strategy to minimize individual risk.

However, the more costly and more effective Test 2 is also more cost-effective (\$182 versus \$200 per life saved). In the real world, therefore, any rational decision maker should view the strategy employing this test to be the optimal choice (whether from the perspective of the group or the individual) and should find a way to cut the budget elsewhere to pay for it. In the same way, we take less expensive vacations, so our children can go to college.

As a result of the unrealistic requirement to spend exactly \$200,000 on one or the other of these tests, selective use of Test 2 in half the population becomes no more costly than uniform use of Test 1 in the entire population, but nonetheless remains both more effective (1,100 versus 1,000 lives saved) and more cost-effective (the same \$182 versus \$200 per life saved). In the absence of any conflict between effectiveness and cost-effectiveness, therefore, one's preference hinges instead on *the perceived fairness of rationing in the face of an unfair constraint*. It's as if we were asked to choose only one of our two children for college so we could continue taking those expensive vacations. No wonder the decision makers in this study were evenly split!

The following modifications introduce the requisite conflict. Assume Test A costs \$200,000 and saves 200 lives (\$1,000 per life saved) versus Test B which costs \$50,000 and saves 100 lives (\$500 per life saved). Here, the effectiveness of Test A is twice as great as Test B, but the cost-effectiveness of Test B is twice as great as Test A. A rational choice now depends on the ethical value assigned to the concepts of "cost," "effectiveness," and "cost-effectiveness." If you value "effectiveness" most highly, then you should choose Test A, and if you value "cost-effectiveness" or "cost" most highly, then you should choose Test B. Alternatively, you could opt for a rationing strategy that randomly selects one person in four for Test A. This too costs \$50,000, but saves only 50 lives at a cost-effectiveness of

$1,000 per life (half as good as Test B). In each case, the subjective perception of fairness is no longer an issue because it is now subsumed within one's prioritization of value.

RISK STRATIFICATION

But we could do even better. Suppose, for example, older males are at the highest risk of death from this disease (by a ratio, say, of 2.5:1 compared to the general population). We can thereby *nonrandomly* stratify the population by employing the more effective Test A in only these older males (approximately one person in four). Compared to random selection, this strategy also costs $50,000, but it saves 125 lives instead of 50 at a cost-effectiveness of $400 per life saved instead of $1,000. Cost is the same, while effectiveness and cost-effectiveness are improved 250%. Such nonrandom selection is the basis for a variety of *risk stratification* strategies [13, 14]. According to these strategies, expensive or risky technology is best targeted to individuals with the highest levels of risk.

Consider the following scenario: Socrates undergoes a routine medical evaluation, in the course of which an LDL cholesterol and high sensitivity C-reactive protein are observed to be elevated. He subsequently undergoes exercise-redistribution myocardial perfusion scintigraphy, which reveals reversible regional hypoperfusion. What, he asks, is his risk for a cardiovascular event, and – more importantly – *what should be done to reduce that risk*?

It is axiomatic in the physical sciences that a complete description of any deterministic phenomenon requires knowledge of the values of the relevant variables and their rates of change over time. So too in clinical practice, where rational therapeutic decisions depend jointly on one's assessment of the current level of risk, its concurrent rate of change, and the ability to reduce that rate of change. Conventional risk stratification schemas nevertheless refer only to the first of this triad.

As appealing as it may sound, the logic behind the concept of "risk stratification" does not stand up to scrutiny. Consider the following argument:

> Any individual at risk will receive benefit from treatment.
> Socrates is at risk.
> Therefore, Socrates will receive benefit from treatment.

Risk stratification is founded on a subtle variation of this otherwise valid argument – one that fallaciously conflates "risk" and "benefit":

> Any group at average risk will receive an average benefit from treatment.
> Socrates is at more than average risk.
> Therefore, Socrates will receive more than average benefit from treatment.

It is but a short step down a slippery socioeconomic slope:

> The more benefit one will receive, the more one should be treated.
> Socrates will receive more benefit than Plato.
> Therefore, Socrates should be treated more than Plato.

> Treating only Socrates will cost less than treating both Socrates and Plato
> Cost should be lessened.
> Therefore, only Socrates should be treated.

As a consequence of this ill-conceived chain of arguments, we should similarly treat only the sickest patients, school only the most ignorant students, and install brakes on only the fastest cars. Clearly, however, *benefit* always trumps *risk*. *All* cars need brakes – not just the fastest. Rational treatment decisions should thereby be based not on a narrow assessment of risk, but on a wider appreciation of clinical benefit [15]. That's the focus of Socrates questions.

This utilitarian emphasis on the individual patient heralds a major shift in ethical dynamics. Until recently, the patient has been accorded a rather remote role in the health care process – one insider going so far as to claim that, "Passengers who insist on flying the airplane are called hijackers!" [16] In our view, patients need not actually fly the health care airplane, but they must have something to say about its cost, construction, course, and destination if we expect them to buy a ticket and board the flight.

ALTERNATIVE STRATEGIC STANDARDS

In this context, "cost-effectiveness" is an attractive criterion upon which to base the practicality of large-scale screening strategies such as that proposed by the SHAPE Task Force. However, the putative standards for its determination are inherently arbitrary, and different standards can lead to different conclusions.

Imagine that a particular disease is associated with a mortality of 12% per year and that Treatment A is known to reduce that mortality to 9% per year at a cost of $2,100 per patient. Imagine further that an alternative Treatment B is available at a cost of $4,200 per patient. Investigators wish to determine the effectiveness and cost-effectiveness of Treatment B versus Treatment A in a head-to-head randomized clinical trial.

In order to calculate the sample size required for this trial, the investigators assume the "minimal clinically important difference" in mortality between A and B to be 25% (a baseline mortality of 9% with A versus 6.75% with B). Using this 25% threshold, a conventional sample size determination (α=0.05 and β=0.2) requires the enrolment of 2,337 subjects in each treatment group over the one-year period of follow-up. The subsequent trial results are summarized in the following 2×2 table:

	Died	Lived
A	210	2,127
B	158	2,179

These results correspond almost exactly with the assumptions used in the sample size determination (a mortality of 9.0±0.6% for A versus 6.8±0.5% for B; p=0.005 using a chi-square test). The observed risk reduction is 25%, with an odds ratio of 0.74 in favor of B (95% confidence interval: 0.59–0.91). On the basis of these data, the investigators conclude that B is superior to A, and that the difference is clinically important with respect to the prespecified 25% threshold.

Cost per life saved. To determine the cost-effectiveness of B relative to A, the investigators compute the *cost per life saved* for each treatment (the *monetary cost* of the treatment times the *number needed to treat* in order to save one life, the reciprocal of the absolute risk reduction). Accordingly, cost-effectiveness of A will equal cost-effectiveness of B under the following condition:

$$\frac{c_A}{m_0 - m_A} = \frac{c_B}{m_0 - m_B}$$

where c_A and c_B are the monetary costs for A and B, and m_0, m_A and m_B are the annual mortalities for nontreatment, and the respective active treatments. If we rearrange this equation and solve for m_B:

$$m_B = \frac{c_A m_0 - c_B \times (m_0 - m_A)}{c_A}$$

Since $m_0=0.12$, $m_A=0.09$, $c_A=\$2{,}100$ and $c_B=\$4{,}200$, then:

$$m_B = \frac{2100 \times 0.12 - 4200 \times (0.12 - 0.09)}{2100} = 0.06$$

This 6% mortality is equivalent to a relative risk reduction of $100\times(1-m_B/m_A)$ or 33.3%. Treatment B is therefore cost-effective relative to Treatment A if the observed risk reduction exceeds this threshold. Because the observed risk reduction was only 25% (and the trial was well powered to detect differences even larger than this), the investigators conclude that Treatment B is not cost-effective. In support of this conclusion, a Bayesian analysis of the data using an uninformative prior [17] shows only a 13% probability that the observed risk reduction exceeds the 33.3% cost-effectiveness threshold.

Cost per year of life saved. Despite the apparent rigor of this analysis, however, it's not the only way to determine cost-effectiveness. Imagine the investigators had chosen to define cost-effectiveness, not in terms of *cost per life saved*, but in terms of *cost per year of life saved*. Instead of calculating the absolute risk reductions employed earlier, they calculate *years of life* as the reciprocal of the individual annual mortalities [18] and determine the *years of life saved* as the arithmetic difference between treated and untreated years of life. Cost-effectiveness is now equal to the treatment's monetary cost divided by the years of life saved (*cost per year of life saved*). Cost-effectiveness of A now equals cost-effectiveness of B under the following (revised) condition:

$$\frac{c_A}{\dfrac{1}{m_A} - \dfrac{1}{m_0}} = \frac{c_B}{\dfrac{1}{m_B} - \dfrac{1}{m_0}}$$

If we rearrange this new equation and solve for m_B:

$$m_B = \frac{c_A m_0 m_A}{c_A m_A + c_B (m_0 - m_A)}$$

As before, $m_0=0.12$ and $m_A=0.09$ and $c_A=\$2{,}100$ and $c_B=\$4{,}200$. Thus:

$$m_B = \frac{2100 \times 0.12 \times 0.09}{2100 \times 0.09 + 4200 \times (0.12 - 0.09)} = 0.072$$

This 7.2% mortality is equivalent to a risk reduction threshold of $100\times(1-m_B/m_A)$ or 20% (versus the earlier 33.3% threshold), and because the observed 25% risk reduction exceeds this new lower threshold, the investigators now conclude that Treatment B is indeed cost-effective. According to Bayesian analysis (again using an uninformative prior), there is a 74% probability that the observed risk reduction exceeds the new 20% cost-effectiveness threshold.

Thus, a seemingly inconsequential difference in the operative standard of cost-effectiveness (*cost per life saved* versus *cost per year of life saved*) causes contradictory conclusions regarding the cost-effectiveness of Treatment B – and because these standards are arbitrary, so too are the associated risk reduction thresholds (33.3% versus 20%). Consequently, these arbitrary criteria should be made explicit, and sensitivity analyses using alternative criteria should be conducted routinely to enhance the credibility of the dependent judgments. This proviso is all the more important when estimates of life expectancy are quality adjusted, because such adjustments are inherently subjective in nature.

IMPLICATIONS AND CONCLUSIONS

Cost-effectiveness analysis is widely viewed as a rational way to balance competing clinical and economic priorities that arise as a consequence of the inevitable disconnect between an individual's wants and the society's willingness to pay for those wants. Advocates of population screening often employ such analyses as justification of their proposals.

At its core, cost-effectiveness analysis is a simple utilitarian moral calculus that quantifies the value of any action as the ratio of the observable bad qualities to the observable good qualities. In the typical health care application, the amount of "bad" is usually quantified in terms of monetary cost and the amount of "good" is quantified in terms of the clinical benefit associated with the saving of lives, life-years, or quality-adjusted life-years.

The conventional threshold of cost-effectiveness is most often taken to be \$50,000 per quality-adjusted life-year. The justification for this singular boundary dates back to a 1980 report on Medicare coverage for treatment of end-stage renal disease (ESRD), which projected the number of such cases would stabilize at around 90,000 patients in 1995 at an inflation-adjusted cost of \$4.5 billion [19]. This translates to a ratio of \$50,000 per life-year (unadjusted for quality).

Although medical economists often say they really don't believe there is anything special about this naïve threshold, they certainly *act* as if they do since they have employed it in more than 250 studies indexed by PubMed. In any event, the \$50,000 threshold is clearly a product of circular reasoning. The procedures that became standards of practice long before we began thinking seriously about their costs were later shown to have cost-effectiveness ratios in the range of \$50,000 or less. Therefore, \$50,000 came to be taken as the putative standard for cost-effectiveness. The reasoning goes something like this:

Renal dialysis is cost-effective.
Renal dialysis costs \$50,000.
Therefore \$50,000 is cost-effective.

While this argument is technically valid – the conclusion following from its antecedents – the premise that renal dialysis is cost-effective is itself assumed, and the entire argument therefore begs the question – assuming just that which is to be proven.

It's no wonder then that Medicare does not consider cost-effectiveness as a criterion in the determination of reimbursement. In so doing, it is acting in full compliance with operative federal law – specifically, with Executive Order 12866 enacted by President Bill Clinton on September 30, 1993: [20]

> *In deciding whether and how to regulate, (federal) agencies should assess all costs and benefits of available regulatory alternatives, including the alternative of not regulating. Costs and benefits shall be understood to include both quantifiable measures (to the fullest extent that these can be usefully estimated) and qualitative measures of costs and benefits that are difficult to quantify, but nevertheless essential to consider. Further, in choosing among alternative regulatory approaches, agencies should select those approaches that maximize net benefits...*

The only reference to cost-effectiveness in this document refers, not to the decision to regulate, but to the design of the regulation once such a decision is made:

> *When an agency determines that a regulation is the best available method of achieving the regulatory objective, it shall design its regulations in the most cost-effective manner to achieve the regulatory objective (so) that the benefits of the intended regulation justify its costs.*

Rather than advising regulators, economists, and insurers to incorporate specific cost-effectiveness criteria into their policy decisions, we propose directly empowering the end users – physicians and patients. Accordingly, we posit three questions based on accepted principles of consumer protection that better address the justification of any proposed health care strategy – questions that any socially responsible health care advocate should be expected to answer:

1. *How many people will it help?* What is the additional number of (quality-adjusted) life-years saved, or events prevented in the total population under consideration? The larger that number, the better the strategy.
2. *How much will it cost?* What is the total additional cost of the proposal? In purchasing a new car, we want to know the actual cost of our purchase, not the cost per month or the cost per mile that the salesman tries to promote to us in a veiled attempt to hide the actual cost from us. The lower the cost, the better the strategy.
3. *How do we plan to pay for it* given competing needs and existing budgetary constraints? We cannot afford blanket coverage for all the "cost-effective" care we might like, and trimming the wasteful "cost-ineffective" care will never make up the difference.

AN EXEMPLARY CARDIOVASCULAR PREVENTION STRATEGY

Let's apply this consumer protection approach to cardiovascular prevention. In our example, we compare an unconditional treatment strategy (treat everyone), against a conditional test-treatment strategy (screen everyone with a test, and treat only those with an abnormal response). Let's assume that the "treatment" is a preventive drug such as a statin, at a cost of about $2 per day ($720 per year), and the "test" identifies an at-risk population at a one-time cost of $100. In the absence of testing or treatment, we expect about 500,000 atherosclerotic events per year in the target adult population of 50 million – an event rate of 1%.

If we treat every one of these adults, we can expect to reduce these events by about 30% based upon available randomized clinical trials. We will thereby prevent 150,000 events at a total cost of $36 billion annually ($720 per patient per year times 50 million patients). The alternative strategy would have us test all 50 million individuals at $100 per patient. Based on Pareto's 80/20 rule [21], we can expect our test to identify 20% of the population (10 million patients) who will suffer 80% of the events (400,000 events) – an event rate of 4%. If we now treat only this higher risk population we will prevent 120,000 events at a total cost of $12.2 billion ($5 billion for testing plus $7.2 billion for treatment). The unconditional treatment strategy therefore costs an additional $23.8 billion, but prevents 30,000 more events. Assuming each event represents a loss of 12.9 life-years [22], the marginal cost-effectiveness of the unconditional treatment strategy is $61,500 per life-year ($23.8 billion divided by 30,000 events divided by 12.9 life-years per event). The more effective strategy (unconditional treatment) is therefore not cost-effective using the conventional $50,000 threshold.

Of course, different parameters would materially change this conclusion. If the cost of treatment could be reduced to $610, for example, the cost-effectiveness ratio for the unconditional strategy would fall below $50,000. In this context, several generic statins are available from Wal-Mart at only $48 ($4 per month). Alternatively, if the test were interpreted using a more discriminatory diagnostic criterion (capable of identifying 10% of the population experiencing 70% of the events, for example), the cost-effectiveness ratio for the unconditional strategy would again fall below $50,000.

But is that really the point? Whatever the costs (and resultant cost-effectiveness ratios), in the end, the unconditional treatment strategy always prevents more events. Testing might save money, but it can't save lives – only treatment saves lives. We'll leave it to the advocates of the alternative testing strategy to justify this tradeoff between cost and benefit, and tell those who might otherwise have been saved that it just wasn't worth the added expense – that it was, dare we say, more cost-effective to let them go.

In the final analysis, the key issues involved in cost-effectiveness decisions are matters of politics, not of science. A proper accounting of marginal costs and benefits – not their ratio – is the more sensible starting point for strategic decisions. We can encourage this new health care ethic through policies that serve to unify the deontological and utilitarian perspectives. To be more specific, (1) we can accredit a suitable categorical imperative, to the effect that the aim of health care is the provision of clinical benefit; (2) we can prioritize alternative strategic options with respect to this deontological maxim using utilitarian models that formally maximize expected clinical benefit (in terms of quality-adjusted survival, for example); and (3) we can empower the most worthy of these options through enlightened evidence-based financial incentives [23].

It's not enough to do our duty; one must do it in the right way!

REFERENCES

1. Carrat F, Valleron AJ. Influenza mortality among the elderly in France, 1980–90: how many deaths may have been avoided through vaccination? J Epidemiol Community Health 1995;49:419–25.
2. Braun MM, Ellenberg SS. Descriptive epidemiology of adverse events after immunization: reports to the Vaccine Adverse Event Reporting System (VAERS), 1991-1994. J Pediatr 1997;131:529–35.
3. Kant, I. *The Critique of Practical Reason* (original publication, 1788). In: *Great Books of the Western World.* Chicago: University of Chicago Press, 1952;42:291–364.
4. Hutcheson F. *An Inquiry into the Origin of our Ideas of Beauty and Virtue; in Two Treatises. I. Concerning Beauty, Order, Harmony, Design. II. Concerning Moral Good and Evil*, 3rd edn. London: J and J Knapton, J Darby, A Bettesworth, F Fayram, J Pemberton, J Osborn, T Longman, C Rivington, F Clay, J Batley, and A Ward, 1729;179–80.
5. Bentham J. *An Introduction to the Principles of Morals and Legislation* (reprint of "A New Edition, corrected by the author," 1823; original publication, 1789). Oxford: Clarendon Press, 1907;31.
6. Mill JS. *Utilitarianism* (original publication, 1863). In: *Great Books of the Western World.* Chicago: University of Chicago Press, 1952;43:445–76.
7. Redelmeier DA, Tversky A. Discrepancy between medical decisions for individual patients and for groups. N Engl J Med 1990;322:1162–64.
8. Krakauer H, Bailey RC. Epidemiological oversight of the medical care provided to Medicare beneficiaries. Stat Med 1991;10:521–40.
9. Diamond GA, Denton TA. Alternative perspectives on the biased foundations of medical technology assessment. Ann Intern Med 1993;118:455–64.
10. Asch DA. From boardroom to bedside: bioethical implications of policy research for clinical practice. J Investig Med 1999;47:273–77.
11. von Neumann J, Morgenstern O. *Theory of Games and Economic Behavior*, 3rd edn. Princeton: Princeton University Press, 1953;504–55.
12. Ubel PA, DeKay ML, Baron J, Asch DA. Cost-effectiveness analysis in a setting of budget constraints. Is it equitable? N Engl J Med 1996;334:1174–77.
13. Pollock SG, Abbott RD, Boucher CA, Beller GA, Kaul S. Independent and incremental prognostic value of tests performed in an hierarchical order to evaluate patients with suspected coronary artery disease: validation of models based on these tests. Circulation 1992;85:237–48.
14. Hachamovitch R, Berman DS, Kiat H, Bairey-Merz N, Cohen I, Cabico JA, Friedman JD, Germano G, Van Train KF, Diamond GA. Incremental prognostic value, risk stratification, and cost-effectiveness of rest/exercise Tl-201/Tc-99m sestamibi SPECT in women and men. Circulation 1996;93:905–14.
15. Diamond GA. Post-infarction risk stratification. Is preventive war winnable? JAMA 1993;269:2418–19.
16. Starr P. *The Social Transformation of American Medicine*. New York: Basic Books, 1982:379–419.
17. Diamond GA, Kaul S. Prior convictions: Bayesian approaches to the analysis and interpretation of clinical megatrials. J Am Coll Cardiol 2004;43:1929–39.
18. Beck J, Kassirer J, Pauker S. A convenient approximation of life expectancy (the "DEALE"). I. Validation of the method. Am J Med 1982;73:883–89.
19. Rettig RA. Implementing the End-Stage Renal Disease Program of Medicare. R-2505-HCFA/HEW, September 1980.
20. Clinton, Bill. Executive Order 12866. Regulatory planning and review. Federal Register September 30, 1993;58:51735.
21. Koch R. *The 80/20 Principle*. New York: Doubleday, 1998.
22. *Statistical Abstract of the United States*. Table 116. Deaths – Life Years Lost and Mortality Costs by Age, Sex, and Cause: 2000 and 2002. U.S. Department of Commerce 2006:92.
23. Diamond GA, Denton TA, Matloff JM. Fee-for-benefit. A strategy to improve the quality of health care and control costs through reimbursement incentives. J Am Coll Cardiol 1993;22:343–52.

46

A Time to Live: Dynamic Changes in Risk as the Basis for Therapeutic Triage

Sanjay Kaul and George A. Diamond

CONTENTS

ABSTRACT

Clinical prognosis depends on the current threat of an adverse event (risk) and on the rate of change of that risk (hazard). Conventional risk stratification nevertheless relies only on the former—on the frequency of adverse events over some arbitrary period of time. In this study, we suggest that prognosis can be assessed more precisely using dynamic models that consider both risk and hazard. We construct one such model based on principles employed in the field of chemical kinetics and demonstrate its clinical relevance by application to the prediction and prevention of atherosclerotic coronary events.

Key words: Atherosclerotic events; Cardiovascular prevention; Dynamic modeling; Hazard; Kinetic modeling; Prognosis; Risk

KEY POINTS

- Prognosis depends on risk and on its rate of change (hazard).
- Risk stratification relies only on the former.
- Dynamic modeling based on both risk and hazard has the potential to refine the assessment of prognosis and therapeutic prevention strategies.
- Just as the physical trajectory of an object depends on its current magnitude of displacement (velocity) and the concurrent rate of change of that displacement (acceleration), the prognostic trajectory of a patient depends on the current threat of an adverse event (risk) and on the concurrent rate of change of that risk (hazard). Conventional risk stratification nevertheless relies only on the former—on the frequency of adverse events over some arbitrary period of time.

From: *Asymptomatic Atherosclerosis: Pathophysiology, Detection and Treatment*
Edited by: M. Naghavi (ed.), DOI 10.1007/978-1-60327-179-0_46

Clinicians have come to apply these casual risk stratification assessments to two alternative pathophysiological models of ischemic heart disease: a physical model, which presumes that the greater the severity of vascular stenosis, the greater the risk of an adverse cardiovascular event [1]; and a biochemical model, which presumes that the greater the severity of inflammation within the atherosclerotic plaque, the greater the risk of the event [2]. Accordingly, the "stenotic" model is used to justify the primacy of aggressive interventional procedures, while the "inflammatory" model is used to justify the primacy of conservative medical management.

Although each model is supported by a body of evidence sufficient to satisfy its adherents, neither has been established to the exclusion of the other. Thus, while exercise-induced myocardial ischemia is well known to have important prognostic utility [3], the therapeutic relief of that ischemia has comparatively little prognostic benefit [4]. In contrast, even though conventional risk factors are less accurate predictors of cardiovascular events [5], medical therapy directed at these risk factors substantially reduces the frequency of these events [6–8].

A unified model that integrates the two perspectives within a common conceptual framework would go a long way toward improving the overall accuracy of prognosis and the effectiveness of therapy. Conventional attempts to do this rely on multivariate statistical regression, but the resultant prediction rules are entirely empirical and offer no assurance that their prognostic assessments correspond with projected therapeutic benefit [9].

QUANTIFICATION OF RISK DYNAMICS

A kinetic model [10, 11] bridges the divide between the "stenotic" and "inflammatory" paradigms in two ways. First, because it quantifies the dynamics of the transitions from one clinical state to another (from nonischemic to ischemic and from noninflammatory to inflammatory), instead of the static correlations among the states (ischemic event rate vs. inflammatory event rate), it predicts changes in risk—hazard—in addition to the level of risk. Second, instead of relying on clinically obscure statistical criteria such as minimization of variance, the kinetic model rests on a consistent and plausible biological foundation (the interplay between ischemia and inflammation).

In technical terms, a kinetic model quantifies the time-dependent transition from state A to state B (denoted $A \rightarrow B$), the states being expressed in terms of absolute or relative prevalence (denoted $[A]$ and $[B]$), and the time dependence being expressed in terms of a rate constant (k) or half-life ($t_{1/2} = \ln 2/k$). The canonical transition of this kind is that of a monotonic exponential decay ($[A] = e^{-kt}$), where $[A] = 1$ at $t = 0$, the rate of change for $[A]$ is inversely proportional to its prevalence, and the rate constant, k, is the hazard:

$$\frac{d[A]}{dt} = -k[A].$$

Assuming that each of the state-to-state transitions leading to a cardiovascular event obeys this simple exponential law, we can construct a biologically plausible kinetic model for the process as shown in (Fig. 1). According to this model, the normative (noninflammatory and nonstenotic) state N can transition reversibly either to the inflammatory state I or to the stenotic state S. The inflammatory state, in turn, can transition reversibly to the stenotic state or irreversibly to the event state E, and the stenotic state can similarly transition reversibly to the inflammatory state or irreversibly to the event state. The associated constants (k_1 through k_8) quantify the empirically observable rates for each transition. These quantitative constants distinguish this model from qualitative phenomenological schemas such as that proposed by Braunwald [12].

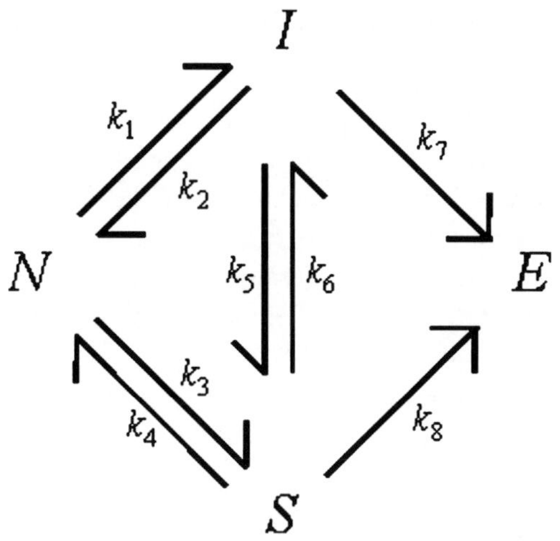

Fig. 1. A kinetic model of atherosclerosis. See text for abbreviations and discussion.

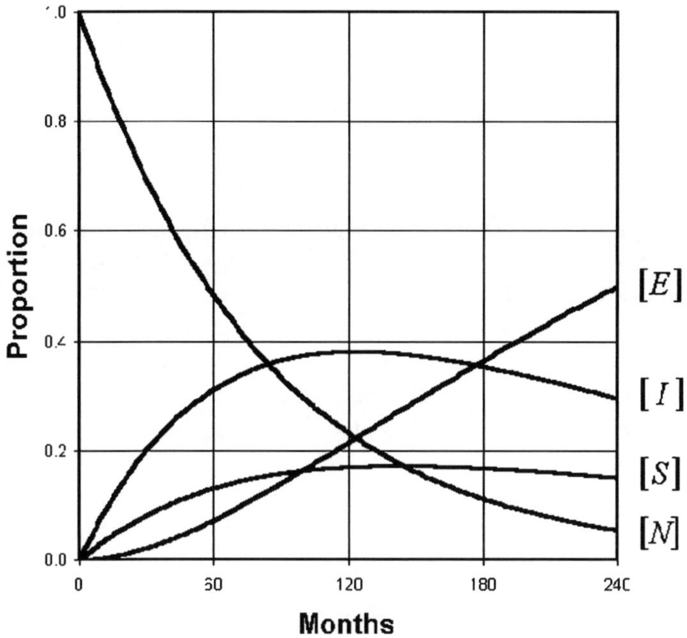

Fig. 2. Time course of atherosclerosis. See text for abbreviations and discussion.

The outcomes predicted by this kinetic model, based on a putative set of rate constants consistent with observational data [13–16], are illustrated in (Fig. 2). In this example, the proportional prevalence of the normative state [*N*] falls as a simple exponential function, while that of the inflammatory [*I*] and stenotic [*S*] states each rise to a broad maximum and then tail off exponentially. As a consequence, event rate [*E*] increases almost linearly.

CLINICAL IMPLICATIONS

The kinetic rate constants employed in this example were derived from population averages and therefore quantify the average hazards for the group. Although this is sufficient for strategic planning, we need to know the specific hazards for each member of the group to conduct case-by-case patient management. Fortunately, the model can be adapted to provide such patient-specific estimates.

Just as chemical rate constants vary with temperature, atherosclerotic rate constants vary with the magnitude of inflammation and ischemia—the greater these magnitudes, the greater the rates. Once these relations are defined, the inflammatory and stenotic markers observed in an individual patient can be used to generate patient-specific rate constants, and these, in turn, can be used to create a patient-specific kinetic model, from which we can derive patient-specific predictions of outcome.

Our kinetic model thereby serves to operationalize SHAPE's conception of the "vulnerable patient" [17]. In this context, the "stenotic" axis of the model might be operationalized in terms of various anatomical surrogates of plaque burden (e.g., coronary calcification scores as markers for the extent of disease), and the "inflammatory" axis, in terms of candidate biochemical surrogates of plaque function (e.g., C-reactive protein and adhesion molecules as markers of disease activity).

Furthermore, the kinetic model resolves the current debate over the role of age and time in coronary risk prediction [18, 19]. This debate stems from a fundamental misunderstanding regarding the underlying dynamics of the prediction process that blurs the distinction between risk stratification and therapeutic triage. The latter depends not only on relative or absolute risk, but also on hazard (its temporal rate of change). Thus, assuming effective therapy is available (a decidedly nontrivial assumption), treatment is well advised (even in low risk individuals) when the hazard is positive (meaning that the risk is currently rising). On the other hand, treatment is ill-advised (even in high risk individuals) when the hazard is negative (meaning that the risk is already falling). The kinetic model formally discriminates between these alternatives; conventional risk stratification models cannot.

In summary, just as one cannot properly assess the dynamic processes resulting in blood flow without simultaneous consideration of pressure and resistance, one cannot assess the dynamic processes resulting in atherosclerotic events without simultaneous consideration of the physics of anatomic stenosis and the chemistry of plaque instability. The kinetic model outlined here thereby promises to replace the superficial practice of risk stratification with a more sophisticated strategy of therapeutic triage. Once prospectively verified, the model would allow one to predict the incremental benefits of treatment strategies directed at stabilization of the atherosclerotic plaque versus restoration of myocardial blood flow.

REFERENCES

1. Gorlin R. Treatment of chronic stable angina pectoris. Am J Cardiol 1992;70:26G–31G.
2. Sheridan PJ, Crossman DC. Critical review of unstable angina and non-ST elevation myocardial infarction. Postgrad Med 2002;78:717–726.
3. Acampa W, Petretta M, Cuocolo A. Nuclear medicine procedures in cardiovascular diseases. An evidence based approach. Q J Nucl Med 2002;46:323–330.
4. Rogers WJ, Bourassa MG, Andrews TC, Bertolet BD, Blumenthal RS, Chaitman BR, et al. Asymptomatic cardiac ischemia pilot (ACIP) study: outcome at 1 year for patients with asymptomatic cardiac ischemia randomized to medical therapy or revascularization. The ACIP investigators. J Am Coll Cardiol 1995;26:594–605.
5. Willerson JT, Ridker PM. Inflammation as a cardiovascular risk factor. Circulation 2004;109:II2–II10.
6. Heart Protection Study Collaborative Group. MRC/BHF Heart protection study of cholesterol lowering with simvastatin in 20 536 high-risk individuals: a randomized placebo-controlled trial. Lancet 2002;360:7–22.
7. Ridker PM, Manson JE, Buring JE, Goldhaber SZ, Hennekens CH. The effect of chronic platelet inhibition with low-dose aspirin on atherosclerotic progression and acute thrombosis: clinical evidence from the physicians' health study. Am Heart J 1991;122:1588–1592.

8. The Heart Outcomes Prevention Evaluation Study Investigators. Effects of an angiotensin-converting-enzyme inhibitor, ramipril, on cardiovascular events in high-risk patients. N Engl J Med 2000;342:145–153.
9. Diamond GA. Future imperfect: the limitations of clinical prediction models and the limits of clinical prediction. J Am Coll Cardiol 1989;14:12A–22A.
10. Diamond GA, Kaul S. From here to eternity. A unified kinetic model for the pathophysiology of atherosclerotic events. Am J Med 2007;120:5–11.
11. Diamond GA, Kaul S. Hazardous to your health. Kinetic foundations of risk stratification and therapeutic triage. Am J Med 2006;119:275.e1–275.e6.
12. Braunwald E. Unstable angina. An etiologic approach to management. Circulation 1998;98:2219–2222.
13. Stefan K, Johann W. The natural course of atherosclerosis. Part I: incidence and progression. Arterioscler Thromb Vasc Biol 1999;19:1484–1490.
14. Libby P. The vascular biology of atherosclerosis. In: Braunwald E, Zipes DP, Libby P, (eds.) Heart disease: a textbook of cardiovascular medicine, 6th ed. Philadelphia: Saunders; 2001:995–1009.
15. Davies MJ. A macro and micro view of coronary vascular insult in ischemic heart disease. Circulation 1990;82(suppl II):38–46.
16. Falk E, Shah PK, Fuster V. Coronary plaque disruption. Circulation 1995;92:657–671.
17. Naghavi M, Libby P, Falk E, Casscells SW, Litovsky S, Rumberger J, et al. From vulnerable plaque to vulnerable patient. A call for new definitions and risk assessment strategies: Part I. Circulation 2003;108:1664–1672, Part II. Circulation 2003;108:1672–1678.
18. Ridker PM, Cook N. Should age and time be eliminated from cardiovascular risk prediction models? Rationale for the creation of a new national risk detection program. Circulation 2005;111:657–658.
19. Vasan RS, D'Agostino RB Sr. Age and time need not and should not be eliminated from the coronary risk prediction models. Circulation 2005;111:542–545.

VI

Treatment of Asymptomatic Atherosclerotic Cardiovascular Disease and the Vulnerable Patients: Systemic Therapies

47 LDL Targeted Therapies

Raul D. Santos, Khurram Nasir, and Roger S. Blumenthal

Contents

Abstract

LDL-cholesterol (LDL-C) levels are directly associated with the prevalence of coronary heart disease. Epidemiological and ecological studies have clearly shown that populations with LDL-C levels significantly lower than those found in western countries have a very low prevalence of coronary heart disease, despite the presence of other risk factors for atherosclerosis. It has been demonstrated that LDL-C reduction with statins not only reduces atherosclerosis progression but can induce its regression, if intensive LDL-C reduction, around 40–50%, is achieved. Most importantly there is a linear relation between LDL-C lowering and cardiovascular disease reduction; for each 1 mmol/L (39 mg/dL) there is ~21% decrease in any major vascular event including death, myocardial infarction, stroke and myocardial revascularization as shown by a meta-analysis involving 90,056 patients who had participated in 14 statin trials. These findings were reinforced by another meta-analysis of more than 27,000 coronary heart disease individuals showing that intensive LDL-C lowering was superior to conventional therapy. Subjects considered to be at high risk by clinical stratification must be treated with intensive LDL-C lowering. Also, it has been proposed that

From: *Asymptomatic Atherosclerosis: Pathophysiology, Detection and Treatment*
Edited by: M. Naghavi (ed.), DOI 10.1007/978-1-60327-179-0_47

asymptomatic subjects not considered at high risk by clinical stratification but otherwise presenting with a high subclinical atherosclerotic burden, must be treated in the same manner.

Key words: Atherosclerosis; Cardiovascular disease; LDL-cholesterol; Lipid lowering therapy; Statins

TOPIC PEARLS

- LDL-cholesterol (LDL-C) levels are directly related with coronary heart disease (CHD) risk. Low LDL-C levels are associated with a low prevalence of coronary disease, irrespective of the presence of other risk factors.
- LDL-C reduction of around 40–50% is associated with the atherosclerotic process-progression, halting, and even its regression. Most importantly there is a linear correlation between LDL-C lowering and CVD reduction; for each 1 mmol/L or 39 mg/dL, there is ~21% decrease in major cardiovascular events as demonstrated in a meta-analysis including 90,056 patients in statin trials.
- Subjects at high clinical risk and possibly those asymptomatic individuals with high atherosclerotic plaque burdens detected by carotid ultrasound, high coronary calcium quantification by computerized tomography or reduced ankle-brachial index must have intense LDL-C reduction irrespective of their baseline LDL-C.

CLINICAL CASE

JBC is a 47 year old white man who presented to a routine medical evaluation complaining that 2 months ago he had suffered a minor persistent chest discomfort. Since his father suffered a myocardial infarction at the age of 50 he went to the emergency room where his physical examination, ECG and cardiac enzymes were normal. He was dismissed with an H2 blocker for possible stomach discomfort. Nowadays JBC has no complaints; he has no time to exercise since he works more than12 h a day, is a little overweight (BMI 25.5 kg/m$^{2)}$, has some abdominal fat (waist measurement 98 cm) and his blood pressure is 130/80 mmhg. He has a fasting glucose of 95 mg/dL, a total cholesterol of 230 mg/dL, triglycerides of 159 mg/dL, HDL-C of 43 mg/dl and a LDL-C of 156 mg/dL. His 10-year CHD risk was 6% according to the Framingham algorithm. He performed a maximal exercise scintigraphy that showed no ECG abnormalities, good blood pressure behavior and attained reading of 13 METS. No changes were found in perfusion or ejection fraction. Further on, he was submitted to coronary calcium quantification by computerized tomography which showed a calcium score of 450 (>75% for age and sex). In spite of the low 10-year CHD risk he was oriented to exercise, and to lose some weight; and was prescribed aspirin, rosuvastatin 10 mg, and ezetimibe 10 mg. He returned after 2 months; he was exercising three times a week, had lost around five pounds and presented an LDL-C of 69 mg/dL and a HDL of 47 mg/dL. The recommendations made for this patient are more aggressive than what is recommended nowadays by the National Cholesterol Education Program (NCEP).

INTRODUCTION

Cardiovascular disease is the leading cause of death in developed countries [1]. Unfortunately tthis epidemic is also spreading to developing countries, as well as to regions where classically coronary heart disease (CHD) was a rarity, like Japan [2].

It is well accepted that patients with established CHD and other high-risk equivalent conditions including diabetes, chronic kidney disease, peripheral arterial disease, and cerebrovascular disease require aggressive intervention in order to reduce risk of recurrent events [3–5]. Unfortunately, sudden death and myocardial infarction are common manifestations of CHD and about two thirds of unexpected cardiac deaths occur without prior recognition of cardiac disease [6]. For these reasons, in the past decade, attention has shifted from a secondary prevention strategy to one focusing on detecting individuals at risk of the first cardiovascular event [7].

Currently there is evidence that the use of imaging techniques to detect subclinical atherosclerotic disease like coronary artery calcium (CAC) quantification by cardiac computerized tomography [8] and carotid intima-media thickness (CIMT) evaluation [9], add to clinical CHD risk stratification. It has been proposed that these techniques be used in addition to risk stratification based on clinical risk scores, in order to improve the detection of asymptomatic individuals at higher levels of risk [10]. Once these subjects are diagnosed intensive risk factor modification, mainly LDL-cholesterol (LDL-C) lowering and aspirin treatment should be instituted, as will be discussed below in this chapter.

LDL-CHOLESTEROL LEVELS AND CORONARY HEART DISEASE – THE EPIDEMIOLOGICAL EVIDENCE

Cholesterol is one of the main components of the atherosclerostic plaque. Circulating LDL infiltrates the vessel wall and is oxidized in the subendothelial space leading to endothelial dysfunction, inflammation, smooth muscle cell proliferation, and atherosclerotic plaque growth [11]. Epidemiological [12–15], as well as ecological [16, 17] studies, have clearly shown that subjects who naturally had lower total and LDL plasma cholesterol levels, had significantly lower rates of CHD deaths despite the presence of other risk factors like hypertension or smoking. Classically, the Ni-Hon-San study [18] showed that Japanese subjects who migrated from Japan to Hawaii and to California showed a graded increase in CHD prevalence, respectively 25.4/1000, 34.7/1000 and 44.6/1000, that was parallel to their total cholesterol levels, 181, 218 and 228 mg/dL respectively, for Japan, Hawaii and San Francisco. Those findings were confirmed by the MRFIT [13] (Table 1), Framingham [14] and by the PROCAM [15] studies. Chen et al. [16], followed from 8 to 13 years 9,021 men and women aged 35–64 from urban Shanghai in China and showed that even for total cholesterol levels significantly lower than those in the MRFIT study and western standards (120–210 mg/dL), there was a significant correlation between cholesterol levels and deaths due to CHD, with the risk increasing 4.5 times from the lower values to the higher with no apparent threshold (Table 2).

Table 1
Total cholesterol levels and relative risk of coronary heart disease mortality in 356,222 men aged 35–57 years: the MRFIT study [13]

Total serum cholesterol (mg/dL)	*Coronary heart disease mortality relative risk*
<182	1
182–202	1.29
203–220	1.73
221–244	2.21
>244	3.42

Table 2
Total cholesterol levels and relative risk of coronary heart disease mortality in 9,021 men and women aged 35–57 in Shanghai, China [16]

Total serum cholesterol (mg/dL)	*Coronary heart disease mortality relative risk*
<137	1
138–160	2.25
160–180	3
>180	4.5

Recently two important studies have strengthened the link between spontaneously lower cholesterol levels and a reduced risk of coronary atherosclerosis [17, 19]. Cohen et al. [17] compared the incidence of CHD events over a 15-year interval in the Atherosclerosis Risk in Communities study, according to the presence or absence of sequence variants in the proprotein convertase subtilisin/kexin type 9 serine protease gene (PCSK9) that are associated with reduced plasma levels of LDL-C. The PCSK9 protein is responsible for degrading the LDL receptor [20], thus, reducing LDL plasma clearance. In Black individuals these mutations were associated with a 28% reduction in mean LDL-C and an 88% reduction in the risk of CHD ($P=0.008$ for the reduction; hazard ratio, 0.11; 95% CI [0.02–0.81]; $P=0.03$). In White subjects a sequence variation in PCSK9 twas associated with a 15% reduction in LDL-C and a 47% reduction in the risk of CHD (hazard ratio 95%CI, 0.50 [0.32–0.79]; $P=0.003$). These benefits occurred in spite of the presence of other risk factors for atherosclerosis.

The second important study was a meta-analysis [19] of 61 prospective observational studies, consisting of almost 900,000 adults without previous disease followed for nearly 12 million/person years, between the ages of 40 and 89 years. The study showed that each 39 mg/dL (1mmol/L) spontaneously lower total cholesterol was associated with about a half (hazard ratio 0.44; 95% CI [0.42–0.48]), a third (0.66 [0.65–0.68]), and a sixth (0.83 [0.81–0.85]) lower CHD mortality in both sexes, at ages 40–49, 50–69, and 70–89 years, respectively. Apparently, in the western developed countries no threshold was found within the range of plasma cholesterol levels in which a lower value did not mean a lower risk of events. Both studies clearly show that spontaneously lower LDL-C levels are associated in the long term with significant reductions in cardiovascular events.

LDL-CHOLESTEROL LOWERING, REDUCTION IN ATHEROSCLEROTIC PLAQUE PROGRESSION AND ATHEROSCLEROSIS REGRESSION

The introduction of HMG-CoA reductase inhibitors or statins for plasma lipid modification treatment in the late 1980s has changed the way cardiology is practiced [3]. Statins exert potent LDL-C lowering effects and also favorably modify HDL-cholesterol, non-HDL-cholesterol as well as triglyceride plasma levels. Furthermore, statins have other favorable effects on inflammation, thrombosis, on smooth muscle cell proliferation, and on progenitor cell mobilization [21] that might influence favorably in the atherosclerotic process.

The effects of LDL-C lowering therapy on atherosclerotic plaque in humans has been evaluated by both invasive [22–26] and noninvasive [27–33] techniques.

Effects of LDL-C Lowering on Coronary Artery Plaque Evaluated by Invasive Methodologies

Angiographic evidence that LDL-C lowering therapy reduces the rate of atherosclerosis progression and induces its regression was obtained in a series of studies conducted in the 1990s [23, 24]. Those studies used coronary quantitative angiography (QCA) to detect the effects of LDL-C lowering in obstructive atherosclerotic plaque progression. LDL-C reductions of approximately 25–30% were associated with modest changes in plaque diameter over 3 years [24]. However, there was a clear linear correlation between attained LDL-C levels and plaque progression ($r^2=0.71$, $P=0.0005$), the higher the level the greater the progression rate. The major benefit of statins relative to placebo was to reduce atherosclerosis progression in coronary artery segments with baseline lesions having <50% diameter stenosis and to reduce new lesion formation as shown in the PLAC I trial [23]. The rate of lesion progression did not differ between treatments in segments with baseline lesions having ≥50% diameter stenosis. These findings suggested that the effectiveness of statin therapy on atherosclerosis progression might be more pronounced in early lesions compared to more advanced ones. This fact has clinical importance and certainly explains some of the favorable effects of statins in clinical CHD events prevention, since roughly 70% of these CHD events originate in lipid-rich, non-obstructive remodeled plaques [34].

The effect of LDL-C lowering therapy on these less obstructive, but otherwise not less dangerous plaques, was confirmed in studies that used intravascular ultrasound (IVUS) technology to verify the effects of more potent statins like atorvastatin and rosuvastatin on plaque size [25, 26]. IVUS was used to compare intensive with moderate statin therapy in the REVERSAL [25] study on patients with angiographic luminal narrowing between 20–50% in one or more vessels and LDL-C levels of 125–210 mg/dL. Intensive therapy with 80 mg atorvastatin produced lower mean LDL-C (79 vs. 110 mg/dL, $P<0.001$) and lower C- reactive protein levels (1.8 vs. 2.9 mg/L) than did moderate therapy with 40 mg pravastatin. IVUS showed that atorvastatin essentially prevented atherosclerosis progression, as the change from baseline over the 18-month follow-up averaged –0.4% in total atheroma volume (95% CI: –2.35 to 1.49%). In comparison, with pravastatin, plaque volume increased by a mean of 2.7% (95% CI: 0.24–4.67%). The difference between treatments in atherosclerosis progression was statistically significant. In the REVERSAL study there was a linear relation between LDL-C level reduction and changes in plaque volume, each 10% LDL-C reduction (0.4 mmol/L or 15 mg/dL) resulted in 1% reduction in atheroma volume. The data pool of the angiographic studies and the REVERSAL trial also showed a linear association between LDL-C levels and coronary minimal luminal diameter ($r^2=0.61$, $P=0.001$) [35]. Apparently an LDL-C ≤67 mg/dL (1.7 mmol/L) was associated with no atherosclerosis progression.

The ASTEROID trial [26] evaluated intensive therapy with rosuvastatin 40 mg/day in a study population comparable to REVERSAL [25]. Rosuvastatin reduced LDL-C by 53% (from 130 to 61 mg/dL) and raised HDL-cholesterol by 15% (both $P<0.001$). Of importance, over the 2-year follow-up period, rosuvastatin induced a median reduction of 0.78- and 6.8% respectively in percent and total atheroma volume vs. baseline ($P<0.001$). The regression in atherosclerosis achieved in ASTEROID is consistent with the linear relationship between the mean achieved LDL-C and median change in atheroma volume seen across IVUS studies ($r^2=0.97$; $P<0.001$). Further analysis from Nichols et al. [36], using a pool of subjects from prospective IVUS, showed that the rate of change in plaque volume was independently associated with LDL-C reduction and HDL-cholesterol increase from the baseline. Substantial plaque regression, defined by a ≥5% reduction in plaque volume, was observed in subjects who achieved LDL-C levels below the mean of 87.5 mg/dL (2.25 mmol/L) and HDL-cholesterol increases above 7.5%. These findings suggest that the benefits of statin therapy on atherosclerosis may be derived mostly from decreases in LDL-C, but also from increases in HDL-C. A post-hoc analysis of the REVERSAL trial [37] showed that some benefit was also attributed to reductions in C- reactive protein levels induced by statin treatment. However, how much anti-inflammatory effects add to LDL-C lowering in plaque regression and especially to clinical events reduction, remains to be determined.

Another important finding from the pool of data derived from IVUS studies [36] is that most of the effects of risk factors modification occurred in the non-calcified portion of the plaque, a fact that justifies the non-favorable effects of LDL-C lowering on CAC progression evaluated by electron beam tomography (EBT) in prospective trials [33, 38]. Besides reduction in plaque volume, statin therapy also reduces the lipid content, and the inflammatory process in atherosclerotic plaques [39].

Taken together, these studies show that moderate LDL-C lowering therapy reduces atherosclerosis progression relative to placebo, and that intensive therapy further reduces progression and induces regression in patients with evidence of CAD. Moreover, LDL-C lowering also induces changes in plaque components that have been associated with plaque instability and clinical CHD events.

Effects of LDL-C Lowering on Atherosclerotic Plaques Evaluated by Noninvasive Methodologies

Carotid Intima Media Thickness (CIMT)

CIMT, evaluated by B-mode ultrasound, can be used as a marker of subclinical atherosclerosis [10]. In a meta-analysis of eight population-based studies, Lorenz et al. [40] showed that every 0.1 mm increase in CIMT in the common carotid artery, increases age- and gender-adjusted risk of myocardial infarction by 10–15% and stroke by 13–18%. There is also evidence that CIMT evaluation can add to clinical risk stratification in dyslipidemic patients. Baldassarre et al. [9] found in a longitudinal study of 1,969 consecutive patients had the maximum CIMT improved the predictability of the Framingham risk score. Patients considered to be at intermediate risk based on the Framingham assessment, were upgraded to high-risk status if the maximum CIMT was above the 60th percentile in men and 80th percentile in women.

Clinical trials confirm the benefits of LDL-C lowering therapy on atherosclerosis progression evaluated by CIMT in subjects with and without previous manifestation of CHD. In the PLAC II study [23], pravastatin 40 mg/day significantly reduced atherosclerosis progression compared with placebo, when changes in CIMT of the common carotid artery were measured over a 3-year period (0.029 vs. 0.046 mm/year, $P=0.03$). A meta-analysis that included that and six other randomized controlled trials found that moderate LDL-C lowering therapy reduced CIMT progression by a mean of 0.012 mm/year (95% CI: –0.016 to 0.007) compared with placebo [41]. The ARBITER study used carotid CIMT to compare intensive statin therapy with atorvastatin 80 mg/day and moderate statin therapy with pravastatin 40 mg/day in 161 patients who met National Cholesterol Education Panel Adult Treatment Panel (NCEP) criteria for lipid-lowering drug therapy [42]. Forty-six percent of the study patients had a history of coronary artery disease. Atorvastatin 80 mg therapy reduced LDL-C more intensively than did 40 mg of pravastatin (76 vs. 110 mg/dL, $P<0.001$). Atorvastatin also reduced carotid CIMT from baseline, whereas it increased in the pravastatin group over the 12-month follow-up (–0.034 vs. +0.025 mm, $P=0.03$).

Imaging studies also show the benefits of statin therapy in patients with no history of clinical events but presenting subclinical atherosclerosis (Table 3). Wiegman et al. [28] have shown that Pravastatin treatment reduced CIMT progression in children with Familial Hypercholesterolemia in comparison with placebo. Compared with baseline, CIMT showed a trend toward regression with pravastatin (mean [SD], –0.010 [0.048] mm; $P=0.049$), whereas a trend toward progression was observed in the placebo group (mean [SD], +0.005 [0.044] mm; $P=0.28$). The mean (standard deviation) change in IMT compared between the two groups (0.014 [0.046] mm) was significant ($P=0.02$). The ASAP trial [27] used CIMT to compare intensive therapy with atorvastatin 80 mg/day, versus moderate therapy with simvastatin 40 mg/day, in 325 patients with familial hypercholesterolemia, LDL-C was reduced respectively by 53 and 44% in atorvastatin and simvastatin groups ($P<0.01$). Atorvastatin reduced mean CIMT by 0.031 mm from baseline during the 2-year study, whereas CIMT increased by a mean of 0.036 mm in the simvastatin group ($P=0.0005$). Mean CIMT was reduced significantly from baseline by atorvastatin in the common carotid (–0.041 mm, $P=0.001$) and internal carotid (–0.032 mm, $P=0.03$) arteries but not at the carotid bulb.

More recently the METEOR trial [29] evaluated the effects of intensive LDL-C lowering therapy with rosuvastatin 40 mg/day vs. placebo on carotid subclinical atherosclerosis, represented by a CIMT of 1.2–3.5 mm in 984 individuals, with either age (mean, 57 years) as the only CHD risk factor or a 10-year Framingham risk score <10%. Study subjects presented moderately elevated LDL-C levels at baseline (120–190 mg/dL, mean, 154 mg/dL). After a 2 year follow-up, rosuvastatin reduced LDL-C by 49%, resulting in LDL-C levels of 78 vs. 152 mg/dL in the placebo group. After treatment, the

Table 3
Impact of statin therapy on measures of subclinical atherosclerosis in asymptomatic patients

Method	*Study*	*Patients*	*Treatment*	*Follow-up*	*Results*
Carotid ultrasound	Wiegman et al. [28]	214 Children with familial hypercholesterolemia	Pravastatin 20–40 mg vs. placebo	2 years	Carotid IMT showed a trend toward regression with pravastatin (mean [SD], −0.010 [0.048] mm; $P = .049$), whereas a trend toward progression was observed in the placebo group (mean [SD], +0.005 [0.044] mm; $P = 0.28$). The mean (SD) change in IMT compared between the two groups (0.014 [0.046] mm) ($P = 0.02$
	ASAP [27]	325 adults with familial hypercholesterolemia	Atorvastatin 80 mg Simvastatin 40 mg	2 years	Difference in mean carotid IMT favoring atorvastatin (−0.031 vs. +0.036 mm; $P = 0.0005$)
	METEOR [29]	984 subjects with low CHD risk according to Framingham evaluation and moderate carotid IMT thickening	Rosuvastatin 40 mg Placebo	2 years	Difference in maximum carotid IMT at 12 sites favoring rosuvastatin; (−0.0014 vs. +0.0131; $P < 0.001$)
MRI	Corti et al. [30]	21 asymptomatic subjects with atherosclerotic plaques in the carotid arteries and the aorta.	Simvastatin	2 years	Significant ($P < 0.01$) reductions in maximal vessel wall thickness and vessel wall area at 12 months (10 and 11% for aortic and 8 and 11% for carotid plaques, respectively), without changes in lumen area. Further decreases in vessel wall thickness and vessel wall area ranging from 12 to 20% were observed at 18 and 24 months
	Lima et al. [31]	27 patients with evidence of atherosclerotic plaques in the aorta	Sinvastatin 20–80 mg	6 months	Plaque volume was reduced from 3.3 ± 0.1.4 to 2.9 ± 1.4 cm [3] at 6 months ($P < 0.02$)
EBT	BELLES [38]	615 postmenopausal women with LDL-cholesterol above NCEP targets	Atorvastatin 80 mg Pravastatin 40 mg	1 year	Change in coronary artery calcium volume scores did not differ between treatments (median 15.1 and 14.3%, respectively for atorvastatin and pravastatin)
	Schmermund et al. [33]	471 subjects with ≥2 risk factors and moderate calcification	Atorvastatin 80 mg Atorvastatin 10 mg	1 year	Change in coronary artery calcium score did not differ between treatments

maximum CIMT measured at 12 sites was essentially unchanged in the rosuvastatin group but increased in the placebo group (–0.0014 vs. +0.0131 mm/year, $P<0.001$). Similarly, the maximum CIMT at the common carotid artery (–0.0038 vs. +0.0084 mm/year, $P<0.001$), carotid bulb (–0.0040 vs. +0.0172 mm/year, $P<0.001$), and internal carotid artery (+0.0039 vs. +0.0145 mm/year, $P=0.02$) favored rosuvastatin over placebo. Taken together, these studies show, similarly to angiographic studies in the coronary tree, that it's possible to modify atherosclerosis course in the carotid arteries with LDL-C lowering therapy in a subject with or without previous manifestation of CHD. Moreover, intensive LDL-C lowering therapy may not only stops disease progression but can induce its regression.

Magnetic Resonance Imaging

Changes in atherosclerotic plaque by statin treatment can be detected in the carotids and in the thoracic aorta by magnetic resonance imaging (MRI). Corti et al. [30] evaluated the effect of simvastatin treatment on atherosclerotic plaque size by MRI, after 2 years in 21 subjects with LDL-C >130 mg/dL. The effects of statin on these atherosclerotic lesions were evaluated as changes versus baseline in lumen area, vessel wall thickness, and vessel wall area by MRI. Maximal reduction of plasma LDL-C by simvastatin 38% was achieved after approximately 6 weeks of therapy and maintained thereafter throughout the study. Significant ($P<0.01$) reductions in maximal vessel wall thickness and vessel wall area at 12 months (10 and 11% for aortic and 8 and 11% for carotid plaques, respectively), without changes in lumen area, have been reported. Further decreases in vessel wall thickness and vessel wall area ranging from 12 to 20% were observed at 18 and 24 months. A slight but significant increase (ranging from 4 to 6%) in lumen area was seen in both carotid and aortic lesions, at these later time points.

Lima et al. [31] showed that changes in atherosclerotic plaques can be detected as early as 6 months after statin treatment. In that study 27 patients were treated with simvastatin 20–80 mg daily. LDL-C decreased by 23% at 6 months from 125 to 97 mg/dL, $P<0.05$. Plaque volume was reduced from 3.3 ± 0.14 to 2.9 ± 1.4 cm^3 ($P<0.02$), whereas luminal volume increase was less accentuated (from 12.0 ± 3.9 to 12.2 ± 3.7 cm^3, $P<0.06$). Plaque regression was significantly related to LDL-C reduction ($P<0.02$), furthermore luminal volume increase was inversely related to LDL-C reduction ($P<0.04$). These results show that atherosclerosis can be reversed in the carotids, coronary arteries and the aorta and that LDL-C lowering by statin treatment is the main drive of these effects.

Coronary Artery Calcification Evaluated by Computerized Tomography

Coronary artery calcification (CAC) detected by computerized tomography is a marker of subclinical atherosclerosis that correlates with coronary plaque burden [8]. Greater CAC values have been found in populations with higher rates of CHD death [43] in comparison with those with lower CHD prevalence and it has been clearly demonstrated in prospective studies that its severity is independently associated with CHD and death risks [44, 45]. Moreover, CAC quantification can add to Framingham risk stratification in predicting CHD events. It has also been shown that not only CAC severity but its progression is a marker of increased risk of CHD events [46].

Callister et al. [32] evaluated the effects of statin treatment on CAC progression in a retrospective study of 149 patients (61% men and 39% women; age range, 32–75 years) with no history of coronary artery disease who were referred for EBT screening. Patients were followed for a minimum of 12 months (range, 12–15). Treatment with statins was used in 70% at follow-up; a net reduction in the calcium-volume score was observed only in the 65 treated patients whose final LDL-C levels were less than 120 mg/dL (3.10 mmol/L) (mean [±SD] change in the score, $-7\pm23\%$; $P=0.01$). Untreated patients had an average LDL-C level of at least 120 mg per deciliter and at the time of follow-up had a significant net increase in mean calcium-volume score (mean change, $+52\pm36\%$; $P<0.001$).

The 40 treated patients who had average LDL-C levels of at least 120 mg per deciliter had a measurable increase in mean calcium-volume score (mean change, +25 ± 22%, $P < 0.001$), although it was smaller than the increase in the untreated patients.

Despite these results, so far randomized prospective trials have failed to demonstrate that LDL-C lowering with statins consistently reduce CAC progression [33, 38] (Table 4).

In the BELLES trial [38] consistently, 615 postmenopausal women with LDL-C above NCEP-defined target levels for their calculated CHD risk were randomly assigned to receive either atorvastatin 80 mg/day or pravastatin 40 mg/day for 12 months. As expected, LDL-C lowering was higher in the Atorvastatin group 47 vs. 25% $P < 0.0001$. Nevertheless, changes in calcium volume scores measured by EBT did not differ significantly between treatments. No relation was seen between changes in LDL-C and calcium volume scores. Similarly, Schmermund et al. [33]compared 80 and 10 mg doses of atorvastatin in 471 patients with ≥2 cardiovascular risk factors and moderate CAC. After pretreatment

Table 4
Updated NCEP ATP III LDL-C goals and cutpoints for Therapeutic Lifestyle Change (TLC) and drug therapy in different risk categories [4]

Risk category	*LDL-C goal (mg/dL)*	*Initiate TLC (mg/dL)*	*Consider Drug Therapy (mg/dL)*[a]
High risk: CHD[b] or CHD risk equivalents[c] (10-year risk >20%)[d]	<100[e] (optional goal: <70 mg/dL)	≥100	≥100[f,e] (<100 mg/dL: consider drug options)[a]
Moderately high risk: 2_ risk factors[g,e] (10-year risk 10% to 20%)[h]	<130[e]	≥130	≥130[e] (100–129 mg/dL; consider drug options)[i]
Moderate risk: 2_ risk factors[g] (10-year[e] risk <10%)[h,e]	<130	≥160	≥160
Lower risk: 0–1 risk factor[j]	<160	≥160	≥190

[a]When LDL-lowering drug therapy is employed, it is advised that intensity of therapy be sufficient to achieve at least a 30–40% reduction in LDL-C levels

[b]CHD includes history of myocardial infarction, unstable angina, stable angina, coronary artery procedures (angioplasty or bypass surgery), or evidence of clinically significant myocardial ischemia

[c]CHD risk equivalents include clinical manifestations of noncoronary forms of atherosclerotic disease (peripheral arterial disease, abdominal aortic aneurysm, and carotid artery disease _transient ischemic attacks or stroke of carotid origin or _50% obstruction of a carotid artery_), diabetes, and 2_ risk factors with 10-year risk for hard CHD _20%

[d]Very high risk favors the optional LDL-C goal of _70 mg/dL, and in patients with high triglycerides, non-HDL-C _100 mg/dL. Optional LDL-C goal _100 mg/dL

[e]Any person at high risk or moderately high risk who has lifestyle-related risk factors (e.g. obesity, physical inactivity, elevated triglyceride, low HDL-C, or metabolic syndrome) is a candidate for therapeutic lifestyle changes to modify these risk factors regardless of LDL-C level

[f]If baseline LDL-C is _100 mg/dL, institution of an LDL-lowering drug is a therapeutic option on the basis of available clinical trial results. If a high-risk person has high triglycerides or low HDL-C, combining a fibrate or nicotinic acid with an LDL-lowering drug can be considered

[g]Risk factors include cigarette smoking, hypertension (BP ≷140/90 mm Hg or on antihypertensive medication), low HDL cholesterol (_40 mg/dL), family history of premature CHD (CHD in male first-degree relative _55 years of age; CHD in female first-degree relative <65 years of age), and age (men ≷45 years; women <55 years)

[h]Electronic 10-year risk calculators are available at www.nhlbi.nih.gov/guidelines/cholesterol

[i]For moderately high-risk persons, when LDL-C level is 100–129 mg/dL, at baseline or on lifestyle therapy, initiation of an LDL-lowering drug to achieve an LDL-C level _100 mg/d L is a therapeutic option on the basis of available clinical trial results

[j]Almost all people with zero or 1 risk factor have a 10-year risk _10%, and 10-year risk assessment in people with zero or 1 risk factor is thus not necessary

with 10 mg of atorvastatin for 4 weeks, 12 months of study medication reduced LDL-C from 106±22 to 87±33 mg/dL in the group randomized to receive 80 mg of atorvastatin (*P*<0.001), whereas levels remained stable in the group randomized to receive 10 mg (108±23 at baseline, 109±28 mg/dL at the end of the study, P=NS). After 12 months, CAC scores increased from baseline by 27% in the atorvastatin 80-mg/day group as compared to 25% in the 10-mg/day group (*P*=0.65). CAC progression showed no relationship with on-treatment LDL-C levels.

The lack of effect of statin therapy on CAC suggests that either this measure of plaque burden may be independent of LDL-C, or other markers affected by statin therapy, or, alternatively, the 12-month follow-up period may have been too short to detect a significant treatment effect. On the other hand as previously discussed, Nichols et al. [36] have recently reported that patients with a greater amount of coronary atheroma calcification are less likely to undergo changes in plaque volume in response to intensive risk factor modification. This finding suggests that CAC identifies subjects at high cardiovascular risk but currently may not be employed as marker to track the effectiveness of statin therapy. However, these results should not discourage the use of statins in subjects considered as high risk as determined by high CAC burdens. Benefits were shown in a post-hoc analysis in the St Francis Heart Study in subjects who had calcium scores >400 [45]. In that study there was a 42% reduction (8.7 vs. 15.0%) in cardiovascular events in subjects who received atorvastatin and aspirin vs. aspirin alone, *P*=0.046).

LDL-CHOLESTEROL LOWERING AND CARDIOVASCULAR DISEASE PREVENTION

The evidence that LDL-C lowering with statins prevents cardiovascular disease comes from more than100,000 patients enrolled in randomized controlled trials, comparing statins with placebo and more recently low dose vs. high dose, or more potent vs. less potent statins [47, 48].

The pre-specified meta-analysis of the Cholesterol Trialists (CTT) [47] involving 90,056 patients that had participated in 14 statin trials, worked with patient level data and clearly showed a reduction in mortality and coronary events during a follow-up of 5 years. There was a linear relation between LDL-C lowering and cardiovascular event reduction. A 12% proportional reduction in all-cause mortality per 39 mg/dL (1mmol/L) reduction in LDL-C [rate ratio (RR) 0.88, 95% CI 0.84–0.91; *P*<0.0001] was obtained. This reflected a 19% reduction in coronary mortality (0.81, 0.76–0.85; *P*<0.0001), There were corresponding reductions in myocardial infarction or coronary death (0.77, 0.74–0.80; *P*<0.0001), in the need for coronary revascularization (0.76, 0.73–0.80; *P*<0.0001), in fatal or nonfatal stroke (0.83, 0.78–0.88; *P*<0.0001), and, combining these, of 21% in any such major vascular event (0.79, 0.77–0.81; *P*<0.0001). The meta-analysis clearly shows that greater LDL-C reductions implicate greater benefits.

Benefits were similar, irrespective of gender, smoking status, blood pressure, diabetes status, previous cardiovascular disease or not. As expected the absolute reduction was greater in higher risk subjects, approximately half the patients needed to be treated in secondary rather than in primary prevention trials. The longer the treatment the greater the benefit, 10% per 39 mg/dL reduction in the first year vs. 20–30% in the following years. There was no increase in cancer deaths or hemorrhagic strokes with LDL-C lowering.

Recently another meta-analysis comprising 27,548 subjects [48] enrolled in secondary prevention studies, the TNT, and IDEAL trials that involved patients with stable CHD, and the PROVE IT–TIMI-22 and A-to-Z in acute coronary syndrome patients, compared conventional with intensive lipid-lowering therapy with statins. The mean attained LDL-C was 75 mg/dL (1.9 mmol/L) in the intensive treatment, vs. 101 mg/dL (2.5 mmol/L) mean in the conventional statin treatment. Intensive

LDL-C lowering was superior to conventional treatment in preventing myocardial infarction or coronary death (16% odds reduction (95%CI 0.77–0.91, $P<0.00001$) and also caused a 16% odds reduction in coronary death and any cardiovascular event (95% CI 0.80–0.89, $P<0.00001$). The 26 mg/dL (0.67 mmol/L) difference in LDL-C levels between intensive and conventional LDL-C lowering fitted the regression line of the CTT meta-analysis [47].

The advent of more potent statins like atorvastatin and rosuvastatin and the development of the cholesterol intestinal blocker ezetimibe has increased the potential of greater LDL-C reduction, to values around 50–70% [49]. These potent medications open a window of opportunity for intensive LDL-C lowering and improved cardiovascular disease prevention.

Whether additional benefits secondary to triglyceride-rich lipoprotein and inflammation, e.g. C-reactive protein lowering as suggested by the PROVE-IT study [50] where patients that benefited the most were those with LDL-C <70 mg/dL and C-reactive protein <2.0 mg/L, as well as HDL-cholesterol raising add substantial benefit to LDL-C lowering, remains to be determined.

CURRENT GUIDELINES FOR CARDIOVASCULAR DISEASE PREVENTION AND LDL-C LOWERING: CURRENT ISSUES AND FUTURE

LDL-C Lowering After the NCEP Guideline Update in 2004

At the end of 2004, the NCEP updated its guideline goals for CHD [4]. In patients with known atherosclerotic disease and aggravating risk factors like diabetes, the metabolic syndrome, low HDL-C, smoking and after an acute coronary syndrome, an LDL-C goal of <70 mg/dL was suggested. For other high risk subjects the LDL-C <100 mg/dL was maintained as was the case for the <130 and <160 mg/dL goals for lower risk subjects. It's important to emphasize that not only the LDL-C goals were reinforced but also the secondary non-HDL cholesterol goals that represent the atherogenic triglyceride-rich lipoproteins. The LDL-C <70 mg/dL was proposed based on the results of the PROVE-IT trial where patients that benefited the most, attained those LDL-C levels [50]. The NCEP also recommended that LDL-C reduction should be in the order of 30–40%. However, it's important to notice that at the time the NCEP was updated, neither the CTT [47] nor Cannon's [48] meta-analysis had been published, and the benefits of greater LDL-C reductions in non-acute coronary syndrome patients were not known.

Considering that usually LDL-C is around 140 mg/dL in patients who suffer a myocardial infarction [14], we believe that an LDL-C <70 mg/dL, that signifies a 50% reduction in LDL-C, must be pursued in those individuals. Moreover, subjects with lower baseline LDL-C levels might be treated, by aiming at not only getting to an LDL-C <70 mg/dL, but also with LDL-C reductions <50%. On the same token, an LDL-C <100 mg/dL for high risk individuals without clinical manifestations of atherosclerotic disease, e.g. diabetics or subjects with calculated CHD risk >20% in 10 years, may not be enough to prevent disease adequately and lower LDL-C values might be necessary, based on the current evidence. However, prospective trials are necessary for this population and also for intermediate risk subjects. Studies like the JUPITER trial [51], that has enrolled 17,802 increased risk subjects based on inflammation, .e.g. a high-sensitivity C- reactive protein levels >2.0 mg/L, with a median LDL-C of 108 mg/dL(2.7 mmol/L), and that receive 20 mg of rosuvastatin that can reduce LDL-C by up to 50% may help to answer this question.

LDL-C Lowering and the SHAPE Guidelines for Cardiovascular Disease Prevention

The SHAPE guidelines for cardiovascular disease prevention [10] will be discussed more deeply in other parts of this book. These guidelines are based not only on clinical risk stratification but also

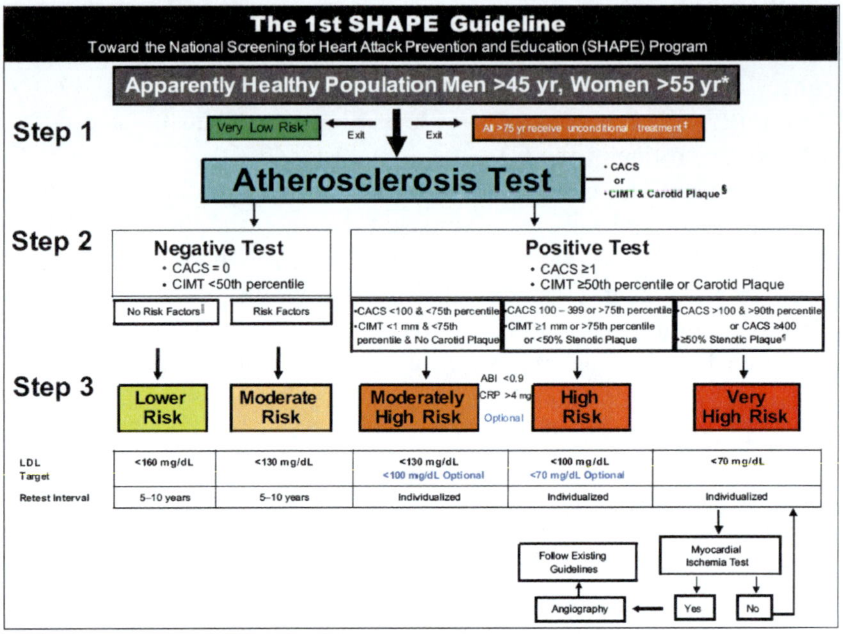

Fig. 1. Recommendations for LDL-C lowering according to SHAPE guidelines [10]

on the detection and evaluation of subclinical atherosclerosis burden (Fig. 1). The premise behind this guideline is that the higher the atherosclerotic plaque burden the higher the risk of clinical events. Consequently, similar to the NCEP guidelines [3, 4], subjects at higher level of risk should be treated more aggressively regarding their LDL-C levels. Furthermore, if started early, a longer term LDL-C reduction could be most effective in preventing cardiovascular events, as seen previously [17, 47].

Individuals with negative tests for atherosclerosis (defined as coronary calcium scores (CACS) = 0, or CIMT <50th percentile without carotid plaque) are classified as lower risk (those without conventional risk factors) or moderate risk (those with established risk factors), and treated as recommended in the NCEP guidelines, with LDL-C targets of <160 mg/dL (4.14 mmol/L) and <130 mg/dL (3.37 mmol/L), respectively. Reassessment is recommended within 5–10 years unless otherwise indicated. Those who test positive for atherosclerosis (CACS ≥1, or CIMT ≥50th percentile or presence of carotid plaque) are further stratified according to the magnitude of atherosclerotic burden into the following risk categories:

(a) Moderately high risk: CACS <100 (but >0) and >75th percentile, or a CIMT <1 mm and <75th percentile (but ≥50th percentile) without discernible carotid plaque. Treatment includes lifestyle modifications and a LDL-C goal of <130 mg/dL (3.37 mmol/L); targeting to 100 mg/dL (2.59 mmol/L) is optional.
(b) High risk: CACS 100–399 or >75th percentile, or a CIMT ≥1 mm or >75th percentile or a carotid plaque causing <50% stenosis. Aggressive lifestyle modifications should be implemented as well as a LDL-C target of <100 mg/dL (2.59 mmol/L); targeting to <70 mg/dL (1.82 mmol/L) is optional.
(c) Very high risk: CACS ≥100 and >90th percentile or a CACS ≥400, or carotid plaque causing ≥50% stenosis. Treatment includes aggressive lifestyle modifications and a LDL-C goal of <70 mg/dL (1.82 mmol/L).

CONCLUSIONS

LDL-C levels are directly associated with the prevalence of CHD. It has been demonstrated that LDL-C reduction not only reduces progression but can induce atherosclerosis regression in the carotid and coronary arteries and in the aorta. Most importantly there is a linear relation between LDL-C lowering and cardiovascular disease reduction. Subjects considered at high risk on clinical evaluation and possibly those who present high subclinical atherosclerotic burden must be treated with intensive LDL-C lowering therapy.

REFERENCES

1. The global significance of cardiovascular disease. In a race against time: The challenging of cardiovascular disease in developing economies . Sacks J ed. The Center for global health and economic development , The Trustees of Columbia University New York, 2004:11–15.
2. Teramoto T, Sasaki J, Ueshima H, Egusa G, Kinoshita M, Shimamoto K, Daida H, Biro S, Hirobe K, Funahashi T, Yokote K, Yokode M. Japan Atherosclerosis Society (JAS) Committee for epidemiology and clinical management of atherosclerosis. Diagnostic criteria for dyslipidemia. Executive summary of Japan Atherosclerosis Society (JAS) guideline for diagnosis and prevention of atherosclerotic cardiovascular diseases for Japanese. *J Atheroscler Thromb*. 2007;14:155–8.
3. Expert panel on detection, evaluation, and treatment of high blood cholesterol in adults. Third report of the National Cholesterol Education Program (NCEP) Expert panel on detection, evaluation, and treatment of High blood cholesterol in adults (Adult Treatment Panel III). Final report. *Circulation.* 2002;106:3143–421.
4. Grundy SM, Cleeman JI, Bairey CN, et al, for the Coordinating Committee of the National Cholesterol Education Program. Implications of recent clinical trials for the National Cholesterol Education Program Adult Treatment Panel III guidelines. *Circulation.* 2004;110:227–39.
5. Fourth Joint Task Force of the European Society of Cardiology and other societies on cardiovascular disease prevention in clinical practice. European guidelines on cardiovascular disease prevention in clinical practice: executive summary. *Eur Heart J.* 2007;28(19):2375–414.
6. American Heart Association. Heart Disease and Stroke Statistics – 2007 Update. Dallas, Texas:American Heart Association; 2007.
7. Grundy SM. Age as a risk factor: you are as old as your arteries. *Am J Cardiol.* 1999;83:1455–7.
8. Budoff MJ, Achenbach S, Blumenthal RS, et al. Assessment of coronary artery disease by cardiac computed tomography. A scientific statement from the American Heart Association Committee on Cardiovascular Imaging and Intervention, Council on Cardiovascular Radiology and Intervention, and Committee on Cardiac Imaging, Council on Clinical Cardiology. *Circulation.* 2006;114:1761–91.
9. Baldassarre D, Amato M, Pustina L, et al. Measurement of carotid artery intima-media thickness in dyslipidemic patients increases the power of traditional risk factors to predict cardiovascular events. *Atherosclerosis.* 2007;191:403–08.
10. Naghavi M, Falk E, Hecht HS, Jamieson MJ et al. SHAPE Task Force from vulnerable plaque to vulnerable patient – Part III: Executive summary of the Screening for Heart Attack Prevention and Education (SHAPE) Task Force report. *Am J Cardiol.* 2006;98(2A):2H–15.
11. Ross R. Atherosclerosis – an inflammatory disease. *N Engl J Med.* 1999;340:115–26.
12. Verschuren WM, Jacobs DR, Bloemberg BP et al. Serum total cholesterol and long-term coronary heart disease mortality in different cultures. Twenty-five-year follow-up of the seven countries study. *JAMA.* 1995;274:131–6.
13. Stamler J, Wentworth D, Neaton JD. Is relationship between serum cholesterol and risk of premature death from coronary heart disease continuous and graded? Findings in 356,222 primary screenees of the Multiple Risk Factor Intervention Trial (MRFIT). *JAMA.* 1986 ;256:2823–8.
14. Castelli WP, Garrison RJ, Wilson PW, Abbott RD, Kalousdian S, Kannel WB. Incidence of coronary heart disease and lipoprotein cholesterol levels. The Framingham Study. *JAMA.* 1986;256:2835–8.
15. Cullen P, Schulte H, Assmann G. The Münster Heart Study (PROCAM): total mortality in middle-aged men is increased at low total and LDL cholesterol concentrations in smokers but not in nonsmokers. *Circulation.* 1997;96:2128–36.
16. Chen Z, Peto R, Collins R, MacMahon S, Lu J, Li W. Serum cholesterol concentration and coronary heart disease in population with low cholesterol concentrations. *BMJ.* 1991;303:276–82.
17. Cohen JC, Boerwinkle E, Mosley TH Jr, Hobbs HH. Sequence variations in PCSK9, low LDL, and protection against coronary heart disease. *N Engl J Med.* 2006;354:1264–72.
18. Robertson TL, Kato H, Rhoads GG, Kagan A, Marmot M, Syme SL, Gordon T, Worth RM, Belsky JL, Dock DS, Miyanishi M, Kawamoto S. Epidemiologic studies of coronary heart disease and stroke in Japanese men living in Japan, Hawaii and California. Incidence of myocardial infarction and death from coronary heart disease. *Am J Cardiol.* 1977;39:239–43.

19. Prospective Studies Collaboration, Lewington S, Whitlock G, Clarke R, Sherliker P, Emberson J, Halsey J, Qizilbash N, Peto R, Collins R. Blood cholesterol and vascular mortality by age, sex, and blood pressure: a meta-analysis of individual data from 61 prospective studies with 55,000 vascular deaths. *Lancet*. 2007;370:1829–39.
20. Lalanne F, Lambert G, Amar MJ, et al. Wild-type PCSK9 inhibits LDL clearance but does not affect apoB-containing lipoprotein production in mouse and cultured cells. *J Lipid Res*. 2005;46:1312–9.
21. Davignon J. Beneficial cardiovascular pleiotropic effects of statins *Circulation*. 2004;109(Suppl 1):III39–43.
22. Blankenhorn DH, Azen SP, Kramsch DM, et al., and the MARS Research Group. Coronary angiographic changes with lovastatin therapy: the Monitored Atherosclerosis Regression Study. *Ann Intern Med*. 1993;119:969–76.
23. Crouse JR III, Byington RP, Bond MG, et al. Pravastatin, lipids, and atherosclerosis in the carotid arteries (PLAC-II). *Am J Cardiol*. 1995;75:455-9.
24. Ballantyne CM, Herd JA, Dunn JK, Jones PH, Farmer JA, Gotto AM Jr. Effects of lipid lowering therapy on progression of coronary and carotid artery disease. *Curr Opin Lipidol*. 1997;8:354–61.
25. Nissen SE, Tuzcu EM, Schoenhagen P, et al, for the REVERSAL Investigators. Effect of intensive compared with moderate lipid-lowering therapy on progression of coronary atherosclerosis. A randomized controlled trial. *JAMA*. 2004;291:1071–80.
26. Nissen SE, Nicholls SJ, Sipahi I, et al, for the ASTEROID Investigators. Effect of very high-intensity statin therapy on regression of coronary atherosclerosis. The ASTEROID trial. *JAMA*. 2006;295:1556–65.
27. Smilde TJ, van Wissen S, Wollersheim H, Trip MD, Kastelein JJP, Stalenhoef AFH. Effect of aggressive versus conventional lipid lowering on atherosclerosis progression in familial hypercholesterolemia (ASAP): a prospective, randomised, double-blind trial. *Lancet*. 2001;357:577–81.
28. Wiegman A, Hutten BA, de Groot E, Rodenburg J, Bakker HD, Büller HR, Sijbrands EJ, Kastelein JJ. Efficacy and safety of statin therapy in children with familial hypercholesterolemia: a randomized controlled trial. *JAMA*. 2004;292:331–7.
29. Crouse JR III, Raichlen JS, Riley WA, et al, for the METEOR Study. Effect of rosuvastatin on progression of carotid intima-media thickness in low-risk individuals with subclinical atherosclerosis. The METEOR trial. *JAMA*. 2007;297:1344–53.
30. Corti R, Fuster V, Fayad ZA, Worthley SG, Helft G, Smith D, Weinberger J, Wentzel J, Mizsei G, Mercuri M, Badimon JJ. Lipid lowering by simvastatin induces regression of human atherosclerotic lesions: two years' follow-up by high-resolution noninvasive magnetic resonance imaging. *Circulation*. 2002;106:2884–7.
31. Lima JAC; Desai MY, Steen H, Warren WP, Gautam S, Lai S. Statin-induced cholesterol lowering and plaque regression after 6 Months of magnetic resonance imaging – monitored therapy. *Circulation*. 2004;110:2336–41.
32. Callister TQ, Raggi P, Cooil B, Lippolis NJ, Russo DJ. Effect of HMG-CoA reductase inhibitors on coronary artery disease as assessed by electron-beam computed tomography. *N Engl J Med*. 1998;339:1972–8.
33. Schmermund A, Achenbach S, Budde T, et al. Effect of intensive versus standard lipid-lowering treatment with atorvastatin on the progression of calcified coronary atherosclerosis over 12 months. A multicenter, randomized, double-blind trial. *Circulation*. 2006;113:427–37.
34. Falk E, Shah PK, Fuster V. Coronary plaque disruption. *Circulation*. 1995;92:657–71.
35. O'Keefe, JR, JH, Cordain L, Harris WH, Moe RM, Vogel R. Optimal low-density lipoprotein is 50 to 70 mg/dl lower is better and physiologically normal. *J Am Coll Cardiol*. 2004;43:2142–46.
36. Nicholls SJ, Tuzcu EM, Sipahi I, et al. Statins, high-density lipoprotein cholesterol, and regression of coronary atherosclerosis. *JAMA*. 2007;297:499–508.
37. Nissen SE, Tuzcu EM, Schoenhagen P, et al, for the REVERSAL Investigators. Statin therapy, LDL cholesterol, C-reactive protein, and coronary artery disease. *N Engl J Med*. 2005;352:29–38.
38. Raggi P, Davidson M, Callister TQ, et al. Aggressive versus moderate lipid-lowering therapy in hyper cholesterolemic postmenopausal women. Beyond Endorsed Lipid Lowering with EBT Scanning (BELLES). *Circulation*. 2005;112:563–71.
39. Crisby M, Nordin-Fredriksson G, MD; Shah PK, Yano J, Zhu J, Nilsson J. Pravastatin treatment increases collagen content and decreases lipid content, inflammation, metalloproteinases, and cell death in human carotid plaques implications for plaque stabilization. *Circulation*. 2001;103:926–33.
40. Lorenz MW, Markus HS, Bots ML, Rosvall M, Sitzer M. Prediction of clinical cardiovascular events with carotid intima-media thickness. A systematic review and meta-analysis. *Circulation*. 2007;115:459–67.
41. Espeland MA, O'Leary DH, Terry JG, Morgan T, Evans G, Mudra H. Carotid intimal-media thickness as a surrogate for cardiovascular disease events in trials of HMG-CoA reductase inhibitors. *Curr Controlled Trials Cardiovasc Med*. 2005;6:3–4.
42. Taylor AJ, Kent SM, Flaherty PJ, Coyle LC, Markwood TT, Vernalis MN. ARBITER: Arterial Biology for the Investigation of the Treatment Effects of Reducing Cholesterol. A randomized trial comparing the effects of atorvastatin and pravastatin on carotid intimal medial thickness. *Circulation*. 2002;106:2055–60.
43. Santos RD, Nasir K, Rumberger JA, Budoff MJ, Braunstein JB, Meneghelo R, Barreiros M, Pereirinha A, Carvalho JA, Blumenthal RS, Raggi P. Difference in atherosclerosis burden in different nations and continents assessed by coronary artery calcium. *Atherosclerosis*. 2006;187:378–84.
44. Greenland P, LaBree L, Azen SP, Doherty TM, Detrano RC. Coronary artery calcium score combined with Framingham score for risk prediction in asymptomatic individuals. *JAMA*. 2004;291:210–5.
45. Arad Y, Spadaro LA, Roth M, Newstein D, Guerci AD. Treatment of asymptomatic adults with elevated coronary calcium scores with atorvastatin, vitamin C, and vitamin E: the St. Francis Heart Study randomized clinical trial. *J Am Coll Cardiol*. 2005;46:166–172.

46. Raggi P, Callister TQ, Shaw LJ. Progression of coronary artery calcium and risk of first myocardial infarction in patients receiving cholesterol-lowering therapy. *Arterioscler Thromb Vasc Biol*. 2004;24:1272–77.
47. Baigent C, Keech A, Kearney PM, Blackwell L, Buck G, Pollicino C, Kirby A, Sourjina T, Peto R, Collins R, Simes R. Cholesterol Treatment Trialists' (CTT) Collaborators. Efficacy and safety of cholesterol-lowering treatment: prospective meta-analysis of data from 90,056 participants in 14 randomised trials of statins. *Lancet*. 2005;366:1267–78.
48. Cannon CP, Steinberg BA, Murphy SA, Mega JL, Braunwald E. Meta-analysis of cardiovascular outcomes trials comparing intensive versus moderate statin therapy. *J Am Coll Cardiol*. 2006;48:438–45.
49. Ballantyne CM, Weiss R, Moccetti T, Vogt A, Eber B, Sosef F, Duffield E; Efficacy and safety of rosuvastatin 40 mg alone or in combination with ezetimibe in patients at high risk of cardiovascular disease (results from the EXPLORER study). *Am J Cardiol*. 2007 ;99:673–80.
50. Ridker PM, Cannon CP, Morrow D, et al, for the Pravastatin or Atorvastatin Evaluation and Infection Therapy – Thrombolysis in Myocardial Infarction 22 (PROVE IT-TIMI 22) Investigators. C-reactive protein levels and outcomes after statin therapy. *N Engl J Med*. 2005;352:20–8.
51. Ridker PM, Fonseca FA, Genest J, Gotto AM, Kastelein JJ, Khurmi NS, Koenig W, Libby P, Lorenzatti AJ, Nordestgaard BG, Shepherd J, Willerson JT, Glynn RJ; JUPITER Trial Study Group. Baseline characteristics of participants in the JUPITER trial, a randomized placebo-controlled primary prevention trial of statin therapy among individuals with low low-density lipoprotein cholesterol and elevated high-sensitivity C-reactive protein. *Am J Cardiol*. 2007;100:1659–64.

48 Antioxidants as Targeted Therapy: A Special Protective Role for Pomegranate and Paraoxonases (PONs)

Mira Rosenblat and Michael Aviram

CONTENTS

ABSTRACT

Increased oxidative stress exists in patients with high risk for atherosclerosis development (hypercholesterolemic, hypertensive, diabetic). This phenomenon is associated with reduced antioxidant status [decreased levels of vitamin E, carotenoids, superoxide dismutase (SOD), catalase, glutathione, and HDL-associated paraoxonase 1 (PON1) activity]. Oxidative stress in atherosclerotic patients exists also in their blood, as well as in arterial wall cells, including macrophages (the hallmark of foam cells in early atherogenesis).

The use of nutritional antioxidants such as vitamin E, carotenoids (lycopene and ß-carotene), and polyphenols (such as those present in red wine, licorice root, or pomegranate) by atherosclerotic patients reduces oxidative stress and attenuates atherosclerosis development. This latter phenomenon is related to protective direct effects of nutritional antioxidants, and to indirect effect by increasing serum HDL-associated paraoxonase activity, which results in the breakdown of specific lipid peroxides.

Key words: Atherosclerosis; Oxidative stress; Macrophages; Antioxidants; Pomegranate; Paraoxonases (PONs)

From: *Asymptomatic Atherosclerosis: Pathophysiology, Detection and Treatment*
Edited by: M. Naghavi (ed.), DOI 10.1007/978-1-60327-179-0_48

TOPIC PEARLS

The use of nutritional antioxidants such as vitamin E, carotenoids (lycopene and ß-carotene), and polyphenols (such as those present in red wine, licorice root, or pomegranate) by atherosclerotic patients reduces oxidative stress and attenuates atherosclerosis development. This latter phenomenon is related to protective direct effects of nutritional antioxidants, and to indirect effect by increasing serum HDL-associated paraoxonase activity, which results in the breakdown of specific lipid peroxides.

OXIDATIVE STRESS AND ATHEROSCLEROSIS

The oxidative modification hypothesis of atherosclerosis proposes that LDL oxidation plays a pivotal role in early atherogenesis. This hypothesis is supported by evidence that oxidized LDL (Ox-LDL) is present in the atherosclerotic lesion and that LDL oxidation takes place in vivo. By using specific antibodies against Ox-LDL, it was demonstrated that elevated levels of circulating Ox-LDL also exist in human plasma from patients with cardiovascular diseases [1]. Furthermore, serum Ox-LDL levels are higher in patients with unstable coronary artery disease (CAD) than in healthy subjects, and correlate with the presence of angiographically documented complicated plaques [2], thus identifying those patients who are at increased risk for future myocardial infarction (MI), independent of other risks. Other serum markers for oxidative stress in CAD patients include urinary 8-isoprostane [2] and plasma advanced oxidation protein products [3]. Elevated serum lipid peroxidation biomarkers in CAD patients were associated with reduced antioxidant status (decreased levels of glutathione, vitamin A, vitamin E, and carotenoids [4]). Among CAD patients, diabetes mellitus (DM) is associated with high risk for developing atherosclerosis and its complications, i.e., stroke, MI, and peripheral vascular disease. Several risk factors have been proposed to explain the increased risk for CAD in DM patients including hyperglycemia, dyslipidemia, accelerated formation of advanced glycation end-products (AGEs), increased oxidative stress, and also genetic factors [5]. Similarly, in patients with renal failure, a positive relationship between oxidative stress and intima-media thickness (IMT) was noted [6].

In hypertensive patients, the increased levels of angiotensin II, the active vasoconstrictor produced by the rennin–angiotensin–aldosterone system (RAAS), were shown to be associated with increased LDL oxidation [7]. The process of LDL oxidation is unlikely to occur in serum in a significant amount, since serum contains high concentrations of antioxidants and metal ion chelators. LDL oxidation is more likely to occur mostly within the artery wall, an environment, which is poor in antioxidants. The identity of the arterial cells responsible for LDL oxidation is uncertain. Macrophages are the prominent cells in early atherogenesis [8, 9], and they can oxidize LDL under atherogenic conditions. Macrophage-mediated oxidation of LDL depends on the balance between prooxidants and antioxidants both in the lipoproteins and in the cells (Fig. 1). Oxidized LDL is taken up by the macrophages at enhanced rate, leading to their conversion into foam cells [8–10]. Furthermore, Ox-LDL was recently shown to induce monocyte-to-macrophage differentiation also in vivo [11]. Macrophage cholesterol accumulation can result not only from increased uptake of modified LDLs, but also from increased cholesterol biosynthesis rate, and/or from decreased rate of HDL-mediated cholesterol efflux from the cells [10]. Oxidative stress in CAD patients exists not only in their serum lipoproteins, but also in their arterial wall cells, including their macrophages. We have previously shown that the increased oxidative stress in macrophages significantly affects their biological activities; these "oxidized macrophages" can oxidize LDL and take up Ox-LDL at enhanced rate [12].

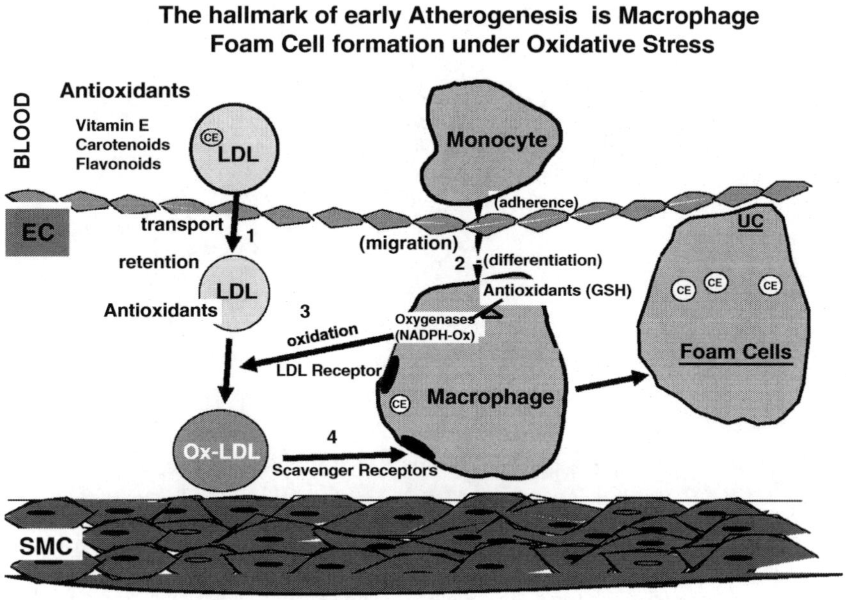

Fig. 1. The hallmark of early atherogenesis is macrophage foam cell formation under oxidative stress. (1) The low density lipoprotein (LDL) particle contains antioxidants mainly vitamin E and carotenoids. Under pathological conditions, the LDL is transported through the endothelium, into the subendothelial space. (2) LDL particles are trapped by proteoglycans, a process called retention. (3) Monocytes from the blood adhere to the endothelium and migrate into the subendothelial space where they are differentiatfed into macrophages. (3) Macrophages can oxidize the retained LDL and convert it into oxidized LDL (Ox-LDL). The extent of macrophage-mediated LDL oxidation depends on the balance between cellular antioxidants (such as reduced glutathione) and oxygenases (such as NADPH-oxidase). (4) Ox-LDL is taken up by the macrophages at enhanced rate via scavenger receptors. (5) Macrophages cholesterol accumulation and foam cell formation. *CE* cholesterol ester, *UC* unesterified cholesterol, *EC* endothelial cells, *SMC* smooth muscle cells, *GSH* reduced glutathione, *NADPH-Ox* NADPH oxidase.

ANTIOXIDANT THERAPY IN CARDIOVASCULAR DISEASES

Since increased oxidative stress was observed in patients with cardiovascular diseases, the use of nutritional antioxidants was suggested for the attenuation of atherosclerosis development [13, 14].

For a compound to be defined as an “antioxidant” it must satisfy at least two basic conditions: (1) When present at low concentration relative to the substrate to be oxidized, it can delay, retard, or prevent auto-oxidation or free radical-mediated oxidation. (2) The resulting compound formed after radical (reactive oxygen species ROS, or reactive nitrogen species, RNS) scavenging must be stable in order to interrupt the oxidation chain reaction.

The oxidation rate of LDL was shown to be reduced by dietary antioxidants intervention in animal models and in humans. The beneficial health effects, attributed to the consumption of fruits and vegetables, are related at least in part, to their antioxidant activity. Dietary antioxidants can inhibit LDL oxidation by several means:

(a) By scavenging free radicals, by chelation of transition metal ions, or by protection of the intrinsic antioxidants in the LDL particle (vitamin E, carotenoids) from oxidation.
(b) By protecting cells in the arterial wall against oxidative damage, and, as a result-inhibition of cell-mediated oxidation of LDL.
(c) By increasing the levels and activity of cellular antioxidants such as: glutathione system, superoxide dismutase (SOD), catalase, or paraoxonases (PONs).

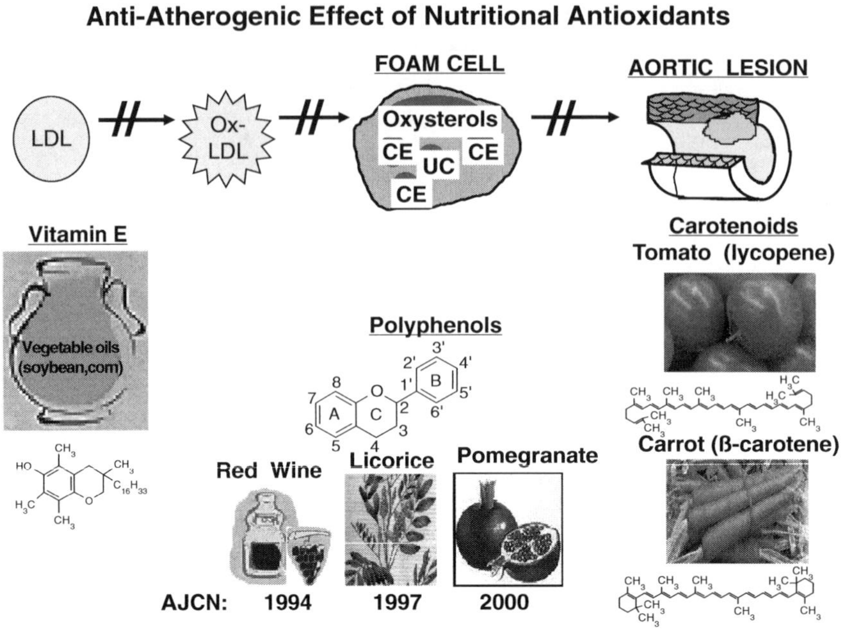

Fig. 2. Antiatherogenic effect of nutritional antioxidants. Three families of antioxidants: vitamin E (present in soybean oil and corn oil), carotenoids (lycopene and ß-carotene), and polyphenols (like those present in red wine, licorice root, or pomegranate) were shown to inhibit low density lipoprotein (LDL) oxidation and its conversion into oxidized LDL (Ox-LDL), to decrease macrophage foam cell formation and to attenuate aortic lesion formation. *CE* cholesterol ester, *UC* unesterfied cholesterol, *AJCN* American Journal of Clinical Nutrition.

EXOGENOUS DIETARY ANTIOXIDANTS

The role of natural antioxidants has been investigated in a large number of epidemiological, clinical, and experimental studies. Human randomized controlled trials, however, were disappointing in contrast to the results obtained in animal studies. This may be related to the fact that natural antioxidants may be effective only in selected subgroups of patients with high levels of oxidative stress (depletion of natural antioxidant defense systems). In addition, the studied dietary antioxidants vitamin E and ß-carotene are much less potent antioxidants and antiatherogenic than the group of polyphenols (which are present at high dose in pomegranate and red wine, Fig. 2).

Vitamin E

Vitamin E (α-Tocopherol) has been proposed to be an important lipid-soluble radical-scavenging antioxidant in cellular and subcellular membranes and also in plasma lipoproteins. Rich sources of vitamin E are vegetable oils, margarine, nuts, seeds, and cereal grains. Vitamin E, however, is not simply a classical antioxidant. It was demonstrated that vitamin E can display neutral, anti-, or even pro-oxidant activity under certain conditions. Vitamin E is regenerated by the water-soluble vitamin C, and also by other coantioxidants, including ubiquinol-10 and a-tocopheryl hydroquinone, which are obtained as part of our diet. Thus, the benefits of vitamin E supplementation together with other antioxidants that act in concert may explain the protection of vitamin-E-rich diet against cardiovascular diseases, more than vitamin E supplements.

Although contradictory findings were reported in the literature regarding vitamin E supplementation, most of the studies demonstrated that populations using vitamin E supplementation are protected against cardiovascular diseases. Alpa-tocopherol supplementation in human subjects has been shown to decrease lipid peroxidation, superoxide production, scavenger receptors (SR-A and CD36) expression, the release of proinflammatory cytokines, and macrophage foam cell formation [15]. Supplementation of alpha-tocopherol and mixed tocopherol to type 2 diabetic patients for 6 weeks resulted in reduced plasma F(2)-isoprostanes. Meta-analysis however showed no evidence of a protective effect for vitamin E on the progression of atherosclerosis [16].

Recently, it was shown that vitamin E supplementation reduces cardiovascular events in individuals with DM that have the haptoglobin 2-2 genotype [17].

Carotenoids

Carotenoids are natural pigments with lipophylic properties, widely distributed in fruits and vegetables, and possess some antioxidant characteristics. β-Carotene and lycopene (which is the open chain analog of β-carotene) are the major carotenoids in human plasma, and they are transported in blood complexed to plasma lipoproteins, mainly to the LDL particle. Supplementation of LDL with β-carotene or with lycopene increases its resistance to oxidation. We have demonstrated that lycopene can indeed act as an effective antioxidant against LDL oxidation in synergism with several natural antioxidants, such as vitamin E, the isoflavan glabridin, and the phenolics rosmarinic and carnosic acid [18]. Dietary carotenoid consumption was shown in epidemiological studies to be associated with reduced cardiovascular mortality. However, intervention trials with carotenoid supplements are still controversial [19]. Low serum levels of carotenoids were associated with an increased risk of subsequent myocardial infarction among smokers, and higher serum carotenoid concentrations were shown to be associated with lower risk of diabetes and insulin resistance in nonsmokers, but not in smokers [20]. An inverse association between carotid IMT and lycopene was observed in patients with essential hypertension and peripheral vascular disease [21]. Furthermore, natural antioxidants from tomato extract reduced blood pressure in patients with grade-1 hypertension [22].

Polyphenolic Flavonoids

Polyphenolic flavonoids constitute one of the largest categories of phytochemicals, most widely distributed among plants, and are integral part of the human diet. Flavonoids compose the largest and most studied group of plant polyphenols, and over 4000 different flavonoids have been identified to date. Flavonoids are powerful antioxidants against LDL oxidation, and their activity is related to their chemical structure. Flavonoids are effective scavengers of hydroxyl and peroxyl radicals, as well as of superoxide anion. Some of them act as antioxidants due to their potent chelation capacity to transition metal ions. Among the different groups of flavonoids, the flavonols, the flavanols, and the isoflavans are the most potent protectors of LDL against oxidation. Furthermore, flavonoids accumulate in macrophages in a time- and dose-dependent manner, and this phenomenon was accompanied by a substantial reduction in the capacity of the flavonoids-enriched cells to oxidize LDL [23]. An inverse association between flavonoids intake and subsequent occurrence of ischemic heart disease, or cerebrovascular disease was indeed shown [24]. In addition to and independent from their antioxidant effect, plant polyphenols demonstrated vasoprotective, antiangiogenic, antiatherogenic, vasorelaxant, and antihypertensive effects.

Licorice

Licorice (Glycyrrhiza Glabra) roots are widely used in Asia as a sweetener or a spice, and it was shown to possess a wide range of therapeutic effects. Glabridin, which is an isoflavan, is the major polyphenol in licorice ethanolic extract (as opposed to the water extract that contains glycerizinic acid). Consumption of licorice ethanolic extract (or glabridin) by humans resulted in an increased resistance of their LDL to oxidation [25]. Similarly, we have shown that glabridin, which is accumulated in macrophages, substantially inhibits cell-mediated oxidation of LDL, superoxide anions release, and the macrophage NADPH oxidase machinery [26]. Structure–function studies revealed that the antioxidant effect of glabridin on LDL oxidation resides mainly in the 2′-hydroxyl group of the isoflavan B ring. The hydrophobic moiety of the isoflavan was also essential in order to obtain the inhibitory effect of glabridin on LDL oxidation, and the position of the hydroxyl groups at the B ring significantly contributes to the ability of glabridin to inhibit LDL oxidation [27].

Red Wine

The grape's skin is a rich source of polyphenols (quercetin, catechin, resveratrol), and thus red wine (unlike white wine), which is prepared by squeezing and storing the whole grape, is a very rich source of polyphenols. Polyphenols from red wine are potent antioxidants and antiatherogenic. In vitro studies demonstrated that polyphenols from red wine are also antiangiogenic, and they suppress human monocyte tissue factor induction [28]. Furthermore, red wine polyphenols, and especially quercetin, stimulate NO-guanylyl cyclase pathway, endothelium-derived hyperpolarizing factor, and entothelin-1, and protect endothelial cells against apoptosis [29]. Epidemiological studies consistently link moderate alcohol consumption with a decreased risk of cardiovascular diseases [30]. Wine consumption by healthy subjects was associated with a significant increase in HDL-cholesterol levels [31], a substantial increase in the resistance of LDL to oxidation [32], and anti-inflammatory effects [33]. Similarly, chronic red wine consumption by hypercholesterolemic postmenopausal women decreased their LDL-cholesterol levels and increased the resistance of their LDL to oxidation [34]. The discrepancy in the extent of LDL oxidation inhibition by red wine consumption could be related to the polyphenol composition of various red wines [35]. The beneficial effects of red wine could be related to both the alcohol and the antioxidant activities of the red wine unique polyphenols [35].

Pomegranate

The pomegranate tree, which is said to have flourished in the Garden of Eden, has been extensively used as a folk medicine in many cultures. The pomegranate fruit contains very potent antioxidants [36]. Pomegranate soluble polyphenols contain hydrolyzable tannins such as the ellagitannin punicalagin, gallic and ellagic acids, as well as anthocyanins and catechins. In vitro studies demonstrated that pomegranate-derived gallic acid, as well as ellagic acid and its unique tannins punicalgin or punicalin and anthocyanins, as well as its unique sugars (which form complexes with the pomegranate phenolics) inhibit LDL oxidation as a result of their free-radical scavenging and metal ion chelation properties [37]. These effects were enhanced when present with other pomegranate polyphenols, as exist in whole fruit [38]. Furthermore, pomegranate juice (PJ) and its purified phenolics or sugars decreased macrophage oxidative stress [37, 39], cholesterol biosynthesis rate, and the extent of Ox-LDL uptake by the cells [40], and these results are associated with PJ effect on oxidation sensitive genes [41]. It was recently demonstrated that pomegranate peels extracts possess similar antiatherogenic properties to PJ, and the flower extract was even more potent [37].

Recent study in healthy human volunteers demonstrated the absorbability of ellagic acid from a pomegranate extract and its ex vivo antioxidant effects [42]. Consumption of PJ by healthy subjects for 2 weeks significantly reduced the oxidation of both LDL and HDL [43]. Studies in patients with carotid artery stenosis (CAS, suffering from a partial blockage in the arteries that supply blood to their brain) who consumed PJ for 3 years clearly demonstrated reduced serum oxidative stress, together with a significant reduction in atherosclerotic lesion size [44]. Similarly, daily consumption of PJ improved stress-induced myocardial ischemia in patients with coronary artery disease [45]. The effect of PJ consumption on blood pressure was also studied. Systolic blood pressure in CAS patients was significantly reduced after PJ consumption for 1 year [44]. Similarly, consumption of PJ by hypertensive patients for only 2 weeks also resulted in a small, but significant, reduction in systolic blood pressure, and in serum ACE activity [46].

In diabetic patients, PJ consumption did not aggravate their diabetic condition, and in fact resulted in a significant reduction in their high oxidative stress, in their serum, as well as in their monocyte-derived macrophages [47].

ENDOGENOUS ANTIOXIDANTS

Glutathione, SOD, Catalase

Cellular antioxidants such as reduced glutathione (GSH), or superoxide dismutase (SOD), or catalase, have an important role in protecting cells against oxidative stress. GSH is the major endogenous antioxidant in mammalian cells, and it is also involved in other cellular functions such as detoxification, amino acid transport, production of coenzymes, and recycling of vitamin E [48]. Furthermore, we have recently demonstrated the antiatherogenic properties of liposomal glutathione [49].

Both SOD and catalase were shown to inhibit Ox-LDL-induced human aortic smooth muscle cell proliferation [50]. Similarly, catalase overexpression attenuated Ox-LDL-induced apoptosis in human aortic endothelial cells [51].

In type 2 diabetic patients with prominent cardiovascular complications, the activities of SOD and glutathione-related enzymes were significantly reduced, and they were negatively correlated with the serum glucose concentration, and the duration of diabetes, and cardiovascular complications [52].

Under oxidative stress, both cellular and serum GSH are converted into oxidized glutathione (GSSG). Serum GSH/GSSG ratio was shown in humans to be an independent predictor of the IMT [53].

Dietary antioxidants can reduce cellular oxidative stress, also secondary to their effect on cellular antioxidants. Experimental data indeed indicated that polyphenols may offer an indirect antioxidant protection by activating endogenous defense systems. Several lines of evidence suggest a tight connection between exogenous and endogenous antioxidants that appear to act in coordinated fashion. Dietary polyphenols can stimulate cellular antioxidant enzyme transcription via antioxidant responsive elements (AREs) which are present in the promoter regions of the related genes [54]. Indeed, in vitro studies demonstrated that the red wine polyphenol resveratrol upregulates SOD [55], catalase, GSH, and gluthathione-related enzymes in cultured aortic smooth muscle cells, or in endothelial cells. High doses of quercetin (another major red wine polyphenol) were also shown to increase GSH concentration and gene expression of Cu/Zn SOD and of catalase in hepatocytes [56].

We have demonstrated that incubation of macrophages with PJ or with the PJ sugar fraction, resulted in an increment in cellular GSH levels [39, 43]. Furthermore, in vivo consumption of PJ by CAS patients increased their lesion GSH levels [44], and consumption of PJ by diabetic patients also increased the GSH levels in the patient's monocytes–macrophages [47].

Paraoxonases (PONs)

The paraoxonase gene family includes PON1, PON2, and PON3 [57]. PONs exhibit a range of activities, including drug metabolism, detoxification of organophosphates (such as nerve agents), and protection against atherosclerosis [57]. PONs are lactonases/lactonizing enzymes, with some overlapping substrates, but their physiological substrates are not known yet [58].

PON1

Most of serum PON1 is HDL associated [58], but low levels of PON1 are also associated with chylomicrons and VLDL, but not with LDL [59]. Apolipoprotein A-I in HDL was shown to stabilize PON1 and to significantly stimulate its lactonase activity [58].

PON1 have two common polymorphisms in the coding region: leucine (L)/methionine (M) at position 55 and glutamine (Q)/arginine(R) at position 192. Previous clinical studies mostly support, but some exclude, a relationship between PON1 polymorphisms and the development of cardiovascular diseases. Furthermore, genetic variation at the PON1 locus has a strong influence on PON1 activity, as well as on carotid IMT. However, serum PON1 concentration and activity are better predictors of the risk for cardiovascular diseases than the PON1 genotype [60]. A negative association was observed between serum PON1 activity and IMT in subjects with CAD [61].

PON1 activity is reduced in type 2 diabetic patients, independent of PON1 genotype, and it correlates with the levels of the patients' plasma Ox-LDL, and with vascular complications [62]. Indeed, PON1 was shown to be inactivated under DM-induced oxidative stress [63]. Smoking in diabetes may be particularly deleterious for PON1, and consequently for the antioxidant capacity of HDL. Furthermore, PON1 activity was found to decrease in parallel to DM duration, and this phenomenon

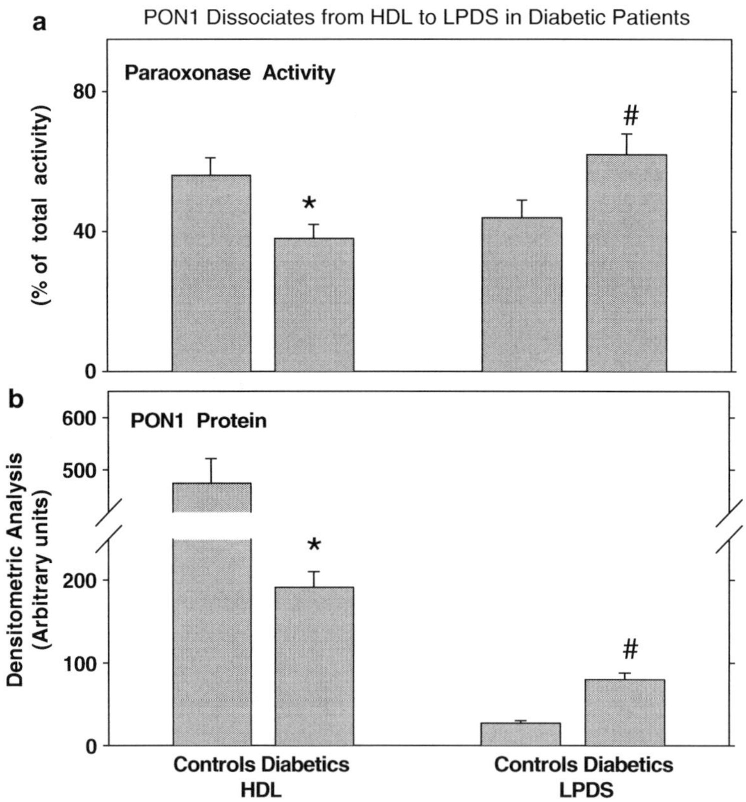

Fig. 3. Paraoxonase 1(PON1) dissociates from high density lipoprotein (HDL) to the lipoprotein-deficient serum (LPDS) in diabetic patients. The HDL and LPDS fractions were isolated from the serum of three healthy subjects (Controls) or from three diabetic patients by density gradient ultracentrifugation. Paraoxonase activity (**a**) was determined in the HDL (HDL-associated PON1) and LPDS fractions (free PON1). PON1 protein was determined by Western blot analysis, and the densitometric analysis of the protein bands is shown (**b**). Results are presented as mean ± SD. *$p<0.01$ Diabetic HDL vs. Control HDL. #$p<0.01$ Diabetic LPDS vs. control LPDS.

may be a factor for acceleration of CAD in DM patients. We have shown that in diabetes, a significant amount of serum PON1 is dissociated from HDL to the lipoprotein-deficient serum (LPDS) fraction (as a free PON1, Fig. 3). Furthermore, we have shown that PON1 in LPDS, unlike PON1 in HDL, is not able to protect against lipid peroxidation and to stimulate macrophage cholesterol efflux [64].

The role of PON1 in atherosclerosis development was demonstrated in studies using mice lacking PON1, or overexpressing PON1. Attenuation of atherosclerosis by PON1 (Fig. 4) can result from its ability to hydrolyze specific oxidized lipids in lipoproteins [65], in arterial wall cells (including macrophages, [66], and in atherosclerotic lesions [67]). PON1 was shown to inhibit cholesterol influx, by reducing the formation of oxidized LDL (Ox-LDL), and its uptake by macrophages. Furthermore, PON1 inhibits cholesterol biosynthesis in macrophages [68] and stimulates HDL-mediated cholesterol efflux from the cells [69]. PON1 activity was also shown to modulate endothelial function in patients with peripheral arterial disease and to reduce monocyte chemotaxis.

Dietary antioxidants can affect PON levels and activities indirectly by reducing oxidative stress, and also directly, by affecting PON's gene expression. In vitro studies demonstrated that antioxidants such as the flavonoids glabridin (from licorice root), quercetin (from red wine), or punicalagin (from pomegranate) when present during LDL oxidation, together with PON1, significantly reduced lipoprotein-associated lipid peroxides content, and preserved PON1 activities, including its ability to hydrolyze Ox-LDL cholesteryl linoleate hydroperoxides [70, 71]. In vitro incubation of HuH7 human hepatoma cell line, with quercetin or with resveratrol, increased PON1 gene expression by an aryl hydrocarbon receptor-dependent mechanism [72].

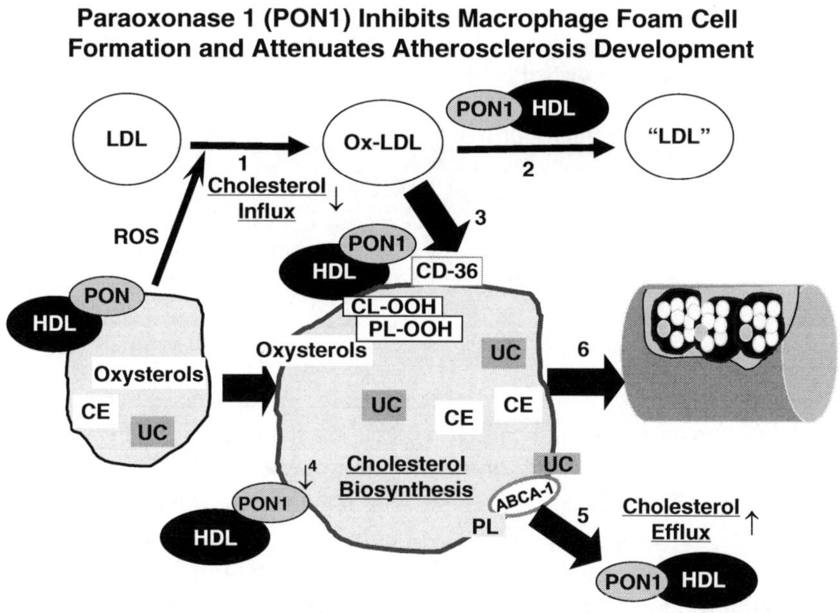

Fig. 4. Paraoxonase 1 (PON1) inhibits macrophage foam cell formation and attenuates atherosclerosis development. (1) High density lipoprotein (HDL)-associated PON1 inhibits macrophage-mediated oxidation of low density lipoprotein (LDL), and its conversion into oxidized LDL (Ox-LDL). (2) PON1 in HDL hydrolyzes oxidized lipids in Ox-LDL, thus converting it to native LDL-like particle ("LDL"). (3) HDL-associated PON1 inhibits cholesterol influx (Ox-LDL uptake) by the macrophages, via the CD-36 scavenger receptor and reduces macrophage oxidative stress. (4) PON1 in HDL inhibits cholesterol biosynthesis in the macrophages, and (5) stimulates HDL-mediated cholesterol efflux via the ABCA1 transporter. (6) All these effects of HDL-associated PON1 lead to attenuation of atherosclerotic lesion development. *ROS* reactive oxygen species, *CL-OOH* cholesteryl linoleate hydroperoxides, *PL-OOH* phospholipids hydroperoxides, *CE* cholesterol ester, *UC* unesterified cholesterol, *PL* phospholipids.

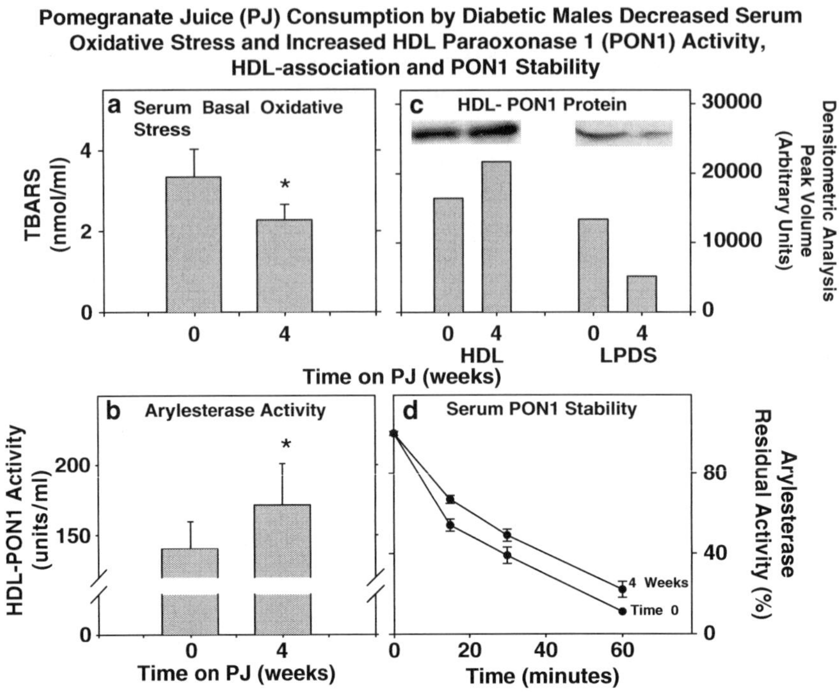

Fig. 5. Pomegranate juice (PJ) consumption by diabetic males decreased serum oxidative stress and increased high density lipoprotein (HDL) paraoxonase 1 (PON1) activity, HDL association, and PON1stability. Ten male patients with type 2 diabetes mellitus consumed pomegranate juice (PJ, 1.5 mmoles of total polyphenols per day) for a period of 1 month. Blood was collected from the diabetic patients (after 12 h of fast) before and 4 weeks after PJ consumption. Basal serum oxidative status was measured by the TBARS assay (**a**). HDL or lipoprotein-deficient serum (LPDS) fractions were isolated from the blood samples of four patients by density gradient ultracentrifugation, and HDL-associated PON1 arylesterase activity was measured (**b**). The HDL fractions (25 μg protein) and LPDS fractions (20 μl) were loaded and run on 10% polyacrylamide gel. PON1 protein band was visualized with mouse antihuman PON1 antibody. Densitometric analysis of a representative experiment of the PON1 bands is shown (**c**). The serum samples were incubated with nitrillioacetate (NTA) for 1 h at 37°C to chelate calcium ions and inactivate the enzyme. Serum PON1 arylesterase residual activity was then measured along the incubation period (**d**). Results are given as mean ± SEM (n=4).

Vitamin C and E intake were also associated with increased paraoxonase activity [73]. Most impressive was the effect of PJ consumption by healthy subjects on stimulating PON1 activity, in association with a reduction in LDL oxidation [43]. PJ administration to patients with CAS for 1 year also resulted in a significant increase in PON1 activity, paralleled by a significant reduction in oxidative stress and in IMT [44]. Furthermore, PJ administration to DM patients resulted in a significant increase in serum and HDL-PON1 activity, and this effect was associated with a reduction in serum oxidative stress [47]. Furthermore, PJ consumption by these patients also increased PON1 binding to the patient's HDL, thus stabilizing the enzyme and improving its activity (Fig. 5).

PON2

Unlike humoral PON1, PON2 is not present in serum. Whereas PON1 is expressed mainly in the liver, but not in arterial macrophages, PON2 is expressed in most tissues, including macrophages [74, 75]. In hypercholesterolemic patients we have demonstrated decreased macrophage PON2 expression [76]. PON2 310 polymorphism was shown to be associated with the presence of microvascular complications in diabetic mellitus [77].

PON2, like PON1, was shown in animal model to have a protective role against atherosclerosis development. PON2 inhibits macrophage-mediated LDL oxidation, and reactive oxygen species (ROS) formation in HeLa and in vascular cells [74, 75, 78]. PON2 expression is upregulated via an NADPH-oxidase – dependent mechanism during monocytes to macrophages differentiation [79]. Upon incubation of J774A.1 macrophages with pomegranate juice, a dose-dependently increased PON2 expression (mRNA and protein), and activity, was noted, paralleled by reduced macrophage oxidative status [80]. These effects could be attributed to the pomegranate unique polyphenols (punicalagin and gallic acid) and are associated with activation of the transcription factors PPAR gamma and AP-1 [80].

Furthermore, PON2 decreases endoplasmic reticulum (ER) stress-induced caspase activation [78]. We have demonstrated that cellular oxidative stress affects macrophage PON2 expression and enzymatic activities in a biphasic U-shape [75, 81].

REFERENCES

1. Mayr M, Kiechl S, Tsimikas S, et al. Oxidized low-density lipoprotein autoantibodies, chronic infections, and carotid atherosclerosis in a population-based study. J. Am. Coll. Cardiol. 2006; 47:2436–2443.
2. Basarici I, Altekin RE, Demir I, et al. Associations of isoprostanes-related oxidative stress with surrogate subclinical and angiographic measure of atherosclerosis. Coron. Artery. Dis. 2007; 18:615–620.
3. Liu SX, Hou FF, Guo ZJ, et al. Advanced oxidation protein products accelerate atherosclerosis through promoting oxidative stress and inflammation. Arterioscler. Thromb. Vasc. Biol. 2006; 26:1156–1162.
4. Polidori MC, Pratico D, Parente B, et al. Elevated lipid peroxidation biomarkers and low antioxidants status in atherosclerotic patients with increased carotid or iliofemoral intima media thickness. J. Invest. Med. 2007; 55:163–167.
5. Renard C, Van Obberghen E. Role of diabetes in atherosclerosis pathogenesis. What have we learned from animal models? Diabetes. Metab. 2006; 32:15–32.
6. Kocak H, Gumuslu S, Ermis C, et al. Oxidative stress and asymmetric dimethylarginine is independently associated with carotid intima media thickness in peritoneal dialysis patients. Am. J. Nephrol. 2008; 28:91-96.
7. Keidar S, Kaplan M, Shapira C, et al. Low density lipoprotein isolated from patients with essential hypertension exhibits increased propensity for oxidation and enhanced uptake by macrophages: a possible role for angiotensin II. Atherosclerosis 1994; 107:71–84.
8. Tiwari RL, Singh V, Barthwal MK. Macrophages: an elusive yet emerging therapeutic target of atherosclerosis. Med. Res. Rev. 2008; 28:483–544.
9. Lusis AJ. Atherosclerosis. Nature 2000; 404:233–241.
10. Aviram M, Rosenblat M. Oxidative stress in cardiovascular disease: role of oxidized lipoproteins in macrophage foam cell formation and atherosclerosis. In: Redox-Genom Interactions in Health and Disease. New York: Dekker; 2003.p. 57–90. Chapter 25.
11. Fuhrman B, Partoush A, Volkova N, et al. Ox-LDL induces monocyte-to macrophage differentiation in vivo: possible role for the macrophage colony stimulating factor receptor (M-CSF-R). Atherosclerosis 2008; 196:598–607.
12. Fuhrman B, Volkova N, Aviram M. Oxidative stress increases the expression of the CD36 scavenger receptors and the cellular uptake of oxidized LDL in macrophages from atherosclerotic mice: protective role of antioxidants and paraoxonase. Atherosclerosis 2002; 161:307–316.
13. Aviram M, Kaplan M, Rosenblat M, et al. Dietary antioxidants and paraoxonases against LDL oxidation and atherosclerosis development. Handb. Exp. Pharmacol. 2005; 170:263–300.
14. Kaliora AC, Deoussis GV, Schmidt H. Dietary antioxidants in preventing atherogenesis. Atherosclerosis 2006; 187:1–17.
15. Singh U, Devaraj S, Jialal I. Vitamin E, oxidative stress, and inflammation. Annu. Rev. Nutr. 2005; 25:151–174.
16. Bleys J, Miller ER, Pastor-Barriuso R, et al. Vitamin–mineral supplementation and the progression of atherosclerosis: a meta-analysis of randomized controlled trials. Am. J. Clin. Nutr. 2006; 84:880–887.
17. Milman U, Blum S, Shapira C, Aronson D, et al. Vitamin E supplementation reduces cardiovascular events in a subgroup of middle-aged individuals with both type 2 diabetes mellitus and the haptoglobin 2-2 genotype: a prospective double-blined clinical trial. Arterioscler. Thromb. Vasc. Biol. 2008; 28:341–347.
18. Fuhrman B, Volkova N, Rosenblat M, et al. Lycopene synergistically inhibits LDL oxidation in combination with vitamin E, glabridin, rosmarinic acid, carnosic acid, or garlic. Antioxid. Redox. Signal. 2000; 2:491–506.
19. Sesso HD. Carotenoids and cardiovascular disease: what research gaps remain? Curr. Opin. Lipidol. 2006; 17:11–16.
20. Hozawa A, Jacobs DR Jr, Steffes MW, et al. Associations of serum carotenoid concentrations with the development of diabetes and with insulin concentration: interaction with smoking: the Coronary Artery Risk Development in Young Adults (CARDIA) Study. Am. J. Epidemiol. 2006; 163:929–937.

21. Gianetti J, Pedrinelli R, Petrucci R, et al. Inverse association between carotid intima-media thickness and the antioxidant lycopene in atherosclerosis. Am. Heart. J. 2002;143:467–474.
22. Engelhard YN, Gazer B, Paran E. Natural antioxidants from tomato extract reduce blood pressure in patients with grade-1 hypertension: a double-blind, placebo- controlled pilot study. Am. Heart. J. 2006; 151:100.
23. Fuhrman B, Aviram M. Flavonoids protect LDL from oxidation and attenuate atherosclerosis. Curr. Opin. Lipidol. 2001; 12:41–48.
24. Knekt P, Kumpulainen J, Jarvinen R, et al. Flavonoid intake and risk of chronic diseases. Am. J. Clin. Nutr. 2002; 76:560–568.
25. Fuhrman B, Buch S, Vaya J, et al. Licorice extract and its major polyphenol glabridin protect low-density lipoprotein against lipid peroxidation: in vitro and ex vivo studies in humans and in atherosclerotic apolipoprotein E-deficient mice. Am. J. Clin. Nutr. 1997; 66:267–275.
26. Rosenblat M, Belinky P, Vaya J, et al. Macrophage enrichment with the isoflavan glabridin inhibits NADPH oxidase-induced cell mediated oxidation of low density lipoprotein. J. Biol. Chem. 1999; 274:13790–13799.
27. Belinky PA, Aviram M, Mahmood S, et al. Structural aspects of the inhibitory effect of glabridin on LDL oxidation. Free. Radic. Biol. Med. 1998; 24:1419–1429.
28. Kaur G, Roberti M, Raul F, et al. Suppression of human monocyte tissue factor induction by red wine phenolics and synthetic derivatives of resveratrol. Thromb. Res. 2007; 119:247–256.
29. Perez-Vizcaino F, Duarte J, et al. Endothelial function and cardiovascular disease: effects of quercetin and wine polyphenols. Free. Radic. Res. 2006; 40:1054–1065.
30. Li JM, Mukamal KJ. An update on alcohol and atherosclerosis. Curr. Opin. Lipidol. 2004; 15:673–680.
31. Hansen AS, Marckmann P, Dragsted LO, et al. Effect of red wine and red grape extract on blood lipids, haemostatic factors, and other risk factors for cardiovascular disease. Eur. J. Clin. Nutr. 2005; 59:449–455.
32. Fuhrman B, Lavy A, and Aviram M. Consumption of red wine with meals reduces the susceptibility of human plasma and LDL to undergo lipid peroxidation. Am. J. Clin. Nutr. 1995; 61:549–554.
33. Estruch R, Sacanella E, Badia E, et al. Different effects of red wine and gin consumption on inflammatory biomarkers of atherosclerosis: a prospective randomized crossover trial. Effects of wine on inflammatory markers. Atherosclerosis 2004; 175:117–123.
34. Naissides M, Mamo JC, Jameas AP, et al. The effect of chronic consumption of red wine on cardiovascular disease risk factors in postmenopausal women. Atherosclerosis 2006; 185:438–445.
35. Howard A, Chopra M, Thurnham D, et al. Red wine consumption and inhibition of LDL oxidation: what are the important components? Med. Hypotheses 2002; 59:101–104.
36. Gil MI, Tomas-Barberan FA, Hess-Pierce B, et al. Antioxidant activity of pomegranate juice and its relationship with phenolics composition and processing. J. Agric. Food. Chem. 2000; 48:4581–4589.
37. Aviram M, Volkova N, Coleman R, et al. Pomegranate phenolics from the peels, arils, and flowers are antiatherogenic: studies in vivo in atherosclerotic apolipoprotein E-deficient mice and in vitro in cultured macrophages and lipoproteins. J. Agric. Food. Chem. 2008; 56:1148–1157.
38. Seeram NP, Adams LS, Henning SM, et al. In vitro antiproliferative, apoptotic and antioxidant activities of punicalagin, ellagic acid and a total pomegranate tannin extract are enhanced in combination with other polyphenols as found in pomegranate juice. J. Nut. Biochem. 2005; 16:360–367.
39. Rozenberg O, Howell A, Aviram M. Pomegranate juice sugar fraction reduces macrophage oxidative stress, whereas white grape juice sugar fraction increases it. Atherosclerosis 2006; 188:68–76.
40. Fuhrman B, Volkova N, Aviram M. Pomegranate juice inhibits oxidized LDL uptake and cholesterol biosynthesis in macrophages. J. Nutr. Biochem. 2005; 16:570–576.
41. De Nigris F, Williams-Ignarro S, Sica V, et al. Effects of a pomegranate fruit extract rich in punicalagin on oxidation-sensitive genes and eNos activity at sites of perturbed shear stress and atherogenesis. Cardiovasc. Res. 2007; 73:414–423.
42. Mertens-Talcott SU, Jilma-Stonhlawetz P, Rios J, et al. Absorption, metabolism, and antioxidant effects of pomegranate (Punica granatum) polyphenols after ingestion of a standardized extract in healthy human volunteers. J. Agric. Food. Chem. 2006; 54:8956–8961.
43. Aviram M, Dornfeld L, Rosenblat M, et al. Pomegranate juice consumption reduces oxidative stress, atherogenic modifications to LDL, and platelet aggregation: studies in humans and in atherosclerotic apolipoprotein E-deficient mice. Am. J. Clin. Nutr. 2000; 71:1062–1076.
44. Aviram M, Rosenblat M, Gaitini D, et al. Pomegranate juice consumption for 3 years by patients with carotid artery stenosis reduces common carotid intima-media thickness, blood pressure and LDL oxidation. Clin. Nutr. 2004; 23:423–433.
45. Sumner MD, Elliott-Eller M, Weidner G, et al. Effects of pomegranate juice consumption on myocardial perfusion in patients with coronary heart disease. Am. J. Cardiol. 2005; 96:810–814.
46. Aviram M, Dornfeld L. Pomegranate juice consumption inhibits serum angiotensin converting enzyme activity and reduces systolic blood pressure. Atherosclerosis 2001; 195–198.
47. Rosenblat M, Hayek T, Aviram M. Anti-oxidative effects of pomegranate juice (PJ) consumption by diabetic patients on serum and on macrophages. Atherosclerosis 2006; 188:68–76.
48. Sies H. Glutathione and its role in cellular functions. Free. Radic. Biol. Med. 1999; 27:916–921.
49. Rosenblat M, Volkova N, Coleman R, et al. Anti-oxidant and anti-atherogenic properties of liposomal glutathione: studies in vitro, and in the atherosclerotic apolipoprotein E-deficient mice. Atherosclerosis 2007; 195:E61–E68.

50. Lin SJ, Shyue SK, Shih MC, et al. Superoxide dismutase and catalase inhibit oxidized low-density lipoprotein-induced human aortic smooth muscle cell proliferation: role of cell-cycle regulation, mitogen-activated protein kinases, and transcription factors. Atherosclerosis 2007; 190:124–134.
51. Lin SJ, Shyue SK, Liu PL, et al. Adenovirus-mediated overexpression of catalase attenuates Ox-LDL induced apoptosis in human aortic endothelial cells via AP-1 and C-Jun N-terminal kinase/extracellular signal-regulated kinase mitogen-activated protein kinase pathways. J. Mol. Cell. Cardiol. 2004; 36:129-139.
52. Colak E, Majkic-Singh N, Stankovic S, et al. Parameters of antioxidative defence in type 2 diabetic patients with cardiovascular complications. Ann. Med. 2005; 37:613–620.
53. Ashfaq S, Abramson JL, Jones DP, et al. The relationship between plasma levels of oxidized and reduced thiols and early atherosclerosis in healthy adults. J. Am. Coll. Cardiol. 2006; 47:1005–1011.
54. Moskaug JO, Carlsen H, Myhrstad MC, et al. Polyphenols and glutathione synthesis regulation. Am. J. Clin. Nutr. 2005; 81:277S–283S.
55. Robb EL, Page MM, Wiens BE, et al. Molecular mechanisms of oxidative stress resistance induced by resveratrol: specific and progressive induction of MnSOD. Biochem. Biophys. Res. Commun. 2008; 367:406–412.
56. Alia M, Mateos R, Ramos S, et al. Influence of quercetin and rulin on growth and antioxidant defense system of a human hepatoma cell lin (HepG2). Eur. J. Nutr. 2006; 45:19–28.
57. Ng CJ, Shih DM, Hama SY, et al. The paraoxonase gene family and atherosclerosis. Free. Radic. Biol. Med. 2005; 38:153–163.
58. Gaidukov L, Tawfik DS. High affinity, stability, and lactonase activity of serum paraoxonase PON1 anchored on HDL with apoA-I. Biochemistry 2005; 44:11843–11854.
59. Fuhrman B, Volkova N, et al. Paraoxonase 1 (PON1) is present in postprandial chylomicrons. Atherosclerosis 2005; 180:55–61.
60. Mackness B, Davies GK, Turkie W, et al. Paraoxonase status in coronary heart disease. Are activity and concentration more important than genotype? Arterioscler. Thromb. Vasc. Biol. 2001; 21:1451–1457.
61. Harangi M, Seres I, Magyar MT, et al. Association between human paraoxonase 1 activity and intima-media thickness in subjects under 55 years of age with carotid artery diseases. Cerebrovasc. Dis. 2007; 25:122–128.
62. Letellier C, Durou MR, Jouanolle AM, et al. Serum paraoxonase activity and paraoxonase gene polymorphism in type 2 diabetic patients with or without vascular complications. Diabetes. Metab. 2002; 28:297–304.
63. Karabina SA, Lehner AN, Frank E, et al. Oxidative inactivation of paraoxonase-implications in diabetes mellitus and atherosclerosis. Biochem. Biophys. Acta. 2005; 1725:213–221.
64. Rosenblat M, Karry R, Aviram M. Paraoxonase 1 (PON1) is a more potent antioxidant and stimulant of macrophage cholesterol efflux, when present in HDL than in lipoprotein-deficient serum: relevance to diabetes. Atherosclerosis 2006; 187:74–81.
65. Aviram M, Rosenblat M, Bisgaier CL, et al. Paraoxonase inhibits high-density lipoprotein oxidation and preserves its functions. A possible peroxidative role for paraoxonase. J. Clin. Invest. 1998; 101:1581–1590.
66. Aviram M, Rosenblat M. Paraoxonases 1, 2 and 3, oxidative stress, and macrophage foam cell formation during atherosclerosis development. Free. Radic. Biol. Chem. 2004; 37:1304–1316.
67. Aviram M, Hardak E, Vaya J, et al. Human serum paraoxonases (PON1) Q and R selectively decrease lipid peroxides in human coronary and carotid atherosclerotic lesions: PON1 esterase and peroxidase-like activities. Circulation 2000; 101:2510–2517.
68. Rozenberg O, Shih DM, Aviram M. Human serum paraoxonase (PON1) decreases macrophage cholesterol biosynthesis: a possible role for its phodpholipase-A_2 activity and lysophosphatidylcholine formation. Arterioscler. Thromb. Vasc. Biol. 2003; 23:461–467.
69. Rosenblat M, Gaidukov L, Khersonsky O, et al. The catalytic histidine dyad of high density lipoprotein-associated serum paraoxonase-1 (PON1) is essential for PON1-mediated inhibition of low density lipoprotein oxidation and stimulation of macrophage cholesterol efflux. J. Biol. Chem. 2006; 281:7657–7665.
70. Aviram M, Rosenblat M, Bisgaier CL, et al. Atorvastatin and gemfibrozil metabolites, but not the parent drugs, are potent antioxidants against lipoprotein oxidation. Atherosclerosis 1998; 138:271–280.
71. Fuhrman B, Aviram M. Preservation of paraoxonase activity by wine flavonoids : possible role in protection of LDL from lipid peroxidation. Ann. N Y. Acad. Sci. 2002; 957:321–324.
72. Gouedard C, Barouki R, Morel Y. Induction of paraoxonase-1 gene expression by resveratrol. Arterioscler. Thromb. Vasc. Biol. 2004; 24:2378–2383.
73. Jarvik GP, Tsai NT, McKinstry LA, et al. Vitamin C and E intake is associated with increased paraoxonase activity. Arterioscler. Thromb. Vasc. Biol. 2002; 22:1329–1333.
74. Ng CJ, Wadleigh DJ, Gangopadhyay A, et al. Paraoxonase-2 is an ubiquitously expressed protein with antioxidant properties, and is capable of preventing cell-mediated oxidative modification of low-density lipoprotein. J. Biol. Chem. 2001; 276:44444–44449.
75. Rosenblat M, Draganov D, Watson CE, et al. Mouse macrophage paraoxonase 2 (PON2) activity is increased whereas cellular PON3 activity is decreased under oxidative stress. Arterioscler. Thromb. Vasc. Biol. 2003; 23:468–474.
76. Rosenblat M, Hayek T, Hussein K, et al. Decreased macrophage paraoxonase 2 expression in patients with hypercholesterolemia is the result of their increased cellular cholesterol content: effect of atorvastatin therapy. Arterioscler. Thromb. Vasc. Biol. 2004; 24:175–180.
77. Mackness B, McElduff P, Mackness MI. The paraoxonase-2-310 polymorphism is associated with the presence of microvascular complications in diabetic mellitus. J. Intern. Med. 2005; 258:363–368.

78. Horke S, Witte I, Wilgenbus P, et al. Paraoxonase-2 reduces oxidative stress in vascular cells and decreases endoplasmic reticulum stress-induced caspase activation. Circulation 2007; 115:2055–2064.
79. Shiner M, Fuhrman B, Aviram M. Paraoxonase 2 (PON2) expression is upregulated via a reduced nicotinamide- adenine-dinucleotide-phosphate (NADPH)-oxidase-dependent mechanism during monocytes differentiation into macrophages. Free. Radical. Biol. Med. 2004; 37:2052–2063.
80. Shiner M, Fuhrman B, Aviram M. Macrophage paraoxonase 2 (PON2) expression is up-regulated by pomegranate juice phenolic anti-oxidants via PPARgamma and AP-1 pathway activation. Atherosclerosis 2007; 195:313–321.
81. Shiner M, Fuhrman B, Aviram M. A biphasic U-shape effect of cellular oxidative stress on the macrophage anti-oxidant paraoxonase 2 (PON2) enzymatic activity. Biochem. Biophys. Res. Commun. 2006; 349:1094–1099.

49 The Multiconstituent Cardiovascular Pill (MCCP): Challenges and Promises of Population Based Prophylactic Drug Therapy for Heart Attack Prevention and Eradication

Michael J. Jamieson, Harvey S. Hecht, and Morteza Naghavi

Contents

Abstract

Risk factors for atherosclerotic cardiovascular disease (CVD) are highly coprevalent but have been poorly identified and treated. The Screening for Heart Attack Prevention and Education (SHAPE) Task Force from the Society for Heart Attack Prevention and Eradication (SHAPE) has proposed a new strategy that recommends screening for subclinical atherosclerosis and implementing aggressive treatment of "vulnerable patients". The Task Force has also envisioned future developments that may shift mass screening strategies to mass prophylactic therapy. The "**Polypill**" concept, introduced by Wald and Law,

From: *Asymptomatic Atherosclerosis: Pathophysiology, Detection and Treatment*
Edited by: M. Naghavi (ed.), DOI 10.1007/978-1-60327-179-0_49

suggests that a combination of statin, low-dose anti-hypertensive, aspirin and folic acid in a single pill taken prophylactically by a high risk population can cut CVD event rates by as much as 80%. In this communication, we review the challenges and promises of such a strategy. "Polypill" is but one of an almost infinite number of possible multiconstituent pills (MCCP). The MCCP concept, although attractive, lacks evidence from randomized controlled trials. The following need to be addressed: credibility of the concept, design and synthesis of such complex pills, pharmacokinetics, pharmacodynamics, bioequivalence, "class" vs. unique properties, interactions, clinical efficacy and safety, regulatory approval, post-marketing surveillance, prescription vs. over-the- counter use, responsibility for initiating and monitoring therapy, patient education, counterfeiting and importation, reimbursement, advertisement, patent protection, and commercial viability. If these issues are favorably addressed, MCCP is poised to dramatically alter the face of CVD prevention, particularly in developing societies. Universal adoption of highly effective, safe, and inexpensive MCCP has the potential to become a major public healthcare initiative in the movement for the worldwide eradication of heart attacks. Nonetheless, in the absence of commercial interests, realizing the promise of MCCP will demand serious attention from national public health policymakers.

Key words: Cardiapill; Cardiopill; Multiconstituent pills; Polyceuticals; Polypill; Preventive/preemptive drug therapy

KEY POINTS

- Most cardiovascular deaths and disability are due to atherosclerosis and hypertension.
- Preemptive population based drug therapies aimed towards prevention and or slowing the progression of atherosclerosis and hypertension can substantially reduce the societal burden of CVD.
- If the challenges described in this chapter are met, multiconstituent pills, such as PolyPill™, with pharmacologic agents that are highly safe, can fulfill such preemptive population-based therapies and save millions of lives.

POPULATION-BASED THERAPY FOR HEART ATTACK PREVENTION

Since the concepts of CVD risk factors and "the sick individual versus the sick population" were put forward by pioneering epidemiologists [1, 2], considerable efforts and major investments have been made to promote and implement population based strategies for the prevention of cardiovascular events. These include dietary guidelines and regulating food industries to lower cholesterol and salt intake, as well as national policies to promote increased physical activity and reduce smoking. Similarly, guidelines for screening and treatment of major modifiable risk factors such as hypercholesterolemia and hypertension have been part of the original strategy for prevention of CVD. However, despite early success, risk factors for atherosclerosis have become increasingly prevalent. For example, in the US more than half of the middle age population has one or more risk factors [3]. Atherosclerotic cardiovascular disease (CVD) – i.e. heart attack and stroke – remains the number one killer in most developed countries and presents a major threat to developing societies. Therefore, newer and more effective strategies are urgently needed.

The discovery of "vulnerable plaque" and its evolution to the broader concept of "the vulnerable patient" [4, 5], have opened new avenues in the field of preventive cardiology.

The Screening for Heart Attack Prevention and Education (SHAPE) Task Force, organized by the Association for Eradication of Heart Attack (AEHA), has issued the SHAPE guideline, introducing a new paradigm for the prevention of acute cardiovascular events [6]. The SHAPE guideline focuses primarily on the detection and aggressive treatment of vulnerable patients – i.e. those individuals with a very high level of risk for a near term event [4, 5].

The SHAPE organization has also envisioned a future era of "*Polypill*"[1] therapy as an "unconditional" [6] population-based strategy for prophylactic therapy of high risk populations without screening, but acknowledged that the time for undertaking such a public initiative has not arrived. In anticipation of such a foreseeable future, we discuss here the challenges and promises of multiconstituent cardiovascular pills (MCCP), including "*Polypill*".

Hypertension, lipid disorders and other risk factors for cardiovascular events are highly coprevalent [7–9]. 30 million US adults have concomitant hypertension and lipid disorders. Even when cardiovascular risk factors are identified, they are infrequently treated to accepted goals. Fewer than 10% with hypertension and lipid disorders are treated to goal for both disorders [10]. That medicines have therapeutic benefits beyond their primary targets is now generally accepted (e.g. the "pleiotropic" benefits of statins beyond cholesterol reduction). The concept of a single, multimechanistic, safe, effective and inexpensive cardiovascular prophylactic that can be taken routinely with minimal professional supervision is certainly attractive and – if realized – has the potential to profoundly impact public health.

"POLYPILL" HYPE OR HOPE?

"*Polypill*" has attracted considerable scientific and media attention, as would any new treatment that purports to abolish atherosclerotic events. The attention is remarkable, since it is based on a theoretical medication that does not, in fact, exist.

Wald and Law first discussed the hypothetical cardiovascular benefits of a single pill that would combine a statin, three antihypertensive agents at half strength, low-dose aspirin, and folic acid [11], based on data from published meta-analyses of randomized trials and cohort studies and a meta-analysis of low-dose aspirin trials (including over 750 trials with 400,000 participants). When taken by everyone over 55 years and by everyone with existing CVD, "*Polypill*" could reduce ischemic heart disease (IHD) events "by 88% (95% confidence interval 84–91%) and stroke by 80% (71–87%). One- third of people taking this pill from age 55 would benefit, gaining on an average about 11 years of life free from an IHD event or stroke. According to the authors, '*Polypill*' would cause symptoms in 8–15% of people" [11].

A subsequent large case-control analysis of 13,029 patients with IHD, conducted in the United Kingdom, generally supports Wald and Law's predictions with respect to three of the components (statin, aspirin and blood pressure lowering drugs). Hippisley-Cox and Coupland found all-cause mortality to be lower in patients taking combinations (of two or three drugs) than in those taking a single agent [12]. In a prescription-event monitoring analysis, Wei et al reached a similar conclusion: two or three, but not necessarily more, seem to be better than one [13].

Rogers' editorial on Wald and Law's paper underlined, how seldom, therapy with these agents is discontinued for pharmacological reasons [14]. Rogers stressed the need for wider debate about population-based preventive strategies in asymptomatic individuals, and the need to integrate pharmacological therapy with societal approaches to modifiable – but often culturally accepted – risk factors, such as smoking, obesity, lipid disorders and hypertension. In addition to those discussed, individual and societal barriers to the provision of evidence-based health (such as health illiteracy, fatalism, inertia, poverty, alternative and folk medicine, and cost containment among others) need to be considered. An individual who fails to understand the concept of preventive therapy, who regards premature cardiovascular death as inevitable, and who cannot afford adequate nutrition, will not be helped by MCCP, including "*Polypill*".

[1] *"Polypill"* is a proprietary name and should be differentiated from the main body of text, as "Polypill" or as *"Polypill"* (in italics, as used in this article). It should not be used in generic fashion as an ordinary word (for example it should not be preceded by the indefinite article nor used in the plural form). A trademark application has been submitted by Professors Wald and Law [US trademark application # 76489257 February 11, 2003. http://www.uspto.gov/; http://tarr.uspto.gov/servlet/tarr?regser=serial&entry=76489257].

The Combination Pharmacotherapy and Public Health Research Working Group of the US Center for Disease Control and Prevention (CDC) has concluded that combination pharmacotherapy may prove especially effective in the developing world, and may have tremendous potential; but that additional study and detailed evaluation are necessary [15].

DEFINITION OF MCCP AND *"POLYPILL"*

The term MCCP is used in the article to refer to multiple component entities in general. "*Polypill*" is only one of an enormous family of multiconstituent entities that could impact CVD. These include pharmaceutical compounds and natural products (including so-called "nutraceuticals" "functional foods", dietary supplements, etc.). Examples of these proliferating entities include "Polymeal", "Cardiopill" "Cardiomeal", and the emerging industry of "Polyceuticals".

Wald and Law's US trademark application refers to "Pharmaceutical preparations used in the prevention and/or treatment of CVD", but this is a narrow definition, given that MCCP can include non-*cardiovascular* components, such as anti-diabetic and anti-inflammatory agents, and non-*pharmaceuticals* such as vitamins (as does indeed the Wald and Law "*Polypill*") and natural products.

Suggested definitions according to mechanism of action and intended therapeutic effect(s) are summarized in Tables 1 and 2.

Table 1
Definition of a Multiconstituent Cardiovascular Pill (MCCP) – by ingredients.

- Single molecules with inherently diverse effects
  - o Established drugs such as Beta-Blockers (central, cardiac, renal, vascular effects), Statins (lipid and nonlipid/"pleiotropic" effects[a]), Calcium Channel Blockers (CCB) (affecting vascular and cardiac muscle)
  - o Developmental compounds e.g. combined PPAR[b] -α, β-/δ, -γ antagonists, other agents with combined effects on lipids, glucose, blood pressure, C-Reactive Protein (CRP) and other inflammatory markers, obesity, smoking cessation and other risk factors – e.g. Rimonabant (Cannabinoid CB1 antagonist) – smoking cessation, lipids, insulin resistance, weight
- Combinations in same "class"[c], same clinical indication
- Combinations outside class, same surrogate indication
  - o Statin + Cholesterol absorption inhibitor; statin + fibrate, aspirin or niacin for lipids; ACEi + CCB; ACEi + ARB, thiazide + other antihypertensive for hypertension
  - o Aspirin + thromboxane receptor inhibitor + clopidogrel-like + oral fractionated factor Xa inhibitor + statin for early prehospital treatment of acute coronary syndrome[2]
- Combinations outside class, different surrogate indications
  - o Statin + CCB (e.g. Caduet® (Amlodipine + Atorvastatin)); Statin + Angiotensin Receptor Antagonist; Statin + folate + aspirin + BP meds (Wald and Law's "*Polypill*")
- Pharmaceutical + "natural"/nutraceutical; OTC products (e.g. cold cures)
- Polymers
  - o Polyaspirin; Poly-para amino salicylic acid
- Polyceuticals (hypothetical)
  - o Combinations with pharmaceutical and nonpharmaceutical constituents

[a]The term "pleiotropic" is loosely used and begs definition outside the scope of this article
[b]*PPAR* Peroxisome Proliferator-Activated Receptor
[c]The concept of "class" effects is simplistic and possibly fictitious, especially in the current context, but the term is used in this article for convenience

[2] Fuster, V – personal communication

Table 2
Definition of a Multiconstituent Cardiovascular Pill (MCCP) – by therapeutic indication(s).

- Combined Over-the-Counter (OTC) products for symptomatic relief
  - No examples currently known
- Combined prescription medications that target several risk factors for the same disease
  - Lipid disorders, hypertension, hyperglycemia – for CHD or ESRD
- Combined prescription medications that target comorbid diseases
  - Rheumatoid arthritis and CHD; Alzheimer's Disease and cerebrovascular disease
- Unscientific or pseudo-scientific combinations
  - Statin + CoQ10

Other definitions and systems for categorizing MCCP are, of course, possible. One might, for example, adopt a contemporary system as preferred by Martindale [16], although conventional classifications (e.g. into antihypertensive, anti-diabetic, lipid lowering agents etc.) may not lend themselves to holistic classification of agents that may not act through traditional surrogates (such as blood pressure and lipids), and whose clinical indications may include less readily measurable outcomes, such as prevention of CVD events and regression of atherosclerosis.

INTEREST IN *"POLYPILL"*

Wald and Law's paper itself, generated considerable interest. A CNN poll conducted after its release found that 95% of 13,070 respondents would take such a "*Polypill*"[3]. A Google™ web search of the terms "*Polypill*" or "Poly Pill" combined with "heart" (to limit false positives) generated more than 10,500 hits (March 2006) and over 30 peer reviewed publications [17–46].

But the recognition that cardiovascular risk factors co-segregate, and increasing interest in multiple risk factor intervention (as promoted in all US and International Guidelines for CVD) that long predates the "*Polypill*" concept, has already spurred the discovery, development and marketing of combinations of cardiovascular drugs with mixed benefits. Examples include combinations of antihypertensives with thiazide diuretics, renin inhibitors with Angiotensin- converting enzyme (ACE) inhibitors and/or Angiotensin Receptor antagonists, and ACE inhibitors with calcium channel antagonists and a statin with a calcium channel antagonist. One ambitious patent[4] describes the combination of an antioxidant, ACE inhibitor, Angiotensin II receptor blocker (ARB), calcium channel blocker (CCB), diuretic, digitalis, beta blocker, a statin or cholestyramine, for "treating or ameliorating arteriosclerosis, atherosclerosis, stiff vessel disease, peripheral vascular disease, coronary heart disease, stroke, myocardial infarct, cardiomyopathies, restenosis, hypertension, isolated systolic hypertension, or heart failure".

[3] http://www.cnn.com/2003/HEALTH/06/26/"Polypill"/index.html posted June 6 2003
[4] US Patent 6,770,663 United States Patent 6770663 "Method for treating fibrotic diseases or other indications utilizing thiazole, oxazole and imidazole compounds". Issued August 3, 2004

RATIONALES FOR MCCP

Clinical

Outcomes

Wald and Law's speculations aside, the true risks and benefits of "*Polypill*" are unknown, and will have to be tested in prospective outcome trials. Whether such trials are ethically or commercially feasible is uncertain. Safety may be the major consideration, as is discussed below. The CDC panel suggested conducting clinical trials and cost effectiveness analysis [12].

Adherence

Adherence with concomitant antihypertensive and lipid lowering therapy is poor. In a retrospective study of a US managed care cohort [47], Chapman found only one in three patients to be adherent to both therapies at 6 months after initiation (adherence defined as filling prescriptions sufficient to cover ≥80% of days with both classes of medications). Improved adherence to combinations (fewer pills to pay for and take) seems self-evident. Patients surely prefer to take one pill rather than six. On the other hand, pill burden may be viewed as endorsing the severity of illness, and may have value in itself. Objective evidence of adherence benefit of combined pills is scarce and published data may be biased in favor of positive studies. Retrospectively querying a commercial pharmacy benefits manager (PBM) database, Dezii found adherence to ACE inhibitor and thiazide diuretic higher with single-pill combinations than with the same two drugs given separately [48]. Taylor and Shoheiber found a modest, 7%, difference in adherence between patients receiving a combination of Amlodipine and Benazepril compared to patients receiving any ACE inhibitor and any dihydropyridine CCB separately [12]. Mismatching of these groups with regard to the particular ACE inhibitors and CCBs taken, and other medications and comorbidities, make it hard to judge the true impact of the combination on adherence. Schwartz et al suggested that simultaneously starting drug therapy for hypertension and lipid disorders leads to better 1 year adherence than when the same therapy is given sequentially, the differences being 11–15% [49].

Potential Impact of MCCP on CVD Screening and Prevention

MCCP has the potential to drive entirely new paradigms for CVD prevention. The widespread availability of cheap, safe, well-tolerated and effective MCCP *with little or no need for medical intervention* could readily lead to the following scenarios:

1. Routine population-based consumption (irrespective of the presence or severity of risk factors) by asymptomatic individuals at high average risk for CV events (e.g. all men and women over 75 as in the SHAPE guideline). Such a scenario makes conventional and emerging risk factor assessment, and screening for asymptomatic disease redundant, but requires governmental oversight and major educational and operational efforts to maximize adherence and safety, and to limit inappropriate usage. The UK's pharmacist-supported "Behind the counter" model[5] facilitates this scenario, but may not find sufficiently wide acceptance in the United States.
2. Individual prescription from a limited MCCP menu, based on physician assessment of risk factors, risk markers and screening tests for disease. The fact that MCCP is available may encourage more screening of asymptomatic individuals than occurs currently.
3. A shift from physician-centered to patient- or consumer-centered care.

[5] "Behind the counter" differs from "Over the Counter" dispensing, in that – whereas neither requires physician prescription – in the former the pharmacist is required to provide information and advice to the purchaser, and to refer to a physician when appropriate.

Routine consumption by concerned individuals at self-perceived modest or higher risk, driven by accessibility to *nonprescription/over the counter* MCCP, potentially includes a near-infinite choice of individualized polyceuticals. Individuals could gauge their risk and decide on therapy based on widely available population-based risk factor calculators, by self-testing of blood pressure, self-sought blood tests for conventional and new risk markers, inexpensive noninvasive surrogate tests for disease (including anatomic imaging, tests of vascular compliance and endothelial function), and by available estimates of benefit. In the future, complex genetic profiling of disease risk as well as safety and efficacy of therapeutic agents, may guide fully individualized "tailored" therapy, also labeled "personalized medicine". These scenarios predict shifts from a conventional provider – patient model of CV disease prevention to a self-affirming model, in which the point of "care" moves from clinics and hospitals to the workplace, pharmacies, fitness clubs (which will seize the opportunity to adopt a true "health club" role), and to even greater reliance than today on the Internet for information and products. This raises the worrying possibility that web-empowered, unregulated commerce in MCCP, coupled with further dramatic increases in importation, counterfeiting and adulteration, will help jeopardize the integrity of US medicines more than what has already occurred[6].

ECONOMIC

Cost-shifting from payers, and from national and state budgets, to the individual, and back to the manufacturers and suppliers will underpin the economic debate around OTC MCCP. Economic factors in a prescription MCCP that may be attractive to Pharma, include:

- Additional revenue (balanced against costs of development, licensing, marketing, sales and post marketing support, and against cannibalization of existing product sales).
- Expanded product portfolio (potentially leading to greater leverage in promotion, contract and pricing negotiations).
- The ability to launch a new product, helping to meet R&D predictions and analyst expectations.
- Expansion of an existing clinical market; development of new markets.
- Commercial advantage over competitors in same class(es) or for same or similar indication(s). An inexpensive MCCP, some or all of whose components have marginal individual market share, may dominate the market in several sectors (e.g. hypertension, lipid disorders, diabetes).
- Extended patent life/delayed loss of exclusivity.

That a successful MCCP should be less expensive than the sum of its components seems intuitive, but – mindful of the significant cost of dispensing fees and copayments, and their less tangible advantages (simplified regimens etc.) – prescription MCCP as costly as or more costly than their parts may well be accepted. Extremely inexpensive MCCP (at prices such as have been suggested for the UK and developing countries) are not likely to be seen as commercially viable. Whether industry will partner philanthropically with governments and non-governmental agencies (especially in developing countries) to develop and distribute cheap CV MCCP, remains to be seen. Certainly, many (often unrecognized) precedent-setting drug assistance programs with substantial public health impact do exist.

[6]Statement of John M. Taylor, III Associate Commissioner for Regulatory Affairs of the FDA, before the Permanent Subcommittee on Investigations, Committee on Governmental Affairs, July 22, 2004; at http://www.fda.gov/ola/2004/importeddrugs0722.html

Table 3
Characteristics of a viable MCCP.

- Commercially viable clinical indication(s). Includes comorbid treatable risk factors, comorbid conditions, conditions with multiple therapeutic targets, conditions amenable to multiple approaches (drugs, vitamins, essential cofactors, other dietary components)
- Existing components with known physico-chemical characteristics
- Pharmaceutically stable when compounded
- Palatable
- Compatible dosing and pharmacokinetics (same time of day, lack of food effect, similar half-lives, similar onset in effect, similar or absent interaction with populations (elderly, children, ethnic groups, renal or hepatic impairment etc.)
- Predictable interactions; lack of negative interaction
- Known or reasonable expectation of efficacy
- Predictable adverse event profiles
- Lack of patent and other legal constraints
- Inexpensive (relative to development and production costs)

WHAT PREDICTS A VIABLE MCCP? (SEE TABLE 3)

Cost

From a Pharmaceutical Industry perspective, promising clinical applications (large target population, chronic therapy) are attractive. The need to recoup R&D and post approval costs, and to retain shareholder value can be critical. In a study conducted by Tufts University's Center for the Study of Drug Development [50], the cost of developing a new drug in the United States was approximately $820 million. But cost considerations have not stalled development and marketing of non "blockbuster" drugs (sometimes defined as $1 billion in annual sales). There are many examples of orphan, niche and "me-too" products.

Daily costs of £0.60 in the United Kingdom, and weekly costs of $6 in India, as have been suggested, are unlikely to spur industry interest. Whether governments will subsidize, reimburse, or drive development and manufacture remain to be seen. The costs and benefits of MCCP need to be balanced against their developmental costs – no easy task. Although CV MCCP might slash the burden of fatal and handicapping CV diseases (perhaps including kidney failure) and might extend productive lifespan, survivors will be exposed to competing risk from other causes of mortality (particularly cancer and infectious diseases), and to an increased burden of chronic diseases such as arthritis, Alzheimer's disease and other potentially debilitating conditions, thus shifting CV disease costs towards non-CV drugs, and to hospital and long-term care.

Characteristics

Characteristics of a promising MCCP are listed in Table 3. Most are self-evident – such as the need for consistent dosing between the ingredients. Combining a statin taken at night with other drugs taken in the morning, or adding a generic t.i.d. ACE inhibitor to a mix of once-a-day agents, makes no sense. Extended release formulations face many obstacles – such as food and other luminal interactions, multiple optimal release sites, pH-dependence, release characteristics of the individual components. The pharmaceutical challenges of synthesizing a pill small enough to be swallowed from as much as a gram, or more, of active compounds with often-incompatible chemistries is less well recognized. Many, or perhaps most, interesting combinations cannot be formulated.

The combination prescription product Pravagard™ PAC (Pravastatin and Aspirin), which has been described as an early "*Polypill*", is in fact simply the presentation in blister pack of Pravastatin tablets and Buffered Aspirin tablets side by side. Whether BMS was unable to combine the two, or elected not to, is not clear.

Notable exceptions, the multivitamin preparations, combine relatively small proportions of vitamins with larger proportions of elemental compounds (in mcg to 100mg+amounts), and of excipients (ingredients other than the active components).

For a brief review, visit http://www.ipecamericas.org/public/faqs.html). Often these pills are large and unpalatable.

MCCP need not be MCC pills. It is not difficult to imagine an era of full-tailored therapy in which patients call, key, swipe, beam, etc., personal data and receive an individualized multi-constituent sachet, gel-cap, dry powder inhaler, cream, lotion, rapidly-dissolving tongue strip, suppository, premixed injection, shake, gum, power bar, or any other imaginable preparation. Auto-tailoring therapy like this is not so farfetched. It revisits the era of the traditional dispensing pharmacist and reminds us that the coffee/tea dispensers and health drink combos of today's service industries often are ahead of medical innovation.

Safety

The risk of drug interactions increases – drug interactions increases at least linearly with the number of interacting drugs – exponentially with four or more interacting drugs [51]. To the extent that many interactions are predictable for a particular MCCP, and recognizing the selection bias in favor of those MCCP with fewest predicted interactions, it still seems ingenuous to predict withdrawal rates in the order of a few percent for any combination of five or six drugs. It will be important to select components with well-recognized minor adverse effects (AEs). Even so, it will be hard to discriminate nonspecific AEs (headache, gastrointestinal symptoms, malaise, etc.) from nondrug-related conditions (most self-limiting). Overlapping AEs (such as those described, and others usually attributed to one type of drug over another – but not always reliably so – such as cough, muscle pains, extremity edema, rashes) will make identification of the "offending" component difficult. Even with a full cabinet of alternative similar MCCPs, the practitioner may be hard pressed to select the appropriate replacement, and may resort to the individual drugs taken singly. Patients may be unwilling to be re-exposed to *any* of the individual components, fearing recurrent unwanted symptoms. Physicians may consider a preliminary trial of the individual components, but such a strategy is not guaranteed to predict tolerability with the combination. The concept of a preliminary trial is at odds with the notion of patient self-directed therapy and would be difficult to enact with over the counter MCCP.

OTHER BARRIERS TO COMMERCIALIZATION

A simple but critical barrier is the potential number of conceivable MCCP combinations. Selecting a cold cure from the many dozens on a Pharmacy shelf is already daunting. Pending the appearance of the omniceutical dispenser, multi-constituent pills could occupy dozens of aisles – entire Pharmacies could be dedicated to multi-constituent pills alone. In a very simplistic calculation, based on the US pharmacopoeia, Wald and Law's cardiovascular "*Polypill*" alone could potentially be marketed in millions of preparations. Taking all possible combinations of 1 of 6 statins, 1 of 10 ACE inhibitors, 1 of 7 thiazide diuretics, 1 of 9 beta-blockers, gives 3780 products. Factoring in 1 of 7 Angiotensin-Receptor Antagonists, 1 of 10 CCBs, 1 of 10 other antihypertensive medications, a folic acid preparation, and an aspirin combination produces more than two million alternatives. That number ignores dose ranges, excipients, other active ingredients (such as fibrates, niacin, cholesterol-absorption inhibitors, thiazolidinediones and other drugs for diabetes, COX-2 inhibitors and other anti-inflammatory compounds; cholesteryl ester transfer protein (CETP) inhibitors and other novel anti-atherosclerosis compounds, drugs for metabolic syndrome, anti-obesity and other compounds in development), other vitamins and other so-called "natural" products. This astronomical total assumes any combination could or would be manufactured – clearly not the case. Nevertheless, the likelihood of commercial success for any single MCCP becomes diminishingly unlikely. A "*Polypill*" explosion more probably will herald a public health Yin-Yang: an era of individualized single-pill OTC polypharmacy – rational and beneficial in many cases, irrational and unsafe in others.

OTHER CHALLENGES

Regulatory

Will regulatory agencies approve based on historical data for the components and limited specific experience for MCCPs themselves, with an emphasis on collecting post marketing safety data in the "real" world? It has been suggested that small studies to confirm bioequivalence, and surrogate markers of efficacy (blood pressure, lipids, etc., and intermediate surrogates such as carotid Intima-Media Thickness (IMT)), may be enough. What might approvable simple surrogate measures look like for non-pharmaceuticals such as folic acid or other vitamins? Will aspirin be subjected to further regulatory scrutiny? Will some constituents (such as vitamins and "natural" products) be subject to less scrutiny than pharmaceuticals? Will MCCP be substantially similar to existing approved products be "grandfathered"? Will "*Polypill*" or other MCCPs be allowed to claim the approved indications and clinical trials from the approved labeling for each of their components? Those debates will continue. One has to assume that regulatory authorities, possibly under an avalanche of MCCP applications, will resist pressure to relax regulations, particularly when judging currently unregulated "natural" constituents.

If these products make the over-the-counter market, and mindful that their possible benefits are substantial and emotive (saving lives, and preventing heart disease and stroke), who will regulate and monitor their advertising for false, misleading and unsubstantiated claims?

BIAS AGAINST COMBINATIONS

The medical community takes a conservative approach to combination therapies and polypharmacy, although in recent years this stance may have relaxed (supported in part by national recommendations such as the reports of the Joint National Committee on Blood Pressure). As discussed above, bias against combinations is rooted in safety concerns about drug–drug and drug–patient interactions, about unfamiliar or untested constituents, the difficulty of identifying which component may be responsible for an apparent AE, and the preference to titrate components individually.

The academic medical community tends to regard combination pills as the nonscientific outcome of marketing strategy, and, therefore, uninteresting; but this ignores the (often hidden) sophistication and innovation in pharmacology and pharmaceutical science needed to develop these products, and the epidemiologic and outcomes data needed to identify clinical benefit.

Primum Non Nocere

Safety being paramount in widespread nonprescription use, the tendency is to approve and market low doses which may not have proven clinical benefit. Merck's Zocor® (Simvastatin) became available over the counter in Britain in the 10 mg strength, despite a lack of evidence of improved clinical outcomes at this low dose. The recommended starting doses of Zocor® in the US are 20 and 40 mg. As the statin component of their "*Polypill*", Wald and Law did suggest Simvastatin 40 mg or Atorvastatin10 mg, both known to improve hard clinical endpoints in large, well-conducted, randomized controlled trials. Wald and Law, however, also recommended half-strength antihypertensive medications in the expectation that clinical benefits would aggregate and AEs would be minimized. This seems intuitive, but is still entirely speculative.

SUMMARY

Risk factors for atherosclerotic CVD are highly co-prevalent but poorly identified and treated. The Screening for Heart Attack Prevention and Education (SHAPE) Task Force from the Society for Heart Attack Prevention and Eradication (SHAPE) has proposed a new strategy that recommends screening for subclinical atherosclerosis and implementing aggressive treatment of "vulnerable patients". The Task Force has also envisioned future developments that may shift mass screening strategies to mass prophylactic therapy. The "*Polypill*" concept, introduced by Wald and Law suggests that a combination of statin, low-dose antihypertensives, aspirin and folic acid in a single pill taken prophylactically by the high risk population can cut CVD event rates by as much as 80%. In this communication, we review the challenges and promises of such a strategy. "Polypill" is but one of an astronomical number of possible multi-constituent pills (MCCP). Attractive as the MCCP concept is, it lacks evidence from randomized controlled trials, and begs numerous questions about the credibility of the concept, the design and synthesis of such complex pills, pharmacokinetics, pharmacodynamics, bioequivalence, "class" vs. unique properties, interactions, evidence of clinical efficacy and safety, regulatory approval, post marketing surveillance, prescription vs. over-the- counter use, responsibility for initiating and monitoring therapy, patient education, counterfeiting and importation, reimbursement, advertisement, patent protection, commercial viability, etc. If these issues are favorably addressed, MCCPs stand to dramatically change the manner in which CVD is prevented, particularly in developing societies. Universal adoption of highly effective, safe, and inexpensive MCCPs has the potential to become a major public healthcare initiative in the movement for the eradication of heart attack worldwide. Notwithstanding, assuming low commercial interest, realizing the promises of MCCPs will demand serious attention from national public health policymakers.

REFERENCES

1. Kannel WB, Dawber TR, Friedman GD, Glennon WE, Mcnamara PM. Risk factors in coronary heart disease. An evaluation of several serum lipids as predictors of coronary heart disease. The Framingham Study. Ann Intern Med. 1964;61:888–99.
2. Rose G. Sick individuals and sick populations. Int J Epidemiol. 2001;30(3):427–32; discussion 433–4.
3. Heart Disease and Stroke Statistics – 2006 Update – American Heart Association, Dallas, TX http://www.americanheart.org/presenter.jhtml?identifier=1928.
4. Naghavi M, Libby P, Falk E, Casscells SW, Litovsky S, Rumberger J, et al. From vulnerable plaque to vulnerable patient: a call for new definitions and risk assessment strategies: Part I. Circulation. 2003;108(14):1664–72.
5. Naghavi M, Libby P, Falk E, Casscells SW, Litovsky S, Rumberger J, et al. From vulnerable plaque to vulnerable patient: a call for new definitions and risk assessment strategies: Part I. Circulation. 2003;108(15):1772–8.
6. Naghavi M, Falk E, Hecht H, Jamieson MJ, Kaul S, Berman D, et al. From vulnerable plaque to vulnerable patient: Part III. Executive summary of the Screening for Heart Attack Prevention and Education (SHAPE) Task Force. Am J Cardiol. Vol. 98, No 2A, 1–15H Available online http://www.aeha.org.
7. Battleman DS, Peterson ED. Estimated prevalence of concomitant hypertension and lipid disorders among US adults. J Manag Care Pharm. 2004;10(2):186.
8. Johnson ML, Pietz K, Battleman DS, Beyth RJ. Prevalence of comorbid hypertension and lipid disorders and associated cardiovascular disease. Am J Manag Care. 2004;10(12):926–32.
9. Ansell BJ. Evidence for a combined approach to the management of hypertension and lipid disorders. Am J Hypertens. 2005;18(9 Pt 1):1249–57.

10. Ford ES, Mokdad AH, Giles WH, Mensah GA. Serum total cholesterol concentrations and awareness, treatment, and control of hypercholesterolemia among US adults. Circulation. 2003;107:2185–9.
11. Wald NJ, Law MR. A strategy to reduce cardiovascular disease by more than 80%. BMJ. 2003;326:1419.
12. Hippisley-Cox J, Coupland C. Effect of combinations of drugs on all cause mortality in patients with ischaemic heart disease: nested case-control analysis. BMJ. 2005;330:1059–63.
13. Wei L, Ebrahim S, Bartlett C, Davey PD, Sullivan FM, MacDonald TM. Statin use in the secondary prevention of coronary heart disease in primary care: cohort study and comparison of inclusion and outcome with patients in randomised trials. BMJ. 2005;330:821.
14. Rogers A. (Editorial) A cure for cardiovascular disease? BMJ. 2003;326:1407–8.
15. Combination Pharmacotherapy and Public Health Research Working Group. Combination pharmacotherapy for cardiovascular disease. Ann Intern Med. 2005;143(8):593–9.
16. Sweetman SC (Ed). Martindale: The Complete Drug Reference, 34rd Edition. Pharmaceutical press, London.
17. Sleight P, Pouleur H, Zannad F. Benefits, challenges, and registerability of the Polypill. Eur Heart J. 2006;27(14):1651–6.
18. Daviglus ML, Lloyd-Jones DM, Pirzada A. Preventing cardiovascular disease in the 21st century: therapeutic and preventive implications of current evidence. Am J Cardiovasc Drugs. 2006;6(2):87–101.
19. Franco OH, Steyerberg EW, de Laet C. The Polypill: at what price would it become cost effective? J Epidemiol Community Health. 2006;60(3):213–7.
20. Wise J. Polypill holds promise for people with chronic disease. Bull World Health Organ. 2005;83(12):885–7.
21. Narayan KM, Mensah GA, Sorensen S, Cheng YJ, Vinicor F, Engelgau MM, Williamson DF. Combination pharmacotherapy for cardiovascular disease prevention: threat or opportunity for public health? Am J Prev Med. 2005;29(5 Suppl 1):134–8.
22. Combination Pharmacotherapy and Public Health Research Working Group. Combination pharmacotherapy for cardiovascular disease. Ann Intern Med. 2005;143(8):593–9.
23. Green LW. Prospects and possible pitfalls of a preventive Polypill: confessions of a health promotion convert. Eur J Clin Nutr. 2005;59(Suppl 1):S4–8.
24. Radziszewska B, Hart RG, Wolf PA, D'Agostino RB Sr, Cutler JA. Clinical research in primary stroke prevention: needs, opportunities, and challenges. Neuroepidemiology. 2005;25(2):91–104.
25. Joshi SR. "Polypill-aspostatinoprilololazide folate" – coprescription for at the risk Asian Indian in chronic non communicable diseases. J Assoc Physicians India. 2005;53:175–8.
26. Fahey T, Brindle P, Ebrahim S. The Polypill and cardiovascular disease. BMJ. 2005;330(7499):1035–6.
27. Robinson JG, Maheshwari N. A "poly-portfolio" for secondary prevention: a strategy to reduce subsequent events by up to 97% over five years. Am J Cardiol. 2005;95(3):373–8.
28. Franco OH, Bonneux L, de Laet C, Peeters A, Steyerberg EW, Mackenbach JP. The Polymeal: a more natural, safer, and probably tastier (than the Polypill) strategy to reduce cardiovascular disease by more than 75%. BMJ. 2004;329(7480):1447–50.
29. Frishman WH, Zuckerman AL. Amlodipine/atorvastatin: the first cross risk factor Polypill for the prevention and treatment of cardiovascular disease. Expert Rev Cardiovasc Ther. 2004;2(5):675–81.
30. Gavras I, Rosenthal T. Combination therapy as first-line treatment for hypertension. Curr Hypertens Rep. 2004;6(4):267–72.
31. Scheen AJ. Management of the metabolic syndrome. Minerva Endocrinol. 2004;29(2):31–45.
32. Franklin BA, Kahn JK, Gordon NF, Bonow RO. A cardioprotective Polypill? Independent and additive benefits of lifestyle modification. Am J Cardiol. 2004;94(2):162–6.
33. Colvin HP. Polypill debate continues: people will always be sceptical. BMJ. 2004;328(7434):289.
34. Willis J. Polypill debate continues: concept is a fascinating thought experiment. BMJ. 2004;328(7434):289.
35. Adler J. Next: the Polypill prescription. Newsweek. 2003;142(23):82.
36. Ramos F. Polypill to fight cardiovascular disease: birthday present was much appreciated.BMJ. 2003;327(7418):808.
37. Assmann G, Cullen P, Schulte H. Polypill to fight cardiovascular disease: interpretation of trial data is optimistic. BMJ. 2003;327(7418):808.
38. Midgley AK. Polypill to fight cardiovascular disease: old joke has element of truth. BMJ. 2003;327(7418):808.
39. Messori A, Santarlasci B, Trippoli S, Vaiani M. Polypill to fight cardiovascular disease: cost effectiveness of statins for primary prevention of cardiovascular events is questionable. BMJ. 2003;327(7418):808–9.
40. Trewby P, Trewby C. Polypill to fight cardiovascular disease: patients before populations. BMJ. 2003;327(7418):807; discussion 809; author reply 809–10.
41. Powlson M. Polypill to fight cardiovascular disease: universal polypharmacy goes against recent beliefs in prescribing practice. BMJ. 2003;327(7418):807–8.
42. Taylor S, Konings A. Polypill to fight cardiovascular disease: now who's playing God? BMJ. 2003;327(7418):807.
43. Sherman FT. Polypill as geri-tonic. Geriatrics. 2003;58(8):7–8.
44. Franco OH, Steyerberg EW, de Laet C. The polypill: at what price would it become cost effective? Epidemiol Community Health. 2006;60(3):213–7.
45. Amarenco P. Polypill strategy vs. prevention clinics for stroke prevention. Cerebrovasc Dis. 2006;21(Suppl 1):35–40. Epub 2006 Feb 13.
46. Blank R, LaSalle J, Reeves R, Maroni J, Tarasenko L, Sun F. Single-pill therapy in the treatment of concomitant hypertension and lipid disorders (the amlodipine/atorvastatin gemini study). J Clin Hypertens (Greenwich). 2005;7(5):264–73.

47. Chapman RH, Benner JS, Petrilla AA, Tierce JC, Collins SR, Battleman DS, Schwartz S. Predictors of adherence with antihypertensive and lipid-lowering therapy. Arch Intern Med. 2005;165:1147–52.
48. Dezii C. A retrospective study of persistence with single-pill combination therapy vs. concurrent two-pill therapy in patients with hypertension. Managed Care. 2000;9(9 Suppl):S2–6.
49. Taylor AA, Shoheiber O. Adherence to antihypertensive therapy with fixed-dose amlodipine besylate/benazepril HCl versus comparable component-based therapy. Congest Heart Fail. 2003;9(6):324–32.
50. DiMasi JA, Hansen RW, Grabowski HG. The price of innovation: new estimates of drug development costs. J Health Econ. 2003;22(2):151–85.
51. Schwartz, JS, McLaughlin T, Griffis D, Arnold A, Pettitt D. Adherence to chronic therapy among patients treated for hypertension, lipid disorders, or both. J Am Coll Cardiol. 2003;41:526.

50 Vaccine for Atherosclerosis: An Emerging New Paradigm

Prediman K. Shah, Kuang-Yuh Chyu, Jan Nilsson, and Gunilla N. Fredrikson

CONTENTS

Abstract

Despite many recent advances, atherosclerotic cardiovascular disease continues to pose challenges to the healthcare system throughout the world. Given the limitations of current athero-preventive strategies, new therapeutic and preventive paradigms need to be explored. This chapter highlights the complex role of the immune system in atherogenesis and the potential athero-protective role of active and passive immunization strategies. Immuno-modulation with a vaccine appears feasible and effective in reducing experimental atherosclerosis, warranting clinical development. Although experimental observations are exciting, many questions about vaccination, such as choice of optimal antigens, choice of most effective adjuvants, the optimal route of administration, durability of effects and safety remain to be answered. However, we remain cautiously optimistic that a vaccine-based approach to manage atherosclerotic cardiovascular disease has the potential to become a part of the armamentarium against cardiovascular disease.

Key Words: Atherosclerosis; Immune response; Immunization; Vaccination

From: *Asymptomatic Atherosclerosis: Pathophysiology, Detection and Treatment*
Edited by: M. Naghavi (ed.), DOI 10.1007/978-1-60327-179-0_50

IMMUNE SYSTEM AND ATHEROSCLEROSIS

Atherosclerosis is now recognized to be a chronic immune-mediated inflammatory disease of the medium and large size arteries. The atherosclerotic lesions contain elements of both innate and adaptive immune system. Examples of these are activated immune cells (macrophages, T-cells, dendritic cells, mast cells), various molecules and cytokines to recruit immune cells, complement, immunoglobulins and "pathogen associated microbial pattern" (PAMP) receptors, such as Toll like receptors and scavenger receptors [1–3].

INNATE IMMUNITY AND ATHEROSCLEROSIS

Recent studies have highlighted the complex role of innate immunity in atherogenesis with both athero-promoting and athero-protective effects [1–3]. Innate immunity provides a rapid but nonspecific defense against pathogens and is orchestrated by an inherited repertoire of pattern recognition receptors. Toll-like receptors (TLR) are a group of pattern recognition receptors of innate immunity that appear to be involved in atherogenesis [4–10]. Activation of TLRs by endogenous or exogenous ligands, leads to transcription of several inflammatory genes and the eventual release of inflammatory cytokines that characterize the acute innate immune response [4, 10]. We and others have reported that members of the TLR family are expressed in murine and human atherosclerotic lesions [5, 6]. Disruption of TLR-signaling pathway, through genetic knockout of TLR-4 or TLR-2 or their downstream signaling adaptor molecule (myeloid differentiation factor 88 or MyD88) in hyperlipidemic mice, reduces atherosclerosis, plaque inflammation and circulating inflammatory cytokines in mice [7–9].These observations establish a link between hyperlipidemia and activation of TLR signaling pathways and its pathogenic role in atherosclerosis. Although the precise endogenous ligand responsible for activation of this pathway in hyperlipidemia is unclear, recent observations have attributed such a role to saturated fatty acids [10, 11].

In addition to the pro-atherogenic effects, innate immunity may also have athero-protective effects. Experimental studies have shown that, certain naturally occurring IgM antibodies against phosphorylcholine head group (PC) on apoptotic cells, produced by a subset of splenic B-cells(B-1 cells), cross react with PC moiety on oxidized LDL, reducing oxidized LDL uptake by macrophages [12–16]. Pneumococcal vaccination was shown to enhance the level of anti-PC IgM antibodies in mice, presumably because the cell wall of pneumococcus contains PC, and this led to reduction of murine atherosclerosis [15, 16]. Recent human studies have, however, failed to show an increase in anti-PC antibodies with pneumococcal vaccination [17, 18]. Active immunization with PC antigen and passive immunization with anti-PC IgM antibody have been shown to have athero-protective effects in hyperlipidemic mice [19, 20] (Fig. 1).

Fig. 1. (**a**) A schematic representation of the potential juxtaposed roles of the innate immune response in atherosclerosis. The protherogenic component of the system is related to mediation of inflammatory signaling by Toll-like receptors and myloid differentiation factor 88, a downstream adoptor molecule. The atheroprotective component is mediated by B1-cell-deived natural antibody to phosphorylcholine head group, which cross-reacts with phosphorylcholine on oxidized LDL chloesterol. *MyD88* Myeloid differentiation factor κB, *Ox-LDL* Oxidized LDL chloesterol, *PAMP* Pathogen-associated molecular patterns, *PC* Phosphorylcholine, *SR* Scavenger receptor, *TLR* Toll-like receptor. (**b**) A schematic representation of the potential juxtaposed roles of the adaptive immune response to specific antigens. The protherogenic component results from T-helper-1 cell and natural killer T-cell activation triggered by the presentation of antigens by the major histocompatibility complex class II or CD1 molecules. The atheprotective component is mediated by the secretion of anti-inflammatory cytokines (interleukin-10 and transforming growth factor b), mediated by T-helper-2, T-helper-3 and regulatory T cells, and antibody response mediated by B cells. *MHC class II* Major histocompatibility complex class II, *NK T cell* Natural killer T-cell, *Ox-LDL* Oxidized LDL cholesterol, *PAMP* Pathogen-associated molecular patterns, *SR* Scavenger receptor, *TLR* Toll-like receptor, *Treg* Regulatory T cells (Reproduced from Shah PK et al. Nature Clinical Practice Cardiovascular 2005 [3]).

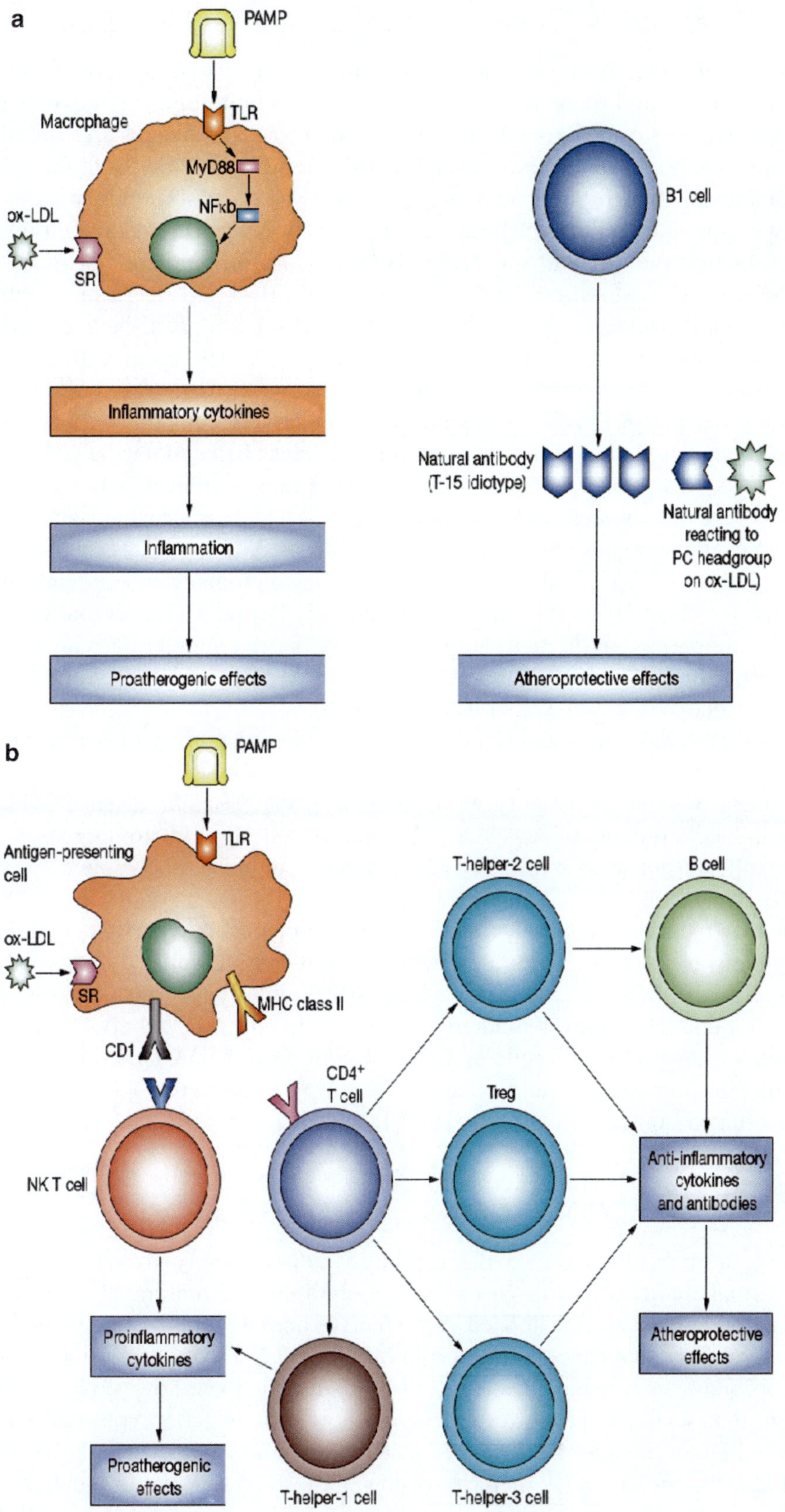
a
PAMP
TLR
Macrophage
MyD88
NFκb
ox-LDL
SR
Inflammatory cytokines
Inflammation
Proatherogenic effects
B1 cell
Natural antibody
(T-15 idiotype)
Natural antibody
reacting to
PC headgroup
on ox-LDL)
Atheroprotective effects
b
PAMP
TLR
Antigen-presenting
cell
ox-LDL
SR
MHC class II
CD1
NK T cell
CD4+
T cell
T-helper-2 cell
B cell
Treg
Anti-inflammatory
cytokines
and antibodies
Proinflammatory
cytokines
Proatherogenic
effects
T-helper-1 cell
T-helper-3 cell
Atheroprotective
effects

ADAPTIVE IMMUNITY IN ATHEROSCLEROSIS

Unlike the innate immune response, the adaptive immune response to various antigens is highly specific, slower to occur and more long lasting through immunologic memory. It is orchestrated by antigen presenting cells (mostly dendritic cells but also by macrophages and B-cells) that process the antigen and present it to CD 4 T-cells through MHC-class II molecules or to CD 8 T-cells through MHC-class I molecules, which along with activation of various costimulatory molecules, result in activation of antigen-specific T cells. T-cell responses provoked by antigen presenting cells may then proceed along various pathways: the Th1 pathway which is largely pro-inflammatory with interferon gamma and IL-12 as the signature cytokines, the Th2 pathway with IL-4 and IL-5 as signature cytokines or Treg (regulatory T-cell) pathway with anti-inflammatory IL-10 and TGF-beta as effector cytokines. In atherosclerosis the predominant response appears to be Th1 which has pro-atherogenic effects [12, 21, 22]. The complexity of the adaptive immune response is further suggested by pro-atherogenic effects of natural killer T (NKT) cells, a subset of CD4 positive T cells that express the natural killer 1.1 receptor and recognize lipid antigens presented by the class I-like molecule CD1 [23]. The role of Th2 pathway is less clear since IL-4 may have pro-atherogenic effects, whereas IL-5 has athero-protective effects [24, 25]. Recent data suggest that Tregs have tolerogenic and athero-protective effects [26–29]. Several subtypes of Tregs have been identified: natural Tregs which are produced in thymus and are CD4+, CD25+, and express Foxp3, have tolerogenic effects and appear to act by depleting effector T-cells of IL-2; Tr1 cells that produce IL-10 and Th3 cells that produce TGF-beta. Tr1 and Tr3 cells are derived in the periphery from naïve T-cells interacting with antigen presenting dendritic cells [30]. Thus, the adaptive immune response may be pro-atherogenic (Th1 biased, NKT cells) or athero-protective (Th-2 biased or Treg mediated).

Several auto-antigens have been identified in experimental and human atherosclerosis. These auto-antigens include oxidized LDL, heat-shock protein 65 and beta-2-glycoprotein 1, and antibodies against these antigens exist in patients with atherosclerotic vascular disease [31]. The immune response to heat-shock protein 65 or beta-2-glycoprotein 1 appears to increase atherosclerosis, whereas an immune response to oxidized LDL generally reduces atherosclerosis in experimental animals [32–39].

Using a bone marrow transplantation strategy, B cell deficiency in hyperlipidemic mice lacking the LDL receptor gene was associated with a reduction of anti-oxLDL antibody and a 30–40% increase in the lesion area, in the proximal and distal aortas [40]. Similarly, adoptive transfer of B cells from donor mice ameliorated the aggravated atherosclerosis in splenectomized apoE knockout mice [41]. Adoptive transfer of naïve CD4+ T cells or CD4+ T cells from MDA-LDL immunized donors into hypercholesterolemic immune-deficient mice resulted in aggravation of atherosclerosis, suggesting CD4+ T cells mediated immunity is pro-atherogenic [21, 22].

VACCINE AGAINST ATHEROSCLEROSIS

Vaccines have dramatically reduced the morbidity and mortality from infectious disease and resulted in the global eradication of diseases such as smallpox and poliomyelitis. In recent years, the utility of vaccination has also been extended to the field of noninfectious diseases such as Alzheimer's disease, multiple sclerosis and cancer. Early observations as far back as 1959 suggested that immunization with lipoproteins may reduce atherosclerosis in animals [42]; however it was not until about 10–15 years ago that scientists began to understand how immunization could affect atherogenesis. Historically native LDL or modified LDL has been the major immunogen used in the active immunization strategy to reduce atherosclerosis. A majority of the studies showed that immunization using native or modified homologous LDL reduces atherosclerosis in hyperlipidemic rabbits and mice using different immunization protocols, routes of administration and adjuvants [35–39]. However the underlying mechanisms and the precise identity of antigens presented by whole LDL or modified LDL remained unclear. Although these early observations suggested the tantalizing possibility that a vaccination strategy could have potential against atherosclerosis, translating such experimental observations to a clinical setting would also pose problems in the case of whole LDL as the antigen, because of the requirement of its isolation in large quantity and the accompanying safety issues. Therefore, to exploit the potential athero-protective effect of LDL immunization, identification of the protective antigenic epitopes in LDL would have provided a major advantage.

Our laboratories at Cedars Sinai Medical Center in Los Angeles, and Lund University in Sweden have focused on identifying antigenic epitopes on Apo B-100, the major protein component of LDL particle [43]. We generated a library of 302 peptide sequences (20 amino acid residues with a five amino acid overlap) spanning the entire structure of human apolipoprotein B100 molecule and screened these peptides against pooled serum from healthy control patients and patients with cardiovascular disease, for antibody titers against native or MDA-modified peptides [43]. Among these peptides, we have identified 102 peptides that are associated with an antibody response in pooled human plasma [43]. In general, the IgM responses were stronger than IgG responses and binding was higher to MDA-modified peptides than to the corresponding native peptides. Some of the peptide sequences, either as peptide mixtures or as a single peptide, when incorporated into a vaccine formulation with alum as an adjuvant, resulted in a 40–70% reduction in aortic atherosclerosis along with a reduction in plaque inflammation [44, 45]. The best athero-protective effects in mice resulted from vaccination with Apo B-100 related peptide sequences, between amino acids 16-35 (P2), 631-650 (P45) and 3136-3155 (P210); and unmodified peptide antigens were more effective than MDA modified antigens in this regard. Such athero protection could be passively transferred to non-immunized mice through adoptive transfer of splenocytes from immunized mice [45], and was associated with increased IgG expression and isotype switch to IgG1, suggesting activation of a Th2 response [44, 45].The precise mechanism(s) by which Apo B-100 peptide immunization produces athero-protective effects remain to be defined, but both an antibody response with Th2 polarization, as well as activation of an athero-protective regulatory T cell response may be involved. In this regard, we have demonstrated that passive immunization using monoclonal IgG antibodies generated against certain Apo B-100 peptide sequence (p45) has profound and rapid athero-protective, athero-regressive and anti-inflammatory effects in murine models of atherosclerosis [46–48]. Interestingly, a recent animal study reported that maternal adaptive immunity to a mixture of MDA-LDL and Cuox-LDL can influence the immune response and reduce atherosclerosis in offspring, indicating transferability of immunity across placenta [49]. If such "transferability" is also present in humans, it could have great clinical implications suggesting the possibility of providing athero-protection to the fetus from the beginning of its development by immunization of the mother.

PASSIVE IMMUNIZATION AGAINST ATHEROSCLEROSIS

Several studies have demonstrated the efficacy of passive immunization using different antibodies to reduce atherosclerosis [46–48, 50–52]. The antibodies used were in the format of IgG, and all studies showed some degrees of reduction in atherosclerosis. As in the case for active immunization, the precise mechanisms by which these IgG antibodies reduce atherosclerosis in animal models remain unclear, yet some observations have suggested that intravenous immunoglobulin confers its immunomodulatory effect via various mechanisms, such as Fc-receptor blockade, neutralization of pathogenic autoantibodies, regulation of complement activities or inactivation of T and B cells [50, 53].

OTHER IMMUNO-MODULATING STRATEGIES

Several observational studies have suggested that influenza vaccination is associated with reduced cardiovascular events, such as myocardial infarction, out-of-hospital cardiac arrest, stroke or incidences of hospital admission [54, 55]. A small randomized controlled trial of influenza vaccination (FLUVAC), further supports the use of influenza vaccination to reduce the risk of cardiovascular mortality in patients with pre-existing atherosclerotic coronary disease [56, 57]. Based on these data, both American Heart Association and American College of Cardiology Guidelines recommend influenza vaccination as a part of secondary prevention measures for patients with cardiovascular disease [58]. The precise mechanism (s) by which influenza vaccination reduces cardiovascular events remains unclear, although blunting of the vascular pro-inflammatory effects of influenza virus infection has been suggested as a potential mechanism [59]. Experimental studies have suggested modest athero-protective effects of pneumococcal vaccination in mice; however, whether similar beneficial effects occur in humans remains unknown. Orally administered DNA vaccine to inhibit plaque angiogenesis has shown athero-protective effects in mice, and a vaccine to inhibit endogenous CETP to raise HDL levels is undergoing further evaluation at this time [60–62]. Whether such immuno-modulating approaches will be safe and effective, remains to be seen.

Tolerance toward a particular antigen can be achieved by prior mucosal (orally or nasally) exposure of such antigen and such exposure is followed by specific suppression of cellular or humoral immune responses to that antigen. The mechanisms include clonal anergy/depletion of T-lymphocytes or induction of CD4+CD25+ Tregs [63]. Heat shock protein, beta-2-glycoprotein I and oxidized LDL are prototypic auto-antigens implicated in atherogenesis. Oral administration of these antigens have been shown to reduce atherosclerosis and inflammation in hypercholesterolemic mice [64–67]. Further evaluation of this approach may also be warranted.

CHALLENGING QUESTIONS AND FUTURE PERSPECTIVES

We believe that active or passive immunization strategy has the potential to emerge as a novel therapy against atherosclerotic vascular disease. However, many challenges exist before the immunization strategy can be tested clinically. We still do not fully understand the mechanisms by which immunization reduces atherosclerosis, hence the choice of optimal immunogens, adjuvants, route of administration and frequency of immunization remain to be defined. Timing of vaccination is another important issue to consider because it would be important to prevent atherosclerosis by immunizing subjects as a primary prevention measure and to slow the progression and/or induce stabilization of existing plaques as a secondary prevention strategy. Limited amount of data shows that immunization favorably changes the composition of established plaques, indicated by decreased plaque inflammation and increased collagen content. Studies to further address this question in detail are required.

Safety of the vaccines will be a major concern for the general public and medical community. A recent example of vaccine safety concern is from a clinical trial of a vaccine against amyloid beta-peptide to prevent Alzheimer's disease. That trial was terminated due to excessive occurrence of meningo-encephalitis presumably because of an adjuvant that may have provoked a Th1 mediated pro-inflammatory response [68]. Studies to investigate whether active (or passive) immunization strategy can induce or exacerbate underlying auto-immune disease or induce immune-complex mediated tissue damage or produce nonspecific immune tolerance and immuno-suppression, will also be needed.

Assessment of the clinical efficacy of immunization is another difficult question to address. It is very likely that the early phases of trials to evaluate immunization efficacy need to rely on the assessment of surrogate end-points such as atherosclerotic plaque burden/plaque composition or phenotype using noninvasive and/or invasive imaging modalities, because atherosclerosis is a chronic disease and it would take a long-term effort and follow-up to detect the effects on hard endpoints, such as death or myocardial infarction. If this initial "proof-of-concept" human trial is successful, long-term trials involving hard end-points and for durability, will also be required.

CONCLUSIONS

The number of patients with atherosclerotic vascular disease continues to grow even in the era of fast advancement in the management of atherosclerotic vascular disease. This fact highlights the need for new therapies. We have provided a brief overview of the complex and conflicting role of innate and adaptive immunity in atherosclerosis, as well as potentially promising immuno-modulatory strategies using active and passive vaccination. The development of such vaccination strategy is still in its infancy and many questions remain to be answered. Based on the existing data, we are cautiously optimistic that there is a potential future for vaccination as a complementary approach to the existing anti-atherogenic management. We sincerely hope that someday an atherosclerosis vaccination strategy (active and/or passive) will become part of our armamentarium to reduce atherosclerotic disease and its complications.

REFERENCES

1. Binder CJ, Chang MK, Shaw PX, Miller YI, Hartvigsen K, Dewan A, Witztum JL: Innate and acquired immunity in atherogenesis. *Nat.Med.* 2002, 8:1218–26.
2. Nilsson J, Hansson G, Shah PK: Immunomodulation of atherosclerosis : implications for vaccine development. *Arterioscler. Thromb.Vasc.Biol.* 2005, 25:18–28.
3. Shah PK, Chyu KY, Fredrikson GN, Nilsson J: Immunomodulation of atherosclerosis with a vaccine. *Nat.Clin.Pract. Cardiovasc.Med.* 2005 Dec;2(12):639–46.
4. Gordon S: Pattern recognition receptors: doubling up for the innate immune response. *Cell.* 2002, 111:927–30.
5. Xu XH, Shah PK, Faure E, Equils O, Thomas L, Fishbein MC, Luthringer D, Xu XP, Rajavashisth TB, Yano J, Kaul S, Arditi M: Toll-like receptor-4 is expressed by macrophages in murine and human lipid-rich atherosclerotic plaques and upregulated by oxidized LDL. *Circulation.* 2001, 104:3103–08.
6. Edfeldt K, Swedenborg J, Hansson GK, Yan ZQ: Expression of toll-like receptors in human atherosclerotic lesions: a possible pathway for plaque activation. *Circulation.* 2002, 105:1158–61.
7. Michelsen KS, Wong MH, Shah PK, Zhang W, Yano J, Doherty TM, Akira S, Rajavashisth TB, Arditi M: Lack of Toll-like receptor 4 or myeloid differentiation factor 88 reduces atherosclerosis and alters plaque phenotype in mice deficient in apolipoprotein E. *Proc.Natl.Acad.Sci.U.S.A.* 2004, 101:10679–84.
8. Bjorkbacka H, Kunjathoor VV, Moore KJ, Koehn S, Ordija CM, Lee MA, Means T, Halmen K, Luster AD, Golenbock DT, Freeman MW: Reduced atherosclerosis in MyD88-null mice links elevated serum cholesterol levels to activation of innate immunity signaling pathways. *Nat.Med.* 2004, 10:416–21.
9. Mullick AE, Tobias PS, Curtiss LK: Modulation of atherosclerosis in mice by Toll-like receptor 2. *J.Clin.Invest.* 2005, 115:3149–56.
10. Bjorkbacka H: Multiple roles of Toll-like receptor signaling in atherosclerosis. *Curr.Opin.Lipidol.* 2006, 17:527–33.
11. Shah PK: Innate immune pathway links obesity to insulin resistance. *Circ.Res.* 2007 Jun 8;100(11):1531–3.
12. Horkko S, Bird DA, Miller E, Itabe H, Leitinger N, Subbanagounder G, Berliner JA, Friedman P, Dennis EA, Curtiss LK, Palinski W, Witztum JL: Monoclonal autoantibodies specific for oxidized phospholipids or oxidized phospholipid-protein adducts inhibit macrophage uptake of oxidized low-density lipoproteins. *J.Clin.Invest.* 1999, 103:117–28.
13. Chang MK, Bergmark C, Laurila A, Horkko S, Han KH, Friedman P, Dennis EA, Witztum JL: Monoclonal antibodies against oxidized low-density lipoprotein bind to apoptotic cells and inhibit their phagocytosis by elicited macrophages: evidence that oxidation-specific epitopes mediate macrophage recognition. *Proc.Natl.Acad.Sci.U.S.A.* 1999, 96:6353–8.
14. Shaw PX, Horkko S, Chang MK, Curtiss LK, Palinski W, Silverman GJ, Witztum JL: Natural antibodies with the T15 idiotype may act in atherosclerosis, apoptotic clearance, and protective immunity. *J.Clin.Invest.* 2000, 105:1731–40.
15. Briles DE, Forman C, Hudak S, Claflin JL: Anti-phosphorylcholine antibodies of the T15 idiotype are optimally protective against Streptococcus pneumoniae. *J.Exp.Med.* 1982, 156:1177–85.
16. Binder CJ, Horkko S, Dewan A, Chang MK, Kieu EP, Goodyear CS, Shaw PX, Palinski W, Witztum JL, Silverman GJ: Pneumococcal vaccination decreases atherosclerotic lesion formation: molecular mimicry between Streptococcus pneumoniae and oxidized LDL. *Nat.Med.* 2003, 9:736–43.

17. Nguyen JT, Myers N, Palaia J, Georgopoulos A, Rubins JB, Janoff EN: Humoral responses to oxidized low-density lipoprotein and related bacterial antigens after pneumococcal vaccine. *Transl.Res.* 2007,150(3):172–9.
18. Damoiseaux J, Rijkers G, Tervaert JW: Pneumococcal vaccination does not increase circulating levels of IgM antibodies to oxidized LDL in humans and therefore precludes an anti-atherogenic effect. *Atherosclerosis.* 2007,190(1):10–1.
19. Caligiuri G, Khallou-Laschet J, Vandaele M, Gaston AT, Delignat S, Mandet C, Kohler HV, Kaveri SV, Nicoletti A. Phosphorylcholine-targeting immunization reduces atherosclerosis. *J.Am.Coll.Cardiol.* 2007 Aug 7;50(6):540–6.
20. Faria-neto JR, Chyu KY, Li XJ, Dimayuga PC, Ferreira C, Yano J, Cercek B, Shah PK: Passive immunization with monoclonal IgM antibodies against phosphorylcholine reduces accelerated vein graft atherosclerosis in apolipoprotein E-null mice. *Atherosclerosis.* 2006, 189:83–90.
21. Zhou X, Nicoletti A, Elhage R, Hansson GK: Transfer of CD4(+) T cells aggravates atherosclerosis in immunodeficient apolipoprotein E knockout mice. *Circulation.* 2000, 102:2919–22.
22. Zhou X, Robertson AK, Hjerpe C, Hansson GK: Adoptive transfer of CD4+ T cells reactive to modified low-density lipoprotein aggravates atherosclerosis. *Arterioscler.Thromb.Vasc.Biol.* 2006, 26:864–70.
23. Tupin E, Nicoletti A, Elhage R, Rudling M, Ljunggren HG, Hansson GK, Berne GP: CD1d-dependent activation of NKT cells aggravates atherosclerosis. *J.Exp.Med.* 2004, 199:417–22.
24. George J, Shoenfeld Y, Gilburd B, Afek A, Shaish A, Harats D: Requisite role for IL-4 in the acceleration of fatty streaks induced by heat shock protein 65 or mycobacterium tuberculosis. *Circ.Res.* 2000; 86:1203–10.
25. Binder CJ, Hartvigsen K, Chang MK et al: IL-5 links adaptive and natural immunity specific for epitopes of oxidized LDL and protects against atherosclerosis. *J.Clin.Invest.* 2004;114:427–37.
26. Mallat Z, Gojova A, Brun V, Esposito B, Fournier N, Cottrez F, Tedgui A, Groux H: Induction of a regulatory T cell type 1 response reduces the development of atherosclerosis in apolipoprotein E-knockout mice. *Circulation.* 2003, 108:1232–7.
27. Pinderski OL, Hedrick CC, Olvera T, Hagenbaugh A, Territo M, Berliner JA, Fyfe AI: Interleukin-10 blocks atherosclerotic events in vitro and in vivo. *Arterioscler.Thromb.Vasc.Biol.* 1999, 19:2847–53.
28. Robertson AK, Rudling M, Zhou X, Gorelik L, Flavell RA, Hansson GK: Disruption of TGF-beta signaling in T cells accelerates atherosclerosis. *J.Clin.Invest.* 2003, 112:1342–50.
29. Ait-Oufella H, Salomon BL, Potteaux S, Robertson AK, Gourdy P, Zoll J, Merval R, Esposito B, Cohen JL, Fisson S, Flavell RA, Hansson GK, Klatzmann D, Tedgui A, Mallat Z: Natural regulatory T cells control the development of atherosclerosis in mice. *Nat.Med.* 2006, 12:178–80.
30. Mallat Z, Ait-Oufella H, Tedgui A: Regulatory T-cell immunity in atherosclerosis. *Trends Cardiovasc.Med.* 2007;17:113–8.
31. Sherer Y, Shoenfeld Y: Mechanisms of disease: atherosclerosis in autoimmune diseases. *Nat.Clin.Pract.Rheumatol.* 2006, 2:99–106.
32. George J, Afek A, Gilburd B, Shoenfeld Y, Harats D: Cellular and humoral immune responses to heat shock protein 65 are both involved in promoting fatty-streak formation in LDL-receptor deficient mice. *J.Am.Coll.Cardiol.* 2001, 38:900–5.
33. George J, Afek A, Gilburd B, Blank M, Levy Y, Aron-Maor A, Levkovitz H, Shaish A, Goldberg I, Kopolovic J, Harats D, Shoenfeld Y: Induction of early atherosclerosis in LDL-receptor-deficient mice immunized with beta2-glycoprotein I. *Circulation.* 1998, 98:1108–15.
34. Dunoyer-Geindre S, Kwak BR, Pelli G, Roth I, Satta N, Fish RJ, Reber G, Mach F, Kruithof EK, de Moerloose P: Immunization of LDL receptor-deficient mice with beta (2) -glycoprotein 1 or human serum albumin induces a more inflammatory phenotype in atherosclerotic plaques. *Thromb.Haemost.* 2007, 97:129–38.
35. Palinski W, Miller E, Witztum JL: Immunization of low density lipoprotein (LDL) receptor-deficient rabbits with homologous malondialdehyde-modified LDL reduces atherogenesis. *Proc.Natl.Acad.Sci.U.S.A.* 1995, 92:821–5.
36. Ameli S, Hultgardh-Nilsson A, Regnstrom J, Calara F, Yano J, Cercek B, Shah PK, Nilsson J: Effect of immunization with homologous LDL and oxidized LDL on early atherosclerosis in hypercholesterolemic rabbits. *Arterioscler.Thromb.Vasc.Biol.* 1996, 16:1074–9.
37. Freigang S, Horkko S, Miller E, Witztum JL, Palinski W: Immunization of LDL receptor-deficient mice with homologous malondialdehyde-modified and native LDL reduces progression of atherosclerosis by mechanisms other than induction of high titers of antibodies to oxidative neoepitopes. *Arterioscler.Thromb.Vasc.Biol.* 1998, 18:1972–2.
38. George J, Afek A, Gilburd B, Levkovitz H, Shaish A, Goldberg I, Kopolovic Y, Wick G, Shoenfeld Y, Harats D: Hyperimmunization of apo-E-deficient mice with homologous malondialdehyde low-density lipoprotein suppresses early atherogenesis. *Atherosclerosis.* 1998, 138:147–52.
39. Chyu KY, Reyes OS, Zhao X, Yano J, Dimayuga P, Nilsson J, Cercek B, Shah PK: Timing affects the efficacy of LDL immunization on atherosclerotic lesions in apo E (-/-) mice. *Atherosclerosis.* 2004, 176:27–35.
40. Major AS, Fazio S, Linton MF: B-lymphocyte deficiency increases atherosclerosis in LDL receptor-null mice. *Arterioscler. Thromb.Vasc.Biol.* 2002, 22:1892–8.
41. Caligiuri G, Nicoletti A, Poirier B, Hansson GK: Protective immunity against atherosclerosis carried by B cells of hypercholesterolemic mice. *J.Clin.Invest.* 2002, 109:745–53.
42. Gero S, Gergely J, Jakab L, Szekely J, Virag S, Farkas K, Czuppon A: Inhibition of cholesterol atherosclerosis by immunisation with beta lipoprotein. *Lancet.* 1959, 2:6–7.
43. Fredrikson GN, Hedblad B, Berglund G, Alm R, Ares M, Cercek B, Chyu KY, Shah PK, Nilsson J: Identification of immune responses against aldehyde-modified peptide sequences in apoB associated with cardiovascular disease. *Arterioscler.Thromb. Vasc.Biol.* 2003, 23:872–8.

44. Fredrikson GN, Soderberg I, Lindholm M, Dimayuga P, Chyu KY, Shah PK, Nilsson J: Inhibition of atherosclerosis in apoE-null mice by immunization with apoB-100 peptide sequences. *Arterioscler.Thromb.Vasc.Biol.* 2003, 23:879–84.
45. Chyu KY, Zhao X, Reyes OS, Babbidge SM, Dimayuga PC, Yano J, Cercek B, Fredrikson GN, Nilsson J, Shah PK: Immunization using an Apo B-100 related epitope reduces atherosclerosis and plaque inflammation in hypercholesterolemic apo E (-/-) mice. *Biochem.Biophys.Res.Commun.* 2005, 338:1982–9.
46. Schiopu A, Bengtsson J, Soderberg I, Janciauskiene S, Lindgren S, Ares MP, Shah PK, Carlsson R, Nilsson J, Fredrikson GN: Recombinant Human Antibodies Against Aldehyde-Modified Apolipoprotein B-100 Peptide Sequences Inhibit Atherosclerosis. *Circulation. 2004*, 110:2047–52.
47. Strom A, Fredrikson GN, Schiopu A et al: Inhibition of injury induced arterial remodeling and carotid atherosclerosis by recombinant human antibodies against aldehyde modified apoB-100. Atherosclerosis 2006; 190:298–305.
48. Schiopu A, Frendeus B, Jansson B et al: Recombinant antibodies to an oxidized low density lipoprotein epitope induce rapid regression of atherosclerosis in apobec-1 (-/-)low density lipoprotein receptor(-/-) mice. *J.Am.Coll.Cardiol.* 2007; 50:2313–8.
49. Yamashita T, Freigang S, Eberle C, Pattison J, Gupta S, Napoli C, Palinski W: Maternal immunization programs postnatal immune responses and reduces atherosclerosis in offspring. *Circ.Res.* 2006, 99:e51–64.
50. Nicoletti A, Kaveri S, Caligiuri G, Bariety J, Hansson GK: Immunoglobulin treatment reduces atherosclerosis in apo E knock-out mice. *J.Clin.Invest.* 1998, 102:910–8.
51. Yuan Z, Kishimoto C, Sano H, Shioji K, Xu Y, Yokode M: Immunoglobulin treatment suppresses atherosclerosis in apolipoprotein E-deficient mice via the Fc portion. *Am.J.Physiol.Heart Circ.Physiol.* 2003, 285:H899–906.
52. Nicolo D, Goldman BI, Monestier M: Reduction of atherosclerosis in low-density lipoprotein receptor-deficient mice by passive administration of antiphospholipid antibody. *Arthritis Rheum.* 2003, 48:2974–8.
53. Sapir T, Shoenfeld Y: Facing the enigma of immunomodulatory effects of intravenous immunoglobulin. *Clin.Rev.Allergy Immunol.* 2005, 29:185–99.
54. Nichol KL, Nordin J, Mullooly J, Lask R, Fillbrandt K, Iwane M: Influenza vaccination and reduction in hospitalizations for cardiac disease and stroke among the elderly. *N.Engl.J.Med.* 2003, 348:1322–32.
55. Madjid M, Naghavi M, Litovsky S, Casscells SW: Influenza and cardiovascular disease: a new opportunity for prevention and the need for further studies. *Circulation.* 2003, 108:2730–36.
56. Gurfinkel EP, de la Fuente RL, Mendiz O, Mautner B: Influenza vaccine pilot study in acute coronary syndromes and planned percutaneous coronary interventions: the FLU Vaccination Acute Coronary Syndromes (FLUVACS) Study. *Circulation.* 2002, 105:2143–47.
57. Gurfinkel EP, Leon de la FR, Mendiz O, Mautner B: Flu vaccination in acute coronary syndromes and planned percutaneous coronary interventions (FLUVACS) Study. *Eur.Heart J.* 2004, 25:25–31.
58. Davis MM, Taubert K, Benin AL, Brown DW, Mensah GA, Baddour LM, Dunbar S, Krumholz HM: Influenza vaccination as secondary prevention for cardiovascular disease. A science advisory from the American Heart Association/American College of Cardiology. *Circulation.* 2006, 114:1549–53.
59. Van Lenten BJ, Wagner AC, Anantharamaiah GM, Garber DW, Fishbein MC, Adhikary L, Nayak DP, Hama S, Navab M, Fogelman AM: Influenza infection promotes macrophage traffic into arteries of mice that is prevented by D-4F, an apolipoprotein A-I mimetic peptide. *Circulation.* 2002;106(9):1127–32.
60. Petrovan RJ, Kaplan CD, Reisfeld RA, Curtiss LK: DNA vaccination against VEGF receptor 2 reduces atherosclerosis in LDL receptor-deficient mice. *Arterioscler.Thromb.Vasc.Biol.* 2007 May;27(5):1095–100. Epub 2007 Feb 15.
61. Chyu KY, Shah PK: Choking off plaque neovascularity: a promising atheroprotective strategy or a double-edged sword? *Arterioscler.Thromb.Vasc.Biol.* 2007 May;27(5):993–5.
62. Davidson MH, Maki K, Umporowicz D, Wheeler A, Rittershaus C, Ryan U: The safety and immunogenicity of a CETP vaccine in healthy adults. *Atherosclerosis.* 2003 Jul;169(1):113–20.
63. Faria AM, Weiner HL: Oral tolerance. *Immunol.Rev.* 2005, 206:232–59.
64. Maron R, Sukhova G, Faria AM, Hoffmann E, Mach F, Libby P, Weiner HL: Mucosal administration of heat shock protein-65 decreases atherosclerosis and inflammation in aortic arch of low-density lipoprotein receptor-deficient mice. *Circulation.* 2002, 106:1708–15.
65. Harats D, Yacov N, Gilburd B, Shoenfeld Y, George J: Oral tolerance with heat shock protein 65 attenuates Mycobacterium tuberculosis-induced and high-fat-diet-driven atherosclerotic lesions. *J.Am.Coll.Cardiol.* 2002, 40:1333–8.
66. George J, Yacov N, Breitbart E, Bangio L, Shaish A, Gilburd B, Shoenfeld Y, Harats D: Suppression of early atherosclerosis in LDL-receptor deficient mice by oral tolerance with beta 2-glycoprotein I. *Cardiovasc.Res.* 2004, 62:603–9.
67. van Puijvelde GH, Hauer AD, de Vos P, van den HR, van Herwijnen MJ, van der ZR, van Eden W, van Berkel TJ, Kuiper J: Induction of oral tolerance to oxidized low-density lipoprotein ameliorates atherosclerosis. *Circulation.* 2006, 114:1968–1976.
68. Orgogozo JM, Gilman S, Dartigues JF, Laurent B, Puel M, Kirby LC, Jouanny P, Dubois B, Eisner L, Flitman S, Michel BF, Boada M, Frank A, Hock C: Subacute meningoencephalitis in a subset of patients with AD after Abeta42 immunization. *Neurology.* 2003, 61:46–54.

VII

Local and Focal Therapies for Stabilization of Vulnerable Arteries and Plaques

51 Drug-Eluting Stents: A Potential Preemptive Treatment Choice for Vulnerable Coronary Plaques

Edwin Lee, George Dangas, and Roxana Mehran

CONTENTS

ABSTRACT

Restenosis, a major limitation of percutaneous transluminal coronary angioplasty, has been dramatically reduced by the use of drug-eluting stents (DES). Because the majority of acute coronary events occur at nonobstructive lesions that are vulnerable, it has been suggested that prophylactic stenting of vulnerable plaques (VP) to prevent further plaque instability, thereby preventing future coronary events, is as a reasonable strategy. The use of DES in treating intermediate coronary lesions has been shown to be safe and effective. Clinical trials evaluating different intracoronary imaging modalities for the detection of VP and to define its association with subsequent coronary events are ongoing. Risk stratification of such intermediate lesions by VP imaging can help to identify appropriate lesions for preemptive treatment in patients who are at high risk for acute coronary events or recurrent events. Such a strategy should help to improve

From: *Asymptomatic Atherosclerosis: Pathophysiology, Detection and Treatment*
Edited by: M. Naghavi (ed.), DOI 10.1007/978-1-60327-179-0_51

outcomes in these patients. Current limitations of DES include the long-term risk of stent thrombosis and the need for prolonged dual antiplatelet therapy. Several other transcatheter-based approaches for the stabilization of VP to overcome the limitations of DES are under development. These include drug-eluting balloons, bioabsorbable stents, photodynamic therapy, and cyroenergy. These improvements in technology hopefully will reduce or eliminate the long-term risk of stent thrombosis associated with DES, thus shifting the risk-benefit ratio toward prophylactic stenting of nonobstructive VP in the future.

Key words: Drug-eluting stents; Vulnerable plaque; Intermediate lesions

KEY POINTS

- The majority of fatal and nonfatal myocardial infarctions (MIs) are triggered by the rupture of vulnerable plaque (VP), frequently at noncritical sites in the coronary tree.
- The ultimate goal of VP treatment is to accurately risk stratify patients and target therapy toward passivating VP, thereby preventing future acute coronary events.
- For drug-eluting stents (DES) to be used as a preemptive therapy for VP, they must confer a healing effect as well as an antirestenotic effect.
- Currently, several catheter-based approaches are under investigation for the stabilization of VP.

DES have dramatically reduced restenosis, one of the major limitations of modern percutaneous coronary interventions (PCI). However, with this advance, new controversy has arisen about the optimal management of incidental stenoses identified during PCI. Previously, these asymptomatic, nonculprit stenoses were treated conservatively due to the risk of restenosis. However, more than 80% of fatal and nonfatal MIs occur at sites that were recently less than 75% stenotic [1], and most cardiac events are triggered by the rupture of vulnerable plaque (VP), frequently found at nonobstructive locations in the coronary tree [2, 3].

The ultimate goal of VP detection is to accurately risk stratify patients and target therapy toward passivating VP, thereby preventing future acute coronary events. Although local treatment of VP is a welcome addition, many events continue to occur in patients receiving the best current medical therapy; even optimal low-density lipoprotein levels do not eliminate all events on follow-up (In the PROVE-IT trial, 22.4% of patients had a coronary event during 2 years of intensive statin therapy) [4]. Therefore, the impact of early VP detection and local therapy would represent a major breakthrough in the prevention of acute coronary events.

IS LOCAL THERAPY FOR VP FEASIBLE?

For local VP therapy to be feasible, one must show the existence and prospective detection of local areas of the vessel that are at increased risk of causing a coronary event. During a dedicated VP conference, Ambrose proposed a set of prerequisites for the use of local therapy for the treatment of VP [5] (see Table 1). Questions to be addressed include: What is the best imaging method

Table 1
Prerequisites for a local approach for the treatment of vulnerable plaque

• Vulnerable plaque can be identified with modern diagnostic imaging methods
• Vulnerable plaque prone to plaque rupture or plaque erosion should be readily identifiable
• The number of vulnerable plaques is known, and the number is limited
• The natural history of a vulnerable plaque has been identified in patients treated with optimal systemic therapies
• A local interventional approach to an asymptomatic VP is proven to reduce future events relative to the best systemic therapy

Modified from [5]

(morphological, functional, or a combination) for detection of VP in the absence of a 'gold standard' since tissue from patients for histological analysis is not routinely available? How many VP areas are present at any one time at a per lesion, per vessel or per patient level? What is the temporal stability of VPs–do some quiesce or heal? What type of imaging will have the greatest predictive accuracy for VP detection and subsequent events? These questions need to be answered with the use of a validated detector of VP before a recommendation can be made for focal therapy, which must be based on data from a randomized trial demonstrating that the focal therapy provides benefits that outweigh the complications associated with the intervention. Such clinical trials of intracoronary VP detection are being planned or are in progress (see Table 2).

Table 2
Summary of prospective clinical trials (in progress or planned) of vulnerable plaques characterized by intracoronary diagnostic devices

Name of trial	*Technique to be evaluated*	*Trial design*	*Types and number of patients to be enrolled*
PREDICTION	Shear stress profiling	Changes in plaque morphology at sites with low shear stress, plus major adverse cardiac events	500 PCI
PROSPECT	IVUS-based plaque composition	Natural history for coronary events	700 PCI ACS
SPECIAL	IVUS-based plaque composition	Lesion progression and natural history for coronary events	2,000 PCI, including 1,000 with repeat IVUS measurements at 12 months
Substudy of PROSPECT	Palpography	Natural history for coronary events?	200 PCI
IBIS-2	Palpography	Assessment of treatment with inhibitor of lipoprotein-associated phospholipase-2; end points are palpography and CRP	450 PCI
Vulnerability Index Program 1	Thermography	Feasibility and tolerability of thermal measurements	160 PCI stable angina
Vulnerability Index Program 2	Thermography	Natural history for coronary events (after vulnerability index program 1)	700 PCI ACS
SPECTACL	NIR spectroscopy	Spectra in patients, followed by natural history for coronary events	2,000 PCI
NIH-funded OCT	Optical Coherence Tomography	Stenosis progression on 18-month restudy	100 PCI

Modified from [18]. *ACS* acute coronary syndrome, *CRP* C-reactive protein, *IVUS* intravascular ultrasound, *NIR* near infrared, *PCI* percutaneous coronary intervention

DOES LOCAL TREATMENT MAKE SENSE WHEN ATHEROSCLEROSIS IS A DIFFUSE DISEASE?

Although atherosclerosis is a systemic disease affecting many arterial vessels, it also has been demonstrated that most cases of fatal MI or sudden cardiac death result from a single occlusive thrombus over a ruptured or eroded plaque, and most have at least 1 or 2 additional VPs [3]. In patients with acute coronary syndromes (ACSs), in addition to the culprit lesion causing the index ischemic event, multiple ruptured plaques are found in addition to these lesions in vessels not related to the acute event. Goldstein et al. [6] reported the presence of additional complex angiographic lesions in one third of patients presenting with ACS. In an angioscopic study, Asakura et al. [7] reported the frequent presence of vulnerable, yellow coronary plaques distant from the culprit lesion in patients with ACS. With the use of IVUS, Rioufol et al. reported that almost 80% of ACS patients have more than 1 ruptured plaque [8], which is in sharp contrast to the commonly held belief of a "single culprit lesion."

The aforementioned studies all support the conclusion that atherosclerosis is a systemic disease with focal manifestations. It also has shown that certain areas of the coronary arteries based on location of culprit lesions are responsible for ACS. It has been shown that most of the lesions causing ACS occur within the proximal 30 mm of the major coronary arteries [9]. The presence of these lesions at focal sites is no coincidence, because these areas also are sites of decreased shear stress and increased numbers of thin-capped fibroatheroma and ruptured plaques [10], which play a critical role in vulnerability. Because VP is localized and the risk of ACS is predictable and associated with a relatively limited length of the artery, it is possible that local therapy at these sites in at-risk patients might be useful for preventing subsequent coronary events.

IS THERE A ROLE FOR STENTING OF INTERMEDIATE CORONARY STENOSES THAT MAY NOT BE FLOW LIMITING?

With the reduction in restenosis achieved by using DES, there is controversy concerning the management of incidental, nontarget lesions, which have been treated conservatively in the past because of the risk of restenosis. The decision whether to treat such lesions to prevent potential future plaque instability is challenging.

The magnitude of risk posed by the progression of such incidental nonculprit lesions was reported by Glaser et al. [11]. In the year following culprit lesion PCI, 6% of patients required clinically driven repeat PCI for nonculprit lesions. More than half of these patients presented with ACS. The majority (87%) of lesions requiring subsequent PCI were reported to be intermediate stenoses during the original PCI. Cutlip et al. [12] also reported that the majority of events in the years after culprit PCI were due to events related to nontarget lesion disease progression. On the other hand, one should take into consideration the potential long-term risks after DES implantation, which may relate either to the DES components themselves or to the required antiplatelet therapy.

IS THERE A RANDOMIZED TRIAL OF TREATMENT OF INTERMEDIATE LESIONS?

The use of stents or angioplasty for lesions causing intermediate stenosis was prospectively examined in the DEFER trial, which used angiography and coronary flow dynamics to assess stenosis significance [13]. Patients with intermediate stenoses not causing a significant reduction in fractional flow reserve were randomly assigned to intervention [angioplasty or bare-metal stent (BMS)] or medical therapy. At 5-year follow-up, rates of cardiac death and MI were low and equivalent between

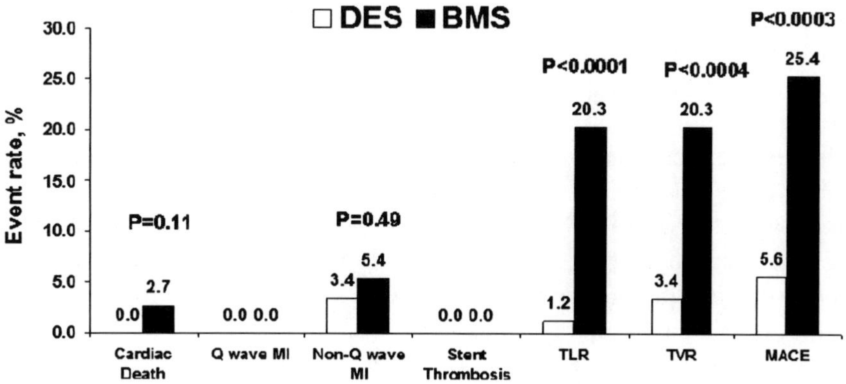

Fig. 1. One-year clinical outcomes of patients with intermediate lesions randomized to drug-eluting stents versus bare metal stents. Modified from [15]. *TLR* target lesion revascularization, *TVR* target vessel revascularization, *MACE* major adverse cardiac events.

patients assigned to medical therapy and those treated with the intervention [14]. The authors concluded that the low risk of MI and cardiac death in this population (<1% per year) did not justify intervention for intermediate stenoses in this group of patients. However, the study excluded patients with more active disease who had sustained an MI; balloon angioplasty without a stent was used in the majority of patients.

The use of contemporary DES for the treatment of intermediate coronary lesions was examined retrospectively in a pooled analysis of clinical trials comparing DES with BMS [15]. At 1-year follow-up, patients treated with DES compared with BMS had lower rates of restenosis, target vessel revascularization (TVR), and major adverse cardiac events, while rates of cardiac death and MI were low and equivalent (Fig. 1). No patients in either group developed stent thrombosis. The favorable safety and efficacy conferred by DES along with the low rates of restenosis in treating intermediate lesions has reignited an interest in strategies to prevent plaque rupture and progression of atherosclerosis.

VP imaging can help risk-stratify such intermediate lesions, and along with defining systemic patient risks [16, 17], can help identify appropriate lesions for local treatment, which should improve outcomes in such patients. The possibility that stenting of intermediate lesions suspected of being vulnerable will be of value should constitute the subject of a prospective clinical trial.

WHAT IS THE ROLE OF DES IN THE TREATMENT OF VULNERABLE CORONARY PLAQUES?

Use of DES in an atherosclerotic rabbit model as a possible treatment for VP has been evaluated. Placement of a DES over VP reduced the size of the lipid core, induced formation of an additional “fibrous cap” over the lipid pool, and caused new healthy neointima formation over the thin shoulders of the plaque [18]. These encouraging animal results will have to be tested clinically to investigate whether the benefits outweigh the risks associated with stenting VP.

At present, there is no clinical evidence supporting the use of DES for the local treatment of VP in nonobstructive lesions. The identification of VP lesions is a critical issue because current VP imaging methods have yet to achieve the goal of characterizing plaque morphology to the degree necessary to correctly identify rupture-prone lesions according to pathological criteria. Thus, the evaluation of promising local treatments for VP (DES, photodynamic therapy and other options) is hindered by the absence of validated diagnostic devices. Much research is underway to identify the optimal combination of imaging and biomarkers to improve diagnosis of VP.

Given these gaps in our knowledge, patients who may potentially benefit from DES treatment of VP include those who are at high risk for acute coronary events (primary prevention) and those who are at high risk for recurrent coronary events (secondary prevention) [16, 17]. These individuals possess VP whose near-term risk of causing ACS is high and for whom the benefits of treatment far outweigh the risks associated with DES. In addition, for local therapies of VP to be effective, systemic treatments must supplement local therapies in treating the "vulnerable patient" and not merely the VP [18, 19]. The theory behind such an approach is similar to some cancer treatments, such as treating breast cancer with systemic chemotherapy plus local radiation.

Besides showing efficacy in clinical trials, local DES therapy of VP also must be cost-effective. Bosch et al. [20] reported a hypothetical catheter-based approach for VP detection in patients with CAD undergoing PCI and treatment of nonstenotic VP with DES. The study showed that treatment prevented many unfavorable events, such as recurrent angina, MIs, and sudden death, which are associated with higher costs and poor quality of life. Even when the catheter VP test had a sensitivity and specificity of 80% with a VP prevalence of 10% or more in the population, this strategy of DES treatment remained cost effective.

IS THERE A "KINDER AND GENTLER" TYPE OF STENT TO BE MADE?

Compared with BMS, DES can markedly reduce neointimal proliferation and restenosis rates, leading to a major reduction in the need for TVR and an improved long-term clinical outcome [21, 22]. However, the potent anti-inflammatory and antiproliferative properties of DES may represent a double-edged sword. DES are coated with antiproliferative drugs that abolish the excessive healing response, but at the same time hinder the healing process that covers the stent struts with endothelial cells [23, 24], thereby impairing normal endothelial function [25] and possibly affecting endothelium-dependent vasomotor function [26]. Other concerns with DES include late malapposition, hypersensitivity reactions [27], and the long-term risk of stent thrombosis [28]. These limitations of DES potentially may be overcome by utilization of bioabsorbable stents.

Bioabsorbable metallic stents provide temporary scaffolding that "disappears" by absorption at 60–90 days after deployment. The concept of PCI with bioabsorbable stents is attractive, since there may be more disadvantages with a permanent coronary stent. Animal studies of bioabsorbable stents show complete and rapid endothelization, low neointima proliferation, minimum inflammatory changes, and complete absorption within 2 months [29–31]. Potential advantages of having the bioabsorbable stent disappear from the treated site may include reduced late-stent thrombosis; if the struts disappear, these foreign bodies (metal and polymer) would not be persistently present. Stent absorption may allow restoration of vasomotion and possibly reduce problems with current stent technology such as stent-strut fracture and a delayed allergy to polymer [27, 28]. The first-in-human experience with a bioabsorbable magnesium stent in 63 patients found them to be safe at 1-year follow-up with no stent thrombosis, MI, or death [32]. However, angiographic restenosis occurred in 48% of patients and overall target lesion revascularization (TLR) was 45% at 1 year. These rates are similar to, or higher than, those reported with balloon angioplasty alone. Nonmetallic bioabsorbable stents that elute the antiproliferative drug everolimus are currently being tested. They may reduce restenosis and TLR rates seen with current bioabsorbable stents. Although bioabsorbable stents are in an early stage of development, they hold promise in overcoming some of the limitations of permanent metallic implants.

Table 3
Other focal intracoronary devices for the treatment of vulnerable plaque

- Photodynamic therapy
- Cryotherapy
- Sonotherapy
- Heating
- Bioabsorbable stents
- Drug-eluting balloons

ARE THERE ANY OTHER LOCAL APPROACHES FOR THE TREATMENT OF VULNERABLE PLAQUES?

Several other catheter-based approaches are currently under investigation to try to stabilize VP before it disrupts, including various types of drug eluting balloons (see Table 3).

It has been hypothesized that percutaneous transluminal coronary angioplasty (PTCA) reinjures arterial segments and leaves a primitive scar behind that is not capable of "growing" atherosclerosis [33]. PTCA typically induces plaque splitting that causes a tissue reaction to cover the plaque. The smooth muscle-rich neointima later transforms into a collagen-rich layer, which results in plaque sealing. The concept of plaque sealing was examined in a post-hoc analysis of clinical trials and registries that showed an unacceptably high 1-year event rate when intermediate stenoses were treated by PTCA [34]. Plaque sealing, however, could be reconsidered in light of drug-eluting balloons [35, 36] as a method to intentionally rupture nonstenotic VP. Compared with DES, PTCA with drug-eluting balloons requires combined dual antiplatelet therapy for 1 month post intervention followed by treatment with aspirin alone. PTCA also would not carry the long-term risks associated with stenting. This concept requires evaluation in randomized trials, however.

Photodynamic therapy has been used to stabilize a specific plaque or an arterial region by selective ablation of macrophages or other targeted cells. This method involves the combination of a chemical photosensitizer and visible light at a specific wavelength to selectively illuminate and activate the photosensitizer, leading to production of radical oxygen species and resulting apoptosis. Motexafin lutetium is a photosensitizer derived from the porphyrin molecule that binds to LDL receptors and is transported into macrophage-rich plaque [37]. In atherosclerotic rabbit model, photoactivation led to a marked decrease in macrophages and a mild reduction in atheroma with no damage to normal tissue. The same agent has been tested in human coronary artery disease in patients undergoing coronary stenting and found to be well tolerated [38].

Cryoenergy as a treatment modality has been shown to reduce restenosis and increase the density of type III collage in balloon-injured porcine arteries [39]. Therefore, cryoenergy might favorably modify VP because it can induce local apoptosis without causing excessive neointimal proliferation. Although intravascular heating and sonotherapy have been considered as possible methods to treat VP, there has been little evidence to support such a strategy.

CONCLUSION

The concept of identifying and treating "vulnerable patients" prone to plaque rupture has been described as the "Holy Grail of cardiology." DES (and the accompanying low restenosis rates) have been shown to be safe and efficacious in treating intermediate coronary lesions. A randomized clinical trial is needed to determine if DES treatment of VP is feasible (i.e., safe and effective). Improvements in stent and balloon technology have led to new devices (bioabsorbable stents and drug-eluting balloons) that may reduce or eliminate the long-term risk of stent thrombosis. This could potentially shift the risk-to-benefit ratio toward prophylactic stenting of nonstenotic VPs in the future. Until then, the theoretical quest for an appropriate local therapy for VP continues.

REFERENCES

1. Falk E, Shah PK, Fuster V. Coronary plaque disruption. Circulation 1995;92:657–71.
2. Kolodgie FD, Virmani R, Burke AP, et al. Pathologic assessment of the vulnerable human coronary plaque. Heart 2004;90:1385–91.
3. Burke AP, Farb A, Malcom GT, Liang YH, Smialek J, Virmani R. Coronary risk factors and plaque morphology in men with coronary disease who died suddenly. N Engl J Med 1997;336:1276–82.
4. Ridker PM, Cannon CP, Morrow D, et al. C-reactive protein levels and outcomes after statin therapy. N Engl J Med 2005;352:20–8.
5. Ambrose JA. In search of the "vulnerable plaque": can it be localized and will focal regional therapy ever be an option for cardiac prevention? J Am Coll Cardiol 2008;51:1539–42.
6. Goldstein JA, Demetriou D, Grines CL, Pica M, Shoukfeh M, O'Neill WW. Multiple complex coronary plaques in patients with acute myocardial infarction. N Engl J Med 2000;343:915–22.
7. Asakura M, Ueda Y, Yamaguchi O, et al. Extensive development of vulnerable plaques as a pan-coronary process in patients with myocardial infarction: an angioscopic study. J Am Coll Cardiol 2001;37:1284–8.
8. Rioufol G, Finet G, Ginon I, et al. Multiple atherosclerotic plaque rupture in acute coronary syndrome: a three-vessel intravascular ultrasound study. Circulation 2002;106:804–8.
9. Wang JC, Normand SL, Mauri L, Kuntz RE. Coronary artery spatial distribution of acute myocardial infarction occlusions. Circulation 2004;110:278–84.
10. Kolodgie FD, Burke AP, Farb A, et al. The thin-cap fibroatheroma: a type of vulnerable plaque: the major precursor lesion to acute coronary syndromes. Curr Opin Cardiol 2001;16:285–92.
11. Glaser R, Selzer F, Faxon DP, et al. Clinical progression of incidental, asymptomatic lesions discovered during culprit vessel coronary intervention. Circulation 2005;111:143–9.
12. Cutlip DE, Chhabra AG, Baim DS, et al. Beyond restenosis: five-year clinical outcomes from second-generation coronary stent trials. Circulation 2004;110:1226–30.
13. Bech GJ, De Bruyne B, Pijls NH, et al. Fractional flow reserve to determine the appropriateness of angioplasty in moderate coronary stenosis: a randomized trial. Circulation 2001;103:2928–34.
14. Pijls NH, van Schaardenburgh P, Manoharan G, et al. Percutaneous coronary intervention of functionally nonsignificant stenosis: 5-year follow-up of the DEFER study. J Am Coll Cardiol 2007;49:2105–11.
15. Moses JW, Stone GW, Nikolsky E, et al. Drug-eluting stents in the treatment of intermediate lesions: pooled analysis from four randomized trials. J Am Coll Cardiol 2006;47:2164–71.
16. Naghavi M, Falk E, Hecht HS, et al. From vulnerable plaque to vulnerable patient–Part III: executive summary of the screening for heart attack prevention and education (SHAPE) task force report. Am J Cardiol 2006;98:2H–15.
17. Young JJ, Phillips HR, Marso SP, et al. Vulnerable plaque intervention: state of the art. Catheter Cardiovasc Interv 2008;71:367–74.
18. Waxman S, Ishibashi F, Muller JE. Detection and treatment of vulnerable plaques and vulnerable patients: novel approaches to prevention of coronary events. Circulation 2006;114:2390–411.
19. Ambrose JA, D'Agate DJ. Plaque rupture and intracoronary thrombus in nonculprit vessels: an eyewitness account. J Am Coll Cardiol 2005;45:659–60.
20. Bosch JL, Beinfeld MT, Muller JE, Brady T, Gazelle GS. A cost-effectiveness analysis of a hypothetical catheter-based strategy for the detection and treatment of vulnerable coronary plaques with drug-eluting stents. J Interv Cardiol 2005;18:339–49.
21. Spaulding C, Daemen J, Boersma E, Cutlip DE, Serruys PW. A pooled analysis of data comparing sirolimus-eluting stents with bare-metal stents. N Engl J Med 2007;356:989–97.
22. Stone GW, Moses JW, Ellis SG, et al. Safety and efficacy of sirolimus- and paclitaxel-eluting coronary stents. N Engl J Med 2007;356:998–1008.
23. Kotani J, Awata M, Nanto S, et al. Incomplete neointimal coverage of sirolimus-eluting stents: angioscopic findings. J Am Coll Cardiol 2006;47:2108–11.
24. Finn AV, Joner M, Nakazawa G, et al. Pathological correlates of late drug-eluting stent thrombosis: strut coverage as a marker of endothelialization. Circulation 2007;115:2435–41.
25. Hofma SH, van der Giessen WJ, van Dalen BM, et al. Indication of long-term endothelial dysfunction after sirolimus-eluting stent implantation. Eur Heart J 2006;27:166–70.

26. Obata JE, Kitta Y, Takano H, et al. Sirolimus-eluting stent implantation aggravates endothelial vasomotor dysfunction in the infarct-related coronary artery in patients with acute myocardial infarction. J Am Coll Cardiol 2007;50:1305–9.
27. Virmani R, Guagliumi G, Farb A, et al. Localized hypersensitivity and late coronary thrombosis secondary to a sirolimus-eluting stent: should we be cautious? Circulation 2004;109:701–5.
28. Finn AV, Nakazawa G, Joner M, et al. Vascular responses to drug eluting stents: importance of delayed healing. Arterioscler Thromb Vasc Biol 2007;27:1500–10.
29. Heublein B, Rohde R, Kaese V, Niemeyer M, Hartung W, Haverich A. Biocorrosion of magnesium alloys: a new principle in cardiovascular implant technology? Heart 2003;89:651–6.
30. Waksman R, Pakala R, Kuchulakanti PK, et al. Safety and efficacy of bioabsorbable magnesium alloy stents in porcine coronary arteries. Catheter Cardiovasc Interv 2006;68:607–17; discussion 618–9.
31. Di Mario C, Griffiths H, Goktekin O, et al. Drug-eluting bioabsorbable magnesium stent. J Interv Cardiol 2004;17:391–5.
32. Erbel R, Di Mario C, Bartunek J, et al. Temporary scaffolding of coronary arteries with bioabsorbable magnesium stents: a prospective, non-randomised multicentre trial. Lancet 2007;369:1869–75.
33. Meier B. Plaque sealing by coronary angioplasty. Heart 2004;90:1395–8.
34. Mercado N, Maier W, Boersma E, et al. Clinical and angiographic outcome of patients with mild coronary lesions treated with balloon angioplasty or coronary stenting. Implications for mechanical plaque sealing. Eur Heart J 2003;24:541–51.
35. Scheller B, Hehrlein C, Bocksch W, et al. Treatment of coronary in-stent restenosis with a paclitaxel-coated balloon catheter. N Engl J Med 2006;355:2113–24.
36. Tepe G, Zeller T, Albrecht T, et al. Local delivery of paclitaxel to inhibit restenosis during angioplasty of the leg. N Engl J Med 2008;358:689–99.
37. Hayase M, Woodbum KW, Perlroth J, et al. Photoangioplasty with local motexafin lutetium delivery reduces macrophages in a rabbit post-balloon injury model. Cardiovasc Res 2001;49:449–55.
38. Kereiakes DJ, Szyniszewski AM, Wahr D, et al. Phase I drug and light dose-escalation trial of motexafin lutetium and far red light activation (phototherapy) in subjects with coronary artery disease undergoing percutaneous coronary intervention and stent deployment: procedural and long-term results. Circulation 2003;108:1310–5.
39. Tanguay JF, Geoffroy P, Dorval JF, Sirois MG. Percutaneous endoluminal arterial cryoenergy improves vascular remodelling after angioplasty. Thromb Haemost 2004;92:1114–21.

52 Intrapericardial Approach for Pancoronary Stabilization of the Vulnerable Arteries and Myocardium

Venkatesan Vidi and Sergio Waxman

CONTENTS

ABSTRACT

Percutaneous intrapericardial drug delivery may be a potential alternative to existing methods of percutaneous revascularization, myocardial preservation, and plaque stabilization.

Because of the natural barrier action of the pericardium, systemic absorption of drugs or biological agents is considerably less than with intravascular routes. This allows for the use of smaller doses of such substances to obtain higher concentrations in the pericardial fluid, prolonging their time of action and exposure to epicardial coronary arteries and myocardium, and increasing their cardiac specificity.

Experimental studies of intrapericardial therapy have demonstrated salvage of infarcted myocardium and treatment of ischemia by angiogenesis, as well as inhibition of restenosis and antiarrhythmic effects, underscoring the potential opportunities of using the pericardial space for therapeutic interventions.

Percutaneous methods to access the pericardial space for drug delivery have been explored and appear to be feasible and well tolerated in preclinical models.

Even though the localized delivery of therapeutic agents into the pericardial space appears to have advantages over other routes of administration, the long-term effects of pharmacobiologic agents injected into the pericardial space are unknown. Further studies are needed to evaluate this approach.

From: *Asymptomatic Atherosclerosis: Pathophysiology, Detection and Treatment*
Edited by: M. Naghavi (ed.), DOI 10.1007/978-1-60327-179-0_52

Key words: Coronary artery disease; Local drug delivery; Pericardial delivery; Pericardium

KEY POINTS

- Percutaneous intrapericardial drug delivery may be a potential alternative to existing methods of percutaneous revascularization, myocardial preservation, and plaque stabilization.
- Because of the natural barrier action of the pericardium, systemic absorption of drugs or biological agents is considerably less than with intravascular routes. This allows for the use of smaller doses of such substances to obtain higher concentrations in the pericardial fluid, prolonging their time of action and exposure to epicardial coronary arteries and myocardium, and increasing their cardiac specificity.
- Experimental studies of intrapericardial therapy have demonstrated salvage of infarcted myocardium and treatment of ischemia by angiogenesis, as well as inhibition of restenosis and antiarrhythmic effects, underscoring the potential opportunities of using the pericardial space for therapeutic interventions.
- Percutaneous methods to access the pericardial space for drug delivery have been explored and appear to be feasible and well tolerated in preclinical models.
- Even though the localized delivery of therapeutic agents into the pericardial space appears to have advantages over other routes of administration, the long-term effects of pharmacobiologic agents injected into the pericardial space are unknown. Further studies are needed to evaluate this approach.

INTRODUCTION

The estimated prevalence of coronary artery disease (CAD) in America was 16 million in 2005. CAD caused one in five deaths in the United States in 2004. The estimated annual incidence of myocardial infarction is 600,000 new events, and despite major advances in the treatment of coronary heart disease, an estimated 320,000 recurrent attacks occur annually [1] in patients who are already known to have CAD. After successful treatment of the initial culprit lesion by a percutaneous coronary intervention (PCI), the incidence of clinical plaque progression requiring additional nontarget lesion PCI is approximately 6% in the next year [2], and in subsequent years, the events rates from nontarget lesions may even be higher than target lesion events (average annual hazard rate 6.3% vs. 1.7%, respectively). Over a follow-up period of 5 years, these nontarget lesion events contribute to a 46.4% overall event rate [3]. These sobering numbers have led to a search for different and improved approaches to stabilize the so-called vulnerable plaques, and justify the growing interest in the possibility of intrapericardial treatment targeted at vulnerable arteries and myocardium. The aim of this study is to highlight the rationale for pericardial delivery and review preclinical data, possible methods of approach, and agents that could be used for pericardial treatment for vulnerable plaques and myocardium.

CASE SCENARIO

This is the hypothetical case of a sedentary 52-year-old man with a 30-pack year history of smoking and family history of premature atherosclerosis, now presenting with a non-ST elevation myocardial infarction. His coronary angiogram (Fig. 1) revealed a 40% stenosis in his mid-right coronary artery (RCA), followed by an 80% stenosis distally, and a 90% stenosis in the posterior descending artery, of which the latter two are considered to be the culprit lesions. His proximal left anterior descending artery had a 60% stenosis, and another 50% stenosis was noted in the mid-portion. The left circumflex artery was noted to have diffuse luminal irregularities. A contemporary treatment plan would include stenting of the two narrowest lesions in the RCA and aggressive medical therapy with aspirin, clopidogrel, a beta-blocker, and an angiotensin-converting enzyme

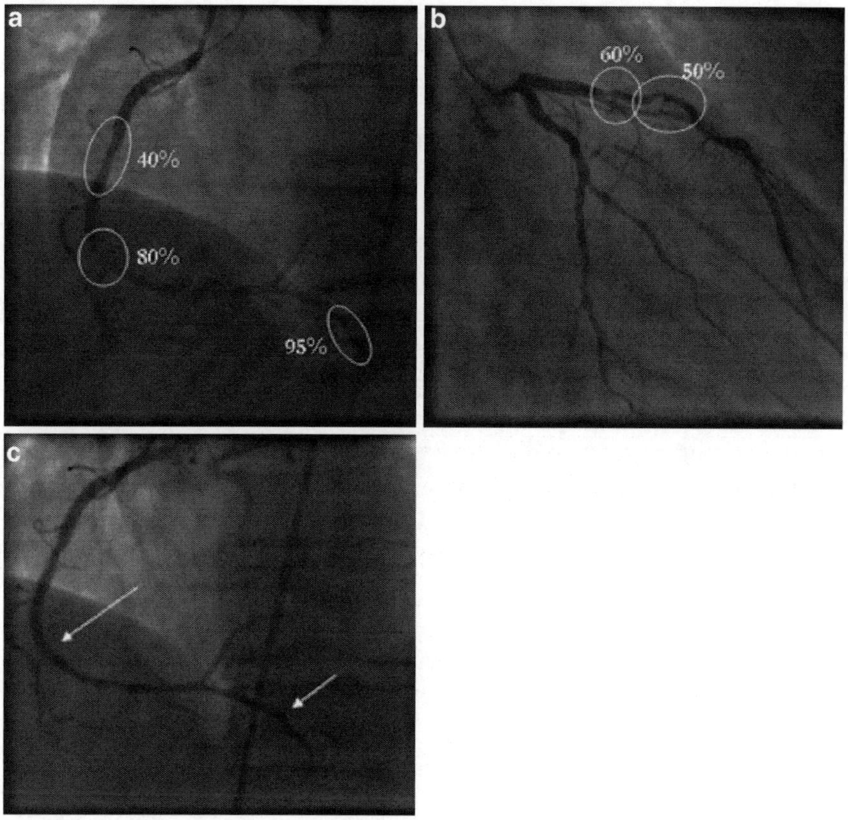

Fig. 1. Coronary angiogram of a hypothetical patient. (**a**) *Left anterior* oblique projection of the *right coronary* artery. There is a 40% stenosis in the mid-portion of the vessel, followed by an 80% stenosis. A 95% stenosis was found in the posterior descending branch. (**b**) *Straight anteroposterior* projection of the *left coronary* reveals a 60% stenosis in the proximal portion of the *left anterior* descending artery, followed by a 50% in its mid-portion. There are diffuse luminal irregularities in the circumflex artery. (**c**) The presumed culprit lesions in the *right coronary* artery have been stented (*arrows*).

inhibitor, aggressive lipid-lowering with a statin, smoking cessation, and exercise. But what about the disease left behind? According to data referred to in [3], this patient, even with optimal therapy, has an 18% risk of a target site event and a 12% risk of a nontarget site event within the first year (cumulative 30% event risk at 1 year). In the subsequent years, the risk of a target site event fell to 1–2%; however, the risk for a nontarget event remains relatively high at 5–7%! If you take into account his initial presentation of an acute coronary syndrome, this patient is likely to have between one and three nonculprit thin-cap fibroatheromas at the time of presentation, which may put him at high risk of subsequent events despite optimal medical therapy. It is possible that in the future, further examination of his coronaries with new imaging modalities may detect high-risk coronary segments which then may justify preemptive treatment with stabilizing local treatments such as stents (drug-eluting, biodegradable), balloon-eluting angioplasty, or photodynamic therapy. The expense and cumulative risk of this approach would need to be carefully analyzed in large cost-benefit studies. But what if the entire coronary tree could be "stabilized" with one treatment that had high specificity and very low toxicity and risk of adverse effects? Intrapericardial delivery of a pharmacologic agent has been proposed as a method that could provide efficient pancoronary therapy using very small concentrations of a drug with minimal systemic absorption.

RATIONALE FOR PERICARDIAL DELIVERY

Intrapericardial delivery of therapeutic agents takes advantage of the pericardial space as a reservoir wherein a drug or a biologic agent will have a prolonged residence time and therefore direct exposure with epicardial, myocardial, and coronary vasculature. The natural barrier action of the pericardium delays and lessens systemic absorption as compared with oral or intravascular routes of delivery. This enables the use of smaller doses of drugs, proteins, or other biologic substances to obtain higher local concentrations in the pericardial fluid prolonging the duration of action of these agents and increasing the specificity to act on target tissues while minimizing untoward systemic effects. Baek et al. [4] reported delayed clearance of radiolabeled substances from the pericardial space which was dependent on their larger molecular weight. However, there are likely to be other factors, such as tissue affinity and hydrophilic properties, which may play a role on the pericardial residence time of a substance.

Evidence for the localizing advantage and barrier action of the pericardium comes from a number of studies. Pericardial administration of fluorescent macromolecules in rats resulted in substance concentrations in pericardial fluid that exceeded 10–30 times those in plasma (Fig. 2) and could be explained by low clearance of these substances in the pericardial fluid, offering a promising strategy for site-specific treatments [5].

Studies by Laham et al. [6] have demonstrated that intrapericardial delivery of fibroblast growth factor (FGF)-2 provides markedly higher myocardial deposition and retention (Fig. 3) and lower

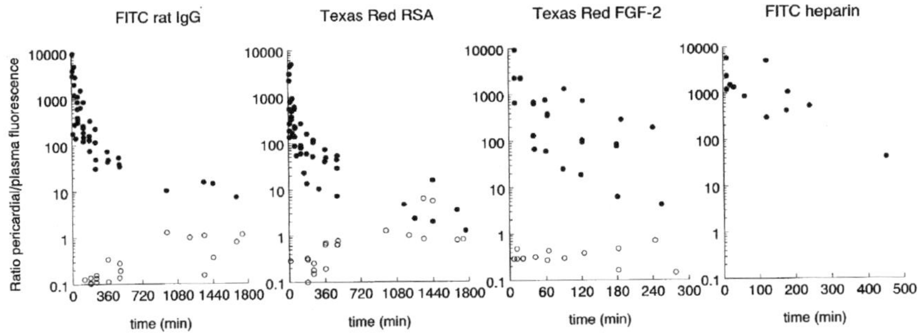

Fig. 2. Ratios of fluorescence measured in pericardial fluid and plasma after intrapericardial (*closed circles*) or intra-arterial bolus injections of fluorescent macromolecules. Rats were given bolus injections of 50 µl intrapericardially or 100 µl intra-arterially, and pericardial fluid and blood samples were collected at various time points and analyzed as described. Data in each graph represent three to six rats. For FITC-heparin, data are lacking for systemic administration because fluorescence of pericardial fluid could not be detected. Reprinted from [5].

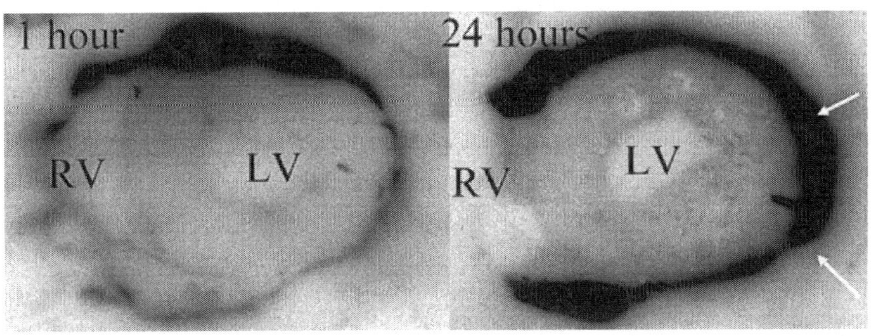

Fig. 3. *Left ventricular* autoradiography at 1 h (*left*) and 24 h (*right*) in an ischemic animal, showing increased uptake at 24 h in all areas, particularly the lateral wall (*arrow*). In addition, there is poor endocardial penetration at both 1 and 24 h. Reprinted from [6].

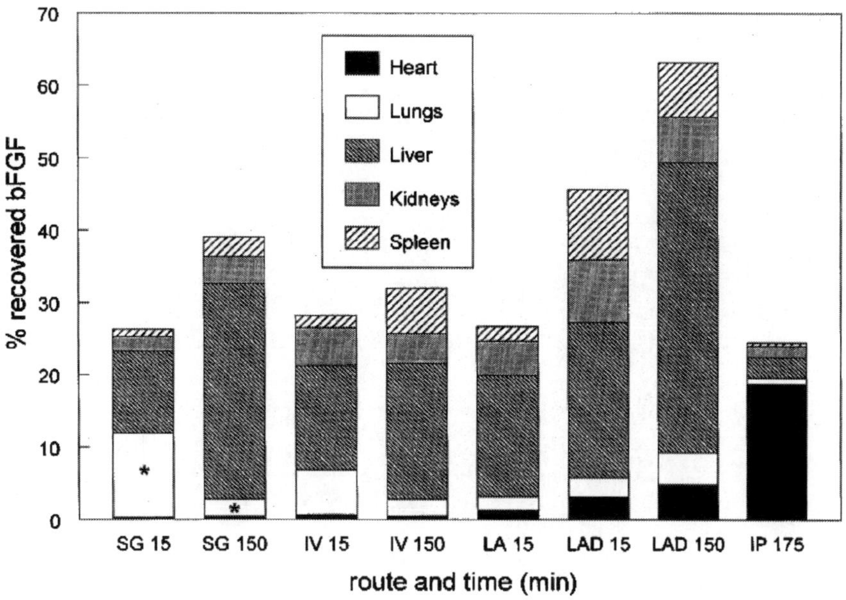

Fig. 4. Comparison of five routes of administration on regional bFGF distribution. Recovered bFGF is expressed as a percentage of the total injected counts. ^{125}I activity was assessed 15 and 150 min after injection. The greatest proportion of bFGF was recovered from liver. Relative myocardial bFGF levels were highest following pericardial and IC_intracoronary LAD administration; intermediate following LA delivery, and lowest after IV and SG administration. There was significant pulmonary bFGF recovery after IV and SG administration; however, bFGF was inhomogeneously distributed after SG delivery. Mean lung bFGF after SG administration represents only an approximation of total lung bFGF because of the marked disparity in bFGF deposition between the injected and the uninjected lung parenchyma. *IV* intravenous; *SG* Swan Ganz; *LA* left atrial; *LAD* intracoronary into the left anterior descending coronary artery territory; *IP* intrapericardial; 15 after 15 min; 150 after 150 min. Reprinted from [8].

systemic recirculation than intracoronary or intravenous delivery at the expense of diminished subendocardial penetration. In another study by the same group [7], intrapericardial delivery of FGF-2 in pigs resulted in functionally significant angiogenesis even with lower doses suggesting that intrapericardial delivery may induce myocardial revascularization by acting on the epicardial layers promoting epicardial collaterals.

Lazarous et al. [8] showed that pericardial administration of basic-FGF was associated with the highest myocardial uptake (19% at 150 min) and was far more effective in achieving high cardiac tissue uptake than intracoronary or left atrial delivery (Fig. 4) and also uptake in extracardiac tissues were minimal with intrapericardial injection compared with other routes of delivery. Stoll et al. [9] reported that while intracoronary delivery of basic-FGF results in a 33,000-fold variability in intramural coronary arterial retention, pericardial administration results in much more uniform intramural concentrations with 10–15-fold variability, which can translate into more accurate and smaller dosing of agents. Redistribution rates were also lower with pericardial delivery (22 h) as compared with endoluminal delivery (7 h), suggesting again prolongation of the residence time of an agent following pericardial delivery and therefore increased potential for myocardial and coronary arterial exposure.

Our group demonstrated that nitroglycerin (NTG) delivered intrapericardially is associated with more prolonged and marked coronary vasodilatation compared with same dose intracoronary administration [10] (Fig. 5). Furthermore, the effects of the pericardial drug were devoid of hypotension, which was observed with the intracoronary route, supporting the idea that potential adverse effects of pharmacologic agents may be reduced when they are administered intrapericardially.

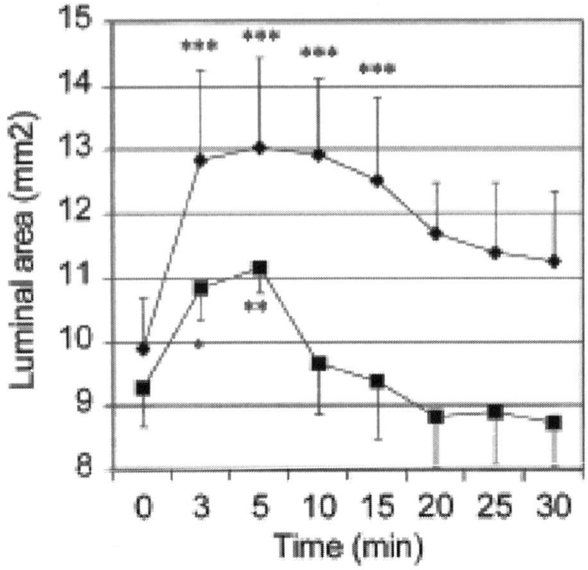

Fig. 5. Bar graph comparing the effects of intrapericardial (*diamonds*) and intracoronary (*squares*) nitroglycerin on *left anterior* descending coronary artery luminal area as assessed by intravascular ultrasound in pigs. The *asterisks* indicate significance with respect to baseline value (***$p<0.001$, **$p<0.01$, *$p<0.05$). The curves were statistically different using two-way analysis of variance ($p=0.03$). Values are presented as means ± standard errors. Reprinted from [10].

Lastly, the intrapericardial approach may also be an effective way of delivering gene therapy. Lazarous et al. [11] administered a replication-deficient adenovirus carrying the cDNA for AdCMV. VEGF165 intrapericardially in a canine model of progressive coronary occlusion. Pericardial delivery resulted in sustained (8–14 day) pericardial transgene expression with VEGF levels peaking 3 days after infection (>200 ng/ml) and decreasing thereafter, with no detectable increase in serum VEGF level. Transfection efficiency was extensive in the pericardium and epicardium, and minimal in the mid-myocardium and endocardium. Although angiogenesis did not occur in this study, it demonstrates the ability to use the pericardium to produce cytokines or other signaling agents that could be effective in achieving localized myocardial or coronary effects. March et al. [12] similarly demonstrated that gene therapy may be possible using the pericardium as a substrate. They instilled adenoviral vectors into the pericardial space of dogs obtaining efficient gene transfer that was mainly localized to the pericardial mesothelium with very little transduction of extracardiac tissues, demonstrating the possibility of pericardial gene transfer as an approach to sustained-release protein delivery. This method can provide the means to generate sufficiently high concentrations of desired gene products, i.e., an angiogenic protein or signal that can then diffuse into the epicardial region to potentially produce a therapeutic biologic effect.

INFLAMMATORY MARKERS IN PERICARDIAL FLUID

Several studies have reported that the pericardial fluid is a rich source of inflammatory mediators involved in myocardial ischemia and vascular regeneration. The presence of these inflammatory markers in the pericardial fluid may provide some insight regarding the pathophysiology of CAD. It is still poorly understood, however, whether these mediators have a functional role through their pericardial concentration, or whether their presence is merely a reflection of the underlying milieu of the myocardium and coronaries. Pericardial fluid levels of paroxonase, an enzyme involved in the degradation of oxidized phospholipids and as such, considered to have an antiatherogenic effect, were found to be low in patients with severe coronary atherosclerosis [13]. Pericardial fluid levels of heart-type fatty acid-binding protein, a small cytoplasmic protein involved in lipid homeostasis which is abundant in heart muscle and has been used as an early biomarker of myocardial infarction, were found to be significantly higher in patients with unstable angina within 24 h of presentation [14]. Pericardial concentration of endothelin-1, a vasoconstricting peptide, has been found to be higher in patients with chronic ischemic heart disease [15]. Basic FGF levels [16], vascular endothelial growth factor (VEGF), and pericardial IL-1b have been found to be higher in patients with unstable angina. Levels of angiostatin, an angiogenesis inhibitor protein, in the pericardial fluid, have been found to be negatively associated with collateral growth in patients with CAD [17]. Future research should be targeted toward these different mediators, as intrapericardial manipulation could be used to target their specific effects in the myocardium and coronaries.

EFFICACY OF INTRAPERICARDIAL DELIVERY: PRECLINICAL DATA

Arrhythmia

There are data about the unique antiarrhythmic effects of intrapericardially administered drugs. Kumar et al. [18] have shown that NTG administered intrapericardially is capable of suppressing ventricular arrthymias and decreasing T-wave alternans magnitude in a porcine model of myocardial ischemia by intraluminal balloon occlusion of the left anterior descending artery. This effect was devoid of the hypotensive effect of systemic NTG. Intrapericardial NTG also significantly blunted the augmentation in left ventricular $dP/dt_{max,}$ an index of contractility, induced by intracoronary dobutamine. This action probably relates to the formation of NO, which is capable of blocking adrenergic profibrillatory influences and improving calcium handling during severe myocardial ischemia.

Moreno et al. [19] reported that the antitachycardic effect of intrapericardial esmolol was significantly prolonged compared with intravenous esmolol (10 min vs. 3 min) in a porcine model. Intrapericardial esmolol did not affect blood pressure or left ventricular dP/dt_{max}, whereas intravenous esmolol significantly and simultaneously decreased blood pressure and contractility. Thus, intrapericardial esmolol suppressed adrenergically induced sinus tachycardia without decreasing contractility or blood pressure.

Xiao et al. [20] have shown in a pig model of ischemia that intrapericardial treatment with docosahexaenoic acid (DHA), an omega-3 fatty acid, significantly reduced infarct size as compared with control animals. In addition, the DHA-treated animals had significantly lowered heart rates and reduced ventricular arrhythmia scores during ischemia, supporting the concept that this route of delivery could represent a novel approach to treating or preventing myocardial infarctions.

Kolettis et al. [21] have shown that intrapericardial delivery of digitalis and procainamide in swine models produces unique electrophysiological properties compared to intravenous administration. QTc interval decreased by 47±23 ms after digoxin intrapericardially and increased by 128±60 ms after procainamide intrapericardially, whereas QTc interval did not change significantly following intravenous administration. QRS duration, while it did not change with intravenous dosing, increased by 17±9 ms and15±4 ms with intrapericardial administration of digoxin and procainamide, respectively. These results underscore the potential of pericardially administered drugs to modulate the ventricular fibrillation threshold in patients thought to be vulnerable to arrhythmic sudden death.

Van Brakel et al. [22] reported that sustained intrapericardial infusion of sotalol and atenolol in rats was associated with pericardial fluid levels that exceeded plasma levels 97 and 134 times, respectively, and resulted in left ventricular tissue drug levels that were 3.8 and 4.7 times higher than intravenous dosing. Intrapericardial sotalol attenuated the dobutamine response curve to a greater extent than intravenous. They concluded that similar antitachycardiac effects can be obtained with intrapericardial delivery at a *10–30-fold lower dose* compared with intravenous delivery. Thus, the beta-blocking properties of sotalol and atenolol can be greatly enhanced by applying them intrapericardially.

Mounting evidence consistently demonstrates that delivery of these substances into the pericardial space could prove valuable both in elucidating fundamental modes of pharmacologic action and in leading to new therapeutic approaches to contain triggers of life-threatening arrhythmias.

Angiogenesis/Myocardial Preservation/CHF

Several studies over more than a decade have shed evidence regarding the efficacy of pericardial delivery for myocardial preservation in response to ischemia. Some of these effects have been associated with a heightened angiogenic response, while some other mechanisms remain unclear.

Uchida et al. [23] reported in 1995 that intrapericardial delivery of basic FGF in a dog model of myocardial infarction induced by coronary embolization was associated with a significant improvement in left ventricular ejection fraction and reduction in infarct size as compared with controls. An increased number of neovessels in the epicardium covering the infarcted area was observed in the animals treated with basic FGF. Around the same time, Landau et al. [24] also reported enhanced new epicardial small-vessel growth in a rabbit model of chronic ischemia. Laham et al. [7] described that a single intrapericardial FGF-2 treatment resulted in significant increases in left-to-left angiographic collaterals and left circumflex coronary artery blood flow in a pig model of chronic ischemia. These benefits were accompanied by improvement in myocardial perfusion and function in the ischemic territory, as well as histologic evidence of increased myocardial vascularity without any adverse effects. Not one of these benefits was seen in saline- or heparin-treated ischemic animals. These studies, along with the study by Xiao et al. [20] on the effect of intrapericardial omega-3 fatty acid to reduce infarct size, would suggest that it may be possible to exert myocardial protective treatments in the setting of ischemia with low doses of pharmacologic agents delivered pericardially.

Our group reported that intrapericardial delivery of autologous endothelial progenitor cells (EPC) in a porcine model of myocardial infarction, induced by prolonged intracoronary balloon-inflation, was associated with preservation of myocardial contractility of the ischemic area at 21 days [25]. Furthermore, the pericardially administered EPC localized in the ischemic area. These findings support further efforts to study the potential of intrapericardial cell therapy with aims to preserve and regenerate myocardium.

The potential advantages of pericardial therapy may not only be confined to ameliorate the effects of acute or chronic ischemia, but also in chronic debilitating conditions such as heart failure. Mathews et al. [26] administered intrapericardial insulin growth factor-I (IGF-I) to sheep with chronic heart failure and found that this mode of therapy resulted in a higher concentration of IGF-I in the myocardium as compared with subcutaneous IGF-I, and was associated with a rapid and sustained increase in left ventricular function, which remained elevated 14 days after cessation of treatment.

Evidence of Local Vascular Action/Modulation (Possible Uses for Vulnerable Plaque/Restenosis)

The earlier-mentioned studies focused on the feasibility of the intrapericardial approach to treat or prevent arrhythmias and to preserve myocardium and left ventricular function in the setting of ischemia or congestive heart failure. The evidence to follow focuses on the localized effect of intrapericardial therapy in the coronary circulation, which can potentially be used for pancoronary modulation of the response to injury or inflammation.

Our group has demonstrated that intrapericardial NTG causes significantly more marked and prolonged coronary vasodilatation as compared with the same dose administered via the intracoronary route, and was devoid of systemic effects of hypotension [10]. Our findings support the localized and potent effects of intrapericardial drugs on the coronary circulation. Hou et al. [27] reported that in a porcine model of coronary overstretch balloon injury, intrapericardial administration of micellar paclitaxel resulted in a significant reduction in neointimal area, maximal intimal thickness, and adventitial thickness for both the low- and the high-dose groups compared with the control group (Fig. 6). Baek et al. [4] showed that perivascular exposure of coronary arteries to the nitric oxide donor, diazeniumdiolated bovine serum albumin, via intrapericardial administration in pigs, reduced the intimal/medial area ratio by up to 50% relative to controls when measured 2 weeks after coronary balloon overstretch injury. They also noted positive remodeling in the treated group, which increased the luminal area relative to control (Fig. 7). Lastly, Hou et al. [28] administered 30% ethanol intrapericardially after overstretch injury of the porcine coronaries and observed significantly reduced neointimal and adventitial thickness as compared with control, and suggested that a similar strategy may be useful and feasible in the setting of coronary angioplasty to prevent restenosis. One can hypothesize one step further that stabilization of plaques and prevention of plaque progression and in some instances, even plaque regression with optimal remodeling, could be achieved with intrapericardial delivery of an ideal pharmacobiologic agent.

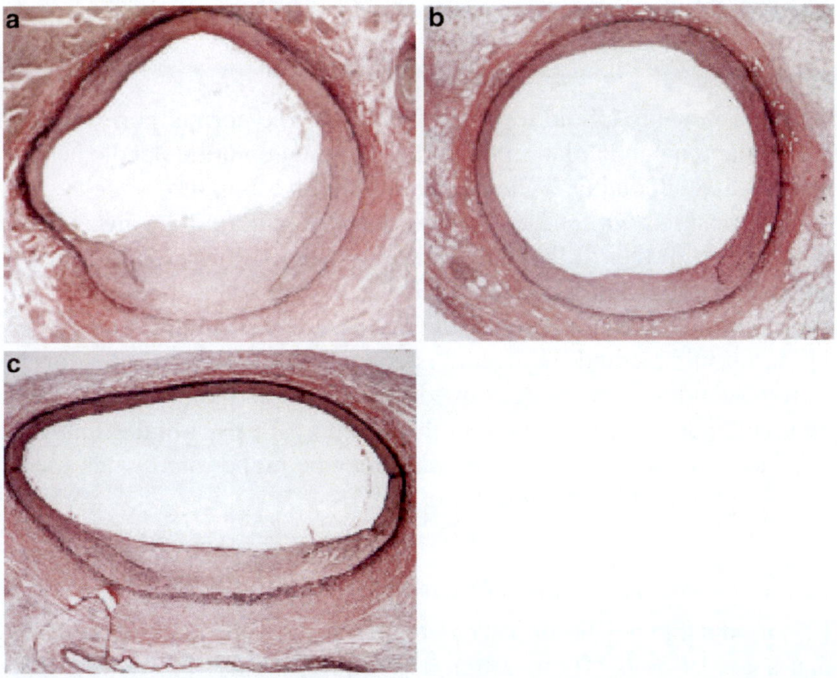

Fig. 6. Effect of IPC paclitaxel delivery on coronary arteries 28 days after balloon angioplasty (Verhoff-van Giesson's staining). (**a**) Untreated artery segment showing intimal proliferation. (**b**, **c**) Treated segments (10 and 50 mg paclitaxel, respectively). Note reduction in neointima and enlarged vessel lumen versus control. Magnification ×25. Reprinted from [27].

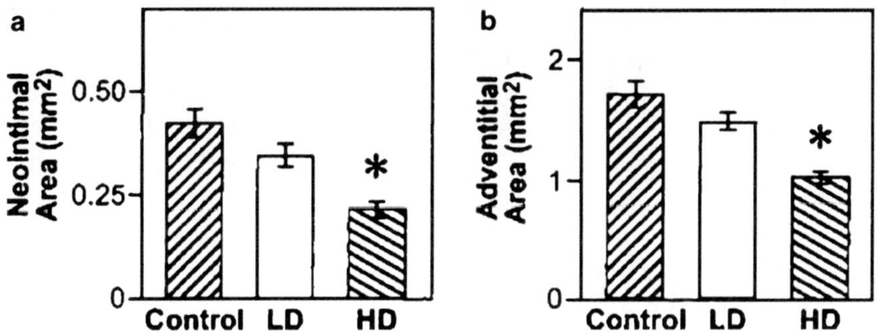

Fig. 7. Dose-dependent inhibition of vascular hyperplasia by NO-releasing protein derivative, D-BSA, injected intrapericardially immediately before angioplasty of porcine coronary artery. Shown are effects of LD (40 mg/pig) and HD (400 mg/pig) D-BSA, as well as of underivatized albumin that releases no NO (control), on development of neointima (**a**), and on proliferation of adventitia (**b**), during 2 weeks after balloon overstretch. *Significantly different from control, $p<0.001$. Reprinted from [4].

APPROACHES FOR INTRAPERICARDIAL DELIVERY

Nonthoracotomy access to the pericardial space has been traditionally restricted to patients with pericardial effusions large enough for a needle or catheter to be inserted safely and reserved for specific treatment or diagnosis of such conditions. Recently, a number of percutaneous methods to access the normal pericardial space have emerged, and they appear to be feasible and well tolerated. Some of these rely on a transvenous route, whereas others use a subxiphoid approach. Although they are in different stages of development, these methods are discussed here in their present form.

Subxiphoid

Sosa et al. [29,30] used a subxiphoid technique to access the normal pericardial space of patients to perform epicardial mapping and ablation. They used a blunt epidural needle advanced under fluoroscopy toward the cardiac silhouette. When a slight negative pressure is felt, contrast medium is injected to corroborate position within the pericardial space and a guidewire is inserted through the hollow needle. A catheter can then follow the wire into the pericardial space. In their series, hemopericardium requiring drainage developed in one of ten patients and three other patients developed minimal retrosternal discomfort and a pericardial friction rub. A similar method was used by Laham et al. in pigs [31], but in this method the needle is connected to pressurized saline. As the needle is advanced and it enters the pericardial space, flow of saline suggests entry into the low-pressure space. Although the subxiphoid approach is feasible in the absence of pericardial effusion, the risk of myocardial or coronary laceration cannot be ignored and may be higher than when the procedure is performed in the presence of a sizable effusion.

Transatrial

Uchida et al. [23] used a thin needle-tipped catheter to inject basic FGF through the right atrial wall into the pericardial space of dogs. Their technique required the use of contrast material to confirm position of the needle in the pericardial space. Verrier and Waxman described the transatrial method for pericardial access [32] in which a guiding catheter is advanced into the right atrial appendage and a wire is used to pierce the atrial wall and advance into the pericardial space (Fig. 8). The wire confirms adequate position in the pericardial space as it conforms to the contour of the heart and secures

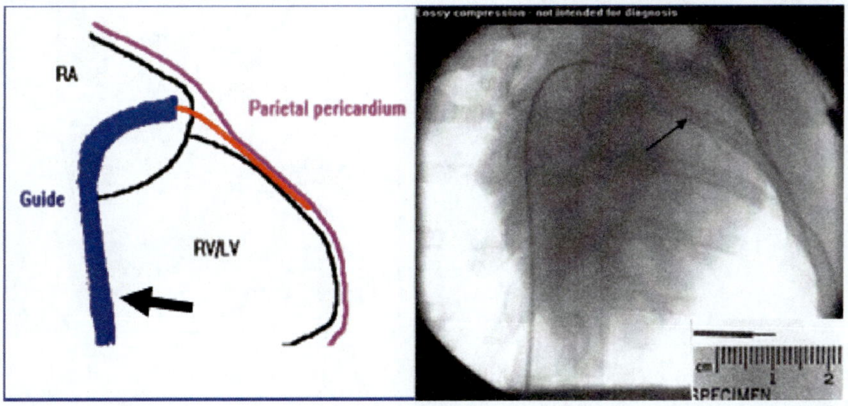

Fig. 8. Fluoroscopic image and corresponding illustration of the transatrial approach to the pericardial space. A guiding catheter (*thick arrow*) is advanced under fluoroscopic guidance into the *right atrial* appendage. A 0.014″ guidewire inside a 0.038″ infusion wire (inset) is used to perforate the atrial appendage. The relatively flexible wires (*thin arrow*) follow the contour of the heart in the pericardial space. The smaller wire is removed, and the infusion wire is used for sampling of pericardial fluid or delivery of a pharmacologic agent.

the point of entry into the pericardial space. A number of catheters can be then introduced over the wire for sampling of pericardial fluid or drug delivery. This method takes advantage of the orientation of the right atrial appendage, directing the wire tangentially to the heart and minimizing the risk of coronary and myocardial laceration. The safety and the feasibility of this system have been demonstrated in the porcine model under normal conditions [33] and in the presence of aspirin therapy and experimental pulmonary hypertension [34], achieving pericardial access consistently in 3–5 min. Necropsy of these animals at 14 days demonstrated healing of the puncture site in the right atrial appendage and no evidence of pericardial inflammation. Thus transvenous methods appear promising and safe for drug delivery. However, because these approaches involve penetration through myocardial tissue, alternative means to access the pericardial space may be required if large catheters are to be used.

Transventricular

March et al. [12] described a percutaneous approach in large animals using a hollow, helix-tipped catheter positioned transmurally across the right ventricular wall. Injection of a mixture of saline and contrast was necessary to confirm position of the catheter tip in the pericardial space (Fig. 9). They described no significant bleeding or electrocardiographic changes up to 3 days after the procedure.

Anterior Mediastinal

Seferovic [35] and Macris [36] reported their clinical experience with a device for accessing the pericardial space via the anterior mediastinum (PerDUCER™, Comedicus Inc, Columbia Heights, MN). The procedure requires accessing the mediastinal space through a subxiphoid incision with a blunt cannula, usually carried out under general anesthesia. A guidewire and a dilator-introducer sheath are inserted, through which the device is introduced to capture the pericardium by applying vacuum (Fig. 10). The pericardium is punctured and a guidewire advanced into the pericardial space, over which catheters can be exchanged. Variable results have been obtained in these studies, mainly limited to difficult access in obese patients, pain at the access site, and mild transient fever. Maisch

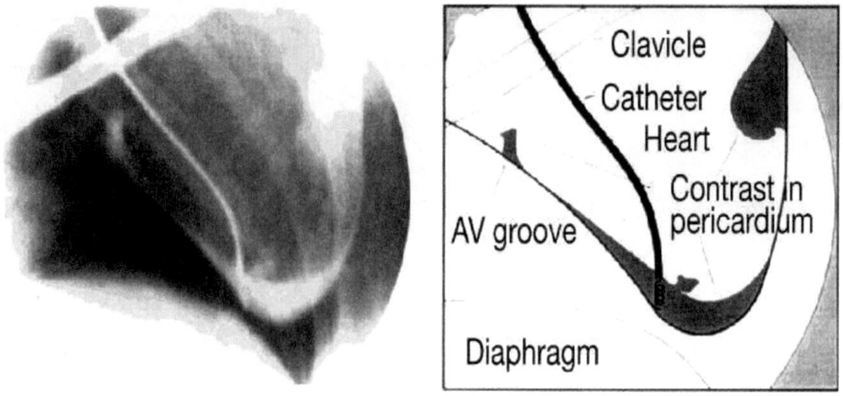

Fig. 9. Flouroscopic image and corresponding illustration of a percutaneous intrapericardial delivery procedure using a transventricular approach. The cardiac silhouette is seen from a *right anterior* oblique projection. A specialized helix catheter has been positioned transmurally in the *right ventricular* wall and contrast has been injected through the catheter to confirm pericardial loculation. Modified from [12].

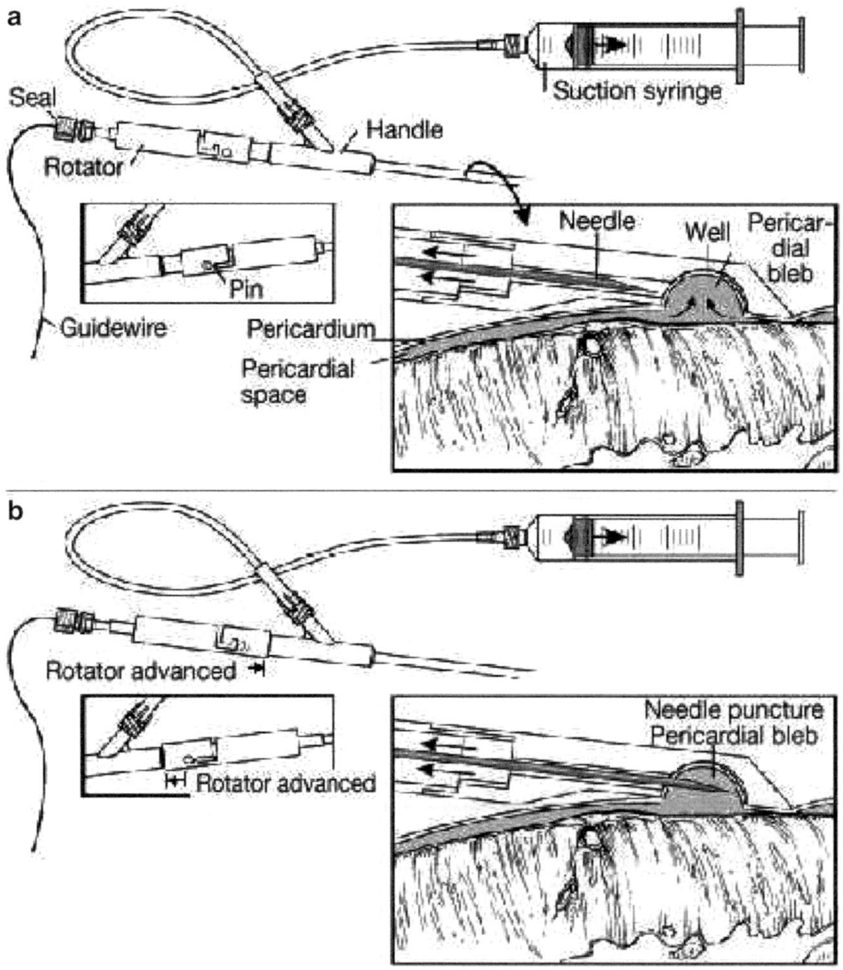

Fig. 10. Illustration of the PerDUCER pericardial access device (Comedicus Inc., Columbia Heights, MN) showing its handle, suction syringe, and cross section (*close-up*) of tip, pericardium and myocardium during capture of the pericardium with suction (**a**) and pericardial puncture with the hollow needle (**b**). The device is introduced in the anterior mediastinal space through a subxiphoid incision. Modified from [36].

et al. [37] reported success with the device using pericardioscopy in both animal and human settings to enable visualization of the portions of the pericardium suitable for puncture with the device. Hou et al. [38] also proved the feasibility and utility of the PerDUCER™ to gain pericardial access in a large series of animals (53 pigs). The procedure was found to be well tolerated by all animals and there were no signs of significant adverse hemodynamic effects. Histologic examination showed no occurrence of epicardial vessel or myocardial damage in this series.

Chronic Delivery Systems: Polymers and Implantables

Whatever approach is used, pericardial access technology is in its early stages of development and it is likely that improvements in design and materials will lead to wider acceptance of this route of drug delivery. The design of access methods needs to take into account that lasting effects may be desirable in certain applications, which may require long acting formulations with polymeric controlled delivery or implantable components for repeated dosing. One of the challenges to either of these possible solutions is the known inflammatory reaction of the pericardium to foreign substances. We demonstrated that pericardial delivery of an *N*-acetyl-glucosamine polymer in a rabbit model was devoid of significant inflammation, thus providing a possible vehicle for the polymeric release of drugs in the pericardial space [39]. The feasibility of maintaining a long-term silicone catheter in the pericardium inserted after thoracotomy has been assessed in a canine model by Bartoli et al. [39]. They reported that indwelling intrapericardial catheters left for more than year were associated with only mild chronic inflammation at the site of entry of the catheter into the pericardium and only minimal inflammation along the length of the catheter, and no inflammation at the posterior pericardium away from the catheter. Their animals were also subjected to myocardial ischemia by coronary artery occlusion to see if CAD would contraindicate long-term pericardial catheterization. They also noted that the chronic access to the normal pericardial space was practicable to deliver and withdraw fluid from within the pericardial space. These observations suggest that nonsurgical intrapericardial catheterization, both short and long term, could be further developed and implemented. The use of "smart" pumps attached to chronic indwelling pericardial catheters could provide continuous access to the pericardial space for both diagnostic and therapeutic purposes.

CHALLENGES AND OPPORTUNITIES

Despite promising initial results of intrapericardial drug delivery, a number of limitations must be addressed. Concerns exist regarding the limited penetration of pericardially delivered agents. into the deeper layers of myocardium and endocardium where, for example, in the case of angiogenic cytokines, ischemia tends to be more severe. Also, in the case of therapies aimed at the coronary arterial tree, the extent to which epicardial fat or atherosclerotic thickening of the arteries may interfere with absorption and transport of an agent is unknown. This may require use of technologies aimed at increasing diffusion gradients, such as iontophorectic delivery systems or use of smaller molecules. Further understanding of the pharmacokinetics of pericardially delivered drugs will be required to address this issue.

The optimal agents and the dosing regimens that are needed to elicit long-lasting effects are unknown. Whether a sustained effect can be achieved with single versus multiple injections needs to be investigated further. If repeated administration is required, chronic pump delivery systems or polymer technology may be used and developed to circumvent this limitation as described earlier.

It also remains to be determined whether a desired effect, such as functional angiogenesis, can be achieved by administration of a signaling protein itself or by gene delivery or manipulation, and whether feedback mechanisms will be required to turn the angiogenic signals "on and off" to prevent potential adverse effects.

Finally, although localized delivery of agents in the pericardial space appears to have some theoretical advantages over more conventional routes, the long-term effects of peptides, genes, cells, or other pharmacologic agents injected into the pericardial space are unknown. In addition, this approach is currently limited by the lack of proven access methods to the pericardial space that are familiar to clinicians, since there is no common need or reason to enter the space. Thus, there is a double challenge inherent to this approach, that is, to prove not only efficacy of intrapericardial therapy, but also the feasibility, safety, and practicality of any access method.

SUMMARY

The pericardial space offers an attractive and effective route of delivering pharmacobiologic material to the heart for treating vulnerable coronary arteries and myocardium. The possibility of localizing delivery of an agent to the target sites while minimizing systemic adverse effects constitutes one of the main advantages of this route of delivery. New percutaneous methods to access the normal pericardial space are now available and will likely facilitate the exploration of this route of drug delivery. Although initial results appear promising, extensive research addressing the issues of myocardial and coronary vascular penetration, pharmacokinetics, ideal agents and optimal dosing is required.

REFERENCES

1. Heart Disease and Stroke Statistics -2008 Update. Available at www.americanheart.org.
2. Glaser R, Selzer F, et al. Clinical progression of incidental, asymptomatic lesions discovered during culprit vessel coronary intervention. Circulation 2005;111:143–149.
3. Cutlip DE, Chhabra AG, Baim DS, et al. Beyond restenosis: five-year clinical outcomes from second-generation coronary stent trials. Circulation 2004;110:1226–1230.
4. Baek SH, Hrabie JA, et al. Augmentation of intrapericardial nitric oxide level by a prolonged-release nitric oxide donor reduces luminal narrowing after porcine coronary angioplasty. Circulation 2002;105;2779–2784.
5. Hermans RJJ, van Essen H, et al. Pharmacokinetic advantage of intrapericardially applied substances in the rat. J Pharmacol Exp Ther 2002;301:672–678.
6. Laham RJ, et al. Intrapericardial administration of basic fibroblast growth factor: myocardial and tissue distribution and comparison with intracoronary and intravenous administration. Catheter Cardiovasc Interv 2003;58:375–381.
7. Laham RJ, Rezaee M, Post M, et al. Intrapericardial delivery of fibroblast growth factor-2 induces neovascularization in a porcine model of chronic myocardial ischemia. J Pharmacol Exp Ther 2000;292:795–802.
8. Lazarous DF, Shou M, Stiber J, et al. Pharmacodynamics of basic fibroblast growth factor: route of administration determines myocardial and systemic distribution. Cardiovasc Res 1997;36:78–85.
9. Stoll H, Carlson K, Keefer L, et al. Pharmacokinetics and consistency of pericardial delivery directed to coronary arteries: direct comparison with endoluminal delivery. Clin Cardiol 1999;22(Suppl I):I10–I16.
10. Waxman S, Moreno R, Rowe K, et al. Persistent primary coronary dilation induced by transatrial delivery of nitroglycerin into the pericardial space: a novel approach for local cardiac drug delivery. J Am Coll Cardiol 1999;33:2073–2077.
11. Lazarous DF, Shou M, Stiber JA, et al. Adenoviral-mediated gene transfer induces sustained pericardial VEGF expression in dogs: effect on myocardial angiogenesis. Cardiovasc Res 1999;44:294–302.
12. March K, Woody M, Mehdi K, et al. Efficient in vivo catheter-based pericardial gene transfer medicated by adenoviral vectors. Clin Cardiol 1999;22(Suppl 1):I23–I29.
13. Hernandez AF, et al. Paraoxonase activity in human pericardial fluid: its relationship to coronary artery disease. Int J Legal Med 1993;105:321–324.
14. Tambara K, et al. Pericardial fluid level of heart-type cytoplasmic fatty acid-binding protein (H-FABP) is an indicator of severe myocardial ischemia. Int J Cardiol 2004;93:281–284.
15. Namiki A, et al. Endothelin-1 concentrations in pericardial fluid are more elevated in patients with ischemic heart disease than in patients with nonischemic heart disease. Jpn Heart J 2003;44:633–644.
16. Fujita M, Ikemoto M, Kishishita M, et al. Elevated basic fibroblast growth factor in pericardial fluid of patients with unstable angina. Circulation 1996;94:610–613.

17. Matsunaga T, Chilian WM, et al. Angiostatin is negatively associated with coronary collateral growth in patients with coronary artery disease. Am J Physiol Heart Circ Physiol 2005;288(5):H2042–H2046.
18. Kumar K, Nguyen K, Waxman S, et al. Potent antifibrillatory effects of intrapericardial nitroglycerin in the ischemic porcine heart. J Am Coll Cardiol 2003;41:1831–1837.
19. Moreno R, Waxman S, Rowe K, et al. Intrapericardial beta adrenergic blockage with esmolol exerts a potent antitachycardia effect without depressing contractility. J Cardiovasc Pharmacol 2000;36:722–727
20. Xiao YF, Sigg DC, et al. Pericardial delivery of omega-3 fatty acid: a novel approach to reducing myocardial infarct sizes and arrhythmias. Am J Physiol Heart Circ Physiol 2008;294:H2212–H2218.
21. Kolettis TM, Kazakos N, et al. Intrapericardial drug delivery: pharmacological properties and long-term safety in swine. Int J Cardiol 2005;99(3):415–421.
22. Van Brakel TJ, Herman JJ, et al. Intrapericardial delivery enhances cardiac effects of sotalol and atenolol. J Cardiovasc Pharmacol 2004;44(1):50–56.
23. Uchida Y, Yanagisawa-Miwa A, Nakamura F, et al. Angiogenic therapy of acute myocardial infarction by intrapericardial injection of basic fibroblast growth factor and heparin sulfate: an experimental study. Am Heart J 1995;130:1182–1188.
24. Landau C, Jacobs AK, Haudenschild CC, et al. Intrapericardial basic fibroblast growth factor induces myocardial angiogenesis in a rabbit model of chronic ischemia. Am Heart J 1995;129:924–931.
25. Saltzman AJ, Choi SW, Dabreo A, et al. Endothelial progenitor cells delivered into the pericardial space incorporate into areas of ischemic myocardium. Circulation 2003;108:4–128.
26. Mathews KG, Devlin GP, et al. Intrapericardial IGF-1 improves cardiac function in an ovine model of chronic heart failure. Heart Lung Circ 2005;14(2):98–103.
27. Hou D, Rogers PI, et al. Intrapericardial paclitaxel delivery inhibits neointimal proliferation and promotes arterial enlargement after porcine coronary overstretch. Circulation 2000;102:1575–1581.
28. Hou D, Zhang P, et al. Intrapericardial ethanol delivery inhibits neointimal proliferation after porcine coronary overstretch. J China Med Assoc 2003;66(11):637–642.
29. Sosa E, Scanavacca M, D'Avila A, et al. Endocardial and epicardial ablation guided by nonsurgical transthoracic epicardial mapping to treat recurrent ventricular tachycardia. J Cardiovasc Electrophysiol 1998;9:229–239.
30. Sosa E, Scanavacca M, D'Avila A, et al. Different ways of approaching the normal pericardial space. Circulation 1999;100:E115–E116.
31. Laham RJ, Simons M, Hung D. Subxiphoid access of the normal pericardium: a novel drug delivery technique. Catheter Cardiovasc Interv 1999;47:109–111.
32. Verrier RL, Waxman S, Lovett EG, et al. Transatrial access to the normal pericardial space: a novel approach for diagnosing for diagnostic sampling, pericardiocentesis and therapeutic interventions. Circulation 1998;98:2331–2333.
33. Waxman S, Pulerwitz T, Quist W, et al. Preclinical safety testing of percutaneous transatrial access to the normal pericardial space for local cardiac drug delivery and diagnostic sampling. Catheter Cardiovasc Interv 2000;49:472–477.
34. Pulerwitz T, Waxman S, Rowe K, et al. Transatrial access to the normal pericardial space for local cardiac therapy: preclinical safety testing with aspirin and pulmonary artery hypertension. J Interv Cardiol 2001;14:493–498.
35. Seferovic PM, Ristic AD, Maksimovic R, et al. Initial clinical experience with PerDUCER device: promising new tool in the diagnosis and treatment of pericardial disease. Clin Cardiol 1999;22(Suppl I):I30–I35.
36. Macris MP, Igo SR. Minimally invasive access of the normal pericardium: initial clinical experience with a novel device. Clin Cardiol 1999;22(Suppl 1):I36–I39.
37. Maisch B, Ristic AD et al. Pericardial access using the PerDUCER and flexible percutaneous pericardioscopy. Am J Cardiol 2001;88(11):1323–1326.
38. Hou D, March KL, et al. A novel percutaneous technique for accessing the normal pericardium: a single-center successful experience of 53 porcine procedures. J Invasive Cardiol 2003;15(1):13–17.
39. Bartoli CR, Akiyama I. Godleski JJ, Verrier RL, et al. Long-term pericardial catheterization is associated with minimum foreign-body response. Catheter Cardiovasc Interv 2007;70:221–227.
40. Waxman S, Sriram V, Ashitkov TV, et al. Safety of poly-N-acetylglucosamine in the pericardial space: a novel vehicle for local cardiac drug delivery. Circulation 2001;104(2):729.

VIII Educations, Life Style Modifications and Non-Pharmacologic Treatments for Primary Prevention and Saving the Vulnerable

53 Dietary Management for Coronary Atherosclerosis Prevention and Treatment

Michel de Lorgeril and Patricia Salen

CONTENTS

ABSTRACT

What are the main complications of coronary atherosclerosis? What is the manner in which people succumb to cardiac death? The most effective way of improving survival in patients with coronary atherosclerosis is to focus prevention on the main fatal complications of coronary atherosclerosis, i.e., sudden cardiac death and chronic heart failure, which mainly results from cardiac pump failure. Are dietary habits implicated in these complications? Should dietary counseling be useful for the prevention of these fatal complications? Several aspects of dietary prevention have been studied in the context of coronary complications. This included omega-3 fatty acids and moderate ethanol (wine) drinking. It is, however, the Mediterranean diet model that has been shown as the most effective one in both epidemiological studies with etiological approaches and in controlled trial. In contrast with cholesterol-lowering treatments that have provided conflicting results (especially in terms of mortality), all the published data about the protective effect of the traditional Mediterranean diet model have been positive, particularly in the prevention of fatal complications.

Key words: Atherosclerosis; Sudden cardiac death; Ventricular fibrillation; Chronic heart failure; Cardiac pump failure; Dietary counseling; Omega-3 fatty acids; Wine ethanol drinking; Mediterranean diet; Alpha-linolenic acid; Fatty fish; Olive oil

From: *Asymptomatic Atherosclerosis: Pathophysiology, Detection and Treatment*
Edited by: M. Naghavi (ed.), DOI 10.1007/978-1-60327-179-0_53

TOPIC PEARLS

- All epidemiological studies have confirmed the results of the *Lyon Diet Heart Study,* showing a striking protective effect of the Mediterranean diet, including protection against fatal complications.
- This is in total contrast to cholesterol-lowering drugs trials, the results of which are conflicting, especially in terms of mortality, and often totally negative.
- The Mediterranean diet, rich in plant and marine omega-3 fatty acids, was shown to be protective in secondary prevention in the absence of effect on cholesterol, whereas recent statin trials in secondary prevention and in CHF patients (CORONA, GISSI-HF) were totally negative.

INTRODUCTION

Subclinical atherosclerosis is a dangerous disease because at any moment during the silent progression of the disease, an acute, and often fatal, complication can occur.

What are the main complications of coronary atherosclerosis? What is the manner in which people succumb to cardiac death? The most effective way of improving survival in patients with coronary atherosclerosis is to focus prevention on the main fatal complications of coronary atherosclerosis, i.e., sudden cardiac death (which mainly results from ventricular fibrillation), and chronic heart failure (CHF), which mainly results from cardiac pump failure.

Are dietary habits implicated in these complications? Should dietary counseling be useful for the prevention of these fatal complications?

Several aspects of dietary habits have been studied in the context of coronary atherosclerosis complications. This included, for instance, omega-3 fatty acids and moderate alcohol drinking. It is, however, the Mediterranean diet model that has been shown as the most effective one in both epidemiological studies with etiological approaches and in controlled trial.

In contrast with most other preventive strategies, including cholesterol-lowering treatment, which provided conflicting results (especially in terms of mortality) and were the subject of intense controversy, all the published data about the Mediterranean diet model have been positive. So far, all studies evaluating the Mediterranean diet have reported highly significant protective effect against complications of coronary atherosclerosis. In the next paragraphs, we will briefly discuss some aspects of that protection.

WHAT THE MEDITERRANEAN DIET PARADIGM IS?

In a recent and very large observational study about the health effects of the Mediterranean diet [1], the authors have concluded that their results provide strong evidence of a beneficial effect on risk of death from all causes in a US population, including deaths due to cardiovascular diseases and cancer, when there is a higher conformity with the Mediterranean dietary pattern . They back their conclusions on previous epidemiological studies conducted in non-US populations and that have reported similar data about the effect of the Mediterranean diet on mortality [2, 3].

However, clinicians must interpret observational studies with caution, and randomized clinical trials remain the golden standard in evidence-based medicine. In fact, the hypothesis that the Mediterranean diet is highly protective was tested in a controlled trial [4, 5]. A 50–70% reduction of the risk of cardiovascular complications was recorded in patients having survived myocardial infarction [4, 5], as well as significantly lower mortality (despite rather small sample size), and fewer cancers were diagnosed during follow-up [5, 6]. Thus epidemiological studies [1–3] confirmed the results of the *Lyon Diet Heart Study*, now a reference study [7] in dietary prevention of cardiovascular diseases.

Interestingly in that trial, there was no difference between groups in the main conventional risk factors, including blood cholesterol, blood pressure, and body weight. This suggested that protection was largely independent from these traditional (conventional) factors. Other biological mechanisms have been proposed [8].

This is the Mediterranean diet paradigm.

In practice now, the diet score used to assess conformity with the Mediterranean dietary pattern in epidemiological studies [1–3] is very naive and does not capture the various practical aspects of the real and various traditional Mediterranean diets. The traditional diet of people living in Lebanon, for instance, is actually very different from that of Sicilians or Portuguese. The 9-point score is certainly useful for epidemiological studies, but of little use to compose meals every day.

Briefly, what must clinicians (and their patients) know?

The Mediterranean diet is characterized by the consumption of:

1. A high variety of raw, sometimes cooked, seasonal vegetables throughout the year, often associated with large amounts of onions, garlic, parsley, rosemary, oregano, thyme and other aromatic herbs.
2. Fruit throughout the year, both fresh and dried (during the summer, for consumption in winter, e.g., apricots and grapes).
3. Various nuts (almonds, hazelnuts), particularly walnuts that are rich in alpha-linolenic acid (ALA), and the main plant omega-3, a major characteristic of traditional Mediterranean diets [4]. There are many other sources of ALA in Mediterranean diets, including many types of salads, such as purslane [9] and products from animals fed with ALA-rich feed, such as linseed (rabbit, eggs and chicken, dairy products).
4. Grains, preferably whole, especially wheat in the form of bread, fermented with natural leaven and sometimes flavored with ALA-rich linseed. The wheat used in traditional Mediterranean diets (like the vegetables and fruit) does not contain pesticides as it is not a product of industrial agriculture.
5. Fatty fish, including anchovy, sardine, mackerel, sea bream and red tuna, all rich in very-long chain (marine) omega-3 fatty acids. Another source of indispensable marine omega-3 fatty acids may be the eggs of linseed-fed chicken, as well as the *fish-like effect of moderate wine drinking* [10].
6. Olive oil, the main edible oil used around the Mediterranean area, low-saturated and rich-monounsaturated. However, the monounsaturated fat-saturated fat ratio used by the epidemiologists does not capture one major lipid characteristic of the Mediterranean diet, which is actually low in omega-6 and rich in omega-3 fatty acids. The omega-6/omega-3 ratio has been proposed as a major component of a healthy diet [11].
7. In contradiction with many experts, Mediterranean populations do traditionally eat dairy products, though made of goat and ewe's milk and not cow's milk. Importantly, these are consumed under the fermented forms of cheese and yogurt, and almost never as milk, butter or cream.
8. Mediterranean populations are not vegetarian. They eat ALA-rich eggs and small amounts of meat, mainly lean meat such as rabbit, chicken and duck. Beef and/or pork are also on the menu in the North of the area, while mutton is the preferred meat for festive meals in the South. It is also important to note that everywhere in the Mediterranean area the diet includes a lot of legumes and is therefore rich in vegetable proteins.
9. Moderate alcohol drinking, essentially during meals, is a major characteristic of the Mediterranean diet. The main alcoholic beverage is wine, particularly red wine, a major source of various polyphenols (actually a mix of ethanol and polyphenols). South of the Mediterranean Sea, the main source of healthy polyphenols is not wine but fermented black tea (a mix of water and polyphenols). Thus most people living in the Mediterranean area are high consumers of various polyphenols whose health effects [12] are still considerably underestimated by scientists and physicians. This is another major item not included in the diet score used by epidemiologists.

The next question, therefore, is whether moderate drinking is protective by itself even when it is not in the context of a Mediterranean diet. This is discussed in the next paragraph.

IS MODERATE DRINKING AN EFFECTIVE WAY TO REDUCE MORTALITY?

Medical and scientific literature shows that moderate drinking (1–2 drinks/day for women and 2–4 drinks/day for men) is associated with a better life expectancy in the general population, as well as in patients with established coronary heart disease (CHD) [13–16].

In the absence of a controlled trial, which is neither technically nor ethically feasible, the main question for physicians remains as to whether the inverse association between moderate drinking and CHD complications is a cause-effect relationship. If it is, what should cardiologists do with their patients who are at risk of dying from CHD?

To discuss this complex issue, which has been the subject of an endless controversy, it is better to focus on patients at high risk of dying from recurrent heart attacks. We do not intend to discuss the alcohol issue in the general population or the established fact that patients at very high risk need an implantable cardiac defibrillator (ICD).

Some scientists and physicians think that most studies reporting alcohol-induced protection are biased. The main bias is called the "sick quitter bias," meaning that non-drinkers (the referent group in most studies) include former drinkers who have recently stopped drinking due to illness. That disease may explain the higher risk among non-drinkers as compared to moderate drinkers. Although previous studies, with light drinkers (rather than non-drinkers) as the referent group, have shown that the "sick quitter bias" is not the main explanation for the protective effect of moderate drinking, a recent study, in which former drinkers were examined separately from long-term abstainers, actually confirmed that protection is still present when only long-term abstainers are included in the referent group [17].

This was an important finding because it strongly supports the cause-effect relationship between moderate alcohol drinking and better survival. However, there were technical limitations in that study, including small sample size (and a small number of former drinkers), a small number of (cardiac) deaths and a quite short follow-up; but these converged to weaken the inverse association between moderate drinking and better survival, and hence further supported a cause-effect relationship. It is, therefore, not unexpected that protection appears to be less significant in a small cohort than in other populations or in meta-analyses where moderate drinking generally results in about 30% less cardiac mortality and a 20% reduction of all-cause mortality [13–16], which is considerable when compared with the effect of drug treatment (see below), and in terms of Public Health.

In addition to the strong epidemiological evidence (and in the absence of clinical trials), another way of evaluating the type of relationship between moderate drinking and survival is to examine the biological mechanisms by which moderate alcohol consumption may reduce the risk of cardiac death and improve survival. Beside the well-known effects of alcohol on HDL-cholesterol, haemostasis (through reduced platelet function and fibrinogen levels) and insulin resistance, recent data indicate that moderate drinking may have a direct protective effect on the ischemic myocardium [18], and may positively interact with omega-3 fatty acids [10] known to be highly protective in secondary prevention, especially against sudden cardiac death (SCD) [19]. These two mechanisms are important to know because they may partly explain why moderate drinking was shown to reduce the risk of SCD [20], a CHD complication which accounts for 65–75% of all cardiac deaths in the US population [21].

Thus, epidemiological and biological studies strongly suggest that moderate drinking results in reduced mortality and better life expectancy in patients with established CHD. In consequence, cardiologists should be very pragmatic and give up ideological postures when considering strategies to protect their high-risk patients from dying of recurrent heart attacks.

What are the evidence-based interventions? Smoking abstention, regular physical exercise, a Mediterranean diet (of which wine drinking is one of the major characteristics) and some drug treatments are certainly effective in reducing mortality, with the additional option of an ICD for patients at very high risk. Regarding drug treatment, anti-platelet agents are obviously protective while the rather modest effect of beta-blockers remains to be confirmed in the era of modern interventional cardiology. To get an idea of the potential of moderate drinking to protect our patients' lives, we must compare it with the effects of intense cholesterol lowering, which has become the cornerstone of prevention for many physicians.

Let us have a look at the high-risk patients tested in recent randomized trials wherein patients had been benefiting from most recent advances in interventional cardiology and associated drug treatment. If we specifically look at the overall mortality outcome (the only endpoint that can be easily verified through National Death Registries), and thus control for potential bias due to tight connections between investigators and sponsors [22], what do we see?

Whereas in the first statin trials in post-infarct patients (4S and LIPID), mortality was indeed reduced, in more recent trials conducted in survivors of a recent infarct (TNT, MIRACL, IDEAL trials for instance) or in patients after a recent stroke (SPARCL trial), or in diabetic patients on haemodialysis (the diabetics with the highest risk of cardiac death, in the 4D trial), the numbers of deaths in the very low cholesterol groups were not significantly different from those in the control groups, despite striking differences in LDL-cholesterol between groups in each trial. When adding all the deaths occurring in these trials (thus excluding the "too small sample size" explanation when analyzing each trial separately), the total numbers of deaths are respectively 1664 and 1670, showing no effect of more intense cholesterol lowering on mortality. We must also keep in mind that in different clinical contexts, such as in primary prevention and in women with CHD, cholesterol lowering has not had any effect on mortality [23].

Thus, cardiologists should be aware that moderate drinking appears to be much more effective than cholesterol lowering (which appears to have no effect at all) to protect the lives of their high-risk and post-AMI patients [13–17]. This is not surprising because cholesterol, contrary to alcohol drinking, is not a mediator of platelet function, coagulation, fibrinolysis, thrombosis, leukocyte function and inflammation, the main mechanisms and pathways by which acute coronary obstruction, myocardial ischemia and SCD occur. Also, unlike alcohol drinking [20], cholesterol lowering does not have any effect on the risk of malignant ventricular arrhythmia and SCD, the main causes of cardiac death [21, 23]. In addition, the hazards of unsafe sex, violence and accident (the main causes of morbidity and mortality due to alcohol among the young as well as among binge and heavy drinkers) are quite unlikely in these middle-aged or aging patients. Finally, cardiologists should remember that moderate drinking is a social lubricant and a major characteristic of the lifestyle, often associated with the feeling of "joie de vivre," especially in Southern Europe. They should keep in mind that they must not only protect the lives, but also preserve the quality of life of their fragile high-risk patients.

Thus, the duty of cardiologists for their CHD patients regarding alcohol consumption would be (1) to identify those at very high risk of cardiac death, for whom there is a clear indication for an ICD; (2) to identify binge and heavy drinkers and explain to them a better way of drinking to protect their lives; (3) to identify non-drinkers (and respect their choice), but also those who abstain because they wrongly believe that even light drinking is bad for their health; (4) to explain to all patients (with or without ICD) that moderate drinking, especially (but not only) in the form of wine, in the context of the traditional Mediterranean diet, is the most effective way to prevent both fatal and nonfatal complications of CHD [24], even in Northern Europe and in old age [25].

Finally, coming back to the Mediterranean diet and to the specific consumption of wine, the next question is whether wine drinking (the preferred beverage of the Mediterranean populations) is superior to other alcoholic beverages for the prevention of atherosclerotic complications. Recent observational data and meta-analysis actually suggest that wine is more protective than beer and spirits [26].

WHAT DO WE KNOW ABOUT DIET AND CHRONIC HEART FAILURE?

The incidence of CHF (chronic heart failure), the common end-result of most cardiac diseases, is increasing steadily despite (and probably because of) considerable improvements in the acute and chronic treatment of coronary atherosclerosis, which is nowadays the main cause of CHF in most countries [27]. In the recent years, most research effort about CHF has been focused on drug treatment, and there has been little attention paid to non-pharmacological management. Some unidentified factors may indeed contribute to the rise in the prevalence of CHF and should be recognized and corrected if possible. For instance, CHF is now seen also as a metabolic problem with endocrine and immunological disturbances potentially contributing to the progression of the disease. Only recently has it been also recognized that increased oxidative stress may contribute to the pathogenesis of CHF. The intimate link between diet and oxidative stress is obvious, knowing that the major antioxidant defences of our body are derived from essential nutrients.

While it is generally considered that a high sodium diet is detrimental (and may result in acute decompensation of heart failure through a volume overload mechanism), little is known about other aspects of diet in CHF in terms of both general nutrition and micronutrients such as vitamins and minerals [28, 29]. In these patients, it is important not only to take care of the diagnosis and treatment of the CHF syndrome itself and for the identification and aggressive management of traditional risk factors of CHD, such as high blood pressure and diabetes (because they can aggravate the syndrome), but also to recognize and correct malnutrition and deficiencies in specific micronutrients.

The vital importance of micronutrients for health and the fact that several micronutrients have antioxidant properties are now fully recognized. These may be as direct antioxidants, such as vitamins C and E, or as components of antioxidant enzymes: glutathione peroxidase, for instance. It is now widely believed (but still not causally demonstrated) that diet-derived antioxidants may play a role in the development (and thus in the prevention) of CHF. For instance, clinical and experimental studies have suggested that CHF may be associated with increased free radical formation and reduced antioxidant defences and that vitamin C may improve endothelial function in patients with CHF. In the secondary prevention of myocardial infarction, in dietary trials in which the tested diet included high intakes of natural antioxidants, the incidence of new episodes of CHF was reduced in the experimental groups. Taken altogether, these data suggest (but do not demonstrate) that antioxidant nutrients may help prevent CHF in post-infarction patients [28, 29].

Other nutrients, however, may be also involved in certain cases of CHF. While deficiency in certain micronutrients, whatever the reason, can actually cause CHF and should be corrected (see below), it is important to understand that patients suffering from CHF also have symptoms that can affect their food intake and result in deficiencies; for instance tiredness when strained, breathing difficulties and gastrointestinal symptoms like nausea, loss of appetite and early feeling of satiety. All of these are mainly consequences, not causative factors, of CHF. Thus the basic treatment of CHF should, in theory, improve these nutritional anomalies. However, since they can contribute to the development and severity of CHF, they should be recognized and corrected as early as possible.

Finally, it has been shown that up to 50% of patients suffering from CHF are malnourished to some degree, and CHF is often associated with weight loss. There may be multiple etiologies to the weight loss, in particular, lack of activity resulting in loss of muscle bulk and increased resting metabolic rate. There is also a shift towards catabolism with insulin resistance and increased catabolic relative to anabolic steroids. Finally, cardiac cachexia is a well-recognized complication of CHF, its prevalence increasing as symptoms worsen, and it is an independent predictor of mortality in CHF patients. However, the pathophysiological alteration leading to cachexia remains unclear and at present, there is no specific treatment apart from the treatment of the basic illness and correction of the associated biological abnormalities.

Thus, an important practical point is that *deficiencies in specific micronutrients* can actually cause CHF, or at least aggravate it [28, 29]. The prevalence of these deficiencies among patients with CHF (and post-infarction patients) is unknown. Whether we should systematically search for them also remains unclear. In particular, we do not know whether the association of several borderline deficiencies that do not individually result in CHF may together result in CHF, especially in the elderly. For certain authors, however, there is sufficient evidence to support a large-scale trial of dietary micronutrient supplementation in CHF.

If we restrict our comments only to human data, things can be summarized as follows. Cases of hypocalcemia-induced cardiomyopathy that can respond dramatically to calcium supplementation have been reported. Hypomagnesemia is often associated with a poor prognosis in CHF, and correction of the magnesium levels leads to an improvement in cardiac function. Low serum and high urinary zinc levels are found in CHF, possibly as a result of diuretic use, but there are no data regarding the clinical effect of zinc supplementation in that context. In a recent study, plasma copper was slightly higher and zinc slightly lower in CHF subjects than in healthy controls. As expected, dietary intakes were in the normal range and no significant relationship was found between dietary intakes and blood levels in the two groups. It is not possible to say whether these copper and zinc abnormalities may contribute to the development of CHF or are simple markers for the chronic inflammation known to be associated with CHF. Further studies are needed to address the point, since the implications for prevention are substantial [28, 29].

Selenium deficiency has been identified as a major factor in the etiology of certain non-ischemic CHF syndromes, especially in low-selenium soil areas such as Eastern China and Western Africa. In Western countries, cases of congestive cardiomyopathy associated with low antioxidant nutrients (vitamins and trace elements) have been reported in malnourished HIV-infected patients and in subjects on chronic parenteral nutrition. Selenium deficiency is also a risk factor for peripartum cardiomyopathy. In China, an endemic cardiomyopathy called Keshan disease seems to be a direct consequence of selenium deficiency. Whereas the question of the mechanism by which selenium deficiency results in CHF remains open, recent data suggest that selenium may be involved in skeletal (and cardiac) muscle deconditioning (and in CHF symptoms such as fatigue and low exercise tolerance) rather than in left ventricular dysfunction [28, 29]. Actually, in the Keshan area, the selenium status coincides with the clinical severity rather than with the degree of left ventricular dysfunction as assessed by echocardiographic studies. When the selenium levels of residents were raised to the typical levels in the non-endemic areas, the mortality rate declined significantly but clinically latent cases were still found and the echocardiographic prevalence of the disease remained high. What we learn from Keshan disease and other studies conducted elsewhere is, therefore, that in patients with a known cause of CHF, even a mild deficiency in selenium may influence the clinical severity of the disease (tolerance to exercise). In a recent small randomized trial in patients with CHF, Witte and colleagues reported a significant improvement of left ventricular function after taking a micronutrient cocktail containing selenium and zinc plus large amounts of homocysteine-lowering vitamins B [30]. Taken together, these data emphasize the importance of interactions between various antioxidant and non antioxidant nutrients in the prevention and treatment of CHF [29].

These data should serve as a strong incentive for the initiation of studies testing the effects of natural antioxidants on the clinical severity of CHF. In the meantime, however, physicians would be well advised to measure selenium in patients with an exercise inability disproportionate to their cardiac dysfunction.

Finally, low whole blood thiamine (vitamin B1) levels have been documented in patients with CHF on loop diuretics and hospitalized elderly patients, and thiamine supplementation induced a significant improvement in cardiac function and symptoms.

Beyond the well known effect of high sodium intake in the clinical course of CHF (and the occurrence of acute episodes of decompensation), another important issue is the role of diet in the development of left ventricular hypertrophy (LVH), a major risk factor for CHF (and also SCD), as well as for cardiovascular and all-cause mortality and morbidity.

The cause of LVH is largely unknown. Whereas male gender, obesity, heredity and insulin resistance may explain some of the variance in LVH, hypertension (HBP) is generally regarded as the primary culprit. Thus, the risks associated with LVH and HBP are intimately linked. Recent data did also suggest that low dietary intake of polyunsaturated fatty acids and high intake of saturated fatty acids, as well as HBP and obesity, at age 50, predicted the prevalence of LVH 20 years later [31]. Although the source of saturated fatty acids is usually animal fat, the source of unsaturated fatty acids in that specific Scandinavian population and at that time was less clear and there was no adjustment for other potential dietary confounders such as magnesium, potassium, calcium and sodium. Thus, this study did not provide conclusive data about the dietary lipid determinants of LVH. However, it does suggest that dietary fatty acids may be involved in the development of LVH and that this "diet-heart connection" may partly explain the harmful effects of animal saturated fatty acids on the heart.

Another "diet-heart connection" in the context of advanced CHF relates to the recent theory that CHF also is a low-grade chronic inflammatory disease with elevated circulating levels of cytokines and cytokine receptors that are otherwise independent predictors of mortality. Various anti-cytokine and immuno-modulating agents were shown to have beneficial effect on heart function and clinical functional class in patients with advanced CHF, suggesting a causal relationship between high cytokine production and CHF. This also suggests that there is a potential for therapies altering cytokine production, in CHF. In that regard, it has been shown that dietary supplementation with n-3 fatty acids (either fish oil or vegetable oil rich in n-3 fatty acid) reduces cytokine production at least in healthy volunteers. An inverse exponential relationship between leukocyte n-3 fatty acid content and cytokine production by these cells was found, most of the reduction in cytokine production being seen with eicosapentanoic acid in cell membrane lower than 1% (of total fatty acids), a level obtained with rather moderate n-3 fatty acid supplementation [32]. However, further studies are warranted to test whether (and at which dosage) dietary n-3 fatty acids may influence the clinical course of CHF through an anti-cytokine effect. Another major component of the Mediterranean diet often associated with n-3 fatty acids is vitamin D. Recent data suggest that vitamin D [33] reduces the inflammatory milieu in CHF patients, and provide some evidence for the involvement of an impaired vitamin D-parathyroid hormone axis in the progression of CHF. Further research is needed to confirm this assumption.

REFERENCES

1. Mitrou PN, Kipnis V, Thiebaut ACM, et al. Mediterranean dietary pattern and prediction of all-cause mortality in a US population. Arch Intern Med 2007;167:2461–8.
2. Trichopoulou A, Costacou T, Barnia C, Trichopoulos D. Adherence to a Mediterranean diet and survival in a Greek population. N Engl J Med 2003;348:2599–608.
3. Knoops KT, de Groot L, Kromhout D, et al. Mediterranean diet, lifestyle factors, and 10-year mortality in elderly European men and women. The HALE project. JAMA 2004;292:1433–9.

4. de Lorgeril M, Renaud S, Mamelle N, Salen P, et al. Mediterranean alpha-linolenic acid-rich diet in secondary prevention of coronary heart disease. Lancet 1994;343:1454–9.
5. de Lorgeril M, Salen P, Martin JL, Mamelle N, et al. Mediterranean diet, traditional risk factors and the rate of cardiovascular complications after myocardial infarction. Final report of the Lyon Diet Heart Study. Circulation 1999;99:779–85.
6. de Lorgeril M, Salen P, Martin JL, Mamelle N, et al. Mediterranean dietary pattern in a randomized trial: Prolonged survival and possible reduced cancer rate. Arch Intern Med 1998;158:1181–7.
7. Kris-Etherton P, Eckel RH, Howard BV, et al. AHA science advisory: Lyon diet heart study. Benefits of a Mediterranean-style, national cholesterol education program/American heart association step I dietary pattern on cardiovascular disease. Circulation 2001;103:1823–5.
8. de Lorgeril M, Salen P. Modified cretan Mediterranean diet in the prevention of coronary heart disease and cancer: An update. World Rev Nutr Diet 2007;97:1–32.
9. Zeghichi S, Kallithraka S, Simopoulos AP, Kypriotakis Z. Nutritional composition of selected wild plants in the diet of Crete. World Rev Nutr Diet 2003;91:22–40.
10. de Lorgeril M, Salen P, Martin JL, Boucher F, de Leiris J. Interactions of wine drinking with omega-3 fatty acids in coronary heart disease patients. A fish-like effect of moderate wine drinking. Am Heart J 2008;155:175–81.
11. Simopoulos A. Importance of the ratio of omega-6/omega-3 essential fatty acids: Evolutionary aspects. World Rev Nutr Diet 2003;92:1–22.
12. Toufektsian MC, de Lorgeril M, Nagy N, Salen P, et al. Chronic dietary intake of plant-derived anthocyanins protects the rat heart against ischemia-reperfusion injury. J Nutr 2008;138:747–52.
13. Ellison C. Importance of pattern of alcohol consumption. Circulation 2005;112:3818–9.
14. Di Castelnuovo A, Costanzo S, Bagnardi V, et al. Alcohol dosing and total mortality in men and women. An updated meta-analysis of 34 prospective studies. Arch Intern Med 2006;166:2437–45.
15. Muntwyler J, Hennekens CH, Buring JE, Gaziano JM. Mortality and light to moderate alcohol consumption after myocardial infarction. Lancet 1998;352:1882–5.
16. Mukamal KJ, Maclure M, Muller JE, Sherwood JB, Mittleman MA. Prior alcohol consumption and mortality following acute myocardial infarction. JAMA 2001;285:1965–70.
17. Janszky I, Ljung R, Ahnve S, et al. Alcohol and long-term prognosis after acute myocardial infarction. The SHEEP study. Eur Heart J 2008;29:45–53.
18. Guiraud A, de Lorgeril M, Boucher F, et al. Cardioprotective effect of chronic low dose ethanol drinking: Insights into the concept of ethanol preconditioning. J Mol Cell Cardiol 2004;36:561–6.
19. GISSI-Prevenzione Investigators. Dietary supplementation with n-3 polyunsaturated fatty acids and vitamin E after myocardial infarction: Results of the GISSI-Prevenzione trial. Lancet 1999;354:447–55.
20. Albert CM, Manson JE, Cook NR, et al. Moderate alcohol consumption and the risk of sudden cardiac death among US male physicians. Circulation 1999;100:944–50.
21. Zheng ZJ, Croft JB, Giles WH, Mensah GA. Sudden cardiac death in the United States, 1989–1998. Circulation 2001;104:2158–63.
22. Bero L, Oostvogel F, Bacchetti P, Lee K. Factors associated with findings of published trials of drug–drug comparisons: Why some statins appear more efficacious than others. PLoS Med 2007;4:e184.
23. de Lorgeril M, Salen P. Cholesterol lowering and mortality: Time for a new paradigm? Nutr Metab Cardiovasc Dis 2006;6:387–90.
24. de Lorgeril M, Salen P, Martin JL, et al. Wine drinking and risks of cardiovascular complications after recent acute myocardial infarction. Circulation 2002;106:1465–9.
25. Strandberg TE, Strandberg AY, Salomaa VV, et al. Alcoholic beverage preference, 29-year mortality, and quality of life in men in old age. J Gerontol 2007;62:213–8.
26. Di Castelnuovo A, Rotondo S, Iacoviello L, Donati MB, De Gaetano G. Meta-analysis of wine and beer consumption in relation to vascular risk. Circulation 2002;105:2836–44.
27. Cowie MR, Mostred A, Wood DA, et al. The epidemiology of heart failure. Eur Heart J 1997;18:208–25.
28. de Lorgeril M, Salen P, Defaye P. Importance of nutrition in chronic heart failure patients. Eur Heart J 2005;26:2215–7.
29. de Lorgeril M, Salen P. Selenium and antioxidant defenses as major mediators in the development of chronic heart failure. Heart Fail Rev 2006;11:13–7.
30. Witte KA, Nikitin NP, Parker AC, et al. The effect of micronutrient supplementation on quality of life and left ventricular function in elderly patients with chronic heart failure. Eur Heart J 2005;26:2238–44.
31. Sundström J, Lind L, Vessby B, et al. Dyslipidemia and an unfavorable fatty acid profile predict left ventricular hypertrophy 20 years later. Circulation 2001;103:836–41.
32. Caughey GE, Mantzioris E, Gibson RA, Cleland LG, James MJ. The effect on human tumor necrosis factor and interleukine-1 production of diets enriched in n-3 fatty acids from vegetable oil or fish oil. Am J Clin Nutr 1996;63:116–22.
33. Schleithoff S, Zittermann A, Tenderich G, et al. Vitamin D supplementation improves cytokine profiles in patients with congestive heart failure: A double-blind, randomized, placebo-controlled trial. Am J Clin Nutr 2006;83:754–9.

54 Management of Preconditioning Physical Activity in a Vulnerable Patient: Getting in SHAPE

Sae Young Jae

Contents

Abstract

Higher levels of physical activity and cardiorespiratory fitness are associated with lower risk of all causes of cardiovascular related mortality in both high and low risk patients. Regular physical activity improves endothelial function, insulin resistance, lipid profiles, blood pressure control, and autonomic function, has antioxidant effects, and reduces psychological stress in vulnerable patients. However, more than one third of the cardiovascular risk reduction related to physical activity cannot be explained by reductions in traditional cardiovascular risk factors. Physical activity also affects novel cardiovascular risk factors such as inflammatory markers. Recent studies have shown that a substantial part of physical activity related to cardiovascular risk reductions may be mediated by direct improvements in subclinical atherosclerosis. Current guidelines recommend 30 min or more of physical activity of moderate intensity like brisk walking on most and preferably all days of the week. Therefore, physical activity management with medical therapy should be utilized to prevent and slow down the progression of subclinical atherosclerosis and reduce mortality in a vulnerable patient.

Key words: Arterial stiffness; Cardiorespiratory fitness; Cardiovascular mortality; Exercise; Physical activity; Subclinical atherosclerosis; Vascular function

From: *Asymptomatic Atherosclerosis: Pathophysiology, Detection and Treatment*
Edited by: M. Naghavi (ed.), DOI 10.1007/978-1-60327-179-0_54

TOPIC PEARLS

- Regular physical activity improves endothelial function, insulin resistance, lipid profiles, blood pressure control, autonomic function, has antioxidant effects, and reduces psychological stress in vulnerable patients.
- Current guidelines recommend 30 min or more of physical activity of moderate intensity like brisk walking on most and preferably all days of the week.
- Physical activity management with medical therapy should be utilized to prevent and slow down the progression of subclinical atherosclerosis and reduce mortality in a vulnerable patient.

CASE PRESENTATION

A 44-year-old man who had participated in recreational physical activity such as walking and cycling twice per week for several years was recently diagnosed with a high risk of cardiovascular disease during his routine medical checkup. He had an increased common carotid artery intima media thickness of 1.3 mm with visible plaque but his Framingham risk score was less than 5%. His doctor recommended intensive control of risk factors and to continue with his exercise program to help prevent a future cardiovascular event. However, he is concerned about what type of exercise is appropriate for his subclinical atherosclerosis.

PHYSICAL ACTIVITY AND CARDIOVASCULAR MORTALITY

Regular physical activity is an important part of primary and secondary prevention of cardiovascular disease as it is associated with reduced cardiovascular mortality [1]. Numerous studies have suggested that higher levels of physical activity and cardiorespiratory fitness are associated with lower risk of all causes of cardiovascular related mortality in both high and low risk patients [2–6]. Conversely, sedentary lifestyle is a major contributor to the development of atherosclerosis and cardiovascular disease. For example, a study of 6,213 men referred for exercise testing over a 6 year period demonstrated that the men with the lowest exercise capacity exhibited a significantly increased cardiovascular death rate (approximately 4.5 times) compared to men with the highest exercise capacity, regardless of the whether the men had been diagnosed with cardiovascular disease or not [7]. Interestingly, exercise capacity was a more powerful predictor of cardiovascular mortality than other established risk factors such as smoking, high blood pressure, high cholesterol, and diabetes. A systematic review of primary prevention in women also suggested that there was a graded inverse association between physical activity and the risk of cardiovascular mortality, with the most active women having a relative risk of 0.67 (95% CI 0.52–0.85) compared with the least active group [8]. Many epidemiological studies provide compelling evidence that regular physical activity and higher levels of cardiorespiratory fitness are associated with a reduced risk of cardiovascular mortality in asymptomatic subjects and patients with metabolic syndrome, obesity, hypertension, and type 2 diabetes [9–11].

The positive effects of high levels of physical activity and cardiorespiratory fitness on cardiovascular mortality extend to patients with cardiovascular disease. There is considerable evidence that physical activity is an important factor contributing to reduced cardiac mortality and hospitalization, and increases quality of life in secondary prevention. A meta analysis suggested that exercise based cardiac rehabilitation programs are associated with a reduction in all cause mortality of 20% and cardiovascular mortality of 26% [12].

EFFECTS OF PHYSICAL ACTIVITY ON CARDIOVASCULAR RISK FACTORS

The effects of physical activity on cardiovascular risk factors are remarkably stable across different ethnic groups and countries. Prior studies showed that physical activity exhibits beneficial effects on traditional cardiovascular risk factors such as high blood pressure, lipid profile, obesity and diabetes.

The American Heart Association's scientific statement [13] states that regular exercise training increases high density lipoprotein cholesterol levels by 4.6%, and decreases triglycerides and low density lipoprotein cholesterol concentrations by 3.5–5%. The effect of exercise training on systolic and diastolic blood pressure reduction averages 3/2 mm Hg in normotensive subjects and 7/6 mm Hg in patients with hypertension. Also, physical activity appears to lower hemoglobin A1c 0.5–1% in patients with type 2 diabetes. Physical activity produces an approximate 30–40% reduction in cardiovascular risk. These powerful effects of physical activity are similar to those associated with antihypertensive and lipid lowering medications.

Recent studies have shown that physical activity also affects novel cardiovascular risk factors such as inflammatory markers [14] and endogenous fibrinolysis [15], which are both strong predictors of cardiovascular events. A number of studies have indicated that exercise reduces inflammatory markers and this reduction is independent of weight change in healthy populations, as well as obese , type 2 diabetes mellitus, and coronary heart disease patients [16–20]. High levels of physical activity are associated with low resting PAI-1 activity and high tPA activity. Furthermore, physically active persons have a greater fibrinolytic activity in response to exercise than inactive individuals [21–23]. Interestingly, a large well designed prospective study suggested that approximately 32% of the observed inverse association between physical activity and cardiovascular events is mediated in substantial part by inflammatory and hemostatic factors [24].

EFFECTS OF PHYSICAL ACTIVITY ON VASCULAR FUNCTION

More than one third of the cardiovascular risk reduction related to physical activity cannot be explained by reductions in traditional cardiovascular risk factors [25]. A substantial part of physical activity related to cardiovascular risk reductions may be mediated by direct improvements in vascular function. It has been suggested that subclinical atherosclerosis may contribute to the pathogenesis of atherosclerosis and increased risk of cardiovascular events in both low and high risk patients. Lifestyle modification programs have been shown to slow down the development of atherosclerosis in asymptomatic individuals at intermediate or high cardiovascular risk [26].

The Los Angeles Atherosclerosis Study [27] examined 500 middle aged subjects free of cardiovascular disease and demonstrated that there was an inverse association between leisure time physical activity and 3 year progression of carotid intima-media thickness. The rates of progression of carotid intima-media thickness in vigorously active subjects (5.5 ± 1.5 microns per year) and moderately active subjects (10.2 ± 1.0 microns per year) were less than that in sedentary subjects (14.3 ± 1.7 microns per year). The Atherosclerosis Risk in Communities Study [28] also suggested that workplace physical activity was inversely related to subclinical atherosclerosis. It is important to note that even though physical activity slowed the atherosclerotic progression, physical activity did not prevent atherosclerotic progression altogether.

Hypertension is strongly associated with cardiovascular mortality and morbidity as well as with target organ damage such as left ventricular hypertrophy and carotid atherosclerosis. Controlling or preventing subclinical target organ damage can prevent further escalation of cardiovascular risk. A cross sectional study demonstrated that higher levels of cardiorespiratory fitness in hypertensive men were less likely to have carotid atherosclerosis independent of established risk factors [29]. Also, an association between high levels of cardiorespiratory fitness and low prevalence of carotid atherosclerosis in middle-aged men has been seen [30]. These cross sectional studies cannot determine causality, and the impact of physical fitness on subclincial carotid atherosclerosis awaits longitudinal evidence.

The lifestyle Heart Trial [31] and other interventional studies showed that lifestyle modification including increased physical activity, dietary changes, smoking cessation, and weight loss can also slow down the progression of coronary atherosclerosis. A 6-month intensive lifestyle modification intervention in patients with type 2 diabetes resulted in improved glycemic control and decreased progression of carotid intima media thickness [32]. The DNASCO study [33] included a 6 year follow-up, showing the group with low to moderate intensity physical activities had a 40% slower progression of carotid IMT than the control group of patients without statin therapy (0.12 mm vs. 0.20 mm, $p=0.02$).

Meyer et al. [34] showed that 6 months of physical exercise in obese children improved carotid IMT and endothelial function and reduced traditional cardiovascular risk factors. There were relative differences between exercise and control groups for maximum IMT of common carotid artery (−8.4 ± 15.8% vs. +0.5 ± 12.8%, $p=0.01$) and carotid bifurcation (−10.9 ± 17.1% vs. +1.5 ± 20.9%, $p=0.015$). This result suggests that earlier intervention of physical activity may be very important for obese children.

So far, only one study has examined the association between physical activity and coronary artery calcium. Desai et al. [35] suggested an inverse association between physical activity levels and prevalence of coronary artery calcium burden in 779 asymptomatic individuals with multiple metabolic risk factors.

Increased arterial stiffness, measured by pulse wave velocity and/or wave reflection, has been shown to be predictive of cardiovascular events [36]. The lifestyle modification program influences arterial stiffness [37]. Several cross sectional studies have revealed that higher levels of physical activity are related to lower arterial stiffness. Generally, aerobically trained individuals have lower arterial stiffness than their sedentary peers [38–40] whereas resistance trained individuals have greater arterial stiffness than their sedentary counterparts [41, 42]. Similarly, acute aerobic exercise reduces arterial stiffness, while acute resistance exercise may increase arterial stiffness [43], but this is not a universal finding. Given these conflicting results between aerobic and resistance training on arterial stiffness, more prospective work is needed. However, recent studies demonstrate that resistance training combined with aerobic exercise [44] or light to moderate intensity resistance exercise (50% of 1 repeated maximal) does not increase arterial stiffness [45, 46]. Therefore, resistance training designed specifically for vulnerable patients that typically employs a low intensity regimen can be used to enhance musculoskeletal health without detrimental cardiovascular effects.

Exercise training also appears to be an effective treatment for intermittent claudication, the primary symptom of peripheral arterial disease [47]. A meta-analysis of exercise training for patients with claudication suggested that exercise training increases the average walking distance to pain onset by 179% or 225 m in patients with intermittent claudication [48].

Several potential mechanisms may explain the effect of physical activity on subclinical atherosclerosis. Regular physical activity improves insulin resistance, improves blood pressure control, improves lipid profiles, has antioxidant effects, improves autonomic function, and reduces psychological stress in vulnerable patients. Particularly, exercise training improves endothelial function through shear stress mediated release of nitric oxide and enhances coronary collateral formation in patients with coronary heart disease [49–52].

Therefore, physical activity may be an effective therapeutic strategy and a highly cost-effective intervention in clinical settings.

RISKS OF PHYSICAL ACTIVITY IN THE VULNERABLE PATIENT

Although the prevalence of physical activity-related adverse cardiovascular events are very low [53, 54], there is a transient increase in the risk of acute coronary syndrome in all patients during acute exercise [55, 56]. This risk is greater in sedentary patients than in patients with a history of regular physical activity [57]. The American Heart Association and the American College of Sports Medicine guideline suggested that all sedentary men over 45 years of age and women over 55 years of age with multiple risk factors should undergo a preparticipation health screening and exercise stress testing with electrocardiogram before initiating a vigorous exercise program [58].

Regular physical activity improves coronary microvascular function. This improvement compensates for the epicardial plaque burden and may negate the ischemic effects of coronary narrowing [59, 60]. Consequently, patients with extensive improvements in coronary microvascular function may not have an abnormal electrocardiogram during an exercise stress test. This phenomenon could explain why the asymptomatic patient may be at increased risk of sudden cardiac events during and after exercise. The vast majority of sudden cardiac deaths in patients older than 35–40 years of age are due to atherosclerotic coronary artery disease [61]. Therefore, vulnerable patients who are going to participate in vigorous exercise training would be considered for subclinical atherosclerosis exams using the coronary artery calcification score or the carotid intima media thickness by ultrasound prior to initiating an exercise program.

EXERCISE PRESCRIPTION FOR VULNERABLE PATIENTS

So far, there have been no physical activity guidelines for patients with subclinical atherosclerosis. Exercise and physical activity in the prevention and treatment of atherosclerotic cardiovascular disease guidelines from the American Heart Association [58, 62], could be effectively used in vulnerable patients. Current guidelines recommend 30 min or more of moderate intensity physical activity (70–85% of the maximal heart rate or 60–75% of the heart rate reserve) like brisk walking on most and preferably all days of the week. Exercise programs should be progressively increased as tolerated. Vulnerable patients also should be encouraged to adopt daily/lifestyle physical activities such as using stairs instead of elevators or escalators, parking their car farther away from their destination, and doing yard work.

The American Heart Association also recommends a prescribed and supervised resistance training regimen to enhance muscular strength and endurance, functional capacity, and quality of life, while reducing progression towards disability in persons with and without cardiovascular disease [63]. The AHA suggests the use of 8–10 repetitions of 50% of 1 repetition maximum for healthy individuals, and 30–40% of 1 repetition maximum with 12–15 repetitions for patients with cardiovascular disease. Resistance training is recommended for a minimum of 2 days per week, with progression to 3 days per week. Advice on physical activity and exercise must take into account the individual's overall fitness levels and the severity of symptoms. However, further information is needed to optimally use physical activity in the management of the vulnerable patient.

In summary, physical activity management with medical therapy should be utilized to prevent and slow down the progression of subclinical atherosclerosis and reduce mortality in the vulnerable patient.

REFERENCES

1. Warburton DE, Nicol CW, Bredin SS. Health benefits of physical activity: the evidence. CMAJ 2006;174:801–809.
2. Blair SN, Kohl HW III, Barlow CE, et al. Changes in physical fitness and all-cause mortality. A prospective study of healthy and unhealthy men. JAMA 1995;273:1093–1098.
3. Bijnen FC, Feskens EJ, Caspersen CJ, et al. Baseline and previous physical activity in relation to mortality in elderly men: the Zutphen Elderly Study. Am J Epidemiol 1999;150:1289–1296.
4. Laukkanen JA, Kurl S, Salonen R, et al. The predictive value of cardiorespiratory fitness for cardiovascular events in men with various risk profiles: a prospective population-based cohort study. Eur Heart J 2004;25:1428–1437.
5. Erikssen G. Physical fitness and changes in mortality: the survival of the fittest. Sports Med 2001;31:571–576.

6. Kokkinos P, Myers J, Kokkinos JP, et al. Exercise capacity and mortality in black and white men. Circulation 2008;117:614–622.
7. Myers J, Prakash M, Froelicher V, et al. Exercise capacity and mortality among men referred for exercise testing. N Engl J Med 2002;346:793–801.
8. Oguma Y, Shinoda-Tagawa T. Physical activity decreases cardiovascular disease risk in women: review and meta-analysis. Am J Prev Med 2004;26:407–418.
9. Church TS, LaMonte MJ, Barlow CE, et al. Cardiorespiratory fitness and body mass index as predictors of cardiovascular disease mortality among men with diabetes. Arch Intern Med 2005;165:2114–2120.
10. Katzmarzyk PT, Church TS, Blair SN. Cardiorespiratory fitness attenuates the effects of the metabolic syndrome on all-cause and cardiovascular disease mortality in men. Arch Intern Med 2004;164:1092–1097.
11. Church TS, Kampert JB, Gibbons LW, et al. Usefulness of cardiorespiratory fitness as a predictor of all-cause and cardiovascular disease mortality in men with systemic hypertension, Am J Cardiol 2001;88:651–656.
12. Taylor RS, Brown A, Ebrahim S, et al. Exercise-based rehabilitation for patients with coronary heart disease: systematic review and meta-analysis of randomized controlled trials. Am J Med 2004;16:682–692.
13. Thompson PD, Buchner D, Pina IL, et al. Exercise and physical activity in the prevention and treatment of atherosclerotic cardiovascular disease: A statement from the council on clinical cardiology (subcommittee on exercise, rehabilitation, and prevent) and the council on nutrition, physical activity, and metabolism (subcommittee on physical activity). Circulation 2003;107:3109–3116.
14. Kasapis C, Thompson PD. The effects of physical activity on serum C-reactive protein and inflammatory markers: a systematic review. J Am Coll Cardiol 2005;45:1563–1569.
15. Lee KW, Lip GY. Effects of lifestyle on hemostasis, fibrinolysis, and platelet reactivity: a systematic review. Arch Intern Med 2003;163:2368–2392.
16. Stewart LK, Flynn MG, Campbell WW, et al. The influence of exercise training on inflammatory cytokines and C-reactive protein. Med Sci Sports Exerc 2007;39:1714–1719.
17. Milani RV, Lavie CJ, Mehra MR. Reduction in C-reactive protein through cardiac rehabilitation and exercise training. J Am Coll Cardiol 2004;43:1056–1061.
18. Church TS, Barlow CE, Earnest CP, et al. Associations between cardiorespiratory fitness and C-reactive protein in men. Arterioscler Thromb Vasc Biol 2002;22:1869–1876.
19. Jae SY, Fernhall B, Heffernan KS, et al. Effects of lifestyle modifications on C-reactive protein: contribution of weight loss and improved aerobic capacity. Metabolism 2006;55:825–831.
20. Jae SY, Heffernan KS, Lee MK, et al. Relation of cardiorespiratory fitness to inflammatory markers, fibrinolytic factors, and lipoprotein(a) in patients with type 2 diabetes mellitus. Am J Cardiol 2008;102:700–703.
21. DeSouza CA, Jones PP, Seals DR. Physical activity status and adverse age-related differences in coagulation and fibrinolytic factors in women. Arterioscler Thromb Vasc Biol 1998;18:362–368.
22. Szymanski LM, Pate RR, Durstine JL. Effects of maximal exercise and venous occlusion on fibrinolytic activity in physically active and inactive men. J Appl Physiol 1994;77:2305–2310.
23. Speiser W, Langer W, Pschaick A, et al. Increased blood fibrinolytic activity after physical exercise: comparative study in individuals with different sporting activities and in patients after myocardial infarction taking part in a rehabilitation sports program. Thromb Res 1988;51:543–555.
24. Mora S, Cook N, Buring JE, et al. Physical activity and reduced risk of cardiovascular events: potential mediating mechanisms. Circulation 2007;116:2110–2118.
25. Green DJ, O'Driscoll G, Joyner MJ, Cable NT. Exercise and cardiovascular risk reduction: time to updata the rationale for exercise? J Appl Physiol 2008;105:766–768.
26. Kadoglou NP, Iliadis F, Liapis CD. Exercise and carotid atherosclerosis. Eur J Vasc Endovasc Surg 2008;35:264–272.
27. Nordstrom CK, Dwyer KM, Merz CN, et al. Leisure time physical activity and early atherosclerosis: the Los Angeles Atherosclerosis Study. Am J Med 2003;115:19–25.
28. Folsom AR, Eckfeldt JH, Weitzman S, et al. Relation of carotid artery wall thickness to diabetes mellitus, fasting glucose and insulin, body size, and physical activity. Atherosclerosis Risk in Communities Study Investigators, Stroke 1994;25:66–73.
29. Jae SY, Carnethon MR, Heffernan KS, et al. Association between cardiorespiratory fitness and prevalence of carotid atherosclerosis among men with hypertension. Am Heart J 2007;153:1001–1005.
30. Rauramaa R, Rankinen T, Tuomainen P, et al. Inverse relationship between cardiorespiratory fitness and carotid atherosclerosis. Atherosclerosis 1995;112:213–221.
31. Ornish D, Scherwitz LW, Billings JH, et al. Intensive lifestyle changes for reversal of coronary heart disease. JAMA 1998;280:2001–2007.
32. Kim SH, Lee SJ, Kang ES, et al. Effects of lifestyle modification on metabolic parameters and carotid intima-media thickness in patients with type 2 diabetes mellitus. Metabolism 2006;55:1053–1059.
33. Rauramaa R, Halonen P, Vaisanen SB, et al. Effects of aerobic physical exercise on inflammation and atherosclerosis in men: the DNASCO Study: a six-year randomized controlled trial. Ann Intern Med 2004;140:1007–1014.
34. Meyer AA, Kundt G, Lenschow U, et al. Improvement of early vascular changes and cardiovascular risk factors in obese children after a six-month exercise program. J Am Coll Cardiol 2006;48:1865–1870.
35. Desai MY, Nasir K, Rumberger JA, et al. Relation of degree of physical activity to coronary artery calcium score in asymptomatic individuals with multiple metabolic risk factors. Am J Cardiol 2004;94:729–732.

36. O'Rourke MF, Staessen JA, Vlachopoulos C, et al. Clinical applications of arterial stiffness; definitions and reference values. Am J Hypertens 2002;15:426–444.
37. Tanaka H, Safar ME. Influence of lifestyle modification on arterial stiffness and wave reflections. Am J Hypertens 2005;18:137–144.
38. Tanaka H, DeSouza CA, Seals DR. Absence of age-related increase in central arterial stiffness in physically active women. Arterioscler Thromb Vasc Biol 1998;18:127–132.
39. Tanaka H, Dinenno FA, Monahan KD, et al. Aging, habitual exercise, and dynamic arterial compliance. Circulation 2000;102:1270–1275.
40. Edwards DG, Schofield RS, Magyari PM, et al. Effect of exercise training on central aortic pressure wave reflection in coronary artery disease. Am J Hypertens 2004;17:540–543.
41. Miyachi M, Donato AJ, Yamamoto K, et al. Greater age-related reductions in central arterial compliance in resistance-trained men. Hypertension 2003;41:130–135.
42. Miyachi M, Kawano H, Sugawara J, et al. Unfavorable effects of resistance training on central arterial compliance: a randomized intervention study. Circulation 2004;110:2858–2863.
43. Heffernan KS, Collier SR, Kelly EE, et al. Arterial stiffness and baroreflex sensitivity following bouts of aerobic and resistance exercise. Int J Sports Med 2007;28:197–203.
44. Kawano H, Tanaka H, Miyachi M. Resistance training and arterial compliance: keeping the benefits while minimizing the stiffening. J Hypertens 2006;24:1753–1759.
45. Casey DP, Beck DT, Braith RW. Progressive resistance training without volume increases does not alter arterial stiffness and aortic wave reflection. Exp Biol Med 2007;232:1228–1235.
46. Casey DP, Pierce GL, Howe KS, et al. Effect of resistance training on arterial wave reflection and brachial artery reactivity in normotensive postmenopausal women. Eur J Appl Physiol 2007;100:403–408.
47. Stewart KJ, Hiatt WR, Regensteiner JG, et al. Exercise training for claudication. N Engl J Med 2002;347:1941–1951.
48. Gardner AW, Poehlman ET. Exercise rehabilitation program for the treatment of claudication pain: a meta-analysis. JAMA 1995;274:975–980.
49. Linke A, Erbs S, Hambrecht R. Effects of exercise training upon endothelial function in patients with cardiovascular disease. Front Biosci 2008;13:424–432.
50. Hambrecht R, Adams V, Erbs S, et al. Regular physical activity improves endothelial function in patients with coronary artery disease by increasing phosphorylation of endothelial nitric oxide sysnthase. Circulation 2003;107:3152–3158.
51. Moyna NM, Thompson PD. The effect of physical activity on endothelial function in man. Acta Physiol Scand 2004;180:113–123.
52. Zbinden R, Zbinden S, Meier P, et al. Coronary collateral flow in response to endurance exercise training. Eur J Cardiovasc Prev Rehabil 2007;14:250–257.
53. Van Camp SP, Bloor CM, Mueller FO, et al. Nontraumatic sports death in high school and college athletes. Med Sci Sports Exerc 1995;27:641–647.
54. Franklin BA, Bonzheim K, Gordon S, et al. Safety of medically supervised outpatient cardiac rehabilitation exercise therapy: a 16-year follow-up. Chest 1998;114:902–906.
55. Siscovick DS, Weiss NS, Fletcher RH, et al. The incidence of primary cardiac arrest during vigorous exercise. N Eng J Med 1984;311:874–877.
56. Thompson PD, Funk EJ, Carleton RA, et al. Incidence of death during jogging in Rhode Island from 1975 through 1980. JAMA 1982;247:2535–2538.
57. Thompson PD, Franklin BA, Balady GJ, et al. Exercise and acute cardiovascular events placing the risks into perspective: a scientific statement from the American Heart Association Council on nutrition, physical activity, and metabolism and the Council on Clinical Cardiology. Circulation 2007;115:2358–2368.
58. Haskell WL, Lee IM, Pate RR, et al. Physical activity and public health: updated recommendation for adults from the American College of Sports Medicine and the American Heart Association. Circulation 2007;116:1081–1093.
59. Mohlenkamp S, Bose D, Mahabadi AA, et al. On the paradox of exercise: coronary atherosclerosis in an apparently healthy marathon runner. Nat Clin Pract Cardiovasc Med 2007;4:396–401.
60. Roberts WO, Maron BJ. Evidence for decreasing occurrence of sudden cardiac death associated with the marathon. J Am Coll Cardiol 2005;46:1373–1374.
61. Maron BJ, Thompson PD, Ackerman MJ, et al. Recommendations and considerations related to preparticipation screening for cardiovascular abnormalities in competitive athletes: 2007 update: a scientific statement from the American Heart Association Council on nutrition, physical activity, and metabolism: endorsed by the American College of Cardiology Foundation. Circulation 2007;115:1643–1655.
62. Thompson PD. Exercise prescription and proscription for patients with coronary artery disease. Circulation 2005;112:2354–2363.
63. Williams MA, Haskell WL, Ades PA, et al. Resistance exercise in individuals with and without cardiovascular disease: 2007 update: a scientific statement from the American Heart Association Council on Clinical Cardiology and Council on nutrition, physical activity, and metabolism. Circulation 2007;116:572–584.

55 Last Chance for Prevention (Acute Prevention): Identification of Prodromal Symptoms and Early Heart Attack Care

Raymond D. Bahr, Yasmin S. Hamirani, and Morteza Naghavi

CONTENTS

ABSTRACT

Atherosclerotic cardiovascular disease is the leading cause of mortality and morbidity in the USA. Millions of dollars are spent each year for research efforts to find the best therapy for reperfusion of acutely closed coronary arteries, which would otherwise lead to acute myocardial infarction (MI). As with other disease states, heart attacks have beginnings. Chest discomfort before severe chest pain represents a clinical ischemia marker, and indicates live myocardium in jeopardy that often precedes

From: *Asymptomatic Atherosclerosis: Pathophysiology, Detection and Treatment*
Edited by: M. Naghavi (ed.), DOI 10.1007/978-1-60327-179-0_55

cardiac arrest or acute MI. The intermittent or stuttering symptoms that precede MI are referred to as "prodromal symptoms." These symptoms correlate with cyclic ST changes and repeated episodes of spontaneous reperfusion and occlusion, occurring during a period of hours or days before the ischemia proceeds to damage. Premonitory, or preinfarct angina, has been associated with improved outcomes in patients with acute MI by providing ischemic preconditioning or opening collateral vessels. Acute MI prevention through prodromal symptoms recognition represents an opportunity for reducing heart attack fatality. In conjunction with the Screening for Heart Attack Prevention and Eradication (SHAPE) initiative, the Early Heart Attack Care program emphasizes prodromal symptom recognition in at-risk populations, facilitating early detection and prevention of fatal heart attacks. Similarly, the strategy behind the chest pain centre movement in the USA is to prepare the hospitals for proper screening of patients suspected of acute coronary syndromes and to detect patients with prodromal symptoms in the community. In the era of the remarkably facilitated communication of Google, iPhone, Facebook, and Twitter, new developments are urgently needed to incorporate information technology into the early detection of prodromal symptoms. An example of such a development is proposed under "http://www.checkmyheart.com" in this chapter.

Key words: Prodromal symptoms; Preinfarct angina; Chest pain centers; Early heart attack care

ABBREVIATIONS

ACS	Acute coronary syndrome
CCU	Coronary care unit
CDU	Clinical decision unit
CHD	Coronary heart disease
CHEPER	Chest pain evaluation registry
CMS	Centers for medicare and medicaid services
CPC	Chest pain centers
CRUSADE	Can rapid risk stratification of unstable angina patients suppress adverse outcomes with early implementation of the American College of Cardiology/American Heart Association Guidelines – National Quality Improvement Initiative registry
ECG	Electrocardiogram
ED	Emergency department
EHAC	Early heart attack care
ER	Emergency room
GUSTO	Global utilization of strategies to open occluded coronary vessels
HCFA	Health care financing administration
MI	Myocardial infarction
MITI	Myocardial infarction triage and intervention
NEJM	New England journal of medicine
NHAEP	National heart attack alert program
NSTEMI	Non ST elevation myocardial infarction
OU	Observation unit
pPCI	Primary percutaneous coronary intervention
SCPC	Society of chest pain centers
SHAPE	Screening for heart attack prevention and education
SHAPE	Society for heart attack prevention and eradication
STEMI	ST elevation myocardial infarction

TIMI	Thrombolysis in acute myocardial infarction
tPA	Tissue plasminogen activator
USPHS	United States public health service

TOPIC PEARLS

- Millions of dollars are spent each year in research efforts to find the best therapy to reperfuse coronary arteries that have suddenly become totally blocked and thus leading to acute myocardial infarction (MI).
- Most heart damage takes place within the first 1–2 h: "Time is Muscle" and even more importantly, "Muscle is Time." Even the best therapy is meaningless if not performed early enough to salvage myocardium. Still, the median time from the onset of symptoms to the opening of occluded coronary arteries is 2½h;it has not changed much in the past decade. Are we barking up the wrong tree? Should we be focused elsewhere?
- Mild chest discomfort, before chest pain sets in, represents a clinical ischemia marker. When this occurs intermittently (stuttering), it is referred to as "prodromal" and indicates live myocardium in jeopardy that often precedes the acute MI.
- Prodromal symptoms have been shown in studies to correlate with intermittent coronary flow, despite the presence of continuous chest pain. Cyclic ST elevation changes can be detected in these patients. The MITI trial provided the first evidence for "acute prevention" of a myocardial infarction: patients treated with thrombolytic therapy in less than 70 min had 1.2% mortality and 40% of these patients had no elevation of cardiac enzymes.
- Prodromal symptoms recognition can reduce the detection time, leading to earlier treatment that could significantly reduce acute MI mortality.
- The observational care provided in chest pain centers can capture prodromal patients. In addition, the observation unit can reduce inappropriate hospital admissions as well as reduce the number of patients with missed myocardial infarctions being sent home from the emergency department.
- Thus, acute prevention of heart attacks can be implemented by identification of patients with prodromal chest symptoms and efficiently screening them outside and inside the emergency rooms.
- In the era of the remarkably facilitated communication of Google, iPhone, Facebook, Twitter, etc., new developments are urgently needed to incorporate the latest information and communication technologies into the early detection of prodromal symptoms. An example of such a development is proposed under checkmyheart.com in this chapter.

INTRODUCTION

Approximately 600,000 fatal heart attacks occur in the USA each year [1]. It is estimated that 8 million patients visit emergency departments (ED) in the USA each year with chest pain. Of these, 2.6 million will have acute cardiac ischemia manifested by a cardiac arrest (490,000), an acute myocardial infarction (AMI) (1.3 million), or unstable angina (810,000) [2]. The remaining 6.4 million represent patients with low probability for ischemia and need to be evaluated for ischemic heart disease [3].

Most of the heart damage occurs within 2 h after the onset of chest pain (Fig. 1). Since the median time of symptom onset to hospital arrival is approximately 2.5 h [5], it is very difficult to bring patients to the hospital early enough to benefit from therapy. It is no wonder that heart attack is the "number one" killer of the adult population in the USA Heart attack remains a cascading event; once the chest pain begins, coronary vessel occlusion is taking place and it is difficult to stop the train of events that follow. Most patients will end up with heart muscle damage that will determine the subsequent hospital course as well as life activities.

Can AMI be stopped early enough to prevent extensive damage? The chain of events underlying a heart attack *is* vulnerable at a crucial step in the ischemic process that provides an opportunity for last minute prevention; that is, "acute prevention."

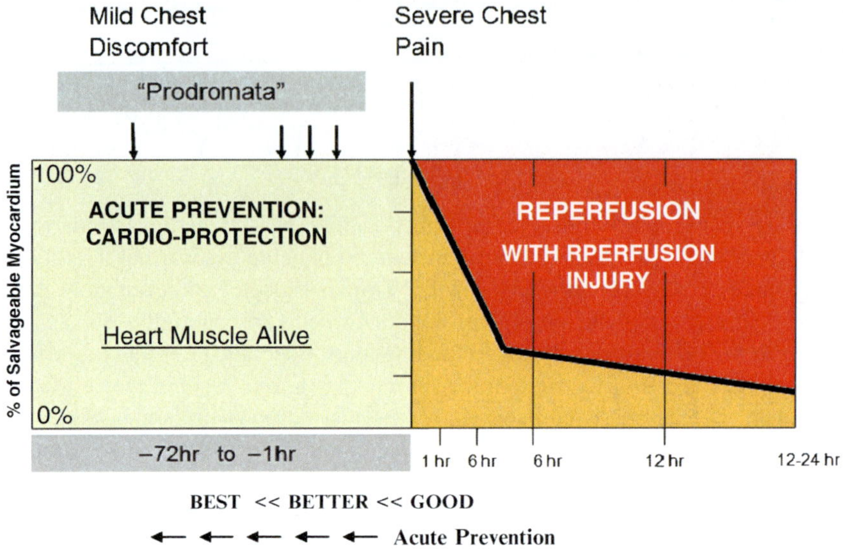

Fig. 1. Chest pain and mortality statistics from onset of chest pain to opening of the artery in the emergency department (adapted from [4]).

EVOLUTION OF HEART ATTACK CARE OVER THE LAST 50 YEARS

Contribution of Coronary Care Units

Figure 55.1 shows the theoretical reduction in heart attack fatality rate from 30% to nearly 0% with implementation of acute prevention. Is this achievable? The answer is "Yes." The mortality for AMI patients treated on hospital wards in the 1960s before Coronary Care Units (CCUs) was approximately 30% [6]. CCUs were able to reduce mortality to 12% [7] with arrhythmia treatment. CCU nurses were allowed to treat malignant arrhythmias through established CCU protocols in the absence of physicians. Further reduction to 10% resulted from hemodynamic monitoring (Swan Ganz Catheter). The major breakthrough was the discovery of thrombolytic therapy to open closed coronary vessels shortly after they have been occluded, with mortality reduction to 6% [8]. Unfortunately, only 1/4 of the MI patients were eligible [9]; the remainder could not be given thrombolytic therapy because of either coming in too late or bleeding related contraindications. Thus mortality in CCUs remained between 8 and 10% in such units.

The watershed moment in heart attack care came when the MI mortality was reduced to 1% in the Myocardial Infarction Triage and Intervention (MITI) trial [10] in which patients were treated with thrombolytic therapy in less than 70 min with the help of a fast response emergency medical system. In fact, 40% of the patients in this 1% mortality group had no cardiac damage as manifested by the absence of a rise in their cardiac enzymes. Thus these patients had 0% mortality. What was the possible explanation for this? It had been known in thrombolytic therapy that the thrombolytic drugs needed about 30 min to open closed coronary vessels [11]. Patients treated within the first hour probably had no cardiac damage due to the fact that the clot was just in the process of forming and easier to dissolve. Thus acute prevention of heart damage was found possible and achievable through early therapy. The question that immediately rose was whether this "Infarctus Interruptus," could be carried out more frequently and more consistently in hospitals throughout the USA

Can We Achieve Last Minute "Acute" Prevention of Heart Attacks Universally?

The answer lies in the realization that all MI are not created equal. Dr. Eugene Braunwald in an editorial in NEJM [12] stated that we all should know that there are two kinds of heart attacks. Those with an abrupt onset AMI and those whose heart attack is heralded by symptoms for hours to days before the total coronary occlusion occurs. The latter had been called "prodromal MI" and had been in the medical literature for over the last 100 years. This "prodromal MI" presentation is characterized by intermittent or stuttering chest discomfort, usually not considered painful or serious enough by the patient to go to the ED. Patients with acute MIs when analyzed as to those with prodromal onset MI vs. those with abrupt onset MI, demonstrated that there was a definite benefit to those patient presenting with the prodromal symptoms. Such patients may even have a longer period of chest pain before heart muscle damage [13] and prodromal unstable angina exists prior to the patient proceeding to prodromal myocardial infarction. Identifying and treating these unstable angina patients may prevent the prodromal myocardial infarction, primarily by educating them to recognize the symptoms (Table 1) and seek early treatment. Numerous studies have reported the existence of prodromal symptoms (Table 2).

What do cardiologist and emergency physicians think about the importance of these prodromal symptoms? Six hundred and fifty eight members of the American College of Cardiology (ACC) and 157 members of the American College of Emergency Physicians (ACEP) were inquired about the existence and the importance of these early chest pain symptoms [14]. Responses to this questionnaire indicated that they recognized the frequent mild chest symptoms before the onset of the severe and prolonged chest pain that is considered characteristic of a heart attack. In most cases, these symptoms were seen frequently in a waxing and waning manner. Eighty one percent felt that such symptoms were significant enough to be clinically important, 81% felt that the general public was unaware of the potential significance of these mild symptoms, and 84% of those responding felt that in most cases there was a significant window of opportunity to permit intervention to minimize myocardial damage.

Table 1
Public education: what is "prodromal angina"? Early symptoms of an impending heart attack

Nonspecific symptoms
Indigestion
Unusual fatigue
Sweating
Nausea
Dizziness
Lightheadedness
Shortness of Breath
Specific symptoms (prodromal angina) usually not perceived as pain
Chest discomfort
Chest pressure
Chest ache
Chest burning
Chest fullness

The word "prodroma" refers to the early symptoms of any illness. For example, a runny nose is one "prodromal" symptom of a cold. "Angina" is the medical term for chest pain or discomfort (pressure, aching, burning, or fullness) that people experience when not enough blood flows to the heart

These mild symptoms may herald the onset of an impending heart attack. Early recognition and response can save lives. Do not wait until chest pain becomes obvious. At the first signs of chest discomfort, seek medical attention

Table 2
Studies showing No. of patients with prodromal symptoms and duration of prodromata

Study	*Year*	*No. of patients included in study*	*Time interval from onset of symptoms*	*Incidence of prodromal symptoms (%)*
Yater et al.	1948	60	3 weeks	10
Mounsey	1951	139	3 months	29
Wood	1961	100	3 months	45
Kinlen	1969	194	1 month	49
Solomon et al.	1969	100	2 months	59
Fulton et al.	1972	121	2 months	44
Alonzo et al.	1975	160	2 months	64
Harper et al.	1979	577	1 month	39
Madsen et al.	1985	166	2 weeks	38

Adapted with permission from: Kouvaras G, Bacoulas G. Unstable angina pectoris as a warning symptom before acute myocardial infarction. Q J Med 1987;64:679–684

Respondents felt that the lack of community response to these "soft symptoms" was due to lack of knowledge as well as denial. Respondents further believed that chest pain and chest discomfort should be considered as "Risk Factors" for acute MI. Although chest pain hysteria and the overburdening of EDs were of concern, 93% agreed that education about prodromal symptoms would result in an increased number of patients with heart attacks being treated earlier. In addition, 87% of those responding agreed that EDs should present a user-friendly attitude to encourage earlier presentation of heart attack and that the patients should be directed to the hospital rather than calling their physician's office for an appointment. Finally, 81% believed that the National Heat, Lung, and Blood Institute should convene a Bethesda Conference to discuss subjects such as mild chest pain as a risk factor and prodromal symptoms recognition of heart attack in the same way as the "golden first hour" is seen in trauma. The Bethesda came to this conclusion:

> The goal of the "Chest Pain ED" movement has been the development of a partnership between emergency physicians and cardiologists in a continuous quality improvement process to enhance delivery of heart attack care through community penetration that links the CPC with an early symptom community awareness program. A major focus of this strategy is addressing reasons for delay when patients are having early symptoms. One focus should be on patients presenting with central chest discomfort, not necessarily perceived as chest pain, as well as those with chest pain. Thus, the CPC movement is a strategy to reduce the time to treatment in patients with evidence of early active ischemic heart disease. The new paradigm, as seen in this light, represents a shift in care to enhance present day management of patients with ischemic heart disease

Strategy and Changing the Direction-Rethinking the MITI trial

The most important outcome of the MITI trial may not have been the mortality reduction with early therapy, but the fact that the performance of hospitals involved in the study fell off after the study. The finding that hospitals were not fully and consistently prepared for treating heart attack patients in the United States was disturbing. The US Public Health Department (USPHS) that played a major role in setting up CCUs throughout the USA in the 1960, was no longer in position to act similarly [15]. Neither the ACC nor AHA was promoting scholarly research and evidence-based medicine. Promoting a national initiative to improve hospital's performances in treating heart attack patients in emergency rooms was not in their domain. This type of approach was left up to the individual hospitals. In many cases, this amounted to random care that occurred often in the midst of many other emergency problems.

The First Chest Pain Center

Just like the CCU effort that had started in a Community Hospital in Bethany, Kansas, there was a similar effort to prepare the emergency department in a Community Hospital for taking care of the heart attack patient. This took place at "St. Agnes Hospital" in Baltimore, MD. St. Agnes had started this in 1981 to reduce cardiac arrest in the community by encouraging patients with chest pain to get in earlier. St. Agnes' performance had not fallen off following its participation in the MITI trial. An important question was then asked. Why are not hospitals ED prepared in a consistent manner for seeing and treating heart attack patients? Why not designate an area in the ER to further evaluate such patients and quickly treat those with chest pain who may be having an active ischemia? To accomplish this they needed to bring together the ER physician and the cardiologist to work closely with the critical care nurses to make this happen. They worked hard at it and they were successful.

THE CHEST PAIN CENTER STRATEGY

The Chest Pain Center Movement

The Chest Pain Center Strategy (Fig. 2) and subsequent movement was based on an early community educational program focusing on prodromal symptom recognition, called "EHAC" for Early Heart Attack Care, initiated by St. Agnes hospital and later by the National Institute of Health – National Heart Attack Alert Program, "Act in Time IN MI" [16]. Between the years 1981 and 1998, the growth of more than 2,500 chest pain centers (CPCs) took place in the USA with many developing outside

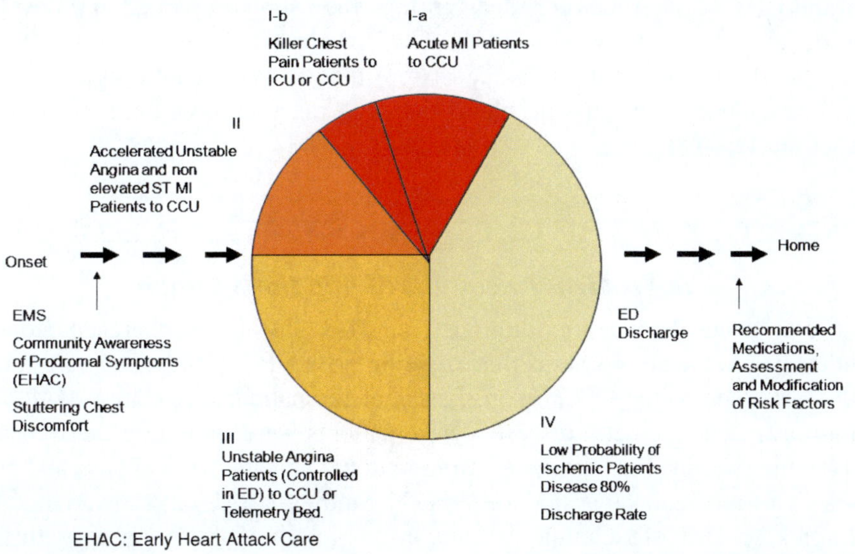

Fig. 2. Patient care strategy and outcomes at chest pain centers; spectrum of mortality in patients with acute myocardial infarction related to time (Adapted from Bahr RD. The chest pain center strategy for delivering community heart attack care by shifting the paradigm of heart attack care to earlier detection and treatment. Prev Cardiol 2002;5:16–22).

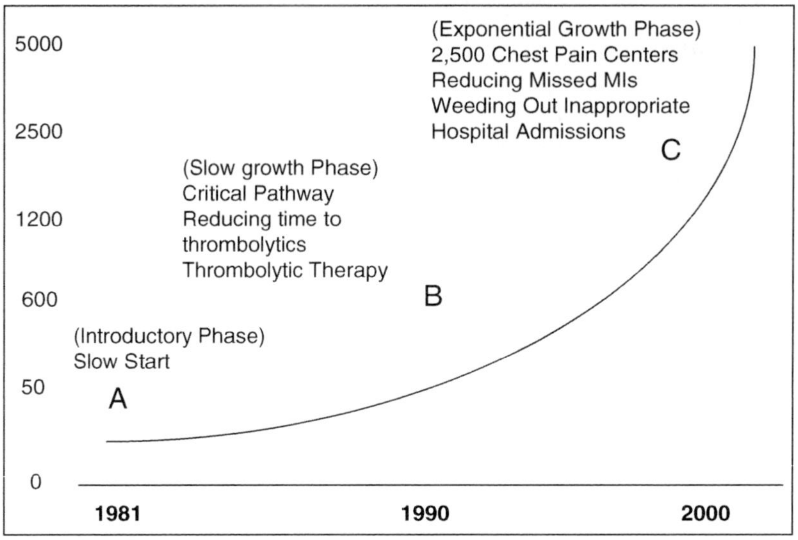

Fig. 3. Growth phases of chest pain centers (Adapted from Bahr RD. The chest pain center strategy for delivering community heart attack care by shifting the paradigm of heart attack care to earlier detection and treatment. Prev Cardiol 2002;5:16–22).

the USA as well (Fig. 3). It made good sense to develop a CPC and to better prepare the hospital to take care of patients presenting with chest pain that may turn out to be an acute MI. It also made even more sense to listen to heart attack patients in the CCU telling about their early symptoms before the event that brought them into the hospital…and to educate the public that it is important to come in with these early symptoms. Growth of CPCs became exponential here. Many of the key personnel from these hospitals toured the CPC at St. Agnes for ideas on how they should proceed and develop. They were however, left to develop their own version of the CPC in a manner similar to how CCUs developed independently in the 1960s. National conferences were held to bring cardiologists, emergency physicians, and critical care nurses to discuss problems that took place in these units, what ideas worked for them and what action steps to take.

ROAD BLOCK IN THIS CHEST PAIN CENTER DEVELOPMENT

The Problem Encountered and the Solution

Through this relationship between cardiologists and ER physicians, there developed a bond that physicians together would tackle problems that arose in those CPCs. Within a short period of time, an observation unit was added to the CPC because 50% of the patients presenting with chest pain were turning out not to have ischemic heart disease. These patients were saturating the EDs and filling beds in the CCU and telemetry units. Patients were admitted to the hospital for 3–4 days and costing the USA 4 billion dollars a year for care that was not needed [17]. Studies carried out showed that this observation unit was able to pick up 15% of ischemic patients in this low probability group with ischemia, while sending 80% of the patients home safely [18]. The CPC allowed more low risk patients to be checked out and opened the door to the community for an educational program about EHAC (Fig. 4).

More and more physicians in cardiology and emergency medicine were joining the CPC effort and at the Third National Congress of CPC in Detroit in 1998, the decision was made to form

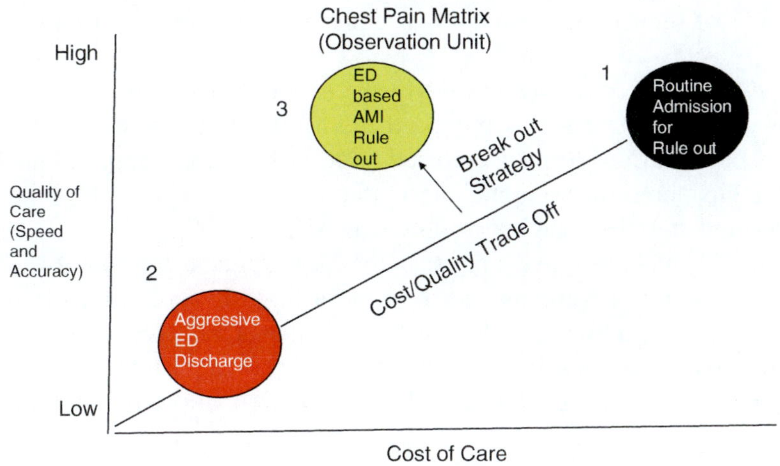

Fig. 4. Reengineering chest pain management – resolves cost quality dilemma.

a new society to help in carrying out the mission of reducing significantly heart attack deaths in the USA This was to be accomplished by preparedness in the ER and focusing on converting patients with late presentation to patients with early presentation through reducing the detection time in the community.

EVIDENCE OF PRODROMAL SYMPTOMS

Prodromal Symptom Recognition of a Heart Attack: The Soft Unstable Angina that Goes Unnoticed Until It Is Too Late

Does the prodromal stage truly exist or is it a myth? If it is real, we need to find it and prove that it is of value and can easily be taught to the Public. We need to link this effort to the CPC in the ED to bring about user-friendly evaluation in this area.

The impetus for the CPC strategy came from listening to patients in the CCU at St. Agnes Hospital that told about their heart attack. In taking the history of a patient in the CCU, it was frequently revealed that the crushing chest pain that brought the patient to the hospital with the acute MI was often preceded by several days of mild chest discomfort that was usually intermittent and lasting for short periods of time. Sometimes it was made worse by activity and this resulted in the patient reducing their activity so as not to have it. Patients would often sit at their desk while at work and hope that the chest discomfort would go away. The chest discomfort would be described as chest fullness, chest burning, chest dullness, chest ache, chest pressure, etc but mild enough to easily go unnoticed by others. Its natural progression would be to become more frequent, last longer in duration, and then get more painful until it became clear that something was seriously wrong and that it was time to push the panic button. Forget the embarrassment CALL AN AMBULANCE NOW!

The astonishing aspect of this was that medical residents were not impressed by this part of the history. They were more interested as to when the "elephant was sitting on the patient's chest"…and look at the beauty of these 10 mm of tombstone elevation in V1–V3! For years, the first author (Dr. Bahr) questioned where was medicine to take advantage of this golden opportunity to prevent deadly MIs? This information on the beginning of a heart attack had been richly described in the literature for many years as the prodromal symptoms of acute myocardial infarction (Table 2). Dack et al. [19] had described this in 46% of their patients in a 1941 study. It even referenced in an article going back to 1926 [20].

Subsequent review of the literature revealed that the occurrence rate for prodromal symptoms was about 40–50% and that these symptoms preceded the acute MI by hours to days to weeks before admission to the hospital. Various terms were used to describe these symptoms such as preinfarction angina, antecedent angina, preceding angina, intermittent angina, waxing and waning angina, winkling and blinking angina, and stuttering angina or stuttering MI.

In 1996, Andreotti [21] had presented a paper in the New England Journal of Medicine (NEJM) on prodromal myocardial infarction patients and the benefit of early reperfusion in these patients with thrombolytic therapy. This was further advanced by Haider et al. [22] who demonstrated that the prodromal chest symptoms were caused by intermittent blood flow and later by Krucoff [23] who showed these patients were having intermittent ST elevation with these symptoms. The pathophysiology was beginning to become clear.

Finding Evidence for the Existence of the Prodromal Symptoms in Major Studies

In the 196 patients enrolled at St. Agnes in the Gusto I Study [24] of 41,021 patients, prodromal symptoms were an important predictor of smaller infarct size and there was improvement in survival at 30 days, 1 year, and 5 years. In patients with minimal or no myocardial damage, 81% had presented with prodromal symptoms. Of these 32 patients, 19 patients were aborted resulting in 0% mortality at 30 days, 0% mortality at 1 year, and 5.9% mortality at 5 years. In these 19 patients, the median time to treatment was 2.72 h, suggesting intermittent coronary blood flow with possible preconditioning (Table 3). In the INTIME-II study [25], 425 patients reported a history of prodromal symptoms. The prodromal group was found to have a smaller infarct size and a lower mortality at 30 days, 6 months, and 5 years (Table 4).

THE HEALTH CARE IMPLICATIONS OF THE CHEST PAIN CENTER ED

The Chest Pain Center ED is not only important in EHAC but now has become a model of urgent care for other medical problems that need rapid assessment and early intervention in the ED. The Centers for Medicare and Medicaid Services (CMS) are now looking into other diagnoses such as stroke, TIAs, heart failure, atrial fibrillation, etc [26]. To accomplish this cost effective care, the chest pain movement is changing the landscape of urgent medical care that will in the future see more patients in the outpatient service (observation) and only the very sick patients in the hospital. The efficiency, cost effectiveness, and reduced hospitalization that take place in these units, is certainly catching the eye of not only CMS but other Insurance Carriers as well.

SHIFTING CHEST PAIN SCREENING TO OUT OF HOSPITAL; NEW STRATEGIES TO CHALLENGE PROLONGED PREHOSPITAL DELAY AND OUT-OF-HOSPITAL SUDDEN CARDIAC DEATH

The rapid proliferation of "Free-Standing" ERs and Urgent Care Clinics (standalone emergency rooms and urgent care centers outside of hospitals mostly) in the past few years has been amazing. This growing business is based on the superior convenience and cost-effectiveness of retail healthcare model vs. traditional hospitals and clinics (where people usually have to wait a long time and are treated less than desired). The retail ER and Urgent Care centers present an opportunity to bring CPCs

Table 3
Summary of results of GUSTO 1

Peak CK MB	*Classification*	*No. of patients*	*No. (%) with prodromal unstable angina*	*Time to treatment (h)*	*30-day death*	*1-year death*	*5-year death*
CK MB <16 U/L 25th, 75th percentiles range	Aborted MI	19	16 (84.2%)	2.72 (2.08, 3.08) 1.08–4.17	0%	0%	1 (5.9%)
CK MB <40 U/L 25th, 75th percentiles range	Aborted MI/minor myocardial damage	32	26 (81.3%)	2.18 (1.37, 3.12) 0.58–3.63	0%	1 (3.1%)	4 (6.3%)
CK MB ≥ 40 U/L (27.2%) 25th, 75th percentiles range	Extreme cardiac injury	163	84 (51.2%)	2.67 (1.95, 3.37) 0.47–8.17	13 (8.0%)	13.0%	40

Data for patients having aborted MI, minor myocardial damage and extensive cardiac injury, categorized by peak CK MB concentration
Adapted with permission from [24]
*$P < 0.1$ for proportional difference between Mi/minor Myocardial damage vs. extreme cardiac injury
Median

Table 4
Summary results of IN TIME – II prodromal symptoms substudy

Mortality/total number in group (%) for abrupt onset acute MI and prodromal unstable angina (UA) patient groups at the different follow up times				
Follow up	*Abrupt onset acute MI*	*Prodromal UA*	*Total mortality*	*Total patients*
30 days	4.6%	3.7%	4.2%	425
6 months	8.0%	4.3%	6.6%	424
5 years	12.7%	10.9%	12.0%	366

Adapted from [25]

outside of hospitals and one step closer to the community. This opportunity can be extremely valuable for solving the long standing dilemma of "delayed arrival" as shown in Fig 1. If access to fast cardiac check up and chest pain screening becomes as easy as access to a shop or a restaurant, many patients with mild prodromal symptoms who otherwise would delay seeking medical care through visiting hospital emergency rooms can be saved from potential fatal heart attacks. Therefore, the combination of Chest Pain Centers and Free Standing ERs or Urgent Care Clinics has merits and must be explored. Furthermore, once mass screening of asymptomatic at-risk population for early detection of high risk individuals (e.g., based on the SHAPE guidelines – screening for heart attack prevention and education) is adopted, those classified as high risk with a high burden of atherosclerotic plaques should be warned to take mild prodromal symptoms seriously. They must be encouraged to visit ERs immediately. To contain cost ramification of ED overuse, CPCs can play a major role. Such centers need not be placed outside hospitals rather than inside "Free-Standing ERs." They can easily screen the high risk patients and route them to hospitals for necessary invasive interventions. They can play the role of "Community Sarcomere" [4] as a link to the hospitals and can assure people that their chest discomfort can be easily screened and managed in collaboration with hospitals if necessary, or safely sent to home after a short stay in the CPC. Current Free Standing ERs do not have a CPC but such a movement is anticipated. Similar innovative strategies are warranted for reducing prehospital delay, a long standing dilemma, which is blamed for high incidence of out-of-hospital sudden death. An example of such new strategies are illustrated in Figs. 5 and 6.

THE RELATIONSHIPS BETWEEN THE VULNERABLE PLAQUE, THE VULNERABLE PATIENTS, AND THE PRODROMAL SYMPTOMS

In reviewing the pathophysiology of the patient with preinfarction angina or prodromal unstable angina, we can see that, if we are to "prevent the event," we need to act early in the ischemic process (Fig. 7) as the underlying and overlying factors interact in the Vulnerable Patient [28,29]. However, this prevention starts after the atherosclerotic plaque begins to rupture. Another way to start prevention is to detect the problem in the plaque event before it gets to the early rupture. Thus, in one instance, we have the vulnerable plaque patients and in the other instance we have what some have termed "the vulnerable plaque." Can the vulnerable plaque be discovered when it has its potential? Nihilists will quickly say "no," but probing research physicians will look at the technology we now have and start a new learning curve to see if discovering the patient with a vulnerable plaque is possible. The approach will at first be considered radical for the moment, but in time hopefully be judged differently.

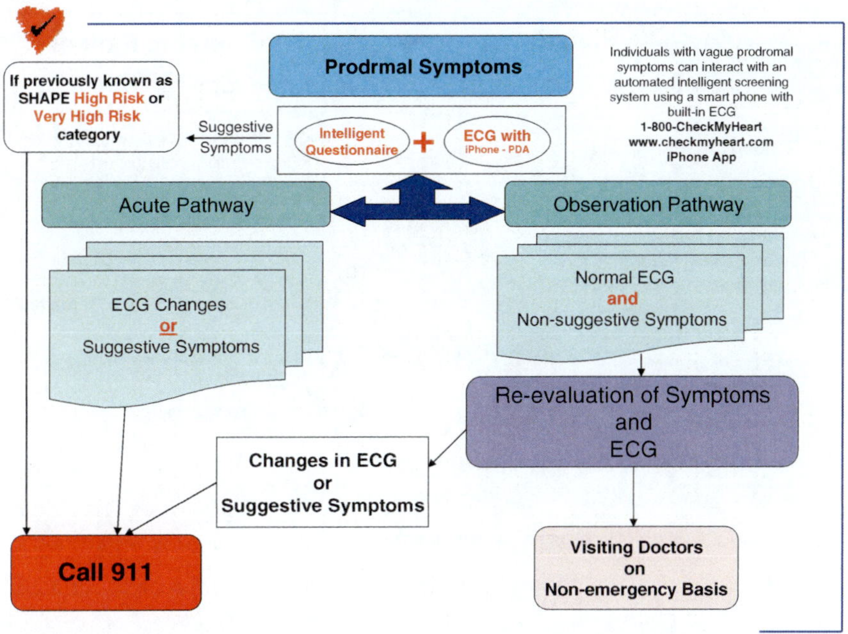

Fig. 5. A new strategy for reducing prehospital delay and out-of-hospital sudden cardiac death.

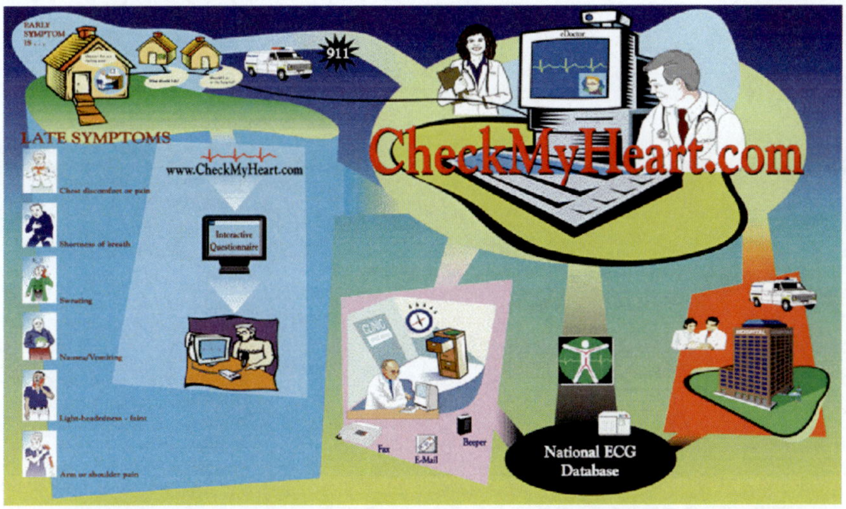

Fig. 6. Modern information and communication technologies should be used for rapid screening and early detection of individuals with mild prodromal symptoms who otherwise would delay seeking medical care. An example of such a system is illustrated.

BARKING ON WRONG TREE

Society for Heart Attack Prevention and Eradication http://www.shapesociety.org (SHAPE) has launched a much needed effort for screening and detection of asymptomatic high risk individuals, that is, the Vulnerable Patient. The SHAPE Task Force, an international coalition of leading cardiovascular researchers, has published the SHAPE Guidelines [30] for early detection and aggressive treatment of the asymptomatic vulnerable patient [31]. The SHAPE Guideline is a new approach based on identi-

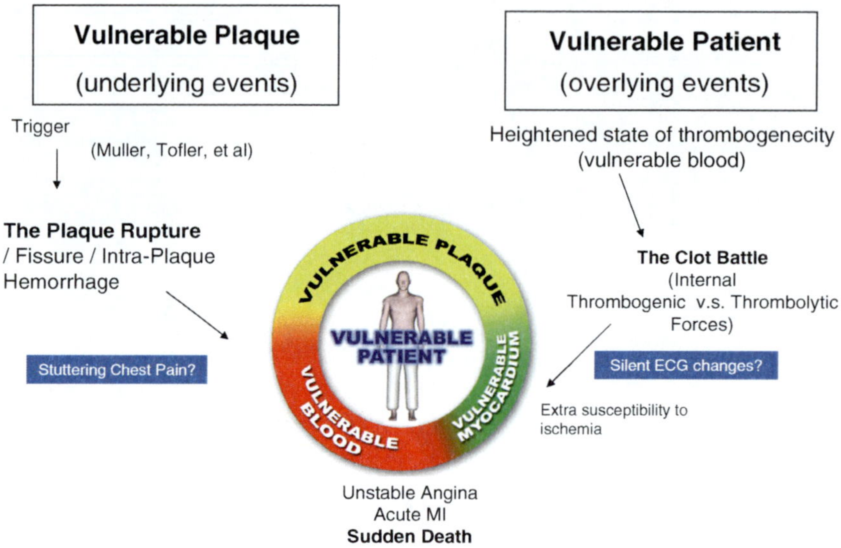

Fig. 7. Relationship of vulnerable plaque to the vulnerable patient before myocardial infarction sets in (adapted from [27]).

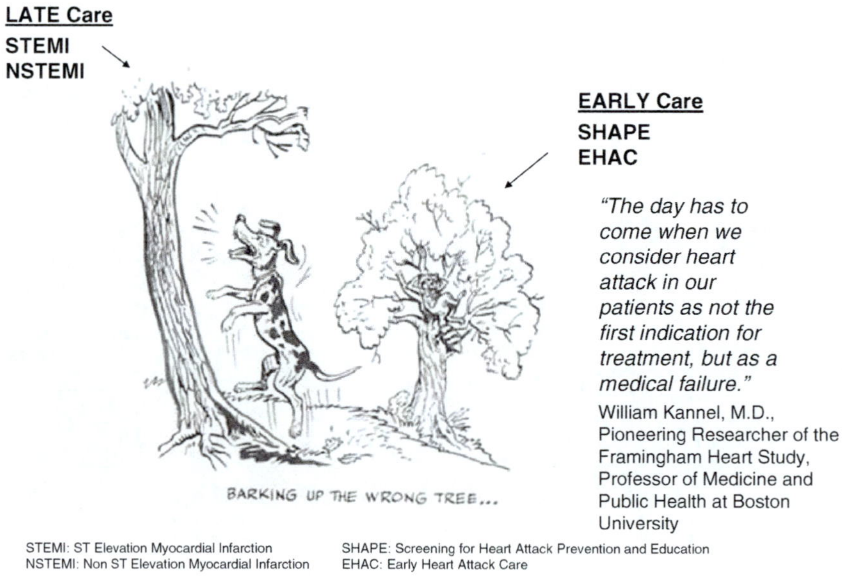

Fig. 8. Cardiovascular healthcare policymakers must shift their attention and investment to primary prevention.

fication of subclinical atherosclerosis using noninvasive imaging tests such as coronary calcium scoring and carotid intima-media thickness as a first step and then incorporating additional information derived from traditional risk factors of atherosclerotic cardiovascular disease. With a functioning Observation Unit in the CPC, there are many low probability patients who turn out not to have an episode of ischemia. These patients, estimated to be about 80% of the ED chest pain patients are discharged. Many are lost to follow up and have been shown to have a higher risk of heart attack These patients should undergo a coronary calcium scan for accurate risk stratification and appropriate therapy and education. While STEMI and NSTEM shaped the treatment of heart attacks in the past decades, SHAPE and EHAC should be the future for primary prevention (Fig. 8).

PRODROMAL CASES

A 62-year-old male woke up with a neck ache and his left arm felt asleep. He called his cardiologist's nurse and asked if he should come in now; she said "No, it is a pinched nerve bothering you." His wife drove him to the emergency department where, after appreciation of the severity of his presentation, he was taken to the cardiac catheterization laboratory, where a totally occluded left anterior descending coronary artery was opened and stented.

A 55-year-old man complained of heart burn and an upset stomach, took some Tums, laid down for a while, and woke up feeling fine. The next morning, he woke up at 2:50 A.M., asked his wife for more "Tums," and said he was not feeling well, and was going to go downstairs for a while. Before he left the room, he turned to his wife and said he felt the same way he did last Thursday, and he had been awake since about 1:10 A.M., and added that his chest felt tight. The family was all sick with "chest colds," so wife was going to give him a few minutes, then check on him. Less than a minute later, she heard him coughing, then heard him collapse. Immediately, the wife ran downstairs, found him on the floor. 911was called but it was too late. The doctors said he died instantly.

A 49-year-old man called his wife – a school teacher to ask if they had any aspirins in the house. Upon asking why he needed them, he mentioned that he had been having indigestion all morning and now was having terrible chest discomfort. The wife rushed home with Aspirin and took him at the hospital. In the emergency department in no more than 10 min, the nurse informed him that his EKG looked good and his blood pressure was fine. As soon as they started walking toward the counter to fill in insurance papers, the husband went into cardiac arrest. The emergency team immediately set to work and within 10 min he was in the heart catheterization lab. The catheterization showed a blockage of the left main artery, angioplasty with stenting was performed.

A 56-year-old female complained of several days of intermittent exertional chest discomfort. She drove herself to her small rural hospital where she was diagnosed with musculoskeletal pain and sent home. Her symptoms continued and she died 12 hours later while talking to her daughter on the telephone.

It is highly likely that, in all of these cases, if the individuals had undergone preventive screening tests based on the SHAPE guidelines (coronary calcium score or carotid IMT), and were aware of their high burden of asymptomatic atherosclerosis, they would not have taken their prodromal symptoms lightly and would have reacted immediately.

CONCLUSION

Atherosclerotic cardiovascular disease manifested by heart attack and stroke has continued to be the number one killer for over 100 years. New strategies are urgently needed to change the status quo. Screening the at-risk population for the detection of asymptomatic atherosclerosis as proposed by the SHAPE Task Force, as well as early detection and rapid response to prodromal symptoms are unmet opportunities that must be considered by cardiovascular healthcare policymakers.

REFERENCES

1. Heart disease statistics:2005 update, Dallas, TX: American Heart Association, 2004
2. American Heart Association. 2001 Heart and Stroke Statistical Update. Dallas, TX: American Heart Association, 2008
3. National Heart, Lung, and Blood Institute. Morbidity & Mortality Chart Book. Bethesda, MD: National Heart, Lung and Blood Institute, National Institutes of Health, 2000
4. Bahr RD. Prodromal symptom recognition of a heart attack. An overlooked phenomenon for recognizing a window of opportunity for early heart attack care. Critic Path Cardiol 2002;1(3):194–206
5. Hwang SY, Ryan C, Zerwic JJ. The influence of age on acute myocardial infarction symptoms and patient delay in seeking treatment. Prog Cardiovasc Nurs 2006;21(1):20–7 doi:10.1111/j.0197-3118.2006.04713.x

6. MacMillan RL, Brown KWG, Peckham GB, Kahn O, Hutchinson DB, Paton M. Changing perspective in coronary care: a five year study. Am J Cardiol 1967;20:451–6
7. Braunwald E. Shattuck lecture – cardiovascular medicine at the turn of the millennium: Triumphs, concerns, and opportunities. New Eng J Med 1997;337:1360–9
8. Weanver WD, Cerqueira M, Hallstrom AP, et al. Pre-hospital-initiated vs. hospital-initiated thrombolytic therapy. J Am Med Assoc 1993;270:1211–6
9. Bar RD. Access to early cardiac care: chest pain as a risk factor for heart attacks and the emergence of early cardiac care centers Maryland Med J 1992;41(2):133–7
10. Weaver WD, Cerqueira M, Hallstrom AP, et al. Prehospital-initiated vs. hospital initiated thrombolytic therapy. The myocardial infarction triage and intervention Trial. JAMA 1993;270:1211–6
11. Emergency department: rapid identification and treatment of patients with acute myocardial infarction. National heart attack alert program coordinating committee, 60 minutes to treatment working group. Ann Emerg Med 1994;23:311–29
12. Braunwald E. Acute myocardial infarction – the value of being prepared. N Engl J Med. 1996;334(1):51–2. No abstract available
13. Shiraki H, Yashikow T, Anzai T, Negishi K, Takahashi T, Asakura Y, Akaishi H, Mitamura H, Ogawa S. Association between preinfarction angina and lower risk of right ventricular infarction. N Engl J Med 1998;338:941–7
14. Bahr, RD, McIntosh, HD. Reawakening awareness of the importance of prodromal symptoms in the shifting paradigm to early heart attack care (EHAC). Clinician 1996;14(4). http://ehacstagnes.org/st-agnes/theclinicianvol14no4/7reawakenmessage.asp
15. Lee TH, Goldman L. The coronary care unit turns 25: Historical trends and future directions. Ann Int Med 1988;105:887–94
16. http://www.nhlbi.nih.gov/about/nhaap/index.htm
17. Weingarten SR, Ermann B, Riedinger MS, et al. Selecting the best triage rule for patients hospitalized with chest pain. Am J Med 1989;87:494–500
18. Gomez MA, Anderson JL, Karagounis LA, et al. An emergency department-based protocol for rapidly ruling out myocardial ischemia reduces hospital time and expense: Results of a randomized study(ROMIO). J Am Coll Cardiol 1996;28:25–33
19. Master AM, Dack S, Jaffe HL. Premonitory symptoms of acute coronary occlusion: a study of 260 cases. Ann Intern Med 1941;14:1155–65
20. Kahn MH Prodromal symptoms in angina pectoris. Am Jr Med Sci 1926;clxxii:418
21. Andreotti F, Pasceri V, Hockett DR, et al. Preinfarction angina as a predictor of more rapid coronary thrombosis in patients with acute myocardial infarction. N Engl J Med 1996;334:7–12
22. Haider AW, Andreotti F, Hackett DR, et al. Early spontaneous intermittent myocardial reperfusion during acute myocardial infarction is associated with augmented thrombogenic activity and less myocardial damage. J Am Coll Cardiol 1995;26:662–7
23. Krucoff MW. Cyclic coronary flow: Defining preinfarction angina at the crossroads of unstable angina and myocardial infarction. Md Med 2001;Spring (Suppl):60–4
24. Bahr RD, Leino EV, Christenson RH. Prodromal unstable angina in acute myocardial infarction: Prognostic value of short and long-term outcome and predictor of infarct size (GUSTO 1 Study). Am Heart J 2000;140:126–33
25. Christenson RH, Leino EV, Giugliano RP, Bahr RD. Usefulness of prodromal unstable angina pectoris in predicting better survival and smaller infarct size in acute myocardial infarction (The InTIME-II prodromal symptoms sub study). Am J Cardiol 2003;92:598–600
26. Bahr RD. Critical pathways in cardiology, the official journal of the society of chest pain centers. Crit Pathw Cardiol 2005;4(1):1–2, Editorial
27. Bahr RD. Value of history in evaluating patients for early myocardial ischemia in observation chest pain centers. Crit Pathw Cardiol 2003;2:104–12
28. Naghavi M, Libby P, Falk E, Casscells SW, Litovsky S, Rumberger J, Badimon JJ, Stefanadis C, Moreno P, Pasterkamp G, Fayad Z, Stone PH, Waxman S, Raggi P, Madjid M, Zarrabi A, Burke A, Yuan C, Fitzgerald PJ, Siscovick DS, de Korte CL, Aikawa M, Juhani Airaksinen KE, Assmann G, Becker CR, Chesebro JH, Farb A, Galis ZS, Jackson C, Jang IK, Koenig W, Lodder RA, March K, Demirovic J, Navab M, Priori SG, Rekhter MD, Bahr R, Grundy SM, Mehran R, Colombo A, Boerwinkle E, Ballantyne C, Insull W Jr, Schwartz RS, Vogel R, Serruys PW, Hansson GK, Faxon DP, Kaul S, Drexler H, Greenland P, Muller JE, Virmani R, Ridker PM, Zipes DP, Shah PK, Willerson JT. From vulnerable plaque to vulnerable patient: a call for new definitions and risk assessment strategies: Part I. Circulation 2003;108(14):1664–72
29. Naghavi M, Libby P, Falk E, Casscells SW, Litovsky S, Rumberger J, Badimon JJ, Stefanadis C, Moreno P, Pasterkamp G, Fayad Z, Stone PH, Waxman S, Raggi P, Madjid M, Zarrabi A, Burke A, Yuan C, Fitzgerald PJ, Siscovick DS, de Korte CL, Aikawa M, Juhani Airaksinen KE, Assmann G, Becker CR, Chesebro JH, Farb A, Galis ZS, Jackson C, Jang IK, Koenig W, Lodder RA, March K, Demirovic J, Navab M, Priori SG, Rekhter MD, Bahr R, Grundy SM, Mehran R, Colombo A, Boerwinkle E, Ballantyne C, Insull W Jr, Schwartz RS, Vogel R, Serruys PW, Hansson GK, Faxon DP, Kaul S, Drexler H, Greenland P, Muller JE, Virmani R, Ridker PM, Zipes DP, Shah PK, Willerson JT. From vulnerable plaque to vulnerable patient: a call for new definitions and risk assessment strategies: Part II. Circulation 2003;108(14):1664–72
30. Naghavi M, Falk E, Hecht HS, Jamieson MJ, Kaul S, Berman D, Fayad Z, Budoff MJ, Rumberger J, Naqvi TZ, Shaw LJ, Faergeman O, Cohn J, Bahr R, Koenig W, Demirovic J, Arking D, Herrera VL, Badimon J, Goldstein JA, Rudy Y, Airaksinen J, Schwartz RS, Riley WA, Mendes RA, Douglas P, Shah PK. From vulnerable plaque to vulnerable patient – Part III: Executive summary of the screening for heart attack prevention and education (SHAPE) task force report. Am J Cardiol 2006;98(2A):2H–15H
31. Meischke H, Ho MT, Eisenberg M, Schaeffer S, Larsen M. Reasons patients with chest pain delay or do not call 911. Ann Emerg Med 1995;25(2):193–7

Index